GENERAL SURGICAL OPERATIONS

DEDICATION

For my wife Peggy,
and for Valentine, Jeremy and Louise

Commissioning Editor: Laurence Hunter
Project Development Manager: Janice Urquhart
Project Manager: Emma Riley
Text Design: Judith Wright
Cover Design: Stewart Larking
Illustration Buyer: Gillian Murray
Illustrator: Ian Ramsden

GENERAL SURGICAL OPERATIONS

FIFTH EDITION

EDITED BY

R. M. KIRK MS FRCS

Honorary Professor of Surgery, Royal Free and University College London School of Medicine, London, UK

Honorary Consulting Surgeon, Royal Free Hospital, London, UK

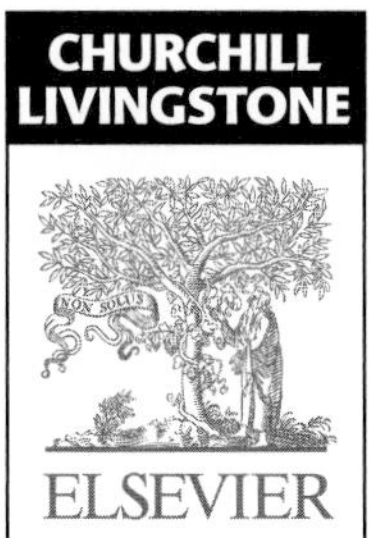

EDINBURGH LONDON NEW YORK OXFORD PHILADELPHIA ST LOUIS SYDNEY TORONTO 2006

CHURCHILL
LIVINGSTONE
ELSEVIER

First edition 1978
Second edition 1987
Third edition 1994
Fourth edition 2000
Fifth edition 2006
Reprinted 2007

ISBN 0 443 10121 3
ISBN-13 978-0-443-10121-2
International edition ISBN 0 443 10122 1
International edition ISBN-13 978-0-443-10122-9

British Library Cataloguing in Publication Data
A catalogue record for this book is available from the British Library

Library of Congress Cataloguing in Publication Data
A catalogue record for this book is available from the Library of Congress

Note

'Knowledge and best practice in this field are constantly changing. As new research and experience broaden our knowledge, changes in practice, treamtnet and drug therapy may become necessary or appropriate. Readers are advised to check the most current information provided i) on procedures featured or (ii) by the manufacturer of each product to be administered, to verify the recommended dose or formula, the method and duration of administration, and contraindcations. It is the responsibility of the practitioner, relying on their own experience and knowledge of the patient, to make diagnoses, to determine dosages and the best treatment for each individual patient, and to take all appropriate safety precautions. To the fullest extent of the law, neither the Publisher nor the editor assumes any liability for any injury and/or damage to persons or property arising out or related to any use of the material contained in this book.'

The Publisher

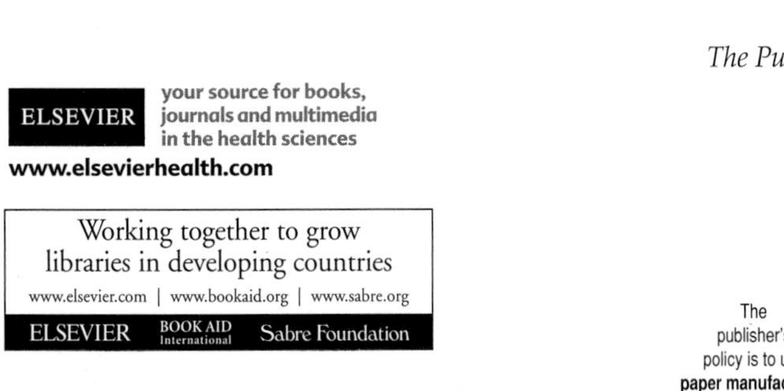

The publisher's policy is to use **paper manufactured from sustainable forests**

Printed in China

Contents

Preface

A good surgeon knows how to operate
A better surgeon knows when to operate
The best surgeon knows when not to operate

Many textbooks are now written to cover an examination syllabus – an abstract of a series of lectures. Excellent operative surgery books are available which aim to do this, with lists of objective, 'black-and-white' steps and bullet points, often containing idealized illustrations. Unfortunately, practical operative surgery does not conform to standardized procedures and this book is primarily aimed at surgeons about to carry out an operation, not merely to describe the 'principles' to an examiner.

In ideal circumstances, surgeons should carry out only operations with which they are familiar and which they perform regularly. There are many places where this cannot be achieved normally; there are likely to be circumstances anywhere in the world where natural disasters, terrorist activities or war overwhelm the available expertise.

In the British Isles, and in many countries, there is partial implementation of specialization; partial because there are insufficient numbers to implement it fully. Surgeons are expected to carry out elective operations exclusively within their sphere of expertise. However, those accepting general surgical emergencies encounter, and may be called upon to provide at least initial diagnosis and care for, conditions outside this range. Older generations were experienced in the generality of surgery, although they might not have been fully up-to-date with current practice in areas outside their normal elective range. Trainees are no longer highly trained in clinical diagnosis throughout the whole range, or familiar with operative procedures. Those trained only within a narrowed field are at an even greater disadvantage in an emergency.

For this reason I have asked the contributors to offer a thorough appraisal of each procedure. Every surgeon must be able to anticipate, recognize and react to unusual findings. These are often subtle and require explanation. They cannot always be listed because their frequency, their importance and their tactical implications are variable.

Past reviewers, usually highly specialized and working in well-staffed large city hospitals, have suggested that it is time to abandon books on the generality of surgery. Meanwhile, in smaller, often understaffed, under-equipped hospitals throughout the world, surgeons working in isolation from specialist colleagues, or in emergency circumstances, are regularly performing a wide range of operations. If they do not perform them, no one will. Progressive diseases are not respecters of tissue planes or the integrity of other systems. Sadly, injuries from motor cars, fires, building collapses, earthquakes, floods, bullets and bombs are not tissue-selective or area-selective. No apparently calm, well-ordered society is immune from natural or man-made disasters.

Authors and editors are often adjured to have a clear targeted readership. It could be argued that my target is too diffuse. True, this book is aimed primarily at a candidate for the Intercollegiate FRCS in General Surgery in Great Britain and Ireland, and equivalent examinations around the world. It is, however, also intended as a vade-mecum for a trained surgeon, anywhere, who is about to carry out an infrequently performed procedure, perhaps in emergency conditions. I therefore hope that it can be a useful reference manual for every surgeon except a highly specialized 'one-procedure' operator. To me, that is a pretty comprehensive target!

As in previous editions, we have used a standardized style, format and headings for easy reference. We offer advice on patient selection and other criteria, preparation, access to the site of operation, recognition of the situation and tactics, how to accomplish the procedure, check that all is well, close and aftercare. Complications are listed, with advice on management. It was tempting to describe and perhaps illustrate unusual specialist instruments, but a person undertaking the operations should be familiar with the required instruments and procedures. There are many deliberate repetitions. A surgeon revising how to proceed through the steps of an operation does not welcome being told to refer to another page, thus we have cut cross-references to a minimum. Because of the need to keep the size and cost within limits, general chapters on preoperative assessment and postoperative complications have been dropped, reluctantly, since relevant factors are discussed for each operation. General care and assessment is discussed in detail in *Clinical Surgery in General* 4th edition, also published by Churchill Livingstone.

Once again my Japanese friends Professors Hiroshi Akiyama FRCS and Harushi Udagawa give a masterly description of oesophagectomy for cancer. Professor Sir Ara Darzi KBE from St Mary's Hospital, London, heads a team of experts in minimal access procedures – a subject to which he has made many contributions. I am once more grateful for six excellent chapters from the Hammersmith Hospital under the careful supervision of Professor Robin Williamson. The description of open biliary operations is particularly important; contemporary trainees are less familiar with the operations than their predecessors, yet they may require to convert minimal access techniques to open surgery, and so require guidance. I am sad to report that my good friend and longstanding colleague Michael Brough became ill during the revision of his chapter on plastic surgery and died. Peter Butler generously stepped in to complete it.

This is a 'What to do' book. You, the reader, should aspire to gain diagnostic, decision-making and operative surgical competence as widely as possible. Do not embark on major procedures unless you have good basic competence. First steps in 'How to do it' are described in *Basic Surgical Techniques* 5th edition, also published by Churchill Livingstone.

Apology

Once again, I apologize to women surgeons and women in general, for the frequent use of the male pronoun. Constant reference to 'he or she' and inappropriate use of plural pronouns are clumsy and irritating. There is no epicene third person pronoun.

R. M. Kirk
2005

Acknowledgements

It has been a great pleasure to work in cooperation with two long-standing friends—Laurence Hunter and Janice Urquhart. I should also like to thank the copyeditor Pru Theaker, the Project Manager Emma Riley, the proofreaders Alison Woodhouse, Ian Ross and Susan Ranson, the illustrator Ian Ramsden and the indexer Linda Swindells.

Contributors

Hiroshi Akiyama MD FRCS(Eng) FACS
Senior Adviser, Toranomon Hospital, Tokyo, Japan

Shaun G. Appleton MS FRCS
Consultant Surgeon, Wycombe Hospital, High Wycombe, UK

Satyajit Bhattacharya MS MPhil FRCS
Consultant Surgeon, Hepatobiliary and Pancreatic Surgery Unit, The Royal London Hospital, London, UK

Michael D. Brough (Deceased)

Kevin G. Burnand MB BS FRCS MS
Professor of Surgery, Guy's, King's and St Thomas's Medical School, King's College London, London, UK

Peter Butler MD FRCSI FRCS FRCS(Plast)
Consultant Plastic Surgeon, Department of Plastic Surgery, Royal Free Hospital, London, UK

C. Richard G. Cohen MD FRCS
Consultant Surgeon, University College Hospitals, London, UK

Richard E.C. Collins MB BS FRCS(Eng) FRCS(Ed)
Consultant Surgeon, Kent and Canterbury Hospital, East Kent NHS Trust, UK

Frank W. Cross MS FRCS
Consultant Surgeon, Royal London Hospital, London, UK

Sir Ara Darzi KBE MD FRCS FACS FRCS(I)
Professor of Surgery and Head of Division, Department of Surgical Oncology and Technology, Imperial College London, St Mary's Hospital, London, UK

Roy W.R. Farrell MA MB BAO BCL FRCSI FRCS
Consultant Otolaryngologist and Head and Neck Surgeon, Northwick Park Hospital, Harrow, UK

Chris Fowler BSc MA MS FRCP FRCS(Urol) FEBU
Professor of Surgical Education and Honorary Consultant Urologist, Barts and the London, Queen Mary's School of Medicine and Dentistry, University of London, London, UK

Nicholas Goddard MB BS FRCS
Consultant Orthopaedic Surgeon, The Royal Free Hospital, London, UK

Gareth Harper MA BM BChir FRCS(Orth)
Consultant Orthopaedic Surgeon, Queen Alexandra Hospital, Portsmouth, UK

Peter L. Harris MB ChB MD FRCS(Eng)
Consultant Vascular Surgeon and Director of Vascular Services, Regional Vascular Unit, Royal Liverpool University Hospital, Liverpool, UK

Michael Hobsley MA MB MChir PhD DSc FRCS
Emeritus Professor, Department of Surgery, University College London Medical School, London, UK

Jonathan D. Jagger MB BS FRCS Do FRCOphth
Consultant Ophthalmic Surgeon, Eye Department, The Royal Free Hospital, London, UK

Long R. Jiao MD FRCS(Eng)
Senior Lecturer, Honorary Consultant Surgeon, Department of Hepatopancreobiliary Surgery, Hammersmith Hospital Campus, Division of Surgery, Anaesthesia and Intensive Care, Imperial College School of Medicine, London, UK

Islam Junaid MB BS FRCS(Ed) FRCS(Urol)
Consultant Urological and Transplant Surgeon, Barts and the London NHS Trust, London, UK

Ajay K. Kakkar MB BS BSc PhD FRCS
Professor and Head, Centre for Surgical Science Barts and The London, Queen Mary's School of Medicine and Dentistry, University of London, Consultant Surgeon St Bartholomew's and Royal London Hospitals Director Designate Thrombosis Research Institute, London, UK

Robin R. Kanagasabay MB BS BSc FRCS(CTh) MRCP
Consultant Cardiothoracic Surgeon, Department of Cardiothoracic Surgery, St George's Healthcare NHS Trust, London, UK

R.M. Kirk MS FRCS
Honorary Professor of Surgery, Royal Free and University College London School of Medicine, London, UK; Honorary Consulting Surgeon, The Royal Free Hospital, London, UK

Iain M. Laws TD MB ChB FDSRCS
Emeritus Consultant, Maxillofacial Surgeon, The Royal Free Hospital, London, UK

Roger J. Leicester OBE MB FRCS(Edin & Eng)
Consultant Colorectal Surgeon, St George's Hospital, London; Endoscopy Tutor, Raven Department of Education, Royal College of Surgeons of England, London, UK

Robert Mason BSc MB ChB ChM MD FRCS(Eng) FRCS(Ed)
Consultant Upper GI Surgeon and Deputy Medical Director, Guy's and St Thomas's Hospitals, London, UK

R.S. Maurice-Williams MA MB BChir FRCS FRCP
Consultant Neurosurgeon, Neurosurgical Unit, The Royal Free Hospital, London, UK

Bridget Mulholland MD FRCOphth
Consultant Ophthalmologist in Cataract and Ocuplastic Surgery, The Royal Free Hospital, London, UK

Stephen J. Nixon MB ChB BSc FRCS FRCP
Consultant Surgeon, Royal Infirmary, Edinburgh, UK

P.A. Paraskeva PhD FRCS
Lecturer in Surgery, Department of Surgical Oncology and Technology, Imperial College London, QEQM Wing, St Mary's Hospital, London, UK

Arthanari Rajasekar MB BS MS(GenSurg) FRCS(Eng) FRCS(Ire)
Consultant Gastrointestinal and Laparoscopic Surgeon, Department of Gastroenterology and Endoscopic Surgery, Sri Gokulam Hospital, Salem, Tamilnadu, India

John A. Rennie MS FRCS
Consultant Surgeon, King's College Hospital, London, UK

Gavin S.M. Robertson MB ChB MD FRCS
Consultant Surgeon, Department of Surgery, Leicester Royal Infirmary, Leicester, UK

T. Rockall MD FRCS
Minimal Access Therapy Training Unit, Royal Surrey County Hospital, Guildford, UK

Keith Rolles MA MS FRCS
Consultant Surgeon, The Royal Free Hospital, London, UK

James M. Ryan MCh FRCS DMCC
Leonard Cheshire Professor of Conflict Recovery, University College London; International Professor of Surgery, USUHS, Bethesda, MD, USA

Richard Sainsbury MB BS MD FRCS
Senior Lecturer and Honorary Consultant Surgeon at the Department of Surgery, University College London, London, UK

Marcus E. Setchell CVO MB BChir FRCSEng FRCOG
Consultant Obstetrician and Gynaecologist, Whittington Hospital, London; Honorary Consultant Gynaecologist, King Edward VII Hospital, London, UK

Arjun Shankar MD FRCS
Consultant Surgeon, University College Hospitals, London, UK

Robert S. Simons QHP(C) MB ChB FRCA FANZCA
Consultant Anaesthetist, The Royal Free Hospital, London, UK

Lewis Spitz MB ChB PhD MD FRCS(Edin) FRCS(Eng) FRCPCH FAAP
Emeritus Nuffield Professor of Paediatric Surgery, Institute of Child Health, University College London; Consultant Paediatric Surgeon, Great Ormond Street Hospital for Children NHS Trust, London, UK

Michael P. Stearns MB BS BDS FRCS
Consultant Otolaryngologist/Head and Neck Surgeon, The Royal Free Hospital, London, UK

Ian D. Sugarman MB ChB FRCS(Ed) FRCS(Paed)
Consultant Paediatric Surgeon, Leeds General Infirmary, Leeds, UK

Justin Tan MB BS MRCS
Academic Department of Surgery, St Thomas's Hospital, London, UK

Jeremy N. Thompson MA MB MChir FRCS
Consultant Surgeon, Chelsea and Westminster and Royal Marsden Hospitals, London, UK

Tom Treasure MD MS FRCS
Consultant Thoracic Surgeon, Guy's and St Thomas's Hospital, London; Professor of Cardiothoracic Surgery, Department of Cardiothoracic Surgery, University of London, London, UK

Matthew G. Tutton BSc MRCS
Specialist Registrar in General Surgery, London Deanery, London, UK

Harushi Udagawa MD DMSc FACS
Head of Gastroenterological Surgery, Toranomon Hospital, Tokyo, Japan

Carolynne Jane Vaizey MD FRCS(Gen) FCS(SA)
Consultant Surgeon, St Mark's Hospital, London, UK

David F.L. Watkin MChir FRCS
Retired Consultant Surgeon, Leicester Royal Infirmary, Leicester, UK

James M. Wellwood MA, MChir(Cantab), FRCS(Eng)
Consultant Surgeon and Honorary Senior Lecturer, Whipps Cross Hospital, London, UK

Douglas E. Whitelaw MB ChB FRCS(Ed) FRCS(GenSurg)
Consultant Surgeon, Luton and Dunstable Hospital, Luton, UK

R.C.N. Williamson MA MD MChir FRCS PhD (Hon)
Consultant Surgeon, Hammersmith Hospital, London; Professor of Surgery, Imperial College, London; Dean, Royal Society of Medicine, London, UK

Marc C. Winslet MS FRCS
Professor of Surgery and Head of Department, University Department of Surgery, The Royal Free Hospital, London, UK

1

Choose well, cut well, get well

R.M. Kirk

CONTENTS

INTRODUCTION

'Choose well, cut well, get well' is a succinct American aphorism summing up the requirements for successful surgery. As in so many complex procedures, the whole is dependent upon every single step. The adage 'Complications are made in the operating room' is not altogether true. Although an incompetently performed operation is likely to bring disaster, it is equally dangerous to perform a skilful but inappropriate procedure on an ill-prepared patient and fail to monitor recovery. The American surgeon Frank Spencer has stated that good surgery is about 20–25% manual dexterity and 70–75% decision-making.[1]

It is worrying that erosion of the master/apprentice system, in which not only explicit knowledge but also tacit wisdom and attitudes that cannot be put into words,[2] has been eroded in surgical training[3] in favour of 'modular' teaching and subsequent assessment. Module (Latin: *modulus*, diminutive of *modus*=measure) has the connotation of teaching by defined, competetence assessable potentially isolated units. There is a danger that the important whole is delegated to secondary importance. As the Gestalt psychologists emphasized at the beginning of the 20th century, the whole is greater than the sum of its parts. We are adjured to apply evidence-based management of patients, but the changes in surgical training are arbitrary. No evidence is presented that overall clinical care of patients is improved by compartmentalizing surgical training. There is a multiplicity of interacting and changing factors at work that affect surgical outcomes.

In the past, the decisions and actions made by physicians and surgeons were rarely questioned. Vogue and idiosyncratic treatments and operations were performed without discussion. The Guy's Hospital surgeon Sir William Withey Gull (1816–1890) stated, 'Make haste and use the new remedies before they lose their effectiveness'.

Public expectations, which were previously low, have risen, driving the medical profession towards greater intraprofessional surveillance, more evidence-based treatments, with review of outcomes. There is corresponding pressure to identify and deal with those who do not maintain acceptable standards. Inevitably, outcome data for individual surgeons is increasingly being collected. Because a surgical operation is a specific event in management, it is too easily, and uncritically, used to compare results between surgeons. We shall need to pay as much attention to the outcome in those patients we decide not to submit to operation, especially since there is now a choice in many traditional surgical fields between effective drugs and treatment using endoscopic and interventional radiological methods.

CHOOSE WELL

Decide

1 The existence of double-blind, controlled clinical trials is well known. Our patients reasonably expect us to choose the correct management for their surgical conditions. Of the treatment methods available, surely, they will say, it is possible, after testing them, to conclude that one is better than the others. Ideally, there should be but one variable, the treatment. Unfortunately, biological variability is so great that very often a conclusive answer cannot be given. The physical and psychological condition of patients and the extent and virulence of diseases make it difficult or impossible to study matched groups of people with matched disease severity. As new methods become available, conflicting evidence emerges about their effectiveness and safety compared with existing methods.

2 Our selection of facts from the available evidence varies as individuals and between surgeons. From the accumulated information, one investigator may be influenced to follow one path, whereas another may direct the focus to other evidence. In reaching a decision about a particular patient, not all pieces of evidence are of equal value. Some features are common to many conditions, but we need to be influenced more by those that are discriminant. As individual surgeons we may be influenced by recent experience, perhaps of a run of successes or disasters, to change our viewpoint.

KEY POINTS Assessing evidence

- When collecting or assessing evidence on which to make a decision, there is a tendency to prefer numerically (digitally) expressed indicators over analogue (continuously variable) evidence. This is natural, because numbers can be compared easily. However, ensure that what is chosen to be measured is valid, and not selected merely because it can be assigned numbers.
- If the results of your investigations conflict with your carefully and confidently obtained clinical findings, trust your clinical judgement.

Moreover, we favour evidence that fits our existing beliefs. A postal questionnaire to surgeons revealed, as one would expect, that those with a declared interest in laparoscopic surgery were more likely to advise their patients to have a laparoscopic hernia repair and to select it for themselves, than those without a declared interest.[4]

3 In some cases we may not have a diagnosis but a clinical feature alone that demands action on our part. This is particularly true for some emergencies, when the exact cause of a life-threatening haemorrhage, cardiorespiratory failure, peritonitis or pyrexia typical of sepsis may not be clear, but urgent treatment is necessary.

4 We cannot concentrate on a single patient in circumstances where many people are ill. This is particularly true in wartime or a civilian disaster. In such cases we must make urgent, sometimes agonizing, decisions. This process of triage (Old French: to pick, select) involves choosing to treat first those whose lives can be saved by quick action, deferring treatment of those with multiple or peripheral injuries. Possible loss of a limb or a special sense is less urgent than cases whose very survival depends on quick, effective action: 'Life comes before limb'.

KEY POINT Rank your priorities

- At intervals review the order of your priorities. They do not remain static.

5 Even in elective circumstances we need to make decisions with incomplete information. We never have all the necessary facts available about the physical and mental state of our patient but make the best guess, based on our general knowledge, the results of appropriately selected investigations and often by intuition.

KEY POINTS 'Intuition'

- Some surgeons get better results than others, although there is no objectively assessable difference in their competence from the average.
- Possibly they analyse their results more critically than others, make better judgements, set higher than average standards.
- The higher ratio of accurate decisions may be based on tacit knowledge, i.e. knowledge that cannot be explicitly stated or objectively identified.
- They are sometimes referred to as 'lucky surgeons'.

6 Success in individual cases does not necessarily indicate good judgement; a robust patient may improve in spite of inappropriate treatment. Conversely, a susceptible patient may deteriorate despite the best treatment.

7 When seeking a solution to a difficult but not urgent problem, take the opportunity to set it aside while you do something else. In some cases you may leave it overnight. There is mounting evidence that the answer to a problem formulates during sleep.[5] It is remarkable how solutions often appear spontaneously, sometimes as a result of viewing the situation from a new point of view. It is also valuable to re-examine, after an interval, the patient who presents with, for example, an acute abdomen as the physical signs can change rapidly.

8 If you reach a decision, regard it as only provisional. Since it is based on incomplete knowledge, you may discover further facts, or the observed effects of your management may suggest that you review and revise the course of action. Too often, initially good management fails because it is inexorably pursued when the circumstances change. Your initial plan is comparable with the *strategy* of a general before battle, but he may need to alter his *tactics* as the battle develops.

KEY POINT Avoid rigid attitudes

- Be flexible. Anticipate, recognize and react to changed circumstances.

9 Attempts to rationalize decisions have resulted in the development of *algorithms*, or standard, step-by-step actions, and *protocols*, which provide a standard approach leading to an expected optimum outcome. Especially in the USA, pressure from managed care organizations and 'stakeholders' (insurers and those who pay the bills) have resulted in *guidelines* and *clinical pathways*, although not all of them have been verified.[6] Such methods have been worked out and evaluated by experts in the particular fields where they can be applied. They do not necessarily fit every circumstance but provide a routine approach that aims to give the best results in most cases. Such methods need to be re-evaluated from time to time as views change with improvements in diagnosis and therapeutics, and in the light of follow-up. *Decision analysis*, another aid in evaluating the best course of action, is discussed later.

KEY POINT Justifiable decisions and actions

- If you are about to make a heterodox decision, ask yourself, 'If my selected course of management fails, can I justify my actions to the patient, to my peers and, most importantly, to myself?'

Remember that all these procedural guides are made to give the best results in the majority of circumstances. They do not fit every situation. For example, when treating major abdominal injuries it is usually possible to stabilize the patient's condition and carry out relevant diagnostic tests. At laparotomy when indicated, you would stop bleeding, explore the whole abdomen, repair all damage and close up. However, you cannot deliberately follow this routine if the patient is bleeding calamitously. You need to recognize that controlling the bleeding is paramount. It may be necessary to pack the abdomen, close it and defer any further action until you have stabilized the patient (see Ch. 3, damage control laparotomy).

10 Do not be too proud to take advice. The very action of arranging and presenting the problem to another person often clarifies it.

11 When you have reached a decision, you must discuss it with the patient, who has the right to participate. However much we try

to offer an objective judgement, it is inevitable that the presentation to our patients is biased. Our decision is the one in which we believe, and inevitably we weight the evidence towards our selected management. There is nothing dishonest about this. Indeed, it would be cowardly not to give positive advice. We have access to the available facts and have to weigh them, reach a decision and place that decision before the patient. It is our professional duty to take responsibility for our decisions and irresolute to place the whole burden on to the patient. This does not, of course, excuse us if we ignore or override the patient's wishes. Patients faced with treatment decisions look at different criteria from us, such as quality of life; our anxieties revolve more closely around survival.[7,8]

DECISION ANALYSIS

1 Decision analysis offers a means of weighing all the factors and possible outcomes.[9] A decision tree is constructed that demonstrates the choice of decisions and possible *outcomes* from each decision (Fig. 1.1).

2 In most cases the probable outcome of operation can be estimated from a study of the relevant literature. However, the outcome of withholding operation in circumstances where it is routinely offered is often not known and must be estimated from reports written before surgery was possible, or from the records of patients who have refused operation.

3 Added into the equation are the value judgements placed by you and the patient on the sequelae of surgical versus conservative management, and the likelihood of benefit from different operations. These subjective values are termed *utilities*. The possibility of curing a threatening condition by major operation has to be placed against the mortality and morbidity associated with it. If the condition is likely to be fatal, life expectation has to be balanced against the quality of life. There are a number of terms used in assessing this. One such is quality-adjusted life-year (*QALY*) expectancy. One year of life in perfect health is 1 QALY; a lower figure is allocated for a portion of a year in perfect health or a full year spent with a disability. Also added in are the economic implications: the *cost–benefit* analysis. Decision analyses have been published for a number of common conditions.

4 The main value of such analyses is in bringing into focus all the possibilities. In the distant past, surgery was often carried out as the last resort. As new methods of management become available, as the effects of various treatments become known, and as the knowledge and desire of patients to participate in the decision-making process increase, so we need to consider and evaluate all the choices.

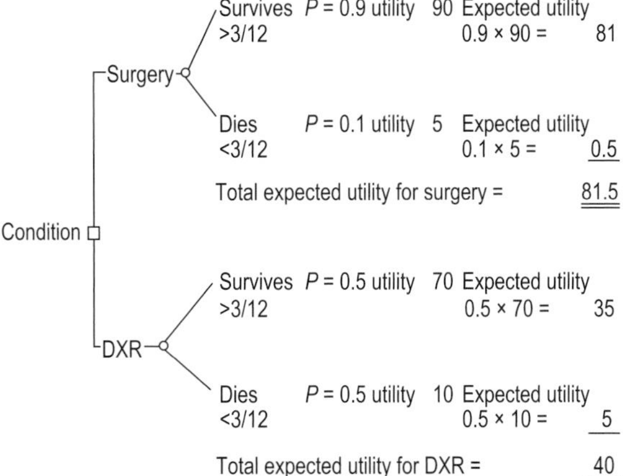

Fig. 1.1 Decision analysis, taking only short-term survival into account. The probability (*P*) of each outcome following surgery or deep X-ray therapy (DXR) is calculated from published results and local experience. The utility of each outcome is given a value between 0 (worst) and 100 (best). The expected utility is the product of probability and utility for each outcome. The sum of the expected utilities for each decision is compared with those of the other decisions. The highest scoring decision offers the best outcome. The square node is a 'decision node'; the circular nodes are 'chance nodes'.

KEY POINTS Responsibility for decision-making

- Investigations, protocols, guidelines, risk and decision analyses are useful but based on generalizations.
- For individual cases, the decision of an experienced clinician must be paramount.[10]

REFERENCES

1. Spencer FC 1979 Competence and compassion: two qualities of surgical excellence. Bulletin of the American College of Surgeons 64:15–22
2. Polanyi M 1958 Personal knowledge. Routledge & Kegan Paul, London
3. Kirk RM 1998 Surgical excellence: threats and opportunities. Annals of the Royal College of Surgeons of England 80(6 Suppl):256–259
4. Williams N, Scott A 1999 Conventional or laparoscopic inguinal hernia repair? The surgeon's choice. Annals of the Royal College of Surgeons of England 81:56–57
5. Nelson L 2004 While you were sleeping. Nature 430:962–964
6. Weiland DE 1997 Why use clinical pathways rather than practice guidelines? American Journal of Surgery 174:592–595
7. Mazur DJ, Hickam DH 1996 Five-year survival curves: how much data are enough for patient-physician decision making in general surgery? European Journal of Surgery 162:101–104
8. Newton-Howes PA, Bedford ND, Dobbs BR et al 1998 Informed consent: what do patients want to know? New Zealand Medical Journal 111:340–342
9. Kirk RM, Cox K 2004 Decision making. In: Kirk RM, Ribbans WJ (eds) Clinical surgery in general, 4th edn. Churchill Livingstone, Edinburgh, pp 144–151
10. Jewell ER, Persson AV 1985 Pre-operative evaluation of the high risk patient. Surgical Clinics of North America 65:3–19

CUT WELL

KEY POINT Competent?

- If operation is indicated, should you perform it? Except in an emergency, avoid carrying out operations that can be better performed by someone else who is available.

Routines

1 Sterile techniques in the operating theatre have been worked out over many years. Most, but not all, have been subjected to scientific evaluation. Although experienced people carry out the correct procedures instinctively, many of us acquire bad habits that go uncorrected. Accept the need to follow strict routines and so be free to concentrate on other aspects of the operation. Question the routines from time to time to decide if they are really valuable. Discuss them with the senior theatre users. Thoughtless disparagement undermines training.

KEY POINTS Achieving success

- Do not rush! Hurried movements result in mistakes and the need to repeat actions. Hand speed does not equate with operative speed. Deliberate, accurate movements are faster than rapid, 'flashy' actions that need to be undone or repeated.
- In an emergency, you may often overcome a dangerous situation, not by rapid action but by intelligently deferring in essential routine procedures.
- **Concentrate on getting everything right first time.**
- A major operation is merely a series of small operations, but a successful outcome depends upon each step being accomplished perfectly.

2 Standardized operative techniques result from the pooled experience of many surgeons. If you are still an assistant, watch carefully and assiduously adopt the accepted and orthodox procedures followed by your chief. You will acquire skills in a natural manner that cannot be transmitted verbally.[1] In this way you will at least have the consolation, if anything goes wrong, that you can justify your actions. Later in your career you may question certain points of technique and have the courage to adopt your own methods, usually a synthesis of points acquired from your teachers.

3 'Set up' standard procedures (e.g. when applying a series of ligatures, suturing and mobilizing structures). Take time to place yourself in the best position; arrange the structures so that you can carry out each manoeuvre in a controlled and natural manner.

4 In the past, most surgeons became competent out of sheer pressure of work so that they eventually learned by overcoming their mistakes. In many countries this is no longer so; for this reason take every opportunity to practise your skills. Skilful operators, like skilful ball-players, are occasionally born. Most of us have to try and emulate them by watching them and practising. Practising differs from mere repetition. Repeating a fixed procedure establishes a series of actions that can be called up without the need for consciously controlling each part of it. While practising, you are consciously observing each part to see if it can be improved. The manner in which skills are improved resembles Bayesian logic, described for elaborate motor tasks by Kording and Wolpert:[2] from previous experience, appropriate action plans are held in the brain—'feed-forward'; while the action is being carried out, sensory feedback is constantly providing information allowing the reaction to be adjusted—'feedback'.

5 Never relax your vigilance over the wound, instruments, swabs and other materials placed into the wound. Use as few swabs as possible and always use the largest ones compatible with the task. Avoid burying all the swab or pack in the wound; leave a portion, or attached tape, protruding to be clipped to the wound towels. There is no single, once-and-for-all action that will prevent articles from being left inside, which brings distress and often tragedy both for the patient and for yourself. Worry about the possibility without a moment's let-up, and accept full responsibility. Check everything, every time. Do not let your acceptance of responsibility prevent you from involving as many others as possible in the check. They may save you from a momentary lapse.

6 Operational failures are a frequent source of litigation. Whenever they occur, do not rush to find a culprit. Try to identify a possible change in the system which, if introduced, will avoid a repetition of the failure. Such an approach is successfully applied within the airlines industry.[3,4]

KEY POINTS Every imperfect action threatens success

- Unless you are intimately familiar with the anatomy, you tend to wander out of the correct tissue plane.
- Even if you know the normal anatomy, disease may have made it abnormal.
- If you handle the tissues roughly they will swell, ooze tissue fluid and heal imperfectly.
- If your haemostasis is imperfect, you leave a potential culture medium for microorganisms.
- If your apposition of anastomoses is poor, they will leak or cause obstruction.
- If your sutures are too tight they will cut out. If they are too slack they will not retain tissue contact.
- If you tie knots slickly but casually they will fail.

7 Whatever decision you made before operation, react to unexpected findings and to difficulties you may encounter. Do not doggedly persist with your original procedure but be flexible in your approach. If appropriate, stop the operation or perform a routine part while turning over the possibilities. Do not hesitate to discuss it with the other people in the operating theatre or seek another opinion directly or over the telephone. Stating the problem to others often clarifies it in your own mind.

HAEMOSTASIS

Prepare

1 Does the patient have a bleeding tendency? If so, did you correct it and arrange for cross-matched replacement blood and clotting factors to be available?

2 If the patient is already bleeding, as following trauma or local disease, are you replacing the lost blood as far as possible? Have you ordered further supplies and, if necessary, fresh frozen plasma?

3 Are you able to identify the site clinically or by suitable investigation? Can you control the bleeding before taking the patient

to the operating theatre? If the bleeding is iatrogenic following inappropriate administration of anticoagulants, has the clotting mechanism been restored?

4 Have you warned the operating theatre staff to prepare the necessary equipment? For calamitous thoracoabdominal bleeding you need very large packs, at least two efficient suckers and vascular surgical instruments.

5 In some cases, operation is not the best method of controlling bleeding. Endoscopy and interventional radiology are sometimes preferable.

Action

1 Bleeding is better prevented than controlled. Whenever possible, seal the tissues with the diathermy before cutting them. Identify, isolate and doubly ligate blood vessels before dividing them, using haemostatic forceps, aneurysm needles, mechanical stapling devices and, if necessary, suture ligation. In some cases it is possible to use cutting diathermy current, an ultrasonic dissector or a laser beam to incise the tissues and at the same time seal the vessels.

2 If you aim to control bleeding following trauma or local disease, do not expose the site until you have everything you need at hand, with efficient suckers tested and working, and packs ready. Intra-abdominal bleeding is reduced as the abdomen distends and becomes tense, but when you perform laparotomy the tension is released and bleeding restarts. Immediately place very large packs into each quadrant of the abdomen. Aspirate residual blood, then gently remove the packs one by one, a little at a time, starting with the ones you suspect are furthest from the bleeding site. You hope to achieve a dry abdomen with the last pack controlling the bleeding point. Cautiously peel away this last pack to identify the bleeding vessels and control them.

3 When you encounter unexpected bleeding, apply pressure from fingers or a swab, maintain it for a few moments while you consider how to control it, and prepare to do so. If the bleeding is calamitous, maintain the pressure for 5 minutes timed by the clock. During the interval allow the anaesthetist to restore blood volume. Muster assistance and any equipment you may require. Often, when you cautiously release compression you discover that the bleeding has stopped or is easily controlled.

KEY POINTS Danger from bleeding

- The greatest danger is usually the result of panic action.
- Whatever you do, avoid panicky stabs with haemostats plunged blindly into a lake of blood.

4 Anticipate oozing from raw surfaces and consider first infiltrating the tissues with a solution of 1:250 000 adrenaline (epinephrine) in physiological saline solution.

5 Small oozing areas can often be sealed by applying gelatin foam, a resorbable mesh graft of polyglycolic acid or by folding the tissue so that the raw surfaces come into contact. If necessary, maintain the contact using a few sutures.

6 Do not rely upon drains when bleeding occurs. It is much better to achieve perfect haemostasis, followed by meticulous removal of all spilt blood.

7 There are times when you cannot control bleeding from a raw area in, for instance, the abdomen. Do not hesitate to pack the area with sterile gauze. Preferably use a long length, folded back-and-forth like a 'jumping jack' cracker. Sometimes the end can be left protruding from the wound; sometimes it is convenient to close the wound over it. In 24–48 hours you may cautiously withdraw the pack, fold by fold. The bleeding has usually stopped. If it has not, or if bleeding continues after packing it, the pack has not been properly placed. Repeat the procedure and ensure that it is effective.

CONTAMINATED WOUNDS

Appraise

- Contamination of healthy tissues with moderate numbers of pathogenic bacteria does not necessarily prevent healing. Even if the organisms invade the living tissues (i.e. infection) they do not always retard healing. The effects depend on the heaviness of contamination, the virulence of the organisms and the viability of the tissues. Large numbers of virulent organisms in tissues with reduced viability, as after burns, may cause cellulitis, abscess, lymphangitis and possible progression to bacteraemia, pyaemia and septicaemia.
- Dirty wounds are often cleaned with 1% cetrimide. This may damage the tissues. Another favoured solution is 3% hydrogen peroxide, which effervesces, but this is out of favour. Simple washing with sterile physiological saline is probably as effective. If there is particulate matter, use a jet from a large syringe. In countries where the water supply is safe, tap water can be used.
- Infection is increased in the presence of slough, which is adherent fibrin, dead tissue and pus. Remove it surgically when it forms a coherent sheet, which usually blackens. The traditional non-surgical method of treating slough is with eusol (Edinburgh University solution of lime). It is particularly used as a local application to deslough areas prior to skin grafting. Eusol has been condemned on experimental evidence that it delays healing, but some surgeons continue to use it. Enzyme mixtures containing streptokinase and streptodornase are not demonstrably more effective than other substances.

KEY POINT Leave no dirt or foreign material

- Thorough, gentle, mechanical cleaning is crucially important.

- The application of local antiseptics to contaminated wounds is controversial. It is safer to apply them only to intact skin around the wound. They damage the tissues as much as they damage the microorganisms. Chlorhexidine as a 0.05% aqueous solution and potassium permanganate as a 0.01% solution are often used. Povidone–iodine 5% solution is valuable against *Staphylococcus aureus*. Acetic acid as a 5% solution helps eradicate *Pseudomonas* spp.

- Locally applied antibiotics are often ineffective. They encourage the emergence of resistant bacterial strains and frequently produce allergic reactions. The only preparation that is generally used is silver sulfadiazine cream to prevent infection of severe burns. As a rule, if antibiotics are needed, give them systemically.
- Meleney's spreading gangrene of the skin of the abdominal wall, necrotizing fasciitis and Fournier's scrotal gangrene result from synergism between micro-aerophilic streptococci and other organisms. Excise the whole of the gangrenous area without delay, to leave no trace of the disease but only healthy clean living tissue. Do not carry out a single excision but repeat it as often as is necessary to eradicate the spreading infection. Remove specimens for bacteriological examination. Give high doses of intravenous antibiotics depending on the likely source of infection until you have been guided by the microbiologist. Crystalline penicillin, metronidazole and third-generation cephalosporins are usual choices.
- Insufficient attention has been paid to the beneficial effects of tissue oxygenation in preventing wound infection. It has been shown, for example, that, when 80% inspired oxygen is given during and for 2 hours following colectomy, the wound infection rate is reduced by 50%.[5] When a wound is closed, the subcutaneous oxygen tension falls.[6] This probably explains the benefits of delayed primary wound closure after injury or contamination.

Action

1. If you suspect contamination (Latin: *contaminen*=pollute, make dirty) or infection (Latin: *in*=into+*facere*=to make; introduction of pathogenic organisms), always start by taking swabs for aerobic and anaerobic culture and tests for antibiotic sensitivity.
2. Do not close a wound that is contaminated, that has ischaemic tissues within it forming a potential source of infection, or one in which body fluids are likely to collect that will form a good culture medium for microorganisms. In case of doubt, insert sutures but delay tying them until you are sure that the wound is clean—delayed primary closure.
3. If there is considerable swelling and tension of the deep tissues, as may occur in cellulitis, burns or following trauma, do not hesitate to release the tension by laying open the constricting tissues, taking care to avoid injury to important structures. In the limbs this is accomplished by making longitudinal incisions through the skin and deep fascia. The term debridement (French: to unbridle) was originally applied to releasing an encircling constriction. It is now commonly and confusingly extended to mean the removal of devitalized or contaminated tissues.
4. Excise from traumatized or infected wounds all dead or dying tissue, in particular muscle that has been crushed, is ischaemic or has been devitalized by the close passage of a high-velocity missile. Remove all foreign material, since it is potentially infected (see Ch. 2). Preserve important structures such as major blood vessels and nerves, remembering that they may be displaced following injury. Do not remove attached bone fragments unless they are grossly displaced. Do not over-aggressively excise damaged skin, especially of the hands and face.
5. In the presence of swelling, where there may be tension after closure, employ delayed primary closure. Leave the wound open, elevate the part if possible and close it when the swelling has diminished.

VIRAL TRANSMISSION

Ensure that you are immunized against hepatitis B (HBV). You remain at risk from hepatitis C (HCV) and from human immunodeficiency virus (HIV). Adapt your technique to protect yourself, your team and patients from risk of transmitting these viruses during your management of them. This applies not just to the operating theatre but to every encounter with patients.[7]

High-risk patients

1. If you suspect that a patient has HBV or HIV, or has overt clinical features suggesting they have AIDS, you should advise them to accept antibody testing. The HIV test must be preceded by counselling.
2. Manage those you consider to have, or who are proven to have, transmissible viral infection such as HBV and HIV in a modified manner. However, they are no longer placed at the end of the operating list and are treated in the usual manner on arrival in the anaesthetic room. The anaesthetist wears eye protection and surgical gloves during induction.
3. Ensure that the operating table is covered with an impervious sheet to avoid contamination of the mattress.
4. Wear eye protection, and a completely impervious gown over a plastic apron that covers impervious boots and overshoes. Wear an impervious mask. Wear two pairs of gloves.
5. After cleaning the skin, apply impervious wound drapes.
6. At the end of the operation, ensure that the 'sharps' container and disposable gowns, drapes and swabs are placed in separate bags to be sent for disposal. Re-usable instruments are placed in containers for separate washing and sterilization. Re-usable gowns and drapes should be soaked in 1% sodium hypochlorite solution before being washed and re-sterilized.

All patients

KEY POINTS Never relax your precautions with any patient

- Employ universal precautions. This means you must use the same safe procedures for every patient, every time.
- Do not delude yourself that the precautions you have taken for 'high-risk' patients protect you from contracting hepatitis virus or HIV. It is the patients you assume not to be infectious that pose the greatest threat to you.
- The most dangerous substances with which you come into contact are human blood, blood products and secretions. The best way to avoid contact with the patient's blood is to avoid spilling it.
- The greatest threats to safety routines are emergency situations.

1 Adopt a standard technique that protects you and your team from contact with the blood and body secretions of all patients at all times.

2 Never allow 'sharps', such as knives, needles, trocars, spikes or hooks, to be passed from hand to hand. Have them placed in a dish. When you use them, take them from the dish and return them to it after use.

3 Avoid contact with the sharp portions of knives and needles. When suturing use a strictly 'no-touch' technique: hold needles in a needle-holder, recover them after they have passed through the tissues with dissecting forceps, from which they are passed back to the needle-holder. Make sure that, as you draw the needle through, you do not injure yourself or anyone in the team. Grasp the thread away from the needle with your fingers (an instrument will damage the thread) and draw it through. This also prevents you from pulling the thread from the swaged needle.

4 Never use your unprotected finger as a guide for a needle or knife, as when penetrating the abdominal or chest wall. Prefer to evert the tissues in order to see the emerging point, or place a flat metal plate over the deeper tissues at risk, or wear a sterile metal thimble on your finger.

5 You must, from time to time, deal with active bleeding. Indeed, the operation may be performed in order to control it. As soon as you have stopped the bleeding, aspirate all the blood. Discard the bloodstained swabs, replace the bloodstained drapes.

6 If your gloves are damaged, change them immediately. If they become heavily bloodstained do not hesitate to change them; as you do so, observe your hands and fingers for blood that may have seeped through a defect, and the elastic cuff of your gown to note if it is bloodstained. If you see such evidence of contact with the patient's blood, rescrub and apply a clean gown and gloves.

7 At the end of the operation, peel off your gloves so they are turned inside out and you can then inspect them for tears. An alternative is first to wash your gloved hands in methylthioninium chloride (methylene blue) solution, then remove your gloves to see if your fingers are stained blue. Inspect your fingers for pricks and cuts.

8 If you have sustained an injury during the operation you should immediately report it to the Occupational Health Officer. At present such injuries are under-reported, and in turn the risks to surgeons and other theatre staff are underestimated.

9 Disposable sharps are carefully placed in a self-locking, disposal carrier.

Surgeon with HIV

A surgeon infected with HIV must cease duties that involve the risk of contact with patients' blood or tissues. This effectively precludes a continuing career in surgery.

Closure

1 Do not close the wound until you have checked that the procedure has been accomplished perfectly, that there is no continuing bleeding and that you have not inadvertently damaged other structures.

2 Did you intend to carry out any ancillary procedure?

3 Have you aspirated any fluid collections?

4 Do you need to insert drains or other apparatus?

5 Can you reduce postoperative pain by carrying out a nerve block? This is particularly valuable for short-stay or day-case patients. Following inguinal herniorrhaphy, consider carrying out inguinal field block using bupivacaine. Do not use more than 100 mg in dilute solution, such as 40 ml of 0.25%. Instillation into the wound of 10 ml of 0.5% (50 mg) plain bupivacaine has been shown to be effective in reducing postoperative pain.

6 Observe the basic principles of surgical closure. Do not leave continuing cause for complications, do not close under tension and attain perfect apposition of the tissues you bring together.

7 Do not use hand-held needles. The risk of skin injuries is probably less with skin staples or clips than with sutured closure. Whenever possible close with subcuticular stitches, preferably of fine absorbable synthetic material that does not require attendance by the patient for removal. Alternatively, use adhesive strips. The newer fibrin tissue adhesives may come into common use.

8 Occasionally the wound needs to be packed because of bleeding that cannot be controlled by any other method. It can occur as a result of an uncorrected or uncorrectable bleeding diathesis, from a localized cause such as a vascular tumour that cannot be removed, or following trauma.

9 An oedematous wound, or one from which superficial tissue is lost, as following trauma or ablative surgery, may be better treated by delayed primary closure after swelling has subsided. After ensuring that the remaining tissues are viable, clean and dry, apply a single layer of non-adherent net, over which apply gauze to seal off the wound.

10 Achieve primary closure of defects using grafts or flaps, for example when bone is exposed or after repairing nerves or blood vessels (see Ch. 36).

Dressings

1 Make sure you know why you are applying dressings and what function they will serve. They may merely protect the wound from damage, prevent the patient from inspecting it or picking at it, protect it from becoming infected or spreading infection elsewhere, soak up exudate, compress the wound to reduce or prevent swelling and act as a supporting corset to reduce tension.

2 Perfectly closed clean minor wounds require no dressing, since they seal within a few hours. Apply a strip of adhesive tape or a varnish if it is necessary to protect the area.

3 If you expect oozing or exudation, apply sufficient sterile gauze to absorb it without 'strike through', ensuring that the gauze is changed before the exudate soaks through and forms a moist pathway for organisms to track down to the wound.

4 If you wish to apply compression, ensure that this is evenly distributed. First apply gauze to absorb any exudate, then evenly laid cotton wool. Do not use the cotton wool as an extra absorbent as it will form a hard, useless cake. Alternatively, use sponge or an inflatable air cushion.

5 It is generally agreed that wounds should not be allowed to dry out. Particularly for wounds associated with burns, cream containing 1% silver sulfadiazine and 0.2% chlorhexidine (Silvzine in the USA and Flamazine elsewhere), is often applied. If you intend leaving the wound open, it is usual to apply a hydrophilic dressing. This will absorb any exudate but should not occlude the wound. Alternatively, apply a single layer of non-adherent net (but not tulle gras which has petroleum jelly that makes the wound soggy), followed by a bulky, absorbent layer of sterile gauze. Some surgeons pack cavities with gauze soaked in flavine emulsion. Do not pack or plug a deep wound as this will seal it from the air. In conflict situations, if all dead and ischaemic tissue and slough and foreign material has been removed and the wound appears clean and healthy, it is often left undisturbed until it is re-dressed 4–5 days later in the operating theatre. Although such wounds usually smell, they can be safely left, provided the patient is well and does not develop signs of sepsis. Of course the dressings must be taken down in the operating theatre if the patient shows features of pain and developing sepsis. In peacetime circumstances and if further removal of dead tissue will probably be required, be prepared to inspect the wounds more frequently.

6 Cavities can also be filled with polymerized foam formed within the cavity. This can be removed for wound cleaning, then washed and re-applied on some exposed areas, as after laying open a pilonidal sinus.

7 To hold dressings in place and exert compression, apply if possible an encircling bandage such as crepe bandage. If you use this method on limbs, always encase the limb with bandage from the extremity up to the site of the wound to avoid producing a garter effect, which would ensue if the bandage were applied only proximally, thus causing venous congestion and distal swelling. Always leave the tips of fingers and toes visible and inspect them regularly to ensure that they are not rendered ischaemic. For the abdomen, many-tailed bandages have been replaced by disposable elastic corsets. Adhesive elastic strips may be applied across the wound under slight tension but they tend to cause excoriation. However, when a wound needs frequent changes of dressing, adhesive strips may be placed on each side of the wound and can be laced together over the dressings to retain them.

REFERENCES

1. Kirk RM 1996 Teaching the craft of operative surgery. Annals of the Royal College of Surgeons of England 78(1 Suppl):25–28
2. Kording KP, Wolpert DM 2004 Bayesian integration in sensorimotor learning. Nature 427:244–247
3. Reason J 1990 Human error. Cambridge University Press, Cambridge
4. Davidson B, Schneider HJ 2004 Audit. In: Kirk RM, Ribbans WJ (eds) Clinical surgery in general, 4th edn. Churchill Livingstone, Edinburgh, pp 428–436
5. Greif R, Akca O, Horn E-P et al 2000 Supplemental perioperative oxygen to reduce the incidence of surgical-wound infection. New England Journal of Medicine 342:161–167
6. Hopf H 2003 Development of subcutaneous wound oxygen measurement in humans: contributions of Thomas K Hunt. Wound Repair and Regeneration 11:424–430
7. Jeffries DJ, Ushiro-Lumb I 2004 The risks to surgeons of nosocomial virus transmission. In: Kirk RM, Ribbans WJ (eds) Clinical surgery in general, 4th edn. Churchill Livingstone, Edinburgh, pp 215–222

GET WELL

- It is not sufficient to carry out the correct procedure perfectly. However well the operation has been performed, the patient has undergone a physiological and psychological disturbance. Your aim must be to help the patient achieve maximum functional recovery and satisfaction with the procedure, as soon as possible. The more ill the patient before operation, the bigger the operation, the greater the risk of complications, in both the short and the long term.
- As a rule you will not carry out all the procedures yourself. Following a general anaesthetic the anaesthetist continues to supervise the general care of patients until they have safely recovered from the effects of the anaesthetic and are in a stable condition (see Ch. 2).
- The recovery room nurses observe the patient and call for assistance as necessary. Nevertheless you must give clear oral and written instructions about the procedure, the likely sequelae and any special observations or actions you require.
- Always make a full record as soon as possible of the operative findings, giving details of the procedure carried out and any special points, such as the insertion of drains. In complicated cases, ensure that drains are labelled; in addition, provide a sketch of the incisions and of attached drains, cannulas or other apparatus, with clear instructions about the management of each one.
- Following a major operation, or one carried out on a poor-risk patient, inform the relatives and the general practitioner as soon as it is convenient, personally or by telephone. It is usually best to defer passing on the full impact of distressing news to relatives until you can speak under less stressful circumstances.

Recovery phase

Regard the patient who has just been submitted to an operation in the same light as one brought into the hospital following an acute illness or trauma.

Monitor

1 Airway, breathing and circulation (ABC) are vital functions to observe during the recovery from anaesthesia.

2 Frequently check the consciousness level of the patient by noting the response to stimuli such as calling the name. In case of doubt, note pupillary and other reflexes and peripheral tone.

3 Do not have a fixed attitude to the amount of pain the patient is likely to suffer. Be willing to administer small, repeated doses of analgesics if the patient recovering consciousness is in pain.[1]

4 In appropriate circumstances check the wound and drains. If blood emerges from an abdominal or chest drain it may be because intra-abdominal or intrathoracic tension has increased as the patient strains. It may also signify that straining has dislodged a ligature. If you suspect that severe bleeding

has restarted, do not hesitate to return the patient to the operating theatre.

5 Restlessness of the patient may have causes other than wound pain. Check that the bladder is not overfull, that the patient is lying comfortably and is not pressed upon by any sharp or hard apparatus.

6 As soon as the patient is responsive, offer information as reassuring as possible about the operation and the present situation.

7 Encourage the wakened patient to breathe deeply, cough and exercise the legs, within the limits posed by the procedure. Moisten the patient's lips or give a mouth wash.

8 Check aspects particular to the patient or the operation. For example, monitor the electrocardiogram (ECG) in patients with cardiac disease, the central nervous system following neurosurgical procedures, the urinary output if renal function is impaired, and the blood sugar in diabetics.

9 Following a general anaesthetic the conscious, stable patient is returned to the ward on instructions from the anaesthetist. The pharyngeal airway is removed before the patient leaves the recovery room. Transfer ill, unstable patients to the intensive care unit.

Intermediate phase

1 Transfer to the ward can be unsettling and uncomfortable.

2 Carefully check airway, breathing, circulation, temperature and other appropriate measurements and record them as a baseline. As the patient recovers, the frequency of monitoring is progressively reduced and stopped.

3 Maintain adequate analgesia. Pain will be reduced if you carried out a field block or instilled long-acting local anaesthetic such as bupivacaine into the wound before closing. The anaesthetist may have inserted an epidural catheter for the instillation of local anaesthetics or opiates. Intramuscular opiates may be titrated, or analgesics may be controlled by the patient. Ensure that the patient's discomfort and pain are reduced to a minimum. Anxiety about respiratory depression or fixed ideas on how much analgesic is needed often leads to inadequate control of pain.

4 Mobilize the patient as quickly as possible, giving breathing and coughing exercises to prevent pulmonary collapse. Encourage leg and foot movement to reduce venous stasis, and frequent changes of posture to prevent pressure sores and allow drainage of the lung bases. Depending upon the operation, aim to have the patient ambulant as soon as possible. In recent years the length of time patients stay in bed after almost all operations has been drastically reduced.

5 Maintain fluid, electrolyte and acid–base balance.[2] This is particularly important in patients who were out of balance before operation, those who must have parenteral intake following, for example, gastrointestinal surgery, and those with renal failure.

6 Following gastrointestinal surgery, aspiration of the digestive tract is usually needed. Check the volume and character of the aspirate.

7 Frequently check the wound and the function of the system subjected to operation.

8 Check the discharge from drains. Most wound drains are removed after 24–48 hours unless they are draining profusely. Chest drains are also removed after 1 or 2 days unless they are draining profusely, or there is a pulmonary leak as evidenced by persistent bubbling through the underwater seal.

9 Insulin-dependent diabetes is usually treated throughout the operation with an infusion of 10% dextrose containing 20 mmol potassium chloride and 300 units of insulin. Approximately 100 ml an hour is given, with frequent checks on blood glucose. It is usually possible to return progressively to the preoperative regime within 2–3 days. Some non-insulin-dependent diabetics need to be given soluble insulin over the operative period but should soon be able to return to their diet or oral islet-cell-stimulant drugs.

10 Long-term drugs often need to be given in a modified form over the perioperative period,[3] and the drugs are restored as the patient recovers. Those on steroid drugs need to have hydrocortisone over the operative period and this is continued, usually in a dose of 100 mg hydrocortisone intravenously by slow infusion every 6 hours, with progressive diminution of the dose so that the preoperative maintenance dose can be restored after 3–5 days. Ensure that there is adequate fluid and salt replacement and urinary output, and monitor the serum electrolytes and blood glucose. Patients with renal failure taking fludrocortisone should have it restarted, preferably within 3–5 days.

11 Patients with prosthetic heart valves who take long-term warfarin will have been given heparin over the operative period, usually as a slow intravenous infusion, controlled by maintaining the activated partial thromboplastin time (APTT) at 1.5–2.5 times normal. After operation, warfarin is restarted, to overlap the heparin; now also check the international normalized ratio (INR).

12 Antidepressant, anxiolytic, anticonvulsant and antiparkinsonian drugs need to be restored. Drugs of abuse, including alcohol and opiates, must also be restored or alternative treatment given.

13 Most patients develop a mild pyrexia during the first 24 hours after operation. If it remains there may be a known reason, but, if not, thoroughly investigate the cause.[4] A swinging pyrexia denotes sepsis and this is most likely to be at the site of operation. Interpret the pyrexia in association with other features, such as the general condition of the patient and any associated circulatory disorder. If you cannot discover the cause, routinely check the possibilities:

- Remember that patients may develop upper respiratory infection, including tonsillitis and ear infections, incidentally. Consider these, especially in young children.
- Clinical examination, chest X-ray and sputum culture may suggest pulmonary collapse, pneumonia or pulmonary embolus. Improvement following inhalations and physiotherapy may confirm a pulmonary cause.
- Apart from the presence of unilateral leg oedema, clinical detection of deep vein thrombosis is unreliable. Clinical evidence of pulmonary embolus may be supported by chest X-ray and ECG.

- Examine the cardiovascular system for features of myocardial infarction and check the ECG and cardiac enzymes.
- Examine the wound and, in the case of abdominal surgery, carefully examine the abdomen and perform a rectal examination. Plain X-ray of the abdomen may reveal air or fluid levels under the diaphragm, dilatation of small and large bowel suggesting adynamic ileus, and thickening of the interfaces between bowel segments—so-called 'layering', which is indicative of peritonitis. Order a white blood cell count.
- Send a midstream urine (MSU) specimen for microscopy and culture.
- Examine intravenous injection and infusion sites for phlebitis.

14 Look at the whole skin surface to exclude raw areas, including pressure sores.

15 Has the patient an artificial cardiac valve? You will have known this before operation and should have given the patient prophylactic antibiotics. Nevertheless, order a blood culture.

16 You may still be uncertain. If you have already sent blood for culture that was unrevealing, send another one: a single specimen may not culture organisms successfully. Re-examine the patient after an interval.

17 If you initiate non-specific supportive treatment and the patient improves, do not assume that the problem is solved. Remain vigilant and anticipate possible deterioration (see Fig. 1.2).

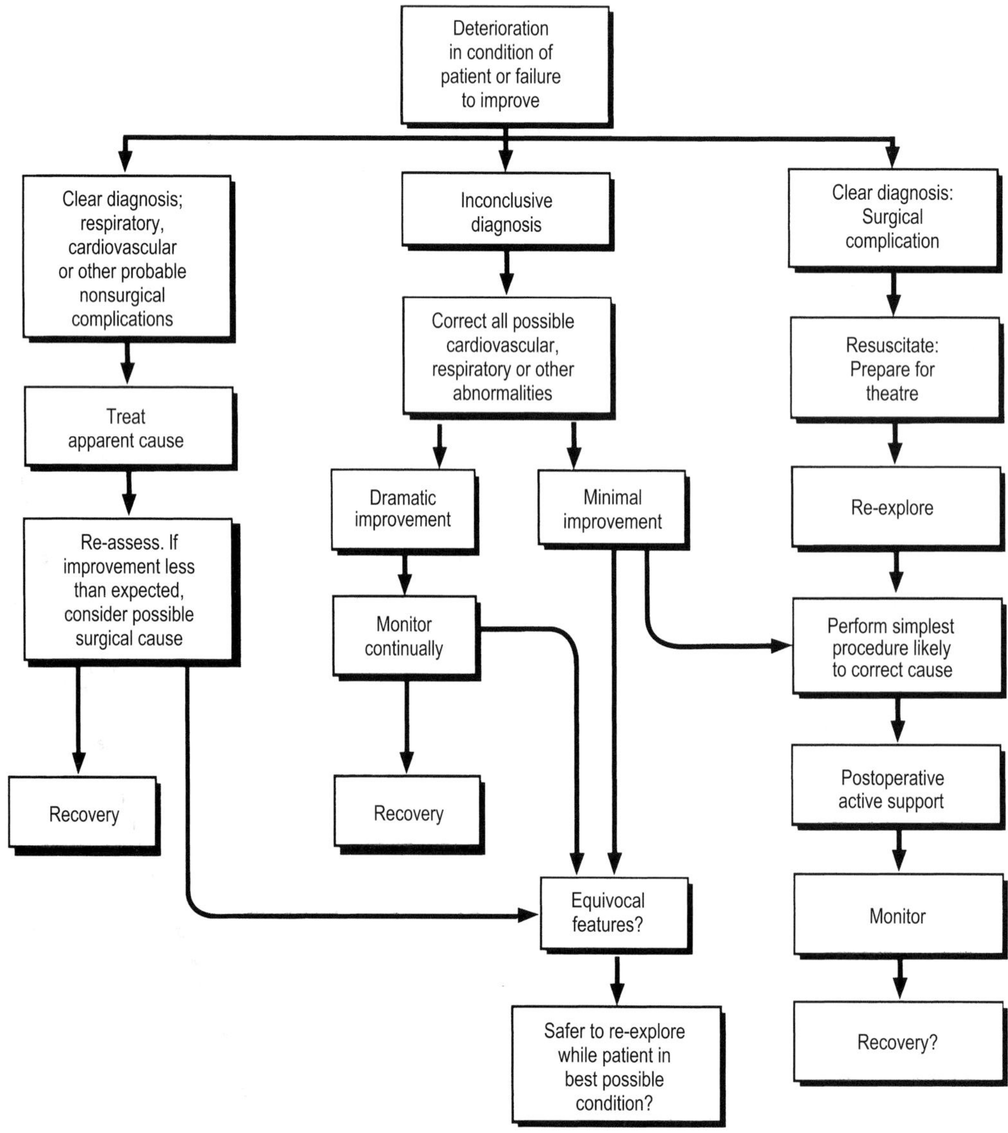

Fig. 1.2 Scheme for management of a patient who develops a complication or fails to recover satisfactorily following an operation. (Adapted with permission from Kirk RM 1990 Reoperation for early intra-abdominal complications following abdominal and abdominothoracic operations. Hospital Update 16:303–310.)

18 Consider what is the likely cause in this patient after the operation that was carried out. Do not order a battery of investigations in the hope that 'something will turn up'. First call in a senior, experienced colleague to examine the patient.

Day case

1 The monitoring of recovery from a general anaesthetic must be as thorough as that of an inpatient. Sedation with benzodiazepines and administration of analgesics may depress respiration, so this must be monitored for 2 hours.

2 The normal assessment of recovery has to be compressed into a shorter period, but ensure that the cardiovascular and respiratory functions are normal before discharge.

3 Check the wound.

4 Fully inform the patient of the procedure, the likely sequelae, danger signs and what to do about them. It is wise to give written instructions for later reference.

5 If a follow-up appointment is to be given, arrange it now.

6 Ensure that those who have had a general anaesthetic or sedation are accompanied home.

7 Record the findings and procedure immediately. Because series of day cases are often arranged, it is easy to confuse the details if they are not recorded individually, between procedures.

Audit

- Remarkable changes have occurred during the last 10 years, and especially during the last 5 years, from changes in public expectation and from media coverage of the complications that developed following the general adoption of minimal access techniques, often by surgeons with minimal training. However, the investigation in 1998 of the results of paediatric cardiac surgery in Bristol brought matters to a head.
- We should all ensure our results are open to scrutiny—not, as formerly, just to our own consciences, but also to our patients and peers.
- Although mortality and morbidity conferences and audit meetings are as yet fairly crude, efforts are being made to grade the severity of acute conditions, such as the modified acute physiology and chronic health evaluation (APACHE II)[5] combination of clinical and laboratory findings. Surgical outcome can be assessed using POSSUM (Physiological and Operative Severity Score for Enumeration of Mortality and Morbidity),[6,7] and this has been used with a modification for the evaluation of vascular surgical operations—the Portsmouth predictor equation.[8]
- Undoubtedly, these methods will be refined so that reliable comparisons will be possible between the likely outcomes following available operations and also of non-operative management.

Follow-up

1 You follow up patients to ensure that they recover without complications, to reassure them, to give further treatment, to assess your own results for comparison with published figures and to detect long-term sequelae.

2 Make sure that you know why each patient is returning to your clinic. If patients attend unnecessarily, the clinic becomes overfilled and those who need attention are deprived of it. Sometimes attendance at the clinic can be averted by allowing patients to write in or telephone when they have a problem or at fixed intervals.

REFERENCES

1. Sodhi V, Fernando R 2004 Management of post-operative pain. In: Kirk RM, Ribbans WJ (eds) Clinical surgery in general, 4th edn. Churchill Livingstone, Edinburgh, pp 357–369
2. Aveling W, Hamilton MA 2004 Fluid, electrolyte and acid-base balance. In: Kirk RM, Ribbans WJ (eds) Clinical surgery in general, 4th edn. Churchill Livingstone, Edinburgh, pp 107–124
3. Tate JJT 2004 Post-operative care. In: Kirk RM, Ribbans WJ (eds) Clinical surgery in general, 4th edn. Churchill Livingstone, Edinburgh, pp 349–356
4. Smith JAR 2004 Complications: prevention and management. In: Kirk RM, Ribbans WJ (eds) Clinical surgery in general, 4th edn. Churchill Livingstone, Edinburgh, pp 373–387
5. Goldhill DR, Sumner A 1998 APACHE II, data accuracy and outcome prediction. Anaesthesia 53:937–943
6. Copeland GP, Jones D, Walters M 1991 POSSUM: a scoring system for surgical audit. British Journal of Surgery 78:355–360
7. Jones HJS, de Cossart L 1999 Risk scoring in surgical patients. British Journal of Surgery 86:149–157
8. Midwinter MJ, Tytherleigh M, Ashley S 1999 Estimation of mortality and morbidity risk in vascular surgery using POSSUM and the Portsmouth predictor equation. British Journal of Surgery 86:471–474

FURTHER READING

Bell D, Shapiro C 1992 The health care worker with HIV infection or AIDS. Clinical Care 4:9–16

Birkmeyer JD, Welch HG 1997 A reader's guide to surgical decision making. Journal of the American College of Surgeons 184: 589–595

Bunker JP, Barnes BA, Mosteller F 1977 Costs, risks, and benefits of surgery. Oxford University Press, Oxford

Clarke JR 1989 Decision making in surgical practice. World Journal of Surgery 13:245–251

Dufour D, Kromann-Jensen S, Owen-Smith M et al 1998 Surgery for victims of war, 3rd edn. IRCR (International Committee of the Red Cross)

Finlayson SRG, Birkmeyer JD 1998 Cost effectiveness analysis in surgery. Surgery 123:151–156

General Medical Council 1988 HIV infection and AIDS: ethical considerations. General Medical Council, London

Greep JM, Siezenis LMLC 1989 Methods of decision analysis: protocols, decision trees, and algorithms in medicine. World Journal of Surgery 13:240–244

Gunning K, Rowan K 1999 Outcome data and scoring systems. British Medical Journal 319:241–244

Kirk RM 2002 Basic surgical techniques, 5th edn. Churchill Livingstone, Edinburgh

Klein R 1989 The role of health economics. British Medical Journal 299:275–276

Royal College of Surgeons of England 1992 A statement by the College on AIDS and HIV infection. Revised March 1992. Royal College of Surgeons of England, London

Spittal MJ, Hunter SJ 1992 A comparison of bupivacaine installation and inguinal field block for control of pain after herniorrhaphy. Annals of the Royal College of Surgeons of England 74:85–88

Thornton JG, Lilford RJ, Johnson N 1992 Decision analysis in medicine. British Medical Journal 304:1099–1103

Timmermans D, Kievit J, van Bockel H 1996 How do surgeons' probability estimates of operative mortality compare with a decision analytic model? Acta Psychologica 93:107–120

UK Health Departments 1997 Guidelines on post-exposure prophylaxis for healthcare workers exposed to HIV. Department of Health, London

UK Health Departments 1998 Guidance for clinical health care workers. Protection against infection with bloodborne viruses. Department of Health, London

UK Health Departments 2000 Hepatitis B infected health care workers. HSC 2000/020. Department of Health, London

Weinstein MC, Finsberg HV (eds) 1980 Clinical decision analysis. WB Saunders, Philadelphia, PA

2

Anaesthesia-related techniques

R.S. Simons

CONTENTS

INTRODUCTION

The topics in this chapter are confined to the practical skill-mix listed above. To obtain a wider understanding of the anaesthetist's contribution to surgical patients, read the relevant chapters in the companion volume: Kirk RM, Ribbans WJ (eds) 2004 Clinical surgery in general, 4th edn. Churchill Livingstone, Edinburgh (an RCS course manual).

These skills, applicable to anaesthetists and surgeon alike include the ability to:

- Evaluate co-morbidities that the patient may have, typically but not exclusively involving cardiovascular, renal, respiratory and metabolic systems.
- Assess preoperative investigations (including blood transfusion requirements) required for surgery in conjunction with the patient's age, co-morbidity and extent of intended surgery.
- Demonstrate proficiency in the ABC (airway, breathing, circulation) of resuscitation.
- Confidently undertake peripheral and central venous access and restore acute and chronic fluid losses.
- Use local anaesthetic techniques to supplant or augment general anaesthesia, including its use in postoperative analgesia.
- Provide effective postoperative pain relief.
- Utilize intensive therapy facilities in a coordinated and efficient manner.

RESPIRATORY SUPPORT

To maintain the heart and the brain,
Give oxygen now and again.
Not now and again, but NOW, AND AGAIN, AND AGAIN, AND AGAIN, AND AGAIN.

(Adapted from a well-known limerick.)

KEY POINT Get oxygen to the brain

- Anoxia damages all organs eventually, but failure of oxygen supply can damage the brain within 3–4 minutes. It is vital that you ensure a patent airway, satisfactory exchange of gases and adequate circulation.

All doctors in clinical practice, regardless of speciality, should receive training and certification in cardiopulmonary resuscitation (CPR) to the level of basic life support (BLS). You should also attend an advanced trauma life support (ATLS) course. Advanced cardiac life support (ALS) requirements are just as simple to learn and perform (see Further reading).

OXYGEN THERAPY

Appraise

Oxygen is vital for metabolism. In the presence of ineffective ventilation, impaired pulmonary gas transfer or low output states, high inspired concentrations may be required to re-store a deficient cellular oxygen supply to normal.

KEY POINTS Give oxygen for:

- All hypoxic states if ventilation, oxygen transfer, or circulation are impaired.
- Intracranial, spinal and chest injuries.
- Postoperatively, especially when ventilation is surgically affected or pulmonary disease co-exists.
- Shock of all types.
- Hypermetabolic states such as shivering and hyperthermia.

Assess

For self-ventilating patients

1 Assess level of consciousness by response to speech or painful stimulus. Assess adequacy of self-ventilation by pulse oximetry, respiratory rate and depth, inspection of abdominal and chest movement, ability to speak. If the patient is unconscious, determine the cause.

2 A clear airway is essential. In patients with altered consciousness (e.g. intracranial damage, drug overdose and profound shock) the airway may be compromised by obstruction in the oro- or laryngopharynx. In the supine patient this is typically caused by the tongue falling back against the posterior pharyngeal wall.

3 In emergencies such as shock, post-arrest and multiple trauma, a high inspired oxygen concentration of 80–95% is desirable. In self-ventilating patients this is best achieved by the use of a 'trauma' or 'non-rebreathing oxygen mask' which has a plastic oxygen reservoir bag incorporating a non-rebreathing valve. Use high oxygen flow rates of 12–15 litres/min.

4 For routine oxygen supplementation postoperatively in the recovery room, or on the ward, use a semirigid, perforated disposable transparent plastic face mask of the Hudson design. Oxygen concentrations reach 30–40% with oxygen flows of 4–6 litres/min.

5 For more precise oxygen therapy, 'fixed-performance' masks such as the Ventimask are recommended. These use the Venturi technique driven by oxygen to entrain air to provide high air flow oxygen-enriched air (HAFOE) of constant composition at flows in excess of the patient's peak inspiratory flow, typically 30 litres/min. Higher oxygen percentage masks will require higher oxygen inflow to achieve this minimum peak flow rate; thus 24%, 28%, 35%, 40% and 60% masks require oxygen flows of 2, 4, 6, 10 and 15 litres/min, respectively. Patients often complain that these masks are noisy and cause drying. Nasal oxygen cannulae are better tolerated by conscious patients for prolonged use, albeit providing lower and less predictable oxygen supplementation. To avoid nasal irritation do not exceed oxygen flows of 2 litres/min.

6 Humidification is essential for oxygen therapy lasting more than 3–4 hours, especially where nasal humidification is bypassed during mouth breathing or by intubation. Humidification is impracticable for nasal cannulae.

7 Standard oxygen therapy masks will not suffice when a patient's ventilatory demands are excessive (e.g. if respiratory rates greater than 25–30 breaths/min and/or oxygen concentrations in excess of 60% are required to maintain adequate arterial saturation). Such demands are best met using a CPAP (continuous positive airway pressure) device which requires a tight-fitting cuffed mask, secured with straps around the head, a PEEP (positive end-expiratory pressure) valve (5–10 cm water) and an oxygen flow in excess of 25–30 litres/min. Such devices are typically managed by outreach teams, respiratory technicians or physiotherapists. The progressive increase in physiological dead space associated with severe gas exchange makes spontaneous ventilation very tiring, and such patients are in any case likely to require tracheal intubation and intermittent positive pressure ventilation (IPPV) if the underlying pathology does not resolve rapidly. Maintain close links with intensive care colleagues when caring for such patients.

8 Patients with acute-on-chronic respiratory failure present a special problem, especially 'blue bloaters' with type II respiratory failure who depend upon a certain degree of hypoxic drive for ventilation. High oxygen concentrations may lead to progressive underventilation. Start with 28–35% 'fixed performance' devices and maintain careful clinical observation of the patient while measuring blood oxygen and carbon dioxide tensions. Deteriorating consciousness level or rising carbon dioxide levels warn of impending respiratory arrest. This process seldom occurs rapidly and ensuring adequate oxygenation clearly takes precedence, especially when the underlying lung pathology is acute and reversible. It may be necessary to institute IPPV if oxygenation remains unsatisfactory. Seek the help of physicians or intensivists skilled in the management of such patients.

9 *Oxygen toxicity* is never a problem during acute resuscitation and occurs only slowly following exposure to high oxygen concentrations for several days. The clinical picture resembles bronchopneumonia, with cough, retrosternal pain, bronchiolar and alveolar exudates. Bronchopulmonary dysplasia may develop, though the condition can resolve if the patient survives the hypoxic episode. In hyperbaric oxygen therapy the condition may evolve within a few hours and convulsions may occur if oxygen levels greater than 2 atmospheres are used.

▶ KEY POINTS Care during oxygen therapy

- Adequate humidification, regular tracheobronchial toilet and physiotherapy are vitally important.
- Anticipate respiratory depression in patients with chronic respiratory disease.
- Oxygen is rapidly absorbed beyond a bronchial blockage causing atelectasis.
- Beware of fire risks.

AIRWAY AND VENTILATORY SUPPORT

Action

In patients with impaired consciousness

1 Remove any dentures and clear the pharynx and mouth of any gross contamination from blood, gastric contents or foreign material. Have available at all times Magill forceps and suction equipment with a semirigid Yankauer handpiece already attached.

2 If trauma has occurred, be suspicious of cervical spine injury. Conduct manoeuvres to ensure airway patency with the head centrally aligned. Do not allow the head and neck to be flexed or extended. Stabilize the head with a firm cervical collar, supports or straps, to prevent axial rotation of the spine.

3 Assess whether simple airway adjuncts, such as the Guedel oropharyngeal airway or soft curved nasopharyngeal tube, will secure patency. Insert a Guedel airway 'upside down' under the upper teeth, then rotate it downwards behind the tongue. After

insertion, continue to support the jaw by jaw lift or jaw thrust. Lubricate a nasopharyngeal airway and insert it into the nose parallel to the hard palate to lie behind the soft palate and tongue. Put a safety pin through the tube to ensure it cannot migrate into the nose.

4 If ventilation is adequate, nurse the patient in the lateral or semiprone recovery position with head dependent to avoid regurgitation and aspiration into the trachea. This posture may be impracticable while you examine, resuscitate or treat the patient, or if spinal trauma is present or suspected.

5 If necessary, reverse the effect of opioid or benzodiazepine drugs with their respective specific antagonists: 0.2–0.4 mg naloxone or 0.3–0.6 mg flumazenil given intravenously.

6 If spontaneous ventilation is inadequate despite the insertion of an oropharyngeal airway, apply the mask (adult sizes 4–6) of a self-inflating bag–mask resuscitator to the nose and mouth (Figs 2.1, 2.2). Hold it securely on the face with one hand while lifting the jaw upwards and forwards, with the airway still in place, and create a tight seal. Try to achieve tidal volumes of 500–800 ml at a rate of 10–15 ml/min. Common problems encountered are an obstructed airway or failure to obtain an adequate seal. If the former is the case, elevate the jaw further and extend the head, provided you do not suspect cervical spine injury. If mask seal is a problem, reapply the mask more evenly or ask an assistant to squeeze the bag while you use both hands to hold it firmly in position.

7 Add oxygen to the bag at 8–10 litres/min to increase the inspired oxygen concentration to 40–60%. Where possible, add a reservoir bag to the resuscitation device. This increases the inspired oxygen level to 80–90%.

8 If you cannot achieve any chest movement, consider the possibility of a foreign body obstructing the hypopharynx, larynx or trachea. Attempt the Heimlich manoeuvre if appropriate and/or use a laryngoscope and Magill forceps to remove the offending foreign body if you can see it at laryngoscopy. If this fails or if severe maxillofacial trauma prevents effective ventilation by conventional methods, prepare for cricothyrotomy as an emergency procedure.

9 *Cricothyrotomy*. Make an incision horizontally in the cricothyroid membrane and insert a suitable hollow device through the membrane into the trachea, below the level of the vocal cords. A 5-mm (internal diameter, ID) tube may be adequate for resuscitation purposes, but presents a high resistance to both inspiratory and expiratory flow. Increased resistance with spontaneous ventilation may induce pulmonary oedema from any forceful negative intrathoracic efforts the patient may attempt. Therefore prefer a 6–7-mm tube if possible and convert it to a formal tracheostomy as soon as practicable. Do not attempt tracheostomy as a primary emergency procedure since it is difficult to perform under emergency conditions in inadequate surroundings on hypoxic patients.

Further considerations

1 Partial or broken dentures, food and foreign debris, blood (active bleeding or clots) and vomited or regurgitated stomach contents represent additional sources of airway obstruction or which may be inhaled into the lungs.

2 Regurgitation with pulmonary aspiration is not uncommon in semiconscious patients and usually develops insidiously. It more commonly occurs in the presence of a full stomach, ileus, pregnancy, hiatal hernia, maxillofacial trauma or muscle relaxants, and may be compounded by air blown into the stomach during mask ventilation. Use cricoid pressure—the Sellick manoeuvre—during resuscitation and intubation to avoid or

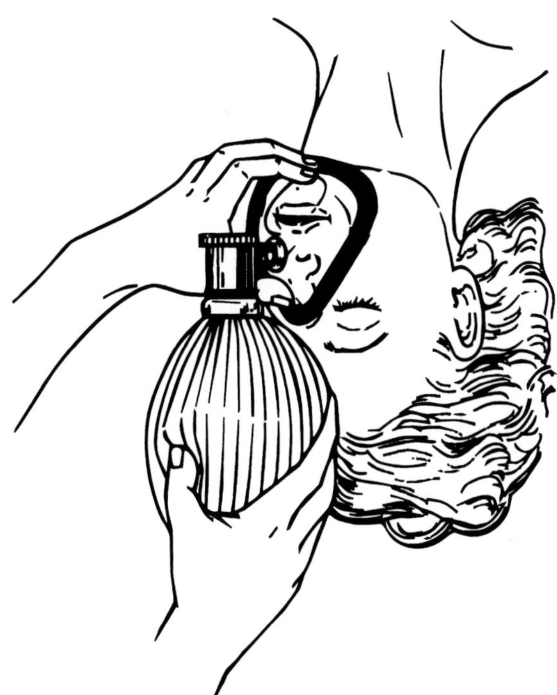

Fig. 2.1 Resuscitation with a bag–valve mask (single-handed).

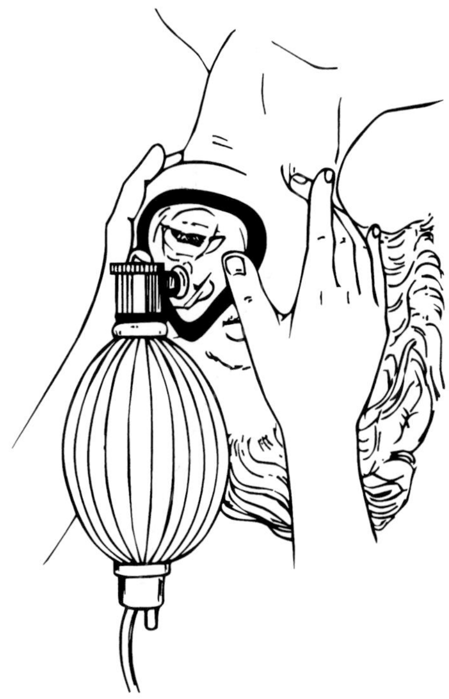

Fig. 2.2 Resuscitation with a bag–valve mask (two-handed).

minimize this risk. Have an assistant press firmly with three fingers straddling the cricoid ring to compress the oesophagus between the cricoid ring and the body of the sixth cervical vertebra.

3 Vomiting, unlike regurgitation, is an active process and usually occurs at lighter levels of unconsciousness. If you observe prodromal retching or vomiting, release cricoid pressure to avoid gastric rupture. Turn the patient quickly into the recovery position with head dependent if possible.

4 The hazard of pulmonary aspiration is accentuated if the aspirate has a pH of less than 3, when the risk of a chemical pneumonitis from acid aspiration (Mendelson's syndrome) is considerable. If you suspect pulmonary contamination, immediately intubate the patient (see below) to secure airway isolation and if possible set aside a suction trap specimen from the lungs or pharynx to measure the acidity of the aspirate with wide-range pH paper (not litmus). Immediately lavage the lungs several times with aliquots of 20–50 ml of saline, using 100% oxygen, large tidal volumes and tracheal suction. The procedure may well avert a full-blown aspiration syndrome, which can develop within 2–4 hours and resemble acute adult respiratory distress syndrome (ARDS). Give broad-spectrum antibiotic therapy. Intravenous steroids and tracheal bicarbonate instillation are of doubtful benefit. Involve anaesthetists or intensivists in the further care of such patients as soon as possible.

KEY POINT Sucker available?

- Always have functioning suction equipment available for unconscious patients.

TRACHEAL INTUBATION

Appraise

1 Achieve competence in tracheal intubation by practising on an intubation training simulator and under supervision by anaesthetists during induction of anaesthesia for routine surgery. It is a useful skill to have when faced with airway emergencies in or out of hospital.

2 Patients tolerate tracheal intubation only at deep levels of unconsciousness, typically associated with general anaesthesia or 'coma'. Intubation ensures the patency of the upper airway, avoiding obstruction from haemorrhage or swelling, and prevents entry of blood, gastric contents, secretions and other foreign matter into the tracheobronchial tree. It is the most effective form of airway isolation when undertaking positive pressure ventilation.

3 When deciding whether an unconscious patient requires tracheal intubation in order to safeguard the airway, be guided by the state of the laryngeal reflexes and the degree of muscle tone. If these are such that intubation is unlikely to be tolerated without great difficulty or sedation, then abandon intubation and use an oral or nasal pharyngeal airway instead.

Prepare

1 *Laryngoscope*. The Macintosh-pattern curved laryngoscope blade is still the most popular and the easiest to learn to use. The standard adult size 3 Macintosh blade is suitable for most patients over 5 years of age, although a size 4 may be required for large males. Check that the laryngoscope bulb and blade are well secured.

2 *Endotracheal tube*. These slightly curved plastic tubes have an ID range of 2.5–10.0 mm in 0.5-mm increments. They are presented as disposable, prepacked items complete with one bevelled end (cuffed above 6.0 mm) and a 15-mm plastic connector lightly inserted into the other end. The tube is stamped with the internal diameter in millimetres near the bevel and the length is often marked in centimetres at the connector end, which requires cutting to length before use. Use 7.0–8.0 mm ID for adult females and 8.0–9.0 mm for adult males. Use cuffed tubes for patients over 7–8 years, uncuffed below that age. A convenient guide to tube diameter can be based on:

- The tip of the patient's little finger; this is a good measure of overall tube size as it closely matches the size of the cricoid ring.
- For children, ID (mm) = [(age in years)/4] + 4.5.

Length for adults ranges from 22 cm for females to 24 cm for males. For nasal intubation add 2–4 cm. A convenient guide to length is gauged by:

- Hold the tube alongside the patient's face, allowing for the curvature in the mouth and measure the distance from lips to cricoid ring; add an allowance for the portion outside the mouth and a safe length in the trachea.
- For children, length (cm) = [(age in years)/2] + 12.

3 *Connections* (Fig. 2.3). Having cut the tube to the recommended length, fit the tapered tube connector tightly into the cut end. The 15-mm end connector is a standard fit for use with a catheter mount to adapt it to a resuscitation device, anaesthetic circuit or ventilator. It also fits directly to a self-inflating bag-valve resuscitator if the catheter mount is not available.

4 Test the cuff of the tube with a few millilitres of air from a 10-ml syringe. Deflate it and apply water-miscible lubricant over the cuffed portion of the tube. Have ready a curved malleable metal stylet or a long gum-elastic bougie to assist in case the intubation is difficult.

5 Test the good working order of the suction equipment. Have available Yankauer semirigid handpieces in addition to a range of plastic suction catheters.

6 Correctly position the patient. Moderately flex the cervical spine by raising the head on one pillow, and then extend the head at the atlanto-occipital joint, as when 'sniffing the morning air'.

7 Inspect the mouth. Remove any dentures and look for loose teeth, crowns or bridges, especially in the upper incisor area, to avoid damaging or dislodging them during intubation.

Action

1 Hold the laryngoscope handle vertical in your left hand with the blade downward and the light shining towards the patient's

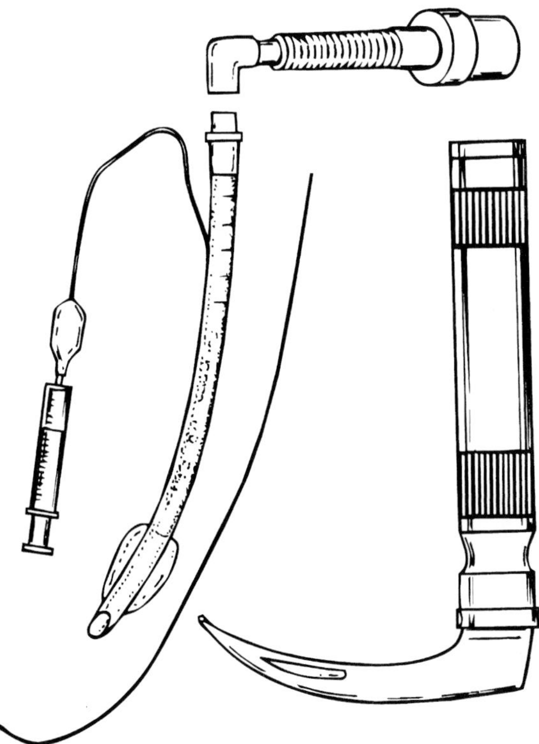

Fig. 2.3 Tracheal intubation equipment: cuffed endotracheal tube with inflation syringe, catheter mount, gum-elastic bougie and laryngoscope.

feet. Open the mouth by gently extending the head with the right hand. Maximum opening can be obtained by placing your right index finger along the line of the upper right premolars and molars, and further extending the head. Avoid damage to the incisors. With the head extended, insert the blade into the right side of the mouth in an arc over the tongue, directing the blade tip towards the uvula. The laryngoscope blade holds the bulk of the tongue out of the way to the left and allows you a clear view down the right side of the mouth. Continue advancing the blade in a gentle curve along the back of the tongue until you see the epiglottis. Then pass the blade anterior to the epiglottis, between it and the base of the tongue, and lodge the tip firmly in the vallecula. The vocal cords may be visible now but it is usually necessary to lift the tongue and jaw together vertically to adequately visualize the glottis. Do not lever on the upper teeth or gums. This causes damage and does not improve the view.

2 If you cannot see the epiglottis, either the laryngoscope blade is not in the midline or it may have passed over the epiglottis into the laryngopharynx. Withdraw the blade to about two-thirds along the tongue and re-advance it.

3 When you see the glottis, hold the tracheal tube near its connector in the right hand, concavity forward, and pass it via the right side of the mouth, so that the tip comes into the midline immediately above the laryngeal opening. Insert the bevel between the vocal cords and slide the tube onwards through the larynx so that the cuff lies below the level of the vocal cords. Hold the tube firmly while gently withdrawing the laryngoscope.

4 To check that the tube is in the correct position, press firmly on the subject's chest. A puff of air emerging from the tube gives some reassurance that it has entered the trachea rather than the oesophagus. Connect it to a ventilating device such as a self-inflating bag or anaesthetic circuit, and apply positive pressure to ventilate the patient's lungs. If you use a cuffed tube, slowly inflate the cuff with an air-filled 10-ml syringe until audible leakage ceases during inspiration; this is typically 3–7 ml. Check for reasonable tension in the pilot cuff. Remove the syringe from the self-sealing Luer-lock valves of the pilot tube.

5 Uniform expansion of the chest indicates correct placement. Confirm correct placement by auscultation with a stethoscope while ventilating the lungs. Also auscultate the epigastrium to ensure the tube was not inadvertently placed in the oesophagus. If one side of the chest expands more than the other then the tube may have passed too far into a main bronchus, usually the right. Deflate the cuff and withdraw the tube until chest expansion is uniform. Re-inflate the cuff. Exclude less frequent causes of unilateral chest expansion such as pneumo- or haemothorax.

6 Secure the tube to the patient's face with strapping or by means of a loop of tape or bandage around the neck, having first knotted it securely around the tube. Avoid constricting the jugular or facial veins by tying too tightly.

? DIFFICULTY

A common difficulty during intubation is an inability to lift the jaw sufficiently forward to expose the glottis fully, or to persuade the tube to follow the curve behind the epiglottis. Bend the tube to increase its curvature and try again. A further option is to pass a lubricated malleable metal stylet into the tube to within 1 cm of the tip, and angulate the tube more sharply. Alternatively, pass a long gum-elastic bougie through the tube so that it protrudes for a few centimetres and angulate the end of this to aid laryngeal entry. In difficult cases, first insert the gum-elastic bougie into the trachea alone and then railroad the tracheal tube over the bougie into the trachea.

Alternative

The laryngeal mask airway (LMA) is very popular with anaesthetists (Fig. 2.4). It has a curved tube with a hollow, soft rubber spoon at one end bearing an inflatable rim. The device is inserted via the mouth into the laryngopharynx, concavity forward, and the cuff is inflated to 'seal' the rim against the laryngeal inlet, so maintaining patency and providing a degree of airway isolation. It is tolerated at lighter levels of consciousness than a standard tracheal tube and may allow positive pressure ventilation, although some leakage is likely. Its ability to isolate the trachea reliably against aspiration cannot be guaranteed, but with practice it is easy to use and is likely to prove a useful adjunct in situations where conventional intubation would be impracticable.

Recent modifications of the device include an intubating LMA and a further device which allows decompression and suction of gastric contents via a venting tube.

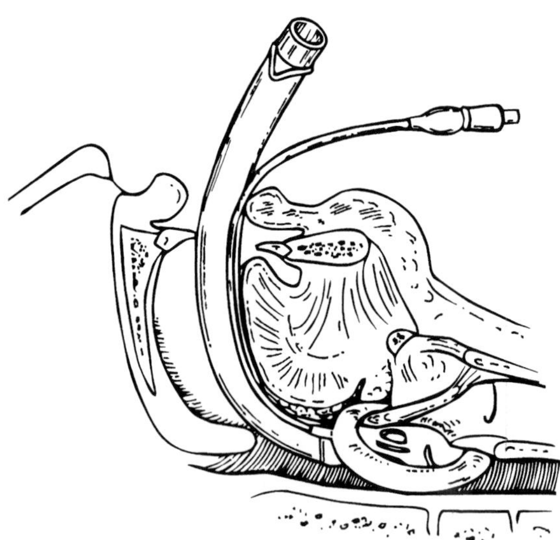

Fig. 2.4 Laryngeal mask airway.

ARTIFICIAL VENTILATION

1 Institute IPPV (intermittent positive pressure ventilation) without delay whenever spontaneous breathing is inadequate to provide effective gas exchange. Room air contains 21% oxygen, and the immediate application of 35–60% oxygen via an oxygen mask is a useful emergency measure to compensate for the hypoxia associated with impaired ventilation while preparing for intubation and ventilation. If breathing is totally absent, immediately institute artificial ventilation.

2 In lay emergency situations, start expired air resuscitation using mouth-to-mouth, mouth-to-nose or mouth-to-airway adjuncts, using the 16% oxygen available in expired air. Mouth-to-mouth ventilation may be hazardous in the presence of oral trauma, and resuscitation equipment for health-care professionals should include self-inflating resuscitation bags with oxygen reservoirs in addition to a range of airway adjuncts: Guedel oropharyngeal airways and soft rubber or plastic nasopharyngeal tubes.

3 Ensure airway patency and ventilate the patient with a bag–mask device. As soon as possible add oxygen from a pipeline or portable cylinder to the inlet valve of the resuscitation bag. At oxygen flows of 6–10 litres/min the inspired oxygen level can be increased from 35% to 80% by adding an oxygen reservoir bag to the self-inflating resuscitator. When using portable oxygen cylinders ensure you have adequate reserves for unexpected delays, especially during transport.

4 Isolate the trachea by passing a tracheal tube or similar device and continue bag–mask ventilation until the patient is connected to a functioning ventilator. Semiconscious patients may need sedation to tolerate airway isolation and IPPV (see below).

KEY POINT Ventilation

- Underventilation is harmful, overventilation rarely so.

5 Aim for a minute volume of 6–8 litres/min in an adult by ventilating at a rate of 10–15 breaths/min with tidal volumes of 500–800 ml. Commence ventilation with 60% inspired oxygen. Inflate the lungs over 1–1.5 seconds and allow 2–2.5 seconds for expiration to occur passively. The expiratory pause is necessary as IPPV raises intrathoracic pressure and impairs venous return.

6 Seek the assistance of anaesthetists and/or intensivists to provide continuing care. Adjust oxygen flow to maintain pulse oximeter saturation readings in excess of 94%, equivalent to arterial oxygen tensions of 11.5–14 kPa (87–105 mmHg). Maintain ventilation to achieve end-tidal carbon dioxide readings or arterial carbon dioxide gases range of 4.0–5.5% (kPa), equivalent to 30–42 mmHg.

7 *Secretions*. Tracheobronchial toilet is necessary during artificial ventilation. Sterility is important. Select sterile disposable catheters with a rounded tip and having several side holes in preference to those with a single end aperture. The latter are traumatic, stick to the tracheal wall and are difficult to advance. Choose a suction catheter that is less than half the tracheal tube diameter (12–14 F in adults) and use it once only. Insert the catheter using sterile gloves or forceps and apply suction intermittently during its withdrawal, avoiding prolonged suction as this causes hypoxia. Collect a sputum-trap specimen for culture initially. A saline nebulizer or repeated saline instillation of 5–10 ml may be useful when secretions are tenacious.

PERIPHERAL VENOUS ACCESS

Appraise

A high-capacity, trouble-free intravenous infusion necessitates one or two large cannulas (16–14FG) in large veins. Venepuncture for this purpose should be a methodical technique. Prepare carefully and do not rush. Gain experience by performing venepuncture on patients with adequate circulation in readiness for the day when your skills are needed for a collapsed, hypovolaemic patient. In such patients your first attempt offers the best chance of success.

Prepare

For the standard percutaneous technique have ready:

- An infusion stand bearing the container of the chosen fluid to which has been attached an intravenous fluid administration set primed to remove air.
- A venous tourniquet (elasticated Velcro band, etc.).
- Swabs for skin cleaning.
- A suitable infusion needle–cannula assembly (see below).
- A 2-ml syringe with a size 25SWG needle for infiltration of local anaesthesia, containing 0.5 ml of 1% plain lidocaine.
- A small sterile disposable scalpel blade.
- A good source of light.
- Adhesive strapping to fix the cannula once inserted.

Action

1 Explain to the patient what is to be done, with reassurance that discomfort will be minimal.

2 Select a suitable vein. The best sites are in the upper limb. Veins of the lower limb are difficult to enter and more liable to spasm and thrombosis. If possible, avoid veins overlying wrist and elbow joints. The best veins are usually found on the radial side of the forearm just proximal to the wrist.

3 Apply a suitable tourniquet to distend the vein without occluding the arterial inflow into the limb. Ask the patient to 'pump' the hand several times. Milk blood from the periphery into the chosen segment or tap the preferred site several times. Ensure good illumination. If necessary, shave the skin over the selected vein; this improves your view of the anatomy, maintains sterility and cause less discomfort when adhesive plaster is subsequently removed. Clean the skin with a suitable cleaning solution such as surgical spirit, isopropyl alcohol or chlorhexidine.

4 In a conscious person minimize discomfort and facilitate venepuncture by using a subcutaneous injection of a small quantity of local anaesthetic.

5 The point of skin penetration should be 0.5–1 cm distal to the point of entry of the vein itself. Select the skin site and inject local anaesthetic solution so as to raise a weal about 4 mm in diameter. Avoid strictly intradermal injection as this distends the skin and makes venepuncture difficult. Allow a short time for the local anaesthetic to work and then penetrate this weal with the tip of a small scalpel blade held vertically. This small skin incision prevents the cannula from being gripped by the skin during insertion and allows more precise entry into the vein.

6 For ordinary purposes choose one of the many proprietary needle-inside-cannula devices (Fig. 2.5). These are disposable and are supplied in a variety of sizes. They generally consist of a flexible, blunt-ended plastic cannula fitting snugly over an inner steel needle whose bevel protrudes slightly beyond the end of the cannula. The distal end of the needle commonly has a transparent flash-back chamber with a semipermeable cap. This cap allows air (but not fluid) to be displaced when blood enters the inner needle and allows visual confirmation of successful venepuncture. Alternatively, remove the cap, attach a 2-ml syringe to the hub of the needle and confirm venepuncture by aspirating blood.

7 Select a cannula–needle assembly of a size appropriate to the size of the chosen vein, the type of fluid to be infused and the desired rate of infusion. For treatment of acute hypovolaemia in adults, one or two 14G cannulas should be inserted (colour code brown). If the veins look too small to accept this size, reduce to a 16G unit (colour code grey).

8 Hold the hub of the unit with the bevel of the needle upwards and insert it at a shallow angle through the small skin incision. Use the thumb of the other hand to stretch the skin so as to keep the vein straight and taut. Advance the tip of the needle up to the vein, keeping it in the long axis of the vein, and enter it from its superficial aspect. Entry is confirmed by the passage of blood back into the flash chamber. Advance the unit a further 0.5–1 cm along the vein to ensure that the tip of the cannula is well into the lumen. Then either hold the hub of the needle steady relative to the skin and slide the cannula down the needle into the vein, or hold the cannula steady relative to the skin and withdraw the needle 0.5–1 cm so as to sheath it within the cannula and then advance the unit as a whole into the vein.

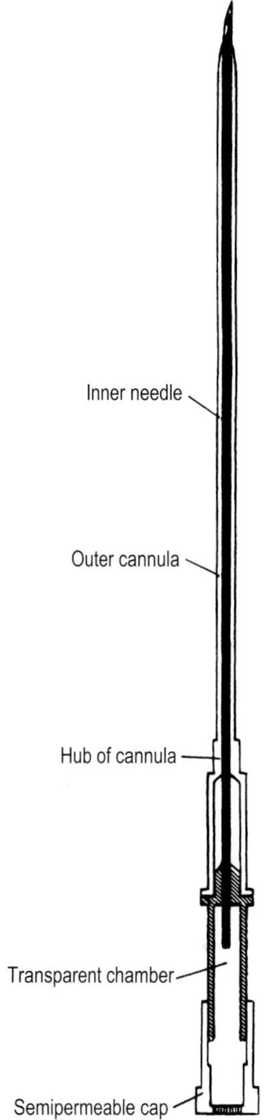

Fig. 2.5 Percutaneous intravenous cannula.

9 Remove the venous tourniquet. Completely withdraw the needle from the cannula, applying pressure over the vein at the point of the cannula tip to prevent blood loss. Attach the infusion set to the cannula and ensure that fluid can flow freely. Form a loop in the drip tubing to protect the catheter from accidental traction. Secure the infusion assembly with a strip of stretchable adhesive placed over the hub of the cannula and adjacent tubing. A splint is not usually needed but may be required if the site of venepuncture is at a joint. In children, secure thoroughly with adhesive plaster but always ensure there is no risk of limb occlusion, especially should venous extravasation occur. Do not bandage so tightly as to impede venous return.

10 With careful and methodical technique it is rarely necessary to use the cutdown method. Nonetheless you should know how to insert a venous catheter by surgical cutdown into the cephalic vein at the wrist, various tributaries at the antecubital fossa, long saphenous vein at the medial malleolus of the ankle and superficial veins in the groin. In an major emergency insert the cut end of a sterile drip-set directly into these larger veins.

KEY POINTS When setting up an intravenous infusion

- Do *not* pressurize rigid containers by injecting or pumping air into them. There is a high risk of air embolus associated with this manoeuvre, especially if your attention is diverted to other problems.
- Do consider using a tap with two giving sets upstream of the warming device so that uninterrupted flow can be maintained during changeover of the fluid bags. When large volumes of fluid have to be infused rapidly, use two or three separate infusion sites.

11 To increase the rate of infusion raise the fluid container as high as possible. Nowadays most fluid containers are collapsible, so apply external pressure to it with a sphygmomanometer cuff or specially designed pressure bag. This is particularly necessary when fluid is being infused through dry or wet warming coils.

12 To avoid thrombophlebitis:
- Use a strict aseptic technique during venepuncture. Cover with a sterile dressing.
- Change the site of infusion every 2–3 days.
- Use non-irritant (Teflon) cannulas in large veins in the upper limbs rather than in the lower limbs.
- When possible avoid dextrose- or potassium-containing solutions in peripheral veins.

CENTRAL VENOUS ACCESS

1 Central venous cannulas or catheters, available as single or multichannel devices of up to four channels (mixed 20–14G size), provide a route for the infusion of fluids, especially veno-irritant medications (e.g. potassium chloride, 50% dextrose, parenteral nutrition) and regulated infusions of inotropes and vasoactive drugs. The resistance in these catheters rather mitigates against their use for rapid intravenous infusion except when large-bore (12G or larger) catheters are used.

2 Central venous access can be gained through the internal jugular, subclavian or femoral veins. Vascular dialysis catheters and tunnelled cuffed Hickman lines can also be inserted through these sites, as can balloon-tipped, flow-directed pulmonary artery (wedge) catheters capable of monitoring mixed venous oxygen saturation, thermal cardiac output and pulmonary capillary wedge pressures (PCWP).

3 Although central venous access may be life-saving, complications occur in 1–5% of patients. Local trauma may occur during insertion, including pneumothorax or haemothorax. Air or catheter emboli are additional hazards. Strict aseptic technique is required during insertion to avoid sepsis, and catheters should be removed when no longer required or if bacteraemia exists or is suspected.

4 *The vein.* For access, use either the internal jugular vein in the neck or the subclavian vein, accessible below the outer two-thirds of either clavicle. Subclavian vein puncture, traditionally the forte of cardiologists, is generally more hazardous than internal jugular access. Current guidelines strongly recommend the use of ultrasound guidance for the insertion of central venous catheters via the internal jugular route, but accept that these may not be readily available in emergency situations.

5 *The catheter.* Two preferred techniques are described. In both, the patient is positioned head-down to distend the veins and avoid the risk of air embolism. Observe acceptable sterile procedures, ranging from a 'no-touch' technique to the use of drapes, gown and gloves:
- For rapid internal jugular cannulation a long (8 cm) version of a standard intravenous cannula-over-needle can be used. The 16G or 14G needle and cannula are advanced together. On aspiration of blood the cannula is advanced and the needle is withdrawn. Under no circumstance should the needle be re-advanced through the catheter when it is in situ as the tip may be sheared off with a risk of central catheter embolization.
- The Seldinger wire technique arguably provides a more controlled means of percutaneous central venous access. Applicable to internal jugular, subclavian and femoral vein puncture, it allows for placement of flexible catheters of varying lengths, and is particularly useful when used in conjunction with ultrasound-guided insertion. Catheters may have single or multiple lumens; these typically vary from 12G to 22G in size, single-lumen 14–16G being the most common. A Seldinger needle or small-bore needle and cannula is first placed in the desired vein and free aspiration of blood is confirmed. Then a flexible guidewire with a floppy straight or J-shaped tip is advanced down the needle or cannula to a position in the superior vena cava (SVC) or right atrium, taking care not to push it so far as to initiate cardiac dysrhythmias. Monitor the ECG continuously during central venous catheterization. Remove the original needle or cannula. Depending on the material and size of the central venous catheter to be used, it may first be necessary to advance progressively larger dilating cannulas over the wire in turn before the final catheter is advanced over the guidewire into the vein. Finally, remove the guidewire. If multiple-lumen catheters are used, pass the wire up the distal lumen only.

Action

Internal jugular vein (Fig. 2.6)

1 With the head turned to the opposite side, the surface markings of the internal jugular vein can be represented as a broad line drawn from the lobe of the ear to the medial end of the clavicle. The vein lies posterior to the external carotid artery in the upper third of the neck, lateral to the common carotid in the middle third and anterolateral to it in the lower third. The vein is overlapped by the sternomastoid in its upper part but lower down

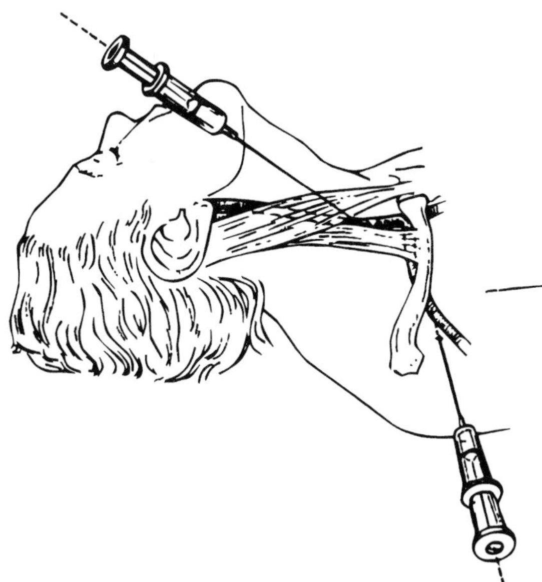

Fig. 2.6 Percutaneous access sites for internal jugular and subclavian vein cannulation.

lies deep on the lateral border of the anterior triangle formed by the sternal and clavicular heads of the sternomastoid and the clavicle below. The right internal jugular vein is sometimes preferred to the left, as on the right the internal jugular veins, innominate vein and superior vena cava are almost in line.

2 Tilt the patient head-down 15–30° in order to distend the vein and reduce the risk of air embolism. Turn the patient's head to the opposite side. It may be possible to palpate the vein deep to the sternomastoid muscle.

3 Observe strict aseptic technique. Thoroughly clean the skin. In a conscious patient use local anaesthesia at the proposed entry site. Palpate the carotid artery and make a small skin incision just lateral to the artery, at the tip of the anterior triangle mentioned above, midway between the ear lobe and the medial end of the clavicle.

4 Using the fingers of the left hand to displace the carotid artery medially, insert the needle at an angle of about 35° to the skin, aiming slightly laterally towards the nipple on the same side. Do not direct the needle tip medially at this stage. A 'give' is felt as the deep fascia is pierced and another as the vein is entered. Reflux of venous blood confirms entry. Advance along the vein a further 1 cm. Check free flow of blood before advancing the guidewire carefully through the needle, depending on the device being inserted. If free movement of the wire is impeded, do *not* pull the guidewire back through the needle. It will be necessary to withdraw the needle and wire as one unit and start again.

Subclavian vein (infraclavicular approach) (Fig. 2.6)

1 The subclavian vein is formed on each side from the axillary vein and runs horizontally behind the clavicle over the first rib to join the internal jugular vein, forming the innominate vein behind the sternoclavicular joint. The subclavian artery lies above and deep to it, and the vein has close relations with the brachial plexus, the dome of the plexus and the thoracic duct on the left. In consequence some users consider subclavian venous access more hazardous than the internal jugular approach, especially on the left side. Nonetheless, catheterization of this vein is quite simple to achieve with a little experience and permits secure comfortable anchoring of the cannula. Ultrasound guidance is less practicable by this route.

2 Tilt the patient head-down 15–30° in order to distend the vein and reduce the risk of air embolism. Thrust the neck forward by means of a pillow or bag of fluid placed centrally along the upper thoracic spine, ensuring that the shoulders 'fall back', allowing good lateral access to the clavicles. Turn the patient's head to the opposite side of proposed cannulation. Clean and drape the area thoroughly and use local anaesthesia if the patient is conscious.

3 The preferred site of access is 1–1.5 cm below the junction of the outer and middle two-thirds of the clavicle. Make a small skin incision, using local anaesthesia if required. Using a saline-filled syringe attached to the intended needle or cannula device, advance the needle behind the clavicle, aiming medially and horizontally towards the ipsilateral sternoclavicular joint. The direction of the needle should thus be slightly headward but remain almost horizontal to the floor to avoid damage to the pleura. Aspirate during insertion to check for successful venepuncture. If unsuccessful, repeat with the needle in a headward direction. If the artery is penetrated, this is usually an indication that the needle direction was too vertical and too high. Withdraw, apply direct pressure and aim in a more superficial and anterior direction.

4 Depending on the chosen device, either remove the needle from the cannula and thread the catheter through the cannula, or advance a guidewire through the needle as described in the Seldinger technique above. Thread the catheter into the required position. You usually need to insert a length of 10–15 cm of catheter into the vein to place the tip within the SVC or right atrium.

Femoral vein

The femoral vein is large and readily accessible at the proximal border of the femoral triangle at the top of the thigh, just medial to the femoral artery. Although traditionally avoided because of danger to the contents of the femoral sheath, access via this vessel may be justified when alternative central vessels are unavailable. Keep below the inguinal ligament to avoid concealed retroperitoneal haemorrhage and preferably use a Seldinger wire technique supported with ultrasound guidance to avoid damage to the femoral artery which often lies below the vein. Unless the catheter tip lies within the thorax, its venous pressure measurements will not accurately represent central venous pressure (CVP), especially in the presence of a distended abdomen. However, any raised inferior vena cava (IVC) pressures measured in these circumstances may reflect the severity of intra-abdominal compartment syndrome and its effect on impaired renal blood flow.

Antecubital vein

Central venous catheterization can be accomplished using a 60-cm catheter inserted via an antecubital vein. This technique is less popular than previously due to the high resistance associated with such a long line. In this technique the radio-opaque catheter is inserted through a cannula (direct insertion through a needle is no longer acceptable) into a suitable antecubital vein and threaded centrally. It is easier to pass a catheter centrally from the cephalic rather than the basilic vein. Long 60-cm catheter kits are variously available. Enter the needle–cannula assembly into the vein as for routine venous cannulation, remove the needle and advance the catheter through the cannula, handling only the sterile sheath to avoid infection.

? DIFFICULTY

When you are inserting an access catheter through the internal jugular or subclavian vein, there may be a hold-up as the tip traverses the fascial layers of the shoulder and root of the neck. Try abducting the arm to aid passage of the catheter into the thorax.

LOCAL ANAESTHESIA

Appraise

1 Operative procedures under local anaesthesia are regularly undertaken in hospitals, clinics and surgeries. Local anaesthetic techniques are particularly well suited for minor operations such as removal of small non-infected superficial lesions and minor surgery of the hands. It may be useful when general anaesthesia is not readily available or is impracticable (e.g. recent ingestion of food). Local anaesthesia is inexpensive as it does not require the specialized staff and facilities that general anaesthesia demands, is relatively safe, causes less systemic upset than general anaesthesia and enables patients to be discharged soon after surgery.

2 More extensive procedures involving large field blocks may not be as safe as general anaesthesia due to the toxic effect associated with the large volume of local anaesthetic required. Moreover, local anaesthesia does not necessarily block the physiological disturbances such as bradycardia and vomiting which arise from autonomic reflexes during some surgical procedures.

3 Local anaesthetic drugs can be administered in various ways according to the required area of analgesia. These include:

- *Topical anaesthesia*: application of local anaesthetics to the mucous membranes of the conjunctival sac, mouth, nose, tracheobronchial tree and urethra.
- *Local infiltration*: direct injection of the anaesthetic into the operative site.
- *Field block*: injection of local anaesthetic around the operative site so as to create an analgesic zone.
- *Individual peripheral nerve blocks*: e.g. ulnar, pudendal, femoral, common peroneal, etc. The extent of the block varies according to the cutaneous distribution the nerve supplies.
- *Regional block*: injection of local anaesthetic around the individual nerves or nerve trunks supplying the region to be operated upon. Where nerves are grouped together as plexuses then several nerves can be blocked at the same time. The brachial plexus is the best known, but the lumbosacral plexus block is occasionally used. The large volumes required for these blocks approach toxic levels.
- *Spinal anaesthesia*: insertion of local anaesthetic drugs directly into the subarachnoid space in small volumes (1.5–3 ml) produces effective sensory and motor block as the nerve roots in this space have negligible covering; low-pressure headache due to cerebrospinal fluid leak is not uncommon following this technique.
- *Extradural block*: injection of local anaesthetic into the epidural or caudal space; these blocks require 4–10 times the volumes used in subarachnoid block because of local diffusion and the presence of dural and myelin covering of the nerve roots. Combined spinal–epidural techniques, pioneered for obstetric anaesthesia, are increasingly popular for their ability to provide effective intraoperative analgesia combined with good postoperative pain relief.
- *Regional intravenous anaesthesia*: injection of a large volume of dilute local anaesthetic into the veins of a previously exsanguinated limb.

Agents

1 Various local anaesthetic drugs are available, of which amino amide derivatives are the most commonly used. Most drugs are marketed in the form of their water-soluble salts, usually the hydrochloride. Before they can act in the body they must dissociate to liberate the free base. Dissociation is inhibited in an acid medium, which explains why analgesia may be unpredictable when local anaesthetics are injected into inflamed tissues.

KEY POINTS Caution when administering local anaesthesia

- Never perform any but the most trivial of blocks single-handed. Serious cardiovascular and neurological consequences can develop suddenly if local anaesthetics are inadvertently injected into the wrong place, while other side-effects or complications may develop some time after the local anaesthetic has been injected. It is desirable to have another competent person who is capable of recognizing and dealing with unexpected problems attending the patient. This is particularly important if the patient is unwell, if concurrent sedation is being administered or if equipment such as a tourniquet is in use. At times another doctor (e.g. an anaesthetist) may be responsible for the patient's care during surgery. Otherwise you are accountable for your patient's safety. You cannot properly observe the patient or treat untoward reactions if you are a single-handed operator–anaesthetist engrossed in the surgery you are performing.
- Do not use local anaesthetic techniques until you are well versed in the relevant aspects of resuscitation. The morbidity and mortality associated with local anaesthesia relate more to the ability of the surgeon to deal rapidly and effectively with unexpected side-effects than to surgical ability.
- Do not attempt to block the ulnar nerve at the elbow or the common peroneal nerve in the leg in unconscious patients. There is a high risk of causing intraneural injury.

2 The duration of action of some local anaesthetics having a low tissue affinity is increased if they are combined with a vasoconstrictor such as adrenaline (epinephrine). This will also reduce the systemic absorption and toxicity of these agents. For infiltration, concentrations of 1 in 250 000 of adrenaline (epinephrine) may be used by the addition of 1 mg (1 ml of adrenaline tartrate 1/1000) to 250 ml of local anaesthetic solution. There is no advantage in using higher concentrations than this. The total amount of adrenaline (epinephrine) injected should not exceed 0.5 mg. Adrenaline (epinephrine) may cause tachycardia and hypertension and should be used with caution in patients with cardiovascular disease and those taking cardiac medication (e.g. beta-blockers). Less toxic vasoconstrictors (e.g. felypressin) are available. Injection of vasoconstrictors is absolutely contraindicated in areas supplied by end arteries (e.g. the fingers, toes and penis) as prolonged ischaemia here may lead to tissue necrosis.

3 The most commonly used agents include:

- *Lidocaine*. This is the most widely used local anaesthetic. It is stable, only moderately toxic, produces no vasodilation and has an onset of action within a few minutes and a duration of action of 60–90 minutes. It is used in concentrations of 4% for topical anaesthesia and concentrations of 0.5–2% for infiltration and nerve blocks. The maximum safe dose is 3 mg/kg body weight when used without adrenaline and 7 mg/kg with adrenaline.
- *Prilocaine*. Chemically related to lidocaine, prilocaine is less toxic but also less potent. Duration of action is less affected by adrenaline (epinephrine) than lidocaine is. Prilocaine is used as a 4% solution for topical anaesthesia and in concentrations of 1–3% for nerve blocks. The maximum safe dose is 10 mg/kg. Excessive doses of prilocaine produce methaemoglobinaemia, which may manifest as apparent cyanosis. Hypoxaemia results if more than 15 mg/kg of the agent is administered. Treatment involves the administration of 1% methylthioninium chloride (methylene blue), 1–2 mg/kg.
- *Bupivacaine*. This agent is two to three times as toxic as lidocaine but about four times more potent. It is used in concentrations of 0.25–0.5% and has a maximum safe dose of 2 mg/kg. It is extensively bound in the tissues and hence has the advantage of a long duration of action (3–12 hours). It has a delayed onset compared to lidocaine, although this may be overcome by mixing bupivacaine and lidocaine together (see Methods below).

Toxicity

1 All local anaesthetics exert toxic effects when given in large doses, and inadvertent intravascular injection, even in small doses, can cause central nervous and cardiovascular disturbances resulting in restlessness, convulsions, hypotension, bradycardia and, in extreme cases, respiratory and cardiac arrest.

2 Management of these toxic effects includes the use of intravenous sedatives with anticonvulsant properties (benzodiazepines or thiopentone), oxygen, intravenous fluids and pressor agents (ephedrine or metaraminol). In extreme circumstances tracheal intubation and artificial ventilation may be necessary. The importance of securing intravenous access before local anaesthesia is commenced is obvious.

3 The conduct of thoracic or lumbar spinal and epidural anaesthesia involves blockade of the T1–L1 sympathetic outflow tracts. This results in vasodilation below the block with compensatory vasoconstriction above this level. If the block reaches above T10, hypotension is likely. Compensatory tachycardia may not occur, especially if a high block affects the T1–T4 outflow or the patient is on beta-blockers or has a pacemaker. For this reason good venous access is important; a preload infusion of 300–500 ml of crystalloid is recommended before such blocks are commenced. Administer a small subcutaneous or intravenous dose of a vaso- and venoconstrictor such as ephedrine, methoxamine or metaraminol before or during the procedure to protect against hypotension.

4 The risk of hypotension is particularly high when pre-existing hypovolaemia is present, during supine hypotension syndrome of pregnancy or when unexpected subarachnoid (spinal) anaesthesia occurs. This latter hazard may arise when an epidural technique is complicated by dural puncture or where an existing epidural catheter perforates the subarachnoid space. Partial or extensive spinal anaesthesia may also occur from misplaced spinal injection during the conduct of pre- or paravertebral blocks. Profound hypotension, unconsciousness and respiratory paralysis can occur. Emergency management involves oxygenation, intubation, ventilation, intravenous infusion and pharmacological support of the cardiovascular system.

Prepare

1 Check that resuscitation equipment is present and in working order and that competent assistance is available if needed urgently. The minimum equipment required is a self-inflating bag with mask and airways, an oxygen cylinder capable of delivering 8–10 litres/min via oxygen mask and resuscitation bag, sedatives to deal with convulsions, intravenous fluids and vasopressors for sudden circulatory failure.

2 Ensure that a quiet environment will be maintained for the duration of surgery. Quiet music may be beneficial but keep casual conversation to a minimum.

3 Take a careful history with particular reference to current therapy, allergies, cardiorespiratory and neurological disease. Examination should include the pulse rate, rhythm and blood pressure. If myocardial disease is suspected have an assistant monitor pulse, blood pressure and ECG throughout the procedure.

4 Explain to the patient what surgery you are proposing to perform under local anaesthesia, check that the correct site (and side) is being operated on and obtain written consent.

5 Explain the sequence of the events that are going to take place, including the initial preparation of the area, the injection of local anaesthetic and the subsequent surgery. Reassure the patient that the pain from any injection will be temporary and that during surgery there should be no pain, although the sense of touch may remain.

6 Study the landmarks of the area carefully before proceeding. Place a catheter in a vein well away from the operative site in case resuscitation is required.

7 Choose local anaesthetic drugs with attention to the likely volume required. 0.5% or 1% lidocaine or prilocaine without adrenaline (epinephrine) is suitable for most infiltrations or nerve blocks, respectively. Calculate the maximum safe dose based on the patient's measured weight. In a 70-kg adult the maximum dose of plain lidocaine is 210 mg (3 mg/kg). As 1% lidocaine contains 10 mg/ml, the maximum safe volume is 21 ml. If larger volumes are required, either reduce these concentrations, add adrenaline (epinephrine) or perform part of the block 15–20 minutes later.

Action

1 Exercise full sterile precautions. Wash hands and arms thoroughly before donning gown and gloves. Prepare the skin with 2% iodine in spirit or 0.5% chlorhexidine in 70% alcohol and cover with suitable drapes. Maintain a sterile environment throughout the procedure.

2 Use fine 25SWG needles for initial intradermal injection of local anaesthesia and 22–23SWG needles for infiltration.

3 When performing local infiltration, inject as the needle is being moved. When injecting round specific nerves this is less practicable. Check by aspiration before injecting to minimize the likelihood of intravascular injection.

4 Be on a constant lookout for untoward reactions. Drowsiness and slurring of speech are early signs of central nervous system toxicity. If you see these prodromal signs stop injecting local anaesthetic and be prepared to initiate urgent treatment.

5 Wait 10–15 minutes after injection for the local anaesthetic to take full effect. Be careful when testing whether a block is working that the patient does not confuse the sensation of pain with that of touch.

6 Warn the patient that there may be some discomfort when the effects of the block begin to wear off.

Methods

1 According to the clinical practice and your confidence, the following procedures may be used. Unless otherwise indicated, use the concentrations of local anaesthetics shown in Table 2.1.

2 Lidocaine and bupivacaine can be mixed to combine the rapid onset of the former with the longer action of the latter. For infiltration anaesthesia, equal volumes of 1% lidocaine (with or without adrenaline (epinephrine)) and 0.5% bupivacaine may be used, providing the combined dose of drugs does not exceed their cumulative toxic level. Amongst anaesthetists, 2% lidocaine and 0.75% bupivacaine have some popularity for use in epidurals to ensure profound sensory and motor block, but such concentrations should not be used routinely.

TABLE 2.1 Use of local anaesthetics

Method	Anaesthetic
Infiltration	0.5% lidocaine, 0.25% bupivacaine
Nerve blocks	1% lidocaine, 1% prilocaine or 0.5% bupivacaine
Epidural	1.5% lidocaine, 0.5% bupivacaine
Spinal	0.5% heavy bupivacaine

Infiltration anaesthesia

- Infiltration anaesthesia provides good operating conditions for the removal of small superficial lesions, such as sebaceous cysts and lipomata. Do not use infiltration anaesthesia in infected sites because of the risk of spreading infection and because adequate sensory block is unlikely to be achieved.
- Follow the general advice on equipment and actions detailed above. 0.5% lidocaine is generally recommended, avoiding adrenaline (epinephrine) where blood supply may be tenuous. Raise a small skin bleb close to the lesion then infiltrate through this bleb, attempting to place the local anaesthetic so that it spreads along tissue planes and the lesion 'floats' in an anaesthetized area.
- Allow an adequate time for the anaesthetic to take effect before commencing surgery.

Superficial and deep cervical plexus blocks

Particularly useful for awake carotid artery surgery, this technique combines deep and superficial plexus blocks. The posterior border of sternomastoid is identified at the C4 level of the thyroid cartilage.

- *Deep*. Place a finger beneath the lateral border of sternomastoid on to the belly of scalenus anterior and move the finger lateral feeling for the interscalene groove. Aim needle downward and medially 10–20 mm in a caudal direction toward contralateral elbow until paraesthesia is felt or the C4 transverse process is contacted. After aspiration test, inject 8–10 ml of solution. Complications include phrenic nerve, recurrent laryngeal and stellate ganglion block.
- *Superficial*. The superficial plexus is blocked by a 10-ml cranial and caudal 'sausage' injection along the posterior border of sternomastoid beneath the first fascial layer.

Interscalene block

1 This block is increasingly popular for shoulder and upper humerus surgery, including continuous postoperative catheter infusion analgesia. The needle passes between the anterior and middle scalene muscles and will achieve a high brachial plexus block.

2 Identify the posterior border of sternomastoid at cricoid level (C6). Place a finger beneath lateral border of sternomastoid on to the belly of anterior scalene muscle. Move finger laterally, separating anterior scalene from middle scalene muscle. Aim for contralateral elbow at a depth of 10–20 mm (maximum). Inject 10–35 ml of solution.

Brachial plexus block

1 Although the roots of the brachial plexus can be blocked by interscalene, supraclavicular or axillary block, the axillary approach is easy to learn and the safest to use for elbow, lower arm and hand surgery.

2 Position a venous tourniquet as high as possible on the upper arm to prevent dissipation of solution from the axillary sheath. Abduct and externally rotate the arm so that the patient's hand is resting near his head. Palpate the axillary artery as far medially as possible between pectoralis major and latissimus dorsi.

3 Raise small blebs of local anaesthesia in the axilla in order to place two 22G needles in the perivascular sheath above and below the axillary artery. Infuse 30–40 ml of 1% prilocaine or 0.375% bupivacaine via the lower needle. The sheath should fill with fluid and drip slowly from the upper needle.

4 It may be necessary to infiltrate some local anaesthetic between the heads of the coracobrachialis to pick up the lateral cutaneous nerve of the arm, which may otherwise escape block.

Elbow blocks

- The *median nerve* can be blocked immediately medial to the brachial artery in the antecubital fossa, 1–2 cm proximal to the intercondylar line.
- The *radial nerve* is best blocked in the cleft between the brachioradialis and the biceps tendon at the level of the elbow joint.
- The *ulnar nerve* can be blocked 1–2 cm proximal to its course in the ulnar groove under the medial epicondyle at the distal end of the humerus.

Wrist blocks

These are particularly useful for minor hand surgery.

- The *ulnar nerve* can be blocked between the flexor carpi ulnaris and palmaris longus tendons, at a depth of 5–10 mm from the skin.
- The *median nerve* is accessible directly lateral to the palmaris longus tendon while the radial nerve can be blocked just dorsal to the radial artery in the anatomical snuff box.

Digital nerve blocks

1 Digital nerves to the fingers and toes pass along the anterolateral line of the phalanx. A digital tourniquet may be used but never use adrenaline (epinephrine).

2 Raise a skin bleb over the dorsum of the proximal phalanx using 1 ml of 1% plain lidocaine. Pass a 23SWG needle through this to deposit about 1–2 ml of the agent on either side of the phalanx. Inject the agent close to the web space to avoid undue distension of the tissues. Unlike infiltration analgesia, nerve blocks may require up to 20 minutes to have an effect.

Lower limb blocks

Nerve blocks of the lower limb involve several major nerves of the thigh and leg, which are technically more difficult to block than those of the upper limb and require large doses of local anaesthetic agent. Surgeons interested in these blocks should consult the texts quoted at the end of the chapter.

- *'3-in-1 block'*. The lumbar plexus is sandwiched between the psoas sheath and quadratus lumborum muscles, and the 3-in-1 block of the femoral nerve, lateral cutaneous nerve of the thigh and obturator nerve with 25–35 ml of solution relies on the spread of local anaesthetic between these muscle planes. The injection site is 1 cm lateral to the femoral artery just below the inguinal ligament. Ultrasound is helpful to avoid perforation of the nearby femoral artery and vein. If only the femoral nerve is effectively blocked, a separate block of the lateral cutaneous nerve of the thigh with 10–15 ml may be required, 1–2 cm below and lateral to the anterior superior iliac spine. Similarly, the obturator nerve may also require a separate injection of 5–10 ml of local anaesthetic into the obturator canal, below and medial to the superior ramus of the pelvis.
- The *sciatic nerve* can be blocked by a posterior approach at a point 3 cm below the midpoint of a line joining the posterior iliac spine and greater trochanter. The nerve lies 6–8 cm deep to the skin at this point. The anterior approach to the sciatic nerve requires a deep injection just medial to the surface marking of the lesser trochanter on the anterior aspect of the thigh.

Knee blocks

- The *common peroneal nerve* block is an extremely useful block for minor surgery to the lateral aspect of the leg and ankle. 5 ml of solution is placed immediately posterior to the head of the fibula on the lateral side of the knee.
- A *tibial nerve* block is appropriate for operations on the lower leg and foot, usually in combination with common peroneal and saphenous nerve blocks, or for incomplete analgesia following epidural or sciatic blocks. 5–10 ml of solution is deposited 1.5–3 cm deep in the middle of a line joining the lateral and middle femoral epicondyles in the popliteal fossa.
- The *saphenous nerve* block at the knee may be used in combination with the above two nerve blocks for operations on the lower leg and foot, or to supplement an incomplete femoral nerve block. 2–10 ml of solution is deposited by subcutaneous infiltration on the anteromedial aspect of the lower leg from the medial edge of the tibial tuberosity backwards to the fleshy margin of the gastrocnemius muscle.

Ankle blocks

Depending on the extent of surgery required, an ankle block will require all or part of the following. Take particular care to avoid the injection of vasoconstrictors into arteries during performance of these blocks.

1 A posterior tibial nerve block behind the medial malleolus, 2–3 ml of solution on both sides of the posterior tibial artery.

2 A deep peroneal nerve block at the front of the ankle just below the level of the lateral malleolus, using 2–3 ml of solution deposited on either side of the dorsalis pedis artery.

3 Subcutaneous infiltration around the ankle 3–4 cm above the malleoli to ensure blockade of the superficial peroneal branches (lateral aspect of the ankle) and saphenous and calcaneal branch (medial aspect of the ankle).

Intrapleural anaesthesia

This technique has been advocated for analgesia following thoracoabdominal surgery or fractured ribs and may prove an effective replacement for the technique of multiple intercostal blocks previously required.

1 Identify the dermatome level on the side of the chest you wish to block. Choose a point above the angle of a suitable rib in the posterolateral line of the chest and raise a bleb of local anaesthetic above the rib. Using sterile gloves, introduce a Tuohy epidural needle just inside the pleural cavity above the rib margin, taking care not to puncture the lung. Remove the stylet and block the hub with a gloved finger to avoid air entering the pleural cavity. Thread an epidural catheter a few centimetres into the cavity. Carefully withdraw the cannula over the catheter, taking care not to cut it, and secure with an airtight dressing. Completely remove the Tuohy needle, replace the Luer-lock assembly and add a bacterial filter to the end.

2 Lay the patient on the side to be blocked and slowly introduce 1% plain lidocaine or 0.5% bupivacaine into the catheter to a maximum of 20–30 ml, depending on patient size. Allow 10–15 minutes in this position before moving the patient.

Caudal (sacral) anaesthesia

This technique of epidural (syn. extradural) anaesthesia is particularly useful for blocking pain associated with pelvic, perineal and lower genitourinary surgery in the L3–S4 distribution, and is commonly used by anaesthetists as an adjunct to general anaesthesia in gynaecological and paediatric urological and hernia surgery. At doses up to 0.5 ml/kg there is negligible effect on the thoracolumbar sympathetic outflow.

1 Lay the patient prone or on his side. The sacral hiatus lies at the tip of an equilateral triangle whose base is a line joining the posterior superior iliac spines. Alternatively, in the laterally positioned patient with legs flexed at right-angles, a line dropped perpendicularly from the line of the femur crosses the sacral hiatus with remarkable consistency.

2 Under sterile precautions a 21–22G needle is introduced cephalad at 45°, lowering and advancing the needle a further 4–10 mm as it 'pops' through the sacrococcygeal membrane. After a negative aspiration test, slowly inject the appropriate mixture to 0.5 ml/kg. Reposition the needle tip if obstruction is felt on initial injection, but abandon if you sense progressive overpressure during injection.

Thoracic and lumbar epidurals, and spinal anaesthesia

For reasons discussed earlier, these procedures should not be performed single-handed, and details of technique are not discussed further in this chapter. The surgeon is encouraged to learn these techniques under guidance and apply them in his or her practice providing adequate assistance is available. Hypotension associated with thoracolumbar sympathetic blockade is common and requires intravenous fluids supplemented with vasoconstrictors if required.

INTRAVENOUS REGIONAL ANAESTHESIA

Appraise

1 The technique is known as Bier's block, having been initially described in 1908 and revised by McHolmes in 1967. A dilute solution of local anaesthetic is injected into the venous system of a limb that has been exsanguinated and is kept isolated from the rest of the circulation. The anaesthetic exerts its action by diffusing from the vascular system into the tissues and thus affecting the terminal branches of sensory nerves. This is a very useful but potentially dangerous block.

KEY POINT Caution when administering Bier's block

- **Never perform this block single-handed. The main danger is failure of the occluding tourniquet and the sudden release of a large amount of local anaesthetic into the circulation.**

2 It is essential for a suitably trained and qualified person to be responsible for the block while another performs the necessary surgery.

3 The block works best in the upper limb. It can be used in the leg, but the larger doses of local anaesthetic needed make its use for this purpose more dangerous.

Method

1 Insert an indwelling 21–23SWG cannula or 'butterfly' needle into a suitable distal vein not adjacent to the operation site. A cannula is preferred as it is less likely to perforate the vein wall during the subsequent stages. Place an additional cannula in another limb in case urgent intravenous access is required for resuscitation.

2 Apply a pneumatic tourniquet to the upper arm. Special double-cuffed tourniquets are commercially available and are preferable to single-cuff devices.

3 Exsanguinate the limb, using an Esmarch bandage or a rubber roller sleeve. If the limb is too painful to tolerate compression, apply an inflatable splint and elevate the limb for 3 minutes.

4 Inflate the upper tourniquet cuff to above systolic pressure, then remove the Esmarch bandage or inflatable splint.

5 Inject local anaesthetic through the indwelling cannula or needle to fill the veins in the occluded limb. Use 0.5% prilocaine or 0.5% lidocaine without adrenaline (epinephrine). The average volume needed for the upper arm of an adult is 40 ml. Do not exceed 4 mg/kg. The local anaesthetic will start to take effect within 5 minutes.

6 Where a double-cuff system is being used, inflate the lower cuff to above systolic pressure after 10 minutes and then release the upper cuff. By this time the arm beneath the lower cuff will be anaesthetized and the patient will not experience tourniquet pain.

7 Throughout the procedure pay constant attention to the degree of inflation of the cuffs. Pneumatic tourniquet cuffs commonly leak. Confusion can arise if the same pump or inflating system is used to inflate both cuffs.

8 At the end of the procedure deflate the cuff, providing at least 20 minutes has elapsed from the time of injection of the local anaesthetic. This allows adequate time for the drug to diffuse from the vessels, and reduces the likelihood of a bolus of anaes-

thetic drug being released into the circulation. As a further precaution against this bolus effect reinflate the cuff quickly after initial deflation, wait a few minutes and deflate again. This can be repeated several times if necessary. This technique is a good one to adopt routinely, especially when using Bier's block in elderly or infirm patients or when short tourniquet times are used.

POSTOPERATIVE ANALGESIA

A review on pain after surgery by the Royal College of Surgeons of England identified that many doctors considered postoperative pain to be an inevitable consequence of surgery and failed to control it adequately. In many countries, in-hospital 'acute pain teams' are responsible for the management of postoperative pain and these are now becoming increasingly common in UK practice.

The financial implications of instituting such a system are considerable, but improvements in pain control and earlier mobilization can be made within the financial constrains of health service practice.

You have an important commitment to minimize postoperative pain and provide leadership to the surgical team (junior staff, anaesthetists, nurses, physiotherapists, etc.) in the way pain control is monitored and managed.

Appraise

1 Failure to relieve pain adequately may have significant repercussions. Pain (real or feared) impairs mobility, and circulation to skin and muscles is reduced. As a consequence, healing is slow and pressure sores may develop with frightening rapidity. The risk of thromboembolic disease is significantly increased in immobile patients. Pain is frequently associated with hypertension and tachycardia, which may exacerbate myocardial ischaemia in susceptible individuals. After abdominal and thoracic surgery, pain will limit respiratory function with attendant risk of hypoxia and chest infection. The return of normal gut motility and absorption may be delayed, resulting in dehydration and the need for extended intravenous therapy. Even after straightforward musculoskeletal operations, pain profoundly limits activity and full function may be delayed for weeks. In financial terms alone, unrelieved pain delays healing, prolongs hospital stay and retards the patient's return to taxpayer status.

2 Analgesia can be achieved using many agents, administered by a variety of routes. The reader is advised to read the chapter on the management of postoperative pain in the companion manual to this book (Kirk RM, Ribbans WJ (eds) 2004 Clinical surgery in general, 4th edn. Churchill Livingstone, Edinburgh, pp 357–369; an RCS course manual) to familiarize himself with the various classes of analgesics available and their methods of delivery.

3 The use of microprocessor-controlled devices for continuous or intermittent intravenous or epidural infusions provide a more consistent pattern of pain relief. Increasingly popular are the use of more complex devices which permit patient-controlled analgesia (PCA), thereby enabling the patient to retain some independent control of their pain. However, these sophisticated techniques do require a good understanding of the pharmacology of the drugs being administered and the complications that may ensue. Regular surveillance during their use must include frequent clinical observation and documentation of the patient's vital signs.

FURTHER READING

Aitkenhead AR, Rowbotham D, Smith G 2001 Textbook of anaesthesia, 4th edn. Churchill Livingstone, Edinburgh

American College of Surgeons Committee on Trauma 1997 Advanced trauma life support for doctors. American College of Surgeons, Chicago, IL

Bersten A, Soni N, Oh TE (eds) 2003 Oh's intensive care manual, 5th edn. Butterworth Heinemann Health, Oxford

Colquhoun MC, Handley AJ, Evans TR (eds) 2003 ABC of resuscitation, 5th edn. BMJ Books, London

Commission on the Provision of Surgical Services 1990 Report of the working party on pain after surgery. Royal College of Surgeons of England/College of Anaesthetists, London

Hahn MB, McQuillan PM, Sheplock GJ 1996 Regional anesthesia. An atlas of anatomy and techniques of anesthesia. Mosby, St Louis, MO

Kirk RM, Ribbans WJ (eds) 2004 Clinical surgery in general, 4th edn. Churchill Livingstone, Edinburgh

Skinner D, Driscoll P (eds) 1999 ABC of major trauma, 3rd edn. BMJ Books, London

3

The severely injured patient

F.W. Cross, J.M. Ryan

CONTENTS

INTRODUCTION

We offer advice on appraising seriously injured patients, including definitive management. Initial management and resuscitation are described elsewhere in this textbook.

However, be aware that your approach to an injured patient is different from that adopted with other surgical illness, in that potentially life-threatening injuries involving the airway, breathing and circulation (ABC) must be corrected as they are diagnosed. You must largely abandon the usual algorithm of taking a detailed history followed by making a detailed clinical examination. For example, damage-control laparotomy as a resuscitative procedure, when the patient fails to respond to transfusion, is now well described. It is occasionally required almost as an initial procedure, leaving other injuries to be dealt with later.

SURGICAL MANAGEMENT

You should, if necessary, be able to carry out life-saving operations on most parts of the body. One test of your judgement is knowing how to modify a standard operation to meet the prevailing requirements. This includes knowing how and when to 'cut corners' safely. The ability to explore a wound successfully is a good test of basic surgical understanding and tissue craft. It is the last stage in diagnosis and at the same time it is the first stage in treating a wound.

In this chapter, we assume that the patient has been fully assessed and resuscitated and you have made a decision to operate. The surgical management of the multiply injured should involve multiple surgical specialists working together.

KEY POINTS Responsibility for early management

- Early management of chest and abdominal wounds, and complex superficial lacerations, falls to general surgeons.
- The management of trauma is truly general surgery.

In many countries, specialist trauma surgeons trained in general surgery, neurosurgery and orthopaedics undertake the definitive management of these patients from admission to discharge. This chapter deals with basic procedures in the head and neck, chest, abdomen and pelvis, whether sustained in civilian or military circumstances. Advanced faciomaxillary, neurosurgical and orthopaedic procedures are dealt with elsewhere in this book.

SOFT TISSUE WOUNDS: GENERAL PRINCIPLES

Exploration of wounds can be a hazardous procedure, especially in the neck. In some situations, if exploration is indicated, you should decide to make a generous incision and achieve control of the major vascular structures as part of the exploration rather than provoke haemorrhage by disturbing the wound with fingers or instruments.

Appraise

1 In this section we describe the principles of wound exploration in general terms, which can be applied to most superficial areas of the body including scalp, face, extremities and superficial wounds of the trunk and perineal area. We give specific instructions for particular problems later in the chapter or elsewhere in the book where appropriate.

2 Learn as much as you can before operation. In particular, examine for potential nerve injury. When there is a penetrating missile injury obtain preliminary biplanar X-rays. They are invaluable, revealing retained missile fragments and providing clues to the missile track. In the abdomen, probing the wound is useless as a means of determining whether or not it enters the peritoneal cavity; the layers move across creating a series of baffles in a different relationship from that at the time of injury.

3 Make sure the anaesthetist is prepared for a prolonged procedure.

4 Manage soft tissue wounds as a formal procedure consisting of clearly defined stages. This is the part most frequently neglected by those with limited or no experience of trauma and war wound surgery. The entry and exit wounds of missile injuries give little indication of the damage that may have occurred to deeper structures. The extent of injury can be detected only by full wound exploration.

5 After exploring limb wounds, carry out thorough wound excision. With very few exceptions, you should leave the wound open. Perform delayed primary closure after 4–7 days.

Prepare

1 Prepare the wounded area and a large enough surrounding area to allow for a necessary but unplanned extension of the skin incision.

2 If possible photograph the injured area or make a sketch; this is particularly useful to pass on to the receiving doctor if you need to transfer the patient.

3 Clean the skin thoroughly with an antiseptic solution of your choice.

KEY POINTS Control bleeding

- Retain pressure dressings over bleeding wounds until the last minute.
- Wounds are usually already contaminated and such dressings rarely contribute to further overall contamination.

Access

1 Identify the extent of visible damage. Knowledge of the force and mechanism of injury and the position of the patient at the time provides added information on the likely extent of the damage.

2 Arrange for adequate assistance, retraction and lighting in order to make a firm assessment.

3 You usually need to enlarge the wound in order to obtain adequate access to damaged structures. Further enlargement may be necessary later during definitive repair.

4 Digital exploration may indicate the direction of the wound but cannot reliably reveal its depth or eventual extent. The most direct way of doing this is usually to incise tissue immediately overlying the track. Bear in mind the site and extent of the resulting wound, particularly if it needs to be extended as part of the definitive procedure, or if it crosses major skin creases. However, cosmesis (the future appearance) is not of primary concern during life-saving surgery. Whenever possible, incise in the long axis of a limb. In some circumstances you may need to make counter-incisions.

Assess

1 Look carefully into the existing wound and identify its extent, if possible without initial dissection.

2 The presence of blood indicates the site of tissue injury. Follow it by retracting the tissues and observing. Do not initially carry out any dissection because it destroys the natural tissue relationships. Defer it as long as necessary.

KEY POINT Anatomy

- You must have knowledge of local anatomy and of possible distortions to perform safely.

3 Explore the wound in layers. Follow any puncture wound through the layers, opening each in turn until you can detect no further penetration. Remember that the tissues may no longer be in the same relationship that they were at the time of the injury, and a penetrating wound may seem to take a different course from that expected. The tissue layers form a series of baffles, as in the abdomen, mentioned above.

4 Identify neurovascular bundles in the wound track and note any damage, but you need not dissect out nerves. The majority of nerve injuries are neurapraxias [Greek: *neuron* (=nerve)+*a* (= not)+*prassein* (=to do)], described by H.J. Seddon as temporary paralysis without degeneration, and recover spontaneously. If a nerve appears to be injured, requiring later exploration, mark its position with a non-absorbable suture.

KEY POINT Nerve injury

- Determine to record in the operation notes the nature and extent of any nerve injury that you detect.

Action

1 Arrest haemorrhage, temporarily compressing the bleeding point with swabs, controlling major vessels proximally and distally with slings or with arterial clamps. Do not apply haemostatic arterial clamps indiscriminately but capture and ligate small bleeding vessels under vision as you encounter them.

2 Do not attempt to explore or repair wounds in the presence of bleeding. It is futile and dangerous.

3 Once you have done this, start by cleaning the wound. Irrigate it with copious quantities of saline followed by aqueous antiseptic. This removes most superficial foreign material and improves visualization. Remove deeper contaminants as the exploration progresses.

4 You need good lighting, intelligent retraction and a bloodless field in order to identify and remove specific foreign bodies, so you should have arranged them before starting. Radio-opaque objects localized with preoperative films may still be difficult to find; if you have intraoperative screening available, it is often helpful. Most glass is radio-opaque. Make sure you can identify the layer of tissue in which the object lies; if you do not, you are not likely to localize the object at all. Approach long narrow objects such as glass slivers or needles from the side rather than end-on, since they seldom leave discernible tracks. It is not necessary to remove every piece of metal or glass visible on a radiograph. Use your clinical judgement: for example, a small piece of smooth-edged windscreen glass left in the face may be safely left undisturbed but vegetable material or slivers of wood form potent sources of chronic infection.

5 Identify and rigorously excise dead muscle, which is pale, non-contractile, mushy and does not bleed when incised.

KEY POINTS Four criteria for muscle excision

- Colour.
- Contractility.
- Consistency.
- Capillary bleeding.

6 Inspect for tendon damage. Tendon repair need not be performed initially. Trim tattered ends and mark them with a non-absorbable suture as for nerves (see above).

7 Now repair any major vessel damage that you had previously noted. Trim damaged vessel ends and carry out a primary

anastomosis wherever possible. Avoid tension; if necessary, mobilize the vessel proximally and distally. It is possible to achieve considerable length by simple mobilization. If this does not work, interpose a graft. If possible use reversed vein because of problems with infection. You may be forced to use a synthetic graft; in this case put antibiotic powder directly into the wound at the end of the operation and cover the repair with healthy muscle. Always repair interrupted major veins at the same time as arteries. Use a plastic shunt to restore the circulation if immediate repair is not possible (see below). Shunt both the damaged artery and vein if possible since venous engorgement of a limb may compromise its viability. For precise details of vascular repair see Chapter 29.

8 Pay particular attention to comminuted bony injuries. Clean contaminated bone but do not remove it if it is still attached to viable periosteum or healthy muscle. Discard small detached bony fragments, which contribute to postoperative wound infection. Carry out orthopaedic fixation after completing vascular repair. In the event of major long bone fractures, allow for the presence of shortening that will be corrected at orthopaedic repair, particularly when you have needed to repair blood vessels.

9 Identify injuries to joints and clean them rigorously. Cover exposed cartilage with at least one layer of healthy tissue, ideally with synovium.

10 Irrigate the wound again at the end of the repair procedure. Secure haemostasis before dressing an open contaminated wound or before closing a clean one.

Checklist

1 Make sure that all dead tissue has been removed, that an open wound is open enough to drain and that haemostasis is secure.

2 Always check distal limb viability before leaving the operating theatre, particularly in the presence of constrictive dressings.

KEY POINTS Delayed primary closure

- Always leave contaminated wounds open.
- This includes the fascia, since damaged muscle deep to fascial layers inevitably swells, potentially causing compartment syndrome.

Open wound

1 Dress an open wound with lightly fluffed gauze to allow free drainage. Avoid tight packing.

Closure

1 Do not close a wound unless you are sure it is recent, clean and healthy. Use delayed primary closure if in doubt. Approximate tissue loosely during closure, never under tension, and in its natural layers. It is seldom necessary to repair muscle, but approximate subcutaneous tissue with absorbable sutures, preferably interrupted, to reduce the risk of tissue fluid collecting in dead spaces.

2 Close the skin with interrupted non-absorbable sutures, trimming the edges where required to reduce bevelling.

3 Consider the use of primary split-skin grafting in addition to suturing at delayed primary closure, particularly when there has been tissue loss.

Postoperative

1 Immobilize the injured soft tissue with cotton wool, conforming bandages and, if necessarily, a splint, even in the absence of bony injury.

2 Keep the limb or other wounded part immobilized as far as possible.

3 Watch for the signs of sepsis outlined in below.

4 Watch for signs of postoperative limb ischaemia or overt haemorrhage.

5 Continue the antibiotic cover started preoperatively.

KEY POINTS Signs of sepsis

- Increasing pain.
- Increasing temperature.
- Soiling of dressings.
- Offensive smell.

SPECIFIC SOFT TISSUE SITES

NECK

1 Blunt injury to the neck rarely requires operative intervention. The cervical collar provides first-aid immobilization. Institute skull traction to decompress the spinal canal if there are neurological signs. If this fails, neurosurgical intervention is needed to decompress it directly. Treat partial section of the cervical spinal cord by early operative decompression and fixation to reduce the amount of residual disability, but this is controversial[1] and it is not indicated for complete section. Seek an urgent neurosurgical referral.

2 Do not explore penetrating wounds that remain superficial to the platysma muscle. If the wound goes deeper, explore it if there is brisk bleeding, an expanding haematoma, haemoptysis or haematemesis, neurological injury, surgical emphysema or an obvious air leak. Do not explore the neck if there is a pneumothorax in the absence of any of these signs. If none of these is present and arteriography and X-ray examination of the pharynx as the patient swallows thin barium are negative, then it is safe to observe the patient. Oesophagoscopy and bronchoscopy are often advised but seldom helpful; in any case, any visible lesion is likely to produce one of the above features.

3 Whilst knife wounds and handgun injuries to the neck may be handled conservatively in the absence of major damage, high-energy-transfer missile wounds often cause extensive disruption and almost always require emergency exploration for the arrest of major haemorrhage.

Action

1 Explore the neck through one of the standard vascular access incisions, either along the clavicle or the anterior border of the sternocleidomastoid muscle, so that you can control the carotid and subclavian vessels if there is sudden bleeding. Be prepared to remove the middle third of the clavicle with a Gigli or air-driven saw to gain better access. You may need to expose injuries to the roots of the great vessels using an additional midline sternotomy (Fig. 3.1).

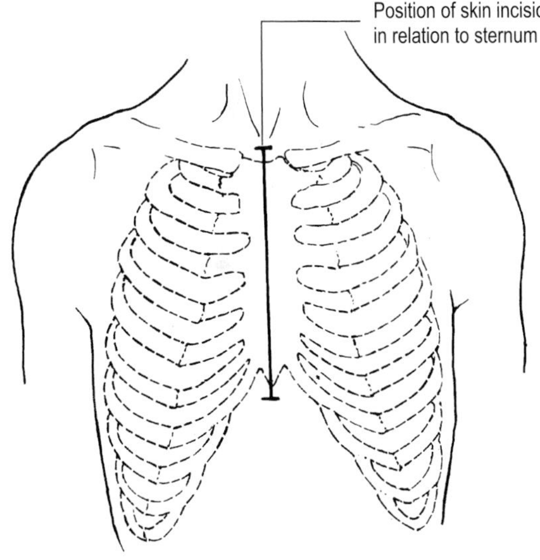

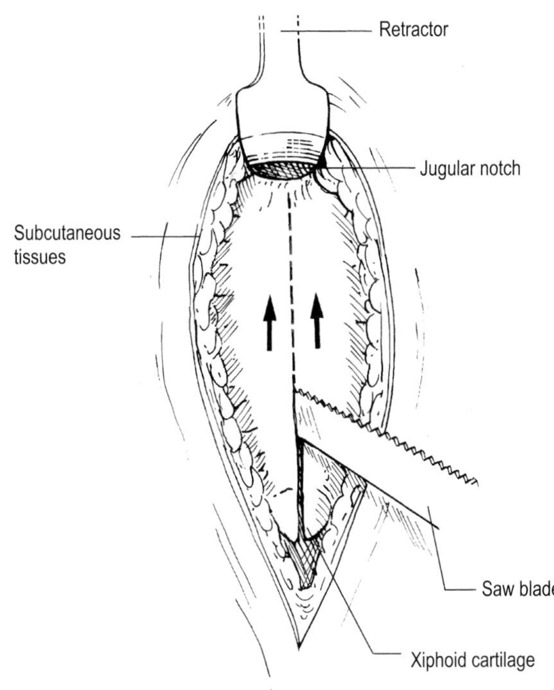

Fig. 3.1 The midline sternotomy for access to all chambers of the heart, the pulmonary vessels and the arch of the aorta. You may use a Gigli saw if you do not have a powered sternal saw available.

2 Haemorrhage from one or other of the major vessels can normally be controlled by simple oversewing, but if the main arteries are contused use a vein patch; alternatively replace a short section with an artificial graft. Always repair the common or internal carotid unless it is actually clotted; in that case there is a risk of embolus to the brain if you disturb the clot. You may safely ligate the external carotid. Haemorrhage from the vertebral artery is usually more difficult to deal with. Obtain access by retracting the carotid sheath medially and developing the prevertebral tissue plane so revealed. You may achieve haemostasis using bone wax and pressure but otherwise control the artery above and below the injury by removing the costal face of the appropriate cervical transverse processes. It is safe to ligate one vessel if the contralateral artery is patent, but in an emergency you may not have had time to obtain an angiogram. Repair the internal jugular veins whenever possible but you may safely ligate all the other neck veins including the facial veins, which often bleed very briskly. Tilting the patient headdown reduces the risk of an air embolus to the heart but also increases the bleeding; try to clamp the vessel on either side of the damaged section before attempting repair.

3 You can normally repair the trachea using a single layer of absorbable material over the endotracheal tube. Defects need to be patched and this is a specialized procedure. Repair the injured pharynx in two layers and drain the wound.

? DIFFICULTY

1. On occasion you explore a neck wound because of severe haemorrhage and you cannot identify any vascular injury.
2. Make a thorough search, exploring the wound to its fullest extent. If you miss a vascular injury and bleeding, the patient is in severe danger.

SURGICAL AIRWAY

Appraise

1 If the airway is obstructed and it is not possible to perform either an orotracheal or nasotracheal intubation you need to create a surgical airway.

2 The commonest indication is severe faciomaxillary injury.

Action

1 Cricothyroidotomy is a relatively safe and bloodless method of securing an airway.

2 It is not recommended in children under 12 years of age because the cricoid cartilage is the sole support for the trachea at this level. Instead employ jet insufflation. Insert a 14G intravenous cannula percutaneously through the cricothyroid membrane and connect this to an intermittent oxygen insufflater, a simple oxygen tube with a Y connector cut into it in series such that oxygen passes through the cannula only when the Y connector is digitally occluded. This procedure leads to a certain amount of carbon dioxide retention so use it for no more than 40 minutes. This buys the time to arrange either an expert

intubation or a formal tracheostomy. There is no need for special positioning of the patient since the cricothyroid membrane is easily accessible.

3 Check the balloon on the cricothyroidotomy tube before starting. Remove any cervical collar. Have an assistant support the neck rigorously between hands or bent knees. A rigid cervical support collar is normally fenestrated and can be replaced after the procedure, passing the airway tube through the fenestration. Identify the cricothyroid membrane between the thyroid and cricoid cartilages and make a 3-cm transverse incision in the skin down onto it. Divide the cricothyroid membrane and enlarge the resulting hole in the trachea with a tracheal dilator or artery forceps. Insert a suitable-sized cuffed adult tracheostomy tube or a purpose-made cricothyroidotomy tube if one is available. Replace the rigid cervical collar.

? DIFFICULTY

1. Keep the cricothyroidotomy incision small, no wider than a stab incision with a large blade. If you make a larger incision you risk damaging the anterior jugular vein, causing a brisk venous haemorrhage. Although you can stop it by pressing on it, prefer to identify, clamp and ligate the cut ends of the vein after you have safely secured the cricothyroidotomy tube. Remember that airway is more urgent than breathing and, if this mishap occurs, ignore the bleeding until the tube is secure in the trachea.
2. Regard tracheostomy as an elective technique, best performed in an anaesthetized, intubated patient. It is a requirement in children. The only real emergency indication in an adult is for penetrating laryngeal trauma with associated damage in the cricothyroid. The technique is described in Chapter 46.
3. When there is an open defect in the trachea, the tracheostomy tube can often be placed in the trachea directly through the wound (Ch. 46).

CHEST

Chest wounds, whether blunt or penetrating, range between trivial and fatal. In war, chest injury is common with a high immediate mortality, usually from mediastinal disruption, open pneumothorax or massive haemothorax. In blunt injury, haemothorax and pneumothorax often accompany falls or other deceleration injuries.

THORACOCENTESIS

Appraise

1 Emergency intervention in chest trauma is largely confined to thoracocentesis for tension pneumothorax, haemothorax or a combination of the two.

2 You should be able to insert an intercostal tube drain gently and painlessly after injecting plenty of local anaesthetic. Unless it is urgent, allow plenty of time, such as 5 minutes, for the local anaesthetic to work.

Prepare

1 As a rule, insert the drain with the patient sitting upright. This may not be possible if the patient is unconscious, with multiple injuries. Thoracocentesis is occasionally required as an emergency if the patient has a tension pneumothorax, but there is usually time to prepare the patient and use an aseptic technique. Use at least a 32G fenestrated (with a side window) chest drain.

2 Identify the incision site in the anterior axillary line, just above the nipple line, in order to avoid diaphragmatic or, particularly on the right, hepatic injury. This leads you to the fifth or sixth intercostal space, which is relatively free of complications. Prepare the chest antiseptic solution. Inject at least 15 ml of 1% lidocaine, preferably with adrenaline (epinephrine) 1 : 200 000, into the skin and deeply and widely into the intercostal muscle.

Action

1 Make a 1-cm transverse incision in the skin and deepen it into the muscle just above the upper border of the rib or you may damage the intercostal vessels.

2 Insert two heavy nylon stitches, one as a mattress suture across the hole (not a purse-string) for closing the hole later, and the other to the side of the incision to secure the drain. Separate the intercostal muscles using scissors or artery forceps, and puncture the parietal pleura. If possible, sweep a finger around the inside of the hole to exclude or separate lung adhesions. If there is a tension pneumothorax there is a brisk gush of air at this point. Select a fenestrated trocar drain, remove the trocar completely, and place the drain gently in the pleural cavity about 6 cm deeper than the most proximal fenestration, using an artery forceps to stiffen the tip. There is no need to introduce the drain to the hilt; expansion of the lung forces both air and blood into its lumen, whatever its position. Under no circumstances use the pointed trocar to force the drain through the intercostal muscle. Connect the drain to a flutter valve or to an underwater seal drain if available (see Ch. 33). Secure it with the previously placed suture and apply a light dressing.

? DIFFICULTY

1. Insertion of the drain through a high interspace in the anterior axillary line is dangerous because of the proximity of hilar structures and the mediastinum.
2. Avoid the mid-axillary line because of the slight but significant risk of injuring an accessory mammary artery which passes down the inside of the chest wall in the mid-axillary position. Although it is present in only 2% of cases, one of us needed to perform a thoracotomy for persisting bleeding following thoracocentesis causing this injury.
3. Do not secure the drain with lengths of 3-inch adhesive plaster; this practice is out of date.

Postoperative

1 Underwater sealed thoracocentesis drains may bubble for days without problems, but persistent drainage of blood is more

serious. Carry out thoracotomy if there is immediate drainage of more than 1 litre of blood, or persistent drainage of more than 250 ml/hour.

PERICARDIOCENTESIS

Appraise

This is occasionally beneficial when managing pericardial tamponade. It is recommended in the Advanced Trauma Life Support (ATLS) core curriculum as an emergency procedure for inexperienced doctors working alone.

Prepare

Prepare the skin with antiseptic solution and identify the xiphoid process. Place electrocardiographic (ECG) chest electrodes; if you touch the myocardium with the needle during this procedure you often see ectopic contraction waves on the monitor.

KEY POINTS Emergency thoracotomy?

- Call for cardiac surgical assistance before starting.
- If the patient requires this procedure to relieve life-threatening tamponade he almost certainly requires an emergency thoracotomy.

Action

1 Introduce a wide-bore needle to the left of the xiphoid process, pointing towards the tip of the left scapula. Aspirate, using a syringe, as you advance the needle. If you obtain blood, attach a three-way tap and 50-ml syringe, to remove larger quantities. Watch the ECG monitor for ectopic activity.

2 The blood is almost always clotted and it is often impossible to remove enough by this technique to relieve the tamponade.[2]

3 Aspiration of blood is not a definitive treatment and the condition will recur.

4 Under these circumstances perform immediate thoracotomy (see Ch. 33).

THORACOTOMY

Appraise

1 Emergency thoracotomy is rarely needed. It is usually indicated for intractable intrathoracic bleeding, as diagnosed by persistent bleeding into the chest drain. The outcome is far better following penetrating trauma than after blunt trauma. Stab wounds usually produce single small lacerations that can be repaired relatively easily. Blunt trauma often causes widespread contusion and laceration which are more difficult to repair.

2 When possible, plan an urgent procedure in the operating theatre. The commonest causes of such bleeding after both blunt or penetrating trauma are damage to the intercostal vessels or lung parenchyma caused either by rib fracture or direct rupture.

3 Mediastinal trauma is less often a cause of bleeding, but when it is, it is much more serious. Lung resection is seldom required in trauma cases; when it is, try to avoid pneumonectomy which carries a high mortality, even in previously fit individuals.

? DIFFICULTY

1. Reserve 'emergency room thoracotomy' for penetrating cardiac wounds in which you perceive that tamponade, or brisk exsanguination through the entry wound, are immediate threats to life.[3] It is indicated only when the vital signs are present on arrival in the emergency room, but are lost despite immediate resuscitative measures.
2. If you can maintain cardiac output, immediately transfer the patient to the operating theatre. Reports from some centres suggest that the results from this procedure are unsatisfactory.[4] Do not carry out this procedure following blunt trauma to the mediastinum or aorta since the damage is nearly always diffuse.

KEY POINTS Indications for formal thoracotomy

- Initial blood loss of more than 1 litre.
- Continued loss of more than 250 ml/hour.
- Cardiac tamponade.
- Other mediastinal injuries.
- Persistent air leak.
- Retained foreign bodies >1.5 cm in diameter.

Prepare

1 Give an anaesthetic if the patient is conscious.

2 The procedure is facilitated if there is sufficient time and the anaesthetist is able to insert a double-lumen tube in order to collapse one lung completely. This is not likely to be feasible during a conflict.

3 Apply antiseptic skin preparation since this takes a few seconds only.

Access

1 To deal with a cardiac injury, make a left anterior approach through the fourth interspace (Fig. 3.2). You can examine the entire surface of the heart through this incision and even deal with stab wounds to the heart from the right of the sternum.

2 If time permits, create a formal posterolateral incision. It provides better access to the posterior mediastinum and it seldom needs to be enlarged. It is convenient for access to the lungs and pleura; carry it out if you suspect that there is injury in addition to, or instead of, a mediastinal injury.

3 A midline sternotomy gives the best access to mediastinal structures (Fig. 3.1). Even if it is available, there is seldom time to carry out the high-resolution computed tomography (CT) needed to exclude other thoracic injury, making this safely possible.

4 If you will also need to perform a laparotomy to deal with penetrating abdominal trauma, use a midline sternotomy. If there is penetrating injury to the abdomen, it is wise to keep the laparotomy separate from the thoracotomy. Isolate the peritoneal cavity from the thoracic cavity for fear of possible faecal contamination of the chest.

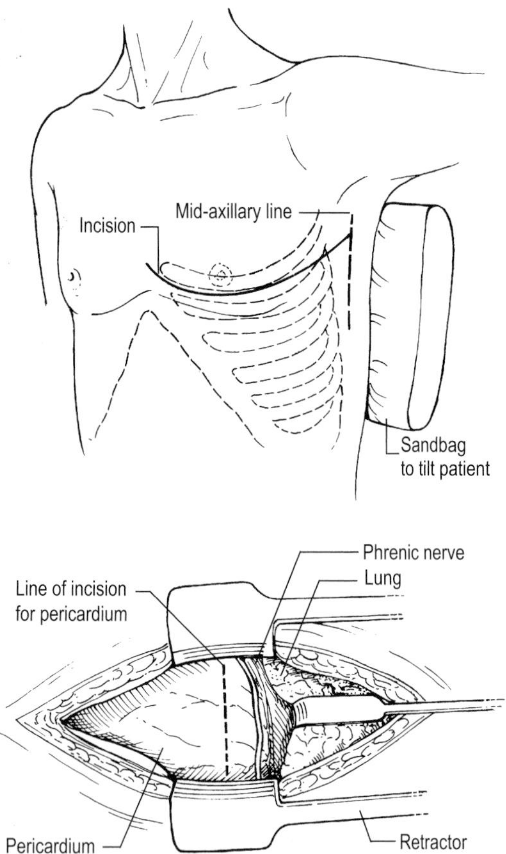

Fig. 3.2 Left anterior thoracotomy, which provides access especially to the left ventricle and pulmonary conus. Avoid the phrenic nerve.

Assess

1 The basic technique for thoracotomy of all types is described in Chapter 33. The description which follows presupposes entry through a posterolateral thoracotomy. Use a large scalpel blade to incise the intercostal muscles and expose the chest cavity and its contents.

2 Insert a rib spreader and examine the thoracic cavity. Evacuate any clot and keep the operative field clear with effective and intelligent retraction and suction. Have the anaesthetist collapse the lung if a double-lumen tube is in place; otherwise have it gently drawn aside with a lung retractor. First examine the chest wall; the majority of haemothoraces among survivors are associated with injury to the intercostal or internal thoracic (mammary) arteries. Next, examine the lung surfaces for lacerations, which may bleed profusely. Finally, turn your attention to the aorta and lung root vessels.

3 Lengthen the thoracotomy wound across the sternum to the contralateral side if you require access to the other lung because of bleeding or an air leak. This 'clamshell' incision (Fig. 3.3) is easier with an anterior thoracotomy than with a posterolateral approach since the medial end of the incision is much higher and the choice of incision may well depend on whether unilateral or bilateral injury is suspected.

4 For access to the heart, incise the pericardium, avoiding damage to the phrenic nerve which runs across the left side of the

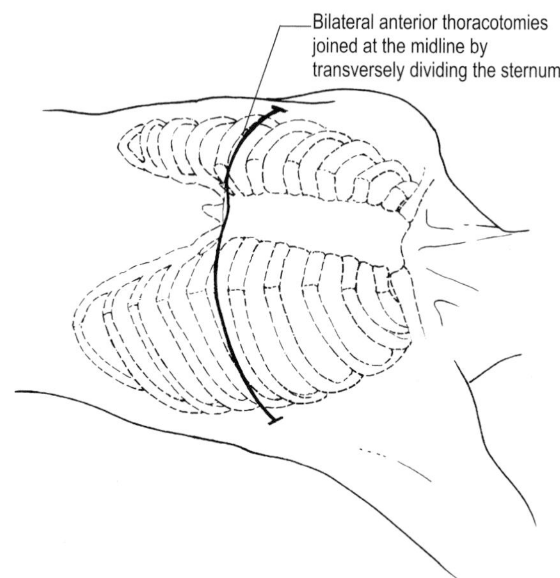

Fig. 3.3 The clamshell incision for access to both thoracic cavities and the mediastinum. The internal mammary (internal thoracic) arteries on both sides need to be cut. Secure both ends of each.

pericardium and is usually obvious. Evacuate the pericardial clot and gently deliver the heart, remembering that excessive traction stops the circulation.

Action

1 First control any bleeding from thoracic wall vessels unless there is massive exsanguination from the pulmonary vessels or aorta; in this case, immediately control the major bleeding by direct pressure. Place a suture around the intercostal bundle or other vessel and tie it down, avoiding, if possible, the intercostal nerve, damage to which leads to postoperative pain. Control minor and moderate tears in the lung parenchyma by oversewing or even simple pressure; bleeding often stops and tears seal spontaneously when the lung is deflated. Control a more extensive tear from a penetrating missile injury by applying clamps on either side of the tear; divide the tissue between them and oversew the bleeding vessels in the exposed wound track (Fig. 3.4). If this is inappropriate because of major hilar vessel bleeding, consider lobectomy or pneumonectomy (see Ch. 33). Be aware that lobectomy and pneumonectomy have poor outcomes when performed by inexperienced operators, so call for expert help if possible. Pulmonary artery tears often extend into the left atrium; repair techniques are beyond the scope of this chapter. If you are working during a conflict you are unlikely to see this major injury at emergency thoracotomy since the mortality is extremely high.

2 Aortic tears or penetrating wounds are difficult to control. Occasionally, if the blood pressure falls, they seal spontaneously. In this case oversew the tear with interrupted, non-absorbable sutures mounted on a round-bodied needle. Control small tears by applying a side clamp such as Brock's or Satinsky's. Control larger tears or transection by proximal and distal cross-clamping, then mobilize the aorta and resect the damaged vessel wall. Carry out a primary repair or insert an interposition tube graft. The superior vena cava (SVC) is much more difficult to repair;

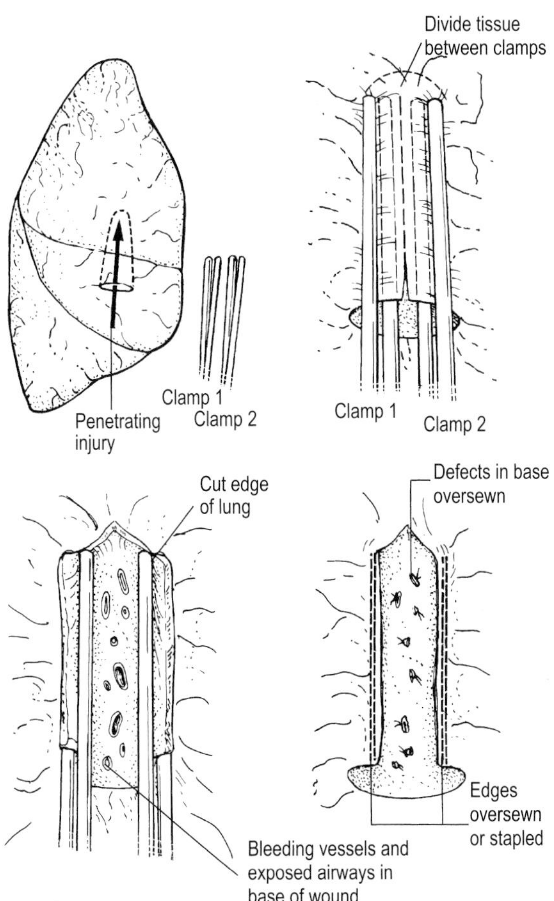

Fig. 3.4 A method for repairing a penetrating injury of the lung with particular emphasis on haemostasis.

it tends to shred when stitched so ask for help from an expert. You almost always need proximal and distal control. In an emergency or when the thoracic wound is contaminated, it is acceptable to oversew the cut ends of the cava.

3 If there is a wound in the heart, place deep sutures in the myocardium using a large curved round-bodied needle, carefully identifying and avoiding the coronary arteries (see also Ch. 33). In order to achieve temporary control of bleeding from a penetrating ventricular wound, insert a collapsed Foley catheter into the ventricle, inflate the balloon and pull it against the inner edges of the defect. Hold the catheter in position with a stitch ligature into the ventricular muscle (Fig. 3.5). The injured right atrium is thin-walled and floppy, so insert full-thickness continuous sutures to bring the wound edges into apposition.

? DIFFICULTY

1. Occasionally a penetrating cardiac injury results in a large tear in one of the cardiac chambers and this presents more severe problems. If you have expert help available, urgently call for the assistance of the cardiac surgery team.
2. A damaged coronary artery bleeds briskly and should be expertly repaired using magnification.

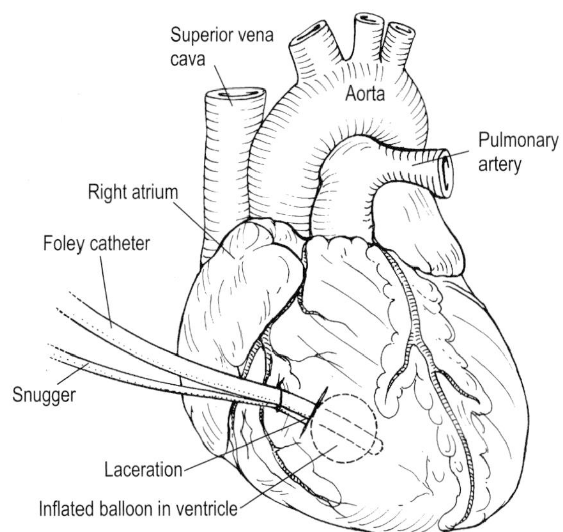

Fig. 3.5 A method for achieving temporary haemostasis in penetrating cardiac trauma, using a Foley catheter.

Checklist

Do not close the chest until you have ensured that all major bleeding has been controlled and that the continuity of all damaged structures has been restored.

Closure

1 The techniques of formal thoracotomy closure in the trauma patient are no different from those used in elective procedures (Ch. 33). Always use wide-bore, larger than 32G, fenestrated chest drains, bearing in mind the possibility of postoperative infection.

2 If the wound is contaminated or infected, leave the skin and subcutaneous layers open. Of course you cannot leave the chest cavity open to drain and this is why the drains are so important.

KEY POINTS Chest drain precautions

- Make sure the drains are properly secured with strong, No. 1, nylon stitches which indent the drain when tied down tightly. It is disastrous if the drains are pulled out inadvertently during transport, particularly during evacuation by air transport.
- Never clamp drains prior to evacuation by air or road; this can easily lead to an unrecognized tension pneumothorax and death.

Postoperative

1 Ensure that the patient is carefully monitored, preferably in a critical care unit. This may be possible even in war and conflict circumstances with robust, field-tested, modern monitoring devices. Probably the most useful device is the pulse oximeter. If the patient cannot maintain an adequate oxygen saturation despite oxygen therapy, you may need to order vigorous

physiotherapy or even assisted ventilation. Always carry out a full, thorough re-examination to exclude a simple correctable cause such as a pneumothorax or haemothorax.

2 If these are excluded, deterioration nearly always results from progressive lung infection with atelectasis which may proceed to the onset of one of the acute lung injury syndromes such as adult respiratory distress syndrome (ARDS)

Complications

1 These include bleeding, infection, continuing air leak and cardiac dysrhythmias. Bleeding is a problem only if it is persistent and profuse (i.e. more than 250 ml/hour). Postoperative bleeding tends to diminish and stop with time, and transfusion if necessary. Re-open the chest only if the patient becomes shocked despite adequate resuscitation.

2 Infection of the thoracotomy incision or of sustained entry and exit wounds is common, particularly if resources are constrained. Employ first principles, including re-opening the wound, draining any pus and giving appropriate antibiotics.

3 Intrathoracic infection usually presents later as an empyema.

4 Continuing air leak is common following lung parenchymal injury. Provided the lung is fully expanded it will stop spontaneously over 24–48 hours. Leaks beyond this point may be associated with previously unrecognized bronchial or even tracheal injury. Consider this if the lung fails to expand despite the presence of two large drains and suction. In the setting of a conflict, you need to evacuate the patient to a specialist centre.

5 The commonest cardiac dysrhythmia following chest injury is atrial fibrillation, which is usually associated with shunting and hypoxia. Ventricular ectopic beats are associated with post-traumatic myocardial ischaemia. Do not forget that older patients may already have an underlying cardiac problem.

TRACHEAL INJURIES

Appraise

1 Injury to the trachea in the neck is open or closed. Open injury is obvious. Closed injury may lead to surgical emphysema in the neck with characteristic crepitus. The trachea is rarely injured in isolation from a penetrating injury. Always investigate the oesophagus (see below). The diagnosis is more difficult following blunt trauma but you must carry out an exploration, if possible preceded by endoscopy.

2 Injury to the trachea and main bronchi in the chest is unusual but leads to a massive air leak. On examination you find only a tension pneumothorax but when you insert a chest drain there is a persistent air leak. If the lung does not re-expand after drainage, suspect a major airway injury, so insert a second chest drain and apply suction to both of them.

Prepare

Secure the airway. Because of the likelihood of damage to other structures including the thyroid and major vessels, seek expert help before embarking on a major exploration and repair.

Access

Injuries in the neck are dealt with locally. Otherwise carry out a posterolateral thoracotomy.

Assess and action

1 These two sections are dealt with together because the extent of injury will determine your technique.

2 Oversew closed injuries to the trachea in the neck, using interrupted absorbable sutures.

3 Open injuries such as those associated with high-energy transfer missiles may be associated with extensive tissue loss, precluding direct primary repair. You may be able only to insert an endotracheal tube into the disrupted trachea, thus securing the airway and closing the leak at the same time. Seek help from an expert.

4 In the chest, oversew a simple tear of the trachea or main bronchus using interrupted non-absorbable sutures. This requires expertise; the consequences of a bronchopleural fistula are lethal. More extensive injury involves the blood vessels, again demanding expert help if available.

5 Hilar near-avulsion probably requires pneumonectomy. You are unlikely to encounter this in the operating theatre since it is usually rapidly fatal.

OESOPHAGEAL INJURY

Appraise

1 This is usually occult. Clinically, you detect subcutaneous surgical empyema in the supraclavicular fossae. Chest X-ray may demonstrate air in the mediastinum. Oesophageal injury is normally associated with other mediastinal injuries, whether blunt or penetrating. Order a Gastrografin swallow X-ray to confirm the diagnosis.

KEY POINT Do not miss oesophageal rupture

- A missed rupture carries the gravest of prognoses.

Prepare

Prepare the patient for a left posterolateral thoracotomy, possibly with a separate neck access incision or a thoracoabdominal extension. Covering antibiotics are essential.

Access

Most of the intrathoracic oesophagus can be reached through the posterolateral incision. Look out for and protect the phrenic nerve crossing the pericardium, and also the descending thoracic aorta, which is also vulnerable.

Assess

A fresh injury is relatively clean and easy to repair. If there is any delay at all, anticipate medastinitis with pleural cavity contamination

Action

1 Dissect the oesophagus free from surrounding structures and introduce slings above and below the site of injury. Repair a fresh injury by approximating the mucosa with interrupted absorbable sutures. This is the most important layer; a second muscular suture adds security to the repair. Drain the injury site and close the chest in the usual way.

2 A contaminated ruptured oesophagus is irreparable. It has the consistency of wet blotting paper. Manage it by draining and isolating it.

3 Drain the site and insert a tube gastrostomy in the stomach.

4 Through an incision through the sternomastoid in the neck, carry out an open formal pharyngostomy, suturing mucosa to skin. This acts as a diversion to keep the saliva out of the mediastinum.

Checklist, closure and postoperative care

1 These are the same as for thoracotomy.

ABDOMEN

LAPAROTOMY

Appraise

1 The conduct of a laparotomy for trauma follows standard guidelines which apply irrespective of whether this is a blunt or penetrating injury. Some techniques may vary depending on the skills and resources available locally.

KEY POINTS Laparotomy is indicated:

- When there is unequivocal clinical evidence of peritonitis.
- When the patient is difficult to resuscitate, requiring continuing intravenous fluids, and bleeding has been excluded in other areas.
- When air is present under the diaphragm or there is evidence of diaphragmatic rupture on the erect chest X-ray.
- When there is a positive diagnostic peritoneal lavage or a CT scan reveals the presence of blood and ruptured solid viscera.
- When there is a penetrating or perforating missile wound in a resource-constrained environment.

2 If an unconscious patient is stable, take advantage of available diagnostic aids. CT scan of the abdomen with contrast injection is considered the best single test, especially when the patient is undergoing a CT scan of the head. Remember, though, that a CT scan of the abdomen performed very soon following injury may not yet demonstrate blood because insufficient has not yet collected in the peritoneal cavity to show unequivocally on the scan.

KEY POINTS Fail to look, fail to diagnose

- Always remember to examine the back.

3 Constantly reappraise the patient's clinical condition. If CT is not available, ultrasound may be useful. If this is also not available, employ diagnostic peritoneal lavage, which remains a reliable tool (Ch. 4).

4 If the patient is not stable, proceed to resuscitative laparotomy without delay.

5 The laparotomy is being carried out because the patient has either shown signs of peritonitis or haemorrhage into the peritoneal cavity, or that a diagnostic test has given a positive result.

6 Penetrating wounds may initially present with few clinical signs but there is always a danger of the patient's condition suddenly deteriorating. Blunt injury giving rise to visceral damage normally leaves tell-tale signs on the abdominal wall such as bruising, abrasion, tyre marks, or seatbelt tattooing.

KEY POINT Exploration of penetrating wounds

- Conventional advice is that all penetrating abdominal wounds should be explored, but this is not necessary provided that:
  —The patient is absolutely stable, with no signs of intra-abdominal injury or shock.
  —You reassess the patient at frequent intervals, every 2 hours if necessary.
  —At the first sign of deterioration such as increasing pulse rate, falling blood pressure or increasing abdominal tenderness, you carry out a laparotomy. Treat such an event not as a failure but as a natural resolution of the equivocal physical signs.

Prepare

1 There is always time to prepare and drape the abdomen properly before laparotomy.

2 Make sure that rapid transfusion of blood or fluids can be started as soon as the abdomen is opened. The abdominal wall often tamponades bleeding and this is released when the abdomen is opened.

3 Warn the theatre staff to have available necessary equipment such as two powerful suckers, adequate numbers of large packs, and vascular instruments if massive bleeding is likely.

4 Cover as much of the patient as possible with heat-reflective blankets to prevent hypothermia. A warm-air blanket is most useful if available. Bleeding patients cool off rapidly even in hot climates.

5 If the patient has not been given prophylactic antibiotics, give an initial intravenous loading dose of a versatile appropriate antibiotic now.

6 Before operation, pass a nasogastric tube into the stomach and a urinary catheter into the bladder.

Access

Explore the abdomen through a midline incision which can be extended in both directions, even into a median sternotomy if necessary.

Assess

Examine all viscera, explore the lesser sac, identify all sources of bleeding and explore all stab wounds to their fullest extent (Ch. 4).

Action

1 Control of haemorrhage is the first priority within the abdomen. Major intraperitoneal bleeding can be a daunting prospect. Have two suckers ready as well as a number of large packs. As soon as the peritoneum has been opened try to identify the general area from which the bleeding is coming and clear away as much clot and free blood as possible to identify the specific source.

2 Treat life-threatening exsanguination from abdominal bleeding by opening the left chest and cross-clamping the aorta. You may leave the clamp in place for a maximum of 45 minutes while seeking and dealing with the vascular injury. In penetrating trauma explore expanding retroperitoneal haematomata to exclude major vessel injury. In blunt trauma, especially that associated with pelvic fractures, leave haematomata alone as exploration may lead to uncontrollable venous haemorrhage. Control bleeding from major abdominal vessels with pressure whilst dissecting around the wound to achieve control above and below the bleeding point. Then repair the vessel with polypropylene sutures. Major damage to aorta and vena cava requires expert assistance during repair.

3 Oversew smaller bleeding mesenteric vessels. Always examine distal bowel afterwards and resect it if you doubt its viability.

4 Repair damaged hollow viscera next, thereby limiting contamination of the peritoneum. Examine both surfaces of the stomach. Oversew tears or penetrating injuries. Watch for doubtful viability of the greater curve if there is a longitudinal tear parallel to it. If you are in doubt, resect it.

5 Explore the area of the duodenum if there is retroperitoneal haemorrhage or biliary discoloration in the region of the duodenum. Mobilize the duodenum by Kocher's manoeuvre to examine its posterior surface. If possible repair it rather than resect it. Most duodenal tears can be repaired primarily or patched with a loop of jejunum. Perform a diversionary gastrojejunostomy and place a T-tube in the common bile duct in addition to the repair if there is extensive duodenal damage. Make sure that you adequately drain the area afterwards. You may need to resect the duodenum if there is severe tissue loss and major concurrent pancreatic trauma, but the morbidity is formidable.

6 Small bowel injuries are easier to deal with than those of the duodenum. It is not uncommon for a single stab wound to traverse several loops of small bowel. Carefully oversew all penetrating wounds or tears with absorbable sutures in a single interrupted layer. Consider resection if there are a large number of tears in a short length of bowel, or if you are in doubt about the viability.

7 Large bowel injury is more likely to require resection. If there is a small penetrating wound only that is less than 6 hours old, particularly on the right side of the colon, prefer to oversew it. A grossly contaminated wound of the right side of the colon can be treated by right hemicolectomy and primary anastomosis. Grossly contaminated left-sided colonic injury is best treated with resection and anastomosis, protected with a proximal colostomy. However, if there is established, generalized faecal peritonitis, choose the safer Hartmann's procedure (Ch. 4). Conservative surgery of large bowel perforation is possible but controversial (Ch. 16). If you are inexperienced, call for advice from a senior colleague.

8 Hepatic tears are often mild and may have stopped bleeding by the time you perform the laparotomy (Ch. 22). Suture major tears using a liver needle, taking care to prevent the needle from moving laterally in the parenchyma and so making the tear worse. If there is substantial haemorrhage from the liver use the manoeuvre described in 1908 by the Glaswegian surgeon J. Hogarth Pringle (1863–1941). Place a non-crushing clamp across the portal triad, with one blade through the foramen of Winslow into the lesser sac. This compresses the hepatic artery and portal vein while you assess and repair the liver damage. If bleeding continues after clamping, it is from the hepatic veins or inferior vena cava (IVC). Do not leave the clamp in place for more than 20 minutes.

9 Major hepatic injury may demand lobectomy. Damage to the retrohepatic IVC can be difficult to reach and control problems. You may need to control the IVC in the chest through a midline sternotomy, then insert a bypass tube from the right atrium to the infrarenal cava, isolating the hepatic veins and retrohepatic cava for repair. Summon expert help. Survival rates from this injury are extremely disappointing.

10 Pack otherwise uncontrollable haemorrhage[5] and re-operate at 24 hours to remove the packs and reassess the position. Repack if the bleeding restarts. There is increasing evidence that a conservative approach to hepatic trauma may be of benefit in up to 20% of cases.[6,7] Whenever possible seek expert help.

11 Splenectomy is the safest approach to the ruptured spleen. Sweep your hand between the diaphragm and the spleen to break down any adhesions and deliver the spleen forwards into the wound. Clamp and divide the gastrosplenic and lienorenal ligaments, avoiding the tail of the pancreas. Resect the spleen and double-tie the pedicles with heavy absorbable ligatures. Control oozing from disrupted adhesions by packing. It usually stops without further attention; if it does not, use diathermy current coagulation.

12 Splenic salvage surgery[8] may spare the patient from splenectomy. It involves applying haemostatic agents to the injury such as microfibrillar collagen or Vicryl mesh bags, together with diathermy coagulation and oversewing of the defect. Conservative management of the ruptured spleen may be successful in up to a quarter of patients.[9,10] This may be a course to pursue in children who are haemodynamically stable; children are far more likely than adults to develop overwhelming post-splenectomy infections. Institute active conservative management (Ch. 23). Do not forget to arrange for immunization against pneumococcus and long-term antibiotics if the spleen does have to be resected.

13 Avoid operating for blunt renal trauma unless there is intractable parenchymal bleeding, signified by gross haemo-

dynamically significant haematuria for more than 24 hours, or a urinary leak, or an expanding perirenal haematoma discovered at laparotomy. It is less often possible to manage penetrating trauma conservatively, but intravenous urography (IVU) and CT are helpful in excluding blood or urine leaks. The IVU demonstrates whether both kidneys are functioning if you need to consider nephrectomy. Always approach the damaged kidney through a midline laparotomy. Other viscera may be damaged and they cannot be dealt with through a loin incision. Oversew contused or penetrated bleeding areas with deep liver sutures. Conserve as much kidney as possible, bearing in mind the end artery anatomy of this organ.

14 Repair injured ureters and bladder primarily, using absorbable sutures. Insert a single layer to the ureter over a double 'J' stent. Insert a double layer into the bladder, over a suprapubic catheter. Urethral repair is described in Chapter 43.

15 Pancreatic injury can be problematic. If the injury is slight and the ducts are intact, stop all bleeding. Do not try to repair the injury but leave a drain down to the injured part. Treat distal injuries involving the duct by distal resection. Injuries to the head of the pancreas involving the duct are more difficult to deal with. Repair the duct or unite it to a jejunal loop. These are specialized procedures (see Ch. 21), so call for experienced assistance if possible.

16 Retroperitoneal access for bleeding can be difficult. Achieve access to the IVC on the right of the abdomen by dividing the congenital adhesions in the right paracolic gutter and sweeping the entire right colon together with the duodenum to the left. You can then control the cava proximally and distally. Injuries to the retrohepatic cava high up at the level of the hepatic veins are particularly difficult to deal with; you may need to insert an excluding shunt within the cava (see above under hepatic injuries). These injuries are nearly always fatal.

17 Expose injuries to the aorta in a manner similar to exposing the IVC. Divide the congenital adhesions in the left paracolic gutter and swing the entire left colon, including if necessary the spleen and left kidney, to the right. In this way you can expose, control and deal with injuries to the suprarenal and coeliac levels of the aorta.

Checklist

1 Check that you have secured haemostasis.

2 Is the peritoneal cavity well washed out, even in cases of recent injury, before you close the abdomen? Also confirm that all the viscera are viable once they have been returned to the abdomen. Make sure they are not under tension.

3 Check that you have placed adequate drains and that they are properly placed and secured to the abdominal wall. Are stoma bags correctly placed, stomata covered with dressings to avoid wound contamination?

Closure

1 Close the laparotomy wound using a mass closure technique, usually with a single layer looped no. 1 nylon thread. You may leave open a grossly contaminated abdomen or one with major retroperitoneal oedema. Cover the wound with wet gauze swabs. Alternatively and probably appropriately, apply a Bogota bag. Open up an intravenous fluid bag, shape it, apply the inner sterile surface over the wound and loosely suture it to the skin edges with a continuous nylon suture. It is a crude but highly effective technique, allowing continuous inspection of abdominal contents and their drainage, and it is particularly useful if you are worried concerning abdominal compartment syndrome or bowel viability (see Ch. 4). It is particularly appropriate when resources are constrained.

2 Leave open associated missile entrance and exit wounds in the abdominal wall. Excise them and leave them for delayed primary closure.

Postoperative

Major abdominal surgery may lead to surprisingly few postoperative problems provided adequate preparation has been carried out beforehand. This is seldom possible in the trauma patient and the immediate postoperative management is crucial. This should take place in a critical care environment and details are beyond the scope of this chapter. Where a resuscitative 'damage-control' laparotomy has been carried out, a subsequent 'second-look' laparotomy is nearly always necessary in order to check tissue viability and to search for and correct injuries missed during resuscitation.

Complications

1 The most important postoperative complication is bleeding. It demands re-laparotomy.

2 Control of bleeding may be simple but can be extremely difficult; there is seldom anything in between. Remember that bleeding may result from clotting deficiency and so is not surgically correctable. Clotting deficiency may be avoided to some certain extent by giving 1 unit of fresh frozen plasma to every 4 units of transfused stored blood, together with calcium gluconate injections to reverse the ethylenediamine tetra-acetic acid (EDTA) in the blood. Platelets are needed once the total transfused volume exceeds 10 units; they must be given even if the platelet count appears relatively normal, as many of these platelets are non-functional. A low body temperature wrecks the clotting system completely, so keep the patient warm.

3 Sepsis is a potent cause of collapse after 48–72 hours. Immediate postoperative temperature increase is nearly always respiratory; actively treat the patient with physiotherapy and appropriate antibiotics, and with suction if the patient is on a ventilator. Progressive abdominal sepsis is relentless in its course and leads to multisystem failure including renal, respiratory and hepatic collapse unless you deal with it surgically by drainage.

▶ KEY POINTS Abdominal sepsis

- Do not ignore progressive abdominal sepsis.
- Urgently re-explore the abdomen to determine the cause and deal with it.

4 Anastomotic leaks are more likely following trauma surgery than after elective operations. You must institute judicious drainage at the initial procedure to provide early warning of a leak. Treat such leaks conservatively. Low-output fistulae usually

respond to a few days without oral feeding and instituting nasogastric aspiration. High-output fistulae need parenteral nutrition and the administration of somatostatin or similar agents. Ideally manage the patient in a critical care environment.

5 The specific management of multi-organ failure is a complex subject requiring expert care and back-up.

DAMAGE-CONTROL LAPAROTOMY

This term describes laparotomy to control massive haemorrhage following abdominal injury. The technique differs little from that described previously.

Appraise

1 Studies in the USA in the 1980s showed a rise in handgun injuries, increasingly with semi-automatic guns; one study showed an average of 2.7 penetrations per patient. An increasing proportion of deaths resulted at the scene. The great majority of deaths were associated with vascular damage and bleeding, although some died later from sepsis and multi-organ failure. Standardized methods of treatment were developed and have been described in this chapter, but, following devastating trauma to the torso, mortality remains high from exsanguination.

2 Exsanguination and resulting hypoperfusion reduces tissue oxygenation, consequent anaerobic metabolism, build up of lactic acid and acidosis. Hypothermia develops at the site of injury, during transfer and on exposure of the body cavities at operation. Coagulopathy develops as a result of the exsanguinations, trauma, acidosis, and also from the effects of the hypothermia on the temperature-sensitive clotting cascade. These three factors combine to increase mortality.

KEY POINTS Exsanguination: the lethal triad

- Acidosis.
- Hypothermia.
- Coagulopathy.

3 Recognition and risk of haemorrhage has been classified according to the lost percentage of blood volume:
- Class I: loss of 0–15% usually does not raise the pulse rate or lower the blood pressure. Delayed capillary refill beyond 3 seconds suggests loss of about 10%.
- Class II: loss of 15–30% usually raises the pulse rate above 100/min with tachypnoea and decreased pulse pressure. Catecholamines increase diastolic pressure.
- Class III: loss of 30–40% markedly raises pulse, tachypnoea, lowers systolic pressure and urinary output and sometimes agitation and confusion.
- Class IV: loss over 40% markedly raises pulse, depressed systolic and sometimes undetectable diastolic pressures, mental depression or loss of consciousness, and cold, pale skin.

4 Since the turn of the 20th century, surgeons have argued over the merits of delayed or immediate repair following haemorrhage control after massive injuries with or without delayed definitive repair. It is impossible to demonstrate which is best and in what circumstances, because no two patients are similar and no two injuries are similar in number, type, situation, structures involved, initial management, delay before reaching a surgeon, or the facilities and expertise available. However, there are circumstances when you must recognize that everything else is secondary to stopping further exsanguinations.

KEY POINTS Priorities

- Never forget why you are operating: to save life.
- Life lost is irrecoverable; sepsis, organ failure may be recoverable.
- Rules are the best compromises for most situations. There are times when you must have the courage and decisiveness to break a rule if your clinical judgement tells you that if you continue trying to achieve perfection now, you will succeed—with a dead patient!

KEY POINTS Identifying patients requiring damage control

Physiological

- Hypothermia.
- Severe metabolic acidosis.
- Coagulopathy.

Pathological

- High-energy injury.
- Penetrating injury.
- Multi-organ injury.

Prepare

1 Damage control laparotomy is required in quite extreme circumstances and leaves little time to prepare.

2 Preparation starts in the emergency department. Warm the patient.

3 Order large quantities of whole blood, fresh frozen plasma, platelets. Provide a blood warmer.

4 Transfer the patient to operating theatre as quickly as possible.

5 There is always time to clean and drape the abdomen. Also prepare and drape the chest; you may need to gain access to the mediastinal structures and descending thoracic aorta.

6 Be willing to defer insertion of urinary catheter and nasogastric tube until the end of the procedure.

Access

1 Initially enter the abdomen through a generous midline incision.

2 Under normal circumstances you can reach most of the left chest and mediastinal contents through a left thoracotomy, but if you are using a midline laparotomy this is not possible. In these circumstances access to the chest is via a transverse ('clamshell') incision (Fig. 3.3), to gain access to the pleural cavities and descending thoracic aorta.

3 To gain access to the heart alone, you can create a midline sternotomy.

4 Patients with severe abdominal injuries often have severe intrathoracic injuries in addition.

Assess

1 The usual indication is multiple penetrating trauma. Assess the abdominal contents in a similar manner as for a standard trauma laparotomy.

2 Convert the procedure into a damage-control laparotomy when the number of injuries are such that control and packing alone are possible, not complete repair. Haemorrhage control is the over-riding need.

3 The presence of a major vascular injury together with two hollow visceral injuries, plus Class III shock, are indications for damage control.

Action

The laparotomy proceeds in three parts. Rotondo[11,12] suggests that a survival rate approaching 60% can be achieved by this approach:

- The initial laparotomy: controlling damage which can be controlled and packing damage which cannot.
- An intensive care unit phase, in which you have a small window of opportunity to correct the metabolic acidosis, haemoglobin and blood clotting.
- A return to theatre, with definitive repair of packed injuries at a second-look laparotomy.

Some patients require more than two laparotomies and eventually a laparostomy with a Bogota bag; you have to decide how much definitive repair is possible within the constraints of the level of shock and the requirement for blood transfusion. You will find that you can repair all the injuries at the second laparotomy in the majority of patients.

Checklist, closure, postoperative

These phases are the same as those described following laparotomy for abdominal injury.

REFERENCES

1. Norrell H 1980 The early management of spinal injuries. Clinical Neurosurgery 27:385–391
2. Knottenbelt JD 1991 University of Cape Town trauma handbook. UCT Press, Cape Town, p 46
3. Demetriades D 1986 Cardiac wounds. Experience with 70 patients. Annals of Surgery 203:315–317
4. Esposito TJ, Jurkovich GJ, Rice CL et al 1991 Reappraisal of emergency room thoracotomy in a changing environment. Journal of Trauma 31:881–887
5. Krige JEJ, Bornman PC, Terblanche J 1992 Therapeutic packing in complex liver trauma. British Journal of Surgery 79:43–46
6. Moore FA, Moore EE, Seagroves A 1985 Nonresectional management of major hepatic trauma. American Journal of Surgery 150:725–729
7. Hollands MJ, Little JM 1991 Non-operative management of blunt liver injuries. British Journal of Surgery 78:968–972
8. Giuliano AE, Lim RC 1981 Is splenic salvage safe in the traumatised patient? Archives of Surgery 116:651–656
9. Gibney EJ 1991 Non-operative management of blunt splenic injury. British Medical Journal 302:1553–1554
10. Khoury HI, Peschiera JL, Welling RE 1991 Non-operative management of blunt splenic trauma: a 10 year experience. Injury 22:349–352
11. Rotondo MF, Zonies DH 1997 The damage control sequence and underlying logic. Surgical Clinics of North America 4:761–777
12. Rotondo M, Schwab CW, McGonigal D et al 1993 Damage control: an approach for improved survival in exsanguinating penetrating abdominal injury. Journal of Trauma 35:373–383

FURTHER READING

American College of Surgeons 1989 Advanced trauma life support course for physicians. American College of Surgeons, Chicago

Anderson ID, Woodford M, deDombal FT et al 1988 Retrospective study of 1000 deaths from injury in England and Wales. British Medical Journal 296:1305–1308

Association for the Advancement of Automotive Medicine 1990 Abbreviated injury scale, revision. Association for the Advancement of Automotive Medicine, Des Plaines, IL

Baker SP, O'Neill B, Haddon W et al 1974 The injury severity score: a method for describing patients with multiple injuries and evaluating emergency care. Journal of Trauma 14:187–196

Boyd CR, Tolson MA, Copes WS 1987 Evaluating trauma care: the TRISS method. Journal of Trauma 27:370–378

Champion HR, Robbs JV, Trunkey LD 1989 Trauma surgery. In: Rob & Smith's operative surgery, 4th edn. Butterworths, London

Champion HR, Sacco WJ, Copes WS et al 1989 A revision of the trauma score. Journal of Trauma 29:623–629

Dalal SA, Burgess AR, Siegel JH et al 1989 Pelvic fracture in multiple trauma. Journal of Trauma 29:981–1002

Demetriades D, Charalambides C, Sareli P et al 1990 Late sequelae of penetrating cardiac injuries. British Journal of Surgery 77:813–814

Driscoll PA, Vincent CA 1992 Organising an efficient trauma team. Injury 23:107–110

Feliciano D, Mattox K, Jordan G 1981 Intra-abdominal packing for control of hepatic haemorrhage: a reappraisal. Journal of Trauma 21; 285-294

Feliciano DV, Burch JM, Spjut-Patrinely V et al 1988 Abdominal gunshot wounds. An urban trauma center's experience with 300 consecutive patients. Annals of Surgery 208:362–370

Fremstad JD, Martin SH 1978 Lethal complication from insertion of nasogastric tube after severe basilar skull fracture. Journal of Trauma 18:820–822

Henderson DK, Fahey BJ, Willy M et al 1990 Risk for occupational transmission of human immunodeficiency virus type 1 (HIV-1) associated with clinical exposures. A prospective evaluation. Annals of Internal Medicine 113(10):740–746

Jeffries DJ 1991 Zidovudine after occupational exposure to HIV. British Medical Journal 302:1349–1351

Jennet B, Teasdale G, Braakman R et al 1976 Predicting outcome in individual patients after severe head injury. Lancet i:1031–1034

Manton WI, Thal ER 1986 Lead poisoning from retained missiles. Annals of Surgery 204:594–599

Mattox KL, Moore WS, Feliciano D 1991 Trauma, 3rd edn. Appleton & Lange, New York

McSwain NE Jr 1988 Pneumatic anti-shock garment: state of the art 1988. Annals of Emergency Medicine 17:506–525

Nuffield Provincial Hospitals Trust 1987 Confidential enquiry into perioperative deaths. The King's Fund, London

Over D, Finch M 1991 The development of new documentation for use in cases of major trauma. Injury 22:139–145

Royal College of Surgeons of England 1988 Commission on the Provision of Surgical Services. Report of the working party on the management of patients with major injuries. Royal College of Surgeons of England, London

Shapiro MB, Jenkins DH, Schwab CW 2000 Damage control: collective review. Journal of Trauma 49: 969–978

Skinner D, Driscoll P, Earlam R J (eds) 1991 ABC of major trauma. BMJ Books, London

Soderstrom CA, Furth PA, Glasser D et al 1989 HIV infection rates in a trauma centre treating predominantly rural blunt trauma victims. Journal of Trauma 29:1526–1530

Teasdale G, Jennet B 1974 Assessment of coma and impaired consciousness. A practical scale. Lancet ii:81–83

Trunkey DD 1989 Report to the Council of the Association of Surgeons of Great Britain and Ireland. British Medical Journal 299:31–33

Trunkey DD 1991 Initial treatment of patients with extensive trauma. New England Journal of Medicine 324:1259–1263

Van Wagoner FH 1961 Died in hospital: a three year study of deaths following trauma. Journal of Trauma 1:401–408

Weiner SL, Barrett J 1986 Trauma management. Saunders, Philadelphia

West JG, Trunkey DD, Lim RC 1979 Systems of trauma care. A study of two counties. Archives of Surgery 114:455–460

Wood PR, Peel WJ, Foley MA et al 1990 Junior medical staff and the assessment of trauma. Annals of the Royal College of Surgeons of England 72:196–198

4

Laparotomy: elective and emergency

R.C.N. Williamson, R.M. Kirk

CONTENTS

INTRODUCTION

The Greek word *laparos* (=soft or loose) was used for the soft part between the ribs and hips, thus the flanks or loins. There were objections in 1878 to the use of 'laparotomy' for incisions through the anterior abdominal wall. Although the term defines only the incision, used on its own it often implies 'exploration of the abdomen'.

Surgeons' attitudes to laparotomy have undergone a marked change within a very few years. This change has brought great benefits but also potential dangers. Formerly, good surgeons took great care to make abdominal incisions of sufficient length to allow full exploration in order to confirm the diagnosis and exclude others, and also to carry out the correct procedure through an adequate exposure. By contrast, many operations are now carried out through restricted incisions. Indeed, certain procedures are routinely performed by the technique of 'minimal access' (see Ch. 5).[1] The change has come about for two reasons: improvements in imaging and laboratory tests have had a beneficial effect on diagnosis, while technical facilities have developed dramatically. It is very difficult to predict the future; we are presently seeing the usual enthusiasm for exploring the limits of minimal access procedures in competition with radiological and other indirect manipulations. Laparoscopy is, of course, available not only as a therapeutic tool but also as a diagnostic tool, particularly for the acute abdomen.[2] However, never forget that most diseases of the gastrointestinal tract primarily affect the mucosa; examining the hollow viscera from within the abdomen laparoscopically or at laparotomy does not replace endoscopic examination where this is possible.

KEY POINT Laparotomy as a part of other investigations

- A continuing danger is the fallacious belief that abdominal exploration will reveal the truth, making preoperative investigation seem unnecessary once laparotomy has been decided upon.

An increasing number of conditions previously treated by operation can now be managed by alternative methods. Uncomplicated chronic peptic ulcer is usually amenable to medical treatment. Selected patients with perforated peptic ulcer can be managed conservatively. Gastrointestinal bleeding can often be successfully treated by endoscopic or radiological methods. Strictures can be dilated effectively with single or repeated balloon dilatation with additional stenting if necessary.

Not only may intra-abdominal examination of hollow viscera fail to reveal intraluminal disease, but you may also miss disease processes that are deeply placed in solid organs. However, intraoperative use of high-frequency, high-resolution ultrasound scanning[2] promises to be a valuable diagnostic tool. Vascular blockage or constriction from atheroma is often difficult or impossible to detect in mesenteric vessels at laparotomy because of pulsatile backflow from patent vessels. Undoubtedly, the best time to make the diagnosis is before operation; this knowledge allows you to plan the best treatment. In some cases adequate preoperative investigation may spare the patient the need for operation, for example by showing advanced neoplasia for which surgical management would be ineffective.

Do not place too much reliance on tests. Results expressed numerically have a sometimes spurious appearance of objectivity. Imaging techniques are operator-dependent and generally have an accuracy of only 80–90%. The most certain method of making a diagnosis remains the taking of a good history, carrying out a careful and thorough examination, followed by carefully selected and interpreted investigations. If these methods fail, the next step is not necessarily exploratory laparotomy. Whenever possible, it is better to repeat the diagnostic process from the start, after an interval. Alternatively, ask a trusted colleague to take a completely fresh view of the problem. Computer-aided diagnosis has improved accuracy in dealing with the acute abdomen. Perhaps the general application of this technique will be valuable in elective surgery to prevent inappropriate laparotomy.

REFERENCES

1. Memon MA, Fitzgibbons RJ Jr 1997 The role of minimal access surgery in the acute abdomen. Surgical Clinics of North America 77:1333–1353

2. Luck AJ, Madden GJ 1999 Intraoperative abdominal ultrasonography. British Journal of Surgery 86:5–16

AVOIDING ADHESIONS

Appraise

1 There have been a number of studies of postoperative adhesions and, particularly, of their consequences.[1,2] Well-known technical factors are extensive trauma, bleeding, infection, foreign material, intraperitoneal chemotherapeutic agents and, especially, ischaemic tissue. In Britain there are 12 000–14 400 admissions each year resulting from abdominal adhesions, and in the USA they account for approximately 950 000 patient-days in hospital.

2 One of the most frequently identified causes is the use of starch glove powder. Swedish hospitals admit at least 4700 patients each year with adhesive small-bowel obstruction, and of these 2200 were operated on to relieve the obstruction.[3] Only a quarter of the responders to a questionnaire used powder-free gloves and less than half of them ever washed their gloves. Those who did wash their gloves used ineffective methods. The Swedish authors also indicated suturing of the peritoneum as a probable cause of adhesion formation.

3 Prefer powderless gloves. If you use starch-powdered gloves, wash off the powder by the effective method of Fraser.[4] Put on the gloves, and carry out a 10-minute surgical scrub using 10 ml of povidone–iodine 7.5% in a non-toxic detergent base (Betadine), which combines with the starch. Now rinse in 500 ml of sterile water for 30 seconds.

4 It is likely that the increasing use of minimal-access techniques will reduce the incidence of adhesions, although the technique has not abolished the problem.[5]

5 Liberal irrigation of the peritoneal cavity with Ringer's lactate solution, before abdominal closure, is said to reduce adhesion formation. In the last few years, adhesion-prevention barriers have been developed that prevent the formation of fibrin bridges. They can be laid between surfaces that are potentially adhesiogenic and are subsequently absorbed. Two cellulose-derived membranes have been approved for clinical use: Interceed (Johnson & Johnson) and Seprafilm (Genzyme).[6]

REFERENCES

1. Ellis H 1997 The clinical significance of adhesions: focus on intestinal obstruction. European Journal of Surgery Supplement 577:7–9
2. Wilson MS, Hawkswell J, McCloy RF 1998 Natural history of adhesional small bowel obstruction: counting the cost. British Journal of Surgery 85:1294–1298
3. Holmdahl L, Risberg B 1997 Adhesions: prevention and complications in general surgery. European Journal of Surgery 163:169–174
4. Fraser I 1982 Simple and effective method of removing starch powder from surgical gloves. British Journal of Surgery 284:1835
5. Tulandi T 1996 Adhesion prevention in laparoscopic surgery. International Journal of Fertility and Menopausal Studies 41:452–457
6. Falk K, Holmdahl E, Halvarsson M et al 1998 Polymers that reduce intraperitoneal adhesion formation. British Journal of Surgery 85:1153–1156

OPENING THE ABDOMEN

Preparation

1 Preferably see the patient in the ward before the premedication is given, or in the anaesthetic room while he is still awake. Check that this is the correct patient by visual identification and inspection of the identity bracelet.

2 Inspect the case notes and make sure that any relevant X-rays are available in theatre. If the lesion is unilateral, be quite certain that the operation will be carried out on the correct side (this should have been marked beforehand). It is inexcusable to neglect these elementary precautions.

3 If the bowel will be opened, or if necrotic or infected tissues are likely to be encountered, ensure that a prophylactic injection of an appropriate antibiotic is given at this stage. The choice depends on the nature of expected organisms, whether aerobic or anaerobic. Remember that facultative organisms must be considered in seriously ill patients.[1–3]

4 Carefully palpate the relaxed abdomen of the anaesthetized patient before making the incision.

5 Make sure that the anaesthetist is prepared for the operation to start. Laparotomy is nearly always performed under general anaesthesia, with endotracheal intubation and an intravenous cannula in situ.

6 Cleanse the skin of the operation area with an antiseptic solution applied on gauze held in long sponge-holding forceps. Appropriate solutions include chlorhexidine (Hibitane) 1:5000), povidone–iodine 10% in alcoholic solution (Betadine), cetrimide 1% and 95% white spirit. Apply the solution along the line of the incision and continue to apply it in a centrifugal manner of increasingly wide circles over a wide area. Do not use an inflammable agent, such as white spirit, if you intend to employ diathermy to the skin or immediate subcutaneous tissues.

7 Apply sterile sheets or drapes and secure them to the skin with towel clips, unless local anaesthetic is being used. Leave exposed a limited extent of the abdomen on either side of the proposed line of incision. Alternatively, clip the drapes to each other, or apply an adhesive plastic sheet over the area, which seals off the skin over the proposed incision, extending over and securing the drapes. The incision will be made through the sheet.

Types of incision (Figs 4.1, 4.2)

1 Plan the incision with care to give:
- Good exposure of the target area and versatility; it may be necessary to extend it.
- Minimal damage to intervening structures.
- Sound, cosmetically acceptable repair.

2 *Midline* incisions transgress the linea alba, the tough and relatively avascular cord that unites the anterior and posterior rectus sheaths. They therefore have the advantages of being relatively quick to make and to close and of provoking less bleeding than incisions that divide muscle fibres. Midline incisions can provide access to most abdominal viscera (Table 4.1). In the upper abdomen you can avoid the falciform ligament by

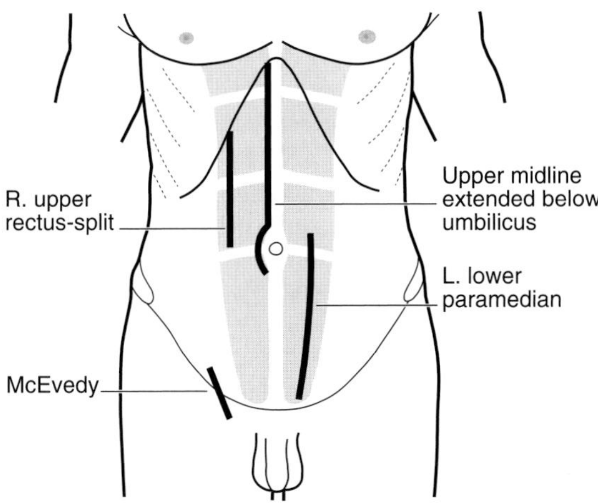

Fig. 4.1 Some vertical laparotomy incisions.

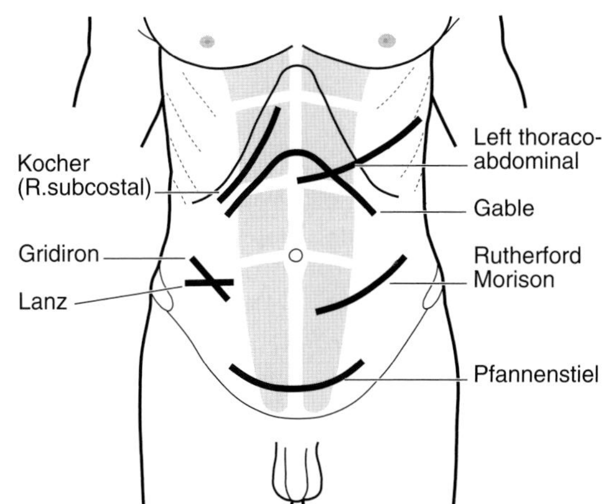

Fig. 4.2 Some transverse and oblique laparotomy incisions.

TABLE 4.1 Incisions to expose the abdominal viscera

Midline	Upper	Hiatus, oesophagus, stomach, duodenum, spleen, liver, pancreas, biliary tract
	Central	Small bowel, colon
	Lower	Sigmoid, rectum, ovary/tube/uterus, bladder and prostate (extraperitoneal)
	Throughout	Aorta
Paramedian (incl. rectus split)	Upper	Biliary tract (right), spleen (left), etc.
	Central	Small bowel, colon
	Lower	Pelvic viscera, lower ureter (extraperitoneal)
Oblique	Subcostal	Liver and biliary tract (right), spleen (left)
	Gable (bilateral)	Pancreas, liver, adrenals
	Gridiron	Caecum–appendix (right)
	Rutherford Morison	Caecum–appendix (right), sigmoid (left), ureter and external iliac vessels (extraperitoneal)
	Posterolateral	Kidney and adrenal (extraperitoneal)
Transverse	Right upper quadrant	Gallbladder, infant pylorus, colostomy
	Mid-abdominal	Small bowel, colon, kidney, lumbar sympathetic chain, vena cava (right)
	Lanz	Caecum–appendix (right)
	Pfannenstiel	Ovary/tube/uterus, prostate (extraperitoneal)
Thoracoabdominal	Right	Liver and portal vein
	Left	Gastro-oesophageal junction, enormous spleen

keeping just to one or other side of the midline when entering the peritoneal cavity. In the lower abdomen remember that the linea alba is less well developed, so take corresponding care to close the wound securely. When necessary, bypass the umbilicus by curving the skin incision and bevelling the underlying cut to regain the midline of the aponeurosis below it.

3 *Paramedian* incisions provide very similar access to the upper, central or lower abdomen. All layers are divided in the line of the vertical skin incision, placed 2 cm to the right or left of the midline, except that the rectus muscle is dissected free and is drawn laterally, thus remaining intact. At the end of the operation allow the rectus muscle to fall medially, covering the line of closure of the peritoneum and, in the upper abdomen, the posterior rectus sheath.

4 *Rectus-splitting* incisions are made 3–4 cm lateral to the midline and divide all the tissues in this line, splitting the rectus muscle and its intersections. They avoid the time-consuming dissection required to free the muscle belly. In theory the medial part of the rectus muscle is denervated and thus rendered atrophic, but in practice the wounds heal strongly. A right upper rectus split provides good access to the gallbladder. Nowadays midline incisions are generally preferred to paramedian or rectus-splitting incisions because they are quicker to create and to close.

5 *Oblique* incisions can sometimes provide good access. The incision described by the Nobel prize-winning Swiss surgeon Theodore Kocher (1841–1917) extends 2 cm below the right costal margin from the midline to the lateral edge of the rectus muscle and exposes the gallbladder. The equivalent left subcostal incision can be used to approach the spleen. In the lower abdomen the incision of Rutherford Morison (1853–1939), who trained with both Lister and Billroth, starts just above

the anterior superior iliac spine and divides all tissues in the line of the external oblique muscle and aponeurosis. The gridiron incision splits each of the three muscle layers of the abdominal wall in the line of its fibres; it therefore seldom gives rise to an incisional hernia. It provides an excellent approach to the appendix and can be enlarged by extending the skin incision in either direction and by dividing the internal oblique and transversus muscles, converting to Rutherford Morison's incision.

6 *Transverse* incisions usually leave the best cosmetic scars and provide adequate exposure, provided they are made long enough. They are therefore best suited for limited exposure in a planned procedure. Ramstedt's pyloromyotomy or transverse colostomy may be performed through a short transverse incision. Transverse laparotomy is useful in children, in certain obese patients and in the upper abdomen when the costal angle is broad. The incision descried by Otto Lanz (1865–1935) of Amsterdam is a horizontal modification of the gridiron incision for appendicectomy and provides the least obtrusive scar at the expense of slightly inferior access. The incision of the Breslau gynaecologist Pfannenstiel (1862–1909) runs transversely above the pubis but just below the hairline. The aponeurosis is divided transversely and reflected above and below, allowing the rectus muscles to be separated vertically in the midline. Gynaecologists then open the peritoneum to gain access to the female reproductive organs, whereas urologists stay in the extraperitoneal plane for retropubic approach to the bladder and prostate.

7 *Angled* incisions provide not a mere slit that can be pulled into an ellipse but a space in the abdominal wall. Combined right and left subcostal incisions joining at the xiphisternum (the 'high gable' incision) enable a large flap to be turned down and provide excellent access for hepatectomy, pancreatectomy and bilateral adrenalectomy. A vertical incision with a T-shaped transverse extension (or vice versa) allows two flaps to be turned back. These incisions take longer to make and repair but can be invaluable for difficult or very extensive operations.

8 *Thoracoabdominal* incisions usually follow the line of a rib and extend obliquely into the upper abdomen. They make light of the cartilaginous cage protecting the upper abdomen. Alternatively, a vertical upper abdominal incision is sometimes converted into a thoracoabdominal approach by extending a thoracic incision in the line of a rib across the costal margin, to join it. Radial incision of the diaphragm towards the oesophageal hiatus (left) or vena cava (right) throws the abdomen and thorax into one cavity and provides unparalleled access for oesophagogastrectomy and right hepatic lobectomy. Thoracolaparotomy may be indicated for removal of an enormous tumour of the kidney, adrenal or spleen.

9 *Posterolateral* incisions for approach to the kidney, adrenal and upper ureter are described in the relevant chapters.

Making the incision

1 Incise the skin with the belly of the knife. Cut cleanly down to the aponeurosis or muscle. Discard the knife.

2 Stop the bleeding. Firmly press each bleeding site with a swab, then remove the swab quickly and pick up the vessel with the minimum surrounding tissue. Use fine-toothed or non-toothed dissecting forceps, which are touched with the diathermy electrode to coagulate the vessel. Alternatively, use diathermy forceps. Bipolar diathermy ensures that current passes only between the two tips of the grasping forceps. In either case, be careful not to burn the skin when coagulating superficial vessels. Capture larger vessels with artery forceps and ligate them with fine absorbable suture material. As you tighten the first half-hitch, have your assistant smoothly release the forceps, removing them when he is confident that you have safely secured the vessel. Complete a reef knot. Have the ligature cut 2–3 mm beyond the knot for small vessels, and 4–5 mm beyond when tying larger vessels.

3 Apply wound towels to the skin edges, if these are to be used. Fix the towels with clips or stitches. Wound towels help to prevent contamination of the wound by the fluid contents of abdominal viscera. If you use them, make sure that, if they become contaminated, they are immediately removed and replaced with fresh sterile towels.

4 Incise the aponeurosis with a clean knife in the line of the skin incision.

5 Cut, split or displace the muscles of the abdominal wall.
- Cut the muscles with a knife or diathermy blade. When cutting the rectus muscle transversely, it helps to insinuate a pair of curved artery forceps beneath the muscle and then divide the fibres on to the forceps. Your assistant picks up vessels running vertically so that they can be ligated or coagulated.
- Split the muscles if the fibres run in the line of the incision or in the gridiron and Lanz incisions.
- In a paramedian approach displace the rectus muscle laterally within its sheath. Cut the tendinous intersection free from the medial part of the sheath and draw the muscle belly laterally.

6 Stop the bleeding with diathermy coagulation or fine ligatures. Control persistent muscle bleeding by inserting a 2/0 absorbable stitch on a round-bodied needle, tying it just tightly enough to stop the bleeding and not so tight that it cuts through the muscle.

7 Open the peritoneum (Fig. 4.3). Pick it up with toothed dissecting forceps and grip the tented portion with artery forceps. Release the artery forceps and reapply to the peritoneum. The change of grip allows the viscera to escape if they are caught by the first application of the forceps. Incise the peritoneum with the belly of the knife. Air enters the abdomen and the viscera fall clear. Insert the blades of non-toothed dissecting forceps and use them to lift the peritoneum clear of viscera. Complete the peritoneal opening with scissors with the deep blade protected between the blades of the dissecting forceps, taking care not to injure the abdominal contents.

REFERENCES

1. Raahave D 1998 Wound contamination and post-operative infection. A review. Danish Medical Bulletin 38:481–485
2. Farber MS, Abrams JH 1997 Antibiotics for the acute abdomen. Surgical Clinics of North America 77:1395–1417

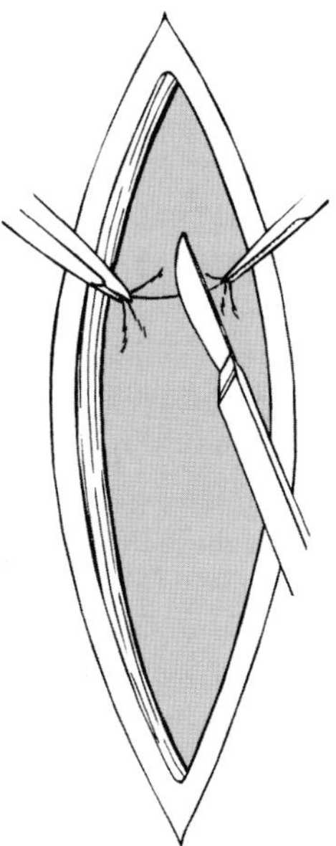

Fig. 4.3 Incising the peritoneum.

3. Bartlett JG 1995 Intra-abdominal sepsis. Medical Clinics of North America 79:599–617

FURTHER READING

Kearns SR, Connolly EM, McNally S et al 2001 Randomized clinical trial of diathermy versus scalpel incision in elective midline laparotomy. British Journal of Surgery 88:41–44

RE-OPENING THE ABDOMEN

Appraise

1 Does the previous incision coincide with the site you would have chosen for present access? If so, re-open it. If not, ignore it and make a new incision in the correct site.

2 Remember that you may require a longer incision than would be necessary for an initial operation.

KEY POINT Old or new incision?

- If the previous incision is convenient there is little advantage in creating a fresh incision. As a rule you will need to dissect off adhesions from within. From a fresh incision you will see them only from one side. Moreover, if the new incision is parallel to the first, there is an intervening denervated panel.

Access through the old incision

1 Make an incision down the centre of the old scar. If the scar is ugly or stretched, excise it as an elongated ellipse.

2 Do not attempt to dissect out a previous paramedian incision, but cut through all the tissues in the line of the skin wound. Do not cut too boldly, because the deeper layers may be defective and you might quickly enter the cavity or even the contents of the abdomen.

3 When opening the peritoneum in the line of the previous incision, remember that viscera may be adherent to its undersurface. Entering the abdomen is greatly facilitated if you extend the wound at one end, so that unscarred peritoneum can be incised first. Alternatively incise the peritoneum slightly to one side of the old incision line.

4 Once the abdomen is opened, carefully extend the incision little by little. Ensure that you identify every structure you cut.

5 Ensure that you leave the abdominal wall and, if possible, the peritoneal lining, intact so that you can achieve a satisfactory closure.

? DIFFICULTY

1. Do not inexorably separate firmly fixed structures through an incomplete incision. Either skirt around them so that they now remain attached to one side of the wound, or open the other end of the wound and approach them from a different direction.
2. Have the wound edge lifted with tissue-holding forceps and encircle the adherent structures to estimate the degree of fixity and the plane of cleavage between them and the original parietal peritoneum. At intervals in the dissection allow the structures to relax, assess progress and start again, possibly from a new approach. Use a scalpel or scissors, remembering never to cut what cannot be seen.
3. If you damage a structure, assess and repair the damage now. Check the repair at the end of the operation.

Access through a new incision

KEY POINT Ubiquitous adhesions

- Although this approach may be initially easier, remember that, after a previous operation, viscera may be adherent to the parietal peritoneum anywhere.

Once the abdomen is opened at a distance from the previous incision, have the intervening abdominal wall lifted with retractors. Arrange for the light to be directed towards any structures attached to the previous scar. If necessary, roll the patient slightly to one or other side, to improve access. Dissect adherent viscera from the undersurface of the old scar, frequently feeling around the other side.

Division of adhesions

1 Separation of adherent viscera from the wound edge has already been described. It can be an arduous and hazardous task, and the small bowel is particularly vulnerable to injury. If you enter the lumen of the small bowel inadvertently, close the defect with two layers of fine absorbable sutures immediately, pausing only to free the damaged loop of bowel to facilitate closure. Try and limit contamination of the wound with intestinal contents by prompt use of the sucker and gauze swabs. If contamination occurs nevertheless, consider lavage of the wound and peritoneal cavity with warm saline.

2 It is not necessary to divide every single adhesion between viscera during every laparotomy; indeed such a policy would often be counterproductive. On the other hand, when the viscera are tangled together it can be difficult to progress with the operation until the normal anatomical relationships have been restored. Learn to recognize thick, fleshy band adhesions that could distort the small bowel and give rise to future symptoms. When operating for adhesion obstruction, it is usually best to take down the adhesions completely and replace the small bowel in an orderly fashion.

3 When dividing intra-abdominal adhesions, vary the point of attack but do not become aimless. Keep in mind the objects of the dissection:

- To allow adequate exploration.
- To permit safe closure without fear of damaging the viscera.
- To prevent subsequent kinking or herniation of the bowel.

EXPLORATORY LAPAROTOMY

Appraise

1 Full exploration of the abdomen was in the past considered a normal part of most operations, provided that it did not result in the spread of infection or malignant disease. If a standard procedure was to be performed, then careful surgeons routinely explored the whole abdomen to ensure that the diagnosed condition was really the cause of symptoms and to exclude incidental conditions that might be noted or demand treatment. The improvement of diagnostic capability (in particular endoscopy) and imaging methods (in particular computed tomography, CT) have eroded this principle. In procedures deliberately planned to be carried out through restricted access, wide exploration is impossible. For example, confidently diagnosed acute appendicitis, perforated peptic ulcer, the creation of a colostomy, the drainage of a localized abscess and the relief of biliary obstruction in patients with advanced pancreatic carcinoma are normally performed through limited incisions.

2 In dealing with emergencies, a clear-cut preoperative diagnosis may not be made and the decision is limited to the need for operation. In this case, exploration may be required to determine the cause of the presenting clinical features.

KEY POINTS Full abdominal examination

- In general, carefully explore the abdomen whenever possible. However, intraoperative use of high-frequency, high-resolution ultrasound promises to be a valuable diagnostic tool, even if the exploration has to be limited. In this way you will acquire a familiarity with the feel of normal structures. One of the most testing clinical decisions is to state that something is normal, so you must know what is the range of normality.
- Once an operation has been carried out, if symptoms continue or fresh features emerge, it is reassuring to know that other serious disease has been excluded.

3 In patients who have extensive carcinoma, adhesions that are unlikely to cause obstruction or a localized abscess that has been adequately drained, obsessive exploration is detrimental.

4 Intraoperative ultrasound scanning promises to be a valuable diagnostic tool. Solid organs such as the liver may contain lesions that are impalpable. Lesions that have been detected by preoperative tests may not be located at operation. Intraoperative ultrasound scanning aids the display or biopsy of such lesions. Within diseased tissues it may be difficult to identify vital structures by conventional means.

5 Exploration of the abdomen is still occasionally carried out as an elective 'final' diagnostic procedure when patients have had inexplicable distressing or sinister symptoms. One such example is a small bowel tumour. Improvement in diagnostic techniques has drastically reduced the indications, but occasionally they are equivocal. The introduction of laparoscopy has reduced the need for diagnostic laparotomy.

6 As previously emphasized, access to the abdominal cavity does not provide direct access to the site of many disease processes, such as the lumen of the bowel, visceral ducts or blood vessels. For this reason do not try to replace careful endoscopy, radiology and other imaging techniques with laparotomy. Some diseases affect the peritoneal surfaces, and some of these can be studied by peritoneal tap or diagnostic laparoscopy.

7 Sadly, patients are still occasionally explored for pain that is referred or which arises in the abdominal wall. Make sure that you have excluded sources of referred pain. If you suspect that the pain arises in the abdominal wall, try the effect of testing for tenderness with the abdominal wall relaxed and then tensed. The tensed muscles protect an internal source of pain from pressure. Tenderness remaining, or even increased, when the muscles are tensed strongly suggests an abdominal wall cause. The diagnosis is strengthened if the injection of local anaesthetic into the tender site gives relief, but warn the patient that the relief will be short-lived.

8 In the presence of unrevealed but clinically suspected intra-abdominal sepsis, time spent waiting for a series of increasingly complex list of investigations can be wasteful. However, CT is invaluable for delineating abdominal abscesses (see Ch. 8).

KEY POINTS The need for laparotomy

- In emergency circumstances, if you are in doubt, use the time during which you are resuscitating the patient to repeat the taking of the history and examination. The features may change!
- When in doubt, trust your clinical acumen rather than 'suggestive' results of investigations, or the results of investigations that are at odds with your clinical findings.

Access

Choice of incision

1 Never forget that the prime function of an incision is to provide safe access. Although important, unsightliness, liability to

herniation and discomfort are side issues. Remember that incisions heal from the sides and not the ends.

2 Open the abdomen over the site of the suspected lesion, so far as the costal margin and iliac crest allow. Use one of the established types of laparotomy incision. Remember that the incision may need to be extended, particularly if you do not have a confident preoperative diagnosis.

3 The choice of incision for a particular operation is listed in Table 4.1 and discussed in the chapter devoted to the relevant organ. The choice may vary according to circumstances. For example, a long incision is appropriate when there is a confident preoperative diagnosis of acute appendicitis, whereas a vertical midline incision provides greater flexibility if the diagnosis is in doubt. In emergency colonic surgery, bear in mind the possible need for an intestinal stoma when selecting the laparotomy incision.

4 In emergency laparotomy for unexplained peritonitis or abdominal trauma, use either a right paramedian incision or a midline incision that skirts the umbilicus. Place the incision more above or more below the umbilicus, depending on the probable site of disease or damage. Incisions that extend on either side of the umbilicus can readily be extended in either direction once the pathology is revealed.

5 Midline incisions are quicker to create (and close) than paramedian incisions, so prefer them in cases of rapid bleeding, such as ruptured spleen or leaking aortic aneurysm.

6 Be prepared to use a previous laparotomy incision if it is conveniently placed or can readily be extended to allow appropriate access. The technique of abdominal re-entry is described in the section above.

Access within the abdomen

1 If, on entering the peritoneal cavity, you find that the incision is likely to provide inadequate exposure, do not hesitate to extend it. If the incision proves to be inappropriate, such as a right Lanz incision for perforated peptic ulcer, close it and start again. Never be too proud to perform one or other of these manoeuvres. Disasters tend to occur when inexperienced surgeons struggle to complete an operation through the wrong incision.

2 Figure 4.4 illustrates ways in which certain common incisions can be extended to deal with unexpected lesions or intraoperative difficulties.

3 Remember that the position of the patient on the operating table can greatly affect exposure, particularly of organs at either end of the abdominal cavity. To approach the pelvic viscera, ask the anaesthetist to tilt the table head-down, a procedure popularized by the Leipzig surgeon Friedrich Trendelenburg (1844–1924). Have the patient tilted head-up (reversed Trendelenburg) for access to the lower oesophagus and diaphragmatic hiatus. Rotating the table away from yourself facilitates an extraperitoneal approach to the ureter or lumbar sympathetic chain on your side. Rotation towards yourself when operating from the patient's right may improve access to the spleen. If you anticipate steep tilts in any direction, secure the patient adequately beforehand, using a pelvic strap and/or a support beneath the heels.

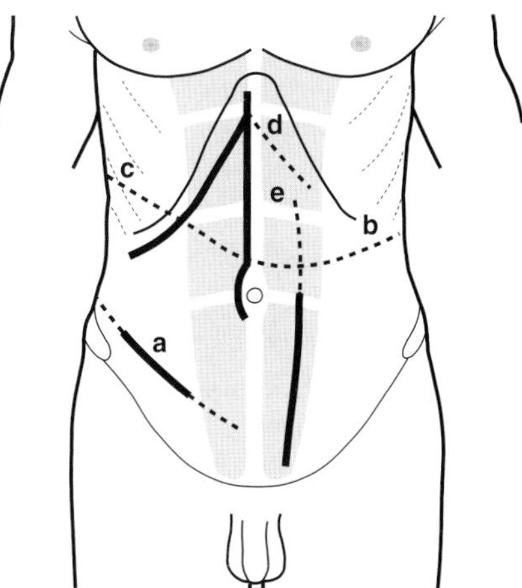

Fig. 4.4 Methods of extending certain abdominal incisions: a, gridiron incision extended laterally and (to a greater extent) medially; b, midline incision with T extension into left upper quadrant to deal with profuse splenic haemorrhage; c, midline incision with T extension into the right chest for ruptured liver; d, Kocher incision with left subcostal extension for major hepatic procedures; e, left lower paramedian incision extended upwards for mobilization of left colic flexure.

4 Nearly every laparotomy requires some retraction of the abdominal wall and adjacent viscera to expose the organ(s) in question. Retraction of the wound edge will assist the initial exploratory laparotomy. When you have assessed the abdominal viscera and determined your operative strategy, insert retractor(s) and instruct your assistant(s) how to hold them. Pack away 'unwanted' organs, principally small-bowel loops, using large gauze swabs to which metal rings have been sewn or large artery forceps attached, to minimize the risk of their being left in the abdomen during closure. The rings or forceps are attached to the packs by tapes, so that they can always hang outside the wound. These packs should be wrung out in warm physiological saline, and they are more effective at restraining the bowel if they are not completely unfolded.

5 Marshal the forces at your disposal carefully. Use of a self-retaining retractor may release an assistant to provide more direct help. Instruments of the DeBakey pattern have an optional third blade, which may help to keep the small bowel out of the pelvis. A sternal retractor is invaluable in operations on the abdominal oesophagus and upper stomach. The instrument hooks under the xiphisternum and is connected to a gantry over the patient's head.

6 Specific manoeuvres are either essential or extremely helpful in the exposure of certain organs. For access to the oesophagus and hiatus, mobilize the left lobe of liver by dividing its peritoneal attachment to the diaphragm. To examine fully the back wall of the stomach and the body of pancreas, you must enter the lesser sac, usually by dividing part of the gastrocolic (greater) omentum. For thorough examination of the duodenum, divide the peritoneum along the convexity of its loop (Kocher's manoeuvre). Displace the small bowel into the upper abdomen to approach the pelvic viscera and out of the abdominal cavity into a plastic bag for operations on the aorta.

Assess

1 If you are not wearing powder-free gloves, wash off the starch powder as described on page 44. Wash blood from the gloves. Deal with established adhesions.

2 Make sure that there are no instruments near the wound except for a retractor for your assistant and a sucker tube available for yourself. It is helpful to have someone in attendance to adjust the theatre light as necessary.

3 Carry out a methodical examination of the abdomen and its contents by feel and, whenever possible, by sight. Always follow the same sequence (Fig. 4.5):

- Right lobe of liver, gallbladder, left lobe of liver, spleen.
- Diaphragmatic hiatus, abdominal oesophagus and stomach: cardia, body, lesser curve, antrum, pylorus and then duodenal bulb.
- Bile ducts, right kidney, duodenal loop, head of pancreas; now draw the transverse colon out of the wound towards the patient's head.
- Body and tail of pancreas, left kidney.

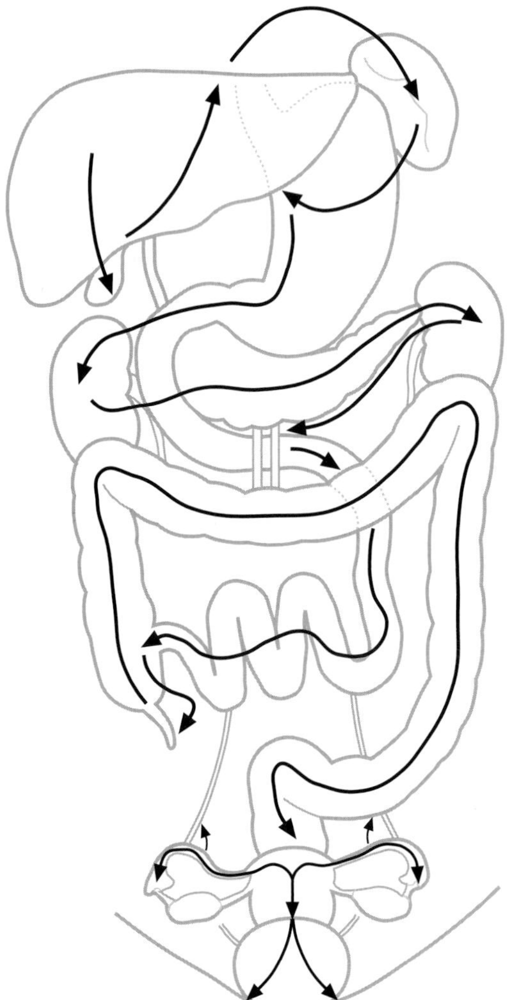

Fig. 4.5 The order of examining the abdominal contents at exploratory laparotomy.

- Root of mesentery, superior mesenteric and middle colic vessels, aorta, inferior mesenteric artery and vein, small bowel and mesentery from ligament of Treitz to ileocaecal valve.
- Appendix, caecum, the rest of the colon, rectum.
- Pelvic peritoneum, uterus, tubes and ovaries in the female, bladder.
- Hernial orifices and main iliac vessels on each side. The ureters can sometimes be seen in thin patients, or if they are dilated.

4 In most *elective* cases, aim to carry out a thorough examination (as above), and record your findings carefully and in detail. These principles are particularly important when laparotomy is the last of a series of investigations to identify the cause of symptoms. Sometimes the incision chosen precludes a complete exploration, for example in interval appendicectomy or pyloromyotomy in infancy. Sometimes the condition found makes further exploration pointless, for example in carcinomatosis peritonei. In this circumstance make a gentle search for the primary tumour, obtain a biopsy from one of the deposits, make sure no palliative procedure (e.g. intestinal bypass) is required and close the abdomen. As a general rule do not touch a malignant tumour more than is essential, for fear of dissemination.

5 In *emergency* laparotomy, immediate action may be required, for example to stop bleeding or close a perforation. Thereafter, proceed to a methodical examination of the other viscera as before, unless the patient's general condition is poor or there is localized infection. Drainage of an abscess should usually be treated as a local condition. Do not forget to note the nature and amount of any free fluid, collecting some for chemical, cytological and microbiological examination. Obtain swabs for bacteriological culture of any potentially infected collection.

Action

1 In deciding the definitive procedure now to be undertaken, you will be guided by your preoperative knowledge of the patient, the extent of disease as revealed at laparotomy and the patient's age and general condition. Options include partial or total resection of an organ, bypass, drainage, exteriorization, closure of perforation, removal of foreign body, biopsy or perhaps no active procedure. In elderly or sick patients, control of the emergency or major elective condition should take precedence over the complete eradication of disease. Once you have formulated a plan of campaign, discuss your intentions with the anaesthetist and intimate how long you are likely to take to carry them out.

2 Be wary of tackling incidental procedures, such as prophylactic appendicectomy, without a clear indication. The chance finding of conditions such as gallstones, diverticula, fibroids or ovarian cysts does not automatically call for action unless they pose an immediate threat to health or offer a better explanation for symptoms than the condition originally diagnosed. The patient's prior consent is unlikely to have been obtained, so any adverse outcome may be more difficult to defend. By contrast, an unsuspected neoplasm should ordinarily be removed, if

necessary through a separate incision, provided the patient's condition allows. Whatever course you adopt, be sure to record all your findings in the operation notes.

3 Remember that the interior of the distal small bowel and the entire large bowel are unsterile. Contents of hollow viscera that are normally sterile such as bile, urine, gastric juice, may also become infected as a result of inflammation and obstruction. Before opening the bowel or other potentially contaminated viscera, isolate them from contact with the wound and other organs. Consider using non-crushing clamps to occlude the lumen, and make sure that you have an efficient suction apparatus to remove any contents that spill. Pack away other structures before opening the viscus and discard the packs once it is closed. Remember that all the instruments used on opened bowel become unsterile; they must therefore be isolated and subsequently discarded. Likewise, change your gloves before closing the abdomen.

4 The danger of infection is one of degree. Healthy tissues can normally cope with a small number of organisms but are overwhelmed by heavy contamination or re-infection. 'It should be axiomatic that reducing bacterial contamination reduces infection.'[1] In patients with impaired local host defences, be sure to obtain culture specimens because they may be growing facultative organisms, particularly if they have had previous antibiotics. *Enterococcus* and *Candida* may be pathogens.[2] Generally, wounds are more susceptible to infection than the peritoneal cavity itself. If there has been gross spillage of infected visceral contents, wash out the abdominal cavity with warm saline and start broad-spectrum antibiotic therapy, but be guided by the microbiologist in case of doubt.[3]

5 Intestinal clamps are of two types: crushing and non-crushing.

- *Crushing* clamps are applied to seal the bowel when it is cut. Payr's powerful double-action clamps are most frequently used, but Lang Stevenson devised a similar clamp with narrow blades. Cope's triple clamps allow the middle clamp to be removed, so that the bowel can be divided through the crushed area, leaving its ends sealed.
- *Non-crushing* clamps have longitudinal ridges and control the leakage of bowel contents without causing irreversible damage to the gut. Lane's twin clamps, which can be locked together, allow two pieces of gut to be occluded and held in apposition for anastomosis. Pringle's clamps hold cut ends of bowel securely, and the lightly crushed segment is so narrow that it can safely be incorporated in the anastomosis.

6 The danger of leaving articles in the abdominal cavity is ever-present, but to do so is inexcusable. Unfortunately, there is no single routine that will entirely guard against this mishap. Always use the minimum number of instruments and the largest swabs, which should remain attached to large instruments lying outside the abdominal wound. Make sure that they are never out of sight. As far as possible, use long-handled instruments for long-term holding, so that the handles protrude from the wound. Involve all your team in guarding against leaving an instrument or swab, even though you must accept the responsibility personally. If the scrub nurse reports a missing swab or instrument while you are closing the abdomen, check the peritoneal cavity once again. If all else fails, obtain an abdominal X-ray before letting the patient wake from the anaesthetic.

KEY POINT Avoid needless procedures

- If this is an exploration for undiagnosed acute or chronic symptoms, or if the expected diagnosis is not confirmed and no cause is found, do not carry out any procedure. Resist the desire to 'do something'. You may give yourself a false sense of security, cause further complications or confuse the diagnosis. Having made sure you have overlooked nothing, close the abdomen and determine to record all your findings.

CLOSING THE ABDOMEN

Assess

1 Before starting to close, make sure that the swab and instrument counts are both correct. Check for haemostasis. Decide whether you need to drain the abdomen (see below). Remove any odds and ends of suture material and replace the viscera in their correct anatomical position.

KEY POINT Avoid needle-stick injury

- Many needle-stick injuries are sustained during abdominal wall closure. Avoid using hand needles. However, even when using curved needles held in a needle holder, there is a danger of injury. A valuable development is the introduction of blunt-tipped (often called 'taper-point') needles, which pass through the tissues but penetrate gloves and skin only if pressed fairly hard against them. Protect yourself. Do not risk acquiring a transmitted viral disease.

2 There are several different techniques for abdominal closure; three are described in the section below. The choice depends upon the type of incision, the extent of the operation, the patient's general condition and your preference. If you are a trainee, as you assist different surgeons, you will learn various technical modifications and develop your own methods of closing the abdomen under differing circumstances. It is a common error among surgical trainees to sew up the abdomen too tightly, for fear it will fall apart. Remember that wounds swell during the first 3–4 postoperative days, oedema will make the sutures even tighter and there is a risk of tissue necrosis and subsequent dehiscence.

3 The most popular method of closure is now a continuous, spiralled, unlocked mass closure of the abdominal wall except for the skin and superficial fascia. The length of suture material used for the aponeurotic layer(s) should be at least four times the length of the incision, although this does not seem critical for lateral paramedian incisions. Place each suture 1 cm from the edge of the wound and 1 cm away from the previous 'bite'.

4 Select a strong non-absorbable suture material for closing the deeper (aponeurotic) layers of the abdominal wall; 1 monofilament nylon on a taper-point, round-bodied needle is very satisfactory in adults. Some surgeons use a doubled length of finer material such as 0 nylon, and run the first stitch through the loop to avoid having a knot at the end of the wound. Synthetic polyglactin 910, polydioxanone or glycomer 631, which are absorbable, have many advocates because they are less likely to produce chronic sinuses than non-absorbable nylon. With a long wound or an obese patient, it may be more convenient to use two lengths of suture, starting at each end and meeting in the middle.

5 There is strong disagreement about the use of tension sutures. Proponents use them if the abdomen is distended or obese, if the wound is infected or likely to become so, if the patient is malnourished, jaundiced, suffering from advanced cancer or has a chronic cough—in short, in any situation where wound healing is prejudiced. It is likely that these sutures have gained a poor reputation because the term 'tension' is often transferred to the tightness of the stitches, albeit that the suture is designed to withstand tension not to create it.

6 Remember that the abdominal wound is the only part of the operation that the patient can see, so take care to produce a neat result. Bury the knots used to tie off the deep sutures, especially in a thin patient. In an uncontaminated wound, aim for close apposition of the skin and a fine linear scar; therefore consider using subcuticular sutures.

Action

Layered closure

1 Some surgeons do not bother to close the peritoneum, especially in a midline incision. There is a view that suturing the peritoneum encourages adhesions in response to the foreign material. Certainly there is little strength to this layer, and a new mesothelial lining develops to cover the defect from within. Where the posterior rectus sheath exists as a separate layer, as in paramedian, transverse and oblique incisions in the upper abdomen, the peritoneum can also be incorporated in the deepest layer of sutures. Use a continuous, unlocked spiral stitch so that the tension can be evenly distributed along the whole suture line.

2 Pick up the edges of the peritoneum and posterior rectus sheath, and apply one pair of artery forceps to these combined layers on each side of the wound and at each end. Make sure that the bowel is not caught. Have the assistant hold up the artery forceps, so that the peritoneum is lifted clear of the viscera as you insert each suture.

3 Starting at one or other end of the incision, take a bite on each side close to the apex and tie the knot securely. Make sure that the needle does not pick up bowel or omentum. Take generous bites with each stitch, and pull up snugly but not tightly, passing it to your assistant to maintain the tension while the next stitch is inserted. Repeated tightening and loosening of the suture has a sawing effect on the tissues and also tends to fray the stitch. After placing four or five stitches and gently and evenly tightening them, insert a finger to confirm that the bowel is free. Tie the knots securely, and do not have the ends shorter than 5 mm.

4 When muscles have been cut or split, unite them with interrupted 2/0 polyglactin 910, polydioxanone or lactomer 9-1 sutures. Tie the sutures just tightly enough to appose the edges. When the rectus muscle is cut transversely, it is not necessary to repair it with sutures because the tendinous intersections limit retraction. Similarly, in a paramedian incision, the rectus muscle falls back into place after closing the peritoneum and no sutures are required. If the muscle does not cover the posterior suture line, draw it medially by inserting stitches through the fibrous intersections and through the medial edge of the rectus sheath.

5 Repair the aponeurosis of external oblique or the anterior rectus sheath using slowly absorbed synthetic or non-absorbable suture such as polyamide. After tying the knot at the end of the incision, cut the end of suture material short and take the next bite from within to without; this manoeuvre will help to bury the knot. Once again, have the assistant maintain an even tension on the thread and avoid pulling up each suture so tightly that you strangle tissue.

6 Ensure that there is no oozing of blood in the superficial layers. Ligate or coagulate any residual bleeding vessels. If the subcutaneous tissues are deep, consider using a few interrupted fine 4/0 absorbable sutures to appose them.

7 Appose the skin edges, using one of several standard techniques. Interrupted sutures are preferable in a contaminated or irregular wound. Mattress sutures help to evert the skin edges slightly and bring together the deeper layers. Suitable suture materials include 2/0 black silk, 2/0 or 3/0 monofilament polyamide or polypropylene; skin clips and adhesive skin strips are alternatives. Some surgeons use a continuous over-and-over or continuous mattress suture routinely.

8 In a clean and straightforward wound, a very acceptable scar results following subcuticular suture, using 2/0 polypropylene. Insert the needle in the line of the incision about 1 cm away from its apex and bring it out through the apex in the subcuticular plane. Now continue along the incision taking small and frequent bites of the subcutis; avoid piercing the skin. When you reach the other end, bring the needle out through the skin about 1 cm beyond the apex of the incision. Tighten the suture material to close the wound and make sure that it runs freely. Fix the suture at each end with tiny lead weights, or tie the ends in a slack loop.

Mass closure

1 This simple, rapid technique can be used routinely or reserved for difficult cases. It is particularly useful when closing an incision through a previous scar, when the layers are often partly fused. The peritoneum and rectus sheaths are closed together, or the linea alba may be closed in one layer without suturing the peritoneum.

2 Insert a continuous running stitch of 1 monofilament nylon mounted on a taper-pointed needle. Place the stitches 1–2 cm from the edges, 1–2 cm apart, catching all the included layers. Monofilament synthetic, slowly absorbable sutures may be successfully used.[1,2]

3 Gently tighten the stitches as you proceed, checking that the bowel is free beneath. Do not let the stitch slip afterwards by getting your assistant to follow-up, but avoid undue tension. Make doubly sure that the bowel is free before tightening and tying the last stitch. Cut the bristly ends of nylon short.

4 Close the skin as for layered closure.

Closure with tension sutures (Fig. 4.6)

1 Tension sutures usually pass through all layers of the abdominal wall, including the skin, so they can be removed subsequently. Alternatively, they may be placed subcutaneously, where they remain permanently. Insert all the interrupted through-and-through sutures and tie them at the end. Use them to supplement a standard closure in poor-risk patients.

2 Use a strong non-absorbable suture material, such as 1 monofilament nylon, swaged to a curved taper-point needle. Take deep bites about 3 cm away from the edge of the wound, incorporating all layers. Be very careful neither to prick the bowel when inserting the stitches nor to trap it when tightening them. If possible, always interpose the greater omentum between the wound and the small intestine to lessen this risk.

3 After inserting each deep tension suture, leave artery forceps attached to both ends of the suture while closing the deeper layers of the abdominal wall. Then tie the tension sutures to appose the skin and subcutaneous tissues. If skin is included, thread each suture over a length of polyethylene or rubber tubing to prevent it cutting in, and be particularly careful not to tie it too tightly. Complete the closure with a limited number of interrupted skin sutures.

4 If healing proceeds satisfactorily, remove the skin sutures 7–10 days postoperatively but leave the tension sutures for a further 2–4 days.

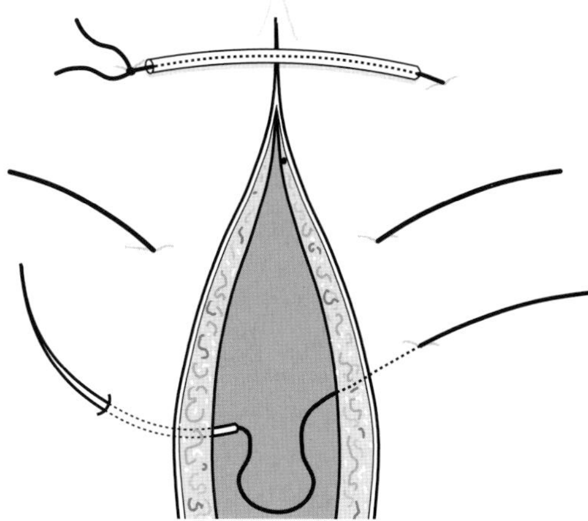

Fig. 4.6 Abdominal closure with deep tension sutures. Strong through-and-through sutures are placed 2–3 cm apart and tied over a protective polyethylene bar (after all sutures have been inserted).

? DIFFICULTY

Closure of the deepest layer may be difficult because the abdominal contents keep bulging through the wound. Inadequate anaesthesia, obesity or intestinal distension are usually to blame. Even after successfully inserting your stitches, they may cut out. Be patient and do not despair.

1. Ask the anaesthetist if the abdominal muscles can be further relaxed.
2. Insert the stitches 2–3 cm from the edges, using a continuous over-and-over or mattress technique. Do not tighten the thread until you have inserted three or four stitches loosely. Now pull up slowly in the line of the incision, while the assistant compresses the abdomen from each side. The assistant should maintain the tension while you insert the next batch of sutures. As the closure proceeds it becomes easier.
3. The bowel is doubly at risk during difficult closures. Consider using a swab on a holder, a length of rubber drain or a 'shoe-horn' depressor laid in the wound to protect the bowel; remove it before completing the closure. Remember to avoid the bowel when placing the final sutures.
4. Brute force brings disaster: dragging the stitches through the tissues under tension acts like a saw, cutting out the stitch. Gentle persistence is most likely to succeed.
5. If a stitch tears out, remain phlegmatic. Insert a mattress suture from within the abdomen, 3–4 cm from the edge, taking a deep bite of tissue.
6. To cover abdominal wall defects or if the edges cannot be apposed without tension, absorbable polyglycolic acid (Dexon) and unabsorbable polypropylene mesh have been inserted to bridge the defect, even in the presence of infection.[3,4]
7. If the intra-abdominal contents will later reduce in volume, do not fight to close the wound. Prefer to wait and perform delayed closure.

Delayed closure

1 If the abdominal cavity is grossly contaminated, as in faecal peritonitis, some degree of wound sepsis is almost inevitable. One option is to close the superficial tissues lightly around a drain. Another is delayed primary suture, leaving the skin and subcutaneous tissue widely open. In either case give parenteral antibiotics and drain the peritoneal cavity. Consider also the possibility of postoperative lavage (see below).

2 Close the musculoaponeurotic layers of the abdominal wall with a continuous monofilament nylon suture. Be particularly careful not to draw the edges together too tightly, because considerable swelling can be anticipated. Superficial to this layer, loosely pack the wound with gauze swabs wrung out in saline.

3 Change the packs and inspect the wound daily. Delayed primary suture can be performed when the patient's condition improves and any wound sepsis has abated.

4 If peritonitis is particularly severe, for example after a major colonic perforation or resulting from infected pancreatic necrosis, it may be appropriate to leave the abdomen completely open as a 'laparostomy'. Make no attempt to close the abdominal wall. Cover the exposed viscera with moist gauze swabs on a polythene (Bogota) bag, and change them every 24–48 hours. In patients who survive, the wound will shrink with time. Late closure of the large incisional hernia may be needed.

5 An alternative to attempted coverage with skin is to apply a clear, sterile plastic sheet after drawing down the omentum, if possible. Over this are laid sump drains. The whole is covered by a double layer of iodophor-impregnated adhesive sheet. This has been successfully used following trauma.[5]

6 Yet another method is to use a zipper, with daily irrigations.[6]

REFERENCES

1. Carlson MA, Condon RE 1995 Polyglyconate (Maxon) versus nylon suture in midline abdominal incision closure: a prospective randomized trial. American Surgeon 61:980–983
2. Cameron AE, Parker CJ, Field ES et al 1987 A randomized comparison of polydioxanone (PDS) and polypropylene (Prolene) for abdominal wound closure. Annals of the Royal College of Surgeons of England 69:113–115
3. Buck JR, Fath JJ, Chung SK et al 1995 Use of absorbable mesh as an aid in abdominal wall closure in the emergent setting. American Surgeon 61:655–658
4. Brandt CP, McHenry CR, Jacobs DG et al 1995 Polypropylene mesh closure after emergency laparotomy: morbidity and outcome. Surgery 118:736–741
5. Sherck J, Selver A, Shatney C et al 1998 Covering the 'open abdomen': a better technique. American Surgeon 64:854–857
6. Sleeman D, Sosa JL, Gonzalez A et al 1995 Reclosure of the open abdomen. Journal of the American College of Surgeons 180:200–204

FURTHER READING

A-Malik R, Scott NA 2001 Double near and far prolene suture closure: a technique for abdominal wall closure after laparostomy. British Journal of Surgery 88:146–147

Nystrom P-O, Wiltman D 2003 Patient to surgeon infections: fact or fiction. British Journal of Surgery 90:1315–1316

ABDOMINAL COMPARTMENT SYNDROME

KEY POINT Compartment syndrome

- Compartment syndrome is a rise in intra-abdominal pressure from a wide variety of causes. It is a potentially fatal condition unless it is correctly diagnosed and managed.

Appraise

1 Peritonitis, intra-abdominal abscess, intestinal obstruction or paralytic abscess, tension pneumoperitoneum, mesenteric venous thrombosis, acute gastric dilatation, intra-abdominal haemorrhage, ascites, large neoplasm, peritoneal dialysis, laparoscopic procedure or abdominal wound closure under tension may all provoke changes labelled 'abdominal compartment syndrome'. Other causes are massive visceral oedema, retroperitoneal haematoma and the need to pack the abdomen as a haemostatic measure.[1]

2 The physiological consequences are a rise in pulse rate and inferior vena cava pressure, with a fall in cardiac output, venous return and glomerular filtration rate. Blood pressure is not usually affected. Intra-abdominal pressure can be estimated via a catheter within the bladder.

Action

1 Do not attempt to close the abdomen formally, or be prepared to re-open it if features develop of rising intra-abdominal pressure.

2 If possible, close the skin after drawing the greater omentum down over the viscera.

3 An alternative is to leave the fascia and skin open and cover the viscera with an absorbable or non-absorbable sheet. One such method is to use a Velcro-like closure (HIDIH Surgical, Doerrebach, Germany).

4 If the underlying condition can be corrected, the abdomen may be formally closed in 2–14 days.

5 A longer delay may result in a defect requiring reconstruction, for example by bilateral advancement of the rectus muscles and fascia and by skin-relaxing incisions to complete the closure.

Drains and dressings

1 Tubular or corrugated drains of plastic or rubber may be inserted either through the end of the wound or through a separate stab hole in the abdominal wall. The inner end of the drain is placed in the region of the operation site to evacuate blood and any other fluid contents from the peritoneal cavity. Fine-bore polyethylene tube drains are now available, which can be screwed to a special trocar for insertion through the abdominal wall. They have many tiny drainage holes, all of which should be placed within the peritoneum, and they can be connected to a vacuum bottle or bag to maintain suction down the tube. Other surgeons prefer to use a silicone tube drain without suction.

2 Other tube drains can be used to drain certain viscera to the exterior during the postoperative period. Again, insert these through a separate stab incision. Examples are a T-tube into the bile duct, a gastrostomy or suprapubic cystostomy catheter and a feeding jejunostomy tube.

3 Stitch the drain to the skin. When possible, insert a large safety pin through the drain to prevent any possibility of it being lost within the abdomen, especially when the drain is shortened prior to removal. If a drainage tube is attached to a closed bag or suction apparatus, tie the stitch securely around the tube.

4 Apply dressings to seal the main wound, with separate dressings over the drain wound. The drain may then be re-dressed, shortened and removed without disturbing the main wound.

5 Opinions differ widely concerning the use of drains following laparotomy. Drains rarely do harm when properly inserted, provided they are removed after about 48 hours if there is no discharge. A closed drainage system should not introduce

infection. Insertion of a drainage tube is no substitute for good operative technique, however. Some generally accepted indications for draining the peritoneal cavity are as follows:

- After operations on the gallbladder, bile duct or pancreas, in case there is leakage of bile or pancreatic juice.
- When there is a localized abscess.
- After suture of a perforated viscus, such as stomach, duodenum or colonic diverticulum, when the tissues are friable. Consider if another operative manoeuvre would give greater safety.
- When there is a large raw area from which oozing can occur. However, do not make insertion of a drain an excuse for failure to control bleeding.
- After operations for severe general peritonitis, even if you have removed the cause.

6 Wound drains are occasionally indicated in very obese patients or grossly contaminated wounds. A thin corrugated drain or a tube suction drain is inserted deep to the skin and subcutaneous tissues and removed after 2–3 days or when it ceases to discharge.

7 Dressings are also controversial. From a bacteriological standpoint it probably makes little difference whether the wound is occluded by a dressing or left open to the atmosphere. Transparent adhesive dressings have the advantage of allowing the surgeon to inspect the wound repeatedly without disturbing the dressing. If a good deal of discharge is anticipated, use dressing gauze and wool. Remember that some patients are sensitive to adhesive strapping.

8 If primary closure of the superficial layers is not possible or is inadvisable because of tension, skin loss or contamination, avoid applying hydrocolloid dressings if the wound could be contaminated with anaerobic organisms.[2]

Lavage

1 The peritoneal cavity has a remarkable ability to combat sepsis. None the less, spillage of contaminated contents, such as faeces or infected bile, may lead to early septicaemia and late abdominal abscess.

2 Where local peritonitis is marked, scrupulously remove all pus and debris from that part of the abdomen. Consider washing out the area with aliquots of warm saline (about 500 ml in toto), sucking out the fluid and inserting a drain. The theoretical risk of disseminating the infection through the peritoneal cavity does not appear to hold true in practice.

3 In generalized peritonitis, thoroughly clean the abdomen with warm saline (1–2 litres or more) at the end of the operation. In very severe cases (e.g. pancreatic necrosis, faecal peritonitis), consider inserting one or two delivery tubes and one or two drainage tubes for postoperative lavage. One drainage tube is placed in the abscess cavity and one in the pelvis; soft, wide-bore, silicone tubes or sump drains are appropriate. Use warmed (37 °C) peritoneal dialysis fluid (Dialaflex 61) with added potassium for lavage, irrigating between 50 and 200 ml/hour depending on the extent of sepsis. Try and obtain a water-tight closure of the abdominal wound and start with small amounts of dialysate (50 ml/hour) overnight, until the peritoneum seals the defects. Postoperative lavage is well tolerated and does not seem to interfere with intestinal motility. Continue the treatment for up to 2 weeks and remove the drains when the return fluid becomes clear.

4 As an alternative to abdominal closure with lavage, the laparotomy incision can be left open in patients with necrotizing pancreatitis or severe faecal peritonitis. The technique of 'laparostomy' is described under laparotomy for acute pancreatitis (Ch. 21).

REFERENCES

1. Schein M, Whittmann DH, Aprahamian CC et al 1995 The abdominal compartment syndrome: the physiological and clinical consequences of elevated intra-abdominal pressure. Journal of the American College of Surgeons 185:745–753
2. Mertz PM, Ovington LG 1993 Wound healing microbiology. Dermatology Clinics 11:739–747

BURST ABDOMEN

Appraise

1 Wound dehiscence results from poor healing, excessive strain on the wound or poor closure technique. In addition, septicaemia, abdominal wound contamination, haematoma or seroma, advanced neoplasia, diabetes, uraemia, jaundice, hypoproteinaemia, steroid or cytotoxic therapy can all impair healing. Abdominal distension from intestinal obstruction, intraperitoneal ascites, unresectable tumour or following loss of abdominal wall may place an excessive strain on the wound closure. However, the remarkably low rate of wound dehiscence reported by some surgeons tends to discount the importance of impaired healing or excess strain. Indict technical failure. The suture material may be incorrectly selected, damaged by crushing or abrasion, imperfectly inserted, overtightened, improperly knotted or trimmed too short at the knots. Layered closure appears to be associated with a higher incidence of burst abdomen than mass closure.[1]

2 Suspect impending wound dehiscence if the patient's abdomen remains silent in the absence of an obvious cause, often accompanied by a low-grade unexplained pyrexia. A premonitory sign is the discharge of slightly bloodstained serous fluid from the wound.

3 Dehiscence usually declares itself 7–14 days postoperatively following straining or the removal of the sutures. The patient feels something 'give' and may partially eviscerate. Burst abdomen is rarely painful; the patient is apprehensive but seldom shocked. The skin may remain healed, but as the patient strains the wound bulges. If the patient is managed conservatively, the skin may remain healed, leaving an incisional hernia.

Prepare

1 Reassure the patient; explain that the wound has given way but can be repaired.

2 Cover the wound with large sterile packs held in place with an encircling bandage or corset or using adhesive, elastic strips.

3 For most patients immediate re-operation is indicated, in which case give the premedication now and pass a nasogastric tube to aspirate the stomach.

4 If there is gross abdominal sepsis with contamination of the wound edges, plan to explore the abdomen, carry out corrective procedures, then pack the wound. Delayed re-suture can be carried out when sepsis is controlled by drainage, further operation, appropriate versatile antibiotics and supportive management of the patient. Alternatively, close the deep part of the wound, leaving the skin closure for later.

Access

1 Have the dressings removed, and make sure they are kept separate from the operative swabs. Have any skin sutures that remain in place removed.

2 Open up the whole incision after preparing the skin and towelling off the area. Remove all suture material while carefully observing whether it has broken or cut out. How large are the suture holes?

3 Change your gloves.

Assess

1 Why has this wound broken down? Collect a bacteriological specimen for aerobic and anaerobic culture. Is the peritoneum partly intact? Where are its edges? Is there any cause for abdominal distension such as free fluid, abscess, blood or other fluid? Determine the cause. Remember that the tissues may be abnormally fragile.

2 Are the abdominal contents normal? Is the underlying small bowel breached or dilated? If free fluid or pus are present or if the bowel is grossly dilated, check the cause.

3 It is inappropriate to re-suture the abdomen unless distended bowel is decompressed, obstruction relieved, ischaemic and necrotic viscera or other tissues excised, septic and foreign material removed and pus drained. If immediate correction is impossible in a very ill patient, consider carrying out what can be achieved now before packing the wound and re-examining the contents after 24–48 hours.

Action

1 Dissect the skin and subcutaneous tissues from the aponeurotic layer on each side to clear 2 cm of aponeurosis or muscle. Similarly, free the omentum and bowel for a short distance on the deep aspect of the wound on each side.

2 Insert deep tension sutures, as described in the previous section. Pass each suture through all layers of the abdominal wall, including the skin. Allow 3–4 cm between tension sutures.

3 Now proceed with mass closure of the peritoneum and rectus sheath or the linea alba. Some surgeons prefer to use interrupted stitches of a strong non-absorbable material. Be certain to take deep bites of tissue, using plenty of suture material, and again avoid tension on the wound. Although recurrent burst abdomen is rare, pulling too tightly on strong thread passed through damaged tissue provokes stitches to cut out.

4 Whether you use continuous or interrupted sutures, take great care not to incorporate the viscera in any of the stitches. If possible, draw the omentum down over the abdominal contents.

5 Now loosely tie the deep tension sutures, once more remembering that they are there to resist tension, not to cause it.

6 Close the skin fairly loosely and consider using a superficial wound drain. In the presence of gross wound sepsis, leave the skin unsutured and place sterile packs on the deep wound closure. Carry out delayed suture when the wound is clean, graft the area, or allow the wound to heal by granulation.

7 A many-tailed bandage or an elastic corset provides extra support.

REFERENCE

1. Niggebrugge AH, Hansen BE, Trimbos JB et al 1995 Mechanical factors influencing the incidence of burst abdomen. European Journal of Surgery 161:655–661

LAPAROTOMY FOR ABDOMINAL TRAUMA

See Chapter 5.

LAPAROTOMY FOR GENERAL PERITONITIS

Appraise

1 The parietal peritoneum is locally irritated by contact with inflamed organs such as the appendix, gallbladder, colon with a segment of diverticulitis, or uterine salpinx. It is irritated by chemical contact from gastric acid, urine, bile, activated pancreatic enzymes, bowel content, blood or foreign materials such as talc and starch. It becomes intensely inflamed by contact with pus or material infected with microorganisms such as infected bile, faecal leakage and bowel content exuding from gangrenous bowel. The features develop over the inflamed area and so may be local or generalized. Adhesion of intestinal loops and omentum may confine the peritonitis so that a localized abscess develops; otherwise the irritant and infected material spreads widely. The magnitude of the contamination is crucial. In a previously healthy person resolution may be rapid and complete, provided the cause does not continue.

2 Peritonitis is easily diagnosed and assessed if it presents conventionally with sharp abdominal pain, worse on moving and breathing, accompanied by tenderness, guarding and rigidity, absent bowel sounds, tachycardia, tachypnoea and pyrexia. The blood granulocyte count rises and there is a shift to the left. There is frequent disturbance of the serum electrolytes. Plain X-ray of the abdomen often shows some dilated bowel loops and, if there has been a leak, free air is usually visible. When intraperitoneal fluid is much increased it produces a ground-glass appearance. Imaging techniques such as ultrasound scan may be helpful in localizing a cause or a mass.

3 The findings are affected by the delay between the onset and your examination. The pain and rigidity often pass off, though the tachycardia and pyrexia continue to rise while blood pressure falls. Always pursue the history of onset of the symptoms. For example, when you see a patient the pain may be generalized, but it may have started suddenly in the epigastrium if a

peptic ulcer perforated, then radiating as the released gastric contents spread through the abdomen. When you first see the patient, the pain and tenderness may be maximal in the right iliac fossa if the contents have tracked down the right paracolic gutter to this site; appendicitis may wrongly be diagnosed unless you ask, 'Where did the pain start?'

4 If the patient becomes septicaemic, the temperature may fall and multisystem failure can develop. Features often change rapidly, so be prepared to repeat the assessment at intervals in case of doubt.

5 Immunocompromised patients such as those suffering from AIDS present particular diagnostic problems including toxic megacolon, which may perforate, or appendicitis caused by cytomegalovirus (CMV). Atypical mycobacterial infection is also reported.

6 Exclude medical conditions that confuse the diagnosis, such as diabetic ketoacidosis, uraemia, sickle cell crisis, Henoch–Schönlein purpura or porphyria.

7 Difficulty is increased when patients who are seriously ill from a medical condition, following trauma or major surgery, develop acute abdominal features. A condition that seems to be increasing in incidence, especially in the intensive care unit, is acalculous cholecystitis. If this is missed, the gallbladder may perforate and produce biliary peritonitis. Ultrasound scan should be diagnostic.

8 Very occasionally generalized peritonitis develops in the absence of any overt visceral disease. Primary peritonitis can occur spontaneously in children and is more common in patients with ascites or nephrotic syndrome or in patients with continuous ambulatory peritoneal dialysis (CAPD). The pneumococcus is one of the more common infecting organisms.

9 Computer-aided diagnosis of the acute abdomen is a valuable and proven method of improving accuracy. It encourages us to try and be specific and not make treatment decisions without defining what we are treating. It acts as an educational tool when we look back on our diagnosis, management and the outcome.

10 Fine catheter aspiration cytology has been recommended for distinguishing between acute inflammatory causes of peritonism and non-specific abdominal pain. A high leucocyte count in the aspirate signals a definite inflammatory lesion. Laparoscopy can also help in equivocal cases of suspected peritonitis but is unnecessary if there is clear evidence of generalized peritonitis. A laparoscopic approach can be used for appendicectomy and closure of perforated peptic ulcer.

Decide

1 In the past, many surgeons made only one decision: whether or not to operate on the acute abdomen. We frequently still have to fall back on the aphorism, 'It's better to look and see than wait and see'. There are times when delay is vacillation and others when precipitate action offers an excuse for not thinking the problem through. None of us always makes the correct decision and the reason is clear—we rarely have all the facts available on which to make an accurate judgement. However, it is often valuable for an individual or a small group to sit down and review what has been discovered, what it means and what should be done about it.

2 Do not make immutable decisions so that you are unwilling to change your mind if new evidence becomes available. When you are in doubt, seek out new evidence by re-examining the patient after an interval. If you make the decision to treat the patient conservatively, remember that this is a provisional decision; if the patient deteriorates or new features emerge, be prepared to explore the abdomen.

3 When your clinical findings and laboratory investigations are at odds with each other, you must ultimately trust your clinical judgement, so ensure that your clinical examination is thorough.

4 The more accurate your diagnosis, the more likely it is that you can spare the patient an unnecessary, and sometimes dangerous, laparotomy. From time to time patients with coronary artery thrombosis and referred epigastric pain are subjected to laparotomy. A simple peritoneal fluid aspiration with cytology or a laparoscopy often spares a patient with extensive carcinomatosis unnecessary and ineffectual surgery. A small perforation of a peptic ulcer can often be successfully treated by vigorous conservative treatment or by laparoscopic suture closure. Improvements in imaging not only aid accurate diagnosis but are valuable in localizing abscesses, for example. If the cause has ceased to act, the abscess can often be drained under scanning control.

Prepare

1 Restore the patient's fluid, electrolyte and acid–base balance intravenously.

2 Pass a nasogastric tube and aspirate the stomach.

3 As far as possible, assess and correct incidental medical conditions, in particular cardiorespiratory disease.

4 Start parenteral antibiotic therapy with a third-generation cephalosporin together with an aminoglycoside and metronidazole. The organisms found within the abdomen are often not those expected, particularly in critically ill patients. *Candida albicans*, *Enterococcus* sp. and *Staphylococcus epidermidis* are more common than most surgeons suspect, so the antibiotic range may need to be broadened.

Access

1 If there are no localizing signs, use a midline or right paramedian incision placed half above and half below the umbilicus. Be prepared to extend it in either direction once the lesion is revealed. Examination of the abdomen under anaesthetic may reveal an unsuspected mass, which helps you to site the incision correctly in the first place.

2 Since acute appendicitis is the commonest cause of peritonitis, use a Lanz or gridiron incision if the diagnosis seems at all likely. The incision can be extended medially or laterally to deal with nearby conditions if the diagnosis proves wrong, or it may be closed and a fresh incision made.

3 Remember that irritant fluids, such as gastric juice, blood and bile, may track around the abdomen. Make sure you establish where the pain first started.

4 If peritonitis follows a recent operation, re-open the previous incision (p. 65).

Assess

1 Note any free fluid or pus and save a specimen for laboratory examination.

2 After a rapid preliminary examination of the abdomen, carry out a methodical exploration.

Action

KEY POINT Keep the main goal in mind

- In all emergency operations and operations carried out on ill patients, never lose sight of the object of the procedure. You are operating for a specific reason. Do not indulge in unnecessary 'heroic' procedures—it is not you who is being heroic. It is the patient who will need to be courageous afterwards. Nevertheless, remember that you must assiduously and fully correct the cause of the condition, though by the simplest and most effective means.

1 Make sure that the incision, the assistance and the instruments available are adequate for the proposed procedure.

2 Resect an inflamed appendix, gallbladder, segment of gangrenous or damaged bowel, perforated neoplasm or diseased Meckel's diverticulum.

3 Repair ruptured small bowel or a leaking suture line from a previous operation. Close a perforated peptic ulcer. Consider definitive procedures such as proximal gastric vagotomy or vagotomy and pyloroplasty only in appropriate patients with a long history of indigestion who are fit and would merit elective surgical treatment before the perforation occurred. Such patients are now rare.

4 Resect a specimen of perforated colon, but be very cautious about restoring intestinal continuity without a proximal diverting colostomy. Resection with exteriorization of the bowel ends is an even safer option. Closure of a perforated sigmoid diverticulum with or without transverse colostomy may be appropriate in a few selected cases, but resect perforated carcinomas if possible.

5 Make sure no dead or ischaemic tissue remains.

6 Remove any foreign bodies from the peritoneal cavity. Consider saline lavage and postoperative drainage if there is gross infection or contamination with intestinal contents. Drain an abscess.

7 Normally take no definitive action if you encounter acute pancreatitis, acute salpingitis, uncomplicated ileitis or primary peritonitis. Consider whether a biopsy (e.g. of a lymph node in Crohn's disease) or bacteriological culture swab from the uterine tube might provide useful information. Acute pancreatitis is recognized by a bloodstained effusion, discoloration of the retroperitoneum and the presence of whitish patches of fat necrosis. In salpingitis, both uterine tubes are reddened, swollen and oedematous, often discharging pus from the abdominal ostia. Regional ileitis produces an inflamed, thickened bowel and mesentery, often covered with exudate. In primary peritonitis no cause can be found; the pus tends to be odourless, and a Gram film may reveal cocci.

8 If there has been extensive contamination, carefully wash out the peritoneal cavity using sterile normal saline at body temperature, repeating this until the aspirate is clear.

9 Some surgeons continue lavage after operation by inserting an inflow catheter and a pelvic sump drain. If you use this method, carefully chart and monitor fluid balance.

10 Drains usually drain for a few hours to drain exudate, although they occasionally drain for much longer.

Checklist

1 Have you achieved the purpose of the intervention? If you have not, and require to re-operate to accomplish something that should have been completed now, the patient's chance of recovery is seriously prejudiced.[1]

2 Ensure that, if there are postoperative sequelae, you can feel confident that it is not the result of some overlooked, correctable lesion.

REFERENCE

1. Anderson ID, Fearon KC, Grant IS 1996 Laparotomy for abdominal sepsis in the critically ill. British Journal of Surgery 83:535–539

FURTHER READING

Chamber A, Lord RSA 2001 Incidence of acquired immune deficiency syndrome (AIDS)-related disorder at laparotomy in patients with AIDS. British Journal of Surgery 88:294–297

Lamme B, Boermeester MA, Reitsma JB et al 2002 Meta-analysis of relaparotomy for secondary peritonitis. British Journal of Surgery 89:1516–1524

Lee FYS, Leung KL, Lai PBS et al 2001 Selection of patients for laparoscopic repair of perforated peptic ulcer. British Journal of Surgery 88:133–136

LAPAROTOMY FOR INTESTINAL OBSTRUCTION

Appraise

1 The diagnosis of intestinal obstruction is not always easy to make, nor is it an automatic indication for operation. The features may be indefinite and sometimes fleeting, so that a once-and-for-all history-taking and examination are often misleading. Classically there are four cardinal features—colic, distension, vomiting and constipation—but the prominence of each of these is affected by the site and type of obstruction.

KEY POINT Repeated examination of a patient with obstruction

- Intestinal obstruction is not a once-and-for-all diagnosis. Examine the patient generally, locally and rectally at intervals to identify localizing features and indications that there may be strangulation, sepsis, perforation or other associated conditions in what appeared to be straightforward mechanical obstruction.

2 Vomiting is early, distension often absent and constipation late if the obstruction is high. The small bowel is most frequently obstructed from adhesions, and most of these are iatrogenic, so carefully ask about and look for signs of abdominal operations. The second most common cause is external hernia. Do not miss one; if you do you will probably submit the patient to laparotomy when a simple local release and hernia repair would suffice. Inexperienced surgeons noting faeculent vomiting assume that this results from low obstruction; on the contrary, aerobic and anaerobic microorganisms rapidly flourish as soon as the normally sterile upper intestinal content stagnates, and it is the effect of these on the bile that produce the faeculent smell and appearance of vomitus. A careful history often reveals premonitory features that help in diagnosis and subsequent management. For example, a long history of diarrhoea, with recent improvement, may suggest 'burned-out' Crohn's disease. Initial conservative management and a confirming small bowel enema can help differentiate adhesive and luminal obstruction.

3 Colonic carcinoma is the commonest cause of large-bowel obstruction, although occasionally the presentation is more in keeping with small-bowel obstruction. It is a tragedy to submit a patient to an emergency laparotomy only to discover that the site of obstruction is at the rectosigmoid junction and could have been relieved from below, thus allowing an elective operation to be planned. However high the obstruction appears to be, perform a rectal examination, sigmoidoscopy and, if indicated, a flexible sigmoidoscopic or colonoscopic examination. You can make the diagnosis of cancer and confirm it by obtaining a biopsy. Diverticular disease causing obstruction may produce a palpable peridiverticular mass. Provided the bowel is functioning and absorbing, low-bowel obstruction may not produce marked distension in spite of the fact that a well-hydrated adult pours 8–9 litres of secretion into the bowel. The picture becomes even more obscure if the obstruction is only partial, as often occurs in the large bowel. Consider a water-contrast enema if colonic pseudo-obstruction is a possibility, for example in a septic or postoperative patient (see paragraph 17 below).

4 Patients occasionally present with vague, irregular abdominal cramps and nausea soon after starting meals. If obstruction is missed, it may be rapidly transformed into adynamic ileus so that the anticipated high-pitched bowel sounds are absent and all that is heard is the occasional lower-pitched splash on respiration, resulting from fluid and air moving in the relaxed, inactive bowel.

5 Plain abdominal X-rays are very helpful. Radiologists often deprecate erect films, stating that supine and lateral films are just as valuable. However, the erect posteroanterior film gives you the best chance of determining the site of obstruction and the confirmatory evidence of air–fluid levels. Look for the caecum if it is distended; this suggests distal obstruction. Ultrasound scans and CT can be useful if you are in doubt. Do not fail to carry out simple laboratory tests to exclude diabetes, ketosis, uraemia, anaemia and blood cell changes that may elucidate the diagnosis and monitor the patient's fitness for operation.

6 Patients presenting with recurring obstruction, sometimes following an initial, often trivial, operation, cause great anxiety. The earlier they are seen, before the bowel is distended, the more likely to succeed is vigorous non-operative management, primarily with nasogastric suction and intravenous fluid replacement. Put a time limit, such as 2–3 days, on conservative management, assuming that the patient's general condition is stable. When oral fluids and then feeding are re-introduced, do not delay operation if features of obstruction immediately recur.

7 Classically, it is possible to distinguish strangulation from simple obstruction because there is residual pain between bouts of colic. Of course there may also be tenderness, but this is often detectable at the site of simple obstruction. There may also be guarding and rigidity in strangulating obstruction but this is frequently a late sign as are increasing tachycardia, pyrexia, hypovolaemic shock, gastrointestinal bleeding and a rising white cell count. These features may also be produced by perforation and infection. Do not delay. Carry out a rapid assessment of the likely cause, correct the patient's fluid, electrolyte and acid–base balance, administer versatile antibiotics intravenously and proceed with exploratory laparotomy.

8 Closed-loop obstruction occurs in both the small and the large bowel in volvulus. Beware of complete distal colonic obstruction with gross distension of the caecum. This finding suggests that the ileocaecal valve is preventing backflow into the ileum, and the distended, ischaemic caecal wall may rupture.

9 Many standard textbooks paint a dramatic picture of the clinical features at the onset of mesenteric vascular occlusion. However, it often presents insidiously with pain, ileus, diarrhoea or gastrointestinal bleeding. Suspect it in a patient with vascular disease, especially with atrial fibrillation, who develops unremitting abdominal pain, often in the absence of any abnormal abdominal findings in the early stages. Search for bleeding or occult blood. Angiography is sometimes helpful in obscure cases. If the condition is diagnosed and treated early, there is the possibility of clearing or bypassing the obstruction and saving part or all of the intestine. The value of thrombolysis and dilatation of vascular stenoses has not been fully assessed.

10 Crohn's disease causes obstruction in at least three ways. When it is active the resultant swelling may obstruct the lumen. Most patients can be managed conservatively. Adhesions between affected segments and other structures may require surgical management if obstruction occurs. Finally, in some patients the disease spontaneously regresses, leaving a stenosed, fibrotic segment causing chronic obstruction and proximal stagnation. Diagnosis is by small-bowel enema. As a rule, surgical treatment of stenosed segments is by resection, but strictureplasty may be used in appropriate cases (see Ch. 14).

11 Radiation enteritis is a progressive vascular and interstitial cellular change, related to the dosage level. It frequently follows gynaecological pelvic irradiation, and the symptoms can be delayed for several years. Although dietary change and steroid treatment may help, conservative measures may fail, yet operative treatment carries quite a high mortality rate because of failure of healing of the anastomosis.

12 Sclerosing peritonitis was initially associated with the beta-blocking drug practolol, which is no longer used. It may be seen following peritoneal dialysis. The small bowel is enclosed in a

caul of connective tissue. Bouts of obstruction sometimes respond to conservative treatment but, if it fails, a difficult operation is needed.

13 Do not ignore the possibility of metabolic causes of adynamic ileus such as uraemia, diabetes, sepsis and drugs—particularly tricyclic antidepressants.

14 Some cases of distal obstruction due to colorectal carcinoma can be relieved using simple enemas or the passage of a well-lubricated rectal tube. This manoeuvre spares the patient an emergency operation and allows you to plan an effective procedure, after full assessment and preparation.

15 Diverticulitis may result in obstruction if there is leakage with a pericolic abscess, peridiverticulitis, or an adherent loop of small bowel. Segmental ischaemic colitis may present as proximal obstruction.

16 Large-bowel volvulus usually affects the sigmoid colon, although the caecum is occasionally affected. Elderly patients are affected in the UK, but in some developing countries it often occurs in younger patients. It may be subacute or fulminating. The abdomen is distended, and on plain X-ray films the hugely distended sigmoid loop appears to fill most of the left abdomen; it is sometimes twisted on itself and described as a 'bent inner tube'. A simple enema or barium enema occasionally relieves the volvulus, or try passing a well-lubricated rectal tube or a colonoscope. Success is rewarded with a gush of gas and fluid faeces. If these measures fail, explore the abdomen to untwist and fix the colon. Conservative management is sometimes followed by recurrence.

17 Pseudo-obstruction is a term applied to apparent mechanical obstruction of the colon for which no cause is discovered at operation. The underlying pathophysiology is not understood but it is sometimes associated with systemic disease and drugs, or disease of the autonomic plexuses, whether external or within the colonic wall. A number of causes have been indicted and may be revealed if a careful history is taken, such as laxative abuse, diabetes, porphyria and psychiatric treatment with phenothiazines. Pseudo-obstruction may also occur in hypothyroidism and systemic sclerosis. Mechanical obstruction can be excluded by using a contrast enema. Alternatively, flexible sigmoidoscopy or colonoscopy can be used. If mechanical obstruction can be excluded, deflate the distended bowel by passing a tube into the colon. Try the effect of prokinetic drugs such as metoclopramide, domperidone or cisapride. Correct fluid and electrolyte balance and ensure that the patient is adequately oxygenated.

18 The development of balloon dilatation of strictures at other sites stimulated their use in the gut for the temporary relief of strictures following Crohn's disease or inoperable malignant strictures. Of course, relief was usually temporary. Now self-expanding stents have been developed that should give longer lasting relief for gastric and small intestinal strictures[1] and colonic strictures.[2,3]

19 Perhaps the most difficult diagnostic problem is postoperative obstruction following abdominal surgery. The history and physical signs are atypical because they are added to the expected postoperative delay in function, discomfort, wound pain, tenderness and a tensely held abdominal wall. The diagnosis is rarely clear-cut in the early stages. The obstruction may be caused by temporary oedema at a recently fashioned stoma, a localized collection of fluid, blood or pus causing adynamic ileus, a segment of bowel rendered ischaemic at the operation, an anastomotic leak or a wound dehiscence. Do not be obsessed by a single facet of the operative technique. Keep an open mind, re-examine the patient regularly and order relevant investigations. Call in a trusted colleague for a second opinion if you remain in doubt.

Prepare

1 It is rarely beneficial to embark on immediate operation. Some conditions respond to conservative treatment, some require further assessment. The condition of the patient must be restored as much as possible, both from the effects of the obstruction and from any underlying disease.

KEY POINT Did you miss the onset?

- It is sometimes said that early intestinal obstruction is usually less important than later obstruction. Too often the more serious late obstruction is the continuing missed early obstruction.

2 Pass a nasogastric tube and examine the volume and colour of the aspirate. If there is a substantial volume, re-examine the abdomen; there may be physical signs that were obscured by the distended stomach.

3 Institute fluid and electrolyte replacement. Remember that there may be large volumes of bowel secretions sequestered in the gut, roughly representing physiological saline with added potassium. Do not try to replace this lost volume at once but, depending upon the degree of dehydration and electrolyte imbalance, plan to correct circulating volume and salt depletion, but avoid overhydration. Monitoring the central venous pressure can be useful, particularly in an elderly patient with co-existing cardiac disease.

4 Institute appropriate antibiotic therapy if the patient is pyrexial; or, as soon as operation is decided upon, at once administer a versatile cephalosporin or an aminoglycoside together with metronidazole.

Access

1 Make a midline incision half above and half below the umbilicus and at least 15 cm long, unless the site of obstruction is known (e.g. strangulated femoral hernia; see Ch. 6). Alternatively, use a right paramedian incision of similar length.

2 If the patient has had a previous operation, incise through the old scar, if it is convenient. Extend one end of the incision so that the peritoneum can be opened where it is unlikely to be adherent (see previous section on re-opening the abdomen).

Assess

1 Aspirate any free fluid after obtaining a bacteriological specimen.

2 Insert your hand and gently explore the abdomen. Identify the caecum; if it is collapsed, the obstruction lies within the small bowel.

3 If the abdomen is grossly distended, lift out all the dilated loops of bowel and wrap them in warm, moist packs. Avoid any drag on the mesentery which could render the exteriorized bowel ischaemic. Have the assistant support the heavy distended coils of bowel.

4 Trace the dilated bowel distally to identify the cause of the obstruction, dividing any major adhesions that you encounter.

Action

Small-bowel obstruction

1 Release the obstruction if possible. Divide adhesions and bands. Reduce an internal hernia or overlooked external hernia or volvulus of the small bowel. If the bowel is grossly distended, empty it before closing the abdomen. In high obstruction a per-nasal or peroral tube can often be manipulated into the bowel from within the abdomen and can be attached to a sucker. Sometimes distal contents can be gently milked proximally and aspirated, after which the tube is withdrawn. Alternatively, insert a seromuscular purse-string suture on the antimesenteric border of the bowel. Insert a sucker through a small stab wound within the purse-string. After emptying the bowel, remove the sucker and tighten and tie the purse-string suture. Reinforce this suture with a second suture.

2 Pause if strangulated bowel has been released. When the blood vessels are constricted the low-pressure veins are occluded first; as arterial blood pumps in, the small vessels distend with blood that stagnates, losing its oxygen. If the constriction is released now, the dark, congested bowel rapidly improves in colour. If constriction continues, however, the distended small vessels rupture and blood leaks into the interstitial tissues, including the subserosa. Do not then expect the colour to improve greatly when the vascular occlusion is released; it will take days for the extravasated blood to be removed. The bowel may still appear purple or black. Provided it retains its sheen and the supplying blood vessels pulsate, it usually survives, although the most metabolically active layer, the mucosa, may ulcerate and possibly form a stricture when it heals. The critical site to examine is the bowel wall where it has been included in the constricting band or ring. It is usually white from ischaemia, but if it soon regains its colour it may safely be left. Any small doubtful area can be invaginated with a few seromuscular stitches. If the colour of the constriction rings fails to improve at all, or if they are green or purple in colour, excise the segment, ensure the remaining bowel ends are well supplied with blood and carry out an anastomosis.

3 Sometimes a knuckle of small bowel that has been trapped in an internal or external hernia will spontaneously reduce itself. If you observe constriction rings, look for the possible site of hernia and try to close the defect. Constriction rings that remain slightly ischaemic may be invaginated by Lembert sutures.

4 Resect the obstructed bowel if there is a neoplasm or if the bowel or its blood supply are damaged. Massive resection may be necessary if the main vessels are blocked; consider embolectomy in selected patients (Ch. 29).

5 Bypass the obstruction if it cannot be removed. Gastroenterostomy relieves pyloric or duodenal obstruction. Duodenojejunostomy bypasses annular pancreas or duodenal atresia. An enteroanastomosis short-circuits an irresectable primary or secondary tumour of the jejunum or ileum (Ch. 14). Obtain a biopsy specimen in all irresectable cases.

6 Break up, push on or remove intraluminal obstruction such as a food bolus, gallstone or collection of worms.

7 Reduce an intussusception (Chs 14, 40). Resect a polyp or other pathological lesion at the apex of the intussusception (usually in adults).

8 Stricture resulting from Crohn's disease is conventionally treated by resection and anastomosis. Unfortunately, you can never be certain that further resections are avoidable. Indeed, some of the patients presenting with obstructive disease have already had previous extensive resections. In recent years a much more conservative policy has become popular, supported by the fact that what appear to be unaffected healthy segments of bowel are already histologically diseased. For this reason, resection of strictures is kept as short as possible, transgressing macroscopically diseased but unstrictured bowel. For short segments, strictureplasty seems to be satisfactory. The procedure is particularly indicated if the stricture is short, if the disease process is not florid—indicating possible 'burned-out' disease—and if the bowel is already short or will be made short by resecting a large length of strictured bowel (Ch. 14). The operation is performed after the fashion of a Heineke–Mikulicz pyloroplasty; the bowel is incised longitudinally throughout the length of the stricture and opened out so that the incision can be closed to produce a horizontal suture line.

9 Sclerosing peritonitis presents a formidable challenge. The caul of adherent connective tissue must be carefully peeled and dissected from the bowel to free it. This is time-consuming but do not try to hurry or the bowel wall may be damaged and there will be considerable oozing of blood from the raw surfaces. The morbidity and mortality rate following the procedure is high, so take every care.

10 If no other relief can be given, be prepared on occasion to create a proximal stoma as a terminal palliative measure, rather than leave a patient obstructed and vomiting without relief.

11 The management of neonatal obstruction is described in Chapter 40.

12 Patients occasionally require repeated operations for adhesive obstruction. Sometimes only a single kink has occurred and can be relieved without carrying out an extensive dissection of the matted bowel, and it is better to deal with this than disturb the adherent but unobstructed segments. If the whole small bowel requires to be dissected because obstruction is at multiple sites, the operations become increasingly difficult. Once the bowel has been freed throughout its length, consider performing a modification of Noble's operation, in which lengths of bowel are folded back and forth in a boustrophedon (Greek: *bous*=ox +*strophe*=a turning), like the course of the plough in successive furrows or the folds of a 'jumping jack' cracker. In Noble's original method the folds were held permanently by suturing

together adjacent segments of bowel using a running seromuscular stitch. This procedure has been largely superseded by the Childs–Phillips method of fixation. A non-absorbable suture is passed on a long straight needle through the folded layers of the mesentery adjacent to the bowel after taking care to avoid the blood vessels. When all the successive layers have been threaded on, the suture is passed back along a parallel track placed close to the bowel and tied to the first end, forming a long loop. Three such looped sutures are placed: one at each end of the folds and a central one. At the end of the operation the bowel on its mesentery resembles a closed, stitched, folded paper fan. There have been a number of modifications: instead of multiple transfixions of all the layers, each of the folded ends alone may be fixed, in the hope of maintaining the conformation.

Large-bowel obstruction

1 Release an external cause of obstruction. Sometimes a loop of small bowel is adherent to an inflammatory diverticular mass and requires release.

2 A diverticular mass may totally obstruct the sigmoid colon. The conventional method of overcoming this problem is to perform loop transverse colostomy with subsequent resection of the diseased segment electively and, at a third stage, close the colostomy. It is not uncommon to be uncertain whether the mass is an inflammatory mass or an obstructing carcinoma. One option is to perform a transverse colostomy and, before carrying out the second-stage resection, to carry out barium enema X-ray, sigmoidoscopy and colonoscopy to determine the cause. Many surgeons prefer to carry out a resection at the initial laparotomy; sometimes only when the specimen is examined histologically is the diagnosis revealed. If a sigmoid colectomy is performed, a temporary terminal iliac colostomy can be formed, and the lower cut end is closed over and dropped back into the pelvis (Hartmann's procedure). There is seldom sufficient length to bring the lower cut end to the surface as a mucous fistula. At a second elective stage continuity is restored. It may be possible in some cases to carry out resection and anastomosis in one stage following on-table orthograde irrigation of the proximal colon to clear it of faeces (see later).

3 Resect an obstructing carcinoma of the caecum, ascending colon or transverse colon, and restore continuity by end-to-end ileocolostomy. Because the contents of the small bowel are fluid, there is little or no danger in carrying out primary anastomosis in this fashion. To achieve a one-stage resection of a carcinoma of the descending colon it is often appropriate to perform an extended right hemicolectomy, including the splenic flexure and descending colon above and including the obstruction, so that a safe ileocolostomy can be carried out.

4 Traditionally, obstructing carcinoma of the sigmoid colon and rectum is treated in three stages, the first stage being transverse colostomy. Subsequently, elective colectomy is performed and finally the colostomy is closed. Occasionally this is still the best choice. However, many patients are elderly and some have a short life-expectation. The three-stage procedure erodes their remaining life, and there is a high failure rate to complete the full restoration to normal function.

5 One of the stages can be avoided by resecting the obstructed segment now and bringing out the upper cut end as a temporary terminal left iliac colostomy. The lower cut end is dealt with by Hartmann's procedure. Occasionally it can be brought to the surface as a mucous fistula, but more frequently it is too short for this and is better closed and dropped back into the pelvis. At a second stage the two ends are prepared and anastomosed to restore continuity. It is easier to identify the rectal stump at separation if the suture ends are left long.

6 If the obstruction is not gross, it is sometimes feasible to carry out primary resection and anastomosis. To protect the anastomosis, carry out either loop transverse colostomy or caecostomy.

7 Resection and anastomosis can be safely completed in one stage provided the obstructed colon can be cleared of faeces. This clearance is achieved by inserting a large Foley catheter into the caecum and running in physiologically normal saline to wash through the colon. At the upper cut end a length of corrugated anaesthetic tubing is tied into the bowel, connected to a large plastic bag, forming a closed effluent system. Saline is run through until there are no faecal masses to be felt and the effluent is clean. The lavage system is taken down and the bowel is joined end-to-end.

8 In gross obstruction, always carefully inspect the caecum, since if it is overdistended it may perforate or develop gangrene and subsequently burst. In case of doubt perform a caecostomy.

9 Bypass an irresectable carcinoma of the right colon by ileotransverse colostomy. Bypass an irresectable carcinoma of the left colon by colocolostomy if possible. Relieve unresectable obstructing carcinoma of the distal colon or rectum by means of a left iliac end colostomy. If you carry out a colostomy above the tumour, bring the lower cut end to the surface as a mucous fistula. If you close it, you have left a closed loop above the obstructing carcinoma.

10 Always obtain a biopsy specimen if you do not resect the carcinoma.

11 Untwist a volvulus. Have a rectal tube in place so that the distended bowel can be deflated. Alternatively, insert a hypodermic needle through one of the taeniae and patiently allow it to release the air. Prevent future twisting by stitching the bowel to the parietes. If the sigmoid colon is gangrenous, exteriorize it by the Paul–Mikulicz method: bring out the gangrenous loop to the surface, leave it for 24–48 hours so that the exit wound is sealed and then excise the loop. At a later stage the parallel afferent and efferent colon can be formally united or the intervening wall can be crushed in the traditional manner using an enterotome. Alternatively, resect the gangrenous bowel now and bring the upper cut end to the left iliac fossa as a terminal colostomy and perform a Hartmann's procedure on the lower cut end, closing it or bringing it to the surface as a mucous fistula.

12 Move on, break up or remove intraluminal obstruction such as a faecalith.

13 Ischaemic colitis that causes obstruction is best resected and the ends brought to the surface, because it is difficult to be sure how much of the colon will survive.

14 Never forget the purpose of this emergency operation. Do not perform any procedure that does not fulfil this purpose.

Closure

1 This can be difficult if the abdomen is distended. Take care to avoid injuring dilated loops of small bowel. Consider inserting tension sutures if abdominal distension is gross.

? DIFFICULTY

1. In the presence of grossly distended bowel, do not flounder within the abdomen through an inadequate incision. Extend the incision and gently deliver the entire small bowel. Consider decompressing the small bowel by means of a special sucker (p. 64). Decompress the upper small bowel by milking contents back up to within reach of the nasogastric tube, and try to manoeuvre this tube through the pylorus into the duodenum or jejunum.
2. Sometimes adhesions prevent easy delivery of the small bowel or produce an apparently inextricable tangle. Such cases can be very testing. Settle down to a prolonged dissection. Make sure that the incision is adequate for you to visualize the restraining bands, which should then be divided. Patiently disentangle all adherent loops and run the whole small bowel through your hands to make sure it is unravelled, and intact.

Aftercare

1 Monitor fluid, electrolyte and acid–base balance in order to determine the intravenous requirements. If recovery is expected to be rapid there is usually no need to provide nutritional requirements.

2 Monitor the volumes of nasogastric aspirate. Have the tube aspirated every 15 minutes for the first hour, then every half-hour for the next hour and subsequently every hour. Many surgeons take inordinate pride in removing the nasogastric tube at an early stage. Following the relief of intestinal obstruction, with extensive handling of the bowel, there is often a prolonged phase of adynamic ileus. Wait until the aspirate falls to less than the intake after oral fluids have started and/or until the patient passes flatus per rectum.

3 Give measured sips of water early and increase them as the aspirate falls. When the volume of aspirate falls below the volume of oral fluids, first ensure that the tube is patent and correctly sited and, if it is, withdraw it.

4 Examine the abdomen frequently to ensure that it is soft, not distending and not tender. Listen for returning bowel sounds. Monitor the passage of flatus and faeces.

5 If the operation was merely for the release of a simple adhesion obstruction, antibiotics need not be given after operation. If there was contamination, continue them until the swab cultures are reported, then make a decision about stopping or changing them.

REFERENCES

1. Yates MR III, Morgan DE, Baron TH 1998 Palliation of malignant gastric and small intestinal strictures with self-expandable metal stents. Endoscopy 30:266–272
2. Arnell T, Stames M, Takahashi P et al 1998 Colonic stents in colorectal obstruction. American Surgeon 64:986–988
3. Baron TH, Dean PA, Yates MR 1998 Expandable metal stents for the treatment of colonic obstruction: techniques and outcomes. Gastrointestinal Endoscopy 47:277–286

LAPAROTOMY FOR GASTROINTESTINAL BLEEDING

Appraise

1 Ideally, manage patients with gastrointestinal bleeding jointly with a gastroenterological physician with whom you have an agreed policy. A high proportion of affected patients are over 60 years of age and many suffer from concomitant disease. Approximately one-third will have taken aspirin or other non-steroidal anti-inflammatory drugs within a few days of the onset of bleeding.

2 The history and the nature of the bleeding may be helpful in determining its site, but can also be misleading. Haematemesis usually results from a lesion in the oesophagus or stomach such as oesophageal varices, cardio-oesophageal mucosal tears (the Mallory–Weiss syndrome), erosive gastritis or gastroduodenal peptic ulcer. However, blood from the upper small bowel may be regurgitated into the stomach and vomited. Melaena (black, tarry stool with a distinctive smell) is associated with gastroduodenal bleeding but is sometimes indistinguishable when it emanates from the right colon. The passage of bright blood from the rectum suggests a distal cause but can follow brisk bleeding from the small bowel or, exceptionally, from the stomach.

3 Never fail to carry out a thorough examination, including rectal examination, proctoscopy and sigmoidoscopy. The availability of more complex methods of investigation sometimes beguiles clinicians into forgetting basic manoeuvres. Consider the possibility that the condition may result from a bleeding or clotting disorder, parasitic infestation, Peutz–Jeghers syndrome or drug therapy. Order appropriate tests. Consider the possibility of the patient suffering from AIDS; although upper gastrointestinal bleeding is relatively uncommon in this condition, it carries a poor prognosis, partly as a result of the concomitant thrombocytopenia.

4 The availability of superb flexible endoscopes has greatly improved diagnostic accuracy. It is fortunate that the vast majority of gastrointestinal bleeding occurs within the range of vision of oesophagogastroduodenoscopes or of the colonoscope. Bleeding outside the range of these instruments is much more difficult to localize. Carry out endoscopy as soon as possible. Be prepared to wash out clot and blood using a large tube passed into the stomach or lower bowel. If you are not expert in passing the instrument or in interpreting the findings, call for appropriate help. Be prepared to repeat the examination if the first attempt was not completely successful or if the clinical picture changes. There is a wide choice of endoscopic methods for controlling bleeding. A popular technique at present is diathermy using an argon beam,[1] but the heat probe, which has been available for 20 years, can give as good results as other methods.[2]

5 Expertly performed contrast radiography helps identify obscure sites of bleeding. In addition to barium meal and enema X-rays,

small-bowel enema can show up lesions that cannot be seen endoscopically.

6 Selective angiography often demonstrates active bleeding from, for example, Meckel's diverticulum, angiodysplasia, haemangioma or leiomyoma. Bleeding generally needs to be occurring at the time of the examination. If the equipment and expertise is available, conditions such as bleeding peptic ulcer may be amenable to transcatheter embolization. If a lesion is identified in a patient about to be operated upon, it may be valuable to leave the catheter in place, keeping it patent with heparin. At operation the theatre lights may be lowered and 1 ml of methylthioninium chloride (methylene blue) injected through the catheter while the bowel is transilluminated. The site is marked with a suture until it can be exposed and dealt with.

7 ^{99m}Tc-labelled red cells demonstrate slow bleeding better than angiography since the labelled blood remains in the bowel and is recorded by the scintigram, but the technique has an appreciable false-negative rate. ^{99m}Tc-pertechnetate is secreted by the stomach or ectopic gastric mucosa in a Meckel's diverticulum.

8 Intermittent obscure bleeding small intestine can be remarkably difficult to identify and localize, but angiography and intraoperative enteroscopy are useful Very rarely it is necessary to create paired temporary loop ileostomies so that endoscopy can be performed as soon as bleeding starts.[3]

9 Haematochezia (Greek: *chezo*=to go to stool, hence bloody stool) can be immensely challenging, even to the point of recommending an occasional 'blind' subtotal colectomy when the source of bleeding can be confidently located in the colon.[4]

10 For bleeding from oesophageal varices see Chapter 22.

Prepare

1 As you assess the patient, initiate appropriate resuscitation. Do not place too much reliance on the initial haemoglobin and haematocrit results because they are affected by physiological blood dilution. Pass a nasogastric tube to aspirate and monitor upper gastrointestinal bleeding. If needed, transfuse blood, estimate your needs in the immediate future and, if operation is necessary, make sure that blood will be available. Have a central venous catheter inserted if the patient is shocked, to monitor volume replacement. Carefully check, and if necessary replenish, clotting factors, particularly if large volumes of blood need to be given.

KEY POINTS Perioperative endoscopy

- Do not take a patient to the operating theatre without also taking the endoscope.
- Be willing to pass the endoscope after the patient is anaesthetized, to confirm the lesion—and confirm that it is still bleeding. On occasion an unnecessary operation can be cancelled or deferred if the bleeding has stopped.
- Intraoperative endoscopy can be invaluable, including operative guidance of an endoscope passed perorally or peranally to localize small-bowel bleeding.

2 If peptic ulcer has been identified as the cause of bleeding, it is appropriate to give H_2-receptor blocking drugs or a proton pump inhibitor. These drugs may work in part because acid inhibits platelet function and haemostasis.

3 The first line of management of oesophageal variceal bleeding is not operative (see Ch. 22). Similarly, endoscopic and angiographic methods are increasingly used to control peptic ulcer bleeding (see Ch. 13). Somatostatin and tranexamic acid are being evaluated.

4 Do not, however, vacillate in patients with bleeding peptic ulcer if they are over the age of 60 years, have concomitant disease, are shocked, have a visible vessel or are bleeding at endoscopy, continue bleeding or have recurrent bleeding. Such patients need an operation.

5 Operations for the control of severe gastrointestinal bleeding require to be performed by experienced surgeons backed by expert anaesthetists and a trained team of assistants. If you are not experienced in this very demanding field, seek help urgently.

Access

Make a midline or right paramedian incision, sited in the upper or lower abdomen according to the preoperative diagnosis or midway if this is uncertain.

Assess

1 Blood in the lumen can be recognized from without owing to the bluish-black coloration of the gut. The distribution of blood in the stomach, small bowel and colon may roughly localize the site of bleeding, but remember that blood can travel for a considerable distance proximal as well as distal to the lesion.

2 Inspect and palpate the alimentary canal from oesophagus to rectum. Note any abnormality, particularly an ulcer crater, tumour, inflammation, petechiae, scarring or a local increase in vascularity. Examine the liver and spleen. Cirrhosis raises the possibility of variceal haemorrhage; splenomegaly might be associated with a clotting defect. If the gut appears normal, remember that haemobilia and pancreatic cysts are rare causes of gastrointestinal haemorrhage.

Action

1 If there is evidence of *upper* gastrointestinal bleeding, concentrate on the stomach, duodenum and jejunum.
- Enter the lesser sac to examine the posterior surface of the stomach. Consider an anterior gastrotomy in the body of the stomach, which can be extended to allow inspection of the entire gastric mucosa. Under-run any bleeding vessels. Options for gastric ulcer include biopsy or local resection plus vagotomy and drainage, and, in fit patients, partial gastrectomy.
- Closely inspect the anterior surface of the pylorus and duodenal cap for petechial haemorrhage and scarring, consistent with active duodenal ulcer disease. A chronic posterior ulcer crater may be palpable. A duodenotomy may need to be extended across the pyloric ring to allow adequate exposure of an ulcer crater. Under-run the bleeding ulcer with

stout non-absorbable sutures, such as 0 silk, and make sure that haemorrhage is fully controlled. Truncal vagotomy and pyloroplasty is the simplest option thereafter.

- If the stomach and duodenal bulb seem normal, turn your attention to the rest of the duodenal loop, duodenojejunal flexure and jejunum. Look for tumours and diverticula in particular. Consider mobilizing the duodenal loop by Kocher's manoeuvre and taking down the ligament of Treitz. Resect the segment of small bowel bearing a bleeding lesion.

2 If there is evidence of *lower* gastrointestinal bleeding, concentrate on the colon and ileum. The site of bleeding can be difficult to identify in the intestine.

- Look for obvious lesions in the colon, including diverticula, arteriovenous malformations and tumours. Sigmoid diverticula are common in the elderly and cannot necessarily be assumed to explain the haemorrhage. Colonoscopy performed by yourself or a colleague during laparotomy may help to reveal a small mucosal lesion. Resect the segment of large bowel bearing a bleeding lesion. If all else fails, consider transverse colostomy; any future episodes of bleeding can then at least be localized to the right or left colon.
- Examine the entire small bowel from ligament of Treitz to ileocaecal valve. Look in particular for Meckel's diverticulum, acquired diverticula of the jejunum or ileum, tumours and ulcers. If examination is negative but you strongly suspect a small-bowel source of bleeding, consider making a mid-enterotomy and passing a flexible colonoscope up and down the small bowel from this point. By inspecting the transilluminated bowel from without and the mucosal surface from within, you may be able to detect a small vascular lesion.

3 There is no indication for 'blind' procedures, such as partial gastrectomy. If the patient is bleeding from the stomach, you should be able to identify it. If you do not identify it, your operation will add to the patient's immediate, and possibly long-term, disability, confuse the clinical picture and give you a false sense of security. If you have done all you can to find the site of bleeding, close the abdomen, carefully record your findings and determine to carry out appropriate further investigations.

KEY POINTS Never forget the purpose of the operation

- The purpose of the operation is to control life-threatening bleeding and prevent it from recurring. Do not perform any procedure outside this purpose.
- Do not, for example, carry out a definitive operation for peptic ulcer, unless it is vital to accomplish your purpose. Chronic peptic ulcer is amenable to non-operative treatment.

REFERENCES

1. Johanns W, Luis W, Janssen J et al 1997 Argon plasma coagulation (APC) in gastroenterology: experimental and clinical experiences. European Journal of Gastroenterology 9:581–587
2. Kumar P, Fleischer DE 1997 Thermal therapy for gastrointestinal bleeding. Gastrointestinal Endoscopy Clinics of North America 7:593–609
3. Irgau I, Reilly PM, Abdel-Misih RZ 1995 Paired temporary loop ileostomies in the localization of small bowel hemorrhage of obscure origin. American Surgeon 61:1099–1101
4. Billingham RP 1997 The conundrum of lower gastrointestinal bleeding. Surgical Clinics of North America 77:241–252

FURTHER READING

Bornman PC, Graham SM, Dunn JP 1999 Complications of peptic ulcer and their management. In: Taylor TV, Watson A, Williamson RCN (eds) Upper digestive surgery: oesophagus, stomach and small intestine. Saunders, London, pp 495–533

LAPAROTOMY FOR EARLY POSTOPERATIVE COMPLICATIONS

Appraise

1 This can be one of the most daunting surgical challenges that we face. Re-opening the abdomen is associated with a sense of guilt and failure. We feel that, if the first operation had been better performed, or if we had chosen a more appropriate procedure—or even, occasionally, an alternative to operation—or prepared the patient better, a second operation would be unnecessary. Having failed once, how can we hope to succeed from a less advantageous position?

KEY POINT The challenge of re-operating for complications

- Do not feel defeated before you begin; this is a testing time, but success will bring all the more sense of accomplishment.

2 Of course, it is best to avoid the risk of complications by always carrying out the correct operations perfectly, but we all make mistakes of judgement and accomplishment. Reduce the risk by asking yourself when you decide on an impulse to do something beyond the simplest procedure whether it is likely to achieve your object, how you will justify your action to the patient, your colleagues and your conscience if a complication develops. Couch and colleagues[1] identified four mistakes of judgement leading to complications:

- Over-optimism ('I can get away with it.').
- Over-aggression ('It is the patient's only chance.').
- Over-perfection: doing more than is necessary ('Better is the enemy of good.').
- Carrying out a major procedure that has come into vogue rather than a simpler and well-tried procedure.

3 The most frequent complication requiring early re-operation is continuing primary haemorrhage, or reactionary haemorrhage that starts up when the patient's arterial or venous blood pressure rises and dislodges an occluding clot in a cut vessel. Secondary haemorrhage occurs after a few days and results from clot digestion by the proteolytic enzymes produced by infecting microorganisms. Early detection of continuing primary or

reactionary haemorrhage is difficult because the pulse and blood pressure may vary during recovery from the operation and anaesthetic for a number of reasons. Awareness of pain, coughing, overfull bladder and vascular dilatation as the patient is warmed can vary the pulse rate and blood pressure. Do not rely upon intra-abdominal drains or intraluminal drains as monitors of bleeding.

4 Haemorrhage, peritonitis or obstruction may occur during the first week after abdominal operation. Pain, tenderness, agitation, abdominal distension, circulatory and temperature changes often produce a confusing picture. Pyrexia may be masked by antibiotic cover. Do not expect the presentation to be classic. For example, unrelieved obstruction may rapidly pass into adynamic ileus. Absent bowel sounds may also indicate a later than expected normal recovery of gut function, intra-abdominal sepsis, impending wound dehiscence or onset of ischaemia. which can develop at any time.

5 If the patient is not making as quick a recovery as expected, look for general as well as abdominal causes. Take down the wound dressings and inspect it. Look for redness and swelling and gently palpate for tenderness. In case of doubt, gently insinuate a needle attached to a syringe through the scar to seek haematoma, seroma or pus. Never fail to carry out a rectal examination.

KEY POINTS Develop and utilize basic clinical skills

- If you are uncertain, repeat the complete examination after an interval; it is remarkable how rapidly the physical findings can change.
- You are most likely to make an accurate assessment if you have acquired experience by always carrying out regular, assiduous postoperative examination of your patients.
- In this way you have learned what is within normal limits and what is suspicious.

6 Use investigations selectively. If you order them indiscriminately, you will merely confuse the diagnosis. Radiology, ultrasound scanning, CT and endoscopy may be very valuable in localizing or excluding pathology. However, whenever clinical findings and investigations are in opposition, trust your clinical judgement. Investigations are not infallible; do not think that results expressed numerically carry added scientific weight.

7 If the postoperative course is not smooth, it is all too easy to identify some part of the operation that causes anxiety. Do not be obsessed with this facet and remain blinded to some unsuspected cause. Unless the need for operation is obvious, correct all possible abnormalities and reassess the patient. Remember that the patient is likely to improve hereafter. The difficult decision you have to make is whether or not the improvement is as much as you had expected. Is there still some aspect that is unsatisfactory? Does the patient begin to deteriorate as soon as the vigorous correction ceases? Figure 4.2 demonstrates the choices. You have no problem in deciding when the diagnosis is clear, but very often the decision has to be made within the grey area of uncertainty.

KEY POINTS Early operation is often wise

- Do not hope for the best. The rapidity with which a patient with sepsis or ischaemic bowel deteriorates is sometimes startling.
- If you suspect that something serious has occurred, do not put off the decision to re-operate by ordering unnecessary investigations.
- In such circumstances remember the aphorism, 'It is better to look and see, than wait and see'.

8 On the other hand, a complication does not inevitably demand immediate operation. A fistula that is draining freely in a patient who is otherwise well is best treated conservatively at first. This policy gives time for the cause to be investigated and the nutritional status of the patient to be corrected and maintained. Provided the effluent continues to reduce in volume, it is best not to rush into operative management.

9 Do not be too proud to call in someone more experienced to carry out a re-exploration. You may feel that since you performed the first operation it is your responsibility to seek and correct whatever has gone wrong. Your first responsibility is to see that the patient has the best chance of recovery.

Prepare

1 It is very rare that you cannot spend even a few minutes improving the patient's general condition before embarking on the second operation.

2 Start versatile antibiotic treatment or prophylaxis. In most circumstances ensure that blood is cross-matched.

3 Have a nasogastric tube passed so that the stomach can be emptied.

4 Warn the theatre staff of the likely findings, procedure and equipment required.

Access

1 Have the dressings and skin sutures removed. Alternatively, wear two pairs of sterile gloves and discard the outer pair after removing the skin sutures yourself.

2 After cleansing the skin separate the wound edges, using the handle of a scalpel. Seek and remove the deep stitches.

3 Open up the peritoneal cavity with care, using a fingertip to break through the partially sealed peritoneal edges.

Assess

1 Note any gas, blood or other fluid, and save a specimen for subsequent microscopy and culture.

2 Display the area of the previous operation to detect bleeding, mechanical obstruction, anastomotic breakdown, infection, ischaemia or necrosis.

3 Continuing haemorrhage demands immediate control. All other conditions are best considered carefully to determine the best course of action. The patient is more likely to succumb to

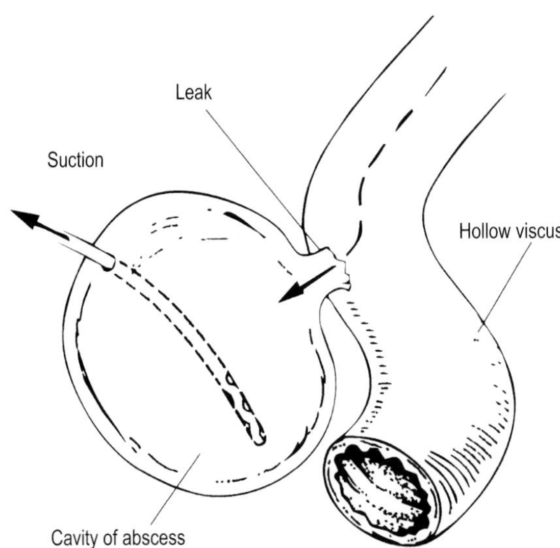

Fig. 4.7 How not to drain an abscess following a leak. The abscess will continue indefinitely unless you drain the leak directly, excise or exteriorize it. (Adapted by permission from Hospital Update.)

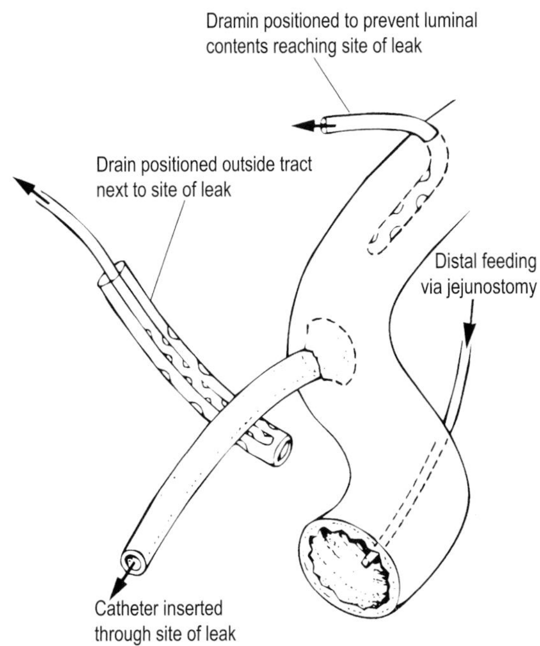

Fig. 4.8 Draining a leak from bowel that cannot be closed, exteriorized or excised. (Adapted by permission from Hospital Update.)

hurried, ineffectual surgery than to deliberate and well-planned corrective measures.

4 Remember why you have re-entered the abdomen. Plan to carry out the simplest effective procedures that will allow the patient to recover. Do not become side-tracked by minor issues.

5 Consider what your reaction would be if the patient does not recover satisfactorily. Will you wish that you had chosen another procedure? If so, why are you not planning to carry out that procedure now?

Action

1 Control bleeding in the most effective way possible and ensure that it will not recur.

2 Consider why an anastomosis has leaked: tension, inadequate blood supply, poor technique, a continuing disease process, impaired wound healing, distal obstruction or a combination of factors? Sometimes it is possible to insert a few sutures to repair a limited leak. Usually it is necessary to re-do the anastomosis completely, perhaps after resecting devitalized tissue and carrying out further mobilization to avoid tension. However, if the gut or duct has been bathed in effluent and pus, the most careful re-anastomosis will fail. In many cases you will do more damage and spread the inflammation. Many small leaks are best accepted. But they must be well drained and, as far as possible, defunctioned. It is inadequate to place a small drain in a large abscess cavity (Fig. 4.7). The leak may continue indefinitely. If you cannot exteriorize or resect or bypass the leak, insert a drain into it, reduce the flow by proximal aspiration or stoma, insert a sump drain near the leak with gentle continuous suction. If possible, institute distal enteral feeding (e.g. through a feeding jejunostomy; Fig. 4.8).

3 Leaking ureteric or biliary anastomoses are best repaired over a stenting tube. If a colonic anastomosis leaks, it is better to bring out each end of bowel as a stoma (or oversew the rectum) than attempt another primary anastomosis. Sometimes a bypass procedure will help to protect a resutured anastomosis (e.g. gastrojejunostomy to bypass a duodenal leak).

4 Correct mechanical obstruction as if this were a first operation. It is particularly important to avoid any distal obstruction (e.g. from adhesions) after refashioning a gastrointestinal anastomosis.

5 Seek the source of infection and control it if possible. Avoid spreading the infection if it is localized. If local sepsis fully explains the complication, it may be best to limit yourself to dealing with it and avoid further exploration. Be careful not to disturb anastomoses that appear to be healing satisfactorily.

6 Evacuate any residual blood, pus or other intra-abdominal fluid and provide adequate drainage to the operation site.

Checklist

1 Have you dealt adequately with the complication?

2 Check the area of the operation thoroughly to ensure that all is well. Memorize exactly your findings and procedure so that you can record the details straight after the operation.

3 It is usually best to explore the whole abdomen to make certain that no other condition is missed, particularly if the local findings do not fully explain the original complications.

4 Replace the viscera in their anatomical position to prevent future mechanical complications.

Closure

1 It is usually best to drain the peritoneal cavity, preferably through a separate stab incision.

2 Use the simplest and most effective means of closing the abdomen. Many surgeons close these wounds like a burst abdomen, using deep tension sutures. Fortunately, like burst abdomens, re-opened wounds seldom break down completely, though superficial separation may complicate infection.

REFERENCE

1. Couch NP, Tilney NL, Rayner AA et al 1981 The high cost of low frequency events. The anatomy and economics of surgical mishaps. New England Journal of Medicine 304:634–637

FURTHER READING

Adams ID, Chan M, Clifford PC et al 1986 Computer-aided diagnosis of acute abdominal pain: a multicentre study. British Medical Journal 293:800–804

Andrews HA, Keighley MRB, Alexander-Williams J et al 1991 Strategy for management of distal Crohn's disease. British Journal of Surgery 78:679–682

Ausobsky JR, Evans M, Pollock AV 1985 Does mass closure of midline laparotomies stand the test of time? A random control trial. Annals of the Royal College of Surgeons of England 67:159–161

Childs WA, Phillips RB 1960 Experience with intestinal plication and a proposed modification. Annals of Surgery 152:258–265

Ellis H 1984 How to do a laparotomy. British Journal of Hospital Medicine 31:437–439

Gallegos NC, Hobsley M 1990 Abdominal wall pain: an alternative diagnosis. British Journal of Surgery 77:1167–1170

Hoffman J 1987 Peritoneal lavage in the diagnosis of the acute abdomen of non-traumatic origin. Acta Chirurgica Scandinavica 153:561–565

Hussain SA 1990 Closure of subcutaneous fat: a prospective randomised trial. British Journal of Surgery 77:107

Irvin TT 1989 Abdominal pain: a surgical audit of 1190 emergency admissions. British Journal of Surgery 76:1121–1125

Jenkins TRN 1976 The burst abdominal wound: a mechanical approach. British Journal of Surgery 63:873–876

Jones PF, Krukowski ZH, Young GG 1998 Emergency abdominal surgery, 3rd edn. Chapman & Hall, London

Kaufman GL Acute abdomen. In: Corson JD, Williamson RCN (eds) Surgery. Mosby, London, pp 3.1–3.13

Kendall SWH, Brennan TG, Guillou PJ 1991 Suture length to wound length ratio and the integrity of midline and lateral paramedian incisions. British Journal of Surgery 78:705–707

Kirk RM 1990 Chronic and recurring abdominal pain. Transactions of the Medical Society of London 105:1–4

Kirk RM 1990 Reoperation for early intra-abdominal complications following abdominal and abdominothoracic operations. Hospital Update 16:303–310

Kirk RM, Stoddart CJ 1986 Complications of surgery of the upper gastrointestinal tract. Baillière Tindall, London

Koruth NM, Krukowski ZH, Youngson GG et al 1985 Intraoperative colonic irrigation in the management of left-sided large bowel emergencies. British Journal of Surgery 72:708–711

Kossi J, Salminen P, Rantala A et al 2003 Population-based study of the surgical workload and economic impact of bowel obstruction caused by postoperative adhesions. British Journal of Surgery 90:1441–1444

Lau WY, Yuen WK, Chu KW et al 1992 Obscure bleeding in the gastrointestinal tract originating in the small intestine. Surgery, Gynecology and Obstetrics 174:119–124

Leaper DJ, Kissin C, Virjee J et al 1991 New diagnostic techniques in the acute abdomen. In: Williamson RCN, Cooper MJ (eds) Emergency abdominal surgery. Churchill Livingstone, Edinburgh, pp 1–20

McCarthy JD 1975 Further experience with the Childs–Phillips plication operation. American Journal of Surgery 130:15–19

O'Dain GN, Leaper DJ 2003 Sequential physiology scoring facilitates objective assessment of revisitation in patients with an intra-abdominal emergency. British Journal of Surgery 90:1445–1450

Parente F, Cernuschi M, Valsecci L et al 1991 Acute upper gastrointestinal bleeding in patients with AIDS: a relatively uncommon condition associated with reduced survival. Gut 32:987–990

Paterson-Brown S 1991 Strategies for reducing inappropriate laparotomy rate in the acute abdomen. British Medical Journal 303:1115–1118

Sawyer RG, Rosenlof LK, Adams RB et al 1992 Peritonitis into the 1990s: changing pathogens and changing strategies in the critically ill. American Surgeon 58:82–87

Silen W 1996 Cope's early diagnosis of the acute abdomen, 19th edn. Oxford University Press, London

Vipond MN, Paterson-Brown S, Tyrrell MR et al 1990 Evaluation of fine catheter aspiration cytology of the peritoneum as an adjunct to decision making in the acute abdomen. British Journal of Surgery 77:86–87

Wheatley KA, Keighley MRB 1990 Peptic ulcer haemorrhage. In: Williamson RCN, Cooper MJ (eds) Emergency abdominal surgery. Churchill Livingstone, Edinburgh, pp 95–109

Williamson RCN, Cooper MJ (eds) 1990 Emergency abdominal surgery. Churchill Livingstone, Edinburgh

5

Principles of minimal access surgery

P.A. Paraskeva, A. Darzi

GENERAL PRINCIPLES OF LAPAROSCOPY

1 Minimal access surgery is intended to cause the least anatomical, physiological and psychological trauma to the patient. The rapid advancements in this type of surgery since the late 1980s have seen the dawning of an age of surgical technological innovation. It would not have been possible without the simultaneous development of improved methods of imaging to replace the traditional 'hands-in' method of open surgery assessment.

2 Along with these developments was the recognition that adequate education and training in minimal access techniques combined with well-considered pre- and postoperative care are essential for successful application of these new approaches.

3 Many surgical and gynaecological procedures are regularly performed using a minimal access approach. Table 5.1 shows examples of the uses of therapeutic laparoscopy. The majority of the discussion in this chapter is related to the basic principles of laparoscopy.

4 Minimal access surgery has implications for the economics of hospitals offering surgical services. Capital equipment is expensive and requires regular servicing to ensure good working standards. Consumables are particularly expensive, and re-use of equipment may prejudice performance. Theatre times are increased initially, although they decrease as surgeons gain experience. Short-stay and 5-day wards with rapid turnover reduce 'hotel' costs, freeing main ward beds and helping to reduce waiting lists.

5 All members of the surgical team need adequate training in the techniques and care of the equipment. This has led to the establishment of minimal access therapy training units (MATTUs) offering basic and higher training courses with availability to senior surgeons trained in open surgery.

KEY POINTS Advantages and disadvantages of laparoscopy

Advantages

- Smaller incisions
- Procedures are less painful and disabling
- Decreased wound-related pathology, such as wound infection
- Decreased tissue trauma
- Decreased physiological insult to the patient when compared to open surgery
- Earlier return to full activity
- Significantly reduced stay in hospital postoperation, leading to cost-effectiveness
- Cosmetic acceptability
- Decreased contact with pathogens such as human immunodeficiency virus (HIV) and hepatitis B virus (HBV)
- The use of video records aid in the art of communication between doctors and with patients and their families. It may also help improve clinical decision-making

Disadvantages

- Lack of tactile feedback from tissues
- Bleeding is difficult to control
- Procedures may take longer, especially on the initial slope of the surgical learning curve
- Technical expertise, advice and specialist equipment are required
- Iatrogenic damage has been a greater problem following minimal access surgery than following traditional open techniques (e.g. bile duct injuries during laparoscopic cholecystectomy)

6 Increasing familiarity with the laparoscopic approach has led to its use in many situations previously contraindicated. Table 5.2 indicates common absolute and relative contraindications for laparoscopy.

Prepare

1 Patients can be admitted on the day of planned surgery. Evaluate and investigate them beforehand to decide whether they can be managed on a day-case basis.

2 Obtain informed consent, including permission to convert to open operation if necessary and quote the likely percentage of conversions. Warn patients of the possibility of experiencing postoperative shoulder tip pain and also of the possibility of developing surgical emphysema. Always explain the commonly occurring risks, how they present and how they are managed. On the other hand, reiterate at this time the likely benefits.

TABLE 5.1 Examples of minimal access operations

General surgery	Gynaecology	Others
Diagnostic laparoscopy Cholecystectomy Choledochoscopy Hernia repair Adhesiolysis Nissen fundoplication Repair of perforated duodenal ulcer Appendicectomy Excision of Meckel's diverticulum Rectopexy Splenectomy Vagotomy Colectomy	Oophorectomy Treatment of ectopic pregnancy Hysterectomy Diagnosis and ablation of endometriosis Ovarian cystectomy Myomectomy Tubal surgery Infertility treatment	Arthroscopy Minimal access urology

3 In the absence of contraindications, arrange antithrombotic prophylaxis such as low-dose heparin and compression stockings. Give prophylactic antibiotics if organs such as the gallbladder are to be removed. Bowel preparation is unnecessary.

4 Some anaesthetists prefer non-steroidal anti-inflammatory drugs rather than opiates as premedication, if necessary with the addition of short-acting benzodiazepines.

5 Equipment:

KEY POINTS Basic equipment for laparoscopy

- Baseline equipment
- Monitor
- Light source
- Insufflator
- Camera
- Diathermy

- Prefer large monitors, with good-quality, high-resolution screens, mounted on mobile trolleys, also containing the light source, insufflator and camera. Position the monitors on either side of the patient, allowing you and your assistants to view them (Fig. 5.1). You should be able to see the light source, usually xenon or halogen, and monitor the light intensity. Ensure that the patient is not at risk of burning.
- The rapid-flow insufflator supplies carbon dioxide to create and maintain the pneumoperitoneum. Have it placed so you can see the display of the intra-abdominal pressure and gas flow in response to preset pressure values. It may also incorporate a gas warmer.
- The video camera head, either a single microchip or a superior three-chip instrument, is attached to the laparoscope to form an electrical–optic interface. The camera is connected by cable to a video processor which interprets and modifies the signal and transmits it to the monitors. Most systems incorporate a 'white balance' function, which can be calibrated to represent the colours accurately.

TABLE 5.2 Contraindications to laparoscopic surgery

Absolute contraindications	Relative contraindications
Generalized peritonitis	Gross obesity. Simple overweight is no contraindication; such patients suffer less from postoperative respiratory complications than they would following open operation
Intestinal obstruction	Pregnancy
Clotting abnormalities	Multiple abdominal adhesions. Provided the first instrument port is inserted by an open technique, laparoscopy can be safely performed on patients with moderate adhesions following, for example, previous surgery
Liver cirrhosis	Organomegaly (enlarged liver or spleen)
Failure to tolerate general anaesthesia Uncontrolled shock Patient refusal	Abdominal aortic aneurysm

- The laparoscope transmits the image using a rod-lens system while the field is illuminated through fibreoptics running alongside the lens. They are usually 10 mm, or less often 5 mm, in diameter, with fields of view of 0° or 30°. For cholecystectomy a 10-mm, 0° laparoscope is usually employed.

KEY POINTS Check

- Check the function.
- Ensure that the camera operator will follow your movements and keep the area of interest in the centre of the field of view.

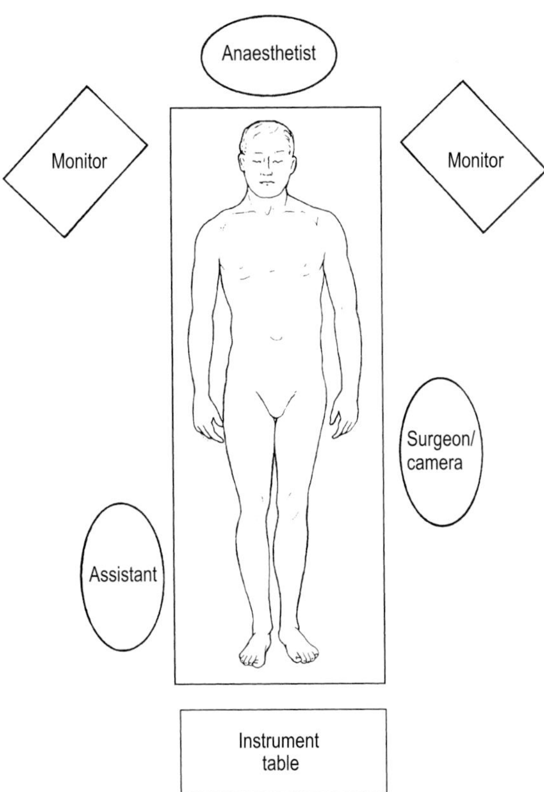

Fig. 5.1 Diagram showing the positioning of the patient, surgeon, assistant and video monitors for a laparoscopic cholecystectomy.

- Warm the laparoscope to prevent fogging of the lens. For the same reason do not insufflate cold carbon dioxide through the same port as the camera.
- Suction and irrigation are carried out through a probe connected to a pressurized reservoir and a suction source, controlled by buttons.
- The ports for insertion of instruments can be disposable or reusable. More expensive disposable ports have the advantage of being sharp, radiolucent and sterile. They may have blunt ends for open induction of pneumoperitoneum, or be fitted with a sharp, spring-loaded trocar with a plastic guard that projects beyond the point as soon as the trocar enters the peritoneal cavity. They are of a range of sizes to accommodate various instruments, but large ports can be fitted with sizers to reduce the lumen. All have attachments to allow insufflation, and valves to prevent gas leaks. Some have collars, allowing them to be secured in position (Fig. 5.2).
- In the closed method of insufflation a Veress needle is inserted. This incorporates a spring-loaded obturator that covers the sharp needle-tip as soon as it enters the peritoneal cavity. It incorporates an attachment to the gas supply (Fig. 5.3).
- A large range of graspers, staplers, dissectors, scissors and diathermy applicators have been developed—either reusable or disposable.

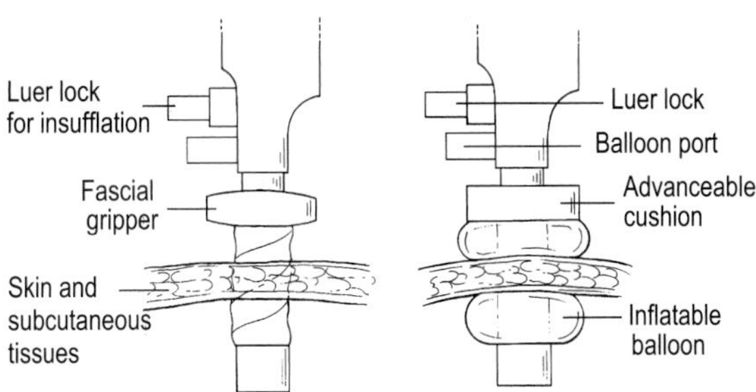

Fig. 5.2 Diagram of two types of laparoscopic port, one with a screw collar and the second with inflatable balloons. Both help to prevent gas leaks around the ports.

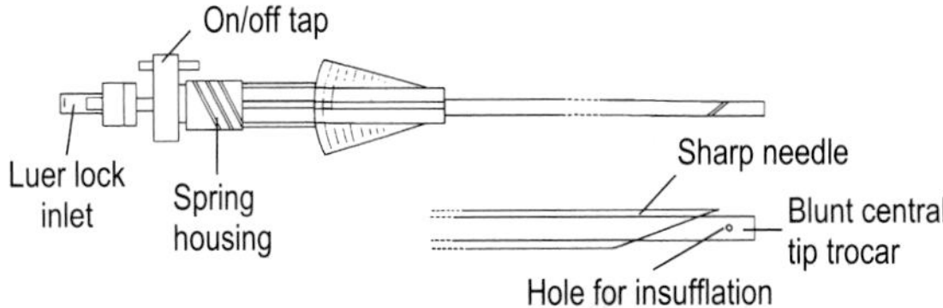

Fig. 5.3 Diagram of a Veress needle showing the device in its entirety, and the spring-loaded tip.

6 The theatre team needs to be trained and efficient, with knowledge of how the equipment functions.

7 General anaesthesia is usually augmented with muscle relaxation, intubation and ventilation so that pneumoperitoneum can be induced without causing cardiorespiratory embarrassment. The anaesthetist monitors abdominal distension and its effect on blood pressure and airways pressure throughout.

Access

1 Induce a pneumoperitoneum. The initial penetration of the abdominal cavity to produce a pneumoperitoneum can be a hazardous task in laparoscopic surgery.

> **KEY POINT Insert instruments carefully**
>
> - Careless insertion of instruments can lead to injury to underlying viscera such as bowel or bladder, or to even deeper structures such as the aorta and the vena cava.

2 Once you have established the first port you can insert additional ports in relative safety. There are open and closed methods of producing a pneumoperitoneum:

- Prefer the safe, open (Hasson) method of port insertion, especially if there has been previous surgery. Make a 1–2-cm infra-umbilical incision, deepening it to the linea alba. Incise the linea alba between two stay sutures and open the peritoneum under direct vision. The stay sutures can be tied together to close the port site at the end of the procedure, by using a box stitch (Fig. 5.4). If you have difficulty locating the linea alba in an obese patient, evert the base of the umbilical stalk upwards, using a clip. This brings the linea alba to the surface (Fig. 5.4a). Insert a finger to sweep away

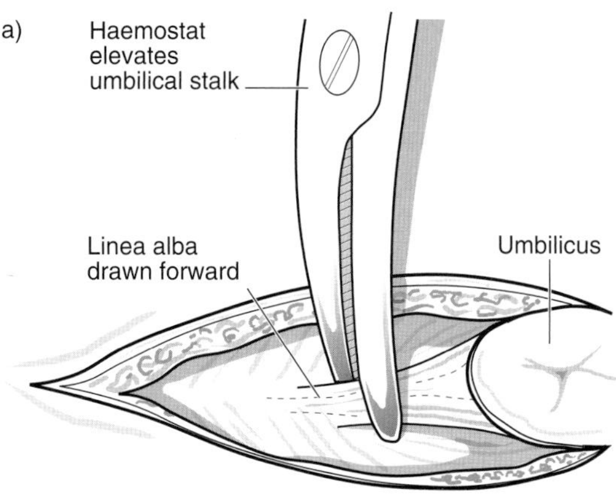

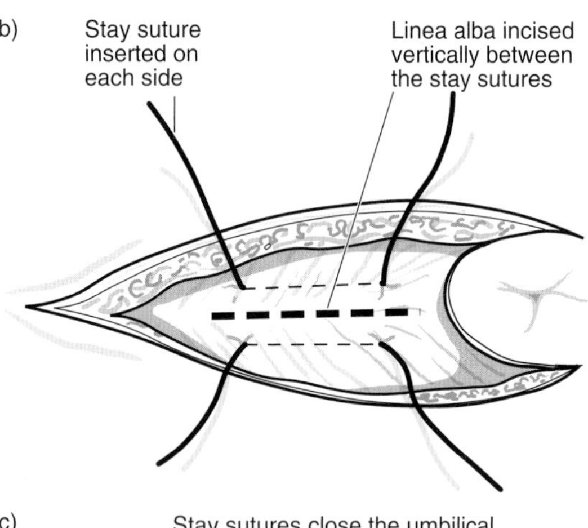

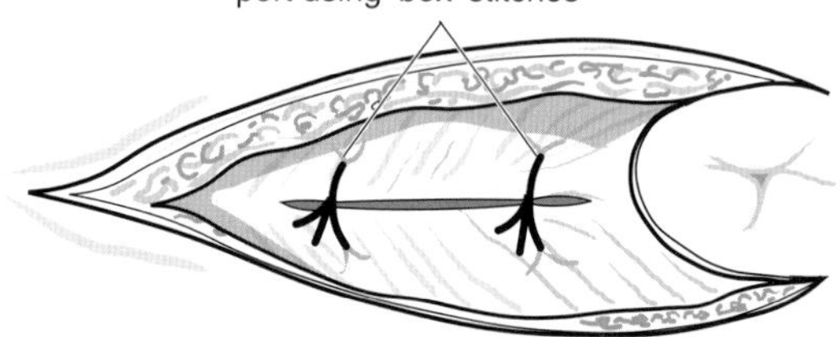

Fig. 5.4 Insertion of a Hasson port just below the umbilicus. (a) Shows the vertical incision made just below the umbilicus, dissected down to the linea alba. (b) Longitudinal absorbable stitches (Vicryl) have been inserted on each side of the midline; the vertical midline incision will be made between them through which the Hasson port will be inserted. (c) On completion and removal of the port, close the defect by tying the sutures across to produce a 'box' or 'mattress' stitch.

any adhesions around the insertion site before introducing a blunt-tipped trocar. Connect the gas supply and establish a pneumoperitoneum. The main disadvantage of this method is the increased incidence of gas leaks around the port. Special ports with sealing balloons have been developed to prevent this.

- The closed (Veress needle) technique is most commonly used. As before, make an infra-umbilical skin incision. Apply a 20–30° Trendelenburg tilt to the patient. Together with your assistant grasp the anterior abdominal wall and lift it up. Insert a Veress needle (Fig. 5.5) perpendicular to the abdominal wall until it penetrates the linea alba and the peritoneum. As soon as a 'give' is felt as the needle enters the peritoneal cavity, direct the needle downwards towards the pelvis to avoid damaging the great vessels.

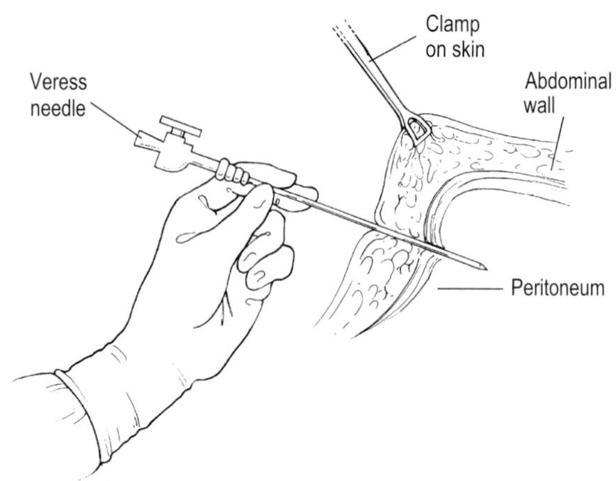

Fig. 5.5 Diagram showing a technique for inserting the Veress needle into the abdominal wall and the layers the needle passes through.

KEY POINTS Check the position of the Veress needle tip

- Is the needle freely mobile?
- Place a drop of saline on the Luer connector of the Veress needle. It should fall freely into the abdomen, where the pressure is subatmospheric.
- Aspirate to check that you do not obtain bowel content or blood.
- Inject 5 ml of saline; it should flow freely through the needle.
- Insufflate gas slowly; if the tip of the needle is within the peritoneal cavity, this should not produce a significant rise in the pressure reading.

? DIFFICULTY

If the intra-abdominal pressure rises above the preset level, an alarm usually sounds. At this point:

1. Stop insufflation.
2. Check port/needle positioning.
3. Check that the gas tubing is not obstructed and that the control taps are on.
4. If there has been too much gas introduced into the abdomen, let some gas out via one of the ports.
5. Liaise with the anaesthetist in case there has been a loss of muscle relaxation.

3 When the abdomen is fully distended and tympanitic to percussion, withdraw the Veress needle and enlarge the superficial part of the incision to accommodate the cannula. Insert a 10-mm trocar and cannula, aiming the tip anterior to the sacral promontory, parallel to the aorta. Use a drilling action from the wrist while lifting up the abdominal wall below the insertion site. Withdraw the trocar, insert the laparoscope and connect it to the insufflator. Observe the view as you insert it to ensure the viscera are not at risk. Inspect the abdomen to identify structures that could be potentially damaged when the other ports are inserted. Secure the port either using a threaded collar or with stay sutures.

4 Insert additional ports under direct vision. You may first infiltrate the tissues with local anaesthetic prior to incision. The sites, size and number are determined by the intended procedure. Each trocar and cannula is inserted while your assistant moves the camera to provide a view so you do not spear the viscera or vessels. Secure the ports with threaded collars or stay sutures.

Assess

1 Now survey the abdomen prior to performing the procedure. Be systematic in identifying landmarks and inspecting the relevant area. Locate the ligamentum teres and falciform ligament. In the right upper quadrant visualize the liver, gallbladder and the underside of the right hemidiaphragm. Now manipulate the laparoscope under the ligamentum teres to look at the left lobe of the liver and the spleen. Change the patient's position to aid visualization by moving the bowel. Inspect both the left and right paracolic gutters, facilitating the exposure by inserting a probe or grasper to manipulate the bowel if necessary.

2 Place the patient in the Trendelenburg position to locate the caecum and appendix. Insert an endoscopic grasper to manoeuvre the bowel while you examine it from distal to proximal. While the patient is in the head-down position examine the pelvis; this is especially important in female patients when they have lower abdominal pain of unknown cause. You can directly visualize the ovaries, uterus and vermiform appendix.

3 In order to inspect organs such as the pancreas, additional manipulation and dissection may be necessary. Diseases such as Hodgkin's can be staged, and masses biopsied.

Diathermy

1 Carefully identify the correct structure. The most common injury results from misidentification and hence burning the wrong structure.

KEY POINT Beware diathermy burns

- Diathermy used during laparoscopic surgery to achieve haemostasis, along with sutures and clips, can cause unrecognized, inadvertent, even fatal injury.

2 Inadvertent activation of the diathermy pedal risks damaging other structures in the abdominal cavity, especially when the electrode is outside the field of view.

3 Faulty insulation, especially when using old instruments subjected to abrasive cleaning, creates a conducting surface other than the electrode to come into contact with a viscus. If burning does not directly cause a perforation, it may lead to autodigestion and perforation at a later date.

4 Current may flow from the active electrode to a contiguous conducting instrument; this is an example of direct coupling. The result is poor function at the active electrode and an unnoticed burn from the second instrument.

5 After use, diathermy electrodes can remain sufficiently hot to cause burns. After use, withdraw the electrode or keep it in view.

6 As in open surgery, diathermy of a pedicle concentrates the current density and so can lead to inadvertent perforation of structures, such as the common bile duct, during laparoscopic cholecystectomy.

7 Alternating currents can pass through insulating materials, as occurs in devices called capacitors. During laparoscopy a capacitor may be inadvertently formed so current induced in a metal port then flows into neighbouring bowel and causes a burn. Avoid capacitative coupling by using a non-conducting electrode. If you are using a metal port ensure that it makes good contact with the abdominal wall. Avoid open-circuit activation, and high-voltage diathermy, such as fulguration.

Closure

1 Before removing the ports, ensure that haemostasis is complete and that there are no free bodies in the abdomen such as spilt gallstones. Remove all laparoscopic instruments and ports under direct vision while checking for port-site bleeding. Make sure no intra-abdominal structures have become trapped in the ports or port sites. Remove the final port slowly, with the laparoscope still inside to finally check.

2 Palpate the abdomen, helping to expel any remaining carbon dioxide, then close the port holes. Identify and grasp the fascia with toothed forceps. Use interrupted absorbable synthetic sutures such as polyglactin 910 (Vicryl) or polydioxanone (PDS). Take care not to pick up bowel with the stitch. Close the skin with either absorbable or non-absorbable sutures.

Postoperative

1 Monitor all patients as following an open laparotomy, with regular observations. Remind them of referred shoulder tip pain from stretching of the peritoneum lining the hemidiaphragms following pneumoperitoneum. Mobilize patients early and encourage them to eat and drink.

2 Most patients can be discharged within 24 hours of laparoscopy; the length of stay increases with more extensive procedures. Some surgeons now perform day-case laparoscopic cholecystectomy.

Complications

Since laparoscopic surgery usually requires a general anaesthetic, patients are susceptible to the usual complications related to this. Table 5.3 lists complications common to laparoscopy and pneumoperitoneum.

TABLE 5.3 Some complications common to laparoscopy and pneumoperitoneum

During pneumoperitoneum induction	Related to port placement	During procedure	Patient-related complications
Damage to viscus or vessels	Damage to underlying structures	Diathermy-related injuries	Obesity: makes operation more difficult, increasing operating time, and may require special instruments
Misplacement of the gas	Be poorly placed	Inadvertent organ ligation or division	Ascites causes oozing from port sites, increasing the risk of port-site damage
Insufflation of the bowel lumen	Haemorrhage	Unrecognized haemorrhage	Organomegaly increases the risk of organ damage
Carbon dioxide embolus and metabolic acidosis may complicate pneumoperitoneum	Herniation		Clotting problems may result in haemorrhage, or conversely in deep vein thrombosis
Over-insufflation of the peritoneal cavity may cause cardiorespiratory problems			Following operation for malignant disease, cancer cells may be transferred to the port site, resulting in metastases

FURTHER READING

Cuschieri A 1989 The laparoscopic revolution: walk carefully before we can run. Journal of the Royal College of Surgeons of Edinburgh 34:295

Darzi A, 2004 Minimal access surgery. In: Kirk RM, Ribbans WJ (eds) Clinical surgery in general, 4th edn. Churchill Livingstone, Edinburgh, pp 237–240

Darzi A, Monson JRT 1994 Laparoscopic inguinal hernia repair. ISIS Medical Media, Oxford

Darzi A, Talamini M, Dunn DC 1997 Atlas of laparoscopic surgical technique. Saunders, London

Hall F 1994 Minimal access surgery for operating room and theatre personnel. Radcliffe Medical Press, Oxford

Hasson HM 1971 Modified instrument method for laparoscopy. American Journal of Obstetrics and Gynecology 110:886–887

Lee VS 1993 Complications of laparoscopic cholecystectomy. American Journal of Surgery 165:527–532

Phillips K 1994 Minimally invasive surgery. British Journal of Theatre Nursing 3:4–8

Phipps JH 1993 Laparoscopic hysterectomy and oophorectomy. Churchill Livingstone, Edinburgh

Reichert M 1993 Laparoscopic instruments, patient care, cost issues. AORN Journal 57:637–655

Rosin RD 1993 Minimal access medicine and surgery: principles and techniques. Radcliffe Medical Press, Oxford

6

Hernias and abdominal wall

D.F.L. Watkin, G.S.M. Robertson

CONTENTS

GENERAL ISSUES IN HERNIA SURGERY

1 Consider whether there is another cause for the patient's symptoms. Groin pain may be due to osteoarthrosis of the hip or a groin strain, rather than the obvious inguinal hernia. Epigastric pain may be biliary colic or a symptom of peptic ulcer and not a consequence of the epigastric hernia.

2 Make sure that patients who come for operation on the day of admission are thoroughly checked beforehand, know what is involved, have consented to operation and understand the circumstances under which it will be performed. They must also know about discharge arrangements.

3 The hernia may not be evident in the anaesthetized patient so it is essential that the site (and side) are marked preoperatively.

4 When prosthetic mesh is to be used for the repair, many surgeons give a prophylactic dose of antibiotic at induction and may use topical antibiotics. This must be administered in operations for strangulated hernia, because the wound may be contaminated.

5 Local anaesthesia is suitable for the repair of many groin hernias and some other hernias but is less well tolerated in young adults, who may require the addition of sedation. There are economic benefits in its use and it is particularly advantageous in the day-case setting and in the elderly. However, it is not devoid of risk and the following general considerations apply:

- The blood pressure, pulse rate and oxygen saturation should be monitored.
- Make sure you know the appropriate procedures for resuscitation in case the patient develops an adverse reaction.
- For effective anaesthesia a sufficient volume is needed; our preference is for 0.5% lidocaine with adrenaline (epinephrine) 1 in 100 000. Alternatively, bupivacaine (0.25%) may be used but it acts more slowly. Some surgeons use a mixture of lidocaine and bupivacaine.
- Decide which local anaesthetic you are going to use for hernia operations and stick to it to avoid confusion.
- Do not exceed the safe dose of local anaesthetic; for lidocaine with adrenaline (epinephrine) this is 70 mg lidocaine per kg, approximating for an average adult to 500 mg, equivalent to 100 ml of a 0.5% solution.
- Clearly record the dose of local anaesthetic and other drugs in the notes.

6 Non-absorbable sutures on curved, round-bodied, eyeless needles should always be used for the repair. Monofilament materials minimize the risk of persistence of a wound infection, polyamide (nylon) and polypropylene being the most popular. Remember that monofilament sutures require extra knots for security. Steel wire is now rarely used because it is difficult to handle.

7 Handle the synthetic monofilament suture material with great care. Do not hold it with instruments, or jerk it when tying knots, or you will seriously weaken it.

8 Do not drag the fine suture through the tissues, since it will cut them, enlarging the holes.

9 Do not tie the sutures too tightly. They will either cut out now or strangulate the tissues and weaken them later and may also increase the risk of troublesome neuralgia.

10 Do not take even bites of the tissues. Although this looks neat, evenly inserted stitches tend to detach a strip of aponeurosis. Therefore take successive bites at differing distances from the edge.

11 Skin closure may be with sutures, clips, staples or adhesive strips. However, a continuous subcuticular absorbable stitch (e.g. polyglactin 910) provides a very neat result and avoids the discomfort and cost of suture removal.

12 Postoperative analgesia is particularly important in day-case work, but also for inpatients discharged the following morning. For patients in whom there is no contraindication (particularly asthma or peptic ulcer), discuss with your anaesthetist the

administration of rectal diclofenac in theatre, but remember that the patient's prior consent is needed. Postoperatively a regular oral dose of diclofenac 50 mg t.d.s. for 2 days, plus co-codamol as required, provides good pain control.

13 Wound complications:

- Bruising and haematoma formation may be reduced by meticulous haemostasis and judicious use of suction drains.
- Wound infection rarely requires more than drainage of any collection. Sinus formation is rare with the use of monofilament sutures but occasionally requires removal of suture knots or mesh.

14 Recurrence appears to be related to technical failures, including missing a hernia and inadequate placement or size of mesh.

15 Outpatient follow-up provides valuable information on wound infections and other local complications such as numbness or pain. It is not feasible to offer the long-term surveillance necessary to monitor recurrence rates.

Use of prosthetic mesh in hernia repair

1 Following the introduction of prosthetic biomaterials for hernia repair in the 1950s and the description by Lichtenstein of their use in groin hernias in the 1980s, their use has become commonplace worldwide. There is little doubt that they often make hernia surgery quicker and easier, reducing recurrence rates. There are now many materials available with several factors influencing choice.[1]

2 Strength/stiffness results not only from the intrinsic strength of the mesh, often related to the density of prosthetic material, but also from the resulting ingrowth of fibrosis which is greater with smaller pore sizes.

3 Flexibility/elasticity: meshes should be flexible enough to conform to the abdominal wall movements on a long-term basis. It is increasingly apparent that current polypropylene meshes may be unnecessarily strong, resulting in pain and the sensation of stiffness when compared with lighter-weight open-weave or compound meshes (Vypro, Ethicon).[2]

4 Size and shape: shrinkage occurs with all prostheses as part of the process of scar maturation. It makes a minimum overlap of the hernial defect by the mesh of 2–3 cm essential for initial fixation and long-term coverage. Various preformed meshes are now available for some hernia sites.

5 Expense in many countries limits the use of mesh.

6 Adhesion formation remains a problem, particularly with intraperitoneal implantation. The use of two-sided meshes with one side engendering tissue ingrowth and the other inhibiting it (DualMesh, Gore) is one way of reducing this risk.

7 Infection: the use of systemic prophylactic antibiotics probably reduces the risk of wound infection.[3] Some meshes incorporate antimicrobial agents.

REFERENCES

1. Schumpelick V, Klinge U 2003 Prosthetic implants for hernia repair. British Journal of Surgery 90:1457–1458
2. Post S, Weiss B, Willer M et al 2004 Randomised clinical trial of lightweight composite mesh for Lichtenstein inguinal hernia repair. British Journal of Surgery 91:44–48
3. Taylor EW, Duffy K, Lee K et al 2004 Surgical site infection after groin hernia repair. British Journal of Surgery 91:105–111

INGUINAL HERNIA

Appraise

1 In the past, indirect hernias were usually repaired; diffuse direct hernias were treated with a truss. Now it is customary to operate on most inguinal hernias. The only reasons not to operate are trivial direct hernias in elderly, inactive or terminally ill patients and those who will not consent. The few who do not have an operation are generally best left without a truss, which is uncomfortable and difficult to manage.

2 In a very obese patient with a large, diffuse direct hernia, defer operation until the patient has lost weight, or consider laparoscopic repair.

3 Local anaesthesia has many advantages for inguinal hernia repair.[1] It is used increasingly, resulting in shorter stay and reduced cost.

4 Bilateral hernias may be repaired at the same time. The results may not be quite so good as when they are repaired separately, but this has to be set against the economic advantage to the patient and the service. Do not hesitate to repair a large hernia on one side, deferring repair of the other side until later. Dose limits preclude local anaesthesia for bilateral repair. Laparoscopic repair is a good option.

5 Many surgeons accept the challenge of repairing recurrent diffuse hernias in obese patients with stretched, fat-infiltrated tissues or with chronic coughs. We are reluctant to do so. These patients are not at risk of strangulation and recurrence is likely following repair. As a trainee, do not embark on these operations.

6 Surgeons often attribute their excellent results to particular details of their technique, but the common factor that produces their success is the perfection with which the procedure is accomplished. For this reason, do not attempt to acquire mastery of all the techniques but become familiar with a small range that will deal with most demands.

7 Individual surgeons have achieved low recurrence rates using sutured methods of repair of the posterior wall of the inguinal canal, bringing the conjoint tendon to the inguinal ligament, with or without a relaxing incision in the rectus sheath (Tanner's slide), or overlapping the transversalis fascia (Shouldice repair). Indeed, the Shouldice Clinic in Toronto has the lowest recorded recurrence rate—less than 1%. Others employed a darn to reinforce the posterior wall. The development of laparoscopic repair of groin hernias in the early 1990s prompted a reappraisal of open technique and overall recurrence rates were found to be approaching 10%. In a systematic review, open mesh repair was followed by fewer recurrences than sutured repair, while the Shouldice repair performed better than other non-mesh methods.[2] The widely used darn repair has been abandoned. The Shouldice method has a relatively long learning curve, so the Lichtenstein mesh repair has been adopted by the majority of surgeons, particularly for training, as it has a similarly low recurrence rate and is simpler. The latter two techniques will be described.

8 Warn the patient of the possible complications of haematoma (especially for large inguinoscrotal hernias), ischaemic orchitis and persistent groin pain.

9 Laparoscopic repair of groin hernias (see Ch. 7) is currently in competition with the open or 'anterior' approach and at this stage there is no clear winner. In clinical trials, the laparoscopic operation has been associated with slightly less postoperative pain and a rather more rapid return to work but higher hospital costs.[3] There is also a very small risk of serious injury to the intestine or the major blood vessels. The open operation has the advantage of being feasible under local anaesthesia. Our, conservative, view is that the majority of primary groin hernias should continue to be repaired by the anterior approach but some patients may choose laparoscopic repair in the interest of a more rapid return to work. The laparoscopic operation is quicker for bilateral hernias, while for recurrent hernias the dissection is in virgin territory, avoiding the need to separate adherent tissue planes in the inguinal canal.

Inspect

1 The diagnosis of groin swellings is notoriously difficult. Experienced as well as inexperienced surgeons make frequent mistakes. Do not accept the diagnosis of the referring doctor, but take a fresh history and carry out a complete examination. Is there another possible cause for the patient's symptoms, apart from the hernia? If a clear history of a reducible intermittent lump in the groin is accompanied by a negative examination, a hernia will be found on exploration; if in doubt consider herniography.

2 Palpation is not the only, or even the most important, method of examination. Look with the patient standing and again with the patient supine. If you see a lump, ask yourself 'Where is it?' If it is reducible, where does it first reappear on coughing or straining? Apart from obstructed and strangulated hernia, a cough impulse may be absent, especially over a femoral hernia in which a small sac is covered by much fatty extraperitoneal tissue. Conversely, a cough impulse is present over Malgaigne's bulgings or a saphena varix.

3 Never fail to examine the scrotum and its contents in male patients. If there is a swelling, ask yourself the fundamental question, 'Can I get above it?' Occasionally undescended testes will be diagnosed and should be addressed at the same procedure.

4 Finally, examine the other hernial orifices.

Prepare

1 Many operations can be performed on a day-case basis in fit people who have good home circumstances. Bilateral procedures (unless done laparoscopically) and operations in unfit or elderly patients or those who live alone require overnight or 48-hour stay.

2 Observe general issues (pp. 75–76).

Local anaesthesia for inguinal hernia repair

1 Follow the instructions for local anaesthesia (p. 75). Remember the maximum dose (e.g. 100 ml of lidocaine 0.5% with adrenaline (epinephrine)).

2 Inject 20 ml along the line of the proposed incision using a fine needle to raise a continuous bleb within the epidermis.

3 Replace the needle with a larger one to inject deeply and along the same line superficial to the anterior wall of the canal.

4 Blunt the needle to improve the 'feel' of passage through the aponeurosis and inject 5 ml of fluid 2 cm above and medial to the anterior superior iliac spine deep to the external oblique to block the iliohypogastric and ilioinguinal nerves.

5 Reserve about half the anaesthetic to inject under the external oblique, around the neck of the sac and into other sensitive areas during the operation.

Access

1 Start the incision a finger's breadth above the palpable pubic tubercle within the skin crease which is often present (as opposed to parallel to the inguinal ligament) and extend this to two-thirds of the way to the anterior superior iliac spine. Incise the fascia to expose the external oblique aponeurosis, ligating and dividing two or three large veins that cross the line of the incision. Avoid cutting into the hernial sac and spermatic cord at the medial end of the incision.

2 Expose the glistening fibres of the external oblique aponeurosis and identify the external inguinal ring, which confirms the line of the inguinal canal.

3 Make a short split with a knife in the line of the fibres of the external oblique aponeurosis over the inguinal canal. Enlarge the split medially and laterally by pushing the half-closed blades of the scissors in the line of the fibres. At the medial end of the split, the external inguinal ring will be opened; be sure to enter the external ring and do not allow the curved blades of the scissors to skirt around outside its crura. Preserve the ilioinguinal nerve lying under the external oblique, to minimize the risk of postoperative numbness and pain.

4 Apply artery forceps to the edges of the aponeurosis and gently elevate each side. As the upper leaf is turned back, look for the arching lower border of internal oblique muscle, with the cord below it. As the lower leaf is everted, sweep loose tissue from the deep surface of the inguinal ligament.

Assess (Fig. 6.1)

KEY POINT Confirm the diagnosis

- Do not rely on preoperative findings of the type of inguinal hernia; determine this during mobilization.

1 Start to mobilize the cord by incising, just above and lateral to the public tubercle, the 'mesentery' of fascia and fibres of cremasteric muscle that extends downwards from the medial part of the conjoint tendon to envelop the cord. Deepen this small incision behind the cord, drawing the latter downwards while passing the index finger from below against the pubic tubercle, to develop a plane to encircle the cord and apply a hernia ring.

2 Now dislocate the cord laterally and downwards by incising the coverings along lines just above and below it. This exposes a direct hernia, which can be freed from the cord.

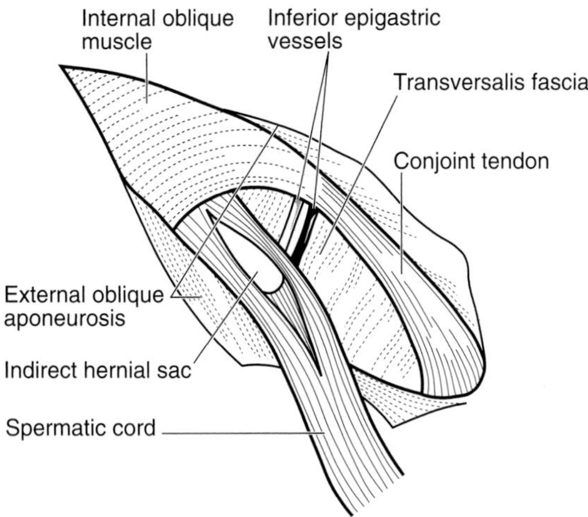

Fig. 6.1 Exposure of the right inguinal canal. The cremasteric fascia is split to show an indirect hernial sac.

3 Carefully divide the fibres of cremaster just distal to the internal ring, ensuring haemostasis.

4 Even though a direct hernia is evident, examine the cord. Normally it is about the thickness of a pencil. It is markedly distended by an unreduced, sometimes adherent, or sliding, hernia. A thickened sac results from a longstanding indirect hernia. Cord lipomata produce thickening, as does an encysted hydrocele of the cord (in females a hydrocele of the canal of Nuck). To exclude an indirect sac, open the spermatic fascia covering the cord and identify the edge of the peritoneum deep to the internal ring.

5 Identify the lower arching fibres of the internal oblique muscle, becoming tendinous at the conjoint tendon, and examine the posterior wall below this. A direct hernia may be a large bulge, a diffuse weakness of the whole posterior wall or, less often, a funicular hernia through a small localized defect (Ogilvie's hernia). If you are in real doubt, ask the anaesthetist to temporarily increase intra-abdominal pressure while you watch for distension and bulging.

6 If there is concern that a femoral hernia may be present, incise the transversalis fascia (as in a Shouldice repair) to expose the upper aspect of the femoral canal. If a femoral sac is present, deal with it as a Lothiesen procedure (see later).

7 The cremasteric vessels pass medially from the inferior epigastric vessels adjacent to the cord. If the internal ring is enlarged it may be necessary to carefully identify, isolate, ligate and then divide the cremasteric vessels to facilitate a snug repair at the internal ring. If they are injured more medially, ligate them proximally and distally to the damage.

Hernial sac

Indirect sac

1 With the left thumb in front, gently stretch the previously mobilized cord over the left index finger, which is placed behind the cord. Make a short split with a knife, in the line of the cord, through the cremasteric and internal spermatic fascial layers. Continue the split proximally to the internal ring using scissors, first with their blades on the flat, separating fascia from deeper layers, then splitting the fascia.

2 Look for the sac. A white curved edge may be seen if the hernial sac is small (Fig. 6.1); if it is large it will be obvious as the fascial layers are separated. Using the point of the scalpel, gently incise the fibres crossing the fundus or the side edges of the sac. Unless it is very adherent it will then be possible to peel the sac out of the cord, with the aid of a few further strokes of the blade. The sac is then dissected back to the level of the abdominal peritoneum, using a combination of wiping with a gauze swab and snipping firm attachments with scissors. Keep the dissection close to the sac and avoid damaging other structures in the cord.

3 Pick up the sac with two artery forceps and open it between the forceps with a knife. Note any contents of the sac and return them to the peritoneal cavity. Adherent omentum may be freed, or ligated and excised.

4 While the empty sac is held vertically by means of the artery forceps, transfix its neck with a polyglactin (Vicryl) suture. Tie the ends of the suture-ligature into a half hitch, completely encircle the neck of the sac and tie a triple-throw knot to ligate the neck of the sac. If contents tend to bulge into the sac, gently hold them back using non-toothed dissecting forceps, sliding them out as the ligature is tightened.

5 Do not let your assistant cut the ends of the ligature. First excise the sac 1 cm distal to the ligature. Examine the cut end to ensure that only sac is seen, it does not bleed and the suture is secure, then cut the ligature yourself. The stump of the sac should retract through the internal ring.

6 Alternatively the sac may, after full mobilization, simply be inverted. The sac need not be ligated for this.

7 If there are large extraperitoneal lipomata, carefully isolate, ligate and excise them but do not try to dissect out all the fatty tissue

Large sac

1 Complete hernias, or scrotal funicular hernias, have no distal edge to the sac as seen at the level of the pubic tubercle. Attempts to dissect out the whole sac cause the scrotal part of the sac and the testis to be drawn into the wound, increasing the risk of haematoma or ischaemic orchitis.

2 Purposefully divide the sac straight across within the inguinal canal. Isolate the proximal portion up to the internal ring, and leave the distal portion open. In this way the dissection is kept to a minimum.

3 If the sac is adherent, open the sac in front and place artery forceps at intervals round the inside as markers. Lift up two forceps, stretch the portion of sac between them, separate the sac from the cord and cut it distal to the forceps. Take the next two forceps and repeat the manoeuvre. Continue in this manner until the proximal circumference of the sac is completely sectioned, with the edges still held in the forceps.

4 After stripping the proximal part of the sac to the inguinal ring, transfix and ligate the neck.

5 Leave the distal part of the sac open.

SLIDING HERNIA

1 In some hernias, retroperitoneal structures slide down to form part of the sac wall, chiefly the sigmoid colon, bladder or caecum. Always be on the look-out for sliding hernia.

2 The slide is discovered when you attempt to empty and free the sac.

3 If the sac is intact, do not open it. If the sac has been opened, mark the fringe of peritoneum on the viscus with artery forceps and close the sac. Ensure that closure is complete.

4 Make sure that neither the organ nor its blood supply was damaged before the true situation was recognized. If the bladder was damaged, repair the wall and remember to insert an indwelling urethral catheter at the end of the operation.

5 The entire hernia sac and sliding viscus should be fully mobilized from the cord and replaced in the abdomen. However, if the sac is inguinoscrotal, divide and close it below the sliding viscus and replace both in the abdomen.

6 Carry out the best possible repair of the posterior wall of the inguinal canal.

HERNIA IN INFANTS

1 Infants' tissues are not suitable for handling by impatient or rough surgeons.

2 Make an incision in the skin crease just above the superficial inguinal ring. The well-developed deep fascia is easily mistaken for the external oblique aponeurosis.

3 The internal and external rings are almost superimposed in infants and it is therefore unnecessary to split the external oblique aponeurosis.

4 Isolate the cord just distal to the external ring, open the external fascial layers of the cord longitudinally and look for the sac. Pick up each layer with two pairs of fine artery forceps and open it between the forceps in the line of the cord. A short sac can be recognized by the white curved distal edge. The easy movement of the slippery internal surfaces of a large sac helps in identifying it. Make sure you are in the correct layer. When the sac is opened, the inner wall is shiny and the tips of the forceps can be passed into the peritoneal cavity.

5 Take great care in dissecting the fragile sac proximally; avoid tearing or splitting it or damaging the inconspicuous and adherent vas deferens. The sight of extraperitoneal fat confirms that the neck has been reached. If the hernia is complete (i.e. it extends down to the testis), do not dissect it distally. Carefully free it circumferentially just distal to the external ring, either from the outside if it is unopened or from within if it is open. Transect the sac, leave the distal end open and dissect the proximal sac. At the external ring, transfix, ligate and divide the neck of the sac. Do not twist the sac, because the vas may be inadvertently twisted with it and damaged.

6 If the external ring has been stretched by a large hernia, narrow it with one or two absorbable synthetic stitches. No other repair is necessary in an infant.

7 Close the subcutaneous layers with fine absorbable sutures. Close the skin with a fine absorbable subcuticular suture.

INGUINAL HERNIA IN WOMEN

1 The approach is similar to that employed in men.

2 The round ligament of the uterus lies in the position of the male spermatic cord. Ligate and excise it at the level of the internal ring to allow closure of the latter.

3 Recognize and isolate the sac, then transfix, ligate and divide it at its neck.

4 If the hernial sac is small, herniotomy is sufficient, combined with closure of the internal ring. For a larger hernia, repair the posterior wall as in a male.

DIRECT HERNIA

1 Always look for an indirect sac.

2 If the direct sac is funicular, resulting from a localized defect in the posterior wall, isolate it, empty it, then transfix, ligate and divide it at the neck. Define the margins of the posterior wall defect. If the hole is small and it can be closed without tension, suture it now, with non-absorbable material on a fine, curved, round-bodied needle.

3 More often the sac is diffuse and associated with a general weakness of the posterior wall; do not open it. If a Lichtenstein repair is to be employed, push it inwards and maintain the invagination by a running suture, of 2/0 polypropylene or polyglactin 910, carried across the stretched transversalis fascia so as to flatten the bulge without tension. The sutures must not bite deeply or the bowel or bladder may be damaged. If a Shouldice repair is to be used, excise any excess of transversalis fascia when preparing the flaps for overlapping.

4 Carry out a suitable repair of the posterior wall of the canal.

COMBINED DIRECT AND INDIRECT HERNIA

1 Such hernias protrude on either side of the inferior epigastric vessels. They are sometimes likened to the legs of pantaloons.

2 In a few cases, a direct funicular sac can be manoeuvred laterally so both sacs emerge lateral to the vessels and can be dealt with together.

3 Do not struggle to achieve this, but deal with each sac separately.

? DIFFICULTY

1. If you cannot find the sac or recognize the tissues, first find the vas deferens, which can be felt as a string-like structure towards the back of the cord. The testicular vessels lie near the vas and, once these are separated, the rest of the cord may be cautiously divided, starting at the front, while keeping in mind that abdominal organs may be encountered. If a structure seems to be the sac, cautiously open it after tenting a portion between two artery forceps. Look for a glistening inner surface and insert a finger to determine if the sac communicates with the peritoneal cavity.
2. *Torn neck of sac?* Carefully free peritoneum from the abdomen to form a new neck.

REPAIR

1 In an infant, child or adolescent with a small indirect hernia, herniotomy is all that is required.

2 If the margins of the internal ring have been stretched by an indirect hernia, narrow the gap in the posterior wall using a non-absorbable suture to approximate the attenuated margins of the transversalis fascia medial to the cord. This is one of the effects of a Shouldice repair.

3 Repairs to the posterior wall in general use are of two types:

- Tissues are brought in from the margins to strengthen the posterior wall. In the classic Bassini repair, the lower fibres of the internal oblique and transversus abdominis muscles, with their medial aponeuroses, are sutured to the inguinal ligament behind the cord. The Shouldice repair is a development of this theme. Other methods, such as Halstead's, which placed the external oblique aponeurosis behind the cord, are now of interest only when found at operation for recurrence.
- Natural or artificial material may be inserted as a sheet to bridge the defect. The insert must be large so as to overlap normal tissue and form a strong fibrous union with it, otherwise the repair will fail. This is exemplified by the Lichtenstein repair. Additionally or alternatively, a mesh 'plug' may be inserted into the defect.[4] The use of a darn of nylon or polypropylene to reinforce the posterior wall has largely been abandoned because of a high recurrence rate.

LICHTENSTEIN REPAIR

The Lichtenstein repair[5] employs a sheet of polypropylene mesh covering the posterior wall of the inguinal canal and extending, for security, over adjacent structures, with a hole to transmit the cord. It is a 'tension-free repair'.

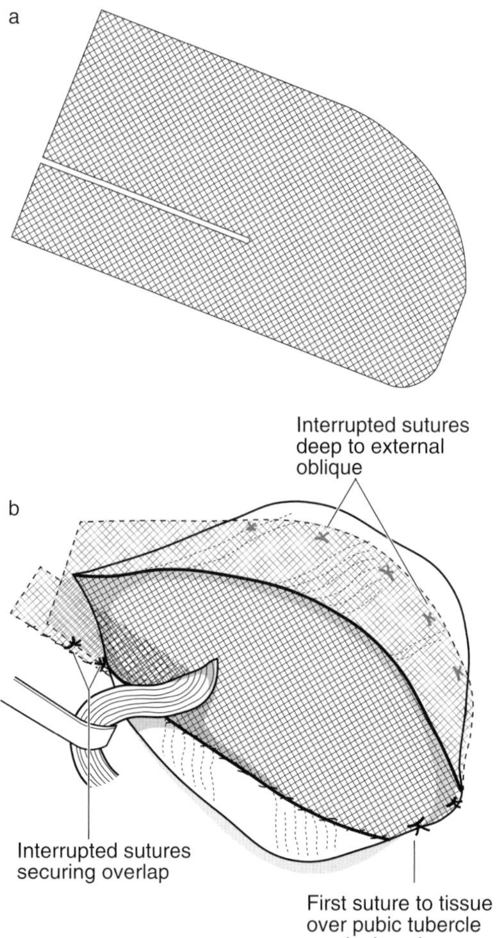

Fig. 6.2 Lichtenstein repair: (a) mesh cut to shape; (b) mesh sutured in place.

Action

1 Expose the inguinal canal and fully mobilize the cord. If there is an indirect sac deal with it as described previously. If there is a substantial direct bulge this may first be plicated so as to invert the excess, but the suture line should be placed so as not to create tension.

2 The mesh should have overall dimensions of 11 cm×6 cm. To accommodate this, the external oblique aponeurosis must be separated from the deeper layers superiorly and medially and from the muscular part of internal oblique laterally to create an adequate pocket to receive the mesh.

3 Prepare the polypropylene mesh as indicated in Fig. 6.2a. The lower medial corner is slightly rounded, the upper medial corner rather more so. The mesh is then incised from its lateral margin, placing the cut one-third of the distance from the lower edge. The cut extends for approximately half the length of the mesh, depending upon the size of the patient; it may need to be extended when the mesh is in place (Step 7). In small patients the upper edge may need to be trimmed slightly.

4 Place the mesh in its final position (Fig. 6.2b). Lift the cord and bring the narrow lower tail through under it, below the internal ring. Then tuck the lateral end under the external oblique; the lower edge of the mesh now lies along the inguinal ligament. Now insert the upper two-thirds of the mesh so that it lies under the external oblique aponeurosis superiorly and medially, ensuring that there is a good overlap on the rectus sheath medially. Tuck the wide upper tail under the external oblique laterally, with its lower edge over the lower tail. Insert your fingers under external oblique superiorly and laterally to ensure that the mesh lies quite flat in the peripheral part of the pocket, though there may be a slight bulge centrally.

5 Start the fixation by passing a 2/0 polypropylene stitch through the mesh and the tissues overlying the pubic tubercle and tying this. Use this to form a continuous suture between the lower edge of the mesh and the inguinal ligament, working from medial to lateral, extending to at least 2 cm lateral to the internal ring. Take irregular bites of the inguinal ligament to avoid splitting it and do not allow the lower leaf of external oblique to roll in and be included in the sutures; if this happens, there will be no external oblique left to close. For the medial part of this suture line it is best to retract the cord downwards. Then as the suture approaches the internal ring, move the cord cephalad and pass the needle under it to continue laterally. When suturing immediately in front of the femoral vessels be careful to take only the ligament and not a bite of a major vessel!

6 If the slit in the mesh is too short it should be extended so that the cord passes directly from the internal ring to the opening in the mesh. A bulky cord may be accommodated by making a small cut in the mesh at right-angles to the slit. If too long a cut has been made, all is not lost; simply shorten the slit with one or two sutures.

7 Overlap the tails of the mesh by bringing the lower edge of the upper portion in front of the lower tail and securing it to the inguinal ligament with two interrupted sutures (or by including it in the lateral part of the continuous suture). The resulting opening in the mesh should be a snug, but not a tight, fit around the cord (Fig. 6.2b).

8 The medial and upper margins of the mesh are then secured with about six interrupted sutures, avoiding the nerves (Fig. 6.2b). These are most conveniently placed 0.5 cm away from the edge, so that the mesh lies flat on the underlying aponeurosis or muscle. The medial sutures are particularly important as there is less overlapping of the mesh there, making it a potential site for recurrence.

9 The mesh repair is now completed. It appears slightly redundant centrally but that does not matter.

KEY POINT Sound repair?

- Provided there is sufficient overlap medially, superiorly and laterally, with a good suture line inferiorly, the fibrosis induced by the polypropylene (Prolene) mesh will produce a sound result.

10 Replace the cord in the inguinal canal.

11 Close the external oblique aponeurosis with a synthetic absorbable suture, starting laterally and ending medially to re-form the external ring snugly but not tightly around the emerging cord. Once again, take care to take bites at unequal distances from the edges, otherwise you will pull from the cut edges a strip of aponeurosis.

12 Appose the subcutaneous fascia with fine absorbable stitches and close the skin wound (see above).

SHOULDICE REPAIR (Fig. 6.3)[1]

The results obtained at the Shouldice Clinic in Toronto are outstanding, with recurrence rates below 1%, but this has not always been the case in other series, probably because the technique is difficult to learn. It has generally been superseded by the Lichtenstein repair, but some surgeons still use it for young adults, or when mesh is unavailable or bowel resection is required.

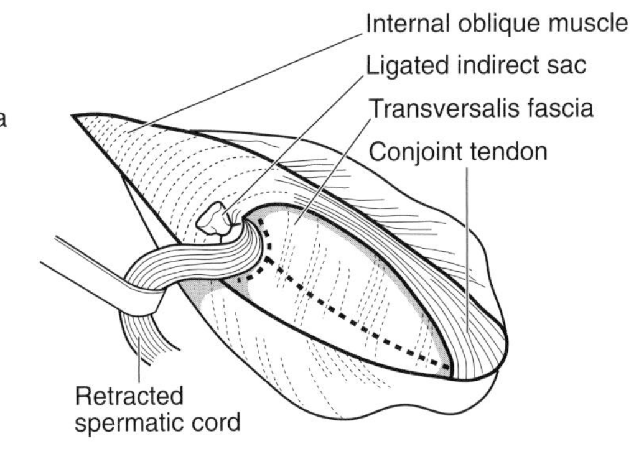

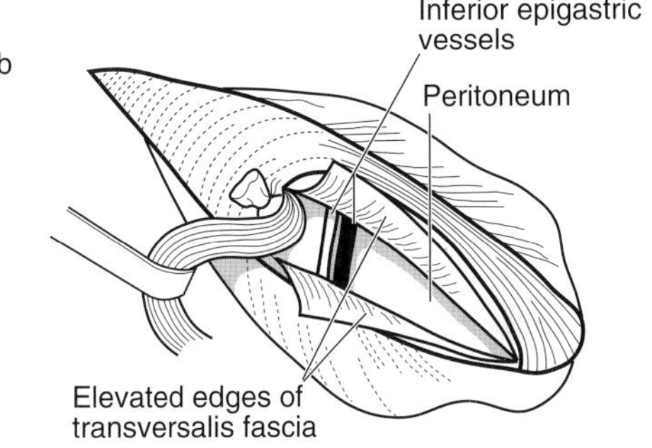

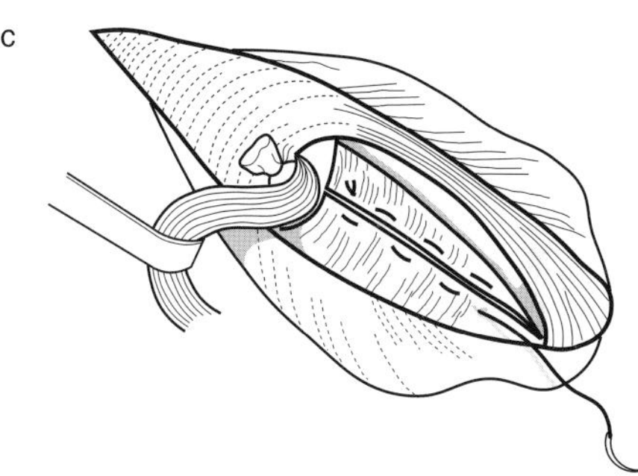

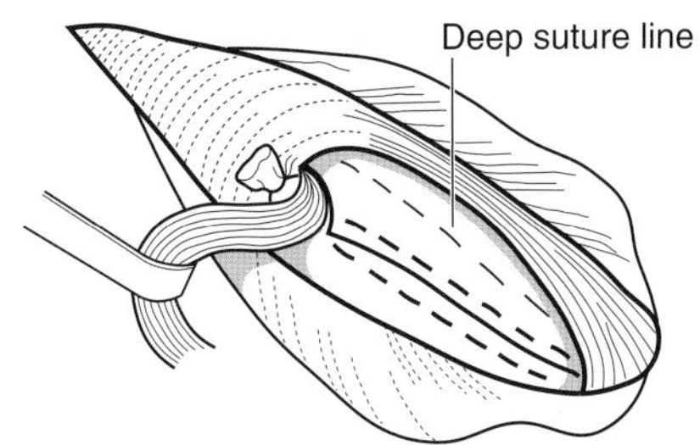

Fig. 6.3 Shouldice repair: (a) the broken line is the incision in transversalis fascia and around the internal ring; (b) the upper and lower flaps have been elevated; (c) the lower flap is sutured to the undersurface of the upper flap; (d) the upper flap is sutured over the lower flap. Finally, the conjoint tendon is sutured to the inguinal ligament.

Action

1 Expose the inguinal canal, mobilize the cord and divide its coverings; if there is an indirect sac deal with it, as described earlier.

2 If there is not a large direct hernia, gently insinuate the closed tips of non-toothed dissecting forceps under the medial edge of the internal ring and pass them medially towards the pubic tubercle, separating the transversalis fascia from the inferior (deep) epigastric vessels. Allow the blades of the forceps to separate by a small amount and insert the deep blade of slightly opened scissors beneath the medial edge of the internal ring, between the forceps blades. Divide the medial edge of the internal ring and continue medially, to split the transversalis fascia as far as the pubic tubercle, halfway between the conjoint

tendon and the inguinal ligament (Fig. 6.3a). Bleeding from small vessels in the fascia often requires diathermy.

3 If there is a large direct hernia, make a spindle-shaped incision in the transversalis fascia, judged so as to preserve suitably sized upper and lower flaps. The intervening, excess, portion of the fascia is then inverted with the hernia.

4 Elevate the upper flap of transversalis fascia from the underlying extraperitoneal tissue, brushing the fat away to expose its shiny white deep surface at the level of the conjoint tendon.

5 If you have not already isolated, ligated and divided the cremasteric vessels close to their origin from the inferior (deep) epigastric vessels when you mobilized the cord, do so now.

6 Separate the lower flap of transversalis fascia down to the inguinal ligament where it continues inferiorly as the femoral sheath (Fig. 6.3b). Take the opportunity to check that there is no femoral hernia.

7 The transversalis fascia will be repaired by overlapping the upper and lower flaps. Bulging of the extraperitoneal tissues into the wound can be prevented by inserting a small dry gauze swab into the extraperitoneal space, removing it just before the first suture line is completed (removal is your responsibility!). Alternatively, a flat retractor or closed sponge-holding forceps can be used to push back the extraperitoneal tissues, being gradually withdrawn as the repair is completed.

8 Lift the upper flap of transversalis fascia and bring to its undersurface the edge of the lower leaf (Fig. 6.3c). Start at the medial end, using a continuous 2/0 monofilament nylon or polypropylene suture. Insert the sutures approximately 3 mm apart, at irregular distances from the lower flap edge. On the upper flap, pick up the more robust white transversalis fascia thickened at the level of the conjoint tendon. As you reach the lateral end, refashion the internal ring snugly around the thinned, emerging cord, taking exceptional care that a ligated indirect sac stump does not slip out.

9 Now fold down the upper flap of fascia transversalis and suture it into the lower flap where it thickens (the iliopubic tract) as it passes under the inguinal ligament (Fig. 6.3d). Suture it securely medially and, at the lateral end, carefully suture it around the medial aspect of the internal ring to reinforce the snug fit around the emerging cord.

10 Further strengthen the posterior wall by suturing the conjoint tendon down to the inguinal ligament. Start medially at the pubic tubercle and work laterally, everting the internal oblique muscle in order to catch the tendinous portion. Take great care, when you reach the internal ring, to snugly enclose it. If the patient is a woman the internal ring and external oblique aponeurosis may be completely closed.

11 Lay the cord back into place and close the external oblique aponeurosis and the wound as described for the Lichtenstein operation.

Postoperative

1 Following repair of inguinal hernia under local anaesthesia, the patient may leave the operating theatre on foot, which is good for confidence.

2 Patients should mobilize immediately after recovery from general anaesthesia. Inpatients generally go home the next day.

3 Activities should be limited only by the patient's comfort.

Complications of inguinal hernia repair

In addition to the complications mentioned in the section on general issues (p. 75), there are others specific to the groin.

1 *Scrotal complications.* Ischaemic orchitis is an uncommon complication presenting as pain and swelling in the first few days after hernia repair. In a proportion of cases it results in testicular atrophy. Damage to the vas should be recognized and repaired at the time of hernia repair. Hydrocele formation is more common after transection of the sac and resorbs spontaneously in most cases. Genital oedema, relatively common in the first 3 days, settles spontaneously, requiring reassurance only.

2 *Nerve injury.* Some degree of transient numbness below and medial to the incision is very common and may persist with little disability. Of much more significance is the incidence of chronic residual pain that occurs in at least 3% of conventional hernia repairs[6] but appears much less common with laparoscopic repair.[7]

3 *Urinary problems.* Bladder injury should be recognized at the time of surgery and treated by primary repair and an indwelling catheter until a cystogram shows healing. Postoperative urinary retention becomes more common with age and after general anaesthesia and usually resolves following a 24-hour period of catheterization.

4 *Impotence.* This is an occasional complaint for which there does not appear to be an organic basis.

RECURRENT INGUINAL HERNIA

Appraise

1 Consider laparoscopic repair to avoid the adherent tissues.

2 For open operations, with a mesh repair, orchidectomy need not be considered but warn the patient of the increased risk of ischaemic orchitis.

Access

1 Incise or excise the previous skin scar.

2 Deepen the incision at a higher level than the previous approach, so that unscarred external oblique aponeurosis is encountered first.

3 Display the external oblique aponeurosis downwards to the inguinal ligament.

4 Re-open the inguinal canal through the scar in the external oblique aponeurosis. Avoid damaging the contents of the canal, which may be adherent.

5 Elevate the upper and lower leaves of the external oblique aponeurosis until you reach unscarred tissue.

6 Isolate the spermatic cord below the pubic tubercle and follow it up to the internal ring. It may lie in an unusual place or be adherent and the vas may have been separated from the vessels.

Assess

1 Look for an indirect recurrence. If a sac is found, isolate it, empty it, then transfix, ligate and divide it at the neck.

2 Look for a direct recurrence. If the recurrence is funicular, isolate it, empty it, then transfix, ligate and divide it at the neck. If it is a diffuse bulge, invert the sac with a running suture to maintain the invagination.

Repair

1 Make a decision regarding the form of repair. A small direct defect may be protected by insertion of a small piece of polypropylene mesh extraperitoneally, either as an underlay or as a 'plug'. For all other inguinal recurrences the Lichtenstein method is the best open repair.

2 For the underlay repair of a small, well-defined direct defect, take a piece of polypropylene mesh 2 cm larger in diameter than the defect. At each quadrant insert a 2/0 polypropylene suture through the intact tissue about 8 mm from the edge of the defect, pick up a small bite of the mesh and pass the needle back out through the intact tissue of the posterior wall, close to the point of entry. Hold the suture with an artery forceps and repeat the manoeuvre at each quadrant of the defect. Then parachute the mesh through the defect into the extraperitoneal space and tie the four sutures. Additionally, suture the edge of the defect to the surface of the mesh with continuous polypropylene.

3 In the 'plug' repair of a small defect, insert a bunched-up piece of polypropylene mesh into the extraperitoneal space and secure it with a few sutures across the open defect.

? DIFFICULTY

The dissection described for a recurrent hernia assumes that the anatomical relationships have not been altered by previous operations. There are several findings that may perplex you:

1. In the Halsted method, the posterior wall was reinforced by closing the external oblique aponeurosis behind the cord, thus superimposing the internal and external rings. A recurrence may appear alongside the cord, leaving the rest of the repair sound. Deal with the sac and define the edges of the stretched ring. This is one circumstance in which it may be best, with the patient's prior permission, to divide the cord so that the ring may be closed, but there will be a 15% risk of ischaemic orchitis.
2. The previous use of a plastic mesh or tantalum gauze insert may result in dense fibrosis, making dissection difficult. Where this is known it is best to arrange for a laparoscopic repair.
3. Recurrences following darns with non-absorbable material are often local defects, suitable for the underlay mesh repair. Leave the sound parts undisturbed.

REFERENCES

1. Glassow F 1984 Inguinal hernia repair using local anaesthesia. Annals of the Royal College of Surgeons of England 66:382–387
2. EU Hernia Trialists Collaboration 2000 Mesh compared with non-mesh methods of open groin hernia repair: systematic review of randomized controlled trials. British Journal of Surgery 87:854–859
3. EU Hernia Trialists Collaboration 2000 Laparoscopic compared with open methods of groin hernia repair: systematic review of randomized controlled trials. British Journal of Surgery 87:860–867
4. Fisher R, Hartley J, Winstanley J et al 1998 Phase II evaluation of the Marlex plug hernia repair. British Journal of Surgery 85(Suppl 1):36
5. Amid PK, Shulman AG, Lichtenstein IL 1993 Critical suturing of the tension free hernioplasty. American Journal of Surgery 165:369–371
6. Courtney CA, Duffy K, Serpell MG et al 2002 Outcome in patients with severe chronic pain following repair of groin hernia. British Journal of Surgery 89:1310–1314
7. Hindmarsh AC, Cheong E, Lewis MNP et al 2003 Attendance at a pain clinic with severe chronic pain after open and laparoscopic inguinal hernia repairs. British Journal of Surgery 90:1152–1154

FEMORAL HERNIA

Appraise

1 It is usually accepted that all femoral hernias should be repaired because of the high risk of strangulation, but there are no absolute rules in surgery. Occasionally a patient is seen who is very old and frail, with an incidentally discovered, longstanding femoral hernia that can reasonably be left alone.

2 One of the reasons for offering surgical repair freely is that the operation can be accomplished easily using local anaesthesia.

3 Be aware of the prevascular femoral hernia; its neck extends laterally in front of the vessels.

4 Try each of the three current open approaches for femoral hernia (Fig. 6.4). They all have merits and they are all safe, provided the operation is skilfully performed. Every surgeon eventually settles upon a favourite approach. We use the low approach for elective operations and McEvedy's for strangulated hernias.

5 Femoral hernias can be repaired laparoscopically, but if diagnosed preoperatively the benefits appear negligible as the low approach does not incise muscle, whereas the laparoscopic dissection proceeds close to the femoral vein, with a theoretical risk of damage.

LOW APPROACH (LOCKWOOD)

Access

1 Make an incision 4–5 cm long in the crease of the groin, below the medial half of the inguinal ligament

2 Cut the superficial tissues over the hernia in the line of the skin incision. Look out for the small veins running into the long saphenous vein; ligate and divide them as necessary.

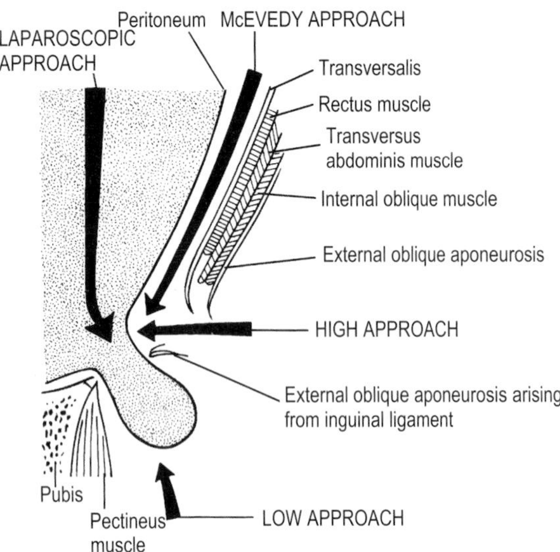

Fig. 6.4 Femoral hernia. A sagittal section through the hernial sac shows the various approaches.

Action

Hernial sac

1 Expose the fat-covered hernial sac. Often, what appears to be a large swelling is mostly extraperitoneal fat, in which lies a small sac. Clean the sac so that it may be traced proximally beneath the inguinal ligament.

2 Cautiously open the sac by incising it while it is held up between two artery forceps. Remember that the bladder may form the medial wall of the sac. Recognize the inside of the sac by seeing free fluid, a glistening surface and contents that may be reduced into the main peritoneal cavity.

3 Pick up the open edges of the sac with three equally spaced artery forceps, then sweep away the external fat to expose the neck, lying between the inguinal ligament anteriorly and the pectineal ligament posteriorly in the same horizontal plane. Note how deeply the neck of the sac lies.

4 Identify the femoral vein lying just laterally and preserve it from damage.

5 Empty the sac, transfix and ligate the neck with 2/0 absorbable suture; it should retract.

6 Excise the sac 1 cm distal to the ligature.

Repair

1 The inguinal and pectineal ligaments meet medially through the arched lacunar ligament. The object of the repair is to unite the ligaments for about 1 cm laterally, without producing constriction of the femoral vein (Fig. 6.5).

2 Use 2/0 monofilament nylon or polypropylene, on a small needle. We find a standard 30-mm round-bodied needle can be shaped to fit into the available space, but avoid damaging the tip. Many use a J-shaped needle.

3 Place a small curved retractor over the femoral vein to protect it and draw it laterally. Insert a stitch deeply into the inguinal ligament and use this to draw the ligament upwards, while the needle is insinuated behind it, to take a good bite of the pectineal ligament. Avoid taking too deep a bite or the needle point will break as it strikes the pubic crest. One, two or three stitches may be used but, for ease of access, insert all the stitches before tying any. As the stitches are tightened, ensure that the femoral vein is not constricted.

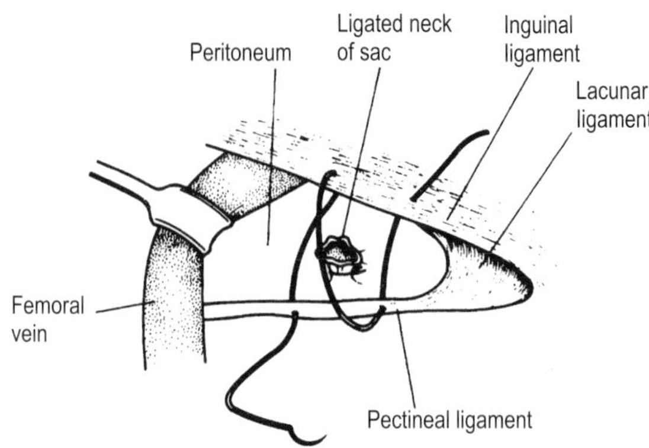

Fig. 6.5 Low approach to right femoral hernia.

4 Alternatively, the femoral canal may be occluded with a 'plug' of rolled mesh, secured with three sutures.[1]

? DIFFICULTY

1. *Can you not identify the sac in the fatty lump?* Remember that most of the lump may be preperitoneal fat. Gently and carefully incise it and separate it. When the peritoneum is incised you can usually see glistening visceral peritoneum or lobulated omental fat. If the sac contains free fluid it appears bluish and may be confused with the appearance of congested bowel. When the sac is carefully incised the fluid escapes, revealing the contents.
2. If you inadvertently tear the neck of the sac, gently free peritoneum from the peritoneal cavity so that it can be drawn down to form a new neck.
3. If the femoral vein is torn, control the bleeding with pressure from gauze packs for 5 minutes. Meanwhile, order blood, arterial sutures, tapes, bulldog clamps and heparin solution, and summon assistance. Expose the vein; do not hesitate to approach it from above and below the inguinal ligament. Apply bulldog clamps and tapes above and below the damaged segment. Insert fine 4/0 or 5/0 sutures set 1 mm apart, 1 mm from the torn edges to evert them and close the hole. Flush with heparin at intervals. Release, then remove the clamps and tapes.
4. It is not possible to suture the whole of a prevascular defect. Insert a piece of mesh and suture the opening medial to the vein.

Closure

1 Unite the subcutaneous tissues with fine absorbable stitches and close the skin, preferably with an absorbable subcuticular suture.

HIGH APPROACH (LOTHIESEN)

Appraise

1 The advantage of this approach is that it can be used for repairing co-existing inguinal and femoral hernias.

2 For femoral hernia alone it has the disadvantage that it damages the inguinal canal and could lead to a subsequent inguinal hernia.

Access

1 Expose the inguinal canal and dislocate the cord, as for operation for inguinal hernia (see p. 77).

2 Incise the transversalis fascia, as in the Shouldice operation.

Action

Hernial sac

1 Identify the neck of the sac and the external iliac vein.

2 Isolate the neck of the sac and gently withdraw the fundus. If there is difficulty, have the lower skin flap retracted downwards, incise the cribriform fascia and isolate, open and empty the sac from below.

3 Ensure that the sac is empty and that the bladder is not adherent, then transfix, ligate and divide the neck of the sac.

Repair

1 With the index finger, feel the margins of the femoral canal. In front is the inguinal ligament, medially the lacunar ligament, posteriorly the pectineal ligament and laterally the femoral vein.

2 Narrow the triangular gap by inserting non-absorbable sutures of 2/0 monofilament nylon or polypropylene between the pectineal ligament and the inguinal ligament.

3 If the upper approach was selected because there is also an inguinal hernia, deal with an indirect sac now.

4 Either close the posterior wall as a Shouldice repair or close the incision in transversalis fascia with a non-absorbable suture and carry out a Lichtenstein repair.

Closure

Close the inguinal canal, subcutaneous tissue and skin as for an inguinal hernia.

McEVEDY'S APPROACH

Appraise

1 We prefer this approach for strangulated hernias as it provides excellent access for assessment of bowel and if necessary for resection.

2 The skin incision, as originally described, left an ugly scar, but this can be avoided by placing it more horizontally.

3 A catheter should be inserted preoperatively, reducing the risk of damage to the bladder.

Access

1 Make an incision from 3 cm above the pubic tubercle running obliquely upwards and laterally for 7–8 cm, crossing the lateral border of the rectus muscle, which lies more vertically. Reflect the skin flaps so as to display the lateral part of the rectus sheath.

2 Incise the lower rectus sheath about 1–2 cm from, and parallel to, its lateral border. The lateral edge may tend to separate into its two anatomical layers.

3 Lift the lateral edge of the sheath and incise the thin transversalis fascia from about 2.5 cm above the pubic tubercle to mobilize the lower lateral edge of the rectus medially. Ligate and divide the inferior epigastric vessels which cross this line low down. The neck of the hernia is now in view as it enters the femoral canal.

Action

1 Retract the lower skin flap and isolate the sac.

2 Reduce the sac, manipulating it from above and below. Open and empty it, then transfix, ligate and divide the neck of the sac.

3 For a strangulated hernia (which is the reason for using this approach), the peritoneum may be opened above the neck to facilitate assessment of the bowel and any necessary resection.

4 Repair the canal from above.

5 Close the incision in the rectus sheath with 0 nylon or polypropylene.

6 Appose the subcutaneous layers and close the skin.

REFERENCE

1. Allan SM, Heddle RM 1989 Prolene plug repair for femoral hernia. Annals of the Royal College of Surgeons of England 71:220–221

STRANGULATED HERNIA

Appraise

1 Most operations listed as strangulated hernia are carried out for painful, irreducible or obstructed hernias. Some hernias reduce spontaneously when the patient is sedated prior to operation, or when anaesthesia is induced.

2 Strangulation results from venous obstruction, a rise in capillary hydrostatic pressure, transudation of fluid, exudation of protein and cells, and eventual arterial obstruction. Alternatively, the pressure of a sharp constriction ring at the neck of the sac may cause local necrosis of the bowel wall.

3 When the diagnosis is made, it is worth trying the effect of reassuring the patient, who is laid supine and told to relax. The head-down position encourages spontaneous reduction. If you are experienced you may try the effect of gentle manipulation to see if the hernia can be reduced, but make sure you do not hurt the patient. There is a slight but real risk that you may reduce the hernia en masse: that is, the hernia remains within the peritoneal sac, the neck of which remains as a constriction, so the strangulation is not relieved.

4 If you can easily reduce the hernia, emergency surgery is unnecessary. Plan for early elective operation.

Prepare

1 Do not rush patients with strangulated hernias to the operating theatre. Make sure you know any reason (such as urinary outflow obstruction or a chest infection) why the patient has developed strangulation now. Identify coincidental disease that may make general anaesthesia and operation hazardous.

2 If strangulation has been present for some time, the patient will require fluid and electrolyte replacement. Some patients, especially with strangulated femoral hernias, do not reach hospital for a few days and by then have a severe biochemical disturbance. They may require up to 24 hours of resuscitation to correct the fluid deficit. This takes priority over the operation. It is likely, in such cases, that bowel in the hernia will already be irreversibly ischaemic, so little is lost by the delay.

Access

1 The approach for inguinal and most other hernias is similar to that for an elective operation.

2 For strangulated femoral hernias McEvedy's incision is preferred, as it provides better access to assess, and if necessary resect, bowel.

3 If the low approach is used and bowel resection proves difficult, have no hesitation in opening the abdomen formally.

Assess

1 If the history was short, the sac will frequently be empty by the time you expose it. The relaxation produced by the anaesthetic often succeeds when other conservative methods have failed to reduce a hernia. There is then no merit in exploring the abdomen. Repair the hernia as though this were an elective operation.

2 If bowel is present in the sac, do not let it slip back into the abdomen but gently draw it down into view. The bowel is likely to have suffered the greatest damage where it was trapped at the neck of the sac.

3 Feel the margins of the neck of the sac with a fingertip.

4 In Richter's hernia, most frequently associated with femoral hernia, a knuckle of the bowel wall is trapped. The bowel lumen is thus not obstructed but the knuckle may become gangrenous and perforate.

▶ KEY POINTS Is the bowel viable?

- If there is a sheen to the bowel wall, if it is pink or becomes pink after release, if the arteries pulsate, if peristalsis is seen, replace the bowel with confidence.
- If the wall is black, green or purple, with no sheen, if there is no pulsation in the mesenteric vessels or it is malodorous, resect it.
- If the bowel is congested, bluish or plum-coloured and still has a sheen, but vascular pulsations cannot be felt, then its viability is doubtful. Remember, however, that blood extravasated subperitoneally cannot be reabsorbed immediately so the colour may not change. Cover the bowel with warm moist packs for 5 minutes and re-examine it. If it has improved in appearance and mesenteric arterial pulsations are palpable it is probably viable.
- The critical areas are the constriction rings at the point of entrapment. These are white when the bowel is first drawn down but may be greenish or black if they are obviously necrotic. Re-examine doubtful rings after an interval to see if the blood supply returns. If it does not, the bowel must be resected. Occasionally it is possible to invaginate and oversew a doubtful ring.
- Experienced surgeons probably resect bowel less frequently than those who are inexperienced. The mucosa is more vulnerable than the seromuscularis to the effects of ischaemia and, if the outer layers survive, the mucosa may slough to leave an annular ulcer. When this heals a constriction may develop. This is the intestinal stenosis of Garré. The patient presents after an interval of weeks or months with incipient small-bowel obstruction. Provided this is recognized, a simple elective resection can be carried out.

5 Maydl's strangulation is very rare. Two loops lie in the sac but the blood supply to an intermediate loop within the abdomen may be prejudiced so that it is gangrenous.

Action

1 If the neck of the hernial sac is constricted, first draw down healthy bowel, then place an index fingertip on each side of the contents, nails facing outwards. Gently dilate the neck of the sac (Fig. 6.6). Make sure the bowel does not slip back. Draw it out

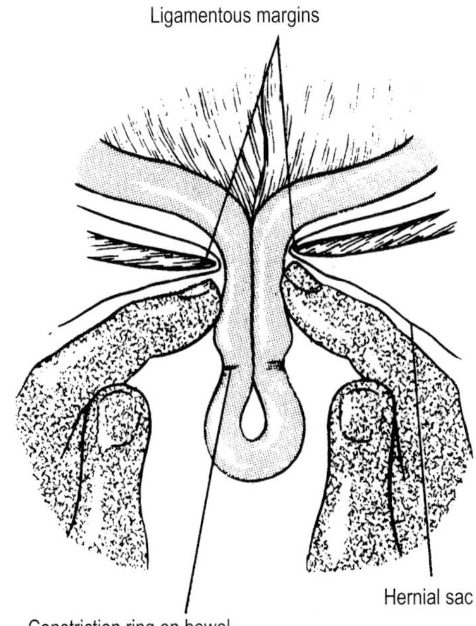

Fig. 6.6 Reducing a strangulated hernia. Healthy bowel is drawn down. The index fingers form a wedge to dilate the ligamentous margins.

to ensure that there is no peritoneal constriction and to expose healthy bowel.

2 If the bowel is viable, return it to the abdomen.

3 If necessary, resect a gangrenous segment of bowel, performing an end-to-end anastomosis.

Repair

After opening the sac and dealing with the contents, repair the hernia as though this were an elective operation, but if possible avoid the use of mesh, for fear of infection.

? DIFFICULTY

1. Sometimes the bulk of tissues contained in the hernial sac makes reduction seem impossible. Provided the margins of the neck are defined, gentleness, patience and persuasion will succeed. If only a little at a time is reduced, do not despair because the reduction must get progressively easier.
2. The McEvedy approach avoids most of the difficulties in dealing with the bowel in a strangulated femoral hernia. When reducing a strangulated femoral hernia from below, it is not necessary to use a bistoury to incise the lacunar ligament; indeed, we find this illogical. Failure to reduce the hernia results from a tight sac neck, not from tight ligamentous margins, which are absent laterally. The femoral vein can be emptied and displaced, producing ample room to reduce the contents.
3. A large mass of fibrotic greater omentum may be adherent within the sac. Do not hesitate to excise the mass, provided the neck of the sac can be isolated, the bowel is not damaged and every blood vessel is safely ligated.
4. If gangrenous bowel slips back into the abdomen and cannot be recovered, repair the hernia, then open the abdomen through an appendix incision, following the terminal ileum proximally until the affected bowel can be delivered, wound protection applied and the gangrenous segment resected.

UMBILICAL HERNIA

ADULT UMBILICAL HERNIA

Appraise

1 Most hernias in adults are para-umbilical, protruding adjacent to the cicatrix. The contents are most frequently omentum, which is often adherent to the interior of the sac.

2 Some adults, especially of African origin, have true umbilical hernias that have been present throughout life.

3 Umbilical hernia is conventionally treated by early operation for fear of strangulation, but small para-umbilical hernias (less than 1 cm) can be left untreated if asymptomatic. However, many patients are grossly obese and elderly, with cardiovascular or respiratory disability and a longstanding hernia that has not been troublesome. Adjure such patients to lose weight and hesitate about offering operation. Ascites may provoke umbilical hernia; find the cause and treat it. In some cases there is extensive malignant disease, when surgery is rarely indicated.

4 Operate on strangulated, painful, irreducible—but not necessarily painless irreducible—hernias and painful reducible hernias, especially those with small, hard margins.

5 The Mayo repair has been widely used, but a mesh repair placed at open operation or laparoscopically has been shown to be preferable.[1]

6 In large hernias which distort the entire umbilicus, the possibility of excising the umbilicus completely should be discussed preoperatively.

Access

1 Make a curved incision in the groove above or below the hernia. If necessary extend the cut transversely outwards on each side, for 2–4 cm.

2 Deepen the incision, identify the aponeurosis and expose it around the adjacent half of the circumference of the hernia.

3 If the hernia is small, preserve the umbilical skin by dissecting it off the hernia as a flap. If the hernia is large, make a spindle-shaped incision to include the umbilicus, excising the stretched skin.

4 Expose 2 cm of aponeurosis around the remainder of the margin of the hernia.

Action

1 Cut through the thinned-out edge of aponeurosis to expose the peritoneum and gradually work round to display the whole circumference of the neck of the sac.

2 Clear the sac of fatty tissue and cut it right round, at least 2 cm distal to the neck if possible. The contents of the sac are less likely to be adherent here than in the fundus, but free them if necessary. Mark the peritoneal edges with artery forceps.

3 If the contents of the sac are free, reduce them. If they are adherent to the fundus of the sac, free them and return them to the peritoneal cavity. If there is a mass of fibrous omentum, excise it with the fundus of the sac but take care to ligate all the bleeding omental vessels and avoid damaging the transverse colon.

4 Separate the peritoneum from the under-surface of the rectus sheath all round, without tearing it.

5 Close the peritoneal neck of the sac with a continuous 2/0 synthetic absorbable suture, producing a transverse linear suture line.

Mesh repair

1 Parachute a piece of polypropylene mesh, 2 cm larger than the defect in each direction, into the extraperitoneal plane and secure it, as described for the underlay repair of a small recurrent inguinal defect (p. 80).

Closure

1 If the skin over the fundus was preserved, pick up the undersurface of the navel with a synthetic absorbable stitch and sew it to the rectus sheath to produce a dimple. Suture the skin as a curved line above or below the newly fashioned umbilicus.

2 If the umbilicus was excised, close the subcutaneous fat and the skin as a transverse suture line.

? DIFFICULTY

1. The hernia may be a true umbilical one, hidden within the cicatrix.
2. Divide the upper or lower edge of the cicatrix to find it.
3. If present, the congenital defect will be obvious and can be closed with interrupted non-absorbable sutures.

INFANTILE UMBILICAL HERNIA

Appraise

1 Most infantile umbilical hernias protrude through the incompletely closed cicatrix. They appear to be more frequent in infants of African origin. Most of them close spontaneously without surgical repair, so wait for 1–2 years. Repair them only if they increase in size.

2 Infants infrequently develop a supra-umbilical hernia. It will not close spontaneously, so repair it locally through a transverse incision sited directly over the defect.

Access for a true umbilical hernia

1 Approach the hernia through a transverse incision curved beneath the everted umbilicus.

2 Preserve the umbilical skin by turning it upwards as a flap.

Action

1 Expose the aponeurosis and the neck of the sac, which is within the cicatrix. The separation is much easier than in acquired hernias.

2 Open the sac, empty it, then close it by suture or transfixion ligature.

Repair

1 Edge-to-edge repair of the aponeurosis is effective.

2 Make sure the peritoneum is separated sufficiently to allow good bites of sheath to be taken, without piercing the peritoneum.

3 Create a transverse suture line using polypropylene or nylon, inverting the knots.

Closure

1 Suture the deep surface of the umbilical skin to the aponeurosis with fine absorbable synthetic material.

2 Close the skin to leave a curved transverse wound, using an absorbable subcuticular stitch.

OMPHALOCELE

Closure should be carried out with the minimum delay after birth; otherwise infection supervenes and the neonate will die (see Ch. 40).

REFERENCE

1. Arroyo A, Garcia P, Andreu J et al 2001 Randomised clinical trial comparing suture and mesh repair of umbilical hernia in adults. British Journal of Surgery 88:1321–1323

UMBILICAL INFECTIONS, TUMOURS, FISTULAS AND SINUSES

Appraise

1 Neglected or imperfectly treated umbilical sepsis, in infants, can progress to septicaemia, distant pyogenic infections, pylephlebitis, liver suppuration and fatal jaundice.

2 An enteroteratoma is the remnant of the vitellointestinal duct forming a raspberry tumour. Cauterize it to destroy the mucosa.

3 Persistent discharge from the umbilicus in infants, children and young adults is likely to be due to a congenital abnormality. An MRI (magnetic resonance imaging) scan may show the connecting track.

- *Congenital faecal fistula* results from persistence of the whole vitellointestinal duct. Faecal staining may be temporary if the fistula closes spontaneously. If there is distal obstruction this must be relieved at the same time as the fistula is closed.
- *Patent urachus* is persistence of the allantois, usually associated with membranous obstruction of the urethra. The urinary obstruction must be dealt with at the time of closing the fistula.

4 In adults, infection is often the result of aggregated keratin forming an 'omphalolith' which can be lifted out of a deep umbilicus without anaesthesia. Persistent omphalitis stimulates granulation tissue, treated by cautery. Recurrent infections may require a minor plastic procedure to reduce the depth of the umbilicus.

5 The umbilicus is a rare site for pilonidal sinus, treated by excision.

6 Endometrioma at the umbilicus classically bleeds at the time of the menses.

7 Squamous epithelioma may develop at the umbilicus and subsequently can involve the inguinal lymph nodes. Excise the umbilicus and, if indicated, carry out bilateral block dissection of the inguinal nodes (p. 94).

9 Secondary carcinoma from the liver or porta hepatis may reach the umbilicus along the ligamentum teres. This presents as Sister Joseph's nodule, first noticed by an observant nun.

10 A port-site metastasis may occur after laparoscopic surgery.

EPIGASTRIC HERNIA AND PORT-SITE HERNIA

Appraise

1 In an epigastric hernia a small knuckle of extraperitoneal fat insinuates itself through a vascular opening in the linea alba. It rarely has a peritoneal sac or contains bowel.

2 Port-site hernias occur after laparoscopic surgery. Repair is similar to that for epigastric hernia

3 Laparoscopic repair is an alternative to the open operation, but for small hernias has no advantages.

Action

1 Make a transverse incision through the skin and deepen it down to the herniated fat.

2 Define the margins of the defect and reduce the hernia. If there is a peritoneal sac, simply invaginate it into the peritoneal cavity.

3 Suture a small (less than 1 cm) defect with a good rim using non-absorbable stitches, inverting the knots. Otherwise place a piece of polypropylene mesh, 2 cm larger than the defect in each direction, in the extraperitoneal plane and secure it, as described for the underlay repair of a well-defined inguinal defect (p. 80).

4 Close the skin, using a synthetic, absorbable subcuticular suture.

SPIGELIAN HERNIA

Appraise

1 Described by Adriaan van der Spieghel (Spigelius) of Padua (1578–1625), herniation is at the lateral margin of the lower rectus sheath and often expands beneath the external oblique aponeurosis.

2 Repair may be by open operation or laparoscopically; the latter facilitates accurate diagnosis.

Action

1 At open operation, make a skin crease incision over the lump and open the external oblique aponeurosis in the line of its fibres, extending the incision medially to open the anterior rectus sheath.

2 Once dissected, invert the sac and develop the preperitoneal space, allowing a check along the lateral edge of the rectus for other defects. Then place a mesh extraperitoneally (p. 80). The layers of the abdominal wall can usually be closed without tension using a 0 Prolene suture.

HAEMATOMA OF THE RECTUS SHEATH

Appraise

1 A sudden strain may rupture one of the inferior epigastric vessels entering the lower rectus abdominis muscle, producing pain. It is more common in patients who are anticoagulated.

2 On the right side, the localized pain and tenderness may be misdiagnosed as appendicitis. However, the patient will not have systemic or gastrointestinal symptoms, pyrexia or leucocytosis. Furthermore, the local tenderness in the right iliac fossa will be greater when the patient puts the muscles under tension.

3 Ultrasound or CT (computed tomography) will confirm the diagnosis; management is then conservative.

4 If you operate thinking the patient has appendicitis and discover a haematoma lying behind the lower rectus muscle, evacuate it. If there is a suspicion of continuing bleeding, isolate and ligate the inferior epigastric vessels in continuity.

ABDOMINAL WALL SEPSIS

WOUND INFECTION

Appraise

1 Wound contamination and haematoma are the major factors leading to wound infection. Following abdominal surgery a variety of organisms may be responsible. Multifilament stitches may perpetuate a wound infection, so monofilament materials are preferred for non-absorbable sutures.

2 Prophylaxis for potentially contaminated wounds comprises perioperative antibiotics, scrupulous haemostasis in the abdominal wall and covering the wound edges with Betadine (povidone–iodine)-soaked swabs or plastic wound protectors.

3 The infection may be a localized wound abscess or an abscess occupying the whole wound, with or without surrounding cellulitis, or there may be cellulitis without an abscess (yet). The wound is hot, red and swollen and the patient is pyrexial and may be toxic.

Action

1 The mainstay of treatment is drainage. Often it is possible to achieve this on the ward by removal of a suture from the softest part of the wound, followed by probing with forceps. If the wound has discharged spontaneously, the opening may need to be enlarged to provide adequate drainage. Where an absorbable subcuticular suture has been used it will need to be cut; this risks inadvertent opening of the whole wound, which can be prevented by insertion of a skin suture (under local anaesthesia) on either side of the site of drainage. Be prepared to open the whole length of the wound for a severe infection. Always send a specimen for bacteriology.

2 Normally, do not administer antibiotics for wound infection unless there is cellulitis or the patient is already septic or at risk from immune deficiency, cardiac disease or prosthetic heart valves.

3 Sometimes when the wound is opened, severe tissue necrosis is discovered. Do not then make the error of leaving a small hole and inserting a drain (see necrotizing fasciitis, below).

4 Following drainage of a wound abscess, a chronic stitch sinus may persist. Explore the sinus with a pair of fine, sterile mosquito forceps, or a sterile crochet hook, to extract the stitch if possible. If the sinus persists, explore it under local or general

anaesthesia to remove the suture material. Usually a knot of non-absorbable suture material will be found; early removal of this may weaken the whole wound, so a delay of up to a year is desirable.

SYNERGISTIC SPREADING GANGRENE

Appraise

1 This is usually named after Meleney, the New York surgeon who described it in 1933. When it affects the scrotum it is called Fournier's gangrene. It may result from the synergistic effects of a number of microorganisms, or from a single organism.

2 The nature of an operation or injury, and the patient's general condition, may predispose to the condition. Exclude diabetes, immunosuppression, uraemia and hepatic disease.

3 It develops as a slowly extending area affecting the whole thickness of the skin. The advancing edge is typically serpiginous and leaves dead, sloughing skin that separates to expose unhealthy granulation tissue.

Action

1 Start the patient immediately on broad-spectrum antibiotics, such as a cephalosporin and metronidazole, pending the result of bacteriology.

2 The essential action in controlling the infection is to excise all the necrotic tissue, exposing healthy, clean tissue. Leave the wound open and dress it frequently, repeating the excision of any developing necrotic tissue.

3 When the infection has been completely controlled, plan to resurface the denuded area with partial thickness skin grafts.

NECROTIZING FASCIITIS[1]

Appraise

1 This spreading gangrene primarily affects the abdominal fascia. It may follow surgical operations or injury. It is predisposed to by general disease, particularly diabetes. Subsequently the overlying skin is also affected, but the skin involvement may not indicate the extent of the fascial infection. The mortality rate is 30%.

2 Management is with broad-spectrum antibiotics and immediate radical excision of all the necrotic tissue to leave healthy living tissue (in the limbs this may involve amputation).

GAS GANGRENE[2]

Appraise

1 Clostridial infection of abdominal wounds is remarkably rare, considering that the organisms can be recovered from normal faeces.

2 The patient rapidly develops pyrexia, toxicity and hypotension.

3 The discolored wound edges are crepitant and may discharge thin pus, described as smelling 'mousy'.

Action

1 Administer 1 million units of benzylpenicillin and continue high doses thereafter.

2 As far as possible, and as rapidly as possible, correct the patient's general condition.

3 Under general anaesthesia radically excise the whole area, back to clean, living tissue. Thoroughly wash the raw area with hydrogen peroxide (20 vols).

4 Hyperbaric oxygen at 3 atmospheres has been recommended.

REFERENCES

1. Ward RG, Walsh MS 1991 Necrotising fasciitis: 10 years' experience in a district general hospital. British Journal of Surgery 78:488–489
2. Darke SG, King AM, Slack WK 1977 Gas gangrene and related infection: classification, clinical features and aetiology, management and mortality. A report of 68 cases. British Journal of Surgery 64:104–112

DESMOID AND OTHER ABDOMINAL WALL TUMOURS

Appraise

1 Desmoid tumours are non-encapsulated tumours that develop in the muscle intersections. They are classified as fibromatoses; connective tissue hyperplasia infiltrates locally, but they do not metastasize. Most occur in women, especially those who have borne children. Remove abdominal wall desmoids completely or they recur.

2 Patients with familial adenomatous polyposis may also develop desmoids within the abdomen; these generally surround the mesenteric vessels and so are irremovable.

3 Carcinoma of intra-abdominal structures may directly invade the abdominal wall. If the tumour is otherwise resectable do not hesitate to excise a portion of the abdominal wall en bloc with the primary neoplasm.

Action

1 Concentrate on excising the tumour with adequate clear margins and depth. In the case of a desmoid tumour do not fail to cut through healthy muscle and connective tissue all the way round.

2 If the abdominal wall is invaded from its deep surface, excise the peritoneum and the deep part of the muscle wall, but leave intact the superficial muscle layer. Do not attempt to repair the defect, which will peritonealize.

3 Close a small full-thickness defect layer by layer.

4 A large defect can often be closed by creating a flap of anterior rectus sheath based on its medial edge to swing to the opposite side, or a layer of lateral muscle may be swung over.

5 If you cannot close the defect with muscle or aponeurosis, the best alternative is to use a myocutaneous flap from the chest or thigh. Unless you are skilled in preparing such flaps, obtain the help of a plastic surgery colleague.

6 If you are completely unable to close the defect, consider inserting a polypropylene mesh or other plastic sheet until you can obtain help and advice.

7 When you cannot close the skin defect by any other means, create a large skin flap based laterally that you can slide over to cover the defect, applying split skin grafts to the donor site.

INCISIONAL HERNIA

Appraise

1 Incisional hernia is a deep disruption of the abdominal wound while the superficial layers remain intact (if the superficial layers also separate then a burst abdomen results).

2 Herniation may occur early, while the patient is still in hospital. More usually it develops during the following months or years.

3 Incisional hernias are associated with careless suturing, the use of rapidly absorbable instead of non-absorbable material, haematomas and infection, the insertion of drains through the main incision and damage to abdominal nerves. Jaundice, malnutrition, obesity, postoperative distension and re-exploration through the same incision after a short interval are other contributory factors, as are steroids and immunosuppression. Laparostomy is another mechanism.

4 Incisional hernias rarely strangulate; therefore do not rush to re-operate. Repairs have a high recurrence rate, reduced by the use of mesh,[1,2] but this increases the risk of persistent infection (MRSA—methicillin-resistant *Staphylococcus aureus*—being particularly troublesome) or intestinal fistula. Careful thought should therefore be given as to the need for operation. We encourage the patient with a wide-necked hernia to try a surgical corset. Some are satisfied with this and avoid an operation.

5 If the patient is overweight, advise reduction before surgery. Ensure that infection has completely resolved before proceeding.

6 If mesh is to be used, give perioperative antibiotic cover.

7 Laparoscopic mesh repair is an alternative, early results showing recurrence rates lower than for open mesh and with less risk of infection (see Ch. 7).[3]

Access

1 Excise the old skin scar.

2 If the skin and peritoneum are fused, excise an ellipse of skin wide enough to expose subcutaneous tissue.

3 Dissect back the skin on each side until unscarred subcutaneous tissue is reached, beyond the margins of the defect.

Action

1 Deepen the incision until aponeurosis or muscle is reached, then work towards the margins of the defect.

2 Dissect the edges cleanly and separate the peritoneum from the deep surface all around (unless placing mesh intraperitoneally).

3 If possible, invaginate the sac with a continuous suture. However, adherent contents and a narrow neck may require that the sac be opened to achieve reduction; if practicable close it.

4 Multiple defects in the abdominal wall ('buttonhole tears') are most conveniently managed by uniting them and repairing the resulting larger defect.

5 The cavity from which the sac has been stripped out often oozes, so meticulous haemostasis is important to minimize the risk of haematoma or seroma formation.

Repair

1 There is no advantage in attempting to define the layers of the abdominal wall.

2 Small defects, less than 4 cm, may be sutured, using non-absorbable material (0 or 1G) but this does introduce tension adjacent to the repair so it is suitable only if the edge is strong.

3 Large defects, or poor tissue, are best repaired with a synthetic patch, to avoid a recurrence rate of 40–50% (refer back to page 76 regarding the properties of these materials). The mesh may be applied at three levels in the abdominal wall[2] as described below (Fig. 6.7). For open operations we prefer the second or third methods on the basis that it is better to patch a bucket on the inside! Wherever it is placed it must extend at least 2 cm beyond the margin of the defect.

4 There are also methods that attach a piece of mesh to each side of the defect and then suture the two together or sandwich the abdominal wall between two layers of mesh.

Action

Onlay patch repair

1 This is the simplest method, placing a patch anterior to the aponeurosis and the defect, which may or may not have been sutured. Polypropylene mesh is most suitable as it is rapidly

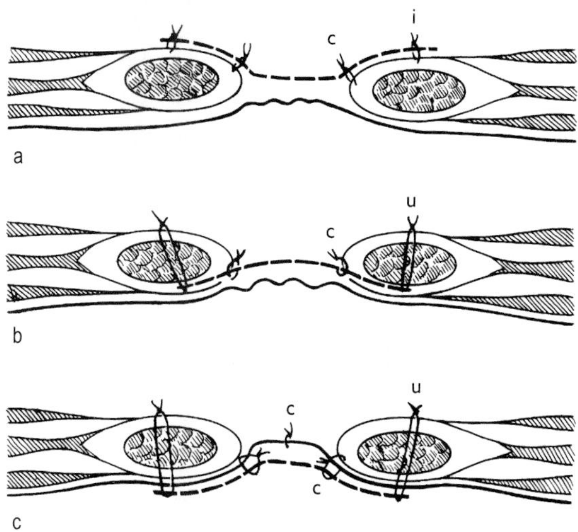

Fig. 6.7 Three alternative levels for placement of mesh in incisional hernia repair: (a) onlay; (b) extraperitoneal; (c) intraperitoneal. Transverse section through abdominal wall. i, interrupted sutures; c, continuous suture; u, 'U' sutures.

incorporated in scar tissue. It should extend 4 cm beyond the edge of the defect.

2 Secure the edge of the mesh with interrupted 2/0 polypropylene sutures at 2-cm intervals, reinforced with a continuous over-and-over stitch.

3 Place another continuous suture to fix the mesh where it lies over the edge of the defect. This is important to prevent herniation of bowel beneath the mesh.

Extraperitoneal mesh repair

1 This is suitable for midline hernias.

2 The peritoneum, plus the posterior rectus sheath if above the arcuate line, is dissected off the posterior aspect of the rectus muscle laterally and from the aponeurosis in the midline, for about 3 cm.

3 Polypropylene mesh will incorporate more rapidly but polyester is easier to position as it can deform on the bias.

4 Cut a piece of mesh 2 cm larger than the defect at each margin.

5 The mesh is drawn into the space deep to the abdominal wall by interrupted 'U' sutures of 2/0 polypropylene at 2-cm intervals. Each passes in through the anterior rectus sheath and rectus, picks up the edge of the mesh and returns to be tied externally.

6 The margin of the defect is then sutured to the surface of the mesh with a continuous over-and-over suture.

Intraperitoneal mesh repair

1 The sac is opened and any adhesions for 4 cm around the rim are freed.

2 Cut a piece of polyester mesh 2 cm larger than the defect in each direction (polypropylene is liable to cause dense intestinal adhesions).

3 Draw the margin of the mesh under the rim of the defect with a series of 'U' sutures of 2/0 polypropylene. These penetrate the peritoneum 2–3 cm from the rim. First place four cardinal sutures and hold them with forceps, adjusting the size of the mesh so that it fits the opening. Then insert more 'U' sutures at 1-cm intervals between one pair of cardinal sutures and tie these. Repeat this for the other three sections.

4 Pick up the mesh and the overlying rim with a continuous over-and-over suture, taking care to avoid the bowel.

Closure

1 Drain the large subcutaneous space with one or two suction drains. The tubing tends to curl up in one corner; prevent this by tunnelling the tube under the fascia at one or two points.

2 Appose the subcutaneous fat.

3 Close the skin with an absorbable subcuticular suture.

Aftercare

1 Leave the drains until the daily loss is less than 30 ml.

2 Any subsequent collection should be aspirated, with sterile precautions.

3 In the event of a wound infection, do not rush to remove the mesh, almost inevitably resulting in re-herniation; it may survive.

REFERENCES

1. Luijendijk RW, Hop WC, van den Tol MP et al 2000 A comparison of suture repair with mesh repair for incisional hernia. New England Journal of Medicine 343:392–398
2. Cassar K, Munro A 2002 Surgical treatment of incisional hernia. British Journal of Surgery 89:534–545
3. Carbajo MA, Martin del Olmo JC, Blanco JI et al 1999 Laparoscopic treatment vs open surgery in the solution of major incisional and abdominal wall hernias with mesh. Surgical Endoscopy 13: 250–252

PARASTOMAL HERNIA

Appraise

1 Stomas leave weak areas in the abdominal wall. The whole area around the stoma may bulge diffusely or a segment of bowel may herniate. In addition, the stoma itself may prolapse.

2 Some parastomal hernias can be accepted, in particular diffuse hernias that are not troublesome since they are unlikely to produce obstruction.

3 Re-siting the stoma, usually on the opposite side of the abdomen, is one approach, but this involves a laparotomy and has a high rate of re-herniation.

4 The best method is to repair the hernia with polypropylene (or Vypro) mesh, either at laparotomy or by a local approach through a curved skin incision lateral to the stoma.

5 The mesh may be placed either extraperitoneally or on the outside of the abdominal wall. Cut a hole in the mesh for the bowel, with a slit to enable it to be inserted without detaching the stoma from the skin. The slit is then sutured. The risk is wound infection, minimized by antibiotic prophylaxis and by sealing the stoma with plastic sheeting.

NON-HIATAL DIAPHRAGMATIC HERNIA

Appraise

1 Neonatal diaphragmatic hernia must be repaired immediately because the lungs cannot expand since the chest cavity is filled with abdominal viscera. It is generally diagnosed on ultrasound before delivery so that specialist paediatric care can be arranged. There is no hernial sac because the defect is the persistent pleuroperitoneal canal—the hernia of Bochdalek (see Ch. 41).

2 Adults occasionally present with acute obstruction within a persistent pleuroperitoneal canal, almost always on the left side. It may also follow thoracoabdominal surgery.

3 Reduction from below is easy, unless the abdominal viscera are adherent within the chest.

Action

Persistent pleuroperitoneal canal (hernia of Bochdalek) in adults

1 By whatever approach is favoured, reduce the abdominal viscera.

2 Trace out the margins of the defect and close it using non-absorbable sutures. The margins usually come together more easily than anticipated.

Hernia of the foramen of Morgagni

1 An abdominal approach is best for this rare hernia, which passes between the costal and xiphoid slips of the diaphragm.

2 Define and repair the defect.

Eventration of the diaphragm

1 A thinned-out leaf of the diaphragm is found, with good muscle at the periphery.

2 Plicate the diaphragm by gathering up a fold and suturing the base of the fold. Lay the fold flat and stitch it down flat, using non-absorbable suture material.

Traumatic hernia

1 An abdominal approach is usually satisfactory and the viscera can be replaced within the abdomen, but a laparoscopic approach is beneficial for postoperative respiratory function in patients who may have lung injury from the trauma.

2 The margins of the defect are nearly always easy to define and repair using non-absorbable suture material.

3 Laparoscopic tensioning of the knots is facilitated by use of braided non-absorbable sutures. Buffers do not appear to be necessary.

OBTURATOR HERNIA

Appraise

1 This is rare. Most occur in females aged over 50 years, and on the right side.

2 Most are admitted with small-bowel obstruction, which, at operation, is discovered to be from an obturator hernia, sometimes of Richter's type. A possible clinical clue is radiation of pain down the inner thigh to the knee. CT is diagnostic.

3 If diagnosed preoperatively it can be repaired laparoscopically by extending the preperitoneal TAPP (transabdominal preperitoneal hernia) or TEP (totally extraperitoneal hernia) dissection inferiorly to include the obturator canal.

Action

1 Assuming the operation is being performed for intestinal obstruction and the small bowel is found to be tethered in the region of the obturator canal, improve the access by carrying the incision down to the pubis. A catheter should already be draining the bladder.

2 Identify the canal with the nerve entering it from the anteromedial aspect; the artery is posterolateral.

3 Gently free the bowel and inspect it to determine if it is viable.

4 Either make no attempt to repair the defect or suture peritoneum over a mesh patch.

LUMBAR HERNIA

Appraise

1 This may emerge spontaneously through the triangle of Petit, bounded by the iliac crest, the posterior edge of external oblique and the anterior edge of latissimus dorsi muscles.

2 Lumbar hernia complicates renal incisions in the loin, drainage of lumbar abscess, trauma or paralysis of the muscles in the lumbar region.

3 Operative repair is rarely required.

GLUTEAL AND SCIATIC HERNIA

Appraise

1 Gluteal hernia emerges above or below the pyriformis muscle through the greater sciatic notch.

2 Sciatic hernia emerges through the lesser sciatic notch.

3 These hernias are usually discovered at exploratory laparotomy for intestinal obstruction and rarely produce a palpable swelling in the buttock.

PELVIC FLOOR HERNIA

This may occur spontaneously, accompanying a cystocele, rectocele or rectal prolapse. It most frequently follows surgery of the pelvic floor, including abdominoperineal resection and hysterectomy.

INTERNAL HERNIA

Appraise

1 Internal hernias present as intestinal obstruction. Most follow abdominal or abdominothoracic operations, the common mechanism being a band adhesion. Intestine may herniate behind an anterior gastroenterostomy, through a transverse mesocolic defect following posterior gastroenterostomy or beside an abdominal stoma if the lateral space is not closed.

2 Internal hernias also occur at anatomical openings, such as the foramen of Winslow or the paraduodenal fossae, and through defects in the falciform ligament, the mesentery or the broad ligament. Think before dividing the 'band', as it may contain an important structure such as the portal triad! After dealing with the bowel the defect must be closed.

BLOCK DISSECTION OF GROIN LYMPH NODES

Appraise

1 Radical groin dissection is carried out for resection of proven or suspected malignant lymph nodes.

2 In general surgery the operation is employed most frequently to excise metastatic melanoma deposits from primary sites in the leg, perineum and gluteal regions.

3 The inguinal nodes may be involved by epidermoid carcinoma of the external male or female genitalia, or of the anal skin. In these cases the nodal dissection is usually accomplished in continuity with excision of the primary lesion.

INGUINAL NODES

Access

1 Make a linear incision, 2.5 cm below and parallel to the inguinal ligament.

2 Alternatively, make a spindle-shaped incision, so that skin overlying involved glands can be excised en bloc.

Action

1 Raise the upper skin flap so that the superficial and deep fascia can be incised 2–3 cm above and parallel to the inguinal ligament to display the lower fibres of the external oblique aponeurosis. Sweep the connective tissues downwards leaving the lower portion of external oblique stripped clean.

2 Dissect the lower flap to reach the fascia lata over the lateral edge of sartorius muscle and incise it here, preparing to sweep it medially with the superficial fascia. Look for, and preserve if possible, the lateral and intermediate cutaneous nerves of the thigh.

3 At the medial border of sartorius muscle, the dissection reaches into the femoral triangle as the femoral nerve, femoral artery and femoral vein are displayed in turn. In the groin, identify, doubly ligate and divide the superficial circumflex iliac, superficial epigastric and superficial external pudendal vessels, to avoid tearing their junctions with the main vessels.

4 Ligate and divide the saphenous vein at the lower extremity of the clearance and again as it joins the femoral vein, so that the segment within the femoral triangle is removed with the specimen.

5 Sweep the superficial tissues and lymph nodes medially as far as possible, then incise the fascia lata vertically over the adductor magnus muscle.

6 The specimen is still attached by the fat and lymphatic tissue entering the femoral canal. Gently draw down the lymph node lying within the canal and remove it with the specimen.

Closure

1 Insert one or two suction drains.

2 Close the skin.

ILIAC NODES

This dissection may be made in continuity with the inguinal node dissection, before or after the groin clearance.

Access

1 For a combined approach, a vertical incision may be made, starting superiorly at the midpoint of a line joining the umbilicus and anterior superior iliac spine and finishing inferiorly at the apex of the femoral triangle. The incision should follow a gentle 'S', lest a future contracture restrict hip movements.

2 Alternatively, iliac node dissection may be carried out laparoscopically.

Action

1 Enter the iliac region through the inguinal ligament, by dividing the ligament over the femoral canal or detaching it from the public tubercle.

2 Incise the external oblique, internal oblique and transversus abdominis muscles 1–2 cm above and parallel to the inguinal ligament, so that the inguinal ligament can be swung laterally.

3 Doubly ligate and divide the inferior epigastric vessels.

4 Sweep up the intact peritoneum from the iliac vessels, making sure that the ureter remains attached to the peritoneum and is thus preserved from damage. Divide the obliterated umbilical artery.

5 Starting in the hollow of the sacrum, sweep out the connective tissue and lymph nodes from the iliac vessels and their branches, including the obturator vessels and nerve. Remove glands along the obturator vessels and nerve and at the obturator foramen.

6 Strip out the loose tissue and lymph nodes from the femoral canal.

Closure

1 Re-attach or repair the inguinal ligament and abdominal muscles. Insert one or more suction drains.

2 Close the skin.

Aftercare

1 Minimize oedema of the leg by elevation, then mobilize in a supporting stocking.

2 Remove the suction drains when the loss is less than 30 ml/day.

FURTHER READING

Fitzgibbon RJ, Greenburg AG (eds) 2001 Nyhus and Condon's hernia, 5th edn. Lippincott, Philadelphia

Kingsnorth AN 2003 Hernias: inguinal and incisional. Lancet 362:1561–1571

Kingsnorth AN, LeBlanc KA 2003 Management of abdominal hernias, 3rd edn. Arnold, New York

Kurzer M, Kark AE, Wantz GE 1999 Surgical management of abdominal wall hernias. Martin Dunitz, London

Macintyre IMC 2003 Best practice in groin hernia repair. British Journal of Surgery 90:131–132

7

Laparoscopic repair of groin and other abdominal wall hernias

J.M. Wellwood, M.G. Tutton

CONTENTS

GENERAL CONSIDERATIONS

Appraise

1 Laparoscopic hernia repair is performed through three short abdominal wounds. The advantages include fewer wound complications, less postoperative pain and for incisional hernias shorter inpatient stays when compared to the open mesh repair. Long-term recurrence rates are similar for open and laparoscopic repair in experienced hands.[1,2]

2 The total extraperitoneal (TEP) approach should not involve entry into the peritoneal cavity, but the transabdominal preperitoneal (TAPP) approach and repair of other abdominal hernias carries a risk of damage to intraperitoneal organs.

3 Laparoscopic repair may be more expensive for the hospital than mesh repair through a standard groin incision.[3]

4 All inguinal hernias may be repaired laparoscopically. Bilateral hernias can be repaired through the same three ports used for unilateral repair. Recurrent hernias after open repair can be repaired laparoscopically without the need to dissect through scar tissue, reducing the risk of inadvertent injury to nerves and vessels.

KEY POINTS Not local anaesthetic

- Laparoscopic repair cannot be satisfactorily performed using local anaesthetic.
- Do not consider it for patients in whom local anaesthesia is medically desirable or requested by the patient.

5 A co-existing femoral hernia may be repaired at the same time as an inguinal hernia using the laparoscopic route. However, laparoscopic femoral hernia repair is not advocated as an alternative to open femoral hernia repair, which is effective with few complications and a rapid recovery.

6 The synthetic mesh placed in the preperitoneal space should extend from the midline medially to a point close to the level of the anterior superior iliac spine laterally, thus covering the whole extent of the inguinal canal including the internal ring and the area medial to the inferior epigastric vessels where direct hernias originate. The mesh will also cover the internal opening of the femoral canal. Mesh, as opposed to sutures, ensures that the repair is tension-free.

7 Anticoagulant therapy is a relative contraindication to laparoscopic repair as bleeding can be more difficult to control than during the open operation. Significant obesity may also contraindicate laparoscopic repair.

8 TAPP repair may be more difficult or even hazardous if there are intraperitoneal adhesions following previous lower abdominal surgery. Furthermore, previous surgery in the preperitoneal space, such as open prostatectomy or procedures for urinary incontinence, may make it hazardous to perform a TAPP or TEP approach. For incisional hernias, the severity of intraperitoneal adhesions must be assessed and, if deemed hazardous, open mesh repair may be preferable.

9 In the TEP approach the operation is carried out in the preperitoneal space and is not therefore technically 'laparoscopic'. The presence of a lower abdominal incision may make the operation difficult or impossible because of adherence of the peritoneum to the muscles and tissues of the anterior abdominal wall. This renders the preperitoneal dissection difficult to perform without making an opening into the peritoneal cavity. This may permit escape of carbon dioxide into the peritoneal cavity making the TEP repair difficult or impossible. Previous appendicectomy does not usually cause this problem. Complete withdrawal of a very large indirect hernia sac may prove difficult by TEP. Simple transection of the sac is likely to allow escape of carbon dioxide gas into the peritoneal cavity, complicating the TEP approach.

Prepare

1 Obtain the patient's signed consent permitting conversion to open repair if necessary. Does the patient with a unilateral

hernia wish you to repair the opposite side should laparoscopy reveal an unexpected (asymptomatic) hernia sac during TAPP but not TEP repair? If so, ensure that this is stated on the consent form.

2 Mark the hernia side with a felt-tipped pen.

3 Do not shave the abdomen.

4 Ensure that the patient empties the bladder before operation. Do not routinely pass a urinary catheter. If preliminary laparoscopic assessment reveals that the bladder is full, pass a catheter before proceeding further with the operation.

5 Place the anaesthetized patient supine on the operating table with arms by the side as they sometimes interfere with the operation if they are folded across the chest.

6 Clean the abdomen with povidone–iodine 10% alcoholic solution or other antiseptic.

7 Drape the whole abdomen to give adequate exposure for the placement of port sites.

8 Choose which side of the patient you wish to stand (Fig. 7.1). We stand on the patient's left for both right and left hernia repair. Alternatively, stand on the opposite side to the hernia. An assistant on the opposite side holds the camera.

9 Position television monitors at the foot of the patient for groin hernias or opposite the surgeon for umbilical or incisional hernias. Although one screen is sufficient, we prefer a second screen for the assistant. The 'scrub' nurse stands on either side and may double as assistant and hold the camera for inguinal hernias (Fig. 7.2). An assistant or the scrub nurse stands on the same side of the patient as yourself for umbilical or incisional hernias.

10 Ensure that you can observe the carbon dioxide insufflator to monitor gas flow and intra-abdominal pressure.

11 Do not have a screen between you and the anaesthetist as this may interfere with your manipulation of instruments.

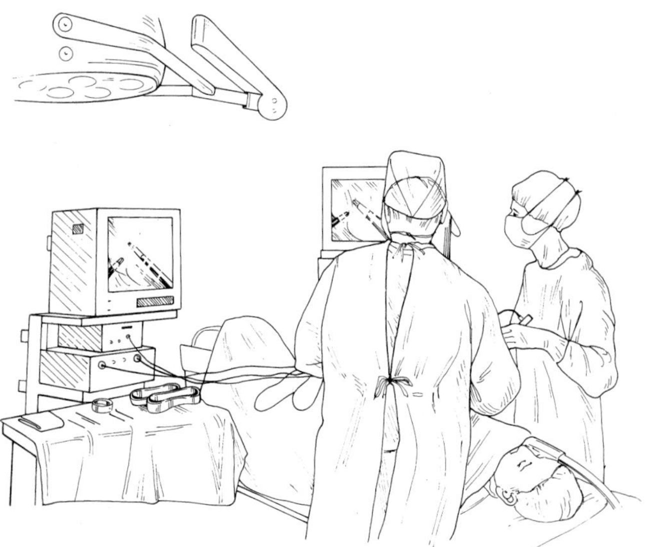

Fig. 7.1 Laparoscopic repair in progress.

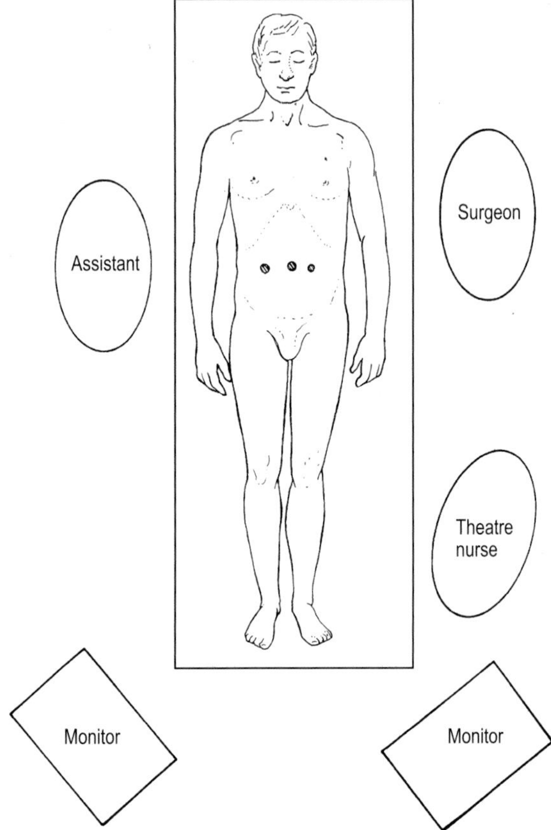

Fig. 7.2 The theatre plan for transabdominal preperitoneal (TAPP) repair.

REFERENCES

1. Douek M, Smith G, Oshowo A et al 2003 Prospective randomised controlled trial of laparoscopic versus open inguinal hernia mesh repair: five year follow-up. British Medical Journal 326:1012–1013
2. Neumayer L, Giobbie-Hurder A, Jonasson O et al 2004 Open mesh versus laparoscopic mesh repair of inguinal hernia. New England Journal of Medicine 350:1819–1827
3. Wellwood J, Sculpher MJ, Stoker D et al 1998 Randomised controlled trial of laparoscopic versus open mesh repair for inguinal hernia: outcome and cost. British Medical Journal 317:103–110

TRANSABDOMINAL PREPERITONEAL (TAPP) HERNIA REPAIR

Access

1 Create a pneumoperitoneum using either an open (Hasan) technique or a closed technique (see Ch. 5). The Hasan technique is safer if there are intra-abdominal adhesions.

2 Make a vertical 1-cm incision from the centre of the umbilicus towards the symphysis pubis. Incise down to the rectus sheath. Open it to enter the peritoneal cavity under direct vision.

3 Insert a 10-mm blunt-tipped trocar and cannula into the peritoneal cavity under direct vision.

4 Attach the lead from the insufflator to the cannula and rapidly create a pneumoperitoneum up to a maximum pressure of 13–14 mmHg.

5 To use a closed technique, make a 1-cm skin incision centred on the umbilicus. Insert a Veress needle aimed towards the sacrum in the midline thus avoiding injury to the large central abdominal vessels. Push the needle through the linea alba and detect a second 'give' as the tip enters the peritoneal cavity. Attach the carbon dioxide insufflation tubing to the needle and insufflate at a low rate, checking that the abdomen is distending uniformly and that the gas flow is unimpeded, as evidenced by low pressure and a high flow. If the pressure is high and the flow is low, check for kinking in the tubing and consider the possibility that your needle is blocked or is not correctly sited in the peritoneal cavity. Insufflate to a maximum pressure of 13–14 mmHg.

6 Insert a 10-mm trocar with cannula through the 1-cm umbilical incision, the instrument again being directed towards the sacrum in the midline in order to avoid the great vessels.

7 First 'white-balance' the video camera. Remove the trocar and pass a laparoscope into the cannula and into abdomen. Direct the laparoscope towards the groin.

8 Adjust the operating table so that the patient is positioned head-down and allow the intestines and omentum to fall away from the groin area to facilitate your view of the hernia orifice.

9 Create two new ports. If you are right-handed, insert a 5-mm trocar and cannula at the level of the umbilicus in the region of the lateral border of the left rectus muscle. Place a 12-mm port in a corresponding position on the patient's right side to be used for scissors and for insertion of the mesh and the stapling device (Fig. 7.3). The left port will be used to grasp the peritoneum and other tissues during dissection. If you are left-handed, you will find it easier to reverse the positions of the 5- and 12-mm cannulas.

Assess

1 If adhesions obscure your view of the inguinal region, divide them carefully using scissors and diathermy. If they are very dense, consider conversion to open hernia repair.

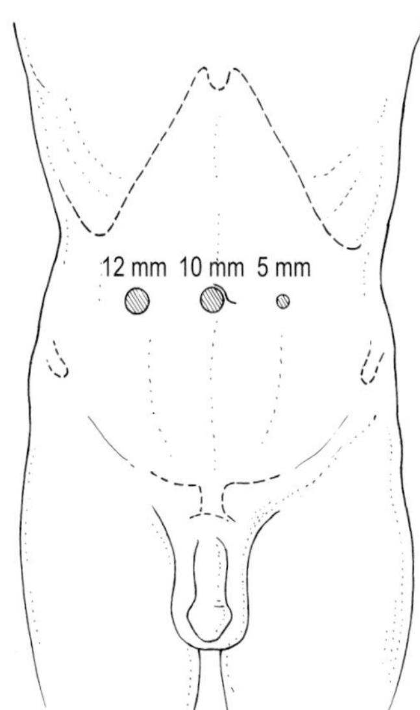

Fig. 7.3 Trocar sites for TAPP repair of left or right inguinal hernia.

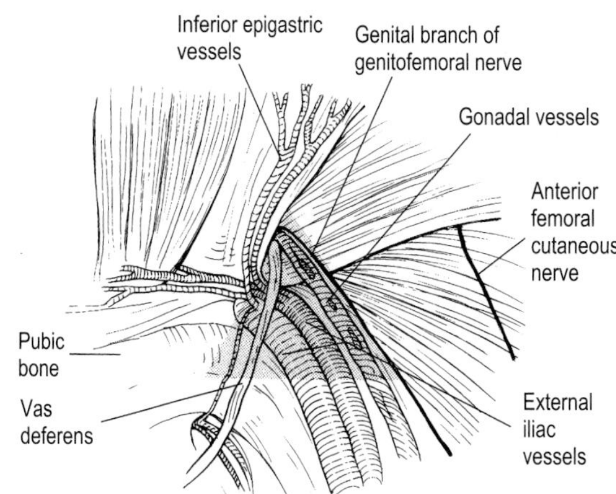

Fig. 7.4 The anatomy of the right groin in relation to TAPP repair. The shaded area has been called the 'triangle of doom' and is bounded by the vas deferens medially and the spermatic vessels laterally. In the floor of the triangle the external iliac vessels can be seen. The femoral nerve is not shown as it is on a deeper plane lateral to the vessels. The genitofemoral and anterior cutaneous nerve of the thigh are shown.

2 Now establish the anatomy as it relates to the hernia (Fig. 7.4). Starting at the midline, identify the bladder and the median umbilical ligament (obliterated urachus) on the inner aspect of the lower abdominal wall. Check that the bladder is not full and catheterize the patient if it is.

3 Moving away from the midline, identify the medial umbilical ligament (obliterated umbilical artery). Immediately lateral to this is the area through which a direct inguinal hernia may pass. Lateral to this, note another ridge, the inferior epigastric vessels that form the lateral umbilical ligament. Lateral to this again is the internal ring through which an indirect inguinal hernia may pass.

4 Moving yet further laterally, compress the abdominal wall at the anterior superior iliac spine and note the lateral extent of the dissection for the TAPP repair.

5 Locate the region of the internal ring by looking for two divergent structures which emerge from it. Passing medially, particularly in thin patients, identify the vas deferens (round ligament of the uterus in females) beneath the peritoneum. Passing laterally from the internal ring is a less distinct ridge caused by the gonadal vessels. Between the diverging vas and the gonadal vessels is the 'triangle of doom' containing the external iliac vessels.

6 Identify whether the hernia is direct (medial to the inferior epigastric vessels) or indirect (lateral to the inferior epigastric vessels).

7 The steps involved in the repair of direct and indirect hernias are essentially the same. However, whereas a direct hernia sac will normally be quite easy to retract, a large indirect hernia sac may be difficult to retract from the scrotum and may need to be divided at or distal to the internal ring. Check that there is not an unexpected hernia on the other side. Now decide whether your repair will be unilateral or bilateral.

8 Don't be alarmed if you find a sliding hernia, as you should not separate the colon from the peritoneal sac. The colon will be retracted with the sac when you are dissecting a preperitoneal pocket in which to place the mesh.

? DIFFICULTY

If you encounter any potentially dangerous and unexpected findings, such as a large iliac artery aneurysm, remove your instruments, deflate the abdomen and proceed to a standard open mesh repair.

Action

1 Ensure that any contents of the hernia sacs are reduced. Omentum adherent to the inside of the sac can be separated with scissors and diathermy. If the contents cannot be reduced laparoscopically, convert to an open repair.

2 Prepare a preperitoneal pocket between the peritoneum and the abdominal muscles in which to place the artificial mesh. The pocket should extend from the midline medially to approximately the level of the anterior superior iliac spine laterally. For bilateral hernias, pockets need to be fashioned on both sides and will become continuous across the midline. A single large mesh or two individual meshes can be used for bilateral hernias.

3 Pick up the peritoneum 1–2 cm above the hernial orifice and make a short incision through the peritoneum using scissors with diathermy attached for haemostasis (Fig. 7.5). Gas may now enter the preperitoneal space and help to lift the peritoneum away from the underlying fascia and muscles.

4 Extend the incision laterally to a level below the anterior superior iliac spine, carefully avoiding the inferior epigastric vessels, and medially into the peritoneal fold of the medial umbilical ligament. It is seldom necessary to fully divide this ligament, which sometimes bleeds.

5 By blunt and sharp scissors dissection (with diathermy), separate the peritoneum below the initial incision away from the underlying fascia and muscle.

6 Deepen the preperitoneal pocket medially and laterally before separating the peritoneum from the internal ring where the peritoneum will be at its most adherent and there will be a risk of injury to the gonadal vessels and the vas deferens.

7 Strip the peritoneum medially downwards and inwards. In the case of a direct hernial sac you will find that it will usually retract out of the hernia orifice with traction and with a little blunt and sharp dissection so that the whole sac is freed from the transversalis fascia. The latter appears as a white fold attached to the sac. Identify the shining white appearance of the superior ramus of the pubic bone and gently strip the tissues downwards away from the pubic ramus, extending the dissection 1–2 cm beyond the midline. The bladder will be seen below and behind the area of dissection.

8 Fashion the lateral part of the peritoneal pocket by stripping the peritoneum downwards and away from the abdominal wall. Below the level of the inguinal ligament, branches of the genitofemoral nerve may be seen lying on the psoas muscle and should be carefully preserved.

9 Now separate the peritoneum, or an indirect sac if present, from the structures at the internal ring (Fig. 7.6). If there is no indirect sac, separate the peritoneum using a mixture of blunt and sharp dissection from the vas deferens or round ligament passing medially and from the gonadal vessels passing laterally from the internal ring. The round ligament is often very adherent to the peritoneum and may be divided.

10 Retract an indirect sac or transect it if it is large. The sac lies anterior to the vas deferens and the gonadal vessels. Retract it progressively from the inguinal canal using a grasper held in the left hand. Control scissors in the right hand for blunt and sharp dissection, to strip away the coverings of the sac. As the dissection proceeds look for the gonadal vessels laterally and the vas deferens medially and dissect the peritoneum away from these structures.

11 A large sac is difficult to reduce, so transect it. Withdraw the sac partially into the abdomen and divide around its circumference,

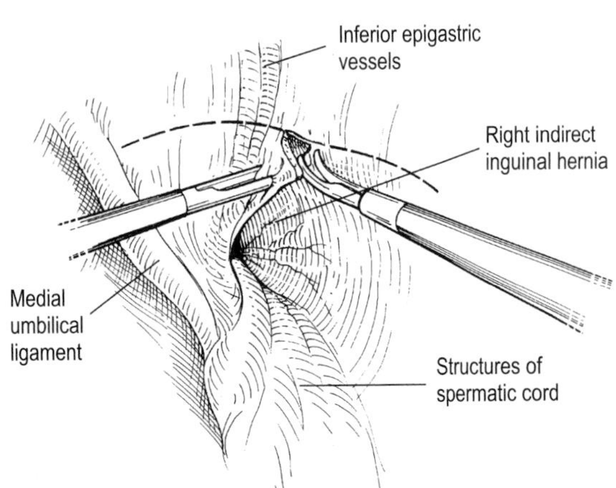

Fig. 7.5 The initial incision of the peritoneum above the internal opening of a right indirect inguinal hernia.

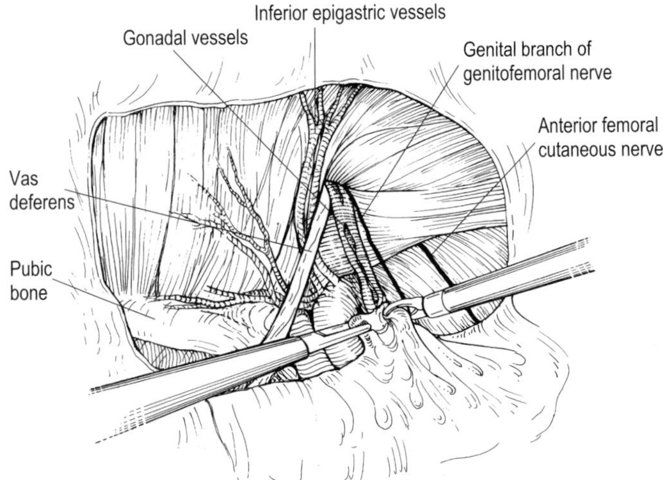

Fig. 7.6 The indirect sac has been withdrawn and the preperitoneal space prepared prior to insertion of the mesh in TAPP repair.

taking care posteriorly where the vas deferens and the gonadal vessels are closely applied. The distal sac will retract back into the inguinal canal. Dissect the transected proximal sac away from the gonadal vessels and vas deferens. Control bleeding with diathermy.

12 Transection of the indirect sac results in a hole in the mobilized peritoneum that will require closure when the mesh has been placed.

13 Now check that the depth of the preperitoneal pocket is sufficient to accommodate a 10-cm deep mesh extending for 15 cm from the midline laterally towards the anterior superior iliac spine. Divide any strands of tissue that would get in the way and prevent the mesh from lying flat (Fig. 7.7).

14 If you are repairing bilateral hernias, repeat the dissection of the preperitoneal pocket on the other side. The resultant pocket extends from one anterior superior iliac spine to the other. It is not usually necessary to divide the peritoneum above the bladder, nor is it necessary to divide either of the medial umbilical ligaments unless access is difficult.

15 Cut the synthetic mesh to the required dimension. For a unilateral hernia this is normally 15 cm × 10 cm. Bilateral hernias can be repaired using two separate 15 cm × 10 cm patches or by one large 28 cm × 10 cm mesh which is stronger but more difficult to place. The latter is more difficult to orientate within the abdomen but is aided by cutting off the corners along one of the long sides of the mesh or by drawing a line on the mesh to indicate the long transverse axis.

16 Take hold of one corner of the mesh with a strong grasper and pass it through the 12-mm port under vision into the region of the pocket you have created.

17 Orientate the mesh so that it covers the groin from the midline to the anterior superior iliac spine within the pocket in front of the peritoneal flap using graspers in each hand. Ensure that the mesh is lying flat and covers the hernial orifice.

18 If bilateral hernias are to be repaired with a 28 cm × 10 cm mesh, pass it behind the midline peritoneum, which has been left undivided, and position it to lie flat and cover the relevant areas on both sides. Alternatively place two 15 cm × 10 cm meshes meeting in the midline.

19 The majority of surgeons staple or suture the mesh in position. Stapling using one of a variety of endoscopic devices is less technically demanding than suturing.

20 Take great care where you put staples. Place three to five staples spaced across the upper border of the mesh, attaching it to the abdominal muscles. Two or three staples may be used to fix the mesh to Cooper's ligament on the superior aspect of the pubic bone medially. No other staples are required (Fig. 7.8).

KEY POINTS Anatomy

- Never staple in the region of the lateral cutaneous nerve of thigh laterally.
- Avoid the area around the femoral vessels and adjacent nerves.
- Staples placed too low have caused serious injury to the great vessels in the 'triangle of doom'. Persistent genitofemoral neuralgia and even femoral nerve paralysis have been reported.

21 Cover the mesh with the peritoneum forming the pocket. Pick up the upper border of the peritoneum with a grasper in the left hand and staple the flap of peritoneum to the abdominal wall, covering the mesh completely. Alternatively, place a running suture between the peritoneum above the mesh and the free peritoneal flap. Ensure complete coverage of the mesh in order to avoid small-bowel adhesion and possible small-bowel obstruction (Fig. 7.9).

22 Repair any hole in the peritoneal covering of the mesh either with staples or by suturing. Such a hole might permit small bowel to pass into the preperitoneal space you have created and give rise to small-bowel obstruction.

Check

1 Check that there is no bleeding. Bleeding from damaged inferior epigastric and gonadal vessels may be controlled using

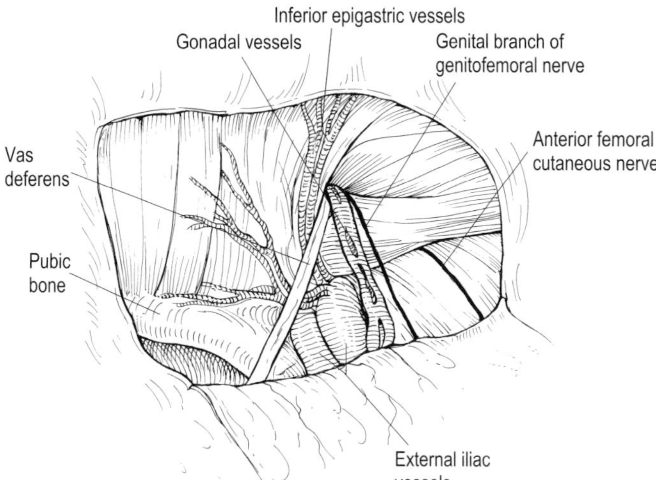

Fig. 7.7 The view during TAPP repair immediately before positioning the mesh.

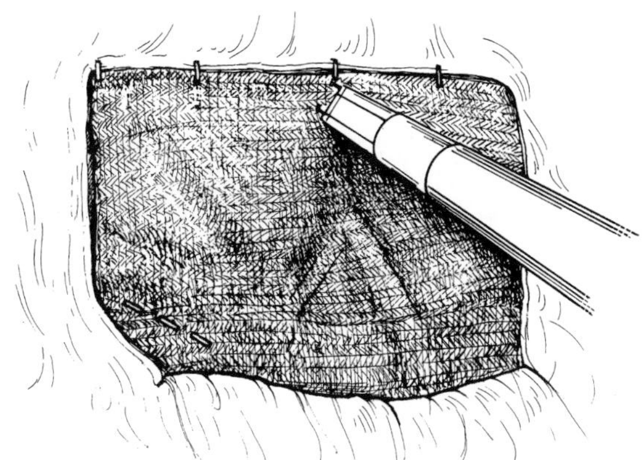

Fig. 7.8 The 15 cm × 10 cm mesh is being stapled into place. Note the three medial staples anchoring the mesh to Cooper's ligament and the pubic bone. Staples are also placed along the superior border of the mesh but nowhere else.

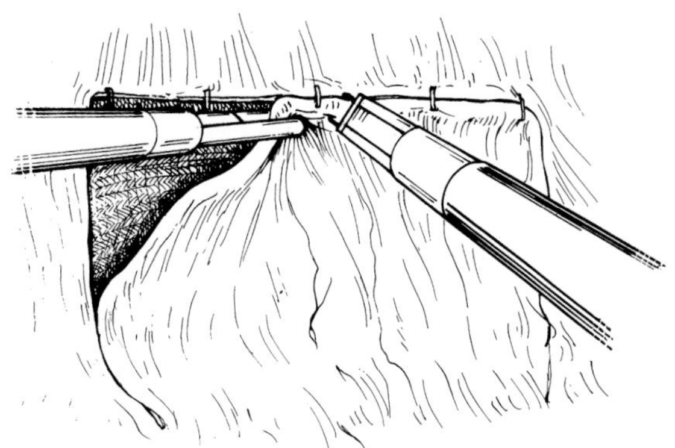

Fig. 7.9 The mesh is being covered completely by replacing the peritoneum.

haemostatic clips. Gonadal injury is unlikely unless previous surgery has been performed, compromising alternative blood supply.

2 Remove any staples that have fallen loose.

3 Check that there are no defects in the peritoneal covering of the mesh. If the peritoneum is thin and tending to tear, staple the margins of the defect in the peritoneum to the mesh, thereby reducing the likelihood of small-bowel herniation.

4 If you have repaired a sliding hernia, carefully check that the colon has not been injured in any way.

5 Disconnect the insufflation and allow the abdomen to deflate.

6 Do not remove the 12- or 10-mm cannulas until the pneumoperitoneum has been evacuated lest a knuckle of small bowel be forced into either of the larger port sites.

7 Remove the 5- and 12-mm cannulas under direct vision and check that there is no bleeding. Control any bleeding and, in the case of unexpected brisk bleeding from the deep part of the port site, pass a Foley catheter into the abdomen through the port site and blow up the balloon. Exert traction on the catheter, thus compressing the port site. The balloon can be left in position and removed later on the ward if necessary.

8 Close the rectus sheath in the 10-mm and 12-mm port sites using 2/0 multifilament synthetic absorbable sutures. Close the skin incisions with polypropylene 3/0 sutures.

TOTALLY EXTRAPERITONEAL (TEP) HERNIA REPAIR

Access

1 Arrange the team around the patient as shown in Figure 7.10. Make a transverse incision exactly 1.5 cm from the midline immediately below the umbilicus on the side of the hernia. Make the incision to the side of the larger of the hernias when bilateral hernias are to be repaired (Fig. 7.11).

2 Deepen the incision to the rectus sheath using small retractors to facilitate dissection.

3 Incise the rectus sheath transversely for about 1 cm.

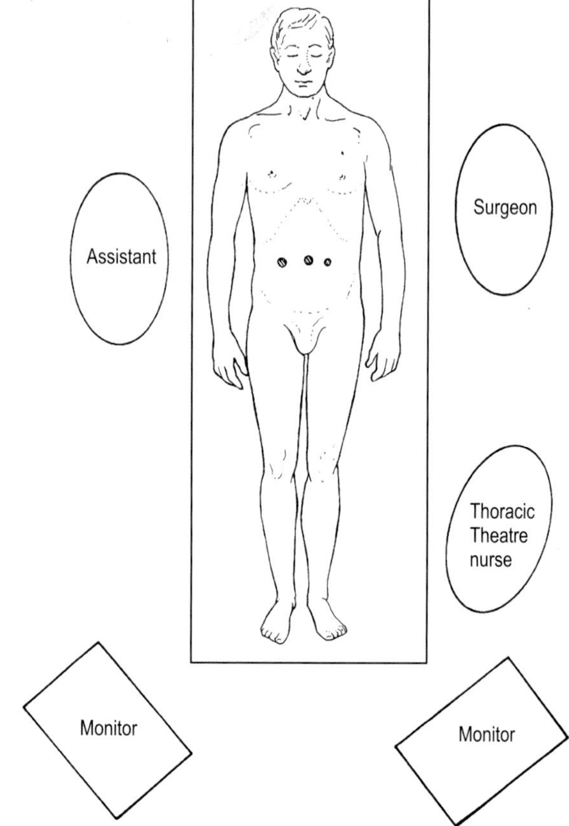

Fig. 7.10 The theatre plan for totally extraperitoneal (TEP) hernia repair.

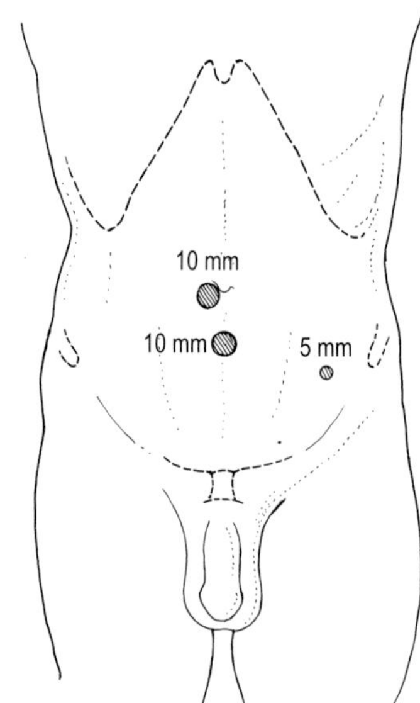

Fig. 7.11 Trocar sites for TEP repair of right inguinal hernia.

4 Identify the medial border of the rectus muscle and retracted it laterally. Access has now been gained to the space within the rectus sheath.

5 In order to fashion a preperitoneal space, pass a 10-mm trocar and cannula with a balloon at its tip into the rectus sheath and guide it downwards until it reaches the pubic symphysis and

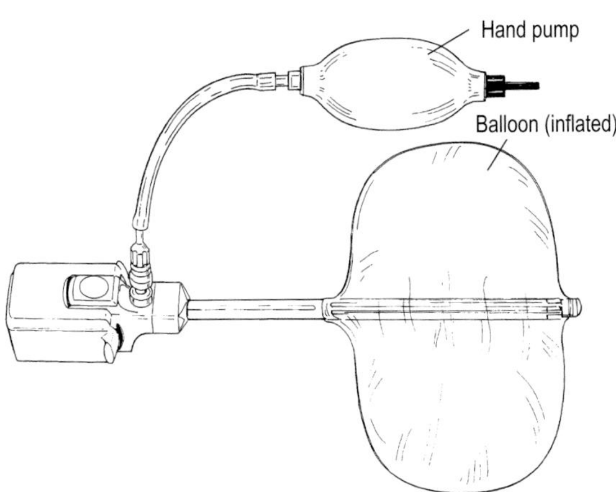

Fig. 7.12 An example of a disposable trocar. Prior to inflation, the balloon is placed through the subumbilical incision and used to initiate the dissection of the preperitoneal space.

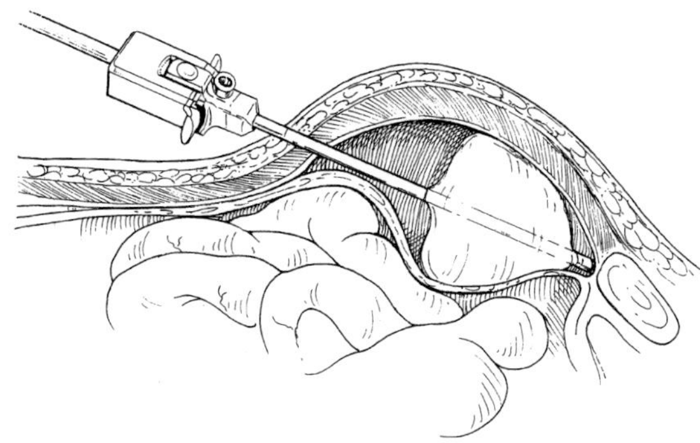

Fig. 7.13 A diagrammatic view of the initial dissection of the preperitoneal space.

then angle the tip to a position just behind the symphysis (Fig. 7.12).

KEY POINT Caution

- Take great care not to angle the cannula in such a way that it might damage the peritoneum and enter the peritoneal cavity, as carbon dioxide gas entering the peritoneal cavity could lead to difficulty maintaining access for TEP repair.

6 Insert a laparoscope into the cannula and maintain the tip of the cannula at a point immediately deep to the pubic bone. Gently inflate the balloon around the end of the cannula until the pubic bone is visible, thereby creating a space between the peritoneum posteriorly and the rectus muscle anteriorly. The lower edge of the posterior rectus sheath can be seen (arcuate line). Inflate the balloon under direct vision and resist the urge to pump the balloon up quickly as this will reduce the likelihood of bleeding. Ensure that the balloon inflates completely. Approximately 20 pumps will be required (Fig. 7.13).

7 Deflate the balloon and withdraw the cannula. Replace the 10-mm cannula with another that has a small retaining balloon at its tip and inflate this so that the balloon sits just inside the rectus sheath (Fig. 7.14). The cannula is designed so that there is very little extension beyond the balloon ensuring that the cannula does not get in the way of the two further cannulas that will be needed. Pass the laparoscope back into position through the umbilical cannula.

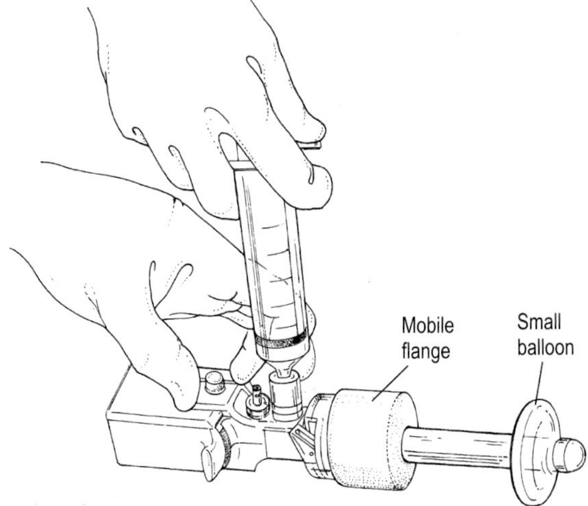

Fig. 7.14 A second disposable cannula used to replace that shown in Fig. 7.12 after the initial preperitoneal dissection has been completed. The small balloon at the tip of the cannula can be inflated to retain the cannula within the preperitoneal space. The mobile flange is passed distally along the cannula so that the abdominal wall is gripped between the distal balloon and the flange. The laparoscope is then passed through the trocar.

8 Attach the carbon dioxide gas lead to the cannula and inflate with carbon dioxide up to a pressure of 8–10 mmHg. Note the partially created pocket in the preperitoneal space. Further dissection is now required.

9 Place a second 10- or 12-mm trocar and cannula under laparoscopic vision in the preperitoneal space already created using a 1-cm midline incision approximately three fingerbreadths below the umbilical cannula at the level where the posterior rectus sheath becomes deficient. This will ensure that the second cannula is placed as high as possible in order to facilitate further dissection of the preperitoneal space, but is not placed too close to the umbilical cannula, which would cause technical difficulties.

Assess

1 Place a blunt-ended 5- or 10-mm dissector in the second (sub-umbilical) cannula and enlarge the preperitoneal space by blunt dissection.

? DIFFICULTY

If gas escapes into the peritoneal cavity via a small hole in the peritoneum, place a Veress needle in the left upper quadrant of the peritoneal cavity to allow gas to escape and prevent distension of the peritoneal cavity, which would obscure the view for TEP repair. Convert to open repair or TAPP repair if a very large tear in the peritoneum prevents completion of TEP repair.

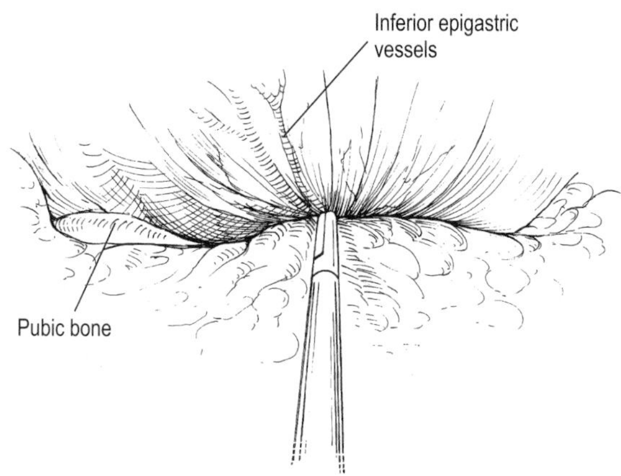

Fig. 7.15 The dissecting instrument is stripping the intact peritoneal sac away from the anterior abdominal wall and the inferior epigastric vessels are in view.

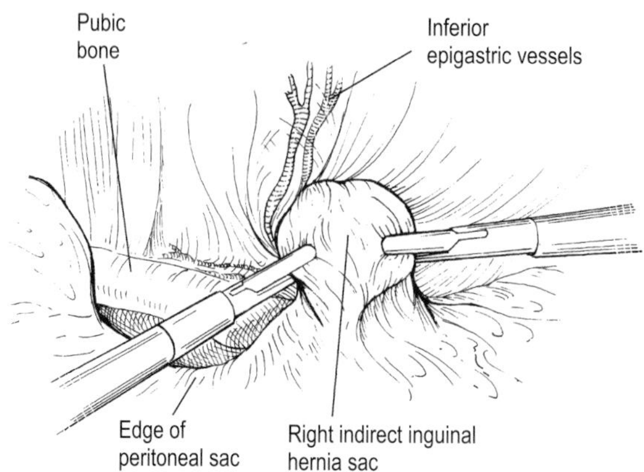

Fig. 7.16 The right indirect inguinal hernial sac is being retracted from the inguinal canal.

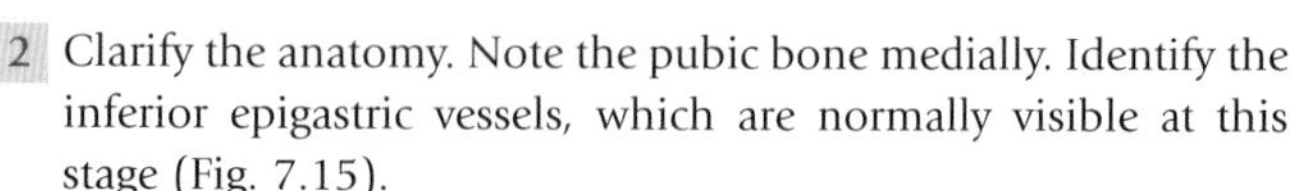

2 Clarify the anatomy. Note the pubic bone medially. Identify the inferior epigastric vessels, which are normally visible at this stage (Fig. 7.15).

3 Strip the peritoneum downward away from the anterior abdominal wall. As in the TAPP repair, do not start at the internal ring but dissect laterally and medially first.

4 Commence the dissection laterally in the region of the anterior superior iliac spine and ensure that the epigastric vessels do not come down with the dissected peritoneal sac but remain up on the anterior abdominal wall.

5 Coagulate small blood vessels and do not rush this phase of the operation.

6 Continue to strip the fat and areolar tissue and the peritoneal sac downwards and backwards in the lateral part of the dissection to reveal a portion of the psoas muscle.

7 Identify the pubic bone medially and gently strip the peritoneum down from this area. The bladder will be seen below the pubic bone near the midline and is gently stripped downwards and backwards. Look for the sac of a direct inguinal hernia, which will be seen attached to the white fold of transversalis fascia.

8 Note an indirect sac as it passes forwards into the internal ring close to the lower end of the inferior epigastric vessels.

Action

1 Create a space for an additional 5-mm cannula by enlarging the preperitoneal pocket by blunt stripping of the peritoneum away from the muscles of the anterior abdominal wall on the side of the hernia.

2 Place the 5-mm trocar and cannula under laparoscopic vision at a point 2 cm medial to the anterior superior spine on the side opposite the hernia. Use this cannula to pass the 5-mm forceps.

3 Retract and free a direct hernia sac by stripping it away from the white fold of transversalis fascia using blunt and occasional scissors dissection. Make sure the sac is completely freed from its coverings and the preperitoneal space can be enlarged below it.

4 Turn your attention to the region of the internal ring.

5 Using a mixture of blunt and, if necessary, sharp dissection carefully dissect the tissues in the region of the internal ring and identify any hernia sac.

6 Grasp an indirect sac with the left-hand grasper and pull it backwards, stripping tissue away from it with the right-hand instrument. As you withdraw the sac place the right-hand forceps beyond the left-hand forceps and further retract the sac with the right hand using the left-hand instrument to strip tissue away from it. Large sacs can usually be withdrawn in this way (Fig. 7.16).

7 As the indirect sac is gradually withdrawn, look for the vas deferens or round ligament (passing medially) and the gonadal vessels (passing laterally). These structures are applied to the deep surface of the peritoneum at the internal ring and more proximally.

? DIFFICULTY

A very large indirect sac may be difficult to withdraw. Although transection of such a large sac with closure of the peritoneal defect may be possible, it may prove technically difficult. In case of technical difficulties convert to an open or TAPP repair.

8 Using blunt and sharp dissection separate the vas deferens and gonadal vessels from the peritoneum of the sac so that the latter can be fully withdrawn (Fig. 7.17).

9 When you have withdrawn the sac fully, strip the peritoneum back further from the internal ring to enlarge the preperitoneal pocket. The edge of the peritoneum should be at least 3–4 cm distant from the internal ring (Fig. 7.18).

10 Avoid injury to the iliac vessels, which lie deep to the triangle between the vas deferens and the gonadal vessels.

11 Prepare a similar pocket in the preperitoneal space on the opposite side if you are repairing bilateral hernias.

12 For unilateral hernias prepare a 15 cm × 10 cm patch of polypropylene mesh. To orientate the mesh correctly mark the long axis of the mesh by drawing a line on it.

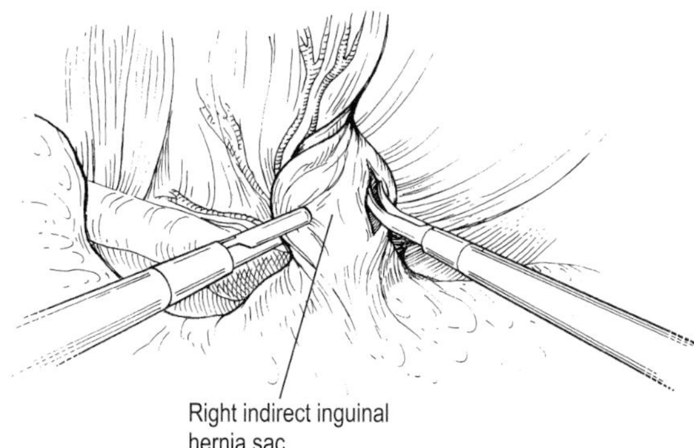

Fig. 7.17 Using a mixture of sharp and blunt dissection, the sac is separated from the vas deferens and the spermatic vessels.

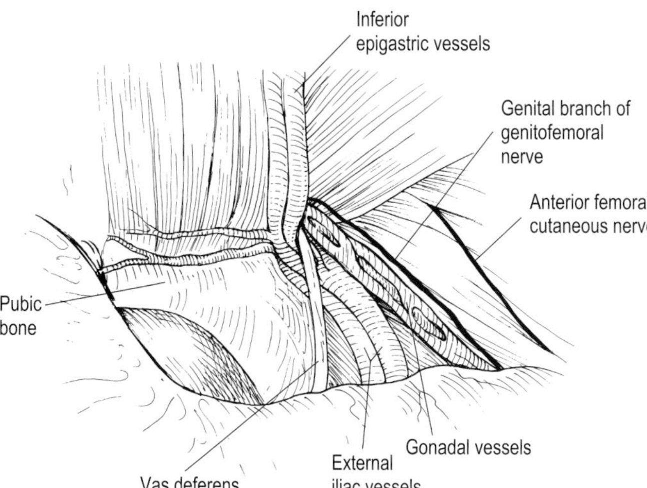

Fig. 7.18 The anatomy of the groin has been displayed and the intact visceral sac has been stripped away from the interior of the groin.

13 Grasp the mesh with forceps and insert it into the preperitoneal space using the midline subumbilical cannula.

14 Position the mesh so that it covers the inguinal region from the midline passing laterally for 15 cm. Ensure that it covers the region of the internal ring, the region medial to the inferior epigastric vessels and the femoral canal and that it reaches the midline. Ensure that the mesh is lying flat against the anterior abdominal wall and on the psoas muscle (Fig. 7.19).

15 Decide if you are going to staple the mesh in position or if you will suture it or leave it unfixed. When staples are used they should only be placed to fix the upper border of the mesh to the abdominal wall and to fix the lower medial part of the mesh to Cooper's ligament or the pubic bone. Do not place staples elsewhere.

16 Place a second mesh in a similar fashion if treating bilateral hernias. It is important that the right- and left-sided meshes overlap the midline. The alternative of a single large mesh may be technically more difficult to place satisfactorily.

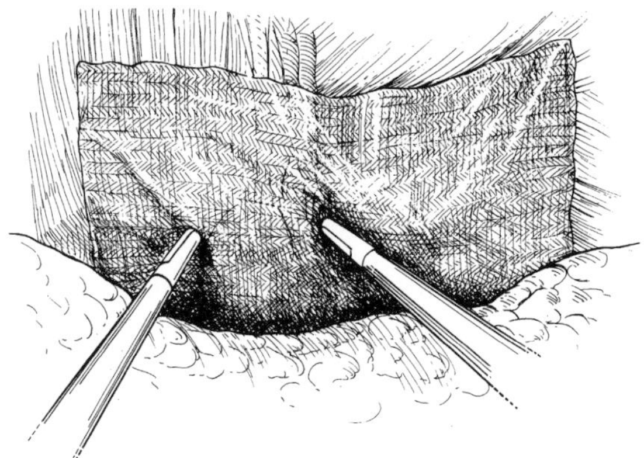

Fig. 7.19 The 15 cm × 10 cm mesh has been placed to cover the hernia defect and extends laterally from the midline. It is being held in place by two forceps as the extra peritoneal space is allowed to deflate. In this case, the mesh has not been stapled in place.

Checklist

1 Check that there is no bleeding and control it with diathermy or clips.

2 Remove any staples that have fallen loose.

3 Disconnect the insufflation and, as the preperitoneal space 'collapses', ensure that the mesh remains flat against the anterior abdominal wall. It is important that the lower edge of the mesh is not lifted up by the peritoneum as the preperitoneal space collapses.

4 Remove the cannulas and check that there is no bleeding. Control brisk bleeding from the depths of a port site by the use of a Foley catheter passed through the port site and inflated.

5 Close the skin incision with a single polypropylene 3/0 suture. The deep layers of the incisions do not require closure after TEP repair.

USE OF INTRAPERITONEAL ONLAY MESH IN LAPAROSCOPIC HERNIA REPAIR

1 Most experience has been gained using an intraperitoneal onlay polypropylene mesh. These meshes in contact with the viscera of the abdominal cavity may adhere to omentum and bowel because of its macroporous nature. However, we have used onlay polypropylene mesh for over 12 years without serious complication. Enterocutaneous or intra-abdominal fistula from intraperitoneal placement of polypropylene mesh appears to be rare even without omental coverage or closure of the peritoneum.[1]

2 Newer materials are available and some composite meshes have been produced. Addition of polyglactin to the polypropylene mesh does not reduce adhesions, although coating with titanium significantly reduces its inflammatory reaction.[2,3] Polytetrafluoroethylene, either on its own or as a composite with polypropylene with the polytetrafluoroethylene side in contact with the viscera, has shown a significantly lower incidence of adhesions both within animal models and in clinical practice.[4,5] The newer meshes cost more than traditional ones.

REFERENCES

1. Vrijland WW, Bonjer HJ 2000 Intraperitoneal polypropylene mesh repair of incisional hernia is not associated with enterocutaneous fistula. British Journal of Surgery 87:1436–1437
2. Scheidbach H, Tamme C, Tannapfel A et al 2004 In vivo studies comparing the biocompatibility of various polypropylene meshes and their handling properties during endoscopic total extraperitoneal (TEP) patchplasty. Surgical Endoscopy 18:211–220
3. Vrijland WW, Bonthuis F, Steyerberg EW et al 2000 Peritoneal adhesions to prosthetic materials: choice of mesh for incisional hernia repair. Surgical Endoscopy 14:960–963
4. Matthews BD, Pratt BL, Pollinger HS et al 2003 Assessment of adhesion formation to intra-abdominal polypropylene mesh and polytetrafluoroethylene mesh. Journal of Surgical Research 114:126–132
5. Koehler RH, Begos D, Berger D et al 2003 Minimal adhesions to ePTFE mesh after laparoscopic ventral incisional hernia repair: reoperative findings in 65 cases. JSLS 7(4):335–340

LAPAROSCOPIC INCISIONAL AND UMBILICAL HERNIA REPAIR USING INTRAPERITONEAL ONLAY MESH

Access

1 Obtain access in an area away from any previous incision and away from the hernia, both of which are usually in the midline. Previous incisions may have adhesions or bowel adherent to them, presenting an inherent risk of damage, so gain access to the abdominal cavity as far back laterally as is safe on the insufflated abdomen. Use either an open (Hasan) technique or a closed technique using a Veress needle. The left subcostal area is often suitable for initial insufflation with a Veress needle.

2 Insert a 5-mm trocar and cannula through the initial incision as described, far back laterally on the abdomen.

3 Remove the trocar and introduce a laparoscope through the cannula into the abdomen.

4 Assess the abdomen and select a suitable position to insert a 5-mm trocar and cannula to the left of the laparoscope and a 12-mm trocar and cannula to the right of the laparoscope, both under direct vision (Fig. 7.20).

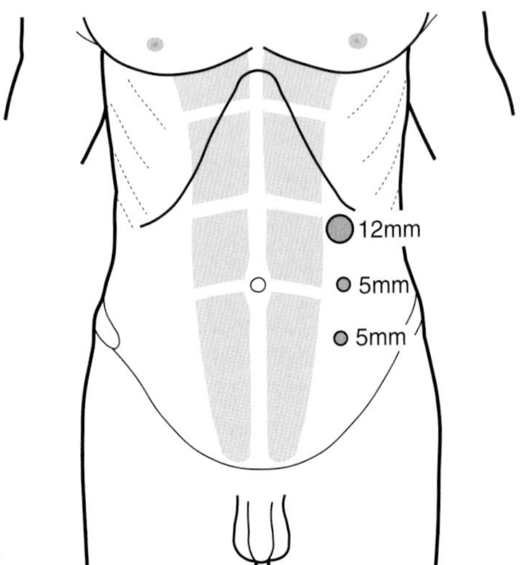

Fig. 7.20 Trocar sites for intraperitoneal incisional hernia repair.

5 Place ports to access midline hernias either on the right or the left of the abdomen depending on your preference. For paramedian incisional hernias insert ports in the opposite side of the abdomen.

Assess

If adhesions obscure your view of the hernia, divide them carefully using scissors and diathermy.

? DIFFICULTY

If initial access to the abdomen is difficult, try placing a 5-mm trocar and cannula in the left subcostal position, then select suitable positions for the lateral insertion of the trocars and cannulas into the abdomen under direct vision.

KEY POINTS Respond to potential difficulties

- Giant incisional hernias and those resulting in a substantial abdominal wall defect are probably better converted to open surgery.
- If adhesions are very dense, consider conversion to open hernia repair.
- Convert to open surgery if bowel is adherent within the hernia.

Continue to divide any adhesions to allow visualization of the anterior abdominal wall for an area large enough to enable placement of a flat mesh of sufficient size.

Action

1 Define the margins of the hernial defect and ensure that any adhesions are cleared for at least 4 cm from the edge of the hernial defect.

2 Reduce the contents of the hernia sac using graspers and diathermy scissors. If this is not possible, convert to an open repair.

3 Leave the peritoneal sac in situ. In patients who have had previous abdominal surgery, it is very difficult to dissect a sufficiently large preperitoneal pocket into which to place a mesh such that it is extraperitoneal.

4 Assess the size of mesh required to give a minimum of a 3-cm overlap of the hernial defect on all sides. Cut the mesh in a square shape to give an equal overlap on all sides. Mark the centre of the mesh with a marker pen to aid orientation inside the abdomen and ensure you position it centrally over the hernia defect.

5 Insert the mesh through the 12-mm cannula. Unfold it, using two graspers, and orientate it centrally over the hernial defect ensuring equal coverage on all sides.

6 Make sure that the mesh lies flat over the abdominal wall. Staple it into position along all sides. If you are inserting a large mesh be willing to apply a second inner row of staples around the defect to fix it securely to the abdominal wall.

Checklist

1 Is the hernial defect well covered with mesh with an overlap of a least 3 cm all round.

2 Check any residual bleeding, using laparoscopic clips if necessary.

3 Remove any staples that have fallen loose.

4 Disconnect the insufflation equipment, allow the abdomen to deflate and remove the cannulas under direct vision.

5 Close the 12-mm port site using a 2/0 multifilament synthetic absorbable suture. Close the skin incisions with polypropylene 3/0 sutures.

LAPAROSCOPIC SPIGELIAN HERNIA REPAIR USING INTRAPERITONEAL ONLAY MESH

Appraise

1 The Belgian anatomist Adrian van der Spieghel (Spigelius) (1578–1625) described the semilunar line. Herniation can develop through defects in the aponeurosis running from the ninth costal cartilage to the pubic spine.

Access

1 Make a 1.5-cm transverse incision about 5 cm above the umbilicus in the epigastrium. Create a pneumoperitoneum using either an open (Hasan) technique or a closed technique.

2 Insert a 5-mm trocar and cannula through the epigastric incision.

3 Remove the trocar and pass a laparoscope into the cannula and into the abdomen and assess the position of the hernia.

4 Create two new ports. Insert a 5-mm trocar and cannula to the left of the laparoscope. Place a 12-mm port in the mid-axillary line to the right of the laparoscope on the side of the hernia. Use 5-mm ports where possible to reduce the risk of port-site hernias.

Assess

1 If adhesions obscure your view of the hernia, divide them carefully using scissors and diathermy.

2 Identify the hernia at the lateral aspect of the rectus abdominis.

Action

1 Reduce any contents of the hernial sac. This is usually easy, but separate any adherent omentum from the inside of the sac with scissors and diathermy.

2 It is usually easy to excise small spigelian hernial sacs since most defects are only 1–2 cm in size.

3 Cut a 10 cm × 15 cm mesh to the required dimension to allow at least 3 cm of coverage on all sides of the defect.

4 Pass the mesh through the 12-mm port with a 5-mm grasper under direct vision.

5 Centre it lying flat on the hernial orifice and staple it into position with three to five staples on each side.

Checklist

1 Control bleeding, using laparoscopic clips if necessary.

2 Remove any loose staples.

3 Disconnect the insufflation equipment, allow the abdomen to deflate and remove the cannulas under direct vision.

4 Close the 12-mm post site using a 2/0 multifilament synthetic absorbable suture. Close the skin incisions with polypropylene 3/0 sutures.

Postoperative

1 The majority of patients undergoing laparoscopic hernia repair can be discharged on the same day. Those undergoing larger incisional hernia repair may require a 2–3-day recovery period because of pain probably caused by friction of the mesh on the peritoneum.

2 Ensure that your operation is secure before recommending same-day discharge.

3 Maximize the chances of earlier discharge by mobilizing the patient early after recovery from the general anaesthetic. Ensure that urine has been passed, the patient can dress himself and that there is someone to provide home-care on the first postoperative night.

4 Provide adequate oral analgesics.

5 Advise the patient to be mobile and return to normal activities as soon as discomfort permits, usually within a week. It is not necessary to restrict activities to prevent recurrence.

Complications of laparoscopic hernia repairs

1 Urinary retention is uncommon and usually resolves spontaneously or following a period of catheter drainage. Elderly men may develop prostatic obstruction requiring urological management.

2 Blue discoloration from skin bruising may develop around the port sites and anterior abdominal wall or scrotum but is painless and resolves spontaneously.

3 Soft, tender groin swellings of serosanginous fluid are common but do not indicate recurrence, resolving slowly and spontaneously. It is seldom necessary to aspirate them. Reassure the patient if they persist for several months.

4 Since the hernial sac is not excised in intraperitoneal onlay repair for incision and umbilical hernia, a cyst may form. Such cysts nearly all disperse within a few months; excise them only if they persist beyond 6 months.

5 Deep vein thrombosis and pulmonary emboli are rare because of the early ambulation.

6 Swelling and redness from infection at the port sites is seldom a major problem.

7 Early or late incisional hernia through a port site following TAPP repair is infrequent and is unlikely if you suture the deep layers of the 10- or 12-mm port sites.

8 Small-bowel obstruction has been reported from adhesion of the small bowel to a poorly covered mesh (TAPP repair) or protrusion of the knuckle of small bowel into a port site or through a defect in the peritoneal covering of the mesh.

9 Aim for a recurrence rate of 1% or less.

10 Peroperative injury to the external iliac vessels has been reported but is entirely avoidable. Treat injury to the inferior epigastric or gonadal vessels by intracorporeal clipping.

11 Injury to the lateral cutaneous nerve of thigh, genitofemoral ranches and the femoral nerve itself results if staples are inserted outside the permitted sites.

12 Injury to the urinary bladder has occurred during dissection of the preperitoneal space but is entirely avoidable.

FURTHER READING

Felix EL, Michas CA, Gonzalez MH 1995 Laparoscopic hernioplasty: TAPP vs TEP. Surgical Endoscopy 9:984–989

Kald A, Anderberg B, Carlsson P et al 1997 Surgical outcome and cost-minimisation. Analysis of laparoscopic and open hernia repair: a randomised prospective trial with one year follow up. European Journal of Surgery 163:505–510

Khoury N 1995 A comparative study of laparoscopic extraperitoneal and transabdominal preperitoneal herniorrhaphy. Journal of Laparoendoscopic Surgery 5:349–355

Kurzer M, Wantz GE (eds) 1999 Surgical management of abdominal wall hernias. Martin Dunitz, London

Lichtenstein IL, Shulman AG, Amid PK et al 2002 Repair of groin hernia with synthetic mesh: meta-analysis of randomised controlled trials. Annals of Surgery 235:322–332

Liem MSL, van der Graaf Y, van Steensel CJ et al 1997 Comparison of conventional anterior surgery and laparoscopic surgery for inguinal hernia repair. New England Journal of Medicine 336:1541–1547

McCormack K, Scott NW, Go PM et al 2003 Hernia Trialists Collaboration. Laparoscopic techniques versus open techniques for inguinal hernia repair. Cochrane Database Systematic Review Issue 1, CD001785

MRC Laparoscopic Groin Hernia Trial Group 1999 Laparoscopic versus open repair of groin hernia: a randomised comparison. Lancet 354:185–190

National Institute for Clinical Excellence 2001 Guidance on the use of laparoscopic surgery for inguinal hernia (Technology appraisal guidance no. 18). NICE, London

Payne JH, Grininger LM, Izawa MT et al 1994 Laparoscopic or open inguinal herniorrhaphy? A randomised prospective trial. Archives of Surgery 129:973–981

Rattner DW 1999 Inguinal herniorrhaphy: for surgical specialists only? Lancet 354:175–176

Slater GH, Hopkins G, Bailey M 2000 Laparoscopic compared with open methods of groin hernia repair: systematic review of randomised controlled trials. British Journal of Surgery 87: 860–867

Stoker DL, Spiegelhalter DJ, Singh R et al 1994 Laparoscopic versus open inguinal hernia repair: randomised prospective trial. Lancet 343:1243–1245

8

Appendix and abdominal abscess

R.C.N. Williamson, D.E. Whitelaw

CONTENTS

APPENDICECTOMY

Appraise

1 The diagnosis of acute appendicitis is essentially clinical. A detailed history and careful examination of the patient carry more weight in making the diagnosis than embarking on radiological investigations, although these investigations can be useful to rule out alternative diagnoses.

2 Although appendicectomy is still the most common reason for laparotomy, remember:
- Young children and the elderly may have atypical presentations of appendicitis and also have a higher mortality and morbidity from this condition.[1]
- Female patients may have a gynaecological cause for pain and tenderness in the right iliac fossa rather than appendicitis. Order a pelvic ultrasound scan and consider carrying out a diagnostic laparoscopy in such cases.
- There is now good evidence that in female patients, appendicitis, even when perforated, does not adversely affect fertility, so you need not perform a mandatory appendicectomy in equivocal cases.[2]
- Although elderly patients do develop appendicitis, consider other pathology such as perforating carcinoma of the caecum and diverticulitis, which may mimic its presenting features. In case of doubt, use a midline incision so you can carry out a full examination of the peritoneal cavity.
- Spiral computed tomography (CT) appears to be the most sensitive imaging technique for diagnosing appendicitis.[3] In view of the cost and radiation dose, reserve this investigation for those in whom a negative laparotomy represents an unjustifiable risk.

3 Tend to treat conservatively a patient with symptoms for 5 or more days in whom you find a mass in the right iliac fossa. Give a 7-day course of intravenous antibiotics such as cefuroxime and metronidazole, withhold oral feeding and replace fluid intravenously. Perform an ultrasound scan to exclude the presence of a large abscess that can be drained percutaneously. Carefully monitor the patient and perform an operation only if:
- The mass, judged by its initially marked margins, increases in size despite antibiotics.
- The patient develops features of bowel obstruction or peritonitis.
- The patient develops worsening toxaemia, or septic shock.

As a rule, order a barium enema X-ray or colonoscopy when the mass has settled, in patients over the age of 40 years, to exclude caecal carcinoma. It has been conventional practice to re-admit patients for 'interval' appendicectomy 1–2 months later, but the number of patients developing recurrent appendicitis is small so it may be justifiable to defer operation indefinitely, after warning fully informed patients to seek medical attention if symptoms recur.

4 Some surgeons carry out diagnostic laparoscopy whenever they suspect appendicitis, proceeding to laparoscopic appendicectomy (see Ch. 9) if the diagnosis is confirmed.

5 Avoid removing a normal appendix incidentally during other operations, such as cholecystectomy. It is a possible cause of complications such as wound infection and subsequent adhesive intestinal obstruction.

Prepare

1 Wound infection is the most common complication following operation for acute appendicitis, so routinely insert a 1-g metronidazole rectal suppository as soon as the decision is made to operate or give 500 mg of metronidazole intravenously at induction of anaesthesia.

2 In patients with clinically severe acute appendicitis who are elderly, have cardiac disease, an implant such as a hip joint replacement, or diabetes, also give cefuroxime prophylactically (1.5 g intravenously).

3 Patients who have a perforated appendix require a full 5-day course of cefuroxime and metronidazole.

KEY POINT Re-examine the abdomen when the patient is anaesthetized

- Intend to re-examine the abdomen when the patient is anaesthetized. You may feel a mass in the relaxed abdomen that was impalpable beforehand. Indeed, it is a valuable general rule before any abdominal operation, and may help you determine the best site for the incision.

Access

1 As a routine employ a Lanz incision in a skin crease. This modification of the gridiron incision transversely crosses McBurney's point—the junction of the middle and outer thirds

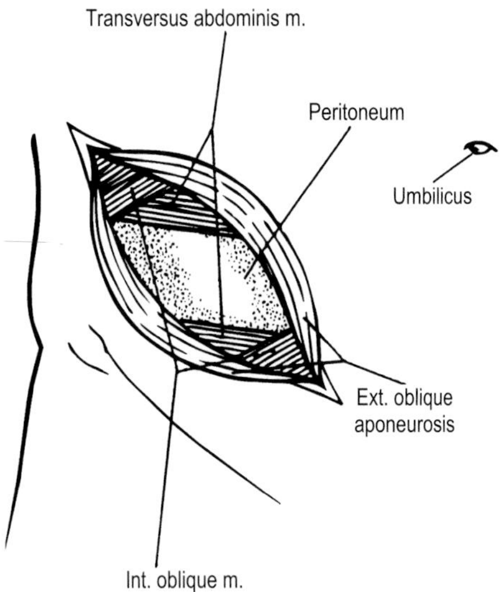

Fig. 8.1 Gridiron incision for appendicectomy. In the Lanz modification the skin incision is transverse but the abdominal muscles are similarly split in the line of their fibres.

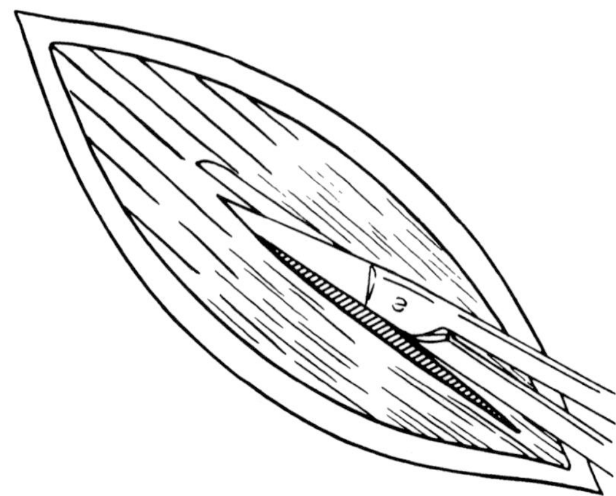

Fig. 8.2 Appendicectomy. Regardless of which skin incision is used, the external oblique aponeurosis is split by pushing partly closed scissors in the line of the fibres.

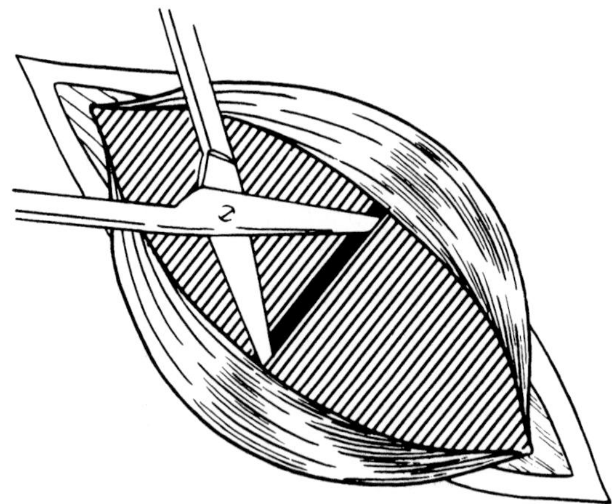

Fig. 8.3 Appendicectomy. The internal oblique muscle is split by opening Mayo's straight scissors in the line of the fibres.

of a line joining the anterior superior iliac spine and the umbilicus. The incision starts 2 cm below and medial to the right anterior, superior iliac spine and extends medially for 5–7 cm. It may be possible to site it lower in a young girl so that the scar lies below the waistline of a bikini swimming costume.

2 Use the traditional gridiron incision, 5–8 cm long, in line with the external oblique fibres if you anticipate the need to extend the exposure (Fig. 8.1). The incision crosses McBurney's point at right-angles to the spino-umbilical line, one-third above, two-thirds below. If necessary, the external oblique muscle and aponeurosis can be split in either direction and the internal oblique and transversus muscles can be cut to convert the incision into a right-sided Rutherford Morison incision (see Ch. 4).

3 If appendicitis is but one of a number of likely diagnoses, prefer a lower midline incision.

Opening the abdomen

1 Incise the skin cleanly with the belly of the knife. Divide the subcutaneous fat, Scarpa's fascia and subjacent areolar tissue to expose the glistening fibres of the external oblique aponeurosis. In the gridiron approach these fibres run parallel to the skin incision.

2 Stop the bleeding. Incise the external oblique aponeurosis in the line of its fibres. Start with a scalpel, then use the partly closed blades of Mayo's scissors (Fig. 8.2) while your assistant retracts the skin edges.

3 Retract the external oblique aponeurosis to display the fibres of internal oblique muscle, which run at right-angles. Split internal oblique and transversus abdominis muscles, using Mayo's straight scissors (Fig. 8.3). Open the blades in the line of the fibres and use both index fingers to widen the split. Provided the scissors are not thrust in violently, the transversalis fascia and peritoneum are pushed away unopened.

4 Stop the bleeding. Have the muscles retracted firmly to display the fused transversalis fascia and peritoneum.

5 Pick up a fold of peritoneum with toothed dissecting forceps and grasp the tented portion with artery forceps. Release the dissecting forceps and take a fresh grasp to ensure that only the peritoneum is held. Make a small incision through the peritoneum with a knife. Allow air to enter the peritoneal cavity, so that viscera fall away. Use scissors to enlarge the hole in the line of the skin incision. Now protect the wound edges with swabs or skin towels.

Assess

1 Look. Is there any free fluid or pus? If so, take a specimen for microscopy and culture for organisms.

2 Find the caecum, identify a taenia and follow it distally to the base of the appendix. Insert a finger and lift out the appendix by pushing from within, not by pulling from without.

KEY POINT Manipulate the inflamed appendix with care

- Never pull on the appendix if the distal end is stuck. If it is gangrenous it will tear and release infected material into the peritoneal cavity. Always improve your view, if necessary by extending the incision.

3 If the appendix is not evident, push your index finger posteriorly until it comes to lie on the peritoneum over the psoas muscle. Then, maintaining contact with the posterior peritoneum, draw your finger to the right until it can go no further. The caecum should now lie between the 'hook' of your finger and the right limit of the iliac fossa, and may be gently pushed out onto the surface. In some cases you may need to mobilize the caecum by incising the parietal peritoneum in the paracolic gutter, in order to raise the caecum on its mesentery, especially if the appendix is adherently retrocaecal. If the caecum is not evident, remember that it sometimes lies quite high, under the right lobe of the liver.

? DIFFICULTY

There is no appendix? In a small number of patients there is no appendix, either because it did not develop or because it has been digested or has atrophied as a result of previous inflammatory disease. In this case, what is the cause of the patient's clinical features? Carry out a search for disease of nearby organs (see below).

4 Confirm the diagnosis: the appendix, or more usually its tip, is swollen, congested, inflamed, even gangrenous, often with fibrin deposition, turbid fluid or frank pus.

? DIFFICULTY

1. If the appendix is not inflamed? Examine its tip to exclude carcinoid tumour, which is usually a yellowish swelling at the tip, since appendicectomy may well be curative. Adenocarcinoma of the appendix demands right hemicolectomy.
2. Examine the caecum, since an ulcer, inflammation or cancer may present as appendicitis. Pass the distal 1.5 m of the ileum and its mesentery through your fingers to exclude mesenteric adenitis, Crohn's disease or Meckel's diverticulum. Palpate the posterior abdominal wall, ascending colon, liver edge and gallbladder fundus and the lower pole of the right kidney. Now feel below into the right rim of the pelvis, the bladder fundus, right iliac vessels and right inguinal region. In females examine the right ovary and fallopian tube, and attempt to feel the uterus and left ovary and tube.
3. Look for features of a distant cause such as bile-stained fluid tracking down from a perforated peptic ulcer, an inflamed gallbladder or a gynaecological cause. Be prepared to close a standard Lanz incision and make a fresh, well-placed incision, rather than struggle to deal with the problem by extending or stretching the incision in the right iliac fossa. The presence of free purulent fluid is an indication to embark on wider examination of the abdominal contents.

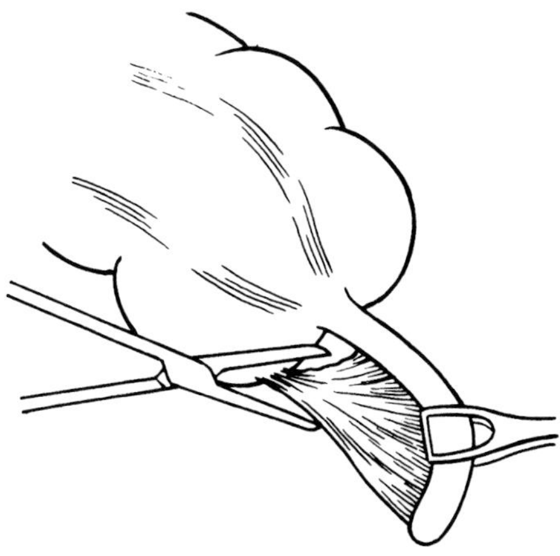

Fig. 8.4 Appendicectomy. Clamping the mesoappendix. The appendix is held up with tissue forceps.

Action

1 Mobilize the appendix from base to tip by gently moving or peeling away adherent structures. Remember that the artery enters from the medial aspect. If the tip is adherent, improve the view. Do not dissect blindly. If necessary, extend the incision. Apply Babcock's tissue forceps to enclose, but not grasp, an uninflamed portion of the appendix, to hold it so you can view the mesentery against the light and identify the artery.

2 Pass one blade of the artery forceps through the mesoappendix and clamp the vessels (Fig. 8.4). If it is thickened, take the mesoappendix in two bites. Divide the mesoappendix distal to the clamp and ligate the vessel gently but firmly with 2/0 polyglactin 910 or similar material, ignoring the slight back-bleeding from the distal cut end.

3 Crush the base of the appendix with a haemostat then replace the clamp 0.5 cm distal to the crushed segment. Ligate the crushed segment with 0 polyglactin 910. Apply a haemostat to the ligature ends after trimming them.

4 Cut off the appendix just distal to the haemostat.

▶ KEY POINT Sterility

- Stop! You have entered the bowel. Place the appendix, held by the Babcock's forceps, together with the knife, into a kidney dish for contaminated articles.

5 Insert a seromuscular purse-string suture of 2/0 polyglactin 910 or similar material, mounted on a round-bodied needle, in the caecum encircling the base of the appendix, at a distance of 10–15 mm from the base. Use the haemostat on the appendix stump ligature to push it in while tying the first half-hitch of the purse-string suture (Fig. 8.5). Gently remove the haemostat before tightening the first half-hitch and then completing the reef knot.

? DIFFICULTY

1. If you cannot carry out the steps of the operation safely you must improve the exposure by extending the wound in the line of the skin incision laterally. Extension of the wound medially may encroach on the inferior epigastric vessels but once you enter the rectus sheath you can retract the rectus muscle medially.
2. If you cannot free the tip of the appendix, it is sometimes helpful to carry out retrograde appendicectomy. Crush, clamp and ligate the base of the appendix before dividing it. Now the base is free you will be better able to follow it to the tip.
3. If the appendix bursts in spite of gentle manipulations, remove it and look to see if a faecalith has escaped. Wash out any freed material using saline lavage and suction. If there has been any contamination, consider inserting a drain into the superficial tissues, since the peritoneal cavity usually copes well with contamination provided the cause is removed.
4. If the base of the appendix is oedematous and fragile, do not attempt to crush it. If possible, carefully ligate it and cut it off 5 mm distally. If it appears unsafe to insert a purse-string, look for a piece of omentum or other peritoneum to draw over the stump and stitch it to a healthy piece of caecal wall.
5. If gangrene extends on to the caecal wall, first apply a non-crushing clamp gently across the bowel to limit contamination. Resect the gangrenous part to reveal healthy wall that can be closed with a suture line. If the hole cannot be closed, insert a large tube drain into the caecum and suture the edges of the bowel to the skin as a caecostomy. The stoma will close spontaneously in most cases, when the tube is removed after a few days.
6. If there is Crohn's disease and the appendix is not inflamed, do not carry out any procedure.
7. If you find an abscess, drain it but do not explore further or pursue a search for a buried appendix within the cavity. It will most probably be destroyed by the inflammatory reaction.
8. In the presence of purulent peritonitis, carry out appendicectomy. Now gently remove pus and debris and drain the wound. Consider copious saline lavage to cleanse the abdomen (see Ch. 4).

Closure

1 Pick up the edges of the peritoneum around the entire incision with fine haemostats to allow easy and safe suturing of the opening with continuous 2/0 polyglactin 910 or similar material.

2 Insert loose interrupted stitches of the same material in the muscle with a continuous stitch to the external oblique aponeurosis to appose but not constrict the tissues.

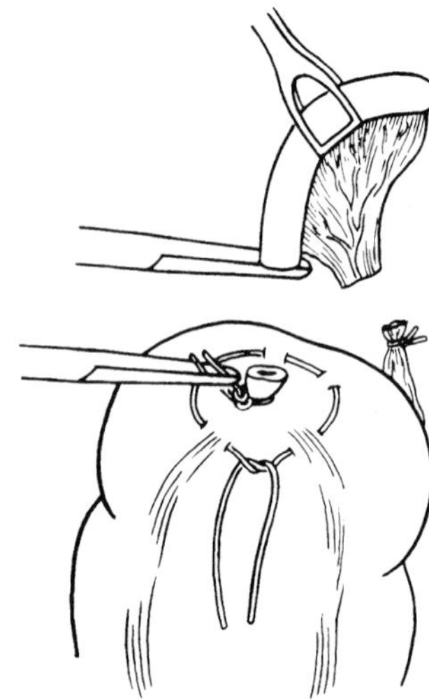

Fig. 8.5 Appendicectomy. The resected appendix, together with the haemostat at its base and the tissue forceps, is placed in a separate dish. The ligated stump of the appendix is invaginated while tying the purse-string suture.

3 Apply povidone–iodine solution to the wound once the peritoneum is closed.

4 Appose the subcuticular tissues with fine sutures in an obese patient and close the skin with a continuous subcuticular suture or clips.

Postoperative

1 In the absence of general peritonitis, start oral fluids and a light diet when the patient is fully awake, as tolerated.

2 If the appendix was perforated, and particularly in a high-risk patient, continue metronidazole suppositories for 5 days and add intravenous cefuroxime 750 mg, 8-hourly.

3 Remove any drain after 2–3 days unless there is still profuse discharge.

4 Monitor the wound if pyrexia develops, and exclude chest and urinary infection.

Complications

1 Wound infection develops occasionally in patients with mild appendicitis but has a higher incidence in those who have had a gangrenous or perforated appendix removed. Anaerobic *Bacteroides* and aerobic coliform organisms are usually responsible. Examine the wound regularly and remove some of the skin suture or clips if there is evidence of infection, to allow any pus to drain.

▶ KEY POINT Explain to the patient what was done

- If you decided not to remove the appendix, ensure that you explain this to the patient. A future clinician, seeing a scar in the right iliac fossa, may wrongly assume that the appendix has been removed and attribute clinical features to other organs.

2 If pyrexia develops, always carry out a rectal examination. Pelvic infection produces localized heat, 'bogginess' and tenderness. Repeat the examination at intervals to detect if an abscess develops and 'points'. Ultrasound or radiological imaging may help if you are uncertain. Finger pressure may release pus but, if not, be willing to aspirate it using a needle inserted through the vagina or rectum. If needle aspiration confirms the presence of an abscess, gently thrust closed, long-handled forceps into the cavity to drain it into the rectum.

3 Reactive haemorrhage is infrequent, but occasionally the ligature falls off the appendicular artery. Return the patient to the operating theatre and re-open the wound to catch and re-ligate the artery.

4 Faecal fistula develops in two circumstances. Either the patient has unsuspected Crohn's disease or in florid appendicitis the appendicular stump or adjacent caecum has undergone necrosis. In the presence of necrosis do not overoptimistically rely on suturing the defect. Prefer to insert a large tube in the hole and suture the margins of the hole to the anterior abdominal wall where the tube emerges. The tube can be removed after a week and the fistula usually heals spontaneously.

REFERENCES

1. Blomqvist PG, Andersson RE, Granath F et al 2001 Mortality after appendectomy in Sweden, 1987–1996. Annals of Surgery 233:455–460
2. Andersson R, Lambe M, Bergström R 1999 Fertility patterns after appendicectomy: historical cohort study. British Medical Journal 318:963–967
3. Paulson EK, Kalady MF, Pappas TN 2003 Suspected appendicitis. New England Journal of Medicine 348:236–242

APPENDIX MASS

Appraise

1 This is usually a late presentation of acute appendicitis.

2 It may result from the adherence of omentum and other viscera to the inflamed appendix. More usually the appendix has ruptured and an abscess has formed, its walls comprising the fibrin-lined omentum and adherent viscera.

3 Antibiotics are commonly given even when there are no clinical features of sepsis and the white cell count is not raised.

4 Provided the patient is well, with no features of sepsis, toxicity or peritonitis, expectant treatment without operation is the preferred management. Mark out the margins of the mass and regularly monitor progress. Provided the marked margins of the mass do not extend and features of toxaemia or peritonitis do not develop, wait for the mass to resolve.

5 Ultrasound scanning or computed tomography (CT) are valuable to confirm the diagnosis and determine whether an abscess is present, which can then be drained percutaneously.[1] If it extends into the pelvis it may be amenable to drainage transrectally under ultrasound guidance.

6 Perform open drainage only if worsening toxaemia or peritonitis develop, or if percutaneous drainage is not feasible or fails.

7 The subsequent management of patients with a resolved abscess remains controversial. Conventionally, the patient is re-admitted for interval appendicectomy after 1–2 months. However, at such operations one frequently finds no evidence of the appendix and, if no interval appendicectomy is undertaken, it is only rarely that recurrent appendicitis develops.[2]

Access

1 Define the mass when the patient is relaxed under anaesthesia.

2 Employ a standard Lanz incision. You may encounter oedema as you reach the deeper layers of the abdominal wall.

3 Alternatively you may enter the abdomen and find the mass on the posterior wall.

Action

1 If you find on entering the abdomen that you are within the abscess cavity, do not rush to explore the wound. Take a specimen of the contents of the cavity for bacterial culture and to determine the antibiotic sensitivity of the contained organisms. Gently and thoroughly aspirate all pus and debris. Explore the cavity with your finger to decide whether it is safe to enlarge the opening without damaging viscera or disrupting the cavity wall.

2 If you gain an improved view you may see the appendix and be able to remove it safely. Sometimes the terminal part has separated and you will need to remove it piecemeal.

KEY POINT The appendix looks normal

- Do not misinterpret the presence of a short, apparently normal appendix. This is the stump left after the distal part has dropped off after a perforation and is lying in the abscess cavity. Look carefully for it and for a causative faecalith and remove both.

3 Sweep your finger round the cavity to identify any loose contents and remove them. Thoroughly aspirate any pus.

4 If you cannot find the appendix or if it is unsafe to open up the abscess cavity, insert a drain, closing the wound layers loosely around it.

5 If, when you open the abdomen, you enter the peritoneal cavity and find a mass lying on the posterior wall, pack it off from the remainder of the abdomen and gently explore it to determine if there is a plane of cleavage into the interior. Remember, inflamed tissues are friable; respond to the findings and be willing to stop if you encounter difficulty.

6 The mass or abscess may lie retrocaecally, retroileally, or within the pelvis. Be prepared to pack off the rest of the abdomen and mobilize the caecum by incising the peritoneum in the paracaecal gutter, so you can gently lift it off the mass. Now explore the mass to decide whether to enter it or leave it.

7 Whether you open the mass or leave it, insert a drain into the peritoneal cavity to provide a track for any pus.

REFERENCES

1. Brown CV, Abrishami M, Muller et al 2003 Appendix abscess: Immediate operation or percutaneous drainage? American Surgeon 69:829–832
2. Dixon MR, Haukoos JS, Park IU et al 2003 An assessment of the severity of recurrent appendicitis. American Journal of Surgery 186:718–722

SUBPHRENIC AND SUBHEPATIC ABSCESS

Appraise

1 An abscess may form following major surgical procedures, operations performed in the presence of infection, or sometimes spontaneously following perforation of a viscus. It could result from a retained foreign body, necrotic tissue, inadequate drainage of blood or contaminated fluid, or an anastomotic leak. The abscess may develop above the liver (subphrenic), below the liver (subhepatic), along either paracolic gutter, between loops of bowel in the mid-abdomen, or in the true pelvis.

2 Reserve the term 'subphrenic' for an abscess lying immediately below the diaphragm. On the right it lies above the right lobe of the liver, on the left it lies above the left lobe of liver, gastric fundus and spleen (Fig. 8.6). Right subhepatic collections may be anterior (paraduodenal) or posterior (suprarenal, Fig. 8.7). Left subhepatic collections may lie anterior to the stomach and transverse colon, or posteriorly in the lesser sac.

3 Suspect the diagnosis if the patient develops rigors, swinging pyrexia, toxicity and leucocytosis. In the presence of a subphrenic abscess the hemidiaphragm may be elevated, as demonstrated on a chest X-ray, and a 'sympathetic' pleural effusion often collects above the diaphragm. You may see a fluid level with gas above if leakage from a viscus or anastomosis has developed, or in the presence of gas-forming organisms. Aspirate a specimen of pus for culture and determination of antibiotic sensitivity. CT or ultrasound scans are valuable means of confirming an abscess, and a radiolabelled white blood cell scan may reveal an occult abscess that is not detectable by other imaging methods.

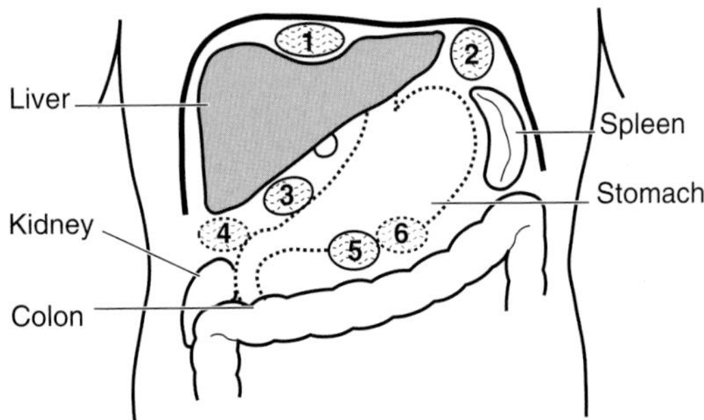

Fig. 8.6 Common sites of abscess above and below the liver: 1, right subphrenic; 2, left subphrenic; 3, right anterior subhepatic; 4, right posterior subhepatic (hepatorenal); 5, left anterior subhepatic; 6, left posterior subhepatic (lesser sac).

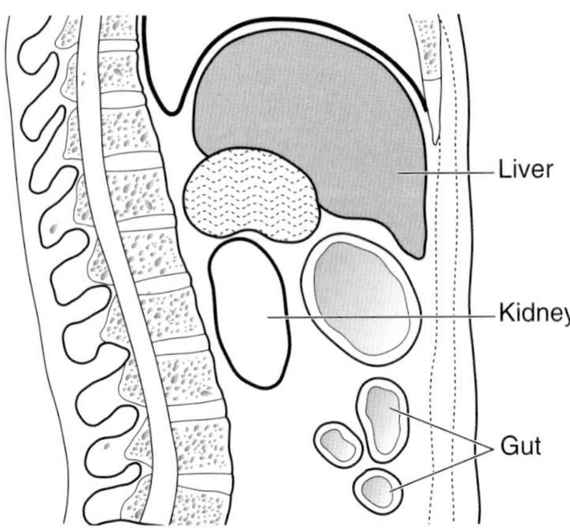

Fig. 8.7 Abscess in the hepatorenal pouch (right posterior subhepatic). This type of posterior collection may be drained by a posterior extraperitoneal approach, through the bed of the 12th rib, or from an anterolateral direction.

4 Once an abscess is identified and localized by clinical signs or imaging methods, insert a percutaneous needle to confirm the presence of pus. Send aspirated material for culture and to be tested for antibiotic sensitivity.

5 The modern, first-line method of dealing with such an abscess should be percutaneous drainage. This is usually effective even for recurrent abscesses.[1] A needle is inserted under ultrasound or CT guidance to avoid damaging adjacent structures. A flexible guidewire is then passed through the needle, which is withdrawn. A bevel-tipped catheter is passed over the guidewire into the cavity and the guidewire is withdrawn. This is the Seldinger technique. This technique may not be successful in obtaining drainage of multiloculated abscesses but these may be successfully drained laparoscopically.[2]

6 Open operation is now rarely necessary for large, loculated or recurrent abscesses and those containing necrotic or inspissated material.

7 The choice of approach depends on the site of the abscess. Ideally, an extrapleural, extraperitoneal approach avoids the possibility of contaminating the peritoneal or pleural cavities. As a rule this is possible only for posterior collections, although a right anterior subphrenic abscess can sometimes be approached extraperitoneally. Multiple or loculated abscess cavities usually demand a transperitoneal approach.

Prepare

Start antibiotic cover against the likely organisms before embarking on operation. Take advice from a clinical microbiologist, especially if you have managed to send a specimen of pus for study.

Action

Posterior approach

1 Place the patient in the full lateral position with the affected side uppermost. Identify the 12th rib and make a 10-cm transverse incision crossing its middle.

2 Cut down on to the rib, incise and elevate the periosteum so you can excise the rib. Incise the bed of the rib cephalad to the middle, to avoid entering the pleural cavity. Divide the origin of the diaphragm and displace the kidney forwards.

3 Feel for the lower edge of the liver and explore below it, using a needle and aspirating syringe to seek out pus. To drain a subphrenic abscess, separate the peritoneum from the undersurface of the diaphragm. When you find it, open the cavity, suck out the pus and debris. Explore it with your finger to avoid leaving necrotic or inspissated material. Now insert a drain.

Anterolateral approach

1 Place the patient supine but with the flank on the affected side elevated by placing a sandbag under the loin.

2 Make a lateral subcostal incision 1 cm below the costal margin and cut through all layers down to, but not including, the peritoneum.

3 Strip the peritoneum from under the diaphragm until you reach the abscess. Open it, and drain it.

4 If you cannot find pus, carefully explore with a needle and finger through the peritoneum and be prepared to enter the peritoneal cavity.

Transperitoneal approach

1 Site the incision according to the site of the abscess derived from the preoperative ultrasound or CT scan.

2 If you are unsure of the site of the abscess or of the cause, carry out a complete exploration of the abdomen (see Ch. 4) before opening up the abscess. This is to avoid the need to carry out an exploration after opening the abscess and risking general contamination. Explore the right and left subphrenic and subhepatic spaces, and enter the lesser sac through an avascular part of the hepatogastric omentum.

3 As soon as you encounter an abscess, pack off the area from the rest of the abdomen.

4 Now open the abscess, suck out the contents and drain the cavity through a separate stab wound in the abdominal wall.

REFERENCES

1. Gervais DA, Ho CH, O'Neill, MJ et al 2004 Recurrent abdominal abscesses: incidence, results of repeated percutaneous drainage, and underlying causes in 956 drainages. American Journal of Roentgenology 182:463–466
2. Lam SC, Kwok SP, Leong HT 1998 Laparoscopic intracavitary drainage of subphrenic abscess. Journal of Laparoendoscopic and Advanced Surgical Techniques Part A 8:57–60

FURTHER READING

Andersson RE 2004 Meta-analysis of the clinical and laboratory diagnosis of appendicitis. British Journal of Surgery 91:28–37

Cooper MJ 1990 Manifestations of appendicitis. In: Williamson RCN, Cooper MJ (eds) Emergency abdominal surgery. Churchill Livingstone, Edinburgh, pp 221–232

Engström L, Fenyö G 1985 Appendicectomy: assessment of stump invagination versus simple ligature: a prospective, randomised trial. British Journal of Surgery 72:971–972

Gillick J, Veayudham M, Puri P 2001 Conservative management of appendix mass in children. British Journal of Surgery 88:1539–1542

Jones PF 2001 Suspected acute appendicitis: trends in management over 30 years. British Journal of Surgery 88:1570–1577

Kirk RM 2002 Basic surgical techniques, 5th edn. Churchill Livingstone, Edinburgh, pp 161–173

Krukowski ZH, Irwin ST, Denholm S et al 1988 Preventing wound infection after appendicectomy: a review. British Journal of Surgery 75:1023–1033

Rao PM, Rhea JT, Rattner DW et al 1999 Introduction of appendiceal CT: impact on negative appendicectomy and appendiceal perforation rates. Annals of Surgery 229:334–349

Silen W 2000 Cope's early diagnosis of the acute abdomen. Oxford University Press, Oxford

9

Laparoscopic appendicectomy

S.J. Nixon, A. Rajasekar

DESCRIPTION OF OPERATION

Appraise

1 Appendicectomy for appendicitis is the most common emergency abdominal operation. A detailed examination of the abdomen and pelvis is not possible. Postoperative morbidity includes wound infection, incisional hernia, deep infection, prolonged ileus, adhesive obstruction, infertility in females and subsequent right inguinal hernia.

2 Laparoscopic appendicectomy is increasingly used. Advantages claimed are decreased wound infection, reduced postoperative pain and accelerated recovery. Laparoscopy allows detailed pelvic and abdominal examination, particularly valuable in young women where preoperative diagnostic accuracy is low. Increased technical difficulty, longer operating times, increased risk of deep infection and increased cost offset these potential advantages.[1–3]

3 Routine use of laparoscopic appendicectomy is debatable on evidence from the surgical literature and depends on your experience.[4,5] However, it may offer particular advantages in women of childbearing age and in obese individuals.

4 The conversion rate and morbidity reported in the literature varies from 0% to 15% and 0% to 18%, respectively.

5 There are no absolute contraindications, and relative contraindications are the same as for other laparoscopic procedures.

KEY POINTS Clinical diagnosis

- In patients with equivocal symptoms and signs, repeated clinical examination is the mainstay of diagnosis.
- Minimize negative laparotomy or laparoscopy rates.

Prepare

1 Obtain informed consent for both laparoscopic and open appendicectomy. Administer metronidazole as a 1-g rectal suppository 1 hour before the operation or give parenteral metronidazole and broad-spectrum antibiotics during anaesthetic induction.

2 Laparoscopic appendicectomy requires general anaesthesia with endotracheal intubation and muscle relaxation.

3 Place the patient supine. In females, the lithotomy position allows peroperative vaginal examination. You and your assistant stand on the patient's left side with the nurse on the right and a monitor at the foot of the table.

4 Catheterize the urinary bladder to reduce risk of injury if there is doubt regarding the recent micturition.

KEY POINTS Examine the abdomen again

- Re-examine the abdomen when the patient is anaesthetized.
- The presence of a mass suggests likely technical difficulty but does not contraindicate trial laparoscopy.

Access

1 Induce pneumoperitoneum, preferably using an open technique, or with a Veress needle. Introduce a 10-mm port at the umbilicus.

2 Insert a 10-mm telescope, inspect the peritoneal cavity and confirm the diagnosis. If you cannot visualize the structures in the right iliac fossa and pelvis, improve access by rotating the patient to the left side with some head-down tilt.

3 Introduce two 5-mm ports, one in the right flank at a distance from the appendix itself and one in the lower midline above the pubic symphysis, avoiding the bladder.

Assess

1 Examine all other pelvic and abdominal organs to exclude ovarian cyst, ectopic pregnancy, pelvic inflammatory disease, cholecystitis, perforated peptic ulcer, Meckel's diverticulum, colonic diverticulitis, Crohn's disease and ischaemic bowel. Your ability to examine abdominal contents is much greater using laparoscopy than by open surgery through a small incision.

2 Identify the appendix which, in early appendicitis, may appear normal if mucosal inflammation has not yet extended to the peritoneum.

3 Plan to remove an apparently 'normal' appendix if you can find no cause for the patient's pain.

Action

1 Your intention is to separate the appendix from its mesentery using diathermy dissection, ideally bipolar if you have it available, starting at the tip and working towards the base where the appendix expands into the caecum, identified by the taenia coli. The appendix mesentery is not removed. If this is a late presentation with advanced inflammation and oedema, this approach may not be possible. You may need to divide the appendix base and mesentery en masse, using a vascular stapler such as the EndoGIA II (Autosuture).

2 Identify the appendix. Hold and elevate its tip using the left-hand grasper. If the tip is not visible, first identify the appendix base and follow this using atraumatic graspers until you reach the tip. Break down inflammatory adhesions using blunt suction dissection. Occasionally, some lateral mobilization of the caecum may be necessary using scissor or hook diathermy dissection.

? DIFFICULTY

1. If you cannot find the appendix, replace the suprapubic port with a 10-mm port.
2. Insert the telescope through this to obtain better views of the base of the caecum and retrocaecal region.

3 With the appendix tip elevated, begin separating the mesentery. Vessels close to the appendix are small and can be divided using diathermy alone, with minimal bleeding. If you cannot control an arterial spurter in this manner you may need to apply a clip, if necessary after replacing the lateral 5-mm port with a 10-mm port. If dissection is difficult, insert a third port in the left iliac fossa. An assistant can hold the mesentery while you hold the appendix, so facilitating the separation.

4 Continue dissecting until you see the base expanding into the caecum. Take care not to injure the caecum with the diathermy.

5 Introduce a Vicryl Endoloop (Ethicon) through the lateral port and place it around the base of the appendix. Place two ties close to the caecum and the third tie approximately 1 cm distal to the first two. Transect the appendix, leaving two ties on the caecum. If the appendix base is friable and oedematous, divide it using a stapler, including some caecal wall if necessary.

6 Do not invaginate or diathermize the appendix stump. Remove any faecal residue from the appendix stump with irrigation. Perform extensive saline irrigation of the right lower abdomen, pelvis and right subphrenic space until you have removed all pus and blood. In case of difficulty, leave a small-bore tube drain into the pelvis.

▶ KEY POINTS Technical considerations

- If you are applying a linear stapler, use a vascular rather than an intestinal cartridge for haemostasis.
- You can reduce costs by tying knots extracorporeally.

7 The appendix base can usually be grasped via the suprapubic port and delivered into the 10-mm umbilical port as you remove the telescope. If this is not possible, replace one of the 5-mm ports with a 10-mm port to aid removal. To prevent contamination, use a retrieval bag if necessary.

▶ KEY POINTS Appendix normal?

- If the appendix looks normal and there is no other accountable pathology, remove the appendix as it may show early appendicitis on histology.
- This also eliminates appendicitis as a diagnosis if the patient has recurrent symptoms.

? DIFFICULTY

1. If the appendix is fixed or lying retrocaecally, place a port in the right upper quadrant of the abdomen to aid mobilization and dissection.
2. Be willing to place the telescope in the suprapubic port to improve your view of the base of the caecum.
3. Do not hesitate to convert the procedure into an open operation if dissection is impossible, if bleeding is uncontrollable, and if you identify or suspect visceral damage.
4. If the appendix is perforated, as soon as possible apply an Endoloop below the perforation, so reducing contamination from leakage of content into the peritoneal cavity. Cut this suture long so that it can be used for retraction. The appendix may be friable and disintegrate if held by forceps. Place the appendix in a retrieval bag to reduce contamination. Use liberal irrigation and suction to remove all purulent fluid from the pelvic, subhepatic and subphrenic spaces. Insert a small tube drain through one of the 5-mm ports, usually to be removed on the next day.
5. If you are experienced you may be able to successfully manage an appendix abscess laparoscopically. When the appendix cannot be identified within an inflammatory mass, you may break down loculations, aspirate as much pus as possible and simply drain the area.
6. If you are in doubt, though, convert to open operation. In such cases, take especial care to avoid inadvertently injuring the intestine, blood vessels or ureter.

Checklist

1 Inspect the pelvic, subphrenic and subhepatic spaces for any collection and use extensive saline irrigation.

2 Check the appendix stump to ensure that it is intact and safely closed.

3 Check for haemostasis and that any applied clips are well secured.

4 Ensure that there is no injury to the surrounding viscera.

5 Remove urinary and gastric catheters if inserted prior to surgery.

Closure

1 Withdraw the accessory ports under vision. Withdraw the telescope and large port.

2 Close the rectus sheath of the 10-mm incision site with Vicryl. Close the skin with Steri-Strip tapes.

3 Infiltrate long-acting local anaesthetic at the port sites.

Postoperative

1 In the absence of general peritonitis allow oral fluids on the first postoperative day.

2 Encourage the patient to get out of bed and walk on the day of operation. Most patients can be discharged on the first postoperative day and almost all by the second.

3 Continue metronidazole and a parenteral antibiotic such as cefuroxime for 3–4 days if there was serious sepsis or contamination, especially in poor-risk patients.

4 If pyrexia develops, check the wounds and exclude chest and urinary infection.

Complications

1 *Bleeding* is one of the most common complications. Possible sources include the inferior epigastric artery, appendicular artery, retroperitoneal vessels or the staple line. You can injure the inferior epigastric artery when introducing the right iliac fossa port. Avoid this by placing the port well lateral to the rectus abdominus muscle. Attempt to identify and control the source of bleeding by re-laparoscopy if possible, before converting to open surgery.

2 *Perforation of the bowel* can occur either from puncture by the trocar, inadvertent electrosurgical injury or slippage of the appendix base loops. If you are an experienced laparoscopic surgeon you may close the perforation laparoscopically. Caecal perforation may be difficult to close laparoscopically, especially when it is inflamed and thick. In these circumstances, convert to an open procedure.

3 Avoid *injury to the bladder* by catheterization and introduce the suprapubic port under direct vision.

4 Postoperative *intra-abdominal and pelvic abscess* occurs in 3–5% of patients and can be detected or confirmed by ultrasound or computed tomography (CT). Perform percutaneous drainage under imaging control.

5 Significant *wound infection* is unusual. Examine the wound regularly and remove the superficial sutures or clips if there is evidence of infection.

6 There are several case reports of *incomplete appendicectomy* leading to recurrent appendicitis. Avoid this problem by carefully identifying the appendix base during dissection.

7 *Incisional hernia* may develop through the trocar site, rarely complicated by a faecal fistula.

8 *Deep venous thrombosis* and *pulmonary embolus* can occur after appendicectomy, especially in the elderly. Reduce the risk by using heparin prophylaxis, although this may increase the risks of bleeding.

REFERENCES

1. Sauerland S, Lefering R, Holthausen U et al 1998 Laparoscopic vs conventional appendectomy: a meta-analysis of randomised controlled trials. Langenbecks Archives of Surgery 383(3–4):289
2. Ortega AE, Hunter JG, Peters JH et al 1995 A prospective randomized comparison of laparoscopic appendectomy with open appendectomy. American Journal of Surgery 169:208–212
3. Tate JJT 1996 Laparoscopic appendicectomy. British Journal of Surgery 83:1169–1170
4. Minne L, Varner D, Burnell A et al 1997 Laparoscopic vs open appendectomy: prospective randomized study of outcomes. Archives of Surgery 132:708–712
5. Klingler A, Henle KP, Beller S et al 1998 Laparoscopic appendectomy does not change the incidence of postoperative infectious complications. American Journal of Surgery 175:232–235

FURTHER READING

O'Reilly MJ, Reddick EJ, Miller WD et al 1993 Laparoscopic appendectomy. In: Zucker KA (ed.) Surgical laparoscopy. Update, St Louis, pp 301–326

Richardson WS, Hunter JG 1997 Complications in appendectomy. In: Ponsky JL (ed.) Complications of endoscopic and laparoscopic surgery. Prevention and management. Lippincott-Raven, Philadelphia, pp 171–176

Internet web site

http://www.edu.rcsed.ac.uk/video_album_menu.htm

10

Oesophagus

R. MASON

CONTENTS

ENDOSCOPY

Appraise

1 Endoscope every patient with dysphagia except when this is fully explained by the presence of neurological or neuromuscular disease.

2 Endoscope patients with suspected disease in the oesophagus producing pain on swallowing (odynophagia), heartburn not responding to simple medication or arising de novo in patients over 50 years, bleeding, or if accidental and iatrogenic damage are suspected.

Prepare

1 Ensure that the endoscope, the ancillary equipment and necessary spares are available, function correctly and are appropriately sterile. The endoscope must be thoroughly prepared between procedures according to the maker's instructions. Fibreoptic instruments, biopsy forceps and similar instruments are scrupulously cleaned using neutral detergent and usually disinfected with 2% alkaline glutaraldehyde. This is capable of eliminating all infective organisms, including HIV. Keep abreast of the literature on methods of sterilization. Initial cleaning is done by hand. Washing and sterilization is performed mechanically in an automatic machine to avoid exposure of endoscopy room staff to glutaraldehyde fumes.

2 Modern gastrointestinal endoscopes are slim, versatile, have remarkably flexible tips and can be passed with pharyngeal anaesthesia alone in most patients. They are safe, relatively comfortable for the patient and allow examination of the stomach and duodenum beyond. Use the end-viewing instrument routinely since it gives the best general view. Through it can be passed biopsy forceps, cytology brushes, snares, guidewires for dilators and needles for injection. Argon plasma coagulation or Nd-YAG laser may be applied through it for the palliation of inoperable neoplasms or for the treatment of Barrett's oesophagus. The technology of endoscopes is steadily improving and the rigid oesophagoscope is, to all intents and purposes, obsolete.

3 Obtain signed informed consent from the patient.

4 Remove dentures from the patient.

5 Except in an emergency have the patient starved of food and fluids for at least 5 hours. In an emergency, especially in patients with upper gastrointestinal haemorrhage who cannot wait 5 hours for the stomach to empty, a crash general anaesthetic with cricoid pressure is the safest means of securing the airway and preventing aspiration.

6 Obtain a preliminary barium swallow X-ray if there is a suspected pharyngeal pouch.

7 Attach a pulse oximeter probe to the patient's finger if sedation is being used, and ensure that there are sufficient staff in the endoscopy room for safe care of a sedated patient.

8 Spray the pharynx with lidocaine solution just before passing the endoscope.

9 In anxious patients, or those in whom intervention (e.g. dilatation) is required, insert a small plastic cannula into a peripheral vein and through it inject slowly 1–2 mg of midazolam until the patient's eyelids just begin to droop. Remember that it takes 2 minutes for the full effect of midazolam to develop.

FIBREOPTIC ENDOSCOPY

1 Lay the patient on the left side with hips and knees flexed. Place a plastic hollow gag between the teeth. Ensure that the patient's head is in the midline and that the chin is lowered on to the chest.

2 Lubricate the previously checked end-viewing instrument with water-soluble jelly.

3 Pass the endoscope tip through the plastic gag, over the tongue to the posterior pharyngeal wall. Depress the tip control slightly so that the instrument tip passes down towards the cricopharyngeal sphincter. Do not overflex the tip or it will be directed anteriorly and enter the larynx. Visualize the larynx and pass the endoscope just behind it.

4 Ask the patient to swallow. Do not resist the slight extrusion of the endoscope as the larynx rises but maintain gentle pressure so that it will advance as the larynx descends and the cricopharyngeal sphincter relaxes. Advance the endoscope under vision,

insufflating air gently to open up the passage. Aspirate any fluid. Spray water across the lens if it becomes obscured. If no hold-up is encountered, pass the tip through the stomach into the duodenum then withdraw it slowly, noting the features. Remove biopsy specimens and take cytology brushings from any ulcers, tumours or other lesions.

5 If a stricture is encountered note its distance from the incisor teeth. Sometimes the instrument will pass through, allowing the length of the stricture to be determined. Always remove biopsy specimens and cytology brushings from within the stricture. If the stricture is benign in appearance gentle dilatation to 12 mm can be attempted if the patient is symptomatic. Dilatation of malignant strictures is not indicated as any benefit is short-lasting and the risk of perforation is high (6–8%). Get biopsies and confirm the diagnosis prior to intervention. If nutritional support is required, fluoroscopic passage of a feeding nasogastric tube can be performed.

KEY POINT Risk of perforation

- Remember that malignant strictures are more easily perforated than benign strictures. This may influence the decision whether to dilate or not. Only dilate if this is important for treatment and then only to 12 mm (36 F).

Assess

1 Note the level of each feature. The cricopharyngeal sphincter is approximately 16 cm from the incisor teeth. The deviation around the aortic arch is 28–30 cm, the cardia lies at 40 cm and here the lining changes abruptly from the pale, bluish, stratified oesophageal epithelium to the florid, pinker, gastric columnar-cell epithelium.

2 Oesophagitis is usually from gastro-oesophageal reflux, but is not necessarily associated with hiatal hernia. Consult a colour chart that illustrates the grades of oesophagitis. Most commonly there are red streaking erosions just above the cardia. Oesophagitis may be seen above a benign stricture. Occasionally, in advanced achalasia one may see a mild diffuse oesophagitis from contact with fermenting food residues. Thick white plaques indicate monilial infection, usually in association with oral involvement. Confirm the diagnosis by taking mucosal scrapings.

3 Sliding hiatal hernia produces a loculus of stomach above the constriction of the crura with a raised gastro-oesophageal mucosal junction. To determine the level of the hiatus, ask the patient to sniff, and note the level at which the crura momentarily narrow the lumen. Reflux and oesophagitis may be visible. A rolling hernia is visible only from within the stomach by inverting the tip of a flexible instrument to view the apparent fundic diverticulum. If the diagnosis is a possibility confirm with a barium study.

4 Frank ulceration in the oesophagus is unusual, but may be due to severe reflux disease. In Barrett's oesophagus the lower gullet is lined with modified gastric mucosa and an ulcer may develop in the columnar-lined segment. In all cases of Barrett's take biopsies of the columnar segment from all four quadrants at 2-cm intervals. In patients with dysplasia even more biopsies are required for accurate assessment. Use 'jumbo' forceps. Ulcerating carcinomas may develop at any level. In most Western countries the majority of cancers are adenocarcinomas and arise in the lower oesophagus in association with Barrett's oesophagus. Take multiple biopsies and cytological brushings from a number of areas of all ulcers.

5 Strictures from peptic oesophagitis or, rarely, ulceration in a Barrett's oesophagus develop at any time from birth onwards, but more frequently occur in middle or old age. Almost always there is a coincidental hiatal hernia. If there is no hernia below the stricture suspect cancer. Also suspect cancer if there is food residue above a stricture. Food residue may also be seen in achalasia and may be the only diagnostic clue. Take multiple biopsies and brushings for cytology. The cause of Schatzki's ring is unknown. It is usually asymptomatic, seen radiologically at the junction between gastric and oesophageal mucosa. Caustic strictures develop at the sites of hold-up of swallowed liquids at the cricopharyngeus, at the aortic arch crossing and at the cardia. Webs or strictures in the upper oesophagus are uncommon. However, it is not unusual to see a patch or ring of ectopic gastric mucosa in the upper oesophagus 1–2 cm below cricopharyngeus, the so-called 'inlet patch'. Stricture may arise from external pressure, of which by far the most common cause is bronchogenic carcinoma.

KEY POINTS Diagnostic appearances

- Remember that it is possible to distinguish benign from malignant lesions from the gross appearances with a high degree of accuracy. Practise this skill, which is particularly useful for triggering speedy reinvestigation of suspicious lesions if biopsies are misleadingly negative.
- Consult a good colour atlas or a CD-ROM. Become familiar with the appearances of early cancer of the oesophagus. Early diagnosis is the best means of improving cure rates.

6 Mega-oesophagus may be seen in achalasia of the cardia, but is now uncommon as most cases are diagnosed long before dilatation takes place. Mega-oesophagus may also be seen in the South American Chagas' disease and in some cases of advanced scleroderma.

7 Pulsion diverticula are related to abnormal oesophageal motility and are seen above the cricopharyngeus muscle (Zenker's diverticulum or pharyngeal pouch) and above segments of presumed spasm. Traction diverticula in the mid-oesophagus develop as a result of chronic inflammation of mediastinal glands, especially from tuberculosis.

8 Oesophageal varices are usually recognized just above the cardia as convoluted varicose veins, which may extend into the upper stomach.

DILATATION OF STRICTURES (Fig. 10.1)

1 Fragile strictures do not always require endoscopic dilatation if the diagnosis is not in doubt or has been confirmed by

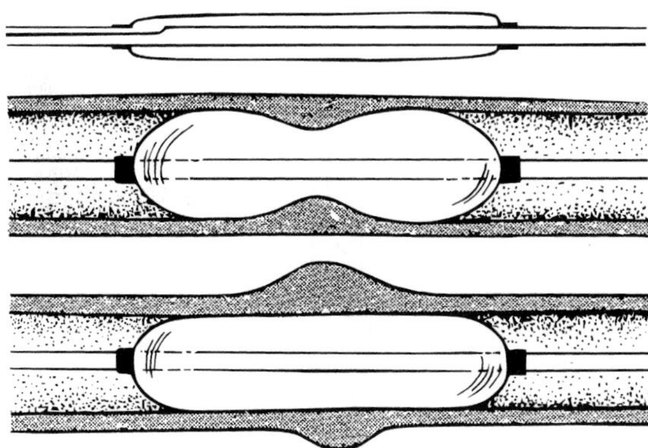

Fig. 10.1 Balloon dilatation. At the top is a balloon collapsed on its introductory catheter. There is a radio-opaque marker at each end of the balloon. In the middle drawing, the balloon is partly inflated within a stricture that has produced a waist. At the bottom, the waist has disappeared as the balloon is fully inflated.

endoscopy. The safest oesophageal dilator is soft, solid food, provided that each bolus contains only aggregated small particles.

2 Record the distance of the stricture from the incisor teeth. If the stricture is short and appears benign, the best means for dilatation is by a through-the-channel balloon. These balloons have a fixed maximum diameter up to a maximum of 2 cm (60 F). Always check for perforation with endoscopy after dilatation. An alternative to these balloon dilatators are soft mercury-laden Maloney dilators. If problems occur inserting them through a tortuous stricture, balloon dilatation using a hydrophilic guidewire inserted under fluoroscopic control should be undertaken.

3 First outline the passage by getting the erect patient to swallow a thin contrast medium. Now introduce a fine, flexible guidewire through a nostril into the oesophagus and negotiate the tip through the stricture using a combination of rotating it and getting the patient to swallow a little water or more contrast medium to outline the passage. Now pass a well-lubricated catheter fitted with a deflated balloon over the guidewire and insinuate it through the stricture. The proximal and distal ends of the balloon have radio-opaque markers so that it can be placed accurately. Carefully inflate the balloon, watching it on the screen. A waist appears at the level of the stricture and as the pressure is gradually increased this disappears. If the patient is apprehensive or complains of discomfort, temporarily stop inflating the balloon.

4 Most strictures can be dilated at a single session, but do not persist unduly in the face of difficulty or discomfort. When the balloon is withdrawn, check to see if there is any blood on it. Now give the patient some contrast medium to swallow and carefully watch it pass through the stricture to ensure that there is no leak.

REMOVAL OF FOREIGN BODIES

Appraise

1 Swallowed articles impact at the sites of narrowing. Objects at the cricopharyngeus muscle are regurgitated but those that pass this point may impact at the crossing of the aortic arch or at the cardia. However, the normal oesophagus is extremely distensible and smooth objects usually pass into the stomach. The most frequent causes of impaction are pre-existing stricture or a sharp foreign body that penetrates the oesophageal wall.

2 Remember that many impacted foreign bodies are radiolucent. Sometimes they are demonstrable on X-rays by giving the patient a drink of water-soluble contrast medium.

3 Most foreign bodies may be removed using a variety of methods in conjunction with fibreoptic endoscopes and an overtube under local anaesthesia with sedation. If a foreign body cannot be removed with modern endoscopic instruments an operation is probably required. Deeply and firmly impacted foreign bodies may require thoracotomy and oesophagotomy to remove them.

4 A smooth foreign body, or a food bolus, may be gently pushed into the stomach. As a rule it will pass through the gut but if it remains in the stomach removal is easier than from the oesophagus.

Action

1 There is a classic repertoire of methods to remove foreign bodies through the rigid oesophagoscope. The grasping forceps are strong and versatile, and can cope with open safety pins and coins. Version and extraction of an open safety pin with the point facing upwards is now part of the folklore of oesophageal surgery. However, the use of the rigid endoscope is not now to be encouraged. There are safer and better methods.

2 Ingenious methods have been used to remove foreign bodies using the end-viewing fibreoptic endoscope. The foreign body may be grasped with forceps or caught with a snare and withdrawn together with the instrument. An external flexible sheath may be pushed over the end of the endoscope tip into which a sharp foreign body can be drawn to protect the mucosa from injury. A variety of snares and grasping forceps should be kept available.

INJECTION OR BANDING OF VARICES

Appraise (see Ch. 22)

1 Recognize these as soft, collapsible, projecting columns in the lower oesophagus sometimes continuing into the gastric cardia.

2 In patients with upper gastrointestinal bleeding who are found to have varices, do not assume that the bleeding is from the varices. A high proportion of such patients have another cause such as peptic ulcer, so always carry out a complete examination.

3 The varices thrombose when injected with ethanolamine oleate warmed to reduce its viscosity. An injection needle is passed down the biopsy channel and 2–5 ml is injected into each varix. The injections are repeated at intervals of 3–4 weeks until the varices are obliterated.

4 Banding of varices has a number of advantages, including better immediate control of active bleeding. A banding device that can fire several bands is loaded into and onto the endoscope. Always

read the instructions on the device. Continuous design improvement is the norm and the device may have changed since you last used it. The varix is identified and then sucked into the banding cap on the end of the endoscope. When a 'red-out' is achieved the bander is fired and the suction released. The band should be seen clearly in the required position. Multiple varices can be ligated at a single session.

INTUBATION OF TUMOURS

Appraise

1 It is not necessary to intubate all strictures that cannot be resected. Malignant strictures that will be submitted to chemo- or radiotherapy may deteriorate temporarily and later expand, so it is worthwhile deferring intubation. Intubation of benign strictures is not recommended unless in exceptional cases in very frail subjects with a limited life-expectancy. Intubation produces a rigid channel through which food must fall by gravity and which can easily become blocked, so reserve its use for patients with real need.

2 The development of expanding metal stents is a considerable advance and has replaced the rigid plastic tube. They provide a larger lumen for swallowing and do not require as much dilatation as semirigid stents such as the Nottingham tube. As a result insertion is safer. Expanding metal stents may be inserted at endoscopy, by radiological screening or by a combination of both methods. They are produced in both covered and uncovered formats.

Insertion of self-expanding metal stent (Fig. 10.2)

1 There are many different designs. Be familiar with the stent, its introducer and the method of deployment. Most expanding stents shorten as they expand and this must be taken into account during insertion. Some stents can be partially deployed and the position adjusted if it is not satisfactory. However, you may have to get it right first time, so be careful.

2 Such stents can be inserted under fluoroscopic or endoscopic control. Fluoroscopy has the advantage of outlining the length and position of the stricture accurately by using a radio-opaque contrast swallow prior to insertion. Dilatation up to 1 cm is usually required prior to stent deployment as described above for dilatation of difficult strictures.

3 Pass the stent with its introducer over the guidewire and into the desired position. An endoscope may be passed alongside the guidewire so that deployment can be checked under vision.

4 Deploy the stent according to the manufacturer's instructions.

5 Correct stent deployment can be checked by endoscopy or contrast swallow. Some stents may be very slow to expand. Expansion may be hastened by dilatation with a through-the-scope balloon.

Aftercare

1 Make sure the patient does not have chest pain, air emphysema in the neck, or a raised temperature. Have a plain chest radiograph taken or perform a contrast swallow.

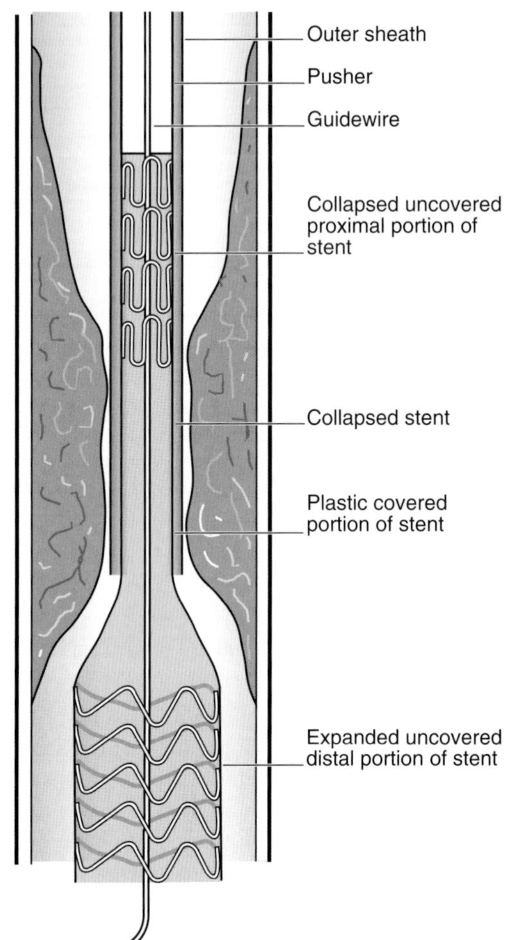

Fig. 10.2 Wall stent: self-expanding metal stent being deployed under fluoroscopic control.

2 If there is evidence of a leak, confirm it and identify the site with X-rays using a water-soluble contrast medium. If an expanding stent is not sealing a leak consider inserting a second stent. Start the patient on broad-spectrum antibiotics and withhold food and fluids until the patient is entirely comfortable and a contrast swallow shows no leak.

3 Following stent insertion, warn the patient against swallowing unchewed food, particularly lumps of meat, fruit skins and stones, and to wash down the food with sips of water. Aerated drinks such as sodium bicarbonate solution (half a teaspoonful in half a glass of water half an hour before meals) or fresh pineapple juice help to wash away adherent mucus that may block the tube.

4 It is now extraordinarily uncommon to fail to intubate a tumour. If it cannot be done, a feeding gastrostomy or jejunostomy may be inserted after full discussion with the patient. This poses ethical and philosophical dilemmas, but these must be faced. However, always remember that the aim of palliation is to improve the quality of remaining life. If a particular therapy will not improve the quality of life in an individual patient, do not use it.

OESOPHAGEAL EXPOSURE

NECK (Fig. 10.3)

1 The cervical oesophagus may be approached from either side. Operations for the removal of pharyngeal pouch, cricopharyngeal myotomy are usually carried out from the left side. For oesophageal anastomosis following resection either side can be used. The right-sided approach minimizes risk of damage to the thoracic duct although this is a rare complication for exposure of the oesophagus and usually occurs as a complication of biopsy of lymph nodes. The left nerve is more likely to be injured during intrathoracic resection or be involved in the malignant process. It is better therefore to expose it to risk of injury rather than the right nerve.

2 The anaesthetized intubated patient lies supine on the operating table with the head turned to the opposite side from which the exploration will be made, resting on a ring with the neck extended. There is no need for complex head towelling, but drapes can be secured with skin staples.

3 Incise along the anterior border of sternomastoid muscle, through platysma muscle, cervical fascia, omohyoid muscle, ligating and dividing the middle thyroid vein to enter the space between the oesophagus, trachea and thyroid gland medially and the carotid sheath laterally. The inferior thyroid artery crosses the space; ligate and divide it laterally only if it interferes with the dissection.

4 Rotate the whole oesophageal–tracheal–thyroid column towards the opposite side, bringing into view the tracheo-oesophageal groove, and display the posterior surface of the oesophagus and lower pharynx. Beware of inserting a Langenbeck's retractor into the tracheo-oesophageal groove since it may well crush the recurrent laryngeal nerve.

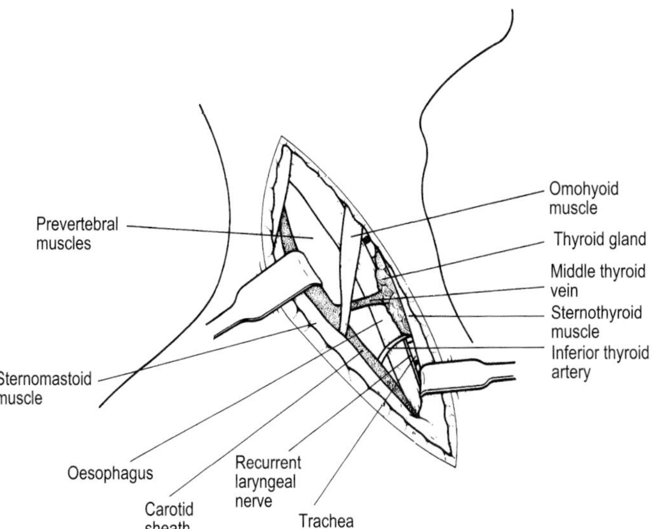

Fig. 10.3 Exposure of the cervical oesophagus on the right side. Sternomastoid muscle and the carotid sheath are drawn laterally. The space between these structures and the midline column of the pharynx and oesophagus, larynx, trachea and thyroid gland is crossed by the omohyoid muscle, middle thyroid vein and the inferior thyroid artery.

5 Mobilize the posterior wall of the oesophagus with blunt dissection. Staying on the muscle wall of the oesophagus come anteriorly and over the front, separating the trachea and recurrent laryngeal nerve anteriorly (Fig. 10.4). It is not necessary to mobilize the nerve and this prevents an ischaemic neuropraxia. Staying on the muscle wall go round the oesophagus on the opposite side retracting the oesophagus laterally. This exposes the prevertebral fascia on the opposite side. A curved forceps can then be placed around the oesophagus and a sling placed. With gentle traction on this the oesophagus can be mobilized by finger dissection staying on the oesophageal wall.

RIGHT POSTEROLATERAL THORACOTOMY (Fig. 10.5)

1 The anaesthetized patient, intubated with a double-lumen tube to allow exclusion of the right lung, lies on the left side. Carry out right posterolateral thoracotomy at the level of the fifth or sixth rib (see Ch. 33).

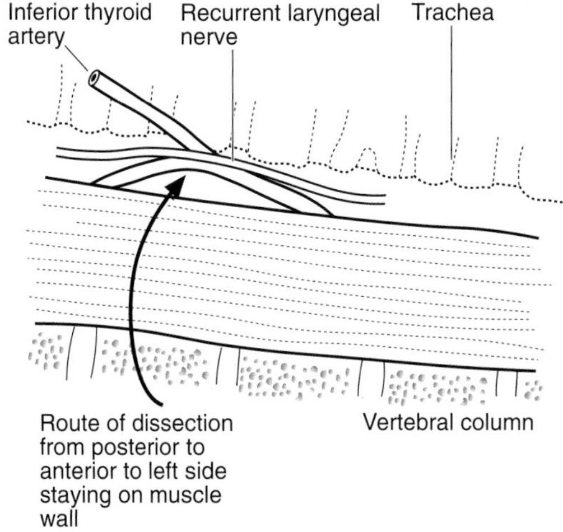

Fig. 10.4 Mobilization of the oesophagus in the neck from the right side preserving the recurrent laryngeal nerve.

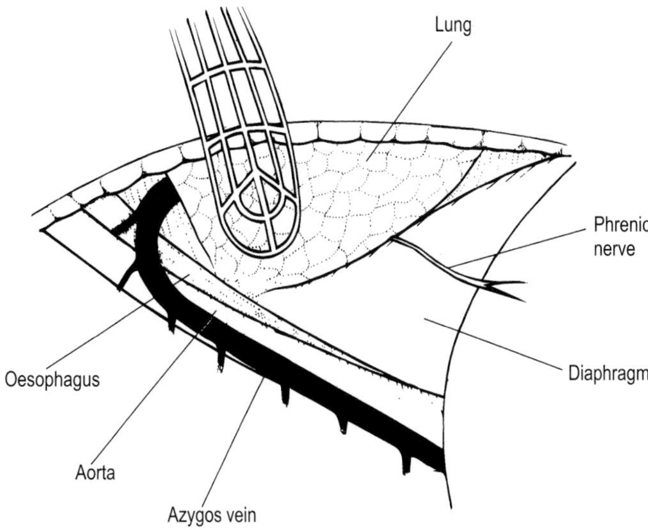

Fig. 10.5 Diagram of approach to the oesophagus through the right pleural space. The right lung is retracted anteriorly.

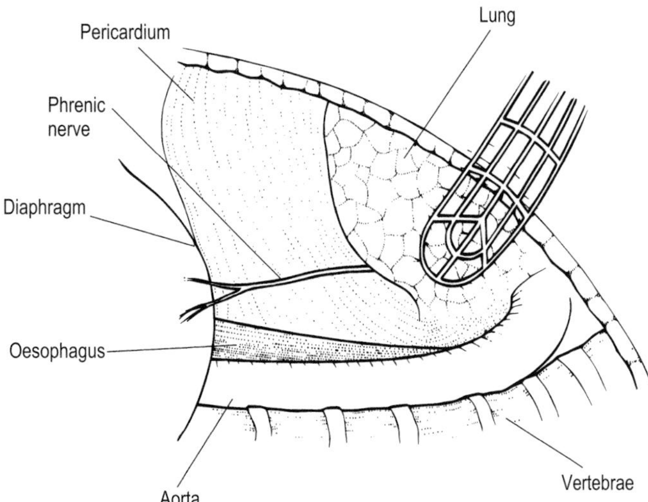

Fig. 10.6 Diagram of approach to the lower oesophagus through the left pleural space. The left lung is retracted anteriorly.

2 Ask the anaesthetist to collapse the right lung. Draw it downwards and forwards to reveal the mediastinal pleura. The oesophagus cannot be seen but the azygos vein can be seen arching over the lung root. Incise the mediastinal pleura, mobilize, doubly ligate and divide the azygos vein. This reveals the oesophagus running posterior to the trachea and lung root. The lower oesophagus is not visible between the left atrium and the vertebral column as it veers to the left. Expose it by dividing the pulmonary ligament until the inferior pulmonary vein is exposed. Then divide the mediastinal pleura anterior to the descending aorta. The upper stomach can be approached after dilating or incising the diaphragmatic crus to enlarge the hiatus.

LEFT THORACOTOMY (Fig. 10.6)

1 The lower thoracic oesophagus may be approached by left thoracotomy at the level of the seventh or eighth rib (see Ch. 33).

2 The left dome of diaphragm or the diaphragmatic crus may be incised to enter the upper abdomen.

LEFT THORACOABDOMINAL APPROACH (Fig. 10.7)

1 The lower thoracic oesophagus and upper stomach are best approached using a combined thoracoabdominal approach (see Ch. 11).

2 Lay the anaesthetized intubated patient on the right side, left leg extended, right leg flexed at hip and knee, both arms flexed with forearms before the face as though performing the hornpipe dance. Allow the patient to lie back with the shoulders at 30° from the vertical. Fix the patient's hips with an encircling band; support the left upper scapula against a padded post.

3 Prepare the skin and drape the area with sterile towels.

4 Start the incision 2.5 cm under the right costal margin in the midclavicular line, carry it obliquely upwards and to the left to cross the costal margin along the line of the seventh or eighth rib, extending to the posterior angle of the chosen rib and up behind the scapula. Deepen the incision to enter the thorax along the line of the rib, cutting and removing 1 cm of the costal

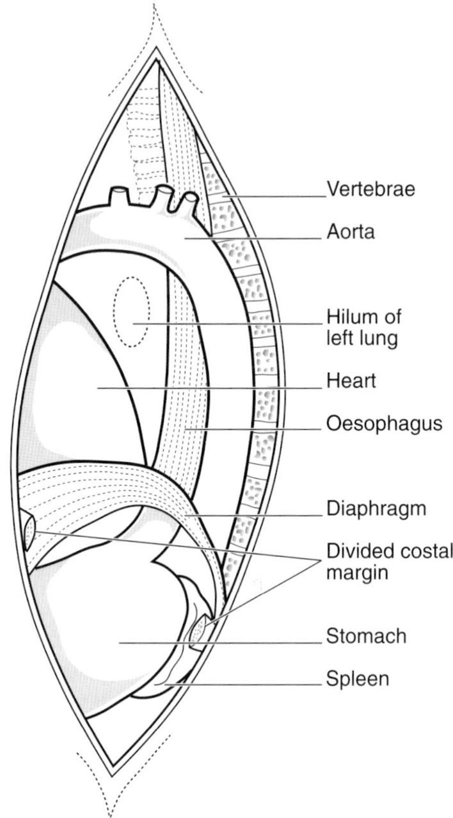

Fig. 10.7 Left thoracoabdominal approach. The diaphragm is divided circumferentially to enable the incision to open. It does not extend to the hiatus. The lung is elevated anteriorly.

margin. Incise the diaphragm peripherally parallel to the chest wall far enough in to enable the chest to be opened but not as far as the hiatus. This method spares the phrenic nerve.

5 In case of doubt make the abdominal or thoracic part of the incision first; assess the condition and now, if indicated, extend it fully.

6 After completing the procedure, close the diaphragm with strong absorbable material. Do not suture the costal margin but resect a wedge of cartilage to enable the ends to lie adjacent. Suture the abdomen in the usual manner. Close the chest after inserting an underwater-sealed drain.

ABDOMINAL (Fig. 10.8)

1 The lower oesophagus is approachable through the abdomen and oesophageal hiatus.

2 The best access, especially in patients with a wide costal angle, is by a roof-top or bilateral subcostal incision. In those with a narrow costal angle an upper midline incision extending to the costal margin is preferable, opening the peritoneum just to the left of the falciform ligament. Ligate the ligamentum teres. Divide it and the falciform ligament.

3 Draw down the stomach while an assistant elevates the left lobe of the liver with a flat-bladed retractor. The lower oesophagus can be felt at the hiatus.

4 If necessary, cut the left triangular ligament and fold the left lobe of the liver to the right.

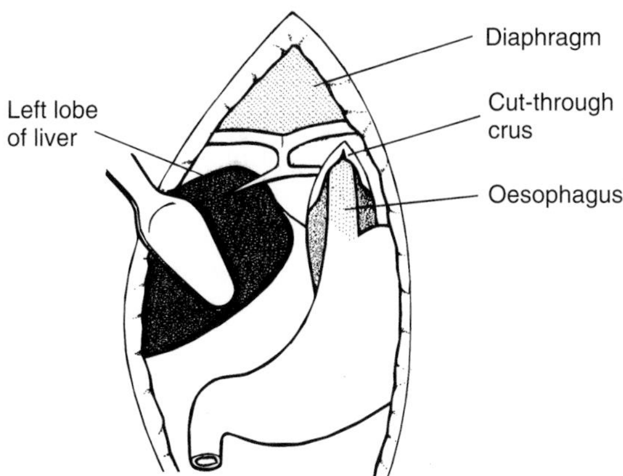

Fig. 10.8 Transabdominal approach to the lower oesophagus. The left lobe of the liver is folded to the right. If necessary, the diaphragmatic crus can be incised anteriorly.

5 To display the lower thoracic oesophagus, transversely incise the peritoneum and fascia over the abdominal oesophagus for 5 cm, preserving the anterior vagal trunk. If greater exposure is necessary insert a finger into the posterior mediastinum. Turn it forwards to separate the pericardium from the upper surface and incise the crus and diaphragm anteriorly for 5–7 cm. In patients of suitable build, the oesophagus can be viewed almost up to the carina of the trachea if the heart is gently elevated with a flat retractor. It is usually unnecessary to close the incision in the crus and diaphragm. The inferior phrenic vein will need to be oversewn.

TRANSHIATAL APPROACH (Fig. 10.9)

1 This encompasses both the abdominal and cervical approaches described above.

2 After division of the diaphragm anteriorly dissect the fat pad off the back of the pericardium. It is common to take the pleura on the left side. Place an anterior resection retraction retractor behind the heart and lift up and towards the head. Take care not to compress the left atrium. Dissect under direct vision to the carina using an harmonic scalpel, dividing the vagi.

3 Mobilize the oesophagus in the neck as described from the left side. After encircling the oesophagus, mobilize it with a finger into the upper mediastinum.

4 Place a tie around the oesophagus low down and produce a mucosal tube as described below. Open the anterior part of the mucosal tube and withdraw the nasogastric tube. Grasp the end of the nasogastric tube and place a tie into it to facilitate bringing it back to the conduit during the anastomosis.

5 Pass the wire of a varicose-vein stripper into the oesophagus and pass it into the stomach. Tighten the tie round the stripper wire distal to its insertion and divide the oesophagus. Place a medium head on the stripper. Gently pull the stripper distally guiding the head into the posterior mediastinum avoiding damage to the adjacent structures. This will invert the oesophagus and deliver it to the abdomen. Vagal strands may prevent full delivery and need division under direct vision from below.

6 To guide the conduit to the neck for anastomosis use a chest drain to avoid rotation.

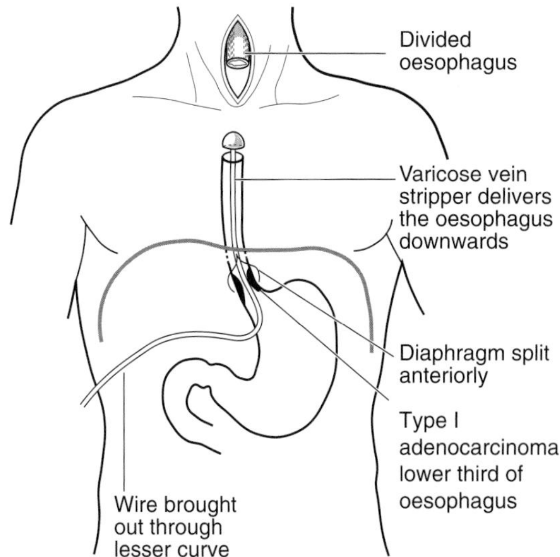

Fig. 10.9 The transhiatal approach, delivering the oesophagus with a varicose-vein stripper.

LAPAROSCOPIC

1 Position the patient supine with the legs flat (for diagnostic or staging endoscopy) or with the legs apart in stirrups, as in rectal surgery (for major procedures, such as antireflux surgery).

2 Induce a pneumoperitoneum using a Veress needle or by an open technique.

3 Insert a 10-mm cannula in the midline approximately one-third of the distance between the umbilicus and the xiphisternum.

4 Liver retraction is best achieved by use of a Nathanson retractor inserted via a small 5-mm incision in the epigastrium. If not available, insert a 5- or 10-mm cannula, depending on what type of liver retractor is used, in the right subcostal region in the midclavicular line. Introduce a liver retractor and lift the left lobe of the liver upwards.

5 The number and position of additional cannulas depend on the procedure to be done and the preference of the operator. Commonly, additional cannulas are placed below the xiphisternum, in the left subcostal region in the midclavicular line and the anterior axillary line (the 'Liege' approach).

6 The oesophagus may then be approached as described in the previous section by dividing the peritoneum over the lower oesophagus. The precise approach to the oesophagus depends on the procedure to be done.

OPERATIVE CONSIDERATIONS

Appraise

1 Most other parts of the bowel are covered with serosa which rapidly forms fibrinous adhesions, sealing small defects and preventing leaks. The oesophagus has no serous coat except on the anterior wall of the abdominal segment.

2 A considerable part of the oesophageal wall is composed of longitudinal muscle. Longitudinally placed sutures thus have a tendency to cut out. The powerful longitudinal muscle produces

shortening of the transected oesophagus when it contracts. Unless this is allowed for, the most carefully placed sutures may be torn out.

3 When the oesophagus is completely relaxed it has a remarkably large lumen. Commonly, the action of the circular muscle makes the diameter appear to be small. However, it can be stretched quite easily by insertion of a Foley catheter and inflating the balloon to facilitate the placement of sutures. If this is not done, closely spaced sutures may become widely separated on stretching, and leakage can easily occur between them.

4 The blood supply to the oesophagus is tenuous when it is mobilized, especially at the lower end.

5 The healthy oesophagus is easily damaged but disease may make it exceptionally fragile.

6 A diseased or partially obstructed oesophagus is contaminated. Prophylactic antibiotics must be given to cover the operation.

7 Although oral feeding may be stopped temporarily following oesophageal surgery, swallowed saliva must still pass through.

8 Intrathoracic oesophageal leakage produces posterior mediastinitis and if the pleura is damaged a pleural collection develops. The best hope for the patient's survival if major leakage occurs is rapid clinical recognition with early re-operative repair and drainage. Minor leaks may be treated conservatively. Place chest drains in all opened chest cavities. Following transhiatal resection even if the pleura is not opened a chest drain in the posterior mediastinum will prevent haematoma collection. A feeding jejunostomy should be placed at operation in all cases for postoperative nutrition and oral intake should not commence until the anastomosis is checked by contrast swallow at 5 days.

KEY POINTS Technical considerations

- Never intubate the oesophagus unnecessarily. Never pass a rigid tube when a flexible one will suffice.
- Never carry out extensive oesophageal mobilization before forming an anastomosis.
- If the oesophagus retracts after division do not grab it with an instrument that may cause damage. Ask the anaesthetist to check the depth of anaesthesia—the longitudinal muscle of the oesophagus is one of the last to relax. The end of the oesophagus will often come easily back into view and stay sutures may be placed.
- Never leave the oesophagus sutured under tension. When joining it to another viscus make sure there will be no traction, even when the oesophagus fully contracts.
- Never attempt an oesophageal anastomosis when access is poor. Improve the view or change tactics.
- Never perform an oesophageal anastomosis when tired. Take a short break if necessary.
- Never use small forceps to grasp the oesophagus. They cause damage. Use forceps with a large surface area and take a firm, but gentle grip. This is much kinder to tissue. Use grasping instruments as little as possible.

Anastomosis

1 The tenuous blood supply of the oesophagus makes it rarely possible to excise a segment, mobilize the cut ends and carry out an end-to-end union, except in neonates. Anastomosis is therefore usually to stomach, jejunum or colon.

2 Sutured anastomoses have been described using many different methods and materials. It is now recognized that single-layer anastomoses with continuous or interrupted anastomoses are best.

3 Circular stapling devices are often useful. Do not assume that perfection automatically follows their use. As with sutures, staplers give results commensurate with the care with which they are used. Which to choose? The stapling device saves a little time. It may allow an anastomosis to be accomplished where suturing is difficult high in the abdomen, under the aortic arch, or high in the thorax; but if it fails, suturing is usually impossible and a higher resection is necessary. The stapling gun has an inevitable crushing effect on the tissues. If a dilated and thickened oesophagus is to be joined to the cut end of bowel, the resulting tissue bulk cannot be accommodated in the staple gun. It is safer to use a sutured anastomosis. Hand suturing is usually preferable in the neck since there may be insufficient bowel accessible below the anastomosis for insertion of the gun.

Sutured anastomosis

1 Have you made sure that the oesophagus and conduit, which may be stomach, jejunum or colon, can be joined without tension and are not twisted? When the oesophagus contracts, the powerful longitudinal muscle causes remarkable shortening. However, longitudinal muscle is of little value in retaining sutures, which easily cut out between the muscle fibres, so the strength of the anastomosis must depend upon the submucous coat and to some extent on the mucosa. To achieve this, when dividing the oesophagus first divide the muscle coat to produce a mucosal tube 1 cm long. Divide this in the middle with one cut leaving the mucosa/submucosa pouting and associated with a little ooze. This is the layer that must be used for the anastomosis (Fig. 10.10).

2 Make sure the hole in the conduit matches the oesophageal lumen when it is slightly stretched. Place the oesophagus and conduit together as they will lie when joined. Avoid traction stitches as they can produce tears in the oesophageal walls. The anastomoses should lie adjacent with no tension.

3 Suture material should be absorbable such as polyglycolic acid, monofilament polyglyconate, polydioxanone or braided polyglactin 910 or braided lactomer 9-1. Use fine material such as 3/0.

4 The argument about continuous versus interrupted stitches continues. Good surgeons obtain good results with both methods. Continuous stitches, having fewer knots that weaken the thread, can, if inserted as an unlocked spiral, appose the tissue accurately without constricting them. Interrupted sutures tied without tension have the advantage that, if one cuts out, those on either side are not necessarily prejudiced. The choice is personal, often the result of following the tenets of an admired teacher. If you use interrupted stitches, those uniting

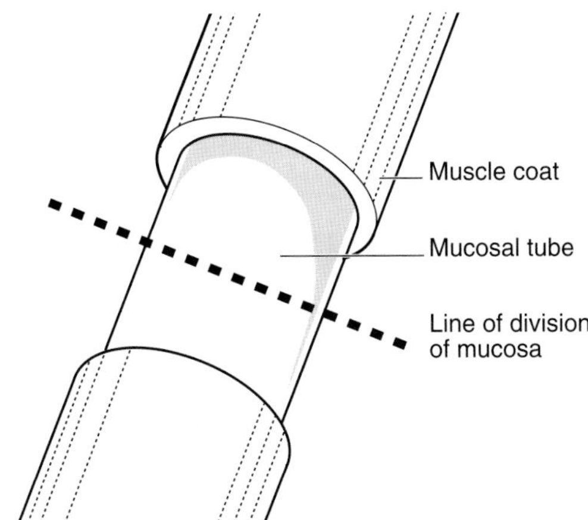

Fig. 10.10 The mucosal tube formed after division of oesophageal muscle.

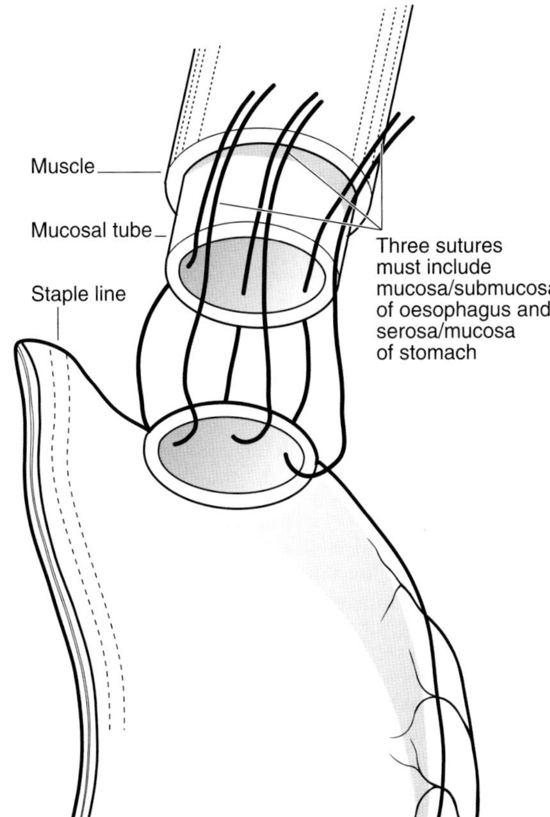

Fig. 10.11 Oesophageal anastomosis. The first three sutures are placed on the posterior wall to enable triangulation.

the posterior walls are tied within the lumen, those uniting the anterior walls are tied on the outer walls.

5 For interrupted sutures, place three loose full-thickness sutures at the middle of the back wall and the angles 3 o'clock and 9 o'clock (Fig. 10.11). Insert further sutures, usually between two or three, again loosely. Make sure that there are no gaps and the sutures include the mucosal layer. When the back wall is complete, tie the sutures leaving those at the angles long. Ask the anaesthetist to pass a nasogastric tube into the conduit and secure. The anterior layer of full-thickness sutures is now placed with knots on the outside. For single-layer anastomosis, it is best to use a double-ended monofilament suture and start at the middle of the back wall. Initial sutures can be placed loose and then tightened. Working from both sides, complete the back wall and introduce the nasogastric tube as before. Complete the anterior wall and tie the suture. Buttress sutures should be avoided; they narrow the lumen and can produce ischaemia.

6 As you draw stitches taut and tie them, remember that there will be some swelling of the tissues within the next few hours. If you have pulled the sutures too tight, they will cut through. Concentrate on placing each suture perfectly. Prefer to cut out and replace any that you are not satisfied with, rather than inserting extra 'bodging' stitches that may merely damage the blood supply. At the end, gently rotate the anastomosis to examine it, but remember that even more important is the integrity of the mucosal apposition.

Stapled anastomosis

1 Make sure that the oesophagus and bowel can be joined together without tension, are not twisted and that both ends have a good blood supply.

2 Transect the oesophagus, muscle first and the mucosa as described above. Insert a purse-string suture using 2/0 Prolene with an over-and-over suture encompassing the mucosal/submucosal layer (Fig. 10.12).

3 Assess the size of the oesophageal lumen by gently opening the jaws of an empty swab-holding forceps. Select the largest size that easily fits the lumen. Do not attempt to force in a larger head as this will split the oesophageal wall. For a non-obstructed oesophagus a 25-mm head usually fits best.

KEY POINT Do not split the oesophagus

- A postoperative stricture is easy to dilate in contrast to a postoperative leak!

4 Open the circular stapling device to its maximum extent, separate the anvil from the spindle and then retract the stem by 'closing' the gun without the anvil. Introduce the anvil into the lower oesophagus. Tipping the anvil sideways may make introduction easier if it is a snug fit. Tighten and tie the previously inserted purse-string suture. Check that the purse-string has

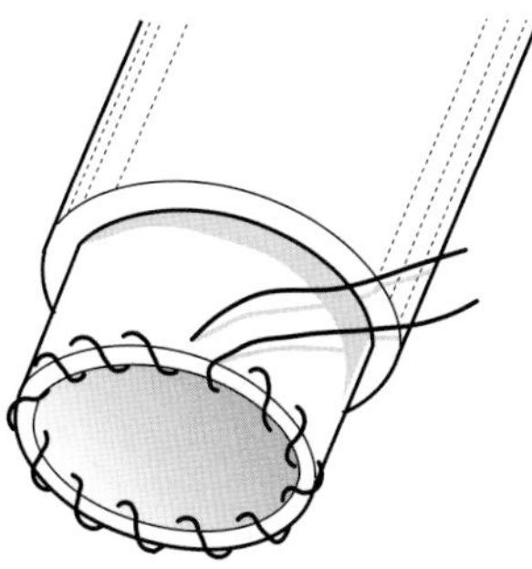

Fig. 10.12 Placement of the purse-string suture with 2/0 Prolene.

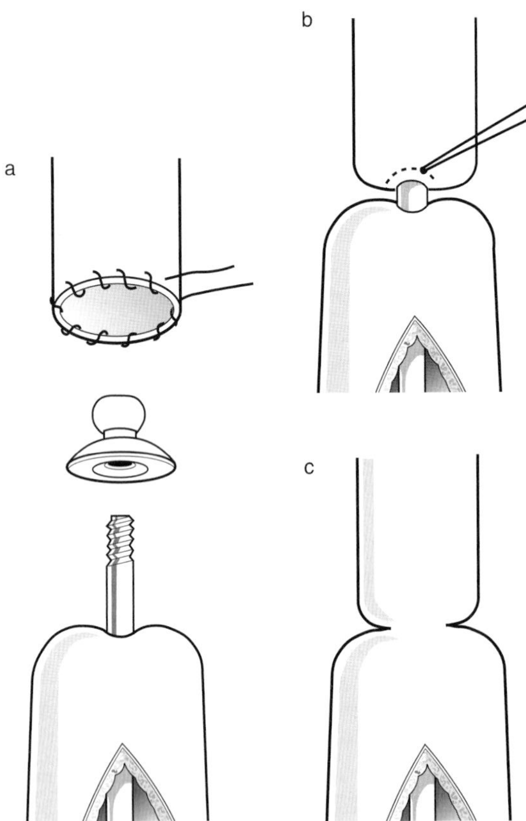

Fig. 10.13 A stapled oesophageal anastomosis: (a) the stapler shaft has been pushed through a hole in the stomach and the anvil is attached so that it can be introduced into the oesophagus; (b) the purse-string suture is tightened; (c) the device is actuated, producing an anastomosis.

drawn the oesophagus close to the stem. If there is a gap, insert a second purse-string.

5 If the stomach is to be used, create a temporary anterior gastrotomy and insert the spindle of the stapler into the fundus at least 2 cm from any suture or staple line. 'Open' the instrument so that its sharp point comes through the stomach (Fig. 10.13). If the jejunum or colon are joined end-to-side, insert the stapler without the anvil head through the cut end; this will be closed later. Protrude the stem through the antimesenteric wall at a suitable point.

6 Attach the anvil on its spindle to the instrument and bring together the conduit and the oesophagus by closing the anvil down on to the cartridge. Check that there is no twisting and that nothing is interposed, nothing is protruding.

7 Release the safety catch.

8 Compress the handles fully and firmly until a definite crunch is felt. The gun has now been 'fired'.

9 Separate the jaws slightly. Gently rotate the device and draw it clear of the stapled anastomosis. Completely withdraw the instrument.

10 Remove the anvil head and check the toroidal ('doughnut'-shaped) oesophageal and viscus cuffs trimmed from the inside of the anastomosis. Make sure they are complete and then place them in fixative solution prior to histological examination.

11 Insert a finger through the anastomosis to check it. If an aspiration tube is to be passed, ask the anaesthetist to pass it now and guide it through the anastomosis with a finger.

12 Close the opening through which the instrument and finger were passed.

13 Carefully check that the anastomosis is complete all the way round and lies without tension.

? DIFFICULTY

1. *The oesophagus splits when a large anvil is inserted.* Trim the split end and perform a sutured anastomosis. If the anastomosis is at the apex of the chest it may be necessary to perform a cervical incision for safe access to the oesophageal stump.
2. *A fragile oesophagus compressed normally within the jaws of the stapling machine is damaged.* The tenuous blood supply may be crushed between the staple carrier and the anvil. The longitudinal muscular wall may be traumatized. Abandon the anastomotic technique and perform a sutured anastomosis.
3. If the anastomosis is imperfect, reinforce the staple line with an encircling suture. Alternatively, abandon attempts to staple the viscera and rely on a carefully sutured anastomosis. Hoping for the best is a recipe for disaster in oesophageal surgery.

OESOPHAGEAL SUBSTITUTES (Fig. 10.14)

1 The alternatives are stomach, colon or jejunum. Jejunum is only applicable to anastomoses to the lower one-third oesophagus in most patients.

2 Both right and left colon can be used. Advocates exist for both, but the best is transverse and left colon based on the ascending branch of the left colic artery. The dogma that there is a vascular watershed at the splenic flexure is false. There is a good marginal artery and it is possible to mobilize a length of bowel which will reach to the floor of the mouth. The right colon is bulky and more difficult to straighten. All colon should be placed isoperistaltically.

3 The stomach is the favoured conduit due to its good vascular supply and adequate length. The conduit is based on the right gastroepiploic artery. The conduit should be a narrow tube 3–4 cm wide based on the greater curvature extending from the fundus to the lesser curve 3–4 cm proximal to the pylorus.

GASTRIC MOBILIZATION

Action

1 Identify the right gastroepiploic artery on the greater curvature of the stomach. Divide the greater omentum outside this arcade. This is best achieved with an harmonic scalpel. Continue this mobilization proximally toward the pylorus taking care not to damage the vessel at its origin where it leaves the gastric wall. Continue dissection towards the fundus of the stomach dividing the left gastroepiploic and short gastric vessels and taking

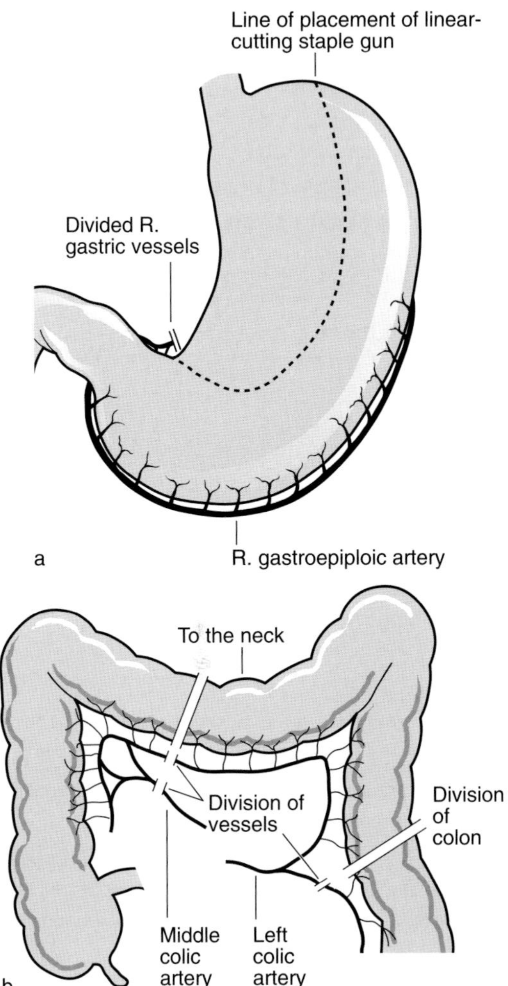

Fig. 10.14 Gastric and colonic oesophageal substitutes and the vascular pedicles on which they are based.

care not to damage the spleen. Dissection is continued to the left crus dividing small vessels to the stomach arising from the splenic artery.

2 The stomach is elevated to display the posterior gastric wall and left gastric pedicle. It is best to do a flush left gastric ligation removing all associated lymph nodes, including those on the common hepatic artery. Dissection is best achieved with bipolar scissors starting on the upper border of the pancreas. The left gastric vein is encountered first and ligated and divided. The left gastric artery is frequently 1 cm behind this and to the right. This should be double-ligated flush to the coeliac axis. The dissection is then continued to the crura which are cleaned of fat and lymphatics.

3 The right gastric artery is divided 3 cm from the pylorus and the gastric tube formed with a series of 'fires' of a TLC 100 linear cutting staple gun. This can be oversewn with a continuous running suture if required. The duodenum is Kocherized to complete mobilization. The gastric tube is usually fashioned in the abdomen and can be hitched to the oesophageal remnant to deliver to the chest or to a chest drain if it is to be delivered to the neck to avoid rotation. Except in cases of pyloric stenosis due to previous duodenal ulceration, there is no need to perform a pyloroplasty.

COLONIC MOBILIZATION

Action

1 Prefer the left colon. Mobilize it by dividing the peritoneum to the left from sigmoid to splenic flexure. Dissect the greater omentum from the colon. The colon can then be elevated and transilluminated to display the blood vessels. The marginal artery can be well visualized. Divide this distal to the ascending branch of the left colic and divide the colon with a linear cutting staple gun.

2 Continue the dissection of the vascular supply proximally, taking care with the middle colic artery which may divide just above its origin. Identify the proximal site of division of colon and transect the colon with a linear cutting stapler and divide the marginal artery. If you doubt the viability then apply vascular clamps before dividing it.

3 Restore colonic continuity between proximal transverse and distal descending colon.

ROUTE OF RECONSTRUCTION

1 The best route for reconstruction is via the oesophageal bed in the posterior mediastinum. Alternatives include substernal and subcutaneous routes for neck anastomoses.

2 Use the substernal route with great caution if colon is the conduit, since it is compressed at the root of the neck, resulting in venous congestion and conduit failure. If you employ this route you should resect the manubrium and first rib to prevent this.

LYMPHADENECTOMY

1 Controversy exists regarding the extent of lymphadenectomy in oesophageal cancer surgery. There is now no role for palliative resection leaving macroscopic disease. Remove all obviously involved nodes with the specimen.

2 As described above, perform coeliac lymphadenectomy as part of gastric mobilization. For transthoracic mobilization and anastomosis, take the para-oesophageal lymphatics with the specimen.

3 For operations through the right and left chest remove the subcarinal glands for accurate staging and, if approaching via the right chest, you can remove thoracic duct. This involves dissecting along the azygos vein to the hiatus taking all the tissue between the vein, vertebral column and aorta. The duct can be clearly seen in this tissue. Double-ligate it at the lower end to prevent chylothorax. If you do not formally dissect it out, for safety place a suture at the level of T10 to encompass all the tissue between aorta, vertebral column and azygos vein after oesophageal mobilization.

TRAUMA, SPONTANEOUS AND POSTOPERATIVE LEAKS

Appraise

1 Swallowed foreign body, stab or missile wounds may immediately rupture the oesophagus, but crush injuries such as those

sustained in road traffic accidents may cause necrosis with late rupture. Incoordinated retching may tear the lower oesophagus, usually just above the hiatus, to the left side; this is Boerhaave's syndrome of 'spontaneous' or postemetic rupture. In some cases the tear is partial thickness, involving mainly mucosa, sometimes extending into the gastric cardia. This is the Mallory–Weiss syndrome and it responds almost always to conservative management.

2 Iatrogenic rupture may follow endoscopy, dilatation of stricture or achalasia, removal of a foreign body, or follow an operation on the oesophagus including cardiomyotomy, vagotomy and resection or bypass.

3 The history of events, complaint of pain, collapse after injury or operation, presence of air emphysema in the neck and on plain radiographs demand radiological study with barium to determine the site, extent and localization of leakage. Barium gives much better imaging than water-soluble contrast and is perfectly safe. Modern water-soluble contrast media are relatively safe, but Gastrografin is hypertonic and should never be used. It is particularly dangerous if aspirated into the trachea. If these tests are negative and suspicion still exists perform endoscopy.

4 Late presentation may produce signs of cellulitis including mediastinitis, pleural effusion, empyema, peritonitis, abscess formation and fistula.

5 Following accidental or violent injury, assess the possibility of other injuries that must be dealt with.

6 Small cervical leaks following instrumental damage usually seal if the patient is fed parenterally for a few days.

7 Treat conservatively tears in the thoracic oesophagus that are detected early, produced at endoscopy or instrumentation, associated with minimal contamination and are contained in the mediastinum. Confirm that the mediastinal pleura is intact with X-rays, using barium. If the mediastinal pleura is breached or if the patient's condition deteriorates following initial conservative treatment, explore the leak. In general, postemetic rupture should be treated surgically as there is significant contamination of the mediastinum.

8 Intrathoracic leaks have a high mortality rate if not treated promptly. The worst results occur if the diagnosis is overlooked and the patient is fed.

9 If the oesophagus is split during dilatation of a carcinoma, immediate treatment is required: either resection or placement of a covered self-expanding metal stent. Remember that such tumours will behave as advanced disease with limited life-expectancy.

CONSERVATIVE MANAGEMENT

1 Stop oral drinking or feeding.

2 Screen a nasogastric tube into the stomach.

3 Institute parenteral fluid replacement and feeding. For a minor leak in a fit patient, fluid and electrolyte replacement may suffice.

4 Administer broad-spectrum antibiotic cover and intravenous proton-pump inhibitors.

5 Do not place a self-expanding metal stent to seal the perforation other than in cases of established cancer. They will not seal the leak and inhibit healing.

6 If the general condition of the patient does not deteriorate, repeat the radiological examination after 7 days. Do not hurry to repeat the examination. This does more harm than good. If the leak is sealed, restart clear fluids orally, proceeding to all fluids, soft solids and full diet.

7 If the mediastinal pleura is breached so that contrast flows into the pleural space, or if the general condition of the patient deteriorates following initial conservative management, explore the leak without delay.

SURGICAL MANAGEMENT

Prepare

1 Resuscitate the patient with intravenous fluids and if necessary cross-match blood.

2 Start treatment with broad-spectrum antibiotic cover.

3 After induction of anaesthesia examine the perforation endoscopically to determine the length of mucosal tear. This is invariably longer than the muscle tear.

Access

1 Left thoracotomy gives good access to the lower oesophagus, right thoracotomy to the mid- and upper oesophagus.

2 If you suspect abdominal injuries use a left thoracoabdominal incision or be prepared to explore the abdomen subsequently.

3 If this is a postoperative leak, good drainage and placement of a T-tube into the hole may suffice (Fig. 10.15). If not, then resection; you should perform proximal oesophagostomy and gastrostomy, with later reconstruction. Local correction and re-anastomosis invariably fails.

4 Expose the oesophagus adequately to allow full assessment of the damage to the oesophagus and related structures.

Assess

1 Is there only a single site of damage? Can you identify healthy mucosa around the whole circumference? If not, extend the hole in the muscle until you can.

KEY POINT Do not underestimate the size of a defect

- Remember that the hole in the mucosa is often larger than the hole in the muscle wall.

2 Are the tissues healthy or ischaemic? Closing defects with unhealthy margins is doomed to failure.

3 Can the defect be repaired? Is there enough tissue for closure without tension?

4 Is there any foreign material? If so, remove it.

5 What is the condition of adjacent structures? Ensure that only healthy tissues remain.

6 If this is a postoperative leak, is the cause evident? What can be learned for future incorporation in your technique?

7 Take a specimen for culture of organisms and tests for antibiotic sensitivity.

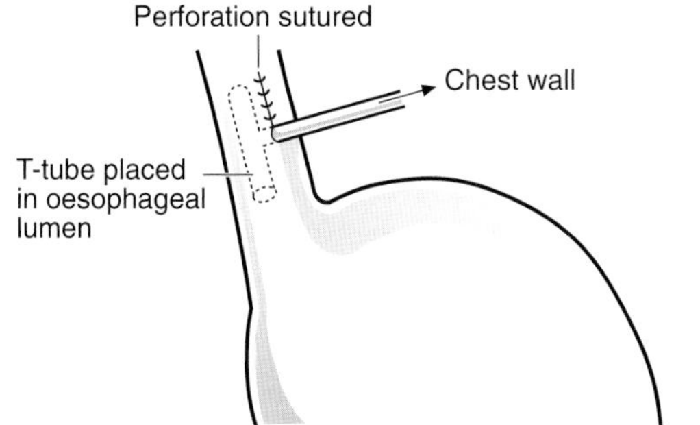

Fig. 10.15 Placement of a T-tube in a spontaneous oesophageal perforation.

Action

1 Remove any foreign material and excise dead or doubtful tissue.

2 Small tears of the cervical oesophagus need no sutures, but it is wise to drain the area. If the tear is large it may be sutured if good access can be obtained. Alternatively, insert a drainage tube through the tear to produce a controlled fistula. Tears of the 'cervical oesophagus' are usually tears of the lower pharynx or perforation of an unexpected pharyngeal pouch.

3 If the defect can be repaired with simple sutures, close it in a single layer using absorbable sutures in one or two layers. Reinforce this if possible with an intercostal muscle flap, a flap of diaphragm or pericardium. Lower oesophageal holes may be reinforced by wrapping with gastric fundus.

4 If the defect cannot be repaired, it may be possible to close it by mobilizing the gastric fundus and suturing the seromuscularis around the margins of the defect. Alternatively, insert a T-tube into the leak to produce a controlled fistula, or resect the oesophagus and perform cervical oesophagostomy and gastrostomy. Reconstruction may be delayed for weeks or months.

5 Facilitate enteral feeding below the leak by performing a jejunostomy.

6 In desperate circumstances isolate a severe leak by disconnecting the oesophagus above and below it, either as a temporary or a permanent measure. Transect the oesophagus in the neck after closing the lower cut end with a ligature and bring out the proximal end to the skin as a temporary cervical oesophagostomy. Transect the oesophagus below the leak. The isolated segment of oesophagus will produce only a little mucus. Never perform an oesophageal anastomosis in an unstable patient. Delayed reconstruction is safer.

Closure

1 Insert underwater-sealed drains to apex and base of the pleural cavity after thoracotomy. One of the drains should be sutured in place in the mediastinum close to the leak.

2 Insert closed suction drains into the neck or mediastinum and upper abdomen if the leak or site of trauma has been approached through the abdomen and hiatus.

3 If you decide to drain a leak, defunction the oesophagus and allow the hole to close spontaneously; place a soft drain close to the hole. If it lies at a distance from the hole, the drain will merely partially empty the large abscess cavity that will form.

Aftercare

1 Continue enteral or parenteral feeding, and antibiotics.

2 Remove chest drains when they cease to drain.

3 Monitor the patient's recovery clinically by progress charts and plain radiographs.

4 Check the repair and healing with a screened barium swallow on the seventh postoperative day. If there is no leak, oral feeding may be started, initially with clear fluids.

5 As drains cease to discharge, remove them. If fresh collections develop, drain them. Percutaneous drainage under computed tomographic (CT) guidance may be useful for secondary collections.

CORROSIVE BURNS

Appraise

1 Corrosives are swallowed accidentally or in suicide attempts during acute depression. Classically, the greatest damage occurs at the sites of hold-up above the cricoid sphincter, at the aortic crossing and above the cardia. The substance burns the mouth, pharynx and larynx; that which passes through the oesophagus into the stomach may remain there and cause ulceration, perforation and severe stricture at the gastric outlet.

2 A particular danger in children is the swallowing of small disc or 'button' batteries, which may release damaging caustic contents. These must be immediately and gently removed endoscopically. It is important not to use instruments that might damage the capsule. Use a snare, but take care not to use excessive force.

3 The mucosa is damaged or destroyed, exposing the deeper layers to any remaining or subsequent passage of corrosive. The wall then becomes friable and liable to rupture, especially if instrumentation is attempted. The oesophageal wall may become gangrenous and rupture spontaneously, resulting in septic mediastinitis.

4 If the oesophagus does not perforate, mucosal regeneration occurs during the next 10–14 days, but wound contraction and contracture often produce rapid and severe, sometimes long, strictures. There is a small long-term risk of carcinoma.

5 Initially exclude hoarseness, stridor and dyspnoea that suggest inhalation of the corrosive. Monitor the blood gases and carry out tracheostomy if the patient has, or develops, respiratory obstruction.

6 Exclude perforation of the oesophagus, which produces back and chest pain, and intra-abdominal perforation with pain, tenderness and guarding. Order plain X-rays of the chest and abdomen.

7 Do not perform a contrast swallow in the acute stage as it may be extremely painful. Early endoscopy is useful in judging the extent and severity of damage. It must be done gently with the minimum of air insufflation.

8 Start broad-spectrum antibiotic cover. Stop oral intake and institute intravenous fluid therapy with subsequent nutritional support.

9 If perforation has occurred or there is extensive necrosis, carry out emergency exploration with a view to oesophagectomy. The decision to restore continuity immediately is an important one. It may be done if the patient is stable and the surviving ends are healthy. If there is any doubt bring the ends of surviving gut to the surface for later union with a suitable conduit.

10 There is no role for steroids in this condition.

11 Do not allow the patient to swallow liquids until you, or another expert, have carried out a radiological or endoscopic examination to confirm that the passage is intact.

12 Anticipate the development of strictures. If they occur, start early treatment with balloon dilators. Do not overdilate the strictures but be prepared to repeat the procedure at gradually lengthening intervals.

13 Sometimes the strictures cannot be dilated, or they recur swiftly, demanding resection and anastomosis or bypass. Occasionally a broncho-oesophageal fistula develops, and this must be defunctioned, initially with a cervical oesophagostomy and gastrostomy. These stomata may be joined later using an isolated segment of colon.

GASTRO-OESOPHAGEAL REFLUX DISEASE

Appraise

1 The continence of the gastro-oesophageal junction is maintained by a combination of anatomical and physiological factors. Elegant anatomical studies have shown a gastro-oesophageal sphincter that corresponds to the high-pressure zone that can be measured by manometry. This area is still known as the lower oesophageal sphincter although, in reality, it is more gastric than oesophageal. The effect of the functioning sphincter is augmented by the muscle of the crura of the diaphragm and by having an intra-abdominal segment of oesophagus that is subject to a degree of external compression. The sphincter, including the diaphragm, is under integrated neurological control and relaxes during swallowing and belching. Stretch receptors in the upper stomach are responsible for relaxation of the sphincter during meals.

2 Gastro-oesophageal reflux disease (GORD) occurs when the function of the lower oesophageal sphincter is impaired. Oesophagitis is a complication of GORD that occurs when the lower oesophagus is exposed to irritant gastroduodenal contents long enough to overcome the normal mucosal protection mechanisms. Hiatal hernia has a variable association with GORD. In general patients with the more severe stages of GORD with oesophagitis tend to have a hernia, but most GORD sufferers do not have a hernia and many of those with a hernia do not have GORD.

3 Careful clinical assessment remains paramount in making the diagnosis and determining its effects on the life of the patient. Endoscopy is valuable to monitor the state of the mucosa and to detect the complication of Barrett's oesophagus, which is a premalignant condition. Norman Barrett (1903–1979), surgeon at St Thomas' Hospital London, described the condition which was later shown to result from persistent acid reflux causing changes in the lower oesophageal mucosal cells, ulceration, strictures and eventual malignancy. If symptoms of reflux cannot be confirmed by endoscopy, 24-hour lower oesophageal pH recording is useful. Assessment of GORD and its complications by radiology is inaccurate and therefore plays little part.

4 The symptoms of reflux may be confused with many disorders causing dyspepsia. Always make an objective diagnosis if surgery is considered.

KEY POINT Discriminate

- Remember that early achalasia produces symptoms that can easily be confused with reflux. Manometry, carried out at the same time as pH recording, excludes achalasia and other motility disorders.
- Remember that many people have dyspepsia in whom a hiatal hernia or gastro-oesophageal reflux can be demonstrated, but the symptoms can be generated elsewhere.

5 Uncomplicated reflux can frequently be managed without surgical treatment. Many patients are overweight. The worst sufferers are sometimes those with good abdominal muscles, such as ex-sportsmen, who subsequently lay down fat that is not obvious, increasing intra-abdominal pressure. Sensible weight loss may cure the symptoms. Smoking, alcohol and fatty foods aggravate the symptoms and are best eschewed. Simple antacid or antacid/alginate preparations may help, but will have been tried long before the patient reaches a surgeon. H_2-receptor antagonists will likewise often have been prescribed. Undoubtedly the most effective medication is a proton-pump inhibitor. Omeprazole, lansoprazole, pantoprazole and rabeprazole all have similar effects although newer drugs such as esomeprazole have a longer duration of action and higher healing rates especially in grade 3 and grade 4 oesophagitis.

6 Consider operation if severe symptoms continue in spite of compliance with medical advice. Be wary of those who will not attempt to lose weight; they frequently put on more weight after operation. Of course, some patients cannot, for a variety of reasons, adhere to an effective regime. Warn the patient that the best reported results are about 85% excellent or good, and that 15% therefore still have symptoms. Be particularly wary of patients who continue to have dyspeptic pain during treatment with an adequate dose of a proton-pump inhibitor. The pain is highly likely to persist after surgery. If in doubt about the effectiveness of a given dose of proton-pump inhibitor, perform 24-hour monitoring of oesophageal and gastric pH to check that acidity is suppressed.

7 The best indication for surgery is persistent regurgitation (volume reflux). This responds poorly to medication and can be remarkably disabling. Beware of offering surgery to patients whose symptoms are well controlled on medical treatment.

8 Barrett's oesophagus is the result of reflux and seems to be increasing in incidence. The role of antireflux surgery in Barrett's oesophagus is unknown and requires investigation. Patients with Barrett's require regular endoscopic surveillance. If persistently severe dysplasia or neoplasia develops then carry out oesophagectomy if the patient is fit enough to withstand it.

9 The most popular antireflux operation is the Nissen circumferential fundoplication. This can be performed by conventional open or laparoscopic surgery through the abdomen. The postoperative result may be marred by dysphagia, 'gas bloat' or change in bowel habit. The operation has been modified to avoid this, by making a short and loose ('floppy') fundic wrap or by performing a 270° wrap (Toupet). Other approaches such as the transthoracic Belsey are rarely used and will not be described further. There is a shift in opinion towards partial fundoplication, but good results may be obtained by either method well done.

10 For complex cases in which there is fixed oesophageal shortening, the Collis procedure may be performed in which a tube is formed from the upper part of the stomach. Anterior and posterior walls of the stomach are sectioned distally from the angle of His and the cut edges are closed, producing a gastric lesser curve extension of the oesophagus and a freed, smaller gastric fundus. A Nissen fundoplication is then performed around the neo-oesophagus. It is very rarely seen, however, and with proper mobilization the oesophagogastric junction can be brought below the hiatus.

11 The vagi should never be divided deliberately as part of an antireflux operation since this risks producing postvagotomy symptoms. If the vagi are cut accidentally, as may well occur during revision operations, a pyloroplasty should not be performed. It is unnecessary and leads to additional side-effects.

12 Some patients with particularly difficult reflux problems complicating previous surgery may be helped by partial gastrectomy and Roux-en-Y reconstruction. However, this is not suitable for treatment of uncomplicated reflux and should not be undertaken lightly.

13 Finally, in extreme circumstances, if the cardia has been severely damaged by disease or surgery the only option may be to resect the oesophagus. Continuity may be restored by transposition of the stomach and anastomosis to the cervical or upper thoracic oesophagus, or by interposition of jejunum or colon.

14 Reflux may complicate cardiomyotomy, surgical damage to the hiatal mechanism and damage to or resection of the cardiac sphincter in the absence of hiatal hernia. The symptoms and effects may be disabling.

TRANSABDOMINAL FLOPPY NISSEN FUNDOPLICATION (Fig. 10.16)

Prepare

1 Do not operate upon an overweight patient until he or she has lost as much weight as possible.

2 Never operate before full investigation has confirmed the diagnosis and excluded other conditions of the upper gastrointestinal tract.

Access (Fig. 10.17)

1 Elevate the head end of the operating table.

2 Use an upper midline abdominal incision, opening the peritoneum to the left of the ligamentum teres and falciform ligament.

3 If necessary, excise the xiphoid process.

4 Use an on-table mechanical retractor to lift the sternum and costal margin to flatten the diaphragm and give good access to the hiatal hernia.

5 Mobilize the left lobe of the liver and fold it to the right.

Assess

1 Explore the abdomen.

2 Look for a sliding hiatal hernia. In fixed hiatal hernia the cardia lies above the hiatus and cannot be drawn down. This indicates oesophageal shortening and a standard Nissen fundoplication cannot be done. A Collis–Nissen operation is required. If the hernia reduces easily and does not tend to spring back into the chest it is safe to proceed with the Nissen operation.

3 In rolling hernia the gastric fundus herniates alongside the gullet into the chest. The cardia may remain in the abdomen or slide into the chest.

Action

1 Resist the temptation to approach the oesophagus as the first manoeuvre. In open surgery it is much easier to perform a Nissen fundoplication if the fundus of the stomach is mobilized first.

2 Divide most of the short gastric vessels that tether the stomach to the spleen. This is best achieved using an harmonic scalpel. There is often a second layer of vessels entering the posterior aspect of the fundus directly from the splenic artery. Divide these also.

3 When the fundus has been mobilized, continue sharp dissection around the hiatus to expose the lower oesophagus and the crural margins. Identify the anterior and posterior vagal trunks and preserve them.

KEY POINTS Dissect with care

- Do not use blunt dissection. This causes bleeding and may damage a friable oesophagus.
- Operate strictly under vision.

4 On the right side, divide the upper portion of the gastrohepatic omentum, to display the right margin of the hiatus. Leave the hepatic branches of the vagus nerve intact, together with an accessory hepatic artery.

5 Trim the sac, consisting of stretched peritoneum and phreno-oesophageal ligament, from the lower oesophagus.

Posterior repair

1 Ask the anaesthetist to pass a 50F Maloney tapered mercury dilator into the stomach. This has a soft flexible tip and can be passed with safety.

2 Displace the gullet forwards and stitch the margins of the hiatus together behind it using 2–4 non-absorbable sutures. Leave a space between the hiatus and the stented oesophagus that will admit a finger. Take care not to overtighten the hiatus to avoid postoperative dysphagia.

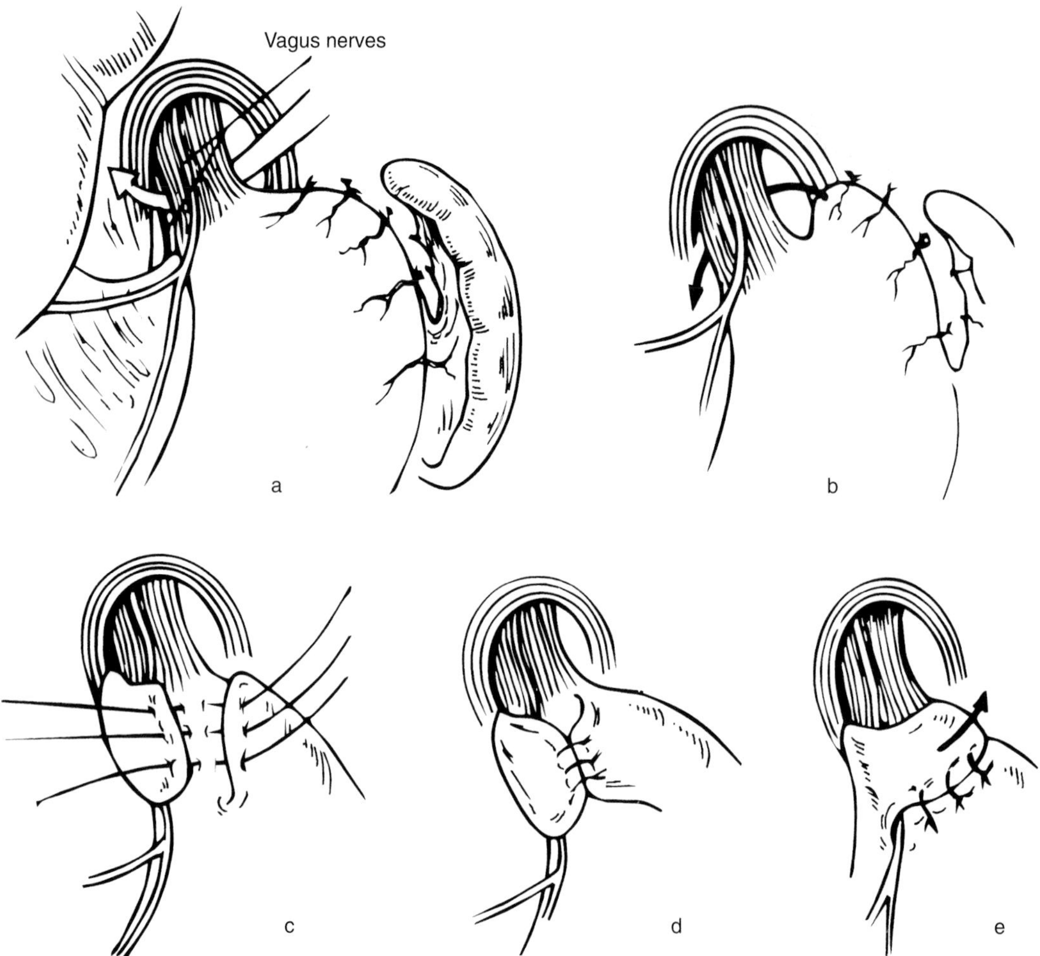

Fig. 10.16 Transabdominal Nissen fundoplication: (a) free the oesophagus in the hiatus, while preserving the vagi and branches; isolate, doubly ligate and divide the upper short gastric vessels; (b) gently fold the freed fundus behind the lower oesophagus to emerge on its right side; (c) insert three or four non-absorbable sutures to pick up the fold, the lower oesophagus and the anterior wall of the stomach to the left of the oesophagus; include the submucosa but not the mucosa; avoid piercing or damaging the vagi; (d) gently tie the sutures; you should be able to insert a finger beneath the cuff so formed; (e) rotate the cuff to the left in order to insert two or three sutures fixing the lower edge of the oesophagogastric junction.

3 Excise the fat pad that lies in front of the cardia. Take care not to damage the anterior vagus when doing this. There are some surprisingly large blood vessels in the pad that must be ligated.

4 Now gently fold the gastric fundus behind the lower oesophagus so that the greater curvature emerges above the lesser curvature. The posterior vagus nerve may be included in the wrap or the wrap may be placed between the posterior vagus and the oesophagus. Both methods have their advocates and are equally acceptable.

5 The fundus of the stomach should fold around the oesophagus with ease and should lie in place when released. If it tends to retract the fundus has not been adequately mobilized.

6 Insert a non-absorbable suture, such as braided polyamide to pick up the upper anterior wall of the stomach on the left of the oesophagus, the lower oesophagus immediately above the cardia and the part of the stomach that has been folded behind and to the right of the oesophagus. Each stitch is deep enough to incorporate the submucosa but not to pierce the mucosa. Tighten the stitch so that the two folds of stomach are brought together in front of the oesophagus. Check that a finger can be passed easily between the wrap and the oesophagus which contains the 56F dilator. The wrap must be really floppy to avoid postoperative dysphagia and gas bloat. Insert a second stitch 1 cm above the first one. The completed fundoplication must not be more than 1 cm long anteriorly. If it is too long, there will be an increased risk of dysphagia and gas bloat. Insert a second row of two sutures over the first two to give added security, but do not lengthen or tighten the fundoplication with these sutures.

7 Resist the temptation to insert extra stitches and hitches. They do more harm than good.

8 Ask the anaesthetist to withdraw the mercury dilator but leave the nasogastric tube.

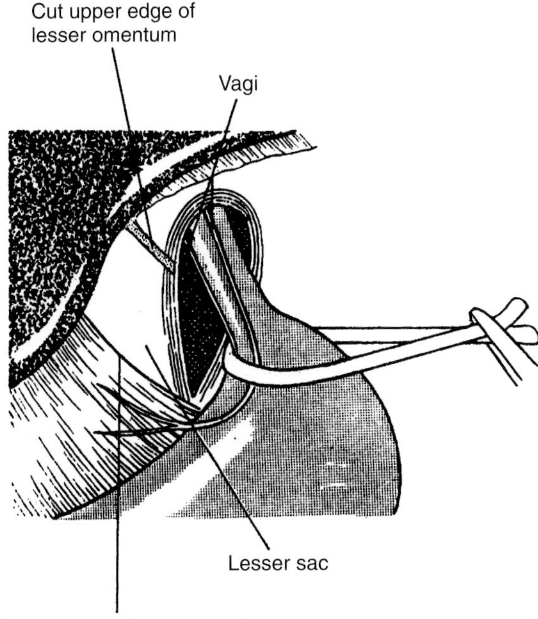

Fig. 10.17 Abdominal approach to the repair of hiatal hernia. The hernial sac has been excised to define the margins of the hiatus, and the upper edge of the lesser omentum has been detached from the diaphragm. Either an anterior or posterior repair may now be performed.

> **KEY POINTS Avoid overtightening**
>
> - Remember, Nissen fundoplication is highly effective in controlling reflux, but it is easy to produce an overcompetent cardia.
> - The wrap must be short and loose. It is impossible to make it too loose.

PARTIAL FUNDOPLICATION

1 In order to reduce the incidence of dysphagia and 'gas bloat', many surgeons favour partial fundoplication. There are various methods, which differ in detail, but the principle is the same.

2 The wrap encircles only 270° of the lower oesophagus. To carry this out, first have the anaesthetist pass a nasogastric tube into the stomach. Mobilize the upper half of the gastric greater curve by dividing at least half the short gastric vessels. Fold the gastric fundus loosely round the lower oesophagus. Insert stitches to produce a wrap not more than 3 cm long, around the lower oesophagus. Each of usually two or three stitches picks up gastric fundus on the right and the oesophagus. A second set of two or three stitches picks up the oesophagus and the left upper stomach, leaving the anterior 90° of oesophagus bare (Fig. 10.18).

3 In the Toupet operation the hiatus is not repaired. Instead, the completed fundoplication is stitched to the crura on both sides.

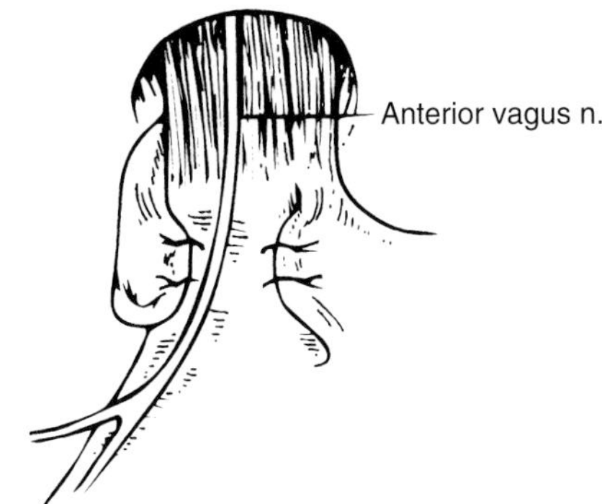

Fig. 10.18 Partial fundoplication, leaving 90° of the oesophageal circumference bare.

LAPAROSCOPIC FUNDOPLICATION

Appraise (see Ch. 12)

The operation is exactly the same in principle as the 'floppy' Nissen. However, the technique is different because of the different access to the organs and because laparoscopic instruments have a different set of disadvantages from those encountered during a conventional approach.

Do not attempt laparoscopic fundoplication unless you are fully competent in the full range of laparoscopic skills.

> **? DIFFICULTY**
>
> 1. If you cannot complete the procedure safely and effectively within a reasonable time, convert to open operation.
> 2. Safety is paramount.

Access

1 Place the patient supine with the legs in Lloyd-Davies stirrups as for a perineal operation.

2 Tilt the operating table 30° head up.

3 Have the anaesthetist pass a nasogastric tube to aspirate the stomach and position a 50F Maloney dilator in the upper oesophagus for subsequent advancement through the cardia.

4 Induce a pneumoperitoneum (see Ch. 5).

5 Place 10-mm cannulas.

Action

Proceed as in Chapter 12.

GASTROPLASTY

Appraise

1 When the oesophagus is shortened by fibrosis it cannot be drawn down into the abdomen, or there is such strong elastic recoil that a conventional antireflux operation will be pulled apart. The Collis gastroplasty creates a tube of upper stomach as an extension of the oesophagus, so that the hiatus can be

closed around it and an effective antireflux operation, usually a Nissen, can be performed without tension.

2 As a general principle in surgery, simple operations are more effective than complicated operations. There are more variables in the Collis–Nissen operation than a simple Nissen and the potential for failure or complications is greater. Do not perform a gastroplasty if it is not necessary. In such cases and in patients with recurrent reflux after failed fundoplication it is better to consider an antrectomy and Roux-en-Y anastomosis.

ROLLING HERNIA

Appraise

1 The gastric fundus may prolapse through the hiatus alongside the oesophagus alone, or alongside a sliding hiatal hernia of the cardia. The fundus may also prolapse through a congenital or acquired defect in the diaphragm near the hiatus.

2 Sometimes the rolling hernia becomes a volvulus of the stomach as the greater curvature increasingly prolapses through the hiatus.

3 Rolling hiatal hernias should always be repaired unless there is a contraindication to an operation. If the patient develops pain, vomiting from entrapment, obstruction or volvulus, operative repair should be performed as a matter of urgency.

4 Occasionally a patient presents as an acute abdominal emergency, nearly always having had previous less severe attacks.

Access

Use an upper midline incision. These hernias can be reduced and repaired through the abdominal route.

Action

1 Identify the gastric fundus disappearing through the hiatus.

2 Reduce the hernia by gentle traction on the stomach. Do not use force or you will tear the gastric wall.

3 When you have completely reduced the stomach, carefully examine its whole circumference by rotating it.

4 In emergency operations for what is in these circumstances often a strangulated hernia, the gastric wall constricted in the crus may be gangrenous in places. Do not immediately get carried away with the desire to carry out a resection. The blood supply is usually intact proximal and distal to the constriction ring. If it is, invaginate the linear gangrenous ring with a running deep seromuscular stitch.

5 Carry out repair of the defect by uniting the crura posterior to the oesophagus, using four or five non-absorbable mattress sutures.

6 Some surgeons insert three or four non-absorbable sutures that fix the gastric fundus to the undersurface of the left diaphragm—a 'fundopexy' (Fig. 10.19).

7 Alternatively, a fundoplication may be performed. Although there is controversy about the need for an antireflux operation, in these circumstances it seems to do little harm, provides good fixation for the stomach and deals with concurrent reflux symptoms.

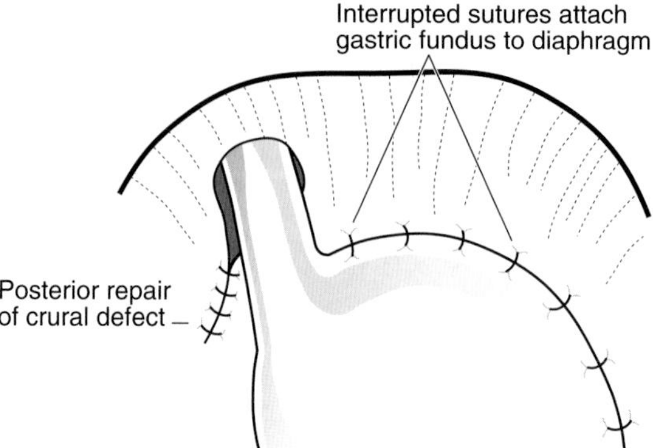

Fig. 10.19 Anterior fundopexy after reduction of gastric volvulus/rolling hiatal hernia. Interrupted non-absorbable sutures anchor the fundus and greater curve to the diaphragm and anterior abdominal wall.

LAPAROSCOPIC REPAIR

Appraise

Laparoscopic repair of a rolling hiatus hernia can be a challenging operation. Do not attempt it if you are an occasional operator for this condition.

Access

1 Place the patient supine with the legs elevated.

2 Insert five cannulas as for an antireflux operation.

Action

1 Elevate the left lobe of the liver and identify the hiatus and the herniated stomach.

2 Gently reduce the stomach into the abdomen.

3 The operation is greatly facilitated by early excision of the hernial sac. Divide the sac at the hiatal margin, pull down and excise the sac taking care not to damage the vagi.

4 Repair the crura posterior to the oesophagus.

5 Some prefer to insert a mesh into the hiatus anteriorly to avoid suturing the crura under tension.

6 Fix the stomach in the abdomen with a fundoplication, if preferred.

SIMPLE LAPAROSCOPIC GASTROPEXY

Appraise

1 Many patients with rolling hiatal hernia are elderly, frail and unfit. They may be severely symptomatic, but not fit for major surgery.

2 If the hernia can be reduced and the stomach straightened out the symptoms of a rolling hernia are relieved and the risk of gastric volvulus is avoided.

3 Simple laparoscopic gastropexy involves minimal surgical trauma and produces surprisingly good results.

Access

1 Place the patient supine with the legs elevated if it is safe to do so. Otherwise operate on the supine patient with the head of the table elevated.

2 Induce a pneumoperitoneum and place cannulas in the following positions: midline above the umbilicus one-third of the distance between umbilicus and xiphisternum; right subcostal, midclavicular; upper midline, below the left lobe of the liver so that the stomach can be sutured to this port site; left subcostal, midclavicular; left subcostal, anterior axillary.

3 Gently reduce the stomach into the abdomen.

4 Insert a non-absorbable suture through the upper midline port leaving the tail of the suture outside the abdomen. Gore-Tex is ideal for this purpose. Take a generous seromuscular bite of the upper stomach at a point that will maintain reduction of the stomach and allow it to be drawn up to the port site when the suture is tied. Bring the needle out of the port and leave the ends long and leave the needle in place.

5 Repeat the above manoeuvre with a suture passed through the left subcostal port.

6 When the sutures have been placed satisfactorily remove the cannulas and deflate the abdomen.

7 Use the sutures to prolapse part of the stomach wall into the two port sites and stitch to the fascia of the abdominal wall.

8 Close the wounds.

ACHALASIA OF THE CARDIA

Appraise

1 Achalasia, in which the lower segment of the oesophagus fails to relax ahead of a peristaltic wave, is probably part of a generalized condition of neuromuscular origin associated with abnormal vagal motor input and myenteric ganglionic degeneration. The failure to relax is associated with a failure of peristalsis above.

2 As achalasia advances there is gradual dilatation of the oesophagus, ending below in a smooth, beak-like entrance into the stomach. Retention of contents within the oesophagus produces oesophagitis, and if the retained food is aspirated the patient may develop respiratory disorders including pulmonary fibrosis. For these reasons do not delay effective treatment.

3 The diagnosis must be confirmed by oesophageal manometry. The aim should be to make the diagnosis at an early stage before the typical X-ray changes appear.

4 Achalasia can be treated using forceful dilatation of the lower oesophagus, or by surgical myotomy of the lower oesophageal sphincter. Injection of botulinum toxin also alleviates the symptoms, but has a relatively transient effect and is not recommended for routine use.

FORCEFUL DILATATION

1 This is carried out on the conscious patient under sedation with midazolam.

2 The procedure is undertaken using a plastic dilating balloon, which is specifically made for treating achalasia, is inelastic beyond a predetermined diameter and ruptures when it is overdistended. Increasing sizes of balloon may be used on successive days. The procedure must be performed under fluoroscopic control whether by an endoscopist or interventional radiologist. A radio-opaque, flexible, soft-tipped guidewire is passed through the cardia and the achalasia dilator is threaded over the guidewire until the radio-opaque markers at each end of the balloon lie above and below the cardia. The balloon is inflated under screening control until the waist, which initially appears at the level of the cardia, disappears. It is usual to start with a balloon of 2 cm in diameter and increase at increments of 0.5 cm until blood is seen on the balloon. It is advisable to check that there is no leakage by getting the patient to swallow contrast medium while screening the oesophagus.

3 This method requires significant expertise and should be carried out by skilled and experienced operators. Do not embark upon dilatation unless you, or others, are available with full surgical facilities in case the oesophagus is inadvertently ruptured.

4 If forceful dilatation has been successful for a reasonable period, such as a few months, it may be repeated. If a second dilatation fails to relieve the symptoms, cardiomyotomy should be advised.

LAPAROSCOPIC CARDIOMYOTOMY

Appraise

1 The aim of cardiomyotomy is to weaken the lower oesophageal sphincter sufficiently to allow food to pass but not to allow gastro-oesophageal reflux. This may be achieved either by performing a limited myotomy with minimal disturbance of the hiatal anatomy or by a more extensive procedure together with an antireflux procedure. Limited myotomy seems the most logical option for most cases. However, if a revision procedure is required, more extensive dissection and an antireflux operation may well be needed.

2 The myotomy should not be carried more than 1 cm on to the stomach because the risk of gastro-oesophageal reflux is increased without improving oesophageal emptying. The proximal extent of the myotomy is not so critical, provided that the short, non-relaxing segment is divided. An oesophageal myotomy of 3–5 cm in length is sufficient.

3 Surgical access for cardiomyotomy may be thoracic or abdominal and there are strong proponents of both. Since myotomy is a limited technical manoeuvre, minimal access techniques are particularly appealing. Laparoscopic cardiomyotomy is probably the procedure of choice provided expertise can be maintained by a sufficient volume of these uncommon cases.

Access

1 Place the patient supine with the legs elevated.

2 Induce a pneumoperitoneum.

3 Place 10-mm laparoscopic cannulas as follows: midline above the umbilicus one-third of the distance between umbilicus and xiphisternum; right subcostal, midclavicular; left subcostal,

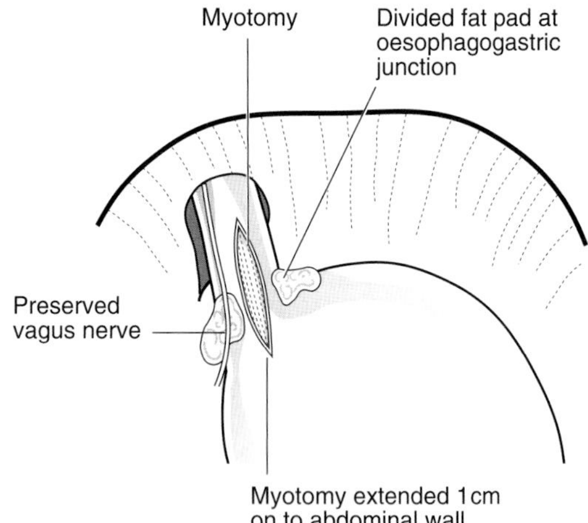

Fig. 10.20 Myotomy for achalasia. The defect can be covered with the gastric fundus to reduce reflux.

midclavicular; left subcostal, anterior axillary. Depending on the instruments that are available, 5-mm cannulas may be substituted for most of the above.

Action (Fig. 10.20)

1 Insert a Nathanson liver retractor through an incision in the epigastrium, deploy it under the left lobe of the liver and retract it upwards.

2 Identify the edge of the caudate lobe as it shows through the almost transparent lesser omentum. Divide the lesser omentum as far proximally as the diaphragm and distally to allow easy exposure of the hiatus. Look for the hepatic branch of the vagus nerve and an accessory hepatic artery, if present. Preserve these structures.

3 Identify the crural muscle on the right side of the hiatus. Divide the peritoneum at the edge of this muscle to open the hiatus. Extend the incision upwards and across the anterior aspect of the oesophagus. Do not take the incision downwards as in an antireflux operation. Disturb the hiatal anatomy as little as possible. It is only necessary to expose the anterior aspect of the oesophagus.

4 Identify the anterior vagus and preserve it.

5 Divide the pad of fat that lies anterior to the cardia. This is vascular and is perhaps the most difficult part of the operation.

6 Use curved, blunt-tipped dissecting scissors to make a small transverse incision through the muscle of the oesophagus, just above the cardia, until mucosa can be seen bulging through. This requires care and patience if the correct plane is to be entered and the mucosa kept intact. Wait until bleeding from the cut muscle subsides. Use a very gentle sucker technique to avoid injury to the mucosa.

7 When the mucosa has been exposed through the initial myotomy it is relatively simple to extend the myotomy proximally for 3–5 cm.

8 Extending the myotomy downwards on to the stomach is more difficult. Make repeated small longitudinal cuts under vision and inspect the mucosa at each stage.

9 Continue the myotomy 1 cm on to the stomach. The gastric mucosa has a different appearance to the oesophageal mucosa and can usually be recognized relatively easily.

10 Ask an experienced assistant to pass a gastroscope into the stomach. Use this to double-check that the myotomy is correctly sited and that the mucosa is intact. If there is any difficulty identifying the anatomical landmarks during the myotomy pass the gastroscope as a guide. It can be extremely useful.

11 If the mucosa is opened during the myotomy it may be repaired laparoscopically provided that the circumstances are ideal. Check the integrity of the repair with the gastroscope. If access to the site of injury is not ideal, or the area is obscured by blood, convert to an open procedure.

12 Close the wounds.

PHARYNGEAL POUCH

Appraise

1 This pulsion diverticulum of Zenker is a mucosal herniation between the transverse and oblique fibres of the inferior pharyngeal constrictor muscle, thought to result from incoordination or achalasia of the cricopharyngeal sphincter.

2 Recommend operation if the patient has dysphagia or regurgitation with the likelihood of aspiration pneumonia.

3 It is now usually treated by transoral stapling in which a linear cutting device both divides cricopharyngeus and opens the diverticulum into the oesophagus (Fig. 10.21). Reserve operation for failures of this technique.

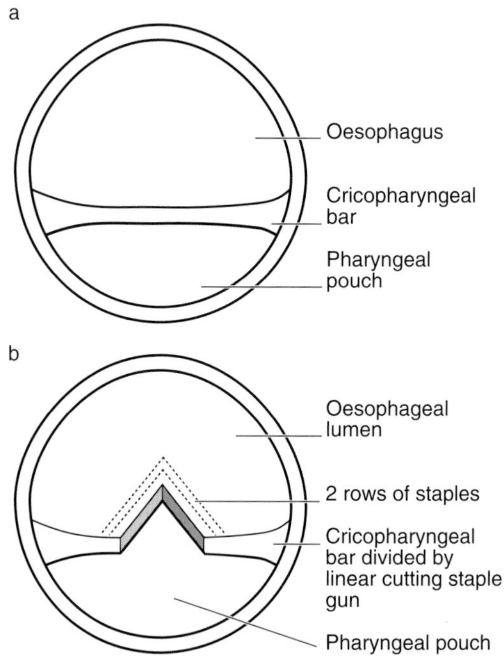

Fig. 10.21 Endoscopic treatment of pharyngeal pouch: (a) the special double-bladed speculum is introduced with the anterior blade in the oesophagus and the posterior blade in the pouch; (b) the bar of cricopharyngeus is divided with an endoscopic linear cutter staple gun.

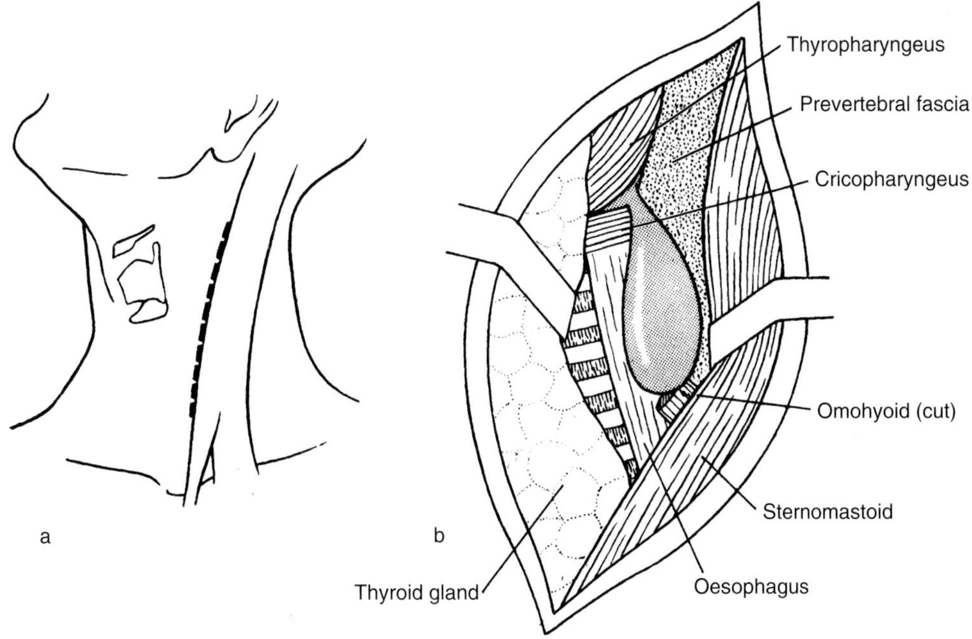

Fig. 10.22 Excision of pharyngeal pouch: (a) head rotated to the right and neck extended, with the incision indicated by a broken line; (b) the pouch and its relations.

Access (Fig. 10.22)

1 The anaesthetized patient, with a cuffed endotracheal tube in place, lies supine with the head on a ring, turned to the right and neck extended. It is helpful to pass an oesophageal speculum and pass a tube or a small mercury dilator into the oesophagus.

2 After preparing the skin and towelling off the left side of the neck, make an incision along the anterior border of the left sternomastoid muscle from the greater horn of the hyoid bone to 5 cm above the sternoclavicular joint. Deepen the incision through the platysma muscle, ligating and dividing the external jugular vein if necessary, and then incise the deep fascia.

3 Identify the carotid sheath and retract it and the sternomastoid muscle posteriorly to view the groove between the carotid sheath laterally and the tracheo-oesophageal column medially.

4 Three structures cross the groove. Identify the belly of omohyoid muscle and divide it. The middle thyroid vein may require double ligation and division but is usually lower. The inferior thyroid artery is lower and deeper than this dissection.

5 Rotate the thyroid gland, larynx, trachea and oesophagus to the right and gently separate the loose tissue in the groove to reach the prevertebral fascia. View the back of the lower pharynx and upper oesophagus to identify the pouch, which lies collapsed against the oesophagus. The neck of the sack lies at the level of the cricoid cartilage.

Action

1 Gently separate the sac from the oesophagus and elevate it from below until it is attached only by the neck. Avoid dissecting away from the sac and in particular keep away from the tracheo-oesophageal groove where lies the recurrent laryngeal nerve.

2 While the sac is still attached, identify the transverse fibres of cricopharyngeus passing just distal to the neck of the pouch. Open the apex of the sac and insert a finger via the sac into the oesophagus. This enables easy identification of the cricopharyngeus, the fibres of which are divided with a scalpel preserving mucosal integrity. Make absolutely sure that no horizontal muscle fibres remain.

3 The most important part of the operation is now completed.

4 A linear 55-mm staple gun is now placed across the neck of the sac to close it and residual sac excised.

5 Alternatively, especially in old people and especially if the sac is small, invert the sac. Stitch the fundus to the prevertebral fascia with one or two non-absorbable sutures so that it is upside down. This prevents the sac from filling.

Closure

1 If the sac has been excised, insert a closed drainage system.

2 Repair the deep fascia and platysma, and close the skin.

Aftercare

1 If the sac has been invaginated or inverted, it is safe to start the patient feeding immediately.

2 If the sac has been excised, start oral fluids after 24 hours. Remove the drain after 2–3 days.

DIVERTICULA

Appraise

1 Traction diverticula result from fibrous adhesion, usually to a diseased, especially tuberculous, lymph node and subsequent contracture. They are rare and do not require specific treatment.

2 Pulsion diverticula result from motility disorders of the oesophagus. Apart from Zenker's diverticulum (pharyngeal pouch), most occur near the lower end of the oesophagus. These rarely require specific treatment. However, the associated motility disorder occasionally demands balloon dilatation or even surgical myotomy. If you need to perform myotomy, excise the diverticulum and close the mucosa. Make sure that the myotomy extends down to the cardia, otherwise there is a high risk of postoperative leakage.

FURTHER READING

Adam A, Ellul J, Watkinson AF et al 1997 A prospective randomised trial of laser therapy and stent placement. Radiology 202:344–348

Adam A, Mason RC, Owen WJ 2000 Practical management of oesophageal disease. Isis Medical Media, Oxford

Agwunobi AO, Bancewicz J 1998 Simple laparoscopic gastropexy as the initial treatment of paraoesophageal hiatal hernia. British Journal of Surgery 85:604–606

Akiyama H 1990 Surgery for cancer of the esophagus. Williams & Wilkins, Baltimore, pp 73–80

Anderson JR 1990 Oesophageal injury: part I. The changing face of the management of instrumental perforations. Gullet 1:10–15

Bate CM, Keeling PWN, O'Morain C et al 1990 A comparison of omeprazole and cimetidine in reflux oesophagitis: symptomatic, endoscopic and histological evaluations. Gut 31:968–970

Coccia G, Bartolotti M, Mitchetti A et al 1991 Prospective clinical and manometric study comparing pneumatic dilatation and sublingual nifedipine in the treatment of oesophageal achalasia. Gut 32:604–606

De Meester TR, Wang CI, Wernly JA et al 1980 Technique, indications and clinical use of 24-hour oesophageal pH monitoring. Journal of Thoracic and Cardiovascular Surgery 79:656–670

Donahue PE, Bombeck CT 1977 The modified Nissen fundoplication: reflux prevention without gas-bloat. Chirurgie et Gastroenterologie 11:15–21

Ellis FH Jr, Gibb SP, Crozier RE 1980 Esophagomyotomy for achalasia of the oesophagus. Annals of Surgery 192:157–161

Fok M, Ah-Chong AK, Cheng SWK et al 1991 Comparison of a single layer continuous hand-sewn method and circular stapling in 580 oesophageal anastomoses. British Journal of Surgery 78:342–345

Friedin N, Fisher MJ, Taylor W et al 1991 Sleep and nocturnal acid reflux in normal subjects and patients with reflux oesophagitis. Gut 32:1275–1279

Gaudreault P, Parent M, McGuigan MA et al 1983 Predictability of esophageal injury from signs and symptoms. A study of caustic ingestion in 378 children. Pediatrics 71:767

Griffin SM, Raimes SA 2001 Upper gastrointestinal surgery, 2nd edn. Saunders

Hallissey MT, Ratliff DA, Temple JG 1992 Paraoesophageal hiatus hernia: surgery for all ages. Annals of the Royal College of Surgeons of England 76:25

Howard PJ, Mher I, Pryde A et al 1991 Systematic comparison of conventional oesophageal manometry with oesophageal motility while eating bread. Gut 32:1264–1269

Hulscher JB, van Sandick JW, de Boer AG et al 2002 Extended transthoracic resection compared with limited transhiatal resection for adenocarcinoma of the oesophagus. New England Journal of Medicine 347:1662–1669

Jenkinson LR, Norris TL, Barlow AP et al A 1990 Acid reflux and oesophagitis: day or night? Gullet 1:36–44

Liu JF, Wang QZ, Hou J 2004 Surgical treatment for cancer of the oesophagus and gastric cardia in Hebei China. British Journal of Surgery 91:90–98

Lordick F, Srein HJ, Peschel C et al 2004 Neoadjuvant therapy for oesophagogastric cancer. British Journal of Surgery 91:540–551

Mason R 1996 Palliation of malignant dysphagia, alternatives to surgery. Annals of the Royal College of Surgeons of England 78:457–462

McFarlane GA 1990 Oesophageal injury: part II. The changing face of the management of ruptured oesophagus: Boerhaave's syndrome. Gullet 1:16–23

Nisson G, Wenner J, Larsson S et al 2004 Randomised clinical trial of laparoscopic versus open fundoplication for gastrooesophageal reflux. British Journal of Surgery 91:552–559

Rokkas T, Sladden GE 1988 Ambulatory pH recording in gastroesophageal reflux: relevance to the development of esophagitis. American Journal of Gastroenterology 88:629–632

Samuelson SL, Weiser HF, Bombeck CT et al 1983 A new concept in the surgical treatment of gastro-oesophageal reflux. Annals of Surgery 197:254–259

Temple DM, McNeese MC 1983 Hazards of battery ingestion. Pediatrics 71:100

Thal AP 1968 A unified approach to surgical problems of the esophagogastric junction. Annals of Surgery 168:542–550

Toussaint J, Gossuin A, Deruttere M et al 1991 Healing and prevention of relapse of reflux oesophagitis by cisapride. Gut 32:1280–1285

Vaz F, Geoghegan J, Tanner A et al 1990 Conservative management of oesophageal perforation following pneumatic dilatation for achalasia. Gullet 1:28–30

11

Oesophageal cancer

H. Udagawa, H. Akiyama, R.M. Kirk

CONTENTS

INTRODUCTION

1 The epidemiology of squamous oesophageal carcinoma is the most varied of any tumour, so that in certain geographical regions there is a very high incidence and in other areas it is rare. It is also well known that squamous cell carcinoma of the oesophagus very often shows multicentric occurrence, including associated head and neck tumours. These suggest that environmental factors are important and many such factors have been postulated, such as smoking, alcohol, dietary nitrosamines, fungal contamination, pickled vegetables, hot tea, gruel and deficiency of certain vitamins and trace elements. A number of benign diseases predispose to its development, including corrosive alkali burns, achalasia, the Paterson–Kelly–Plummer–Vinson syndrome and a history of irradiation. In addition, Barrett's oesophagus clearly increases the risk of the development of adenocarcinoma. Many investigators have reported that adenocarcinoma of the lower oesophagus and gastric cardia is rapidly increasing in Western countries, although it is not clear if this increase is due to the increase of gastro-oesophageal reflux disease (GORD; gastro-esophageal, hence GERD in the USA) and Barrett's oesophagus. The autosomal dominant condition tylosis (Greek: *tylos*=callus) results in hyperkeratosis of the skin, papillomas and eventually carcinoma of the oesophagus.

2 The oesophagus runs from the neck through the thorax and into the abdomen. Apart from the cervical region, the oesophagus is divided into upper, middle and lower thirds, although the abdominal segment is sometimes considered separately. Approximately half of all squamous carcinomas develop in the middle third of the thoracic oesophagus. A much larger number of adenocarcinomas develop in the lower third in Western countries.

3 The tumour spreads circumferentially and longitudinally within the mucosa (intraepithelial spread), and spreads also in the submucosa and the muscle layer continuously or sometimes apart from the main tumour (intramural metastasis). It invades the trachea, bronchi, lungs, thoracic duct, recurrent laryngeal nerves, pericardium and aorta. This tumour notoriously spreads to the lymph nodes, not just locally but also at a considerable distance. Detailed, mainly Japanese, studies have shown that even upper-third carcinomas may be associated with nodal metastases inside the abdomen, while lower-third tumours involve the supraclavicular nodes in a significant proportion of patients. Despite the histopathological variation, lymphatic tumour spread should be assumed to occur according to the location of the main tumour and its depth of invasion. Haematogenous spread is relatively late, and affects the liver, lungs and bones.

4 Because of its insidious development, many patients present with advanced disease, complaining of dysphagia, weight loss, substernal or back pain, aspiration pneumonia or hoarseness. Supraclavicular lymph nodes may be palpable on presentation. The prognosis at this stage is very poor.

5 In Japan, a large number of asymptomatic squamous cell carcinomas are detected through endoscopic examinations at the time of routine health checks, and many of them are treated with endoscopic mucosal resection. According to the Japanese nationwide study, such local treatment is highly curative as long as the tumour invasion is limited to the epithelium and lamina propria mucosae.

6 The diagnosis is strongly suggested if contrast radiography demonstrates a long, irregular stricture. However, early lesions produce only slight or even no mucosal irregularities on contrast barium swallow films. The diagnosis is confirmed by endoscopy with biopsy. The technique of Lugol's iodine staining is very useful, because the unstained mucosa is abnormal, including carcinoma, oesophagitis, ectopic gastric mucosa and Barrett's epithelium. Biopsy specimens should be taken from all suspicious lesions, whenever there is an irregularity or a colour change. Take a number of biopsy specimens and record the levels at which they are taken. Do not take many biopsy specimens from one lesion particularly when the lesion seems to be a candidate of endoscopic mucosal resection, because biopsies often result in submucosal fibrosis and may make later endoscopic mucosal resection difficult.

7 If the cytological brushings and biopsy specimens are reported to be normal but you suspect carcinoma, repeat the examination, and go on repeating it until you are absolutely sure that you are not missing a cancer. Cancers located in the cervical and the thoracic inlet oesophagus are most difficult to detect. They are very often overlooked by otolaryngologists, radiologists and endoscopists. The effort of endoscopists to observe the oesophagus as high as possible including oesophageal inlet and hypopharynx, particularly when the examiner pulls out the scope, is crucial in eliminating misdiagnosis.

8 Of the available imaging methods, the most valuable are double-contrast barium swallow, abdominal and cervical

ultrasonography, computed tomography (CT), endoscopic ultrasonography and magnetic resonance imaging: The last three methods show the tumour size, invasion of contiguous structures and extent of lymph node involvement. Conventional endoscopic ultrasonography images the normal oesophageal wall as 5–7 concentric layers. Recent high-frequency ultrasound machines (both conventional endoscopic ultrasonography and small ultrasound probes passed through the instrumentation channel of an endoscope) can generate 20–30-MHz sound waves and can visualize a nine-layered structure, allowing the depth of penetration to be estimated with an accuracy approaching 90%. Ensure that CT scans include the upper abdomen and also the lower half of the neck, since enlarged lymph nodes that are not easily palpable may otherwise be missed. One should remember at the same time that lymph node size is not sufficient information for the detection of metastasis because micrometastasis is very common and because reactive hypertrophy of lymph nodes without metastasis is also not rare. Perform bronchoscopy, using a flexible instrument, in patients with middle- and upper-third tumours, to determine if there is invasion of the trachea or bronchi.

9 Preoperative staging can now be attempted, using the TNM classification of the International Union against Cancer (Table 11.1).

10 Carry out a careful assessment of the patient to exclude or confirm the presence of incidental disease, particularly that of the cardiovascular and respiratory systems.

11 Recent advances in the field of chemoradiotherapy are rapidly changing the therapeutic scheme of this disease. Although surgery remains the standard measure of treatment for lesions where R0 resection is possible, an increasing number of patients, particularly those with advanced disease, are treated with chemoradiation as the first mode of treatment.

12 The 'sentinel node concept', which is already applied clinically in the surgery of breast cancer or malignant melanoma, is being vigorously investigated in the area of the oesophagus in Japan. Although the concept has not been proved to be feasible, if it were, it would change surgery of oesophageal cancer in the earlier stage drastically.

TABLE 11.1 TNM classification for oesophageal carcinoma (International Union against Cancer, 2002)

T (primary tumour)

TX	Primary tumour cannot be assessed
T0	No evidence of primary tumour
Tis	Carcinoma in situ
T1	Tumour invades lamina propria or submucosa
T2	Tumour invades muscularis propria
T3	Tumour invades adventitia
T4	Tumour invades adjacent structures

N (regional lymph nodes)

For the cervical oesophagus **these are the cervical nodes**
For the intrathoracic oesophagus **these are the mediastinal and perigastric nodes, excluding the coeliac nodes**

NX	Regional lymph nodes cannot be assessed
N0	No regional node metastasis
N1	Regional node metastasis

M (distant metastasis)

MX	Distant metastasis cannot be assessed
M0	No distant metastasis
M1	Distant metastasis

For tumours of lower thoracic oesophagus:

M1a	Metastasis in coeliac lymph nodes
M1b	Other distant metastasis

For tumours of upper thoracic oesophagus:

M1a	Metastasis in cervical lymph nodes
M1b	Other distant metastasis

For tumours of mid-thoracic oesophagus:

M1a	Not applicable
M1b	Non-regional lymph node or other distant metastasis

The classification is based on clinical findings, endoscopic and imaging assessment and/or surgical exploration.

Appraise

1 Because oesophageal carcinoma is so often advanced at the time of diagnosis, some surgeons feel that treatment should be palliative. The arguments then range over the options for palliation. This deprives the patients who might be cured of the opportunity to benefit from a radical approach. Our experience of over 20 years of extensive lymph node dissection proves that even patients with 'distant' lymph node metastases regarded as M1 in the TNM system still have a chance of being cured by surgery. With the recent advance of non-surgical treatments, some T4 tumours have also become candidates for radical operation after neoadjuvant therapy.

2 Except in a few areas, oesophageal carcinoma is not a common disease. Unless patients are referred to a specialist centre, the clinicians who see them have relatively little past experience on which to base management decisions. It has also been shown that surgeons who regularly perform oesophageal operations achieve lower mortality rates and better results than occasional operators.

3 There is general agreement that radical resection is indicated in otherwise fit patients with early lesions that have invaded the submucosa, the muscle layer and even the adventitia, provided they have no detectable nodal involvement (T1/2/3 N0). Many but not all surgeons would perform resection in such patients, even if the regional nodes are involved (N1). However, there are different opinions about what constitutes radical resection.

4 There is even more disagreement about the treatment options for patients with more advanced tumours that involve adjacent structures (T4), have more extensive nodal involvement (M1a, and some lymphatic M1b), or have metastases (M1b with organ metastasis). Resection or bypass surgery is promoted as achieving the best palliation, especially with regard to dysphagia. Radiotherapy (external beam or intracavity, including concurrent chemoradiotherapy), chemotherapy, stenting, Nd-YAG or argon laser therapy and laser-activated photodynamic therapy

are all claimed to be beneficial alone or in combination. In recent reports, concurrent chemoradiotherapy has been shown to be more effective than single-modality treatments. A surgeon working alone is unable to evaluate the various claims that are made. For this reason, work in association with your radiotherapy and oncology colleagues or refer your patients to a specialist centre.

5 Adequate resection of oesophageal carcinoma requires a tumour-free margin to completely avoid the development of recurrent malignant dysphagia. Because of the frequent existence of intraepithelial spread, intramural metastasis and multicentric occurrence, precise preoperative diagnosis is of the utmost importance. Some surgeons send specimens from the upper and lower cut ends for frozen-section histology, but this does not entirely rule out the possibility of a 'skip' lesion. Palliative surgery must never mean inadequate longitudinal excision. It is tragic to submit a patient to such a high-risk operation only to watch the early recurrence of distressing dysphagia, which was the presenting feature. It is better to perform wide bypass, irradiation, laser excision or dilatation and stenting.

6 Do not make your decision without first discussing the possibilities and problems with the patient and, when appropriate, with the relatives. You must take into account the physical fitness and the psychological and philosophical attitudes of the patient. If you have obtained your patient's confidence, you will usually be entrusted with making the decision.

Prepare

1 Discuss the possibilities with the patient, since cooperation is essential to the success of major procedures.

2 Restore the dysphagic patient to a good nutritional state with soft oral foods and an elemental fluid diet, introducing a fine nasogastric tube into the stomach if necessary. Parenteral intravenous alimentation is another very useful option, but enteral feeding is more effective. Nowadays, the concept of 'immunonutrition' is attracting significant attention.

3 Enteral feeding of any kind is precluded for 4–5 days after operation. Set up a central venous line before operation to augment the nutritional intake.

4 Make sure that the best possible cardiorespiratory state is achieved with physiotherapy, blood replacement and correction of serum protein and electrolytes. Smoking should be stopped as early as possible. Order 2–3 units of cross-matched blood. Collecting 800 ml of the patient's own blood for autotransfusion is very useful to avoid allogenic blood transfusion. We also prepare cryoprecipitate from the patient's own blood to apply it to the operative field as fibrin glue.

5 Ensure that the oesophagus, stomach and colon are empty. Have a nasogastric tube passed when anaesthesia is induced. If the colon may be used for reconstruction, have it cleaned with 1 or 2 days of low residual diet and administration of oral intestine cleaning solution on the day before surgery.

6 Arrange for prophylactic antibiotic cover to be started intravenously as the operation begins. Second- or third-generation cephalosporins have been used routinely.

7 Arrange for prophylaxis against deep venous thrombosis. Application of pneumatic cuffs to the lower extremities during and for several days after operation is most effective. Start continuous intravenous administration of heparin (100–150 units/kg/day) from immediately after the operation until the patient is mobile.

8 Arrange for urethral catheterization and monitor hourly urine output during and after the operation.

9 Administration of a small dose of a corticosteroid (methylprednisolone, 250 mg) at 2 hours prior to operation is recommended by some authors to prevent the release of cytokines, which may lead the patient to ALI (acute lung injury) or ARDS (adult respiratory distress syndrome).

RESECTION OF CARCINOMA OF THE LOWER OESOPHAGUS

Appraise

1 Our routine operation for carcinoma of abdominal oesophagus and the cardia is resection of the lower thoracic oesophagus together with a cuff of the gastric cardia or entire stomach followed by jejunal interposition or Roux-en-Y reconstruction. This is done through the left thoracoabdominal approach. Primary oesophageal carcinoma of the lower thoracic oesophagus needs right thoracotomy for lymph node dissection.

2 You will nearly always find that the resection needs to go higher than you had planned. Technically, you can carry out anastomosis behind the carina, or even higher, through this approach. In doubtful cases, choose the right-sided approach, or bluntly dissect and resect the remaining upper thoracic oesophagus and then make an anastomosis in the neck between the cervical oesophagus and the gastric remnant or colon brought up retrosternally or posteromediastinally.

Access

1 Place the anaesthetized, intubated patient on the right side, with the left shoulder rotated back against a support attached to the operating table, or use a self-retaining mat (Fig. 11.1).

2 Open the left upper abdomen obliquely along the line of the sixth or seventh intercostal space, starting in the midline halfway between the umbilicus and the tip of the xiphisternum and extending to the left costal margin. The sixth intercostals space is more suitable when the lesion has substantial extension in the thoracic oesophagus, and lower mediastinal lymph node dissection is planned. Palpate the liver and the pelvis to detect distant spread. Determine the fixity of the cardia and feel for extensive lymph node involvement that would make resection useless. In very advanced cases, laparoscopic observation of the abdominal cavity may prove peritoneal dissemination and avoid useless laparotomy.

3 If resection seems feasible, cut across the costal margin and elongate the skin incision toward the posterior axillary line along the aimed intercostals space. Open the chest cutting along the lower attachment of the intercostals muscles. Even in elderly patients with fixed ribs, sufficient length of separation of intercostals muscles from the rib will allow adequate access.

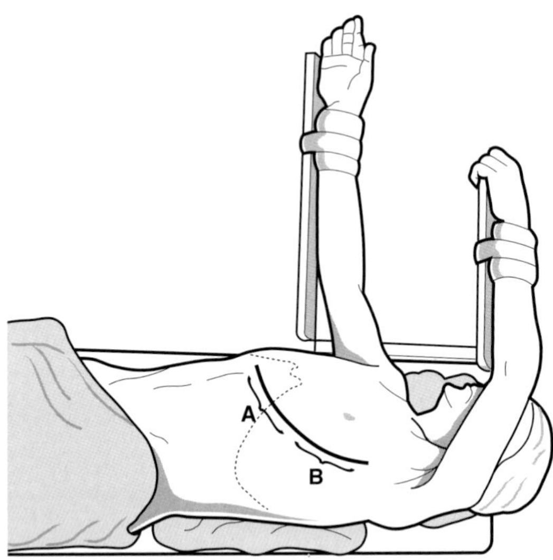

Fig. 11.1 Left thoracoabdominal approach to the lower oesophagus. Line A is for initial abdominal exploration. When the tumour is resectable, the incision is extended (line B). (Modified with permission from Akiyama H 1990 Surgery for cancer of the esophagus. Williams & Wilkins, Baltimore.)

4 Cut the diaphragm radially 10–15 cm towards the right crus. Even in very advanced case with direct tumour invasion to the crural muscle, you can get the safe surgical margin with circular resection of the muscle around the hiatus. It is usually unnecessary to cut through the diaphragm.

5 Insert a self-retaining rib retractor and gently open it in stages.

6 Stop all bleeding meticulously.

7 Anchor the edge of the incised diaphragm to the edge of the skin incision so that the left lung will not prolapse and interfere with the operative field during the intra-abdominal procedure.

KEY POINT Ensuring a good view

- Anchoring the edge of the incised diaphragm is helpful not only to prevent the left lung from interfering with the operative field but also to get a better view of the spleen and the fornix by flattening the dome of the left diaphragm.

Assess

1 Determine the extent of spread to the gastric cardia and glands along the left gastric vessels and around the coeliac axis.

2 Even if the stomach and associated glands appear to be uninvolved, remove the left gastric area (see Fig. 11.8), including the root of the left gastric artery. If the cardia or upper stomach is widely involved, prefer total gastrectomy.

3 If the tumour is fixed, or if there are multiple hepatic or intraperitoneal metastases, resection is inappropriate. Be willing to carry out an adequate longitudinal resection in a fit patient with a resectable tumour and not-too-extensive lymph node or liver metastases. Treat unresectable lesions by bypass, taking the stomach, jejunum or colon well above the tumour and joining it to the oesophagus in the chest or the neck. In Britain, gastro-oesophageal anastomosis in the neck is associated with the name of Kenneth McKeown of Northallerton. For fixed, extensive, obstructing tumours in high-risk patients, dilatation and insertion of an expandable metallic stent is the treatment of choice. Tube jejunostomy is also recommended for supplementary nutrition.

Resect

Abdominal procedure

1 Open the lesser sac, dissecting the greater omentum from the transverse colon and severing the avascular portion of the gastric lesser omentum.

2 Ligate and cut each artery and vein of the stomach at the root according to the planned resection procedure.

3 Cut the stomach (for proximal gastrectomy) or the duodenal bulb (for total gastrectomy) with a linear stapling device.

KEY POINT Distal pancreatectomy and splenectomy?

- If the lymph nodes along the splenic artery are highly suspicious of metastasis or the tumour has directly invaded to the surface of the distal pancreas, distal pancreatectomy and splenectomy assures en bloc resection of the tumour. Distal pancreatectomy and splenectomy is also recommended when 'omental bursectomy' is planned.

4 Remove the anchoring stitch from the diaphragm and pass a tape through the hiatus. Pull the tape down to get good exposure of the left thoracic cavity.

Thoracic procedure

1 Gently free the lower lobe of the left lung, dividing the pulmonary ligament, taking care not to injure the pulmonary vein.

2 Locate the lower thoracic aorta and incise the mediastinal pleura just anterior to it. Dissect the anterior surface of the aorta. Ligate and cut the proper oesophageal arteries, which are rather rarely found in the lower mediastinum. Elevate and pull forward the lower lobe of the lung to display the posterior mediastinum.

3 Incise the mediastinal pleura just posterior to the pericardium. Gently mobilize the lower oesophagus, leaving the mediastinal adipose tissue on the oesophageal side and taking care not to accidentally injure the azygos vein and the thoracic duct on the left side. If you injure the thoracic duct, cut and ligate it to prevent postoperative chylothorax. If necessary, excise the posterior pericardium and a portion of the right pleura after warning the anaesthetist that the right chest is open.

4 Decide the level of oesophageal transection and do not mobilize too high above this point. Too extensive mobilization (5 cm or more) of the oesophagus will result in ischaemia of the oesophageal stump.

5 Gently grasp the oesophagus with Akiyama's oesophageal clamp or a right-angled vascular clamp and transect the oesoph-

agus below it. Remove the specimen for histological examination. At least 2 cm of normal oesophagus should be removed above the oral margin of the tumour. Intraoperative iodine staining and immediate frozen section examination should be carried out if the oral margin is uncertain.

Unite (Fig. 11.2)

1 Design the mesenteric incision line under transillumination to obtain the longest jejunal loop. The second or third jejunal artery is usually most suitable as a feeder. Cut the jejunum between two clamps and put the anal cut end up retrocolically through the hiatus to the oesophageal stump.

2 Place a running purse-string suture at the oesophageal stump. Apply a circular end-to-end stapling device from the jejunal cut end to make an end-to-side (functionally end-to-end) oesophagojejunostomy. Close the open jejunal stump manually or use a linear stapling device. Add seromuscular sutures to bury the inner suture line. Insert a nasogastric tube though the anastomosis.

3 If the distal stomach is preserved, bury the line of staples in the gastric remnant with seromuscular stitches. Cut the elevated jejunum 20 cm below the hiatus, while preserving the feeding vessels. Make an anastomosis between the distal end of the jejunal segment and the gastric remnant. This anastomosis can be created at the tip of the greater curvature of the gastric remnant or on the anterior gastric wall. Then form another end-to-end jejunojejunal anastomosis below the mesocolon to complete the reconstruction.

4 Following a total gastrectomy, Roux-en-Y reconstruction is a possible choice instead of jejunal interposition.

KEY POINT Roux-en-Y reconstruction

- If you create a Roux-en-Y method, unite the afferent jejunal segment from the ligament of Treitz, on the patient's left side of the elevated jejunum that will be anastomosed to the oesophagus. Otherwise, the afferent jejunal loop may prolapse to the left side through the space behind the raised segment of jejunum and can then produce a complicated bowel torsion.

5 If the gastric remnant is long enough, intrathoracic oesophagogastrostomy is also a choice of reconstruction. Addition of an antireflux procedure is usually recommended. Cervical oesophagogastrostomy is also possible.

6 Heineke–Mikulicz pyloroplasty was done routinely for a long time when the distal stomach was preserved. However, omitting it only results in early-stage gastric stasis even without complete lack of vagal control of antral peristalsis and pyloric ring function. In long-term follow-up, such patients without pyloroplasty show fewer episodes of bile regurgitation.

7 Make sure there is no tension on the anastomoses, and no twisting or kinking of the bowel.

Checklist

1 Make sure the intrathoracic anastomosis is perfectly fashioned and there is no evidence of tension or ischaemia. An intrathoracic leak is often fatal.

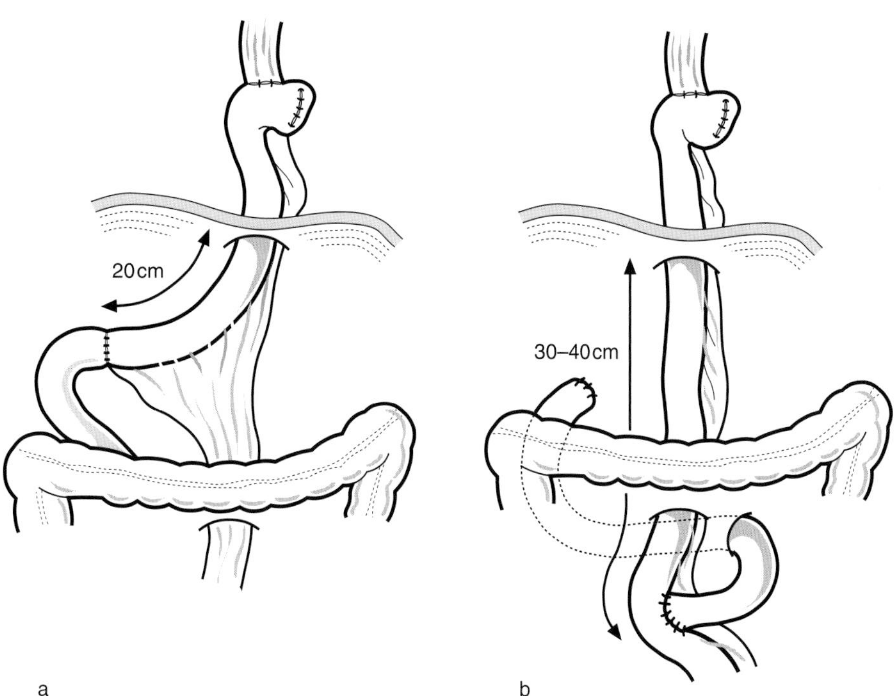

Fig. 11.2 Standard reconstructive methods after resection of lower oesophagus and stomach: (a) jejunal interposition; (b) Roux-en-Y reconstruction. (Modified with permission from Akiyama H 1990 Surgery for cancer of the esophagus. Williams & Wilkins, Baltimore.)

2 Has all the bleeding stopped?

3 Close all the defects of the mesentery and mesocolon in order to avoid internal herniation. Fix the organ that was elevated for reconstruction to the hiatus if there is a risk of prolapse into the thoracic cavity. Do not tighten the hiatus unless it was widened during the tumour resection. When you perform hiatal narrowing, make sure that the hiatus is still loose afterwards.

Closure

1 Insert an underwater-sealed drain into the left pleural cavity through a separate stab incision near the costophrenic angle in the posterior axillary line.

? DIFFICULTY

1. There are wide variations in the extent of resection and the mode of reconstruction. It is most important to make sure that the anastomosis remains free from recurrence. Therefore, never skimp on tumour resection to facilitate anastomosis.
2. *Has the tumour proved to be irremovable?* A bypass operation usually preserves patency longer than oesophageal stenting and is functionally superior as long as it is done safely.
3. If the lesion is very extensive, abandon attempts to resect or bypass it.
4. If the respiratory function of the patient is too poor for left thoracotomy and the upper margin of the tumour is only 2 or 3 cm higher than the level of the hiatus, a transhiatal approach can be considered. Cut the central tendon of the diaphragm anterior to the hiatus so that you can achieve wide exposure of the lower posterior mediastinum. Take care not to place excessive compression on the heart when using this approach.

2 Close the diaphragm using a continuous interlocking suture. The last 4–5 cm is closed with interrupted sutures from abdominal side. Leave them unknotted until the incised intercostal space has been approximated with two thick, absorbable threads through both ribs.

3 Close the abdominal wound in your usual manner.

4 Close the chest wound, including the external oblique muscle and serratus anterior muscle above and below.

OPERATIONS FOR THORACIC OESOPHAGEAL CARCINOMA

INTRODUCTION

1 The two-step operation of Ivor Lewis is the classic method for dealing with mid-oesophageal carcinoma. Many surgeons still employ this as their standard procedure for all oesophageal carcinomas.

2 Newer and more radical techniques are also applied these days. They include the extensive (three-field) lymph node dissection promoted by Akiyama and other Japanese surgeons. Some surgeons have started performing VATS (video-assisted thoracic surgery) oesophagectomy. They claim that they can perform the same radical operation, but many other surgeons are not convinced.

3 It is not safe to embark on any of these advanced techniques after simply reading a description. However, all the advanced techniques were developed as the result of step-by-step revision of older methods, so there should be many clues for surgeons who try to make their operations more radical.

4 On the other hand, the more limited procedure of transhiatal oesophagectomy is still also applied combined with adjuvant therapy and is claimed to be equally effective by its advocates.

IVOR LEWIS RESECTION FOR MID-OESOPHAGEAL CARCINOMA

Appraise

1 This operation is the source of other newer and more radical operations. Therefore, the essential points of the Ivor Lewis operation are all included in other newer techniques. Only the general concept of the operation and a few specific points are presented here.

2 The first step is the abdominal operation, in which the whole stomach is mobilized for reconstruction leaving the right gastric and gastroepiploic vessels as feeding and draining vessels. The second step is the thoracic operation, involving oesophageal resection and reconstruction using pulled-up stomach as an oesophageal substitute. An oesophagogastrostomy is made intrathoracically. This is performed with an end-to-end circular stapling device or side-to side application of the linear stapling device and is rarely performed manually these days.

3 By careful positioning of the patient, it is possible for two surgical teams to work simultaneously, placing the upper part of the patient in the position for right thoracotomy, with the pelvis almost flat on the operating table. The position may thereafter be adjusted by tilting the table.

4 Carry out a full Kocher's mobilization of the head of pancreas and duodenal loop, because oesophageal reconstruction is usually done after closure of the abdominal incision.

RADICAL CURATIVE SURGERY: EXTENSIVE LYMPH NODE DISSECTION (AKIYAMA)

Appraise

1 Japanese surgeons have been performing extensive lymph node dissection for about 20 years, and it has also been done recently by some surgeons in North America and Europe. The operative mortality is satisfactorily low and the 5-year survival rate exceeds 50% for those who undergo a curative (R0) resection. These good results are often attributed to differences

between countries in the type of tumour, population screening procedures, the build of the patients, and stage migration due to extensive lymph node dissection itself (Will Rogers phenomenon), but there is no good evidence that such factors play a part.

2 Skinner proposes and advocates his 'en bloc dissection' as a variation of such radical surgery. The essential concept of his operation is wide resection of tissues surrounding the oesophageal tumour, including mediastinal pleura, azygos vein, thoracic duct and pericardium. It is particularly important for tumours with infiltrative growth beyond the adventitia. These days, such tumours are regarded to be candidates of neoadjuvant chemoradiation. To obtain negative surgical margin for local control and to accomplish extended lymphadenectomy for regional control are different but equally important targets for real R0 resection.

3 This extensive operation has been developed on the basis of investigation of the extent of lymphatic tumour spread, and careful attention to detail in planning and performing the operation has made it feasible. We do not take an inflexible attitude towards the extent of either oesophageal or lymph node excision. We try to match the operation to the site and extent of tumour growth and to the likelihood of invasion and spread to the lymph nodes.

4 Reliable preoperative assessment of the tumour by endoscopy, conventional ultrasound of the neck and abdomen, endoscopic ultrasound and CT is mandatory.

5 Although this preoperative assessment is helpful in detecting spread, it does not reveal micrometastases, so radical dissection must encompass what appears to be normal tissue.

6 Modern imaging techniques have made an initial abdominal exploration unnecessary in most patients. If uncertainty exists concerning resectability and curability in the abdomen, start with the abdominal procedure. In such cases, the cervical and abdominal parts of the operation can be completed first (reconstruction-first approach). The order of mediastinal dissection and reconstruction is interchangeable so this is not a major problem.

THORACIC PROCEDURE

Access

1 Place the anaesthetized, intubated patient on the left side using a self-retaining mat.

2 Make a right thoracotomy incision in the fourth intercostal space. Anterolateral thoracotomy is chosen in order to preserve the right latissimus dorsi muscle.

3 Cut the intercostal muscles with electrocautery along the upper margin of the fifth rib from a point lateral to the internal mammary artery to a point lateral to the sympathetic trunk.

4 Apply two self-retaining rib retractors in a crossed fashion to produce a square window for access to the right thoracic cavity.

KEY POINTS Separating the ribs

- When inserting the self-retaining rib retractor, gently and gradually open it.
- When it becomes too tight, leave it for a few minutes and try again. In this way you improve the access without causing unnecessary rib fractures.
- When the chest cage is very stiff, initially cut the lower (fifth, for thoracotomy through the fourth intercostal space) costal cartilage near the sternocostal joint. This facilitates safe widening of the window. If this is insufficient, be prepared to cut a rib near the neck, above or below the incision, to allow adequate access. The cut rib can be fixed at the time of wound closure using an absorbable hydroxyapatite intracostal implant.

5 Free the lower lobe of the lung dividing the right pulmonary ligament.

Assess

1 Rule out tumour implantation. Any suspicious nodules should be sent to the pathologist for frozen section diagnosis.

2 Check whether the main tumour is fixed to the surrounding organs. If direct invasion is suspected, carefully dissect the tumour from the organs around it. The trachea, left main bronchus and descending aorta are the most important organs to be checked. Lung, pericardium, azygos vein, thoracic duct and diaphragm are organs that can be easily resected together with the oesophagus. When the tumour is fixed to the pericardium, cut into the pericardiac space at a tumour-free site and check that the involved portion of the pericardium can be completely resected.

Action (Fig. 11.3)

1 Incise the mediastinal pleura vertically over the right vagus nerve on the lateral tracheal wall. Elongate the pleural incision upward to the level of the subclavian artery. Identify the origin of the right recurrent laryngeal nerve and gently dissect it upward. The area behind this is the lower portion of the right recurrent laryngeal lymph node chain, which is a very frequent site of lymph node metastasis. You can dissect this lymph node chain until the lower pole of the right thyroid lobe is encountered, but it is safer to leave the upper half untouched and dissect it from the neck (Figs 11.4, 11.10).

2 Dissect the anterior and posterior ends of the azygos arch, ligate and cut it. Be sure that the right bronchial artery, which lies below the azygos arch, is not included (Fig. 11.4).

3 Identify the right bronchial artery, which is usually the main branch from the third right intercostal artery. Ligate and cut the (third) intercostal artery peripheral to the origin of the right bronchial artery so that you can safely retract the mediastinum anteriorly without tension on the bronchial artery (Figs 11.4, 11.5).

4 Identify the thoracic duct running on the surface of the descending aorta anteriorly to the origin of the right intercostal bronchial artery. Dissect it upward and downward for en bloc

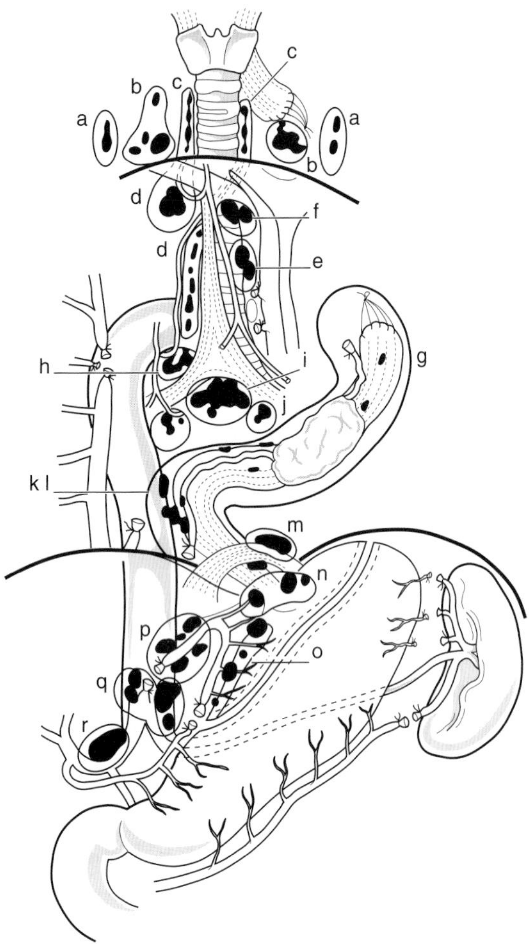

Fig. 11.3 Extent of resection and lymph node dissection of the standard radical oesophagectomy with extensive lymph node dissection for thoracic oesophageal carcinoma. Nodes to be dissected are in solid black. The mediastinal part is the lateral view. a, deep lateral cervical nodes; b, deep jugular nodes; c, cervical portion of recurrent nerve chain; d, thoracic portion of recurrent nerve chain; e, (right) pretracheal nodes; f, brachiocephalic artery nodes; g, upper para-oesophageal nodes; h, infra-aortic arch nodes; i, subcarinal nodes; j, sub-bronchial nodes; k, mid-para-oesophageal nodes; l, lower para-oesophageal nodes; m, diaphragmatic nodes; n, paracardiac nodes; o, lesser curvature nodes; p, left gastric artery nodes; q, coeliac trunk nodes; r, common hepatic artery nodes. Area k and l includes para-aortic nodes and thoracic duct nodes. (Modified with permission from Akiyama H 1990 Surgery for cancer of the esophagus. Williams & Wilkins, Baltimore.)

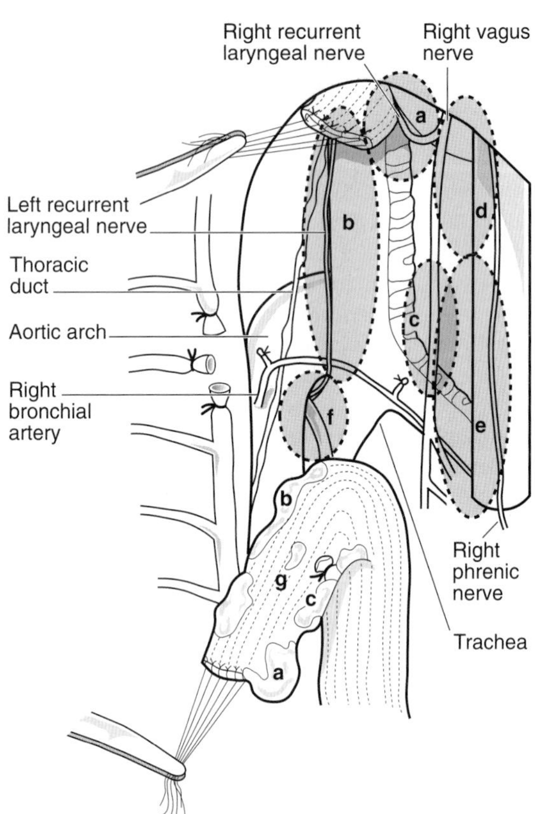

Fig. 11.4 Superior mediastinum in the course of lymph node dissection viewed from the right side. Thoracic duct is preserved, and the third intercostal artery arising from its common trunk with the right bronchial artery is divided. Nodes indicated by dotted ellipsoids are to be dissected. Metastasis is rarely seen in the late stage in lower pretracheal nodes (e), so they are preserved to maintain tracheobronchial circulation when the tumour is located in the lower third of the oesophagus or the tumour is in the early stage. a, right recurrent nerve nodes; b, left recurrent nerve nodes; c, right tracheobronchial nodes; d, pretracheal nodes, upper one-third (brachiocephalic nodes); e, pretracheal nodes, lower two-thirds; f, left tracheobronchial nodes (subaortic arch nodes); g, para-oesophageal nodes.

resection with the oesophagus. It runs over the vertebral bodies behind the oesophagus, lying between the azygos vein on its right and the aorta on its left in the middle and inferior mediastinum. The thoracic duct is preserved when the tumour is T1 or when the patient has liver cirrhosis.

5 Dissect the lymph nodes below the bilateral main bronchi and the carina, preserving the peripheral branches of the right bronchial artery and the bilateral pulmonary branches of the vagus nerves. The plane between the oesophagus and pericardium leads to glands that must be resected. Ligate the branches of other bronchial arteries from the anterior aspect of the subcarinal nodes if they are encountered (Fig. 11.5).

KEY POINTS Thoracic duct

- If you are not be able to preserve the thoracic duct without producing injury or stenosis, prefer to ligate it at its lower end in the thorax.
- Beware, though, that ligation of the thoracic duct produces marked retroperitoneal oedema and rapidly progressing decrease in the circulating plasma volume during the early postoperative period.
- This augmented third space accumulation of extracellular fluid causes an overload to circulatory and respiratory organs within the subsequent 2 or 3 days.

6 Dissect the plane between the membranous portion of the trachea and the upper thoracic oesophagus. Take care not to dissect too close to the tracheal wall in order to maintain the microvascular circulation and prevent tracheobronchial injury.

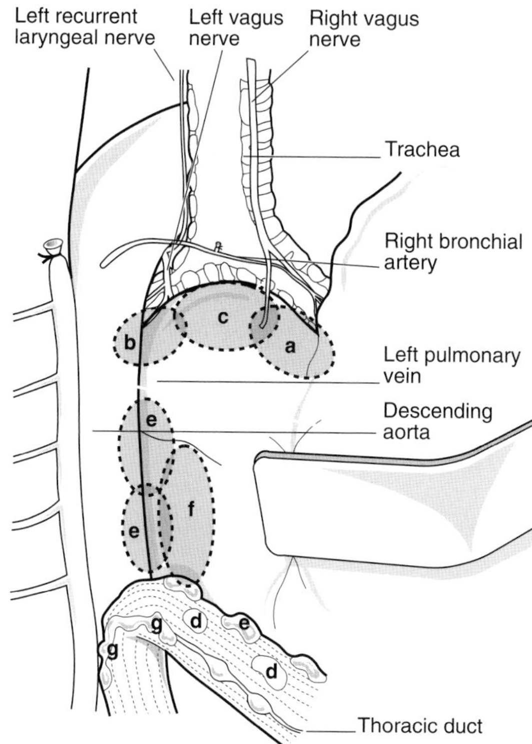

Fig. 11.5 Middle mediastinum in the course of lymph node dissection viewed from the right side. Bilateral oesophageal branches of the vagus nerves are transected. The thoracic duct is resected with the oesophagus. a, right sub-bronchial nodes; b, left sub-bronchial nodes; c, subcarinal nodes; d, para-oesophageal nodes; e, para-aortic nodes; f, pulmonary ligament nodes; g, thoracic duct nodes.

7 Anchor the upper thoracic oesophagus as high as possible using tape. Sharply dissect the soft tissue on the left lateral side of the trachea so that the fascial structure over the left subclavian artery is denuded. This dissection plane meets the space already made from the posterior side of the oesophagus in mobilizing the thoracic duct.

8 Identify the left recurrent laryngeal nerve in the soft tissue dissected from the left lateral side of the trachea. Sharply cut out the recurrent nerve and dissect en bloc the left paratracheal nodes (left recurrent laryngeal nerve nodes) remaining attached to the oesophagus.

KEY POINT Protect the recurrent laryngeal nerve

- Golden rules for avoiding injury are:
  —Gentle manipulation of the nerve.
  —Very slight traction to straighten it.
  —Close sharp dissection of the nerve without electrocautery.

9 Transect the thoracic oesophagus at its upper end. Temporarily close both cut ends manually. Cut and ligate the thoracic duct behind the upper thoracic oesophagus at its upper end in the thorax.

10 Dissect the nodes around the oesophagus, pulling the oral cut end of the oesophagus downward past the arch of preserved right bronchial artery. Several proper oesophageal arteries that arise from the descending aorta need to be ligated and cut. Completely dissect the nodes in the posterior mediastinum so that the left lung can be observed through the thin left mediastinal pleura and the descending aorta is denuded widely to its left lateral margin (Fig. 11.5).

11 Ligate and cut the lower end of the thoracic duct. Dissect the soft tissues around the hiatus and visualize the crural muscles (Fig. 11.6).

12 Go back to the superior mediastinum again and dissect the pretracheal nodes and subaortic arch nodes (Fig. 11.4). Also dissect the left tracheobronchial and subaortic arch nodes (Fig. 11.4).

13 Cover the fully mobilized oesophagus with nodes attached using a rubber sac in order to avoid possible scattering of tumour cells and loss of some nodes when the oesophagus is pulled out later from the thoracic cavity.

? DIFFICULTY

1. If you cannot find the right recurrent laryngeal nerve, also search for it from the medial aspect. The left recurrent laryngeal nerve can be identified on the left lateral surface of the dissection plane when the soft tissue on the left side of the trachea is dissected en bloc. If you go into this soft tissue directly to identify the nerve, it might retract itself anteriorly behind the left posterior edge of the tracheal cartilage. If there are two or more candidates, follow them proximally (downwards). Only the true left recurrent laryngeal nerve arises from the left vagus trunk and runs around the lower surface of the aortic arch. Do not cut any suspicious structure until you are quite sure that you have found the correct one.
2. The right bronchial artery can be sacrificed when it is too thin to preserve or too close to the tumour. However, it is safer to preserve it if you plan extensive lymph node dissection in the superior mediastinum. If you have sacrificed the right bronchial artery, you should avoid too-extensive dissection of the subaortic arch space so as not to sacrifice the left bronchial arteries.
3. Transection can be done at the lower end of the thoracic oesophagus when the upper margin of the tumour is so high that simple transection at the upper end cannot obtain a safe surgical margin (discussed under the cervical procedure).

Checklist

1 Has all the bleeding stopped? Most bleeding points may be on the dissected oesophagus, which has to be left in the thorax for a while.

2 Are the lower end of the thoracic duct and its small branches completely ligated? An unligated small branch arising from the left can also cause postoperative chylothorax.

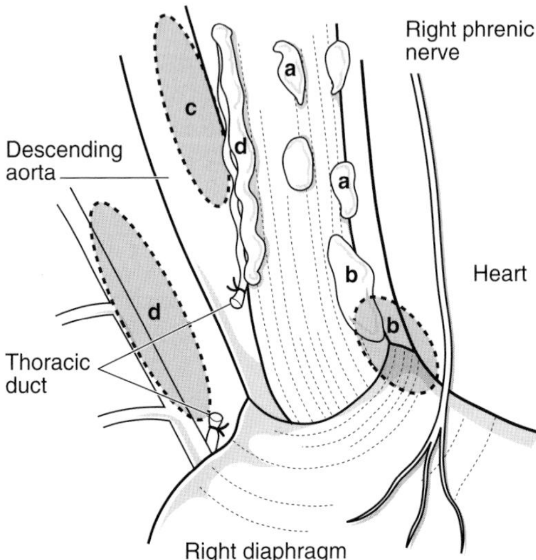

Fig. 11.6 Inferior mediastinum in the course of lymph node dissection viewed from the right side. The thoracic duct is resected with the oesophagus, and its lower end in the thoracic cavity is ligated and cut. a, para-oesophageal nodes; b, supradiaphragmatic nodes; c, para-aortic nodes; d, thoracic duct nodes.

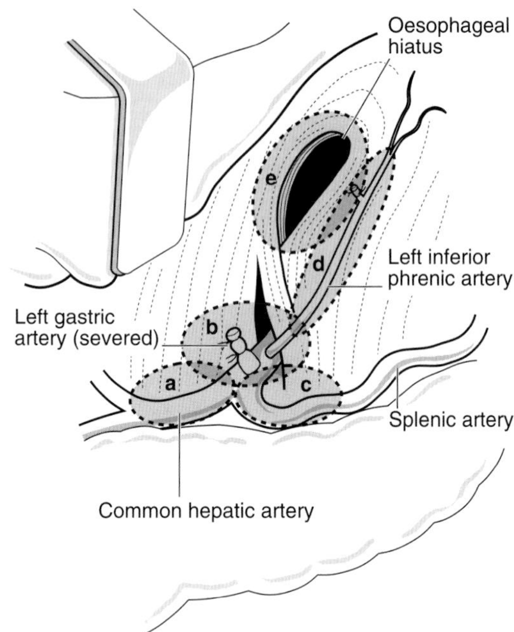

Fig. 11.7 Upper abdomen in the course of lymph node dissection. a, common hepatic artery nodes; b, coeliac nodes; c, proximal splenic artery nodes; d, inferior phrenic artery nodes; e, hiatal nodes.

3 If the left mediastinal pleura is opened, suck out all the fluid that has accumulated in the left pleural cavity during right thoracotomy.

4 If pulmonary injury occurred during the thoracic operation, repair it meticulously with manual suturing, ligation, linear stapling and fibrin glue. A new product of synthetic sheet of collagen with fibrinogen and thrombin on one side is very effective to control difficult air leakage and persistent bleeding.

Closure

1 Insert an underwater-sealed drain into the right pleural cavity through a separate stab incision in the seventh or sixth intercostal space in the posterior axillary line.

2 Approximate the incised intercostal space with two thick, absorbable sutures through both ribs.

3 Close the chest wound, including the pectoralis and serratus anterior muscles above and below.

ABDOMINAL AND CERVICAL PROCEDURES

Access

1 Move the patient to a supine position with the neck extended.

2 Make an upper median laparotomy incision for the abdominal operation and a collar incision for the cervical operation. These two operations are started simultaneously by two separate teams.

Assess: abdominal procedure

1 Determine the extent of spread to the lymph nodes along the left gastric vessels and around the coeliac axis.

2 Also check for para-aortic lymph node involvement. Peritoneal dissemination, which occurs when tumour seeds from the main lesion or massively metastatic lymph nodes, should also be excluded. Such advanced tumour growth should be suspected as a result of preoperative assessment, and a 'reconstruction-first' method should be employed.

Action: abdominal procedure

1 The basic manoeuvres applied around the root of the left gastric artery are very similar to Japanese D2 dissection for gastric cancer. We routinely dissect the nodes on the common hepatic artery, the root of splenic artery and the nodes around the coeliac axis (Fig. 11.7).

2 After complete mobilization of the stomach by dividing the left gastroepiploic, short gastric, posterior gastric and left gastric vessels, while dissecting the nodes mentioned above, cut the phreno-oesophageal ligament and carefully pull out the oesophagus from the thorax with lymph nodes attached. Cover the oesophagus with a towel.

3 Find the highest point by the 'pinching up' technique (Fig. 11.8). Design the resection line for the stomach by connecting the points where the vessels from the left gastric artery enter the gastric wall so that the pericardiac nodes and the nodes in the left gastric area are all removed. Resection is done along this line with two or three applications of a linear stapling device. The suture line is covered with interrupted seromuscular stitches.

KEY POINT Gastric circulation

- Take care to avoid injuring the right gastric vessels. They are very fragile, are easily torn, and bleed when pulled downwards. Although they are safely sacrificed in most cases, try not to injure them to preserve better circulation of the gastric remnant.

Technical point

Nowadays, hand-assisted laparoscopic surgery (HALS) can also be applied to oesophageal operations. The smaller laparotomy wound, about 7 cm in length, reduces postoperative pain. Although a standard lymph node dissection can be performed using HALS, we do not apply this procedure to patients with evident abdominal lymph node metastases, for fear of tumour implantation.

? DIFFICULTY

1. When another abnormality of the stomach has been detected preoperatively, such as an ulcer scar or early gastric cancer, try to include such lesions in the resected portion.
2. You can endoscopically place clips around the lesion preoperatively, or you can make a longitudinal incision in the gastric wall near the lesser curvature to observe the lesion directly and perform intraoperative mucosal resection.
3. If the stomach is not suitable for oesophageal reconstruction, ileocolon is the next best choice.

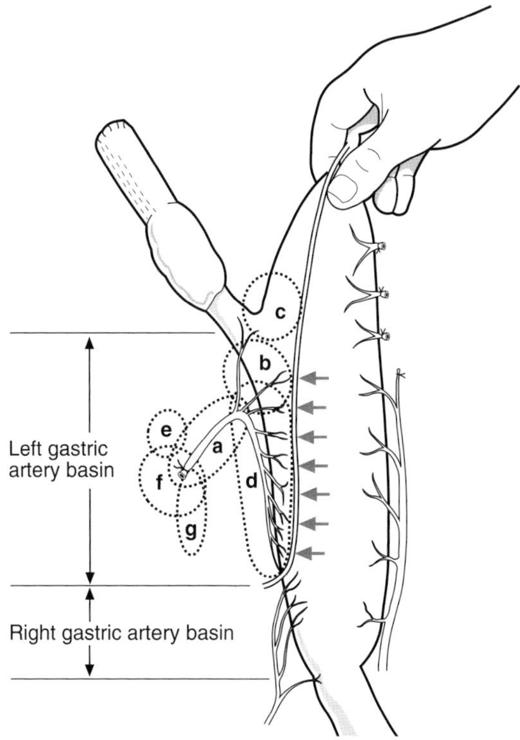

Fig. 11.8 'Pinching-up' technique to select the 'highest point'. Resection is done along the line connecting the points (short arrows) where the vessels of the left gastric area enter the gastric wall. Take care not to injure the right gastric vessels by traction. Nodes indicated by a–g are dissected. a, left gastric artery nodes; b, right paracardiac nodes; c, left paracardiac nodes; d, left lesser curvature nodes; e, proximal splenic artery nodes; f, coeliac nodes; g, common hepatic artery nodes.

Action: cervical procedure

1 Mobilize the bilateral sternomastoid muscles widely. Separate the clavicular part from the sternal part, and place tapes around each muscle. Supraclavicular dissection can be achieved by pulling these tapes laterally and medially without cutting any muscle head (Fig. 11.9).

2 The area to be cleared extends from the cervical oesophagus laterally to the lateral supraclavicular nerve and from the level near the laryngeal promontory down to the subclavian vein and apical pleura (Fig. 11.9). More than 90% of cervical lymph node metastases arising from tumours of the thoracic oesophagus are located within the triangle defined by the bilateral omohyoid muscles and subclavian veins.

3 Lymph nodes lateral to the common carotid arteries are dissected out first. Areolar tissue and lymph nodes are cleared away from the posterior surface of the platysma, to the anterior, middle and posterior scalene muscles, the thyrocervical trunk and its three branches. The phrenic and vagus nerves are identified and preserved. The omohyoid muscle is sacrificed.

4 The cut end of the thoracic duct is drawn up into the neck on the left side and its entry into the junction of the internal jugular and subclavian veins is ligated and cut.

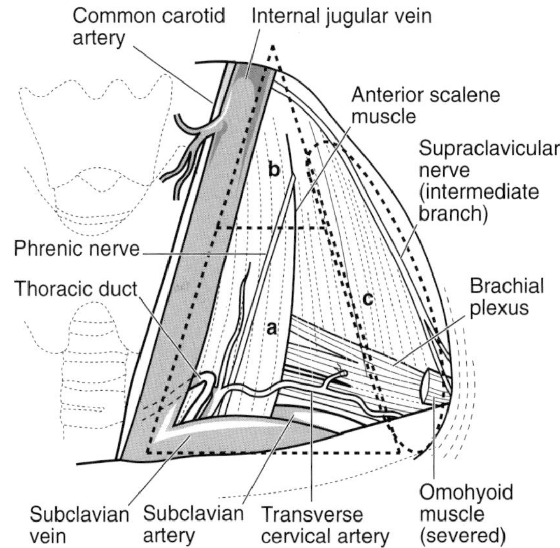

Fig. 11.9 Lymph nodes to be dissected in the cervical procedure except the paratracheal nodes. The thoracic duct is preserved. a, supraclavicular fossa nodes; b, deep jugular nodes; c, lateral cervical nodes.

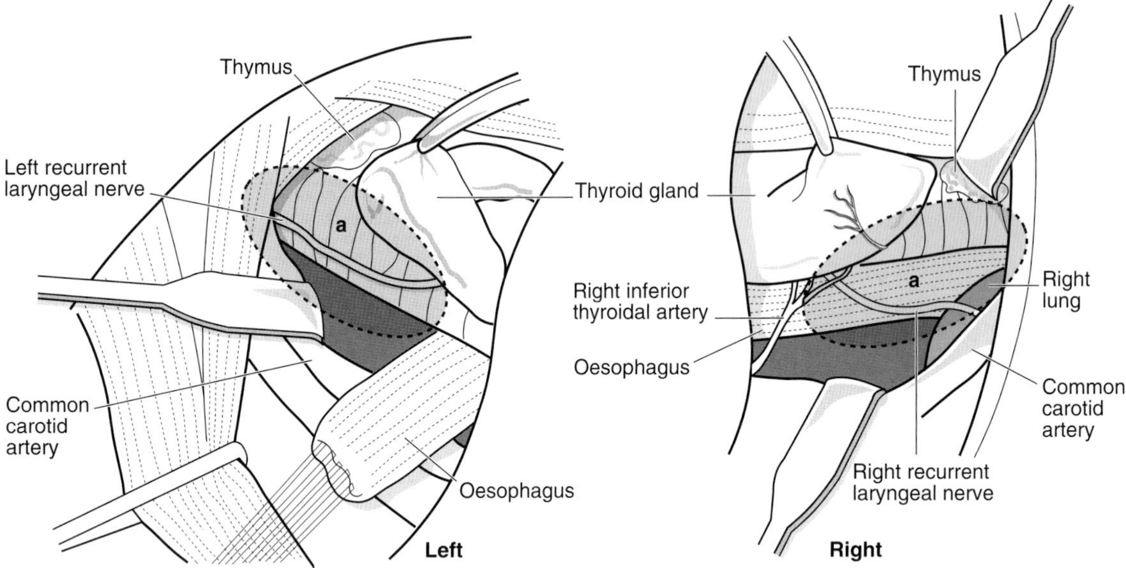

Fig. 11.10 Completion of lymph node dissection in bilateral cervical paratracheal area. a, cervical recurrent nerve nodes (paratracheal and para-oesophageal nodes).

5 Now dissect out the lymph nodes along the carefully preserved recurrent laryngeal nerves. They may be very small, but are liable to contain micrometastases. Make sure that the paratracheal dissection plane of the thoracic operation and the cervical operation are completely continuous on both sides (Fig. 11.10).

KEY POINTS Recurrent laryngeal nerve and thoracic duct

- Be aware that metastatic nodes tend to be located posterior to the recurrent laryngeal nerve on the right, and anterior to the nerve on the left. Performing left paratracheal dissection is easier when the upper oesophageal stump is pulled out to the left with the left recurrent laryngeal nerve lying in front, and the left strap muscles are transected at their lower end.
- When you preserve the thoracic duct in the intrathoracic procedure, you must identify its entry to the left cervical venous angle. Make sure that it is not injured or stenosed in the neck. If it has been injured, ligate it at its lower end through the abdominal wound where it lies behind the right crural muscle.

RECONSTRUCTION

Appraise

As is well known, there are three possible routes for oesophageal reconstruction: antethoracic (subcutaneous), retrosternal and posterior mediastinal. There are pros and cons for each route. You should select one of them by considering all the relevant possibilities. Our standard procedure for advanced thoracic oesophageal carcinoma using the retrosternal route is presented here.

Action

1 The cervical oesophagus should be dissected from the surrounding tissue to obtain enough length for anastomosis. The left sternohyoid and sternothyroid muscles are transected with electrocautery near their heads. Then the retrosternal space behind the sternal incisura is bluntly opened with a finger.

2 In the abdominal operating field, close the oesophageal hiatus with three interrupted sutures. Place the gastric remnant with the suture line on the dorsal side of the patient. Fix two tapes of different colours on each side near the tip with suture-ligatures.

3 Make a retrosternal tunnel using blunt finger dissection and a long, delicately curved, flat, flexible intestinal retractor with a hole at the tip. Ligate the two coloured tapes on the same side of the retractor through the hole at the tip.

4 Then pass the retractor through the retrosternal tunnel again and catch the two tapes in the neck. Bring the tip of the gastric remnant up to the neck by pushing from the abdominal side and gently pulling on the tapes in the neck. Take care to avoid rotation of the gastric remnant in the tunnel, using the coloured tapes as a guide.

5 Oesophagogastrostomy is done manually with two layers of 5/0 silk or absorbable monofilament thread. Pass a nasogastric tube for decompression.

? DIFFICULTY

1. When the oral margin of the main tumour is high, or there are multiple lesions or intramural metastasis is suspected near the cervical oesophagus, the upper margin of the oesophagectomy should be determined using the cervical operating field.
   - The oesophagus should have been divided at a lower level in the thorax. Pull out the thoracic oesophagus to the left cervical area with nodes attached, and cover it with a towel. Then dissect the cervical oesophagus from the surrounding tissue to as high a level as possible. Cut up the cricopharyngeal part of the inferior pharyngeal constrictor muscle on the left posterolateral side for better exposure and, more importantly, to facilitate postoperative swallowing function.
   - Incise the oesophagus longitudinally on the contralateral side of the suspected lesion. The lumen can be opened easily when you cut the wall over a nasogastric tube.
   - Wipe the mucosal surface gently with a dry soft cotton ball, then spread Lugol's solution evenly over the mucosa with a cotton ball. All the unstained mucosa should be included in the resected segment. Remember that submucosal spread cannot be ruled out by this technique. This should be checked by pathological examination of frozen sections.
2. If the gastric remnant is too short for cervical anastomosis, add Kocher's mobilization. If this is not enough, cut the peritoneum over the hepatoduodenal ligament transversely near the duodenum and carefully cut the restraining lesser curve strands of lesser omentum that prevent the curvature from straightening. The gastric remnant can be stretched longer if it has been made narrower, but the circulation is uncertain.

▶ KEY POINT Preventing gastric prolapse

- If you choose the posterior mediastinal route for reconstruction, slightly pull down the elevated stomach and fix it to the crural muscles after completing the cervical anastomosis. This prevents the gastric remnant from prolapsing into the right thoracic cavity.

Check

Has all the bleeding in the neck and the abdomen stopped? The supraclavicular fossa is a very frequent site of postoperative re-bleeding. Most frequently, re-bleeding is from the cut end of a small branch of the transverse cervical artery, the posterior surface of the sternomastoid muscle, or a small branch of the inferior thyroid artery.

Closure

1 Insert a pair of silicone cylinder drains 5 mm in diameter with multiple holes or longitudinal grooves, through small incisions on the anterior chest surface. Pass them into the dissected supraclavicular fossae through the two heads of sternomastoid muscle on both sides and connect them to the closed low-pressure suction bag.

2 Close the cervical collar incision in the same airtight manner as after a thyroid operation.

3 Close the abdominal wound in your usual manner except that, when the retrosternal route has been chosen for reconstruction, the peritoneal incision line is not sutured at the most cephalic 10 cm so that the elevated stomach is not constricted.

RESECTION OF THE THORACIC OESOPHAGUS WITHOUT THORACOTOMY

Appraise

1 Palliative resection of the oesophagus may be achieved by combined transhiatal abdominal and cervical approaches.

2 We believe that this procedure should be restricted to high-risk patients in whom standard thoracotomy is impossible, or you will deprive some patients with potentially curable disease of the chance to undergo a more radical resection.

3 Another good indication for this procedure is dysphagic patients with resectable oesophageal carcinoma who have distant nodes involved or organ metastases but otherwise have a reasonable life-expectancy. It also offers a convenient means of providing a gastric conduit following pharyngolaryngectomy. When there are widespread or multiple superficial mucosal cancers for which endoscopic mucosal resection is impractical, this is also a good procedure, although the indication of this procedure to such superficial mucosal cancers has been decreasing as the technique of endoscopic mucosal resection has been revised. The technique can also occasionally be employed for recurrent dysphagia following radiotherapy, adenocarcinoma of the cardia and lower oesophagus, intractable benign stricture, incapacitating motility disorders and irrevocable damage following trauma.

4 Take into account all the advantages and disadvantages before you perform this procedure on oesophageal malignant disease. There are many other options for palliation including bypass surgery, indwelling expandable metallic stent, palliative (chemo-)radiation and simple feeding gastrostomy.

5 Do not embark upon this technique unless you have an intimate knowledge of the mediastinal anatomy and are competent to carry out a formal thoracotomy if necessary. Clumsy and ignorant blunt dissection can lead to calamitous bleeding or tearing of the fragile posterior membrane of the trachea or bronchi, with disastrous results.

6 Orringer and colleagues claim that this approach, together with radiotherapy or chemoradiotherapy, can be an acceptable alternative to other methods of radical oesophagectomy. However, we can see no prognostic benefit in this approach compared

with the results obtained by our method of oesophagectomy with extensive lymphadenectomy. Anyway, no trial has been done to compare neoadjuvant therapy plus transhiatal oesophagectomy with radical oesophagectomy.

Access

1 Place the anaesthetized, intubated patient supine, with the head turned moderately to the right, and insert a small folded sheet beneath the scapulae to extend the neck.

2 Approach the abdomen through an upper midline incision.

3 Video mediastinoscopy from the hiatus is useful.

4 Make a neck incision along the lower anterior border of the left sternomastoid muscle. Cut platysma, dissect the medial border of sternomastoid muscle and cut the omohyoid muscle and the middle thyroid vein. This gives you entry to the space between the common carotid artery and the left lateral surface of the trachea and the thyroid gland.

Assess

1 Explore the abdomen to assess the intra-abdominal spread and operability. Do not commit yourself to resection until you are sure that the procedure is feasible and you can achieve it safely.

2 If the tumour involves the stomach, safe resection below this may preclude an oesophagogastric anastomosis in the neck. You may be able to get a safe surgical margin by performing palliative resection of the lower thoracic oesophagus containing the main lesion together with proximal or total gastrectomy through a widened oesophageal hiatus, followed by jejunal interposition or Roux-en-Y reconstruction. Alternatively, colon or an ileocolon conduit can be safely brought up to the neck. If the tumour is advanced or the patient is unfit, consider inserting a stent to relieve dysphagia. In the absence of dysphagia, do not feel under pressure to 'do something'. Be prepared to simply close the abdomen.

Action

Abdominal procedure

1 If resection is feasible, mobilize the left lobe of the liver and fold it to the right (Fig. 11.11).

2 Incise the peritoneum and the transversalis fascia over the front of the oesophageal hiatus. Insert a finger into the posterior mediastinum and separate the pericardium from the upper surface of the diaphragm. Incise the central tendon of diaphragm forwards for 7–8 cm from the hiatus, while ligating and dividing the inferior phrenic vessels.

3 Assess the extent of the tumour in the lower oesophagus.

4 Mobilize the lower oesophagus keeping well clear of the tumour and excising a cuff of diaphragmatic crus, posterior pericardium, mediastinal pleura, and posterior connective tissue as necessary. The oesophagus can be mobilized under vision almost up to the level of the tracheal carina. Carefully avoid excessive compression of the heart, which might cause hypotension, tachyarrhythmia and even cardiac arrest in patients with cardiovascular risk factors.

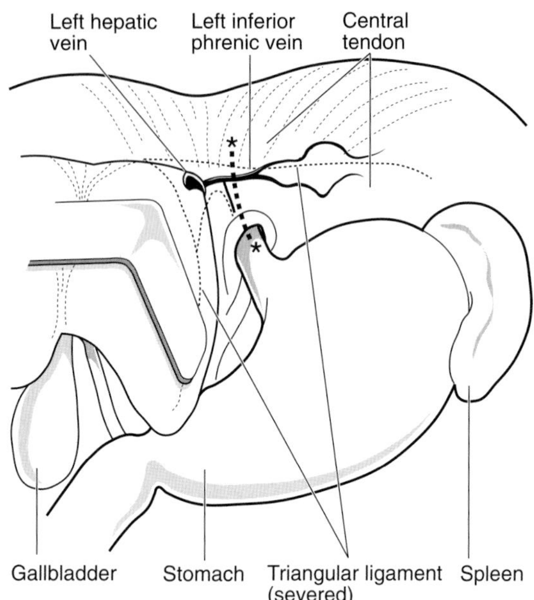

Fig. 11.11 Incisional line (*---*) of the diaphragm for widening of the hiatus.

5 Now proceed close to the oesophagus, carefully separating it from the back of the trachea. Hook the branches of the vagus nerves within the flexed index and middle fingers, and cut them using long scissors within the protection of the fingers.

Cervical procedure

1 Access is increased, if necessary, by transecting the strap muscles on the left. Median sternotomy or excision of the medial clavicle, a portion of the first rib and a half of the manubrium sterni on one side will very efficiently widen the operative field, but it is usually not necessary unless large tumour, primary or metastatic, interferes with the access.

2 Expose the left lateral surface of the cervical oesophagus behind the trachea. The longitudinal fat pad along the posterior margin of the tracheal cartilage contains the left recurrent laryngeal nerve. Sharply dissect this fat pad from the oesophagus and enter the space between the membranous portion of the trachea and the anterior surface of the oesophagus. Widen this space upward and downward. Dissect the posterior surface of the cervical oesophagus from the prevertebral fascia. Place a tape around the oesophagus just on its right lateral surface to avoid injury to the right recurrent laryngeal nerve. Care should also be taken not to compress the left recurrent laryngeal nerve on the left lateral tracheal surface.

3 Continue freeing the oesophagus downwards into the superior mediastinum. Final mobilization is best achieved by inserting the index finger of one hand through the neck and passing the other hand up from the abdomen through the posterior mediastinum.

Resect

1 Remove the nasogastric tube.

2 Apply a ligature (or a linear stapling device) around the cervical oesophagus as low as possible.

3 Transect the oesophagus above the ligature, sterilize the tip and allow the lower ligated cut end to retract into the mediastinum. A tape should be connected to the oesophageal stump to guide pulling up the oesophageal substitute later.

4 In the abdomen, transect the upper part of the stomach in the same manner described for extended lymph node dissection (p. 148), because early recurrence around the elevated stomach should be avoided. Cover the suture line with seromuscular stitches.

5 Remove the specimen for histology.

6 Insert a basal or apical underwater-sealed drain whenever the pleural cavity has been breached. The necessity of this pleural drainage is only temporally as long as the lung was not injured.

Unite

1 If the gastric remnant can be used as the conduit, mobilize it in the same manner as other techniques. Ensure that the tip of the gastric remnant will reach the neck by laying it on the chest wall. Bring up the gastric remnant to the neck through one of the three possible routes (usually posterior mediastinal) and unite it to the cervical oesophagus.

2 The alternatives were already discussed under 'Assess'.

OESOPHAGEAL BYPASS

1 Resection may not be possible, or may be contraindicated because the tumour is too extensive. Bypass is preferable to stenting in patients with a prognosis of months rather than weeks. Bypass does not preclude radiotherapy, and the conduit lies at a distance from the field of irradiation.

2 The mobilized stomach may be raised above the unresected tumour when the left thoracoabdominal operation or the Ivor Lewis operation is planned. The anastomosis above the tumour can be fashioned after transection of the oesophagus and closure of the cut lower end or, if there is no fistula, it can be made in the lateral wall of the oesophagus without transection. If possible, leave the lower oesophagus in continuity with the stomach. Sometimes it is necessary to divide the lower oesophagus to free the stomach, so that it can be joined well above the tumour.

3 Kirschner's operation (the total bypass of the thoracic oesophagus with stomach) is preferable to bypass unresectable middle-third lesions. Mobilize the stomach through the abdomen. You can transect the oesophagus at the cardia and use the whole stomach, but our preference is to prepare the stomach as described for extensive lymph node dissection (p. 148) but without the 'pinching up' technique so as not to pull up the stomach with metastatic lymph nodes. The bypass route can be made retrosternally or antethoracically. In order to make the antethoracic route, elevate the skin at the upper end of the wound. Use long-handled scissors to create a track 7–10 cm wide in the subcutaneous tissue over the sternum and manubrium with a combination of blunt and sharp dissection. Mobilize the cervical oesophagus through an incision in the side of the neck (we prefer the left side) in the same manner as that described for resection of the thoracic oesophagus without thoracotomy (p. 152), and use this incision to complete the subcutaneous track into the neck. Grasp the oesophagus with a clamp as low as possible in the mobilized cervical oesophagus. Transect the oesophagus above the grasped level, close the lower cut end, and allow it to retract into the superior mediastinum. Gently manoeuvre the stomach through the subcutaneous track by a combination of pushing and traction. Avoid tension and twisting of the organ. Now anastomose the upper cut end of the oesophagus to the upper surface of the drawn-up stomach.

4 It is often said that you can safely leave the oesophagus after closing both ends of a segment containing an unresectable tumour. However, this holds true for only a certain period of time, so internal or external (tube) drainage is necessary when the continuity of the oesophagus and the lower gastrointestinal tract cannot be maintained, unless there is a large fistula with the tracheobronchial tree. This can be achieved by simply inserting a drainage tube from the lower cut end, or anastomosing the lower end to a Roux loop of jejunum. We prefer tube oesophagojejunostomy with Witzel jejunostomy on the anal side (Fig. 11.12).

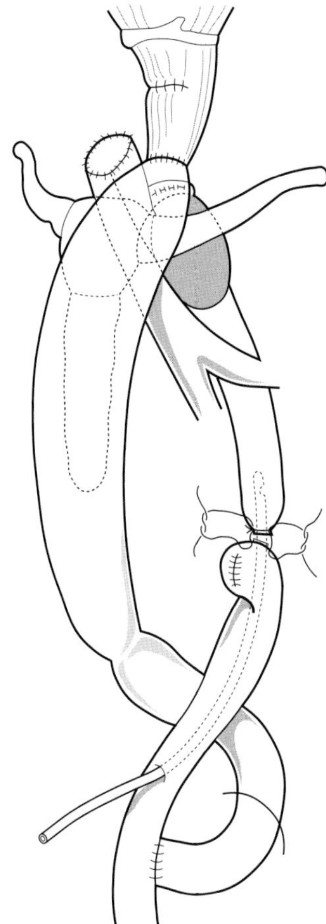

Fig. 11.12 Diagram of oesophageal bypass with laryngectomy. Drainage of the isolated oesophagus is accomplished by a simple technique of tube oesophagojejunostomy. Two sites of purse-string sutures around a thin drainage tube are approximated with a few additional stitches. (Modified from Udagawa H 1991 Esophageal bypass with laryngectomy: a method of palliation for nonresectable upper esophageal carcinoma. Diseases of the Esophagus 4:63–70.)

5 Carcinoma at or near the cardia can be bypassed using a Roux-en-Y loop of jejunum that is taken up subcutaneously or retrosternally to the neck, but mobilization of such a long segment of jejunum is difficult. A segment of colon (see below) taken out of circuit is usually more easily fashioned into a conduit between the cervical oesophagus and the distal stomach.

6 When the tumour is too high to get enough length of cervical oesophagus for anastomosis, often with impending higher airway obstruction or recurrent laryngeal nerve palsy, oesophageal bypass with laryngectomy (Fig. 11.12) is a possible means of palliation.

COLONIC REPLACEMENT OR BYPASS OF THE OESOPHAGUS

Appraise

1 The colon usually has a good marginal blood supply (Fig. 11.13) and it makes an excellent oesophageal replacement.

2 An antiperistaltic loop can be created by swinging up the mobilized left colon after dividing the left colic vessels, so that it is supplied through the middle colic vessels. Because it does not always function well, this method should be the last alternative.

3 An isoperistaltic loop of right colon can be swung up, based on the middle colic vessels, after dividing the right colic and ileocolic vessels. The bulky caecum is brought to the neck after closing the terminal ileum and carrying out appendicectomy. The caecal bulk soon diminishes. 15–20 cm of terminal ileum can also be used for reconstruction or bypass. In this situation, the right colic vessels may be preserved and you can expect an antireflux function of the ileocaecal valve. Perfusion of the ileum should be carefully examined because the peripheral vascular connections between the ileocolic and the right colic vessels are poor in some patients.

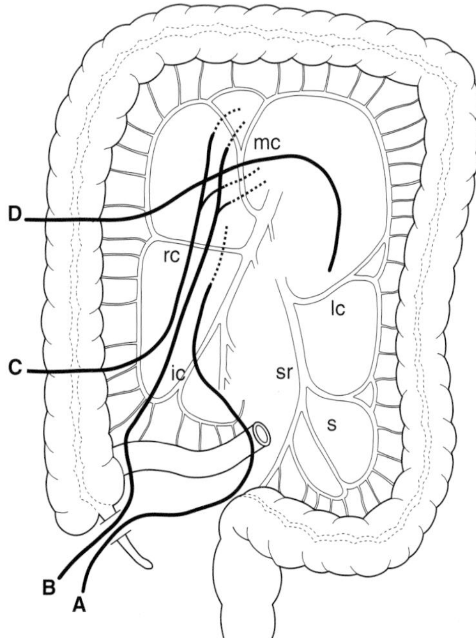

Fig. 11.13 Cutting lines for oesophageal reconstruction or bypass with isoperistaltic colonic segment. Additional separation of the vasculature along the dashed lines is possible unless it spoils the circulation of the segment. We routinely begin with A, shifting step by step to B, C and D according to the circulatory state of the tip and the length of the segment. ic, ileocolic, rc, right colic; mc, middle colic; lc, left colic; S, sigmoidal; Sr, superior rectal artery.

4 An isoperistaltic loop can be fashioned based on the left upper colic vessels.

5 If the tip of the elevated colon shows poor arterial circulation or bad venous return and microvascular technique is available, addition of an arterial or venous anastomosis of the once sacrificed colonic vessels to a suitable cervical vasculature can save this difficult situation.

Prepare

The colon must be prepared beforehand by feeding the patient with low residual diet or liquid meal for preoperative 1–2 days and by administering oral intestine cleaning solution on the day before surgery. No prophylactic antibiotics are given.

Action

1 Carefully study the anatomy of the marginal vessels.

2 Any bypass route for a colon segment, particularly when the right colon is used, should be designed to be wider than for gastric pull-up.

3 Mobilize the caecum, ascending colon and right transverse colon on to the primitive mesentery. Check for vascular continuity by inspecting the mobilized mesocolon against a light. In case of doubt, gently apply bulldog clips to the blood vessels at the intended sites of division and an intestinal clamp on the terminal ileum for several minutes, and then check the colour and circulation. Do not commit yourself to colonic bypass with an ischaemic or congested segment of colon. Remember, the venous drainage is as important as the arterial supply.

4 Doubly ligate and divide the ileocaecal vessels near their origin from the superior mesenteric vessels. Do not divide the right colic vessels at this stage, because it is often unnecessary. Then divide the ileum at the point about 20 cm (depending on the pattern of mesenteric vasculature) proximal to the Bauhin's valve with linear stapling device. Apply seromuscular stitches to the distal cut end of the terminal ileum. Check the length of the ileocolic segment placing it on the anterior chest wall. The right colic vessels can be divided if greater length is required. Swing the caecum upwards and gently push and pull it along the prepared track. Carefully avoid violent traction on the root of the draining vein when you are pulling up any colonic segment. Anastomose the caecum or terminal ileum to the cervical oesophagus in an end-to-side fashion.

5 Meticulously divide the marginal vessels for 3 cm at a suitable point on the transverse colon for distal anastomosis, while avoiding injury to the vascular arcade. Divide the transverse

colon at the centre of the devascularized segment. Anastomose the proximal cut end of the colon to a suitable organ (i.e. distal stomach, duodenal bulb or side of the jejunal loop brought up antecolically), depending on the situation. Then anastomose the proximal cut end of the terminal ileum to the distal cut end of the transverse colon.

KEY POINTS Small-bowel complications

- Ischaemic contraction of the bowels may be observed when the ileocolic vessels are divided in patients with poor vascular arcade between the right colic and ileocolic vessels, This is usually resolved with gradual vascular dilatation. If you can find palpable or visible pulsation of the ileocolic trunk after 10–20 minutes of observation, it is a reliable sign that the arterial perfusion to the ileocolic arterial basin is sufficient. If you are not sure yet, take off the ligature of the ileocolic artery. If there is good backflow, you can safely continue the procedure. If there is not, it is safer to cut off the ileocolic arterial basin or to consider cervical vascular anastomosis.
- It is only the antimesenteric wall of the ileum that is necessary for the oesophago-ileostomy in the neck. Furthermore, the real distance via the retrosternal tunnel is shorter than the distance you can measure on the body surface. These mean that the length of the mesentery required for ileocolic pull-up is not as long as one may imagine. Therefore avoid unnecessary division of right colic vessels by precisely estimating which vessels must be divided.
- If you carry out end-to-side colonojejunostomy, as mentioned for Roux-en-Y reconstruction, place the afferent loop on the patient's left side, that is the same side as the ligament of Treitz. If you do not, the anastomosis may undergo torsion when the fluid accumulates in the afferent loop, possibly causing bowel obstruction.

6 Close the mesenteric window to prevent internal herniation. Close the diaphragm or anterior abdominal wall slackly around the colon so that it is not constricted. Ensure that the bowel and blood vessels are not twisted and are not under tension before closing the incisions.

7 Belsey has described the use of an isoperistaltic loop of transverse colon based on the left colic vessels. If necessary, the left branch or even the right branch of the middle colic artery can be divided.

Checklist

1 Ensure that bleeding and oozing from the many raw surfaces has been controlled before closing the wounds.

2 Have all the anastomoses been performed satisfactorily? Leakage of an anastomosis including colon leads to fatal complications. If you have even a slight doubt, you should do it again.

Aftercare

1 Following major oesophageal surgery, the patient should remain in the intensive care unit for at least 24 hours, so that cardiorespiratory, renal and cerebral functions can be monitored with early correction of any abnormalities. After extensive radical oesophagectomy, it takes much longer for pulmonary function to be restored, so it is advisable to keep the patient in intensive care for 3–4 days. Some patients benefit from initial mechanical ventilation via an endotracheal tube. Arrange for regular chest X-rays to ensure full pulmonary expansion. Order chest physiotherapy and aspiration of bronchial secretions either orally, through the endotracheal tube, or using a flexible bronchoscope.

2 Order adequate regular analgesics, and continue antibiotics and prophylaxis for venous thrombosis.

3 Aspirate the visceral tube regularly but, as bowel function recovers, the tube may be used for feeding if its position has been checked radiographically. After 7–9 days, screen the patient following a swallow of water-soluble contrast to exclude anastomotic leakage. Withdraw the tube and start oral feeding, progressing to solids over a day or two. Then stop parenteral feeding. If a jejunostomy was created, give small volumes of dilute fluid as soon as bowel sounds return, gradually increasing to larger volumes of full-strength feeds until oral feeding is established. The jejunostomy catheter can be left for several months for supplementary feeding.

4 Remove the chest drains after 48–72 hours unless fluid is being produced. If a drain fails to function and intrapleural fluid or air persists, do not hesitate to insert further suitably placed underwater-sealed drains.

5 Study the pathologist's report carefully. Is adjuvant radiotherapy or chemotherapy justified?

ADJUVANT TREATMENT

1 Although squamous carcinoma, and indeed adenocarcinoma, responds to external beam therapy, the effect of such adjuvant treatment on the prognosis is questionable. Most controlled trials of preoperative radiotherapy have failed to show any prognostic benefit. Radiotherapy has been used instead of surgery in some series and Pearson reported results as good as those obtained with surgery, especially for mid- and upper oesophageal tumours.

2 Brachytherapy (intracavity irradiation with caesium-137 or iridium-192) offers certain advantages, notably that the radiation is concentrated on the tumour. A guidewire is inserted endoscopically or under fluoroscopy and an external applicator tube is passed over the guidewire to straddle the tumour. Pellets of caesium or iridium, stored in a safe source, are then pneumatically transferred into the applicator and are transferred back at the end of treatment. This is an effective way to increase local control rate of radiotherapy. However, care should be taken because severe local tissue damage may lead to perforation if the tube positioning was not appropriate.

3 Endoscopic Nd-YAG laser therapy is valuable for palliation of dysphagia but it often has to be repeated to alleviate dysphagia and to maintain patency.

4 Photodynamic therapy involves giving sensitizing drugs, usually haematoporphyrin derivatives or phthalylcyanates, which are retained by tumour cells. When exposed to certain light wavelengths, these agents produce cytotoxic substances such as singlet oxygen. The light is usually delivered via optical fibre, but there is little tissue penetration, so the activity is mainly confined to the surface of lesions.

5 Chemotherapy has been tried, alone or in a variety of combinations. Cisplatin has been combined with 5-fluorouracil, and this combination (FP) is still regarded as the standard regimen. Many other drugs such as Adriamycin, etoposide, vindecine and recently paclitaxel, docetaxel and irinotecan have also been tried usually in combination with diamminedichloroplatinum or FP. Postoperative chemotherapy had been thought to lack scientific evidence in survival benefit, but a recent Japanese multicentric phase III trial with FP successfully showed significant prolongation of disease-free survival.

6 The concept of neoadjuvant treatment was proposed in 1981. Since then, a variety of preoperative treatments have been tried. Among them, concurrent chemoradiotherapy has attracted wide attention and many trials of neoadjuvant chemoradiotherapy are still ongoing. The general rules of treatment might be rewritten in the near future as a result although many surgeons still think that surgery is the standard treatment as long as R0 resection is possible. The indication of neoadjuvant (preoperative) chemoradiotherapy should be investigated in regard to tumour stage and the pattern of combined surgical treatment. It is often claimed that neoadjuvant chemoradiotherapy does not increase the risk of a subsequent operation. However, this claim remains controversial.

7 Chemoradiotherapy is also applied as a definitive treatment not only to non-resectable advanced tumours but also to earlier stage tumours as the main therapeutic measure in treatment intending organ preservation. However, chemoradiotherapy is still a kind of local therapy, with a wider influence than local resection and narrower than extensive lymph node dissection, and its late adverse effects are not fully understood. It is very often found that most tumour cells are destroyed, but a small nidus in a certain part or in lymph nodes located outside the radiation field contains metastasis. The salvage operation for the recurrent tumour after definitive chemoradiotherapy is not easy and the postoperative quality of life is often poor.

8 Now that we have many treatment options for oesophageal cancer, the most important point to remember is rational individualization of treatment, combining two, three or more modalities. Many researchers are trying to find a rational way of this individualization by applying techniques of molecular biology and genetics. More experimental treatments are also being tried in several centres, such as adoptive immunotherapy and gene therapy.

KEY POINTS Decision-making and patient consent

- Informed consent is a first priority in modern society
- Because many different modes of therapy are available and effective against oesophageal cancer, you need to give patients the best information possible. You must, therefore, be fully aware of the vast field of oncology.
- With the easy availability of information technology, you can remain aware of the very latest knowledge in the field.
- Remember that 'evidence-based medicine' is based on an imaginary average patient only. You must take into account all the unique conditions of each individual patient and offer the treatment option that you decide is the best for your patient.

FURTHER READING

Akiyama H 1980 Surgery for carcinoma of the esophagus. In: Current problems in surgery. Year Book Publishers, Chicago

Akiyama H 1990 Surgery for cancer of the esophagus. Williams & Wilkins, Baltimore

Akiyama H, Udagawa H 1999 Surgical management of esophageal cancer: The Japanese experience. In: Daly JM, Hennessy TPJ et al (eds) Management of upper gastrointestinal cancer. Saunders, London, pp 200–225

Akiyama H, Udagawa H 2002 Total gastrectomy and Roux-en-Y reconstruction. In: Pearson FG, Cooper JD et al (eds) Esophageal surgery, 2nd edn. Churchill Livingstone, New York, pp 871-879

Akiyama H, Tsurumaru M, Udagawa H 1988 Imaging techniques. In: Delarue NC, Wilkins EW Jr, Wong J (eds) Esophageal cancer. Mosby, St Louis, pp 53–68

Akiyama H, Tsurumaru M, Ono Y et al 1991 Transoral esophagectomy. Surgery, Gynecology and Obstetrics 173:399–400

Akiyama H, Tsurumaru M, Udagawa H et al 1997 Esophageal cancer. In: Current problems in surgery. Mosby, St Louis

al-Sarraf M, Martz K et al 1997 Progress report of combined chemoradiotherapy versus radiotherapy alone in patients with esophageal cancer: an intergroup study. Journal of Clinical Oncology 15:277–284

Ando N, Iizuka T, Ide H et al 2003 Surgery plus chemotherapy compared with surgery alone for localized squamous cell carcinoma of the thoracic esophagus: a Japan Clinical Oncology Group Study—JCOG9204. Journal of Clinical Oncology 21:4592–4596

Cuschieri A 1991 Invited introduction. Treatment of carcinoma of the oesophagus. Annals of the Royal College of Surgeons of England 73:1–3

Dimick JB, Pronovost PJ et al 2003 Surgical volume and quality of care for esophageal resection: do high-volume hospitals have fewer complications? Annals of Thoracic Surgery 75:337–341

Earlam R 1991 An MRC prospective randomized trial of radiotherapy versus surgery for operable squamous cell carcinoma of the oesophagus. Annals of the Royal College of Surgeons of England 73:8–12

Endo M 1993 Endoscopic resection as local treatment of mucosal cancer of the esophagus. Endoscopy 25:672–674

Flores AD, Stoller JL et al 1988 Combined primary treatment of cancer of the esophagus and cardia by intracavity and external irradiation. In: International trends in general thoracic surgery 4. Mosby, St Louis, pp 368–377

Fujita H, Kakegawa T, Yamana H et al 1995 Mortality and morbidity rates, postoperative course, quality of life, and prognosis after extended radical lymphadenectomy for esophageal cancer.

Comparison of three-field lymphadenectomy with two-field lymphadenectomy. Annals of Surgery 222:654–662

Herskovic A, Martz K et al 1992 Combined chemotherapy and radiotherapy compared with radiotherapy alone in patients with cancer of the esophagus. New England Journal of Medicine 326:1593–1598

Hurt RL 1989 Management of oesophageal carcinoma. Springer-Verlag, London

Ilson DH, Bains M, Ginsberg RJ et al 1997 Neoadjuvant therapy of esophageal cancer. Surgery and Oncology Clinics of North America 6:723-740

Isono K, Sato H, Nakayama K 1991 Results of a nationwide study on the three-field lymph node dissection of esophageal cancer. Oncology 48:411–420

Jamieson GG 1988 Surgery of the oesophagus. Churchill Livingstone, Edinburgh

Japanese Society for Esophageal Diseases 2004 Guidelines for clinical and pathologic studies on carcinoma of the esophagus, 9th edn. Preface, general principles, part I. Esophagus 1:61–88

Japanese Society for Esophageal Diseases 2004 Guidelines for clinical and pathologic studies on carcinoma of the esophagus, 9th edn. Part II. Esophagus 1: (in press)

Khoury GA 1991 Squamous cell carcinoma of the oesophagus: 10 years on. Annals of the Royal College of Surgeons of England 73:4–7

Kitagawa Y, Fujii H, Mukai M et al 2002 Intraoperative lymphatic mapping and sentinel lymph node sampling in esophageal and gastric cancer. Surgical Oncology Clinics of North America 11:293–304

Kodama M, Kakegawa T 1998 Treatment of superficial cancer of the esophagus: a summary of responses to a questionnaire on superficial cancer of the esophagus in Japan. Surgery 123:432–439

Krasna MJ, Tepper J 2000 The role of multimodality therapy for esophageal cancer. Chest Surgery Clinics of North America 10:591–603

Mathisen DJ 1995 Ivor Lewis procedure. In: Pearson FG et al (eds) Esophageal surgery. Churchill Livingstone, New York, pp 669–676

Matthews HR, Powell DJ, McConkey CC 1986 Effect of surgical experience on the results of resection for oesophageal carcinoma. British Journal of Surgery 73:621–623

Murata Y, Suzuki S, Ohta M et al 1996 Small ultrasonic probes for determination of the depth of superficial esophageal cancer. Gastrointestinal Endoscopy 44:23–28

Orringer MB 1995 Transhiatal esophagectomy without thoracotomy. In: Pearson FG et al (eds) Esophageal surgery. Churchill Livingstone, New York, pp 683–701

Osugi H, Takemura M, Higashino M et al 2003 Learning curve of video-assisted thoracoscopic esophagectomy and extended lymphadenectomy for squamous cell cancer of the thoracic esophagus and results. Surgical Endoscopy 17:515–519

Pearson JG 1977 The present status and future potential of radiotherapy in the management of esophageal cancer. Cancer 39:882–890

Raijman I, Siddique I, Ajani J et al 1998 Palliation of malignant dysphagia and fistulae with coated expandable metal stents: experience with 101 patients. Gastrointestinal Endoscopy 48:172–179

Refaely Y, Krasna MJ 2002 Multimodality therapy for esophageal cancer. Surgical Clinics of North America 23:1851–1858

Rutgeerts P, Vantrappen G, Broeckaert L et al 1988 Palliative Nd:YAG laser therapy for cancer of the esophagus and gastroesophageal junction: impact on the quality of remaining life. Gastrointestinal Endoscopy 34:87

Shimada H, Okazumi S, Matsubara H et al Effect of steroid therapy on postoperative course and survival of patients with thoracic esophageal carcinoma. Esophagus 1:89–94

Skinner DB 1983 En bloc resection for neoplasms of the esophagus and cardia. Journal of Thoracic and Cardiovascular Surgery 85: 59–71

Skinner DB 1991 Atlas of esophageal surgery. Churchill Livingstone, New York

Sobin LH, Witteind Ch (eds) 2002 International Union Against Cancer. TNM classification of malignant tumors, 6th edn. Wiley, pp 60–71

Thomas RJ, Abbott M, Bhathal PS et al 1987 High-dose photoirradiation of esophageal cancer. Annals of Surgery 206:193

Tytgat GNJ, Tio TL 1990 Techniques for staging oesophageal cancer. Gullet 1:4–9

Udagawa H 1991 Esophageal bypass with laryngectomy: a method of palliation for nonresectable upper esophageal carcinoma. Diseases of the Esophagus 4:63–70

Udagawa H, Akiyama H 2001 Surgical treatment of esophageal cancer: Tokyo experience of the three-field technique. Diseases of the Esophagus 14:110–114

Urba S 2002 Combined modality therapy of esophageal cancer: standard of care? Surgical Clinics of North America 11:377–386

Urschel JD, Vasan H 2003 A meta-analysis of randomized controlled trials that compared neoadjuvant chemoradiation and surgery to surgery alone for resectable esophageal cancer. American Journal of Surgery 185:538–543

Urschel JD, Ashiku S, Thurer R et al 2003 Salvage or planned esophagectomy after chemoradiation therapy for locally advanced esophageal cancer: a review. Diseases of the Esophagus 16:60–65

Laparoscopic Nissen fundoplication

A. Darzi, P.A. Paraskeva

DESCRIPTION OF OPERATION

Appraise

1 Gastro-oesophageal reflux disease (GORD; GERD, gastro-esophageal, in the USA), which often results from irreversible injury to the lower oesophageal sphincter, is not always responsive to medical therapy or recurs after stopping treatment. Persistent heartburn and regurgitation may be complicated by nocturnal choking, aspiration pneumonia, oesophageal stricture and oesophageal mucosal changes and ulceration described in 1950 by the London surgeon Norman Barrett (1903–1979).

2 Confirm reflux with 24-hour pH monitoring. If manometric studies reveal ineffective lower oesophageal sphincter and oesophageal body peristalsis, some form of antireflux procedure is necessary. The motility disorders are often secondary to the reflux and will not respond to prokinetic or prolonged acid-reduction medication.

3 A 'loose' Nissen, partial fundoplication such as the Toupet, a Hill procedure or Belsey mark IV are suitable. Laparoscopic Nissen fundoplication produces results comparable with open fundoplication but benefits from the minimally invasive approach.

KEY POINTS Preoperative considerations

- Adequate consent: conversion to open surgery, 'gas bloat' syndrome, recurrence of symptoms, other options.
- Previous gastroscopy.
- Barium swallow.
- 24-hour pH monitoring, oesophageal manometry.

Prepare

1 Perform laparoscopic fundoplication under general anaesthesia with endotracheal intubation.

2 Place the patient supine while you stand on the right side. Your assistant stands on the patient's left. The second assistant, who will hold the liver retractor and the camera, stands next to you on the patient's right.

3 Alternatively, use a modified lithotomy position with the patient's knees flexed only 35°, thus allowing free manipulation of the instruments. You then stand between the patient's legs and have easy access to the instruments. Have 20–30° of reverse Trendelenburg (head-up) tilt so that the viscera and fat fall into the pelvis under gravity, so improving the exposure of the hiatus (Fig. 12.1).

Access

1 Create a pneumoperitoneum using a Veress needle or by an open Hassan entry.

2 Place the ports as demonstrated in Figure 12.2.

KEY POINT Siting of trocars

- Do not place the trocars too low, or the instruments inserted through them will prove to be too short to reach up to the hiatus.

3 Insert the first port, which accommodates the camera, well above the umbilicus; insert subsequent ports under direct vision, angling them towards the hiatus. The angulation permits left lateral retraction of the oesophagus and downward retraction of the stomach, both of which are essential for safe accomplishment of the procedure. Use 10-mm ports for all, thus providing access for large instruments.

4 Introduce a liver retractor through the right subcostal port. This may be hand-held or attached to a mechanical holder secured to the table (Fig. 12.3).

5 Retract the stomach and oesophagus with a grasper or Babcock's forceps introduced through the left subcostal port in the anterior axillary line.

6 Ensure perfect haemostasis using diathermy coagulation. Vision is obscured by even a small amount of bleeding because the blood accumulates in the hiatus, in spite of the patient being in the reversed Trendelenburg position.

? DIFFICULTY

1. Obesity makes safe entry into the abdomen difficult, so carefully observe the insufflator flow-rate and pressure. If the readings are outside the safe range (see Ch. 5), employ the Hassan technique.
2. You need an experienced first assistant, since exposure is difficult, even though the patient is placed in a steep reverse Trendelenburg position.

Action

1 First expose the distal oesophagus by dividing the gastrohepatic ligament from about the level of the left gastric artery to the hiatus (Fig. 12.4).

2 Stay close to the liver and avoid the hepatic artery; damage to it produces significant bleeding. You now see the right crus of

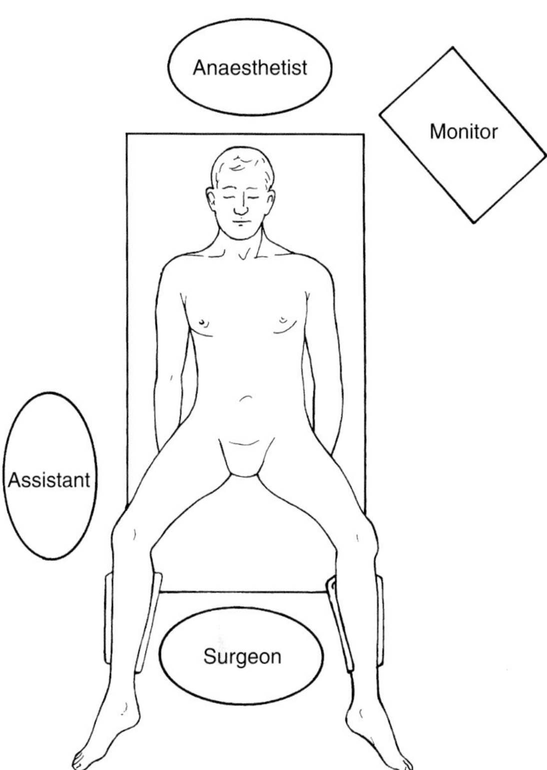

Fig. 12.1 The theatre set-up for a laparoscopic Nissen fundoplication.

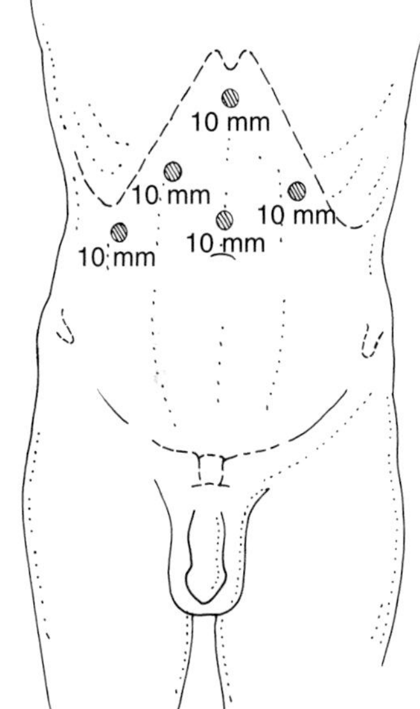

Fig. 12.2 The positions for the placement of ports for a laparoscopic Nissen fundoplication.

the diaphragm, even in obese patients, provided the liver and stomach are correctly retracted.

3 Now completely expose the crural structure, exposing the landmarks for safe posterior dissection of the oesophagus. Use hook diathermy or scissors to skeletonize the hiatus (Fig. 12.5).

4 Take especial care to expose the most posterior aspect of the left crus in order to create the posterior window safely. When the

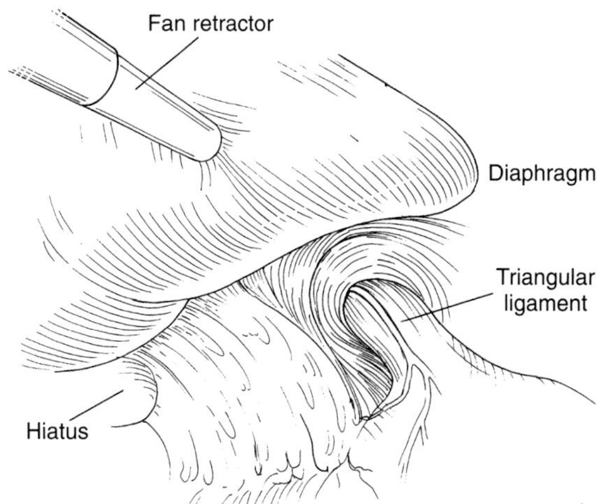

Fig. 12.3 Liver retracted by a laparoscopic fan retractor inserted into a right-sided port to enable the left lobe of the liver to be lifted from the field of view to reveal vital anatomical landmarks.

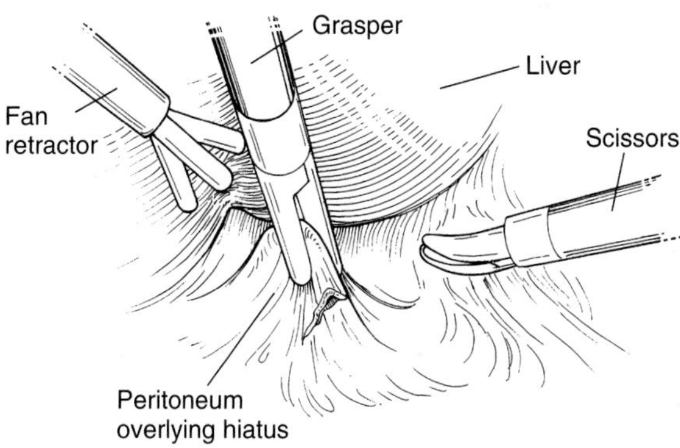

Fig. 12.4 Division of the gastrohepatic ligament.

crural muscular fibres are fully exposed, blunt dissection of the oesophagus can be safely accomplished from the lateral and anterior aspects.

5 If a hiatal hernial sac is present, deliver it during the exposure of the muscle fibres.

KEY POINT Avoid damaging the oesophagus

- Never grasp the oesophagus for retraction throughout the procedure.

6 Prepare to create a window posterior to the oesophagus. First ensure that the posterior left crus is completely dissected; it is 1 mm wide and has a firm consistency when you feel it with your right-handed blunt grasping forceps as they sweep inferiorly, following left lateral and anterior retraction of the oesophagus. In thinner patients the posterior crus presents as a visible ridge of tissue covered by para-oesophageal fat, provided retraction is correct. The left crus can also be identified by looking for the posterior vagus nerve as it curves over the structure.

7 You are at risk of gastric or oesophageal perforation if you dissect too inferiorly to the gastric wall, or too anteriorly to the gastro-oesophageal junction.

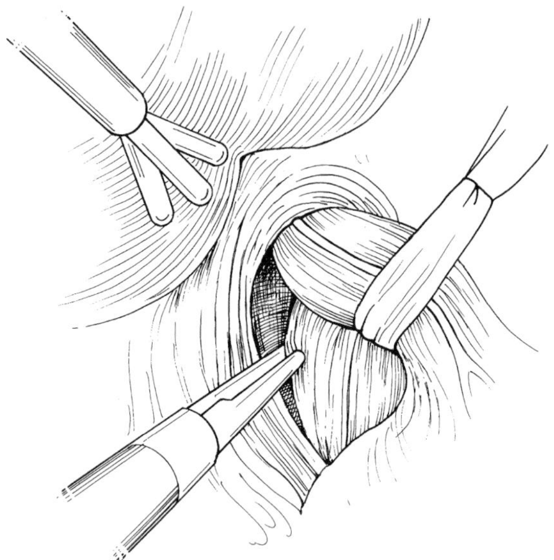

Fig. 12.5 The method of skeletonizing the hiatus to reveal the left crus.

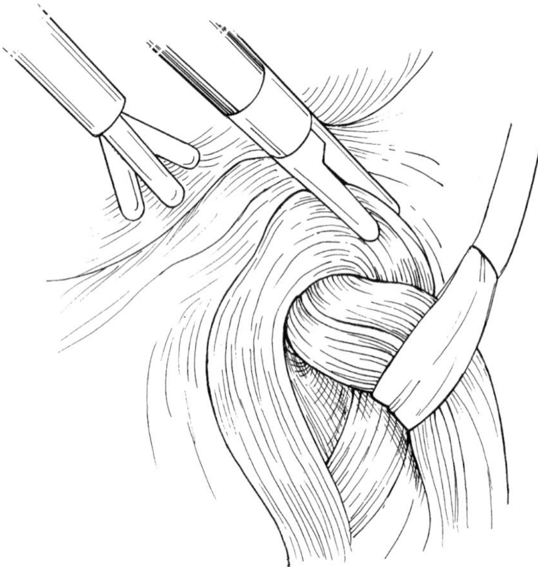

Fig. 12.6 The creation of a posterior window for the fundal wrap.

8 Sweep the posterior vagus nerve inferiorly, using gentle blunt dissection. The window can then be created by exposing the muscle fibres of the posterior left crus (Fig. 12.6). Position it safely 2 mm below the lower edge of the exposed oesophagus, at the level of the left crus, and within 1 mm of the inferior edge of the posterior crus.

9 Now create a window posterior to the oesophagus. Make this just below the left crus and above the posterior gastric fundus. Use the two 5-mm closed grasping forceps to produce a small opening. Avoid injuring the diaphragm. Continue until you have created a fine peritoneal tissue plane. When you have broken through the membranes, you see the spleen or gastric fundus. We now place a Penrose drain tube around the distal oesophagus as a retractor.

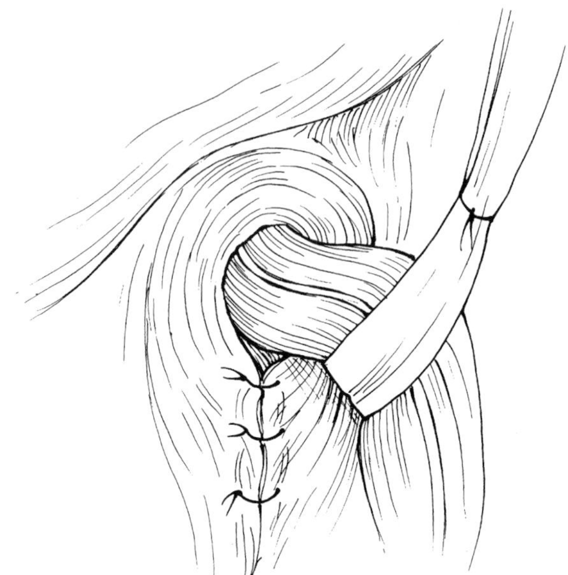

Fig. 12.7 Securing the reduced stomach in the abdomen by closing the hiatus of the diaphragm with sutures.

? DIFFICULTY

1. Peri-oesophageal scarring, secondary to penetrating ulcers, and stricture formation are usually, but not always, predictable.
2. If you have difficulty identifying the posterior aspect of the oesophagus, have a 40F bougie passed intermittently.
3. Do not dissect blindly. If you cannot confidently identify the posterior left crus and the posterior vagal branch, convert to open laparotomy.

10 In order to secure the wrap in the abdomen, you must close the hiatus by suturing the crura together. We use a 2/0 coated, braided polyester (Surgidac) on a curved needle. Take care to avoid injuring the posterior wall of the oesophagus when you place sutures in the left crus (Fig. 12.7).

? DIFFICULTY

1. Although posterior closure of the crura is easily accomplished in the case of small hernias, it may be difficult in a patient with a large para-oesophageal hiatal hernia. If necessary, carry out anterior repair with mesh reinforcement.
2. Fundoplication can be carried out to prevent reflux after widely mobilizing the oesophagus.

11 The right crus is thinner than the left so include its lateral peritoneal covering to prevent the stitch from tearing out. Two deeply placed stitches are usually sufficient, tied intracorporeally. After placing them, have a 60F dilator passed into the stomach to prevent you tying the sutures too tightly.

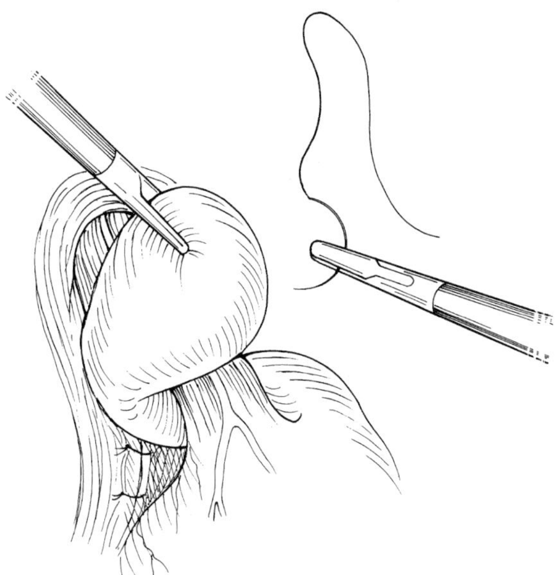

Fig. 12.8 The mobilized fundus is pulled through the posterior oesophageal window and sutured.

12 Greater curvature mobilization is currently a matter of debate. In some circumstances it allows the consistent formation of a loose wrap. Intend to divide the gastrosplenic ligament for 10 cm from the angle of His. Have the first assistant use an atraumatic, finely serrated 5-mm grasping forceps, in order to avoid tearing fatty tissue or the short gastric vessels. You hold the stomach so that the ligament is horizontal and under tension. Divide small amounts of tissue at a time, using harmonic scalpel scissors (Ethicon Endosurgery). Apply two clips on each side of vessels to be divided, but without skeletonizing the vessels, using an automatic clip applicator.

13 You are now ready to perform the fundoplication. Remove the liver retractor from the right subcostal port and replace it with a Babcock clamp. Elevate the oesophagus and, under direct vision, insert the Babcock clamp through the window until you can see it on the left side of the oesophagus. Grasp the greater curve of the stomach approximately 5–7 cm from the angle of His and draw it to the right behind the oesophagus but anterior to the posterior vagus nerve (Fig. 12.8).

14 The nerve helps to hold the wrap in place. Avoid a spiral wrap, which can include the body of the stomach in the left limb of the wrap. Carefully choose the appropriate position for the left limb suture. Try to have the limbs in continuity so that traction on one limb moves the other.

15 Place a full-thickness suture through the stomach but include only the muscular wall of the oesophagus to avoid the risk of postoperative oesophageal leakage. Incorporation of the oesophageal suture is important because it helps to secure the wrap. Prefer intracorporeal knot-tying since it makes it possible to maintain tension as the suture is tied over the 60F bougie.

? DIFFICULTY

1. Avoid the risk of perforation by refraining from applying excessive traction on the anterior stomach. If it does occur, repair it by inserting laparoscopic sutures, provided the extent of injury is clearly visible. If not, convert to open laparotomy.
2. Delayed greater curve perforation at the angle of His may follow excessive use of diathermy. Evade the possibility by using the most up-to-date ultrasonic dissector available for dissection in this area.
3. Posterior oesophageal perforation is a vexing problem. To avoid the danger of missing it following a difficult posterior dissection, test for it by having the oesophagus inflated after you have introduced sterile water to cover the area, so you can watch for bubbles. Attempt laparoscopic closure only if you are very experienced; otherwise, convert to open laparotomy.

Closure (Fig. 12.9)

Remove ports under direct vision. Do not pass a nasogastric tube unless you suspect injury to the stomach or oesophagus.

Postoperative

1 Order a postoperative Gastrografin swallow. X-ray selectively if you encountered any difficulties, but not routinely.

2 Encourage the patient to drink fluids after 6 hours. A sloppy diet can be taken within 24 hours.

3 Most patients can be discharged home within 48 hours with instructions to maintain the sloppy diet for the first 4 weeks.

4 Have the port-site sutures removed 1 week after the operation.

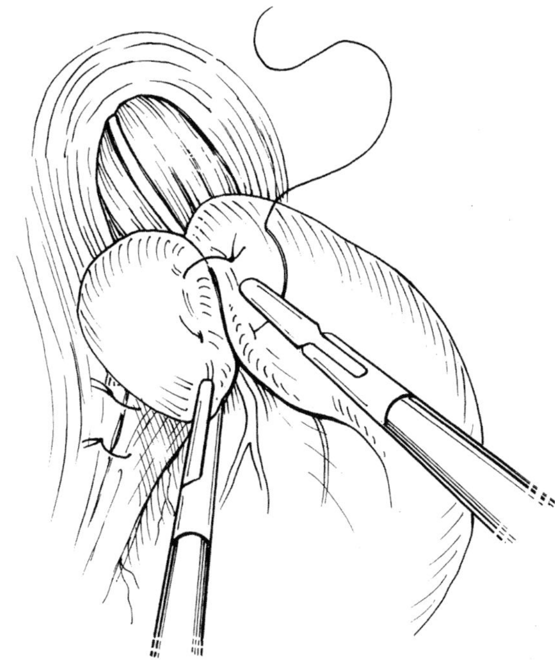

Fig. 12.9 The completed laparoscopic Nissen fundoplication.

FURTHER READING

Anavari M, Allen C, Borm A 1995 Laparoscopic Nissen fundoplication is a satisfactory alternative to long term omeprazole therapy. British Journal of Surgery 82:938–942

Cadiere GB 1994 La chirurgie anti-reflux: indication, principe et apport de la coelioscopie. Revue Medicale de Bruxelles 15:25–30

Cuschieri A, Hunter J, Wolfe B et al 1993 Multicenter prospective evaluation of laparoscopic antireflux surgery: preliminary report. Surgical Endoscopy 7:505–510

Dallemagne B, Weerts JM, Jehaes C et al 1991 Laparoscopic Nissen fundoplication: preliminary report. Surgical Laparoscopy and Endoscopy 1:138–143

EAES 1994 EAES guidelines: training and assessment of competence. Surgical Endoscopy 8:721–722

Huang SM, Wu CW, Hong HT et al 1993 Bile duct injury and bile leakage in laparoscopic cholecystectomy. British Journal of Surgery 80:1590–1592

Jamieson GG, Watson DI, Britten-Jones R et al 1994 Laparoscopic Nissen fundoplication. Annals of Surgery 220:137–145

Peters JH, Ellison C, Innes JT et al 1991 Safety and efficacy of laparoscopic cholecystectomy. Annals of Surgery 213:3–12

Pitcher DE, Curet MD, Martin DT et al 1994 Successful management of gastroesophageal reflux disease with laparoscopic fundoplication. American Journal of Surgery 168:547–554

Reid DB, Winning T, Bell G 1993 Pneumothorax during laparoscopic dissection of the diaphragmatic hiatus (letter). British Journal of Surgery 80:670

Schlumpf R, Klotz HP, Wehrli H, Herzog U 1994 A nation's experience in laparoscopic cholecystectomy: prospective multicentre analysis of 3722 cases. Surgical Endoscopy 8:35–41

Schnieder J, Koehler RH, Brams DM et al 1995 A standardised approach to teaching the laparoscopic Nissen fundoplication. Surgical Endoscopy 9:240 (abstract)

Swanstrom L, Wayne R 1994 Spectrum of gastrointestinal symptoms after laparoscopic fundoplication. American Journal of Surgery 167:538–541

Watson DI, Jamieson GG, Devitt PG et al 1995 Para-oesophageal hiatus hernia: an important complication of laparoscopic Nissen fundoplication. British Journal of Surgery 82:521–523

Watson DI, Jamieson GG, Mitchell PC et al 1995 Stenosis of the esophageal hiatus following laparoscopic fundoplication. Archives of Surgery 130:1014–1016

Weerts JM, Dallemagne B, Hamoir E et al 1993 Laparoscopic fundoplication: detailed analysis of 132 patients. Surgical Laparoscopy and Endoscopy 3:359–364

Zucker KA, Bailey RW, Gadacz TR et al 1991 Laparoscopic guided cholecystectomy. American Journal of Surgery 161:36–44

13

Stomach and duodenum

M.C. Winslet

CONTENTS

ENDOSCOPY

Appraise

1 Diagnostic endoscopy using flexible fibreoptic endoscopes has become so easy that even inexperienced clinicians can safely pass the instrument and interpret most abnormalities. Certainly all gastrointestinal operators should be familiar with the use of the endoscope.

2 Endoscopy does not compete with radiology but is complementary to it. Consider endoscopy whenever there is any possibility of a lesion lying within its scope. It often provides authoritative diagnosis because of the facility to remove guided biopsy specimens or cytological brushings.

3 It is no longer ethical practice to operate on a patient for suspected oesophagogastroduodenal disease without carrying out endoscopy when this is available, even when the diagnosis seems certain. Occasionally, diagnoses made by radiology and other means prove to be fallacious, or other, unsuspected, lesions are discovered in addition to or instead of the expected one. Conversely, many patients are spared operations because an expected condition is excluded.

4 Endoscopy is mandatory before operations for gastrointestinal bleeding. Even when the exact site of bleeding is not seen, it is often possible to exclude suspected lesions.

5 Following previous gastric surgery, radiology may be difficult to interpret and endoscopy allows the mucosa to be studied visually and by histology of biopsy specimens.

6 During an operation when an unexpected diagnostic difficulty is encountered, an endoscope can be passed down to allow examination of the interior of the upper gastrointestinal tract by the surgeon or a colleague.

7 When strictures are encountered they may be dilated using bougies or balloons. Malignant strictures may be enlarged using the Nd-YAG laser, before passing the endoscope through them to view the viscus beyond. The endoscope tip can be reversed to view the stricture from below to ensure that no damage has been sustained. If necessary, a splinting tube may be impacted in the stricture to prevent it from recurring.

8 Polyps may be snared and the base can be coagulated with diathermy current. With some double-channelled instruments, the polyp can be steadied with forceps while the snare is accurately placed.

9 With specially designed instruments it is possible to cannulate the ampulla of Vater for biliary and pancreatic duct radiology after injecting radio-opaque medium, or aspirate fluid for cytology. A diathermy wire can be used to perform sphincterotomy at the ampulla. Stones can be removed using a modified Dormia basket or a Fogarty-type balloon. They can be fragmented with shock waves. A stricture of the bile duct can be dilated using bougies or angioplasty-type balloons. It can then be cannulated with an indwelling drainage tube leading through the obstruction into the duodenum.

10 Percutaneous endoscopic gastrostomy has replaced operative gastrostomy for most purposes.

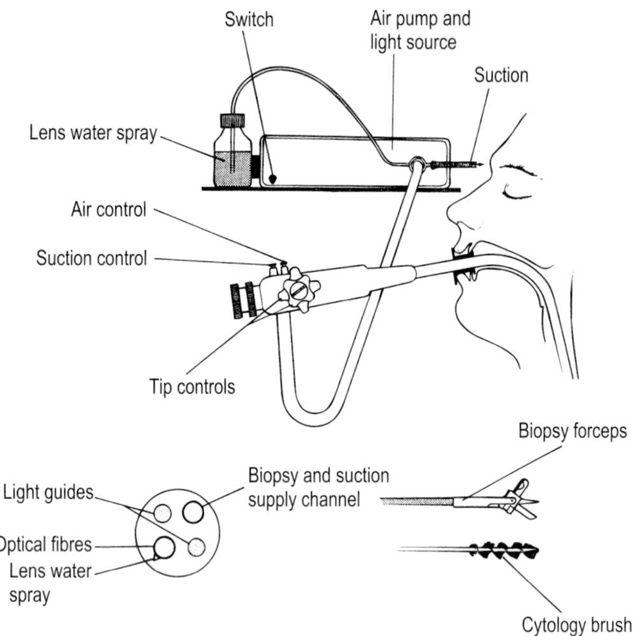

Fig. 13.1 Flexible fibreoptic endoscopy.

Prepare

1 The easiest endoscope to pass is a slim end-viewing instrument originally designed for paediatric use, but other types offer wider suction and biopsy channels through which larger forceps can be passed for biopsy, grasping foreign bodies, or snaring polyps. The very flexible ends of end-viewing endoscopes make them very versatile, but side-viewing instruments are of value in special circumstances, notably when cannulating the ampulla of Vater (Fig. 13.1).

2 Make sure that the instrument, light source, suction apparatus, biopsy forceps and air insufflation pump all work satisfactorily and that the instrument has been sterilized according to the manufacturer's recommendations. Sterilization of instruments during an endoscopy list demands careful organization to guard against transmission of microorganisms such as *Salmonella* spp, *Pseudomonas aeruginosa* and *Mycobacterium* as well as hepatitis B virus (HBV) and human immunodeficiency virus (HIV). Thorough cleaning is followed by immersion in 2% alkaline activated glutaraldehyde or 10% succine dialdehyde for a minimum of 4 minutes. Since these substances are toxic, irritant and may cause allergic reactions, the endoscopes must be thoroughly washed afterwards.

3 Obtain written, informed consent from the patient, highlighting the indications for the procedure and the potential complications.

4 The patient takes no food or fluids for 6 hours. In an emergency, attempt endoscopy even if the patient has had a recent meal, but there is a higher risk of aspiration. It is prudent to have an anaesthetist in attendance.

5 Apply protective gloves and spectacles before starting the procedure.

6 Ensure that the patient has no dentures. Anaesthetize the pharynx with an aerosol spray of 4% lidocaine. For simple diagnostic endoscopy, adequate sedation can usually be obtained by giving diazepam (Valium) 10 mg or midazolam (Hypnovel) 2.5 mg through an indwelling cannula over a period of 1–2 minutes just before passing the instrument. Give further increments of sedative if necessary and, if the procedure becomes painful, give small doses of pethidine. Monitor all patients using a pulse oximeter and administer oxygen if necessary. Elderly or infirm patients given analgesics and sedatives are at risk of hypoxia, especially during prolonged procedures. If peristaltic activity is excessive, give hyoscine butylbromide (Buscopan) 20–40 mg through the indwelling cannula.

7 Insert a plastic mouthpiece between the patient's teeth or gums through which the instrument will slide easily. Smear the endoscope shaft with water-soluble lubricant. Secretion and mucus are less likely to adhere to the lens if it is smeared with silicone liquid and lightly polished to leave a thin film.

8 The patient may be laid on the left side, with no pillow but with the head steadied by an assistant who maintains neck flexion, discouraging the patient from extending his neck which tends to make the instrument pass into the larynx. The patient's pronated left hand lies on the right chest, the right hand grasps the edge of the bed. Both knees and hips are flexed. Alternatively, the patient may lie supine but with the head of the bed raised.

9 Before passing the instrument, carefully inspect any barium meal radiographs to assess potential difficulties and pinpoint areas requiring special attention.

Access

1 Slightly flex the tip of the instrument. Pass it through the mouthpiece, over the tongue, keeping the flexed tip strictly in the midline pointing towards the cricopharyngeal sphincter. As the tip reaches the sphincter there is a hold-up. Ask the patient to swallow. The tip will be slightly extruded, and do not resist this, but suddenly the obstruction disappears as the sphincter relaxes and the instrument can be smoothly passed into the stomach after unflexing the tip.

KEY POINTS Be cautious

- Do not use force.
- Never advance the endoscope blindly.

2 Look down the instrument and concentrate on safely passing the instrument through the oesophagus and stomach and into the duodenum, noting incidentally if there is any abnormality. Insufflate the minimum of air to open up the passage. Hold the eyepiece with the left hand, adjusting the tip controls with the left thumb. Hold the shaft of the endoscope with the right hand close to the patient's mouth, advancing, withdrawing and rotating it as necessary. When the gastric angulus is passed, flex the tip to identify the pylorus. Advance the tip, keeping the pylorus in the centre of the field until the tip slips through.

3 The side-viewing endoscope has a rounded tip which makes it easier to negotiate the pharynx. If there is any doubt about the free passage, always examine the patient first with an end-viewing endoscope. Become familiar with the tip control and

angle of view before passing it. When it has passed into the stomach, rotate it to bring into view the relatively smooth, straight lesser curve which ends at the arch of the angulus, below which can be seen the pylorus in the distance. Angle the instrument up towards the roof of the antrum while advancing the instrument. The view of the pylorus is lost momentarily as the tip slips through into the duodenum. Paradoxically, if the shaft is slightly withdrawn, the instrument is straightened and the tip advances further into the duodenum. Rotate the shaft to bring the medial duodenal wall into view and, as the instrument enters the second part of the duodenum, the ampulla of Vater is usually seen as a nipple, often with a hooded mucosal fold above it.

Assess

1 Withdraw the end-viewing instrument in a spiral fashion to bring into view the whole circumference of the duodenum and stomach. Withdraw the side-viewing endoscope whilst rotating it 180° either side to view the whole circumference. Do not overinflate the stomach and duodenum with air. In the duodenum and distal stomach, keep the endoscope still and watch the peristaltic waves form and pass distally, to estimate the suppleness of the walls and exclude rigidity from infiltration or disease. With the tip of the end-viewing instrument lying in the body of the stomach, flex it fully while gently advancing the shaft to bring the fundus and cardia into view. Flex the side-viewing instrument to produce the same view. From just above the cardia the end-viewing instrument displays the pinchcock action of the diaphragmatic crura at each inspiration. If gastric mucosa is seen above this, there is a sliding hiatal hernia. The gastric mucosa is pink and shiny; at the crenated transition to the thinner and more opaque oesophageal squamous mucosa, the colour becomes paler and sometimes slightly bluish. Islands of pink gastric mucosa may be seen above the line of transition.

2 If the view disappears, withdraw the instrument and insufflate a little air. If the lens is obscured, clean it with the water jet or wipe it against the mucosa to free it of adherent mucus.

3 Look out for inflammation in duodenitis, gastritis and oesophagitis. As a rule, the mucosa appears florid and reddened, but endoscopy is uncertain and biopsy specimens should be removed when in doubt. In atrophic gastritis the distal mucosa is thinned and translucent so that submucosal vessels are visible through it. In gastric atrophy, associated with pernicious anaemia, the fundic mucosa is particularly affected, being flat and featureless. Menetrier's hypertrophic gastritis results in strikingly florid mucosal folds, as may the fundic mucosa in the Zollinger–Ellison syndrome. Primary gastric lymphoma, or secondary involvement of the stomach with systemic lymphoma, has no specific diagnostic features. The mucosa may be hypertrophic and ulcerated, with multiple foci.

4 Peptic ulcers usually display a basal slough, but adherent mucosa may simulate a crater. Healed ulcers typically appear flat and white, with radiating mucosal folds. Diverticula, seen usually high on the gastric lesser curve, have healthy mucosa entering the mouth of the diverticulum. Mallory–Weiss tears show a ragged, often bleeding edge in the mucosa at the cardia.

KEY POINT Cellular diagnosis

- Never fail to remove cytology brushings and biopsy specimens for examination.

5 Tumours are typically elevated and malignant ulcers have raised, everted edges. Gastric polyps may be single or multiple, and can be mucosal or submucosal, such as leiomyomas and leiomyosarcomas, which frequently have healthy mucosa overlying them. Lymphomas—sometimes with mucosal hypertrophy, sharply differentiated from normal mucosa—may reveal no histological abnormality on biopsy, since they tend to spread in the submucosa. They may produce multiple shallow ulcers, or ulcers with raised edges. By the time tumours become obvious they are usually well advanced and the best time to recognize them is in the early pre-invasive stage. Any slight irregularity of the mucosa is suspicious, whether it is a localized depression, plateau, cobblestone irregularity or ulcer, especially if this is an unusual site for a peptic ulcer. In cases of reflux, peptic ulcer disease or dyspepsia remove a sample to be tested for *Helicobacter* (Clotest).

6 Oesophageal varices, seen in portal venous hypertension, appear as tortuous, sometimes bluish, projections into the lumen of the lower oesophagus and may continue into the gastric fundus or are occasionally visible only in the upper stomach. Do not assume in patients who have gastrointestinal bleeding that visible varices are necessarily the site of bleeding.

7 Pyloric stenosis may prevent the passage of the instrument into the duodenum and it is sometimes impossible to assess whether the obstruction is from benign duodenal ulceration, a mucosal diaphragm in the distal stomach or neoplastic infiltration.

8 Previous gastric surgery distorts the anatomy, and preliminary radiological examination is helpful. A stoma or pyloroplasty allows bile to reflux into the stomach. The mucosa around a stoma is often florid. Stomal ulcers usually develop just distal to the anastomosis and the instrument can be passed through it to view them. Recurrent gastric and duodenal ulcers are usually easy to see but remember that carcinoma appears to occur more frequently following previous gastric surgery for peptic ulceration.

9 Bleeding from the upper gastrointestinal tract can often be localized at endoscopy. If possible use an instrument with a wide-bore channel through which efficient suction can be applied. If necessary rotate the patient to bring the site of bleeding uppermost, so that it is not hidden at the bottom of a pool of blood and other gastroduodenal contents. If the source of bleeding cannot be found, remember that the examination can be repeated. If an operation is to be performed, this can be carried out just prior to surgery.

10 Always ensure that endoscopy can be repeated during an operation for upper gastrointestinal bleeding. It is sometimes invaluable in locating the bleeding site while avoiding extensive gastrotomy or gastroduodenotomy.

Action

1 Remove biopsy specimens under vision from any suspicious sites, including tumours, the edges of ulcers, irregularities of the

mucosa and suspected inflammation. Take specimens from different places, preferably from each quadrant of an ulcer. If lymphoma is a possibility, take multiple deep biopsies, since the disease often spreads in the submucosa. Place the specimens in carefully labelled separate pots containing formol saline fixative for histological examination.

2 Cytological diagnosis is extremely helpful. Pass the brush through the biopsy channel and rotate it against the suspicious area. Agitate the brush in a separate jar of fixative; this will be subsequently centrifuged and the cells stained and examined.

3 Polypoid lesions can be caught in a snare for removal and histological examination. If the polyp has a broad base ensure that this is completely caught and, if bleeding is likely, coagulate the base with the diathermy before it is removed.

4 Foreign bodies can be grasped with forceps, snared or caught in a modified Dormia basket for withdrawal. An external tube may be slid over and pushed beyond the endoscope tip to enclose a sharp foreign body as it is withdrawn to protect the mucosa from damage.

5 Bleeding oesophageal varices can be injected under direct vision, using sclerosant solution injected through a long needle passed down the biopsy channel (see Ch. 22). Bleeding ulcers may be coagulated by spraying on thrombogenic substances or using the diathermy point. Argon gas laser or a solid state Nd-YAG laser may be used to coagulate the bleeding vessel by energy release at the point of contact. Since laser light is absorbed by blood clot this must first be gently washed away with a fine water jet. The depth of laser light penetration is crucial: too superficial and the effect is lost, too deep and the resulting necrosis penetrates the wall. For this reason, laser light coagulation must be performed by a skilled, experienced operator.

6 *Endoscopic retrograde cholangiopancreatography* (ERCP). A cannula can be passed through a special side-viewing endoscope for insertion in the bile and pancreatic ducts to obtain radiographic pictures following the injection of radio-opaque medium. The ampulla and lower bile duct can be slit with a diathermy wire, and stones can be removed with a modified Dormia basket. A stricture can be dilated from below followed by the insertion of a prosthetic indwelling plastic tube to maintain a passage. These techniques require special training and equipment.

7 Oesophageal dilatation can be carried out with bougies, balloons or by Nd-YAG laser destruction of tissue. The lumen may be held open by inserting a stent (see Ch. 10).

Postoperative

1 Lay a heavily sedated patient on the left side, slightly face-down, under the care of a trained nurse who will watch him until he recovers fully. If he has any respiratory obstruction this must be overcome; chest physiotherapy will help him to cough up his retained secretions. Do not allow any fluids or foods to be given until the patient is fully recovered and until the effect of pharyngeal anaesthesia has worn off, usually 4 hours.

2 Carefully clean and check the instrument.

PERIOPERATIVE CARE

Preoperative

1 Patients are admitted the day before operation for clinical assessment and routine check of blood count, blood urea, serum electrolytes and chest X-ray for those who have pre-existing disease, those who smoke or those over 40 years of age. If there is suspicion of cardiac disease, order an electrocardiogram (ECG).

2 Explain the intended operation to the patient and obtain informed, signed consent. Detail the risks as well as the benefits.

3 Institute prophylaxis against deep venous thrombosis according to agreed protocol dependent on procedure risk classification.

4 The patient receives no food for 6 hours and water only for 2 hours before operation. If there is evidence of gastric retention, then the stomach should be emptied the day before operation by passing a nasogastric tube for aspiration. Such patients should have an intravenous infusion set up to ensure that they are not dehydrated or electrolytically depleted.

5 Patients with gross pyloric stenosis are best admitted a few days before operation, both to ensure that the stomach is empty and because they are starving. Pass a large-bore gastric tube and siphon off the gastric contents. Run in 300 ml of water at a time through a funnel and siphon it off repeatedly until the efflux is clear. Repeat this daily or twice daily as necessary. Set up an intravenous infusion to replace the loss of electrolytes, correct the disturbed acid–base balance and provide nutritional support since the patient will not be able to absorb oral foods immediately after operation. Do not forget to give vitamin C and other vitamins.

6 Have the patient routinely catheterized with strict aseptic precautions.

7 Ask the anaesthetist to pass a nasogastric tube as soon as anaesthesia is induced.

8 For straightforward elective operations, some surgeons would not give prophylactic antibiotics, but for emergency surgery such as perforated or bleeding ulcer, carcinoma, or pyloric stenosis, give a bacteriocidal antibiotic such as a first- or second-generation cephalosporin before the operation starts and continue it if there is contamination.

Action

1 Although the contents of the healthy stomach are virtually sterile, this is not so in the presence of disease and especially if there is any gastric stasis, as in pyloric stenosis, carcinoma of the stomach and re-operative gastric surgery.

2 Adopt a routine of performing as much dissection as possible before opening the stomach, then isolate the area using added towels of distinctive colour. Keep within the isolated area during the part of the operation that requires the gut to be opened and use a limited number of instruments that are kept separate. Sometimes, in spite of careful preoperative preparation and aspiration of the indwelling nasogastric tube, the stomach is distended with content. In this case, after isolating the area, make

an incision into it that will just allow the sucker tube to be inserted and empty it before proceeding; otherwise, the area is likely to be flooded with foul, retained gastric content. Following this, apply non-crushing clamps to occlude the lumen to prevent further efflux. When the stomach or bowel is closed, discard the special towels and the instruments and change into fresh, sterile gloves to continue the operation.

3 The stomach is well supplied with blood and tolerates extensive mobilization without risk to its blood supply. However, this rich blood supply can lead to bleeding from the suture line so a haemostatic over-and-over stitch is preferable to a Connell type of stitch, unless the blood vessels are first picked up individually and tied or coagulated.

4 The duodenum is fragile and does not tolerate tension or vigorous mobilization. However, the Kocher manoeuvre often renders it mobile and prevents tension (see Fig. 13.3). Rather than anastomose it under tension, be prepared to close it and perform gastroenterostomy if this is possible.

Aftercare

1 Have the patient's condition monitored carefully until he recovers from the anaesthetic. In particular, note his colour, respiration, pulse rate and blood pressure. The blood pressure is taken every 15 minutes for the first 3 hours and then half-hourly until it is stable. Have the wound checked regularly to ensure that there is no bleeding.

2 See that the urinary output is checked hourly. Following major operations, an indwelling catheter is necessary so that urinary output can be monitored. It can be removed as soon as the patient has recovered and is active.

3 Order nasogastric tube aspiration to be recorded every hour. It may be gently aspirated every 4 hours if there is a high output. If gastric aspirate is recorded as nil, suspect that the tube is either in the wrong place or blocked. Remove the tube when the amount aspirated is less then the oral intake and the aspirate is clear, provided the patient is comfortable, with a soft abdomen, passing flatus per anum and has bowel sounds. Try to remove the nasogastric tube early in patients with respiratory problems, if necessary restricting oral fluid intake. It is very difficult to cough with a tube irritating the pharynx.

4 Order intravenous fluids remembering that sodium retention is frequent following operations and that, provided the patient started in fluid and electrolyte balance, only lost electrolytes need be replaced. Provided also that renal function is good, then, if sufficient fluid is given, small imbalances will be compensated. For the 1 or 2 days that are required before adequate oral intake is achieved, a previously fit patient need be given only glucose for his metabolic needs. Establish at once an intravenous feeding regime on a previously undernourished patient or one who has required an oesophageal anastomosis and will not be able to take adequate oral feeding for several days. Since enteral feeding is safer and cheaper than parenteral feeding, consider placing a feeding jejunostomy tube or inserting a fine nasoenteric feeding tube at the time of operation in such patients.

5 On the morning after operation, allow 30 ml of water each hour, increasing to 60 ml the second day and 90 ml the third day, when normal intake can be resumed and intravenous fluid replacement stopped. Following many operations, especially when the stomach and duodenum have not been opened, this regime may be speeded up so that the morning after operation the nasogastric tube can be removed and oral fluid intake allowed in increasing amounts depending on the patient's tolerance and general condition. Withhold oral fluids following gastric operations with oesophageal anastomosis but allow the patient to have mouthwashes. It is not possible to prevent a little fluid and saliva from being swallowed, but as a rule wait for 4–5 days after operation, then check the intactness and adequacy of the anastomosis radiologically using water-soluble medium such as Gastrografin before commencing oral fluids and proceeding gradually to full diet.

6 Modern attitudes to activity following abdominal surgery are more liberal than previously. Allow the patient to sit out of bed the morning following operation and have him walking a little during the next day or two, depending upon his general condition. The help of a cheerful physiotherapist in encouraging the patient to breathe deeply, cough up retained sputum and move freely is of enormous value in preventing the patient from remaining static in bed. The use of epidural anaesthesia greatly facilitates such early mobilization.

ACCESS IN THE UPPER ABDOMEN

Do not attempt difficult manoeuvres in the upper abdomen unless there is an adequate view. As a rule, routine exposures are satisfactory, but in occasional patients the view is severely restricted.

GASTRIC CARDIA

1 Tilt the whole patient slightly head-up.

2 Use an upper right or left paramedian or midline incision, opening the peritoneum to one or other side of the falciform ligament. Start the incision at or alongside the xiphoid process and carry it vertically down for 20 cm, skirting the umbilicus. Alternatively, for better cosmesis, use a paramedian skin incision but open the abdominal wall in the midline.

3 Transverse and oblique incisions do not provide adequate access except in those with a wide costal margin, but they may be combined with vertical incisions to form a flap. An inverted 'V' incision offers good access since the apex of the 'V' can be folded down and sutured to the lower abdominal wall.

4 Carefully place retractors and ensure that the operating theatre light is correctly focused and aimed. To gain access under the diaphragm, use a retractor that elevates the lower sternum and costal margin. Such retractors are attached to a frame fixed to the operating table.

5 Mobilize the left lobe of the liver if this interferes with the view. Insert the fully pronated left hand with the index and middle fingers passing on each side of the left triangular ligament to draw down the lobe. Cut the ligament from its free edge towards the right with long-handled scissors, avoiding damage to the subphrenic vessels and left hepatic veins. Fold the lobe to the right, cover it with a gauze pack and have it held out of the way with a large curved retractor. Remember to replace it carefully at the end of the operation.

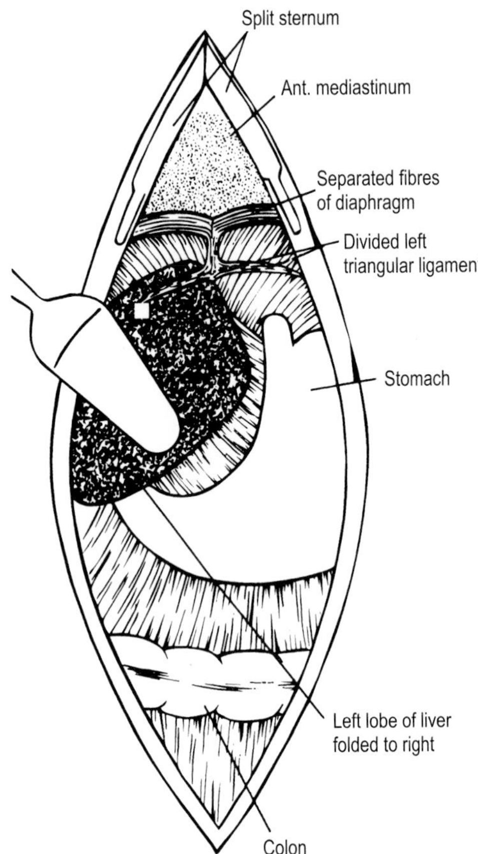

Fig. 13.2 Access in the upper abdomen.

6 Carry the whole depth of the incision right up to the xiphisternum or into the angle between it and the costal margin. Do not hesitate to excise the xiphisternum using bone-cutting forceps, after dissecting off the two diaphragmatic muscle slips from its under-surface (Fig. 13.2).

7 If access is still inadequate, particularly for oesophageal anastomosis, consider performing thoracotomy.

KOCHER'S DUODENAL MOBILIZATION

Appraise

1 This manoeuvre (Fig. 13.3) raises the head of the pancreas contained within the duodenal loop into its embryological midline position, restrained by the structures in the free edge of the lesser omentum above, the superior mesenteric vessels below, and the body and tail of the pancreas to the left.

2 The head and neck of the pancreas can be examined from behind and palpated between fingers and thumb. The lower end of the common bile duct can be palpated and sometimes seen, although it is usually buried within the pancreatic head. The duodenum and especially the ampullary region can be palpated. Duodenotomy allows inspection of the interior of the duodenum. If the incision is placed at the level of the ampulla this can be seen and palpated for tumours or stones. Biopsy, excision of ampullary neoplasms, sphincterotomy, sphincteroplasty, and cannulation or instrumentation of the bile and pancreatic ducts can be carried out under vision.

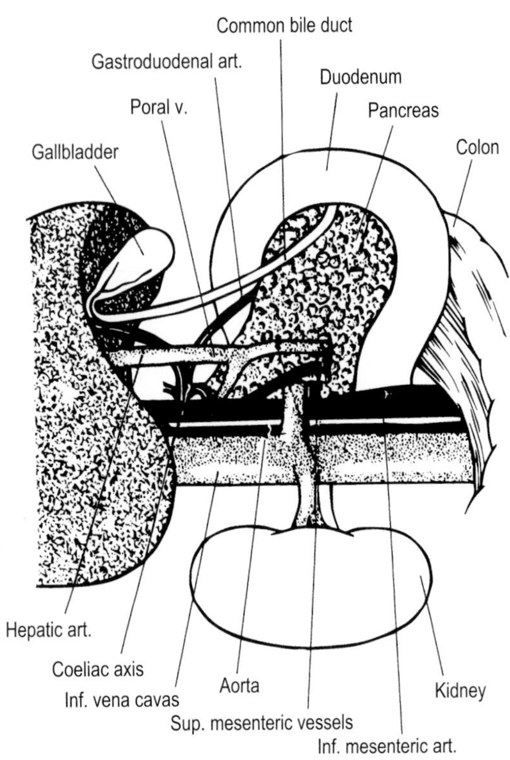

Fig. 13.3 Kocher's duodenal mobilization, as seen from the right side of the patient.

3 Mobilization is essential for excision of the pancreatic head and duodenal loop in Whipple's pancreatoduodenectomy.

4 Elevation of the duodenal loop and pancreatic head reveals the inferior vena cava when performing portocaval anastomosis or major hepatic resections.

5 The manoeuvre is particularly valuable in gastroduodenal operations. Pyloroplasty can be performed easily and the extremities of the gastroduodenal incision can be brought together without tension. In gastrectomy, the proximal duodenum is easily dissected and can be closed or united to the stomach with ease. Full mobilization is an essential step when the stomach is drawn up for gastro-oesophageal or gastropharyngeal anastomosis.

Action

1 If incomplete mobilization is sufficient, as for palpating the lower end of the bile duct or the pancreatic head or for the purpose of carrying out pyloroplasty and gastrectomy by the Polya method, then it may be sufficient to elevate only the superior part of the duodenal loop and pancreatic head. Insinuate a finger into the aditus to the lesser sac and gently split the floor of the foramen downwards, allowing the finger to separate the upper duodenum and pancreas from the inferior vena cava. Extend the mobilization by continuing the split with scissors or diathermy blade, downwards, just outside the convexity of the duodenal loop.

2 For full mobilization, have your assistants draw the hepatic flexure of the colon downwards, the right edge of wound outwards and the duodenal loop to the left.

3 Incise the peritoneum and underlying fascia of Toldt for 5 cm, placing the incision 1 cm from and parallel to the convex border of the second part of the duodenum.

4 Insinuate your fingers beneath the descending duodenum and pancreatic head. A natural plane of cleavage opens up between the embryological layers which were present when the duodenum was freely suspended in the peritoneal cavity.

5 Having defined the plane, cut the peritoneum and fascia upwards, just outside the duodenal convexity, into the mouth of the aditus to the lesser sac, meanwhile lifting the proximal duodenum forward with a finger, so protecting the inferior vena cava from damage. The dissection is easy and can be carried out by splitting with the finger except in the presence of severe scarring as from severe duodenal ulceration.

6 Continue the peritoneal and fascial split below, taking care to avoid damaging the right colic vessels which must be pushed downwards with the hepatic flexure of the colon and mesocolon, to release the junction of the second and third parts of the duodenum.

7 Continue the separation of the pancreas and duodenum across the aorta where it is tethered below by the superior mesenteric artery and its pancreatic branches. The structures in the free edge of the lesser omentum restrain it superiorly.

8 When the appropriate procedure is completed, carefully check the pancreatic head, duodenal loop and the bed from which the structures have been mobilized, before laying them back in place.

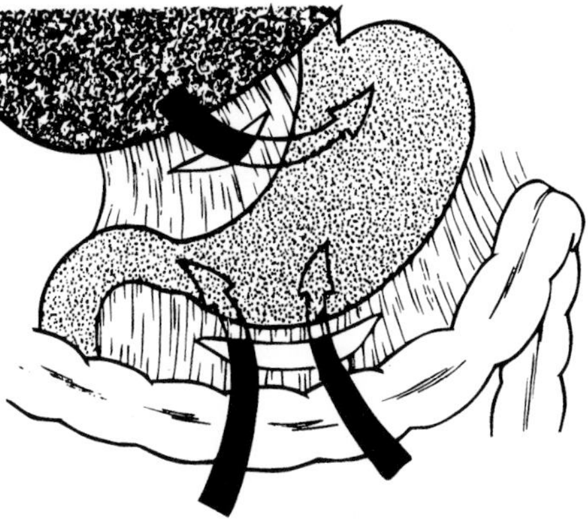

Fig. 13.4 Approaches to the posterior surfaces of the stomach and duodenal bulb, through the gastrohepatic and gastrocolic omenta.

EXAMINATION OF THE STOMACH AND DUODENUM

1 Did you make a firm diagnosis before operation? Mucosal lesions within hollow organs are best assessed from within the lumen by radiology and endoscopy, not by examination of the exterior at operation.

2 Look at the exposed stomach. Is it distended as may be seen in pyloric obstruction? Is the musculature hypertrophied as seen in longstanding partial obstruction? The serous surface may be inflamed and oedematous, or scarred and puckered with petechiae overlying an ulcer. It may be covered with miliary tubercles in tuberculous peritonitis, or metastatic deposits of tumour. The thickened rigid appearance of 'leather-bottle' stomach may be accompanied by serosal extension, giving an appearance resembling crystallized sugar adherent to the serosa.

3 Feel for the lower oesophagus and diaphragmatic crura. Sometimes there is an obvious invagination of the gastric cardia through the diaphragmatic hiatus. If the normal anatomy can be restored by applying traction to the lesser curve of the stomach, this is a sliding hiatal hernia. If the cardia cannot be drawn down, there is a fixed hiatal hernia which may be primary or may be secondary to disease in the posterior mediastinum. There may be a gap between the crura into which the fingers can be inserted but the stomach remains fixed within the abdomen. Gently grasp the gastric cardia between finger and thumb and see if it can be slid through the hiatus into the chest. Record an asymptomatic hiatal hernia discovered incidentally when carrying out another procedure but do not repair it. Palpate the fundus of the stomach. If it disappears through the hiatus into the posterior mediastinum, this is a rolling hernia which may cause obstructive symptoms. If the patient has complained of this then consider repairing it, depending upon the severity of the symptoms, the extent of herniation, the fitness of the patient and the severity of the proposed operation.

4 Examine the body and lesser curve of the stomach for evidence of ulcers and ulcer scars. Ulcers and healed scars are often palpable and visible, and former ulcers can sometimes be detected by pinching the stomach along the lesser curve. Normal mucosa can be felt to slip away from your fingers but it may be tethered at the site of a healed ulcer. The stomach can be palpated most readily by making holes through avascular parts of the lesser and gastrocolic omenta so that fingers can be passed behind to feel the two layers of gastric wall against the thumb placed anteriorly (Fig. 13.4). The scar of an undetected posterior gastric ulcer may be adherent to the pancreas, but there are normally flimsy adhesions across the lesser sac between the stomach and pancreas. If preoperative endoscopy is required, the anaesthetist or an assistant may be asked to pass the endoscope, but it is usually best to leave the operation temporarily and pass the instrument, reach a decision and re-scrub, put on a fresh sterile gown and gloves and continue the operation. If this is not possible, carry out gastrotomy, preferably in the middle of the anterior wall of the stomach at the level of the suspected ulcer or other lesion and evaginate the lesion through the gastrotomy for visual assessment, biopsy or excision. Alternatively, it can be opened along the greater curvature in order not to compromise any subsequent resection, nor to endanger the lesser curve's integrity if you decide to perform ulcer excision and highly selective vagotomy. The gastrotomy may then be closed either because no further action is necessary or prior to carrying out gastrectomy if a hitherto unsuspected chronic gastric ulcer is causing the patient's symptoms. In poor-risk patients, gastric ulcer may be treated by ulcer excision. Vagotomy is now seldom used when most patients with benign ulcers can be treated successfully with antibiotics and proton-pump inhibitors.

5 Look and feel for neoplasms. These will in nearly all cases have been diagnosed and thoroughly staged by the TNM system

before operation. Staging is by computed tomographic (CT) scanning, endoluminal ultrasound and, in selected cases, laparoscopy. Carcinoma is most frequently seen, although lymphosarcoma, reticulum-cell sarcoma, leiomyoma and leiomyosarcoma are not rare, and adenomatous polyps may be felt. Carcinoma may produce a tumour within the stomach, or be felt as an ulcer with raised margins. Remember that early gastric cancers may be impalpable.

KEY POINT Biopsy all gastric ulcers

- Regard all gastric ulcers as malignant until proved, by biopsy, to be benign.

An apparently benign ulcer may have developed malignant characteristics. Extensive submucosal infiltration produces the rigid 'leather-bottle' stomach, often with penetration of the serosa producing a crystallized sugar appearance with beaded irregular blood vessels. If carcinoma is suspected, proven or unexpectedly encountered, do not touch it but examine the prerectal pouch, the ovaries in the female, the remainder of the peritoneal cavity, the root of the mesentery and the liver to assess the degree of spread before palpating the primary tumour, so that malignant cells are not carried around on the gloves. Feel the local glands along the greater and lesser curves, and through holes in the avascular portions in the lesser and gastrocolic omenta assess the degree of posterior infiltration into the pancreas and the involvement of glands around the coeliac axis and along the superior border of the pancreas. When, in some cases, the diagnosis remains in doubt, gastrotomy should be performed with the removal of a specimen for frozen-section histology and then closed. On the basis of the report and the operative assessment, decide on the immediate action. If a distal carcinoma appears to be totally resectable, carry out radical distal gastrectomy. An apparently curable proximal carcinoma is ideally treated by radical total gastrectomy. This may be carried out through a left thoracoabdominal incision and the abdominal incision can be extended to the left after the patient has been turned onto the right side, has had the skin prepared and fresh sterile towels have been applied. Alternatively, for tumours at the cardia, an Ivor Lewis right thoracoabdominal approach gives good access and permits adequate proximal clearance of the tumour. Midgastric tumours can sometimes be adequately excised by abdominal total gastrectomy. Carry out palliative resection or exclusion gastrectomy if inoperable distal carcinoma threatens to cause obstruction or is the source of recurrent bleeding or anaemia.

Completely excise adenomas since histology may reveal malignant changes. Sometimes they are multiple and gastrectomy may be more appropriate. Benign tumours such as angioma and lipoma require merely local removal. Leiomyoma cannot be differentiated at operation, or even by frozen-section histology, from leiomyosarcoma. Excise it with a healthy margin, but only time will tell whether it is benign or malignant. Leiomyoblastoma is less frequently seen and is usually benign. Lymphoma may be primary gastric or nodal in type. Primary gastric lymphoma is associated with only regional lymphadenopathy. In nodal lymphoma there may be splenic and hepatic involvement. It may be difficult to diagnose before operation and frozen-section histology at the time of operation may be valuable in case of doubt. Even if the tumour is extensive it is worth excising as much as possible to leave the minimum tumour bulk for subsequent radiotherapy and chemotherapy and to minimize the risk of perforation.

6 Examine the pyloroduodenal region. The pyloric ring can be picked up between the index finger and thumb of both hands, but the mucosal ring may be smaller than the muscular ring. To check this, invaginate the anterior antral wall through the pylorus on an index finger and invaginate the anterior duodenal wall back into the stomach in a similar manner. If there is obstruction, look again at the stomach. Is it dilated? Is the muscular wall hypertrophied? Look and feel for duodenal ulcer, remembering that the majority of ulcers lie in the bulb, although they may be in the postbulbar region or further distally, especially in the Zollinger–Ellison syndrome. Sometimes an ulcer crater can be palpated, sometimes there is gross and incontrovertible scarring and narrowing, together with pseudodiverticulum formation but there may be minimal scarring, a few petechial haemorrhages—which could be iatrogenic—or there may be nothing abnormal to see or feel. Of course the diagnosis should have been made endoscopically before operation. Occasionally endoscopy has failed because the tip of the instrument could not negotiate the narrow or distorted pyloroduodenal canal. If doubt remains, could a small endoscope be passed by the anaesthetist and the tip negotiated through manually to allow the interior to be viewed? Alternatively, create a small prepyloric gastrotomy and examine the interior with a finger, or by placing small retractors within the pyloroduodenal canal. A mucosal diaphragm that is soft and easily stretched can be dilated, or conventionally treated by pyloroplasty.

7 Diverticula of the stomach are most frequently found on the upper lesser curve, sometimes produced by traction from a leiomyoma. If no primary lesion is present, leave an asymptomatic diverticulum alone. Pseudodiverticula of the duodenum develop when chronic duodenal ulcer causes distortion. The most frequent duodenal diverticulum is not seen unless it is sought for since it lies close to the ampulla, protruding into the pancreas which must be mobilized by Kocher's manoeuvre to approach from posteriorly. It rarely causes symptoms and should normally be left alone.

SUTURING AND STAPLING THE STOMACH AND DUODENUM

SUTURES

1 Strong, reliably absorbed synthetic materials that elicit minimal inflammatory reaction have been introduced. Finer thread can be safely used, thus introducing less foreign material. Some of the earlier synthetic materials did not have the handling properties of traditional materials but this is no longer so. There is a wide choice of sutures. As with all sutures, these recently introduced materials are severely weakened by crushing, abrasion and rough handling, especially when drawing them through the tissues and tying knots.

Braided polyglycolic acid and monofilament polyglyconate retain their tensile strength reliably for longer than catgut does.

Polydioxanone also retains its tensile strength for longer than catgut does and, because it degrades by hydrolysis, there is relatively little inflammatory response during absorption. Braided polyglactin 910 has good handling qualities with slow absorption. For use in the gastrointestinal tract 3/0 or 4/0 has adequate strength.

Some surgeons still insert an outer non-absorbable layer. As an alternative to silk or linen thread, non-absorbable 3/0 or 4/0 braided polyamide may be used, but slowly absorbing synthetics are probably better.

2 Innumerable papers have been written about the best ways of suturing stomach and intestine. Should we use interrupted or continuous, one layer or two, simple through-and-through or complex stitches, including or excluding the mucosa, inverted or edge-to-edge? It is obvious from listening to, and reading the papers of, the advocates, that all the methods are successful. There is but a single common factor and that is the care with which sutures are inserted and tied. If you bring together the edges of stomach or bowel that have a good blood supply, are not under tension and are apposed carefully with sutures that do not strangulate the included tissue, they will heal. Many of us continue to use the methods we learned whilst training, because they have demonstrably worked, even though we accept that they may no longer be in vogue. The one layer that must always be included in the stitches, as shown by Halsted, is the submucosa.

Since all the methods work provided they are employed carefully, it seems logical to employ a single-layer edge-to-edge apposition, allowing each component of the gut wall to join directly to the same component on the opposite edge. Preference for interrupted or continuous stitching is constantly argued. Interrupted stitches have the advantage that, if one cuts out, others remain, and, if they are tied too tightly, the intervening tissue that is not enclosed will survive and unite. Continuous unlocked stitches produce a spiral that does not strangulate the tissues yet allows the tension to be evenly distributed; they withstand much greater distraction of the edges than do interrupted stitches.

3 The risk of needle-stick injury with transmission of hepatitis B virus (HBV), hepatitis C virus (HCV) and human immunodeficiency virus (HIV) is ever present. Invariably hold all needles with instruments and when the points emerge they must be captured with forceps, not with fingers. Whenever possible employ blunt-pointed needles.

LIGATURES

- As with sutures, ligatures are applied using the finest possible materials, although silk and linen are still popular because of their excellent handling properties. Metal clips are reliable to clamp blood vessels but they easily catch in swabs and can be dragged off. One instrument applies two clips side by side and cuts between them, for dividing vascular tissue. Unless they offer advantages in saving time, prefer to tie ligatures, which are more versatile.
- Absorbable synthetic clips have also come into use and may become more commonly used.

STAPLES

- The development of reliable instruments for joining bowel has potentially great value in gastroduodenal surgery. However, they are not as versatile as sutures. If you are a trainee, by all means learn to use stapling instruments but more importantly take every opportunity to master the accurate placement of sutures.
- There are two overriding indications for using stapling instruments. The first is when the difficulties of suturing, perhaps because of inadequate access that cannot be improved, make stapling safer. The second is when speed is essential, perhaps during a major operation.

GASTROTOMY AND GASTRODUODENOTOMY

Appraise

1 Gastric, gastroduodenal and duodenal incision allows the interior of the bowel to be examined to confirm, biopsy or treat a suspected lesion such as an ulcer, tumour or source of bleeding.

2 Gastrotomy allows access from below to the lower oesophagus. Strictures are often dilated more safely from below than from above.

Access

1 As a rule, open the stomach on the anterior wall midway between the greater and lesser curves.

2 To recover a tube or dilate the gullet, open the proximal stomach only sufficiently to pass a finger or bougie or for the prosthetic tube to emerge.

3 For the purpose of diagnosis, start with a small incision, 3–4 cm long, the proximal end of which is 5–6 cm from the pylorus. This incision ensures that the intact pylorus or mucosal diaphragm can be examined and it may be unnecessary to destroy the pyloric muscular ring. The incision can be extended proximally or, if it becomes necessary, distally through the pyloric ring onto the anterior wall of the duodenal bulb.

4 To view the interior, first aspirate all the contents. Retractors may be placed to hold open the stomach so that it can be examined by adjusting the theatre light to shine through the opening. The stomach can be manoeuvred manually to bring different parts of the interior into view. Frequently the gastric wall can be evaginated through the incision so that it can be examined and any lesion excised or biopsied. If the pylorus is not too narrow, small retractors may be placed in to allow the duodenal bulb to be viewed, and, if it is wide, an unscarred duodenal bulbar wall may be evaginated through it on a finger. If there is difficulty in viewing the duodenum to exclude or confirm disease, a per-oral endoscope may be introduced through it. Sometimes when fibreoptic endoscopy is ineffective before operation, perhaps resulting from inability to evacuate the gastric contents, the stomach may be emptied and endoscopy can then be performed. The gastrotomy can be temporarily occluded with a clamp to allow the stomach to be inflated but as a rule the

stomach can be held open to allow endoscopy to be accomplished without the need for inflation.

Closure

1 Close a gastrotomy in one or two layers, leaving a longitudinal suture line.

2 It is conventional practice to close a gastroduodenotomy as a Heineke–Mikulicz pyloroplasty. This may be accomplished using a single edge-to-edge row of sutures, a two-layer invaginating suture or with a row of staples. However, this destroys the pyloric metering function and, if truncal vagotomy is not carried out, it may be preferable to carefully close the incision to create a longitudinal scar, bringing the edges together without invagination in a single layer, taking care to appose the pyloric edges perfectly. If highly selective vagotomy is performed, close the gastroduodenotomy longitudinally, to preserve the sphincter. Cover the suture line with a layer of omentum as an extra precaution.

3 Use ingenuity to incorporate the gastrotomy in plans for other procedures. A distal gastrotomy may be incorporated in a gastroenterostomy. The proximal part of a long gastroduodenotomy may be closed longitudinally and the distal part converted into a pyloroplasty if necessary. If gastrectomy is intended, temporarily close the gastrotomy with stitches or staples to keep soiling to a minimum.

PYLOROMYOTOMY

Appraise

1 Pyloromyotomy for infantile pyloric stenosis is described in Chapter 40.

2 Adult hypertrophic pyloric stenosis is rarely discovered as a cause of gastric retention. It is not known whether or not this represents undiagnosed infantile pyloric stenosis.

3 Following vagotomy for duodenal ulcer, pyloromyotomy may have a beneficial effect in preventing gastric retention if there is no organic stenosis, although most surgeons have not sufficient confidence in the method to employ it routinely. Pyloromyotomy is sometimes carried out following oesophagectomy with oesophagogastric anastomosis, in the hope of preventing gastric retention. Failure of the stomach to empty is more likely to result from gastric atony following the inevitable gastric vagotomy in the absence of pyloric stenosis. However, most surgeons employ pyloroplasty to compensate for the postvagotomy gastric atony.

Assess

Endoscopy should have been performed before operation, but, if this was not possible, pick up the pylorus and feel the thickness of the muscular ring. Assess the size of the mucosal channel by attempting to invaginate the anterior antral wall and the anterior duodenal wall through the pylorus on the tip of an index finger.

Action

1 Grasp the pylorus between finger and thumb of the left hand to steady it (Fig. 13.5).

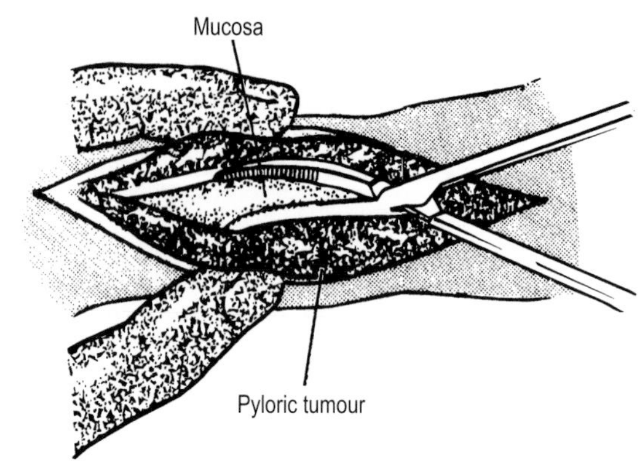

Fig. 13.5 Pyloromyotomy.

2 With a scalpel, incise the seromuscularis along the middle of the anterior antral wall from 1 cm proximal to the thickened segment and carefully extend it distally across the pylorus onto the anterior duodenal wall for 1 cm. The duodenal wall at the fornix is very thin, so take care not to incise into the lumen.

3 Deepen the incision through the thickened muscle of the distal antrum until the mucosa bulges into the split. Make sure all the muscle fibres are divided. The final split may be accomplished by grasping the wall on each side of the split with dry gauze swabs and separating the edges, to allow mucosa to bulge freely along the whole of the incision.

4 Carry the split distally to the pylorus and carefully divide all the circular muscle fibres here, again taking care to expose but not damage the mucosa of the first part of the duodenal bulb. Lift the muscle fibres free of the mucosa with closed fine non-toothed dissecting forceps, allow the forceps blades to open and then cut the fibres between them.

Check

1 Make sure all the fibres have been cut.

2 Gather some gastric air into the segment with the pyloromyotomy, to distend the mucosa so that it bulges into the split. Watch carefully for any leaks. It is no disaster to find a leak and carefully close it with fine stitches on eyeless needles. It may be disastrous to miss a leak.

OPERATIVE GASTROSTOMY

Appraise

1 Gastrostomy offers a valuable method of feeding patients who are unable to swallow because of oesophageal obstruction, bulbar palsy and other causes. Patients with mechanical obstruction who will have reconstructive surgery utilizing the stomach as a conduit should not normally have a temporary gastrostomy since this will interfere with subsequent reconstructive surgery. They are better served by a jejunostomy.

2 As a rule gastrostomy is intended as a temporary measure. When all else fails, do not hesitate to offer it after discussion with the patient.

3 Gastrostomy offers a means of providing gastric aspiration without nasogastric intubation, valuable in patients who have respiratory difficulties and those who cannot tolerate the presence of the tube in their pharynx, during the postoperative recovery period from gastric operations.

4 Duodenal fistula can be treated using a gastrostomy. Two tubes are passed through it. The end of one lies at the site of the leak, kept on continuous aspiration to reduce the rate of flow through the track. A second, longer tube passes into the bowel at least 30 cm beyond the fistula, for enteric feeding.

5 A number of operative techniques have been described. Stamm's gastrostomy is almost universally used now and is described below. The tube passes through the abdominal wall and enters the stomach through a small stab wound. The hole is prevented from leaking by invaginating it using a series of purse-string sutures so that it resembles a non-spill inkwell. Witzel's gastrostomy is similar, but leakage is prevented by laying the emerging tube along the stomach wall and covering it by suturing over it ridges of gastric wall so that it lies in a tunnel. The Depage–Janeway gastrostomy employs a flap of stomach formed into a tube which is brought to the skin surface to create a permanent conduit.

6 Operative gastrostomy is often unnecessary following the advent of percutaneous endoscopic gastrostomy.

Access

1 Gastrostomy can be accomplished under local anaesthesia if necessary. Mix 20 ml of 2% lidocaine with 80 ml of physiological saline for injection. After preparing and towelling off the skin area, inject 20 ml intracutaneously along a vertical line from 1 cm above the left costal margin over the middle of the left rectus muscle, downwards for 8–10 cm. With a longer needle, inject a further 20 ml into the subcutaneous tissues and anterior rectus sheath. Now inject deeper into the posterior rectus sheath and preperitoneal tissues. When the peritoneum is pierced, resistance to injection suddenly disappears. Allow a small volume to enter the peritoneal cavity.

2 Incise the skin vertically downwards from the costal margin for 6–8 cm, cutting through all the tissues into the peritoneum in the same line. Inject additional local anaesthetic into the posterior rectus sheath and preperitoneal connective tissue before incising the peritoneum.

Action

1 Insert retractors and adjust the light to identify the stomach and draw out a portion of the mid-stomach using tissue forceps.

2 After towelling off the area, make a stab wound as high as possible on the anterior wall, midway between the greater and lesser curves. Aspirate the gastric contents with a sucker tube. Insert the end of a 20–24F soft latex catheter for 7–10 cm with the tip directed towards the pylorus (Fig. 13.6).

3 Insert a purse-string suture on an eyeless needle 0.5 cm from the tube and, as it is tightened and tied, push the edges of the stab wound inwards. Tie the ends of the suture around the tube to fix it. Insert a second purse-string 0.5 cm outside this to invaginate it and, if necessary, a third.

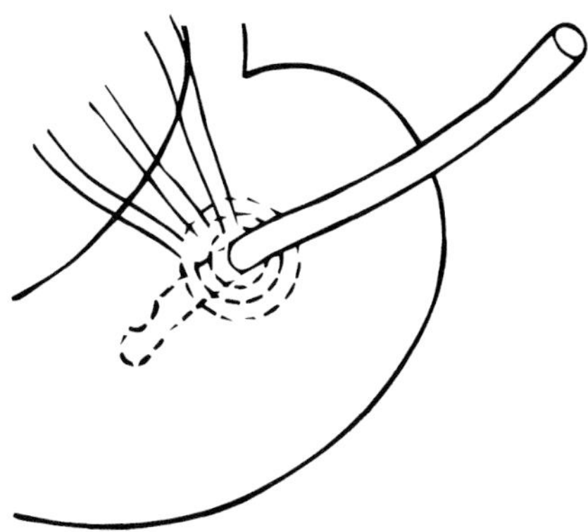

Fig. 13.6 Stamm gastrostomy.

4 Hold the edges of the upper part of the abdominal wound everted and suture the stomach around the gastrostomy to the peritoneum under the edges so that the tube emerges through the upper end of the wound.

Closure

1 Close the remainder of the wound in layers. Insert an extra skin stitch at the upper end of the wound and tie it around the emerging tube to fix it.

2 Apply wound dressings.

3 Test the patency of the gastrostomy by injecting 30 ml of sterile water, then temporarily spigot it.

PERCUTANEOUS ENDOSCOPIC GASTROSTOMY

Appraise

1 Although formal gastrostomy can be carried out under local anaesthesia with minimal risk and distress to the patient, percutaneous endoscopic gastrostomy is a safe and convenient alternative.

2 The commonest application is for intragastric or enteral nutritional support in the presence of, for example, bulbar palsy. Another indication is to enable prolonged gastric aspiration to be performed, especially in those who cannot tolerate nasogastric intubation. This may be necessary in protracted gastric stasis and in the management of duodenal fistula.

3 Do not attempt this method if the patient has an impassable oesophageal stricture, or previous upper abdominal surgery that produces adhesions preventing expansion of the stomach to contact the anterior abdominal wall, or a partial gastrectomy. Gross ascites or sepsis make the procedure dangerous so formal gastrostomy or jejunostomy is preferred. Portal venous hypertension, coagulopathy and gastric ulcer or tumour at the elective site of gastrostomy are also contraindications. Gross obesity may make the procedure difficult.

4 There is a choice of methods, and some excellent commercially produced kits are available. The tubes are approximately 20F in size. I shall describe a simple pull-through technique that is popular.

Prepare

1 Administer intravenous sedation according to protocol.

2 Lie patients who can tolerate it supine. Alternatively, pass the endoscope with the patient lying on the left side and then roll the patient into the supine position.

3 Give a single intravenous injection of a versatile antibiotic. It is advisable to give an intragastric antibiotic in the presence of gastric neoplasm, ulcer, or if the patient is taking regular H_2-receptor antagonists or proton-pump inhibitors.

Action

1 Pass an end-viewing endoscope into the stomach. In the presence of an oesophageal stricture it may be necessary to dilate it using bougies or a balloon, and then introduce a paediatric endoscope. Pass the tip into the distal stomach.

2 Inspect the stomach and duodenum to exclude any condition that would contraindicate gastrostomy.

3 Gently inflate the stomach to distend it.

4 Have the abdomen exposed and the room lights dimmed.

5 Turn the endoscope tip towards the anterior abdominal wall. The light should be visible through the gastric and abdominal walls.

6 Have the abdominal operator indent the anterior abdominal wall with a finger placed where the endoscope light is seen most brightly. The indentation should be visible from within the stomach.

7 Pass a polypectomy snare through the biopsy channel of the endoscope (Fig. 13.7a).

8 If you are the abdominal operator, prepare the skin, infiltrate the chosen puncture spot with 0.5% lidocaine into the skin and abdominal wall, then make an incision in the skin sufficiently large to allow the passage of the gastrostomy tube.

9 Pass a needle carrying a smooth, closely fitting plastic cannula through the abdominal wall into the stomach. A standard intravenous catheter is usually employed.

10 If you are the endoscopist, manoeuvre the loop of the snare over the cannula (Fig. 13.7b). The needle is withdrawn by the abdominal operator and either a flexible wire or a strong thread is passed through the cannula into the stomach.

11 Withdraw the snare from the end of the cannula under vision, in order to grasp the thread or wire that protrudes from the end of the cannula into the stomach (Fig. 13.7c). While the abdominal operator holds the other end of the thread or wire, withdraw the endoscope, snare and trapped thread or wire out through the mouth.

12 Attach the emerging thread or wire to the tapered end of the gastrostomy tube (Fig. 13.7d). The bulbous or inflatable end of the gastrostomy tube will remain in the stomach, pulling it against the abdominal wall.

13 Apply lubricant to the gastrostomy tube.

14 Draw upon the thread or wire emerging from the abdominal cannula while guiding the tapered tip of the gastrostomy tube through the patient's mouth and into the oesophagus and stomach. Eventually the tapered tip is drawn against the cannula tip, extruding it. As you continue to pull, the tapered end of the gastrostomy tube will emerge through the gastric and abdominal walls (Fig. 13.7e).

15 Re-pass the endoscope into the stomach and observe the enlarged end of the gastrostomy tube as it is drawn up against the gastric wall. In some tubes the end is shaped so that it expands automatically; in others, a balloon is expanded by distending it with air or fluid through a side channel. Make sure that the tension on the gastrostomy tube is not sufficient to cause gastric mucosal blanching.

16 Withdraw the endoscope.

17 Cut off the tapered end of the gastrostomy tube and ensure that the expanded end is inflated if it is of this type, and seal the side-tube inflation channel.

18 The tube must be fixed to hold the stomach against the abdominal wall. Most kits contain a fixation base that fits over and holds the gastrostomy tube, having an expanded flat surface that lies against the abdominal wall (Fig. 13.7f).

Aftercare

1 Feeding with suitable varied fluids can usually start after 24–48 hours.

2 Monitor the patient to ensure that there is no chest infection, since reflux and aspiration pneumonia is a well-recognized complication.

3 Check the gastrostomy site since infection is frequent.

4 Leakage around the gastrostomy catheter may develop spontaneously or in the presence of gastric outlet obstruction.

5 Some gastrostomy tubes can be removed by deflating the expanded end and drawing them through the abdominal wall. Others require endoscopic withdrawal.

JEJUNOSTOMY

It is possible to pass a longer, narrower tube through the gastrostomy tube after it is in place. This can be advanced through the pylorus, either spontaneously, under radiographic control or endoscopically, into the duodenum and jejunum. In this way a jejunostomy is created for distal enteral feeding.

PERFORATED PEPTIC ULCER

Appraise

1 Record the patient's age, blood pressure and the presence or absence of serious associated disease such as cardiac, respiratory or renal failure. Fully resuscitate the patient before performing the operation.

2 Perforation of other viscera such as colon or gallbladder may be confused with gastroduodenal perforations. If you are in doubt, proceed as though this were a peptic ulcer perforation but be willing to close the incision and make a better sited one if the need arises. This is preferable to making a compromise incision.

3 Not all patients who have a perforated peptic ulcer should have an operation. Patients seen within 8 hours, in whom a

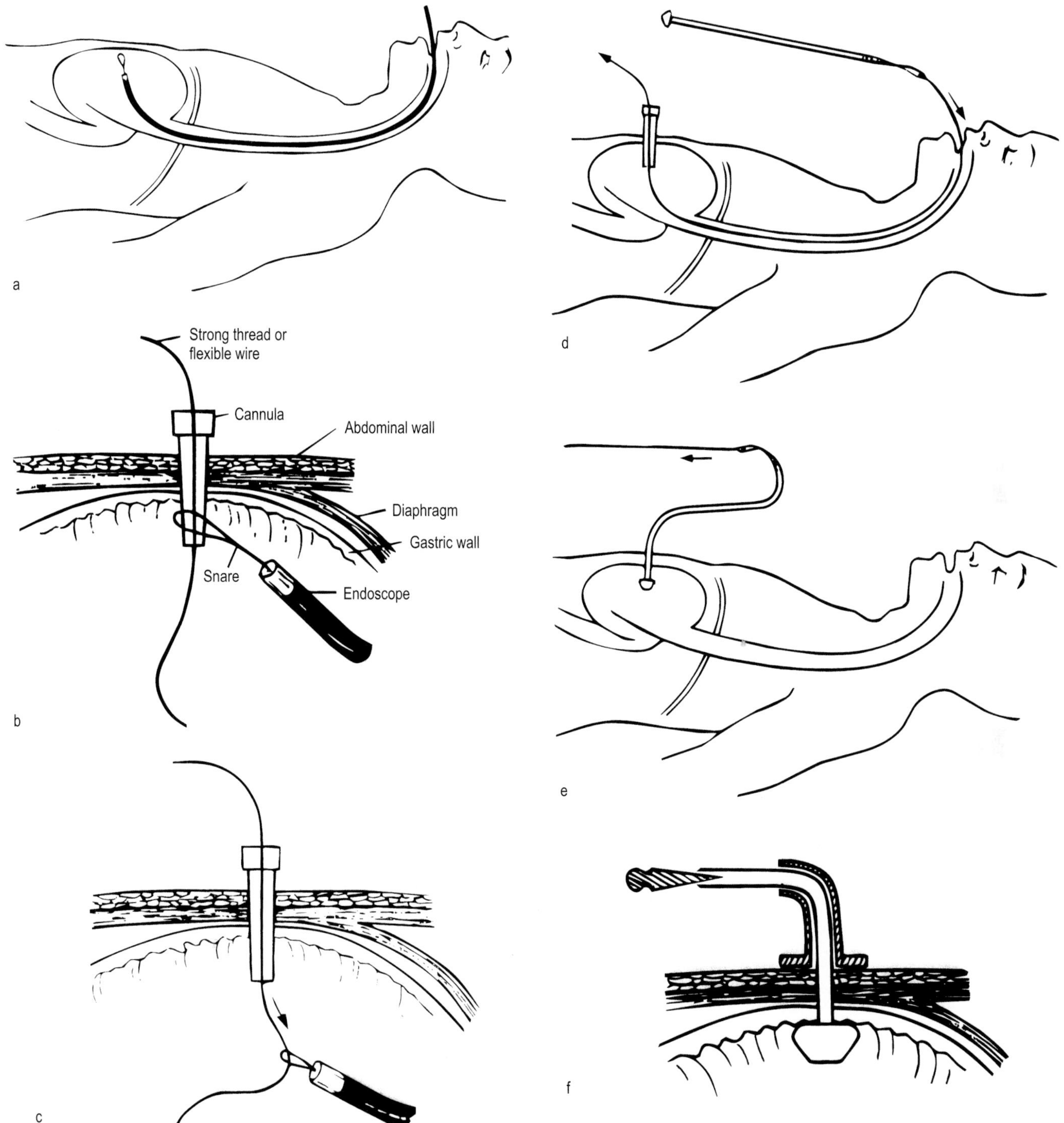

Fig. 13.7 Percutaneous endoscopic gastrostomy: (a) the stomach is distended through the endoscope; a wire snare protrudes from the end of the endoscope; (b) strong thread or wire passed into the stomach; (c) thread or wire snared for withdrawal through the mouth; (d) the tapered end of the gastrostomy tube is fixed to the strong thread or flexible wire; (e) the gastrostomy tube has been pulled through the pharynx, oesophagus and stomach; the bulbous or inflatable end is about to be drawn against the anterior gastric wall; (f) the gastrostomy tube in position.

confident diagnosis is made, and who are haemodynamically stable, may be treated conservatively. Ensure that the tip of an 18F nasogastric tube is accurately placed in the most dependent part of the stomach. A disadvantage is that peritoneal toilet cannot be performed. Proceed to operation at once if the patient develops pyrexia, tachycardia, pain, distension or increasing intraperitoneal gas on X-rays. A few patients develop intraperitoneal abscesses if there has been significant leakage and soiling. Nasogastric suction, parenteral feeding, systemic antibiotics and chest physiotherapy are instituted, and operation is resorted to only if the patient fails to improve or deteriorates.

4 Is definitive surgical treatment of a perforated duodenal ulcer justified as an emergency procedure? Many papers have been written to show that definitive surgery is as safe as simple suture. However, it has been shown that some patients following simple suture never have any serious subsequent dyspepsia, some have recurrent dyspepsia that does not require elective surgery and some require elective or emergency surgery. No-one can predict to which group an individual patient belongs when he is admitted with a perforated peptic ulcer.

The main justification is if a fit patient has perforated within an hour or two before being admitted, who would have been offered elective surgery for disabling and uncontrollable symptoms prior to the perforation and the operation to be carried out would be the one you would choose electively. You as the surgeon, your team and the available facilities must all be appropriate.

5 Perforated gastric ulcer carries a higher mortality than perforated duodenal ulcer, because the patients are, on average, older and less 'fit' generally. Most gastric ulcer perforations are successfully managed by simple suture after excising a specimen from the edge for histology. Sometimes they are difficult to close and demand gastrectomy including the ulcer. If there is doubt about the nature of the ulcer, treat it as though it is benign, remove a biopsy specimen from the edge and, if malignancy is demonstrated histologically, carry out the appropriate operation 2 weeks later as an elective procedure. If the ulcer cannot be sutured but is of doubtful origin and frozen-section histology is equivocal or cannot be arranged, then carry out gastrectomy as though this is a benign ulcer and be prepared to re-operate to carry out an elective radical procedure 2 weeks later. The added risks of performing a radical operation are not justified without confirming the diagnosis.

KEY POINTS Equivocal gastric carcinoma?

- In case of doubt treat it as benign until proven.
- Half-hearted cancer operations prejudice subsequent treatment.

6 Bleeding associated with perforation demands control of both complications. A bleeding perforated gastric ulcer is conventionally controlled by distal gastrectomy including the ulcer. Bleeding is rarely a complication of anterior perforating duodenal ulcer but if there is a co-existent bleeding posterior duodenal ulcer, the anterior perforation can be incorporated into a gastroduodenotomy. Insert non-absorbable stitches into the base of the posterior ulcer to control the bleeding and then close the gastroduodenotomy as a pyloroplasty. Complete the procedure with vagotomy, which is normally truncal, but it may be highly selective if the patient is fit and you are adept.

7 Perforated gastric carcinoma may be amenable to the same operation as would be carried out electively. If not, consider suturing it or plugging the defect with omentum and re-operating electively 2 weeks later after the patient has been brought to the best possible condition. Sometimes inadequate resection is forced upon the surgeon. If so, consider whether this can be corrected later by a more adequate operation.

8 The diagnosis has been confirmed through the laparoscope and followed by repair using sutures, staples or a plug. This may become an accepted method of diagnosis and treatment.

Access

Use a midline or right paramedian incision from the xiphisternum to the umbilicus, 10–12 cm long.

Assess

1 Remove all instruments from the field with the exception of a retractor for your assistant and the sucker tube for yourself.

2 Aspirate any free fluid after collecting a specimen for laboratory examination. Gastric juice is usually bile-stained.

3 Examine the duodenal bulb and the stomach, especially along the lesser curve. If necessary, open the lesser sac of omentum through the lesser or gastrocolic omenta to view the posterior gastric wall.

4 Remember that multiple perforations can occur.

5 Always locally excise or remove a biopsy specimen from the edge of a gastric ulcer.

6 If you cannot find the perforation after a diligent search, explore the whole abdomen, if necessary extending the incision downwards. Examine in particular the gallbladder and sigmoid colon. If you are still puzzled, consider the possibility of Boerhaave's syndrome (spontaneous rupture of distal spontaneous oesophagus).

7 If you are a surgeon in training and find yourself in difficulty either because of failure to discover the cause, or indecision about the best course of action, or because the required procedure is beyond your capabilities, do not hesitate to contact your chief for advice and assistance.

KEY POINTS Treat the emergency condition—that is why you operated

- Your function at this emergency operation is to perform the simplest procedure that will correct the catastrophe.
- If you do more than this, will you be able to justify it to yourself and others if the patient succumbs?

Simple closure

1 Place two or three parallel sutures of 3/0 synthetic absorbable material on eyeless needles through all coats, passing in 1 cm proximal to the ulcer edge and emerging 1 cm distal to the ulcer (Fig. 13.8). Do not pick up the opposite wall as this will obstruct the lumen. When all the sutures are in place, mobilize a tongue of omentum, place it over the perforation and tie the sutures just tightly enough to hold it in place.

2 Insert further sutures to reinforce the obturating action of the omentum to ensure that it is adequately sealed.

3 Even when closure seems secure, do not hesitate to suture omentum over it.

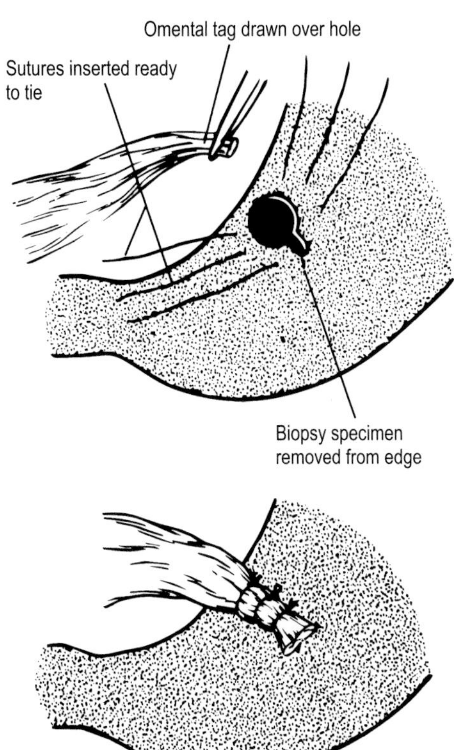

Fig. 13.8 Suture of a perforated peptic ulcer.

4 Aspirate any free fluid from above and below the liver, from within the lesser sac, the right paracolic gutter and from the pelvis.

Checklist

1 Re-examine the closure of the perforation.

2 Aspirate in the collection areas once more.

Drain?

1 If the perforation was sutured without delay, if the closure is secure and peritoneal toilet was adequate, drainage is unnecessary.

2 Make sure the insertion of a drain does not replace careful technique.

ELECTIVE SURGERY FOR PEPTIC ULCER

Appraise

1 Medical treatment has become the mainstay with potent antacids, atropine-like drugs, liquorice extracts, mucosal-coating substances, histamine H_2-receptor-blocking drugs and H^+,K^+-ATPase inhibitors. The elimination of *Helicobacter pylori*, using so-called triple therapy of a proton-pump inhibitor combined with two antibiotics such as clarithromycin and metronidazole, reduces the relapse rate. Most patients can be controlled with these powerful and safe agents and the only people who may require operation are the minority who cannot be controlled medically, who cannot or will not take the required treatment, or who develop complications of the ulcer.

2 The operation that was in vogue in the 1960s and 1970s was proximal gastric vagotomy, known also as highly selective vagotomy. Some centres report high rates of recurrence after long-term follow-up but variations in recurrence rates probably reflect variations in completeness of parietal cell denervation and are thus dependent on the skill of the surgeon. An adjunctive operation to overcome gastric retention is unnecessary if there is no evidence of impending pyloroduodenal stenosis resulting from the chronic ulcer scarring. If there is, some surgeons dilate the canal through a prepyloric gastrotomy using Hegar-type dilators or a finger, or by invaginating the anterior duodenal and gastric antral walls through the stenosed canal on an index finger tip—a manoeuvre introduced by Jaboulay. If the stenosis in confined to the bulb, a longitudinal incision can be made through it without impinging on the pyloric ring, closing it as a transverse suture line after the manner of a pyloroplasty; hence it is called a duodenoplasty. A few surgeons still prefer truncal vagotomy combined with pyloroplasty, gastroenterostomy or distal gastrectomy to improve gastric emptying.

3 Gastric ulcer was treated more aggressively by surgeons in the past than was duodenal ulcer. Many surgeons adopt a fixed policy of carrying out endoscopy and biopsy to confirm that this is initially a benign ulcer, then give the patient a 6–8-week course of medical treatment followed by a check endoscopy. If the ulcer is healed, operation is deferred. If the ulcer is not healed, or if it soon recurs, then surgical treatment is recommended. This more aggressive treatment stems partly from anxiety about the possibility of early malignancy or impending change and partly from the pragmatic knowledge that chronic gastric ulcers are less likely than chronic duodenal ulcers to become quiescent.

Gastric ulcers sometimes develop in patients taking non-steroidal anti-inflammatory drugs (NSAIDs). Misoprostol, a prostaglandin analogue, appears to reduce this tendency.

The operation of choice for gastric ulcers is a Polya partial gastrectomy, including the ulcer in the specimen.

4 Postbulbar duodenal ulcers are quite frequently seen in certain countries, especially southern India, but are relatively uncommon in Western countries. They are often severe and stenosing so that operation may be recommended for fear of incipient obstruction. Proximal gastric vagotomy is effective if the lumen is still widely patent; if it is not, then add gastroenterostomy, thus retaining the vagal supply to the gallbladder, pancreas and small intestine.

5 Zollinger–Ellison syndrome associated with hypergastrinaemia, usually from G-cell hyperplasia or gastrin-secreting tumour in the pancreas, generally produces peptic ulcers in usual sites. If an ulcer lies in an unusual site, or if there are multiple ulcers and especially if the ulcer is in the upper jejunum, suspect the Zollinger–Ellison syndrome (see p. 206).

6 Oesophageal peptic ulceration occurs when gastric acid refluxes into the oesophagus where the squamous mucosa is unresistant to acid attack. This develops most frequently as a result of hiatal hernia but can occur in the absence of herniation of the

stomach into the chest. A less frequent cause of peptic ulcer in the oesophagus is the condition of Barrett's oesophagus. This appears to be acquired although it used to be called 'congenitally short oesophagus'. The gastric mucosa invades the oesophagus and the oesophagogastric mucosal junction moves progressively upwards; an ulcer sometimes develops just above the junction. There is a greatly increased risk of developing adenocarcinoma of the distal oesophagus (see Ch. 10).

VAGOTOMY

The various types of vagotomy are now seldom used in the elective treatment of peptic ulceration, because of the success of medical treatment with antibiotics and potent antacids. Proximal gastric, or highly selective vagotomy is preferable to truncal vagotomy and 'drainage' because side-effects such as dumping and diarrhoea are fewer in incidence and less in severity.

▶ KEY POINT 'Blind' vagotomy

- Never embark on elective vagotomy without confirming the diagnosis of peptic ulcer.

TRUNCAL VAGOTOMY

Appraise

1 Per-hiatal truncal vagotomy was formerly indicated for the management of uncomplicated duodenal ulcer when the full range of medical treatment had been tried and failed to control the symptoms. It is normally accompanied by pyloroplasty or gastroenterostomy to improve the rate of gastric emptying, so-called drainage procedures. Pyloroplasty (see p. 181) is simple to perform unless the patient is very obese with a deep abdomen and with a fixed, very scarred pylorus. Anterior juxtapyloric gastroenterostomy is convenient if pyloroplasty is difficult to perform and has the advantage that it is not irrevocable.

2 Truncal vagotomy may be used when controlling gastroduodenal bleeding from peptic ulcer. At such operations the main task is to stop the bleeding, but the secondary task is to prevent bleeding from recurrent or persistent ulcer.

3 In the surgical management of recurrent peptic ulcer truncal vagotomy is best combined with partial gastrectomy.

4 Truncal vagotomy combined with a 'drainage' operation is sometimes advocated for the definitive management of a perforated duodenal ulcer. The improvement in medical management of uncomplicated duodenal ulcer urges conservatism.

5 Truncal vagotomy and a drainage operation is often effective treatment for chronic gastric ulcer in an unfit patient, but gastrectomy including the ulcer is preferred treatment whenever possible.

Access

1 Use a midline incision 20 cm long, skirting the umbilicus.

2 Mobilize the left lobe of the liver, folding it to the right, to obtain a good view.

3 In an obese patient with a high diaphragm try the effect of tilting the patient 25–30° head-up.

4 Insert a retractor fixed to the table, to elevate the sternum.

Assess

1 Explore the whole abdomen. Remember that patients with proven peptic ulceration may have incidental conditions such as gallstones or colonic carcinoma which might help to explain their symptoms.

2 Examine the stomach and duodenum and note the effects of the ulcer in distorting the duodenum and fixing it, so that you may make a decision about the easiest and safest adjunctive operation.

▶ KEY POINTS Favour simple and safe procedures

- There is little difference between the results of the various operations.
- Do not perform a difficult procedure regardless of other considerations.

Action

1 Make sure there is a nasogastric tube in place, as a guide to the line of the gullet at the oesophageal hiatus.

2 While an assistant grasps the lower anterior wall of the stomach and draws it down, identify the hiatus by feeling for the nasogastric tube. Open the peritoneum transversely, avoiding the inferior phrenic vessels. Beneath this is the phreno-oesophageal ligament. Open this and enlarge the incision to 3–4 cm. You can now pass the closed scissors anterior to the gullet into the posterior mediastinum. If you cannot, you have not yet opened the phreno-oesophageal ligament. Thorough mobilization of the distal oesophagus is the key to the achievement of complete vagotomy.

3 Look out for the anterior vagal trunk lying in front of the oesophagus (Fig. 13.9) and separate it upwards for 5 cm and downwards to where it gives off the hepatic and gastric body branches, continuing as the anterior nerve of Latarjet. Transect it where it breaks up below, crushing the distal stump to occlude the small vessels running with it. Place a curved Moynihan clamp across it as high as possible and transect it just below the clamp, then remove the clamp. This is a 'vagectomy' and ensures that the whole trunk is removed but does not guarantee that vagotomy is complete, since fine branches may come off higher up and bypass the 'vagectomy'.

4 Encircle the lower gullet with the right forefinger and thumb. There is a 'mesentery' behind the gullet in which lies the posterior vagal trunk (Fig. 13.10). Pass the middle finger to the left of the gullet and push this 'mesentery' to the right so that the nerve trunk can be identified. Separate the oesophagus from the vagus and burst through the mesentery behind the vagus. As the trunk is traced down, part of it passes backwards to the coeliac plexus (Fig. 13.11), part continues downwards as the posterior nerve of Latarjet and branches leave to reach the body of the stomach. Crush and cut the nerve below and again as high as

possible to remove a segment of nerve to insure against leaving a separate branch intact.

5 Search for missed, separate branches around the whole circumference of the oesophageal wall. They feel like tight threads and should be divided. Make sure that there is no damage to the oesophagus and that all the bleeding is controlled.

6 Repair the horizontal defect in the hiatus using two or three non-absorbable sutures.

7 Carry out the selected adjunctive procedure of pyloroplasty, gastroenterostomy or gastrectomy.

? DIFFICULTY

1. Access can be very difficult in obese patients. Do not proceed if you do not have an adequate view. Tilt the patient head-up, remove the xiphoid process, mobilize the left lobe of the liver and fold it to the right. If the view is still restricted, do not hesitate to split the sternum in the midline. The only danger is of embarking on vagotomy without being able to see properly and control what is done.
2. The assistant's hand drawing down the stomach may be in the way. Make a hole in an avascular part of the upper lesser omentum, pass curved forceps behind the fundus of the stomach and push them through the gastrophrenic ligament near the angle of His. Draw a rubber tube through the hole as a sling to exert traction without distorting or obscuring the cardia.
3. *Damage to the oesophagus?* Repair the hole carefully, using all-coats sutures followed by a muscle coat stitch. Leave a nasogastric tube in the stomach.
4. *Cannot find the vagi?* Clumsy opening of the phreno-oesophageal ligament may lead to inadvertent anterior vagotomy. Carefully open the peritoneum and phreno-oesophageal ligament until the oesophagus can be seen encircled above by the diaphragmatic crus. The cut anterior trunk will be seen lying on the oesophagus. Alternatively you will see that the anterior trunk has been displaced to one side.
5. The posterior vagal trunk does not always lie close to the oesophagus. If it cannot be felt, carefully display the oesophagus emerging through the crus. The vagal trunk may be seen lying against the muscle of the crus. If you are a surgeon in training and cannot find the vagi, call for advice and assistance. Otherwise remember that more than half of patients treated surgically by gastroenterostomy will be cured of their symptoms. An experienced surgeon may carry out Polya gastrectomy in appropriate circumstances.

PROXIMAL GASTRIC VAGOTOMY

Appraise

- This operation is otherwise known as highly selective vagotomy.

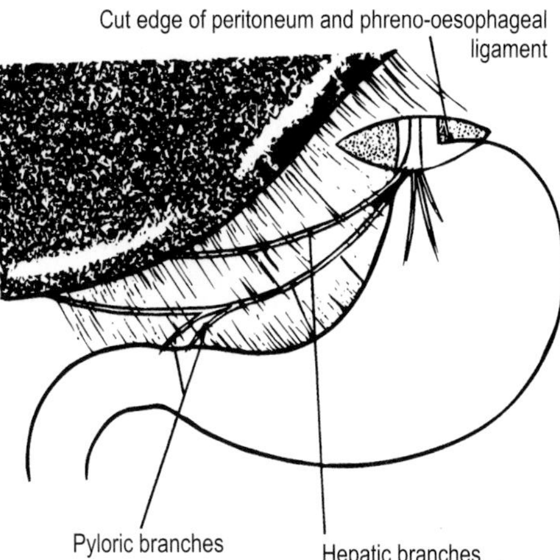

Fig. 13.9 Truncal vagotomy. Exposure of the anterior nerve; the distribution of the nerve is indicated.

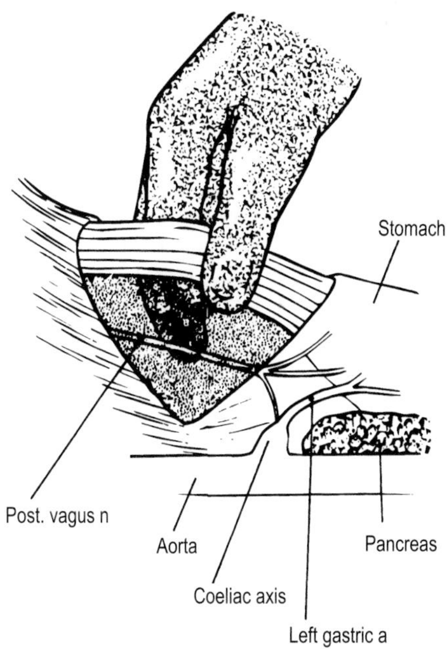

Fig. 13.10 Truncal vagotomy. Exposure of the posterior nerve as seen from the right side of the patient. While the gullet is encircled by the right thumb and forefinger, the right middle finger pushes the 'mesentery' containing the dorsal nerve to the right.

- Proximal gastric vagotomy aims to denervate only the acid-secreting proximal part of the stomach, leaving the alkali-secreting antrum, with its muscular pumping action, still innervated. Thus gastric acid secretion is reduced but gastric emptying is usually unimpaired. The addition of a drainage operation can be dispensed with in most patients in the absence of pyloroduodenal stenosis.

Access

Use an upper midline or paramedian incision, skirting the umbilicus, 20 cm long.

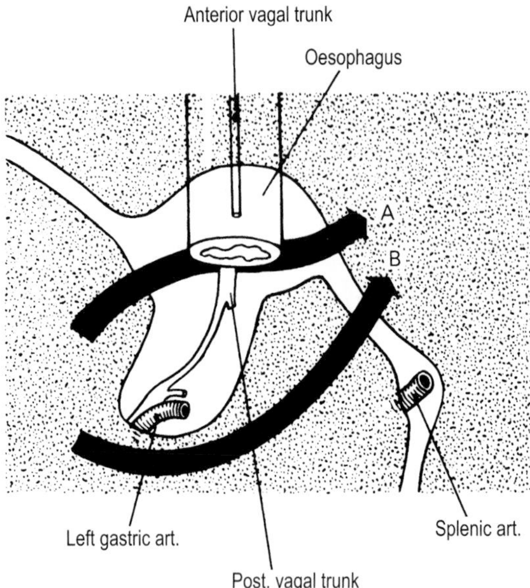

Fig. 13.11 Diagram of peritoneal reflections from the posterior abdominal wall. The posterior vagal trunk is gathered along path A but not along path B.

Action

1 Make a hole through an avascular area in the mid-portion of the gastrocolic omentum. While the stomach is lifted forwards, carefully and completely separate the flimsy attachments of the stomach to the pancreas, watching out for, and preserving, the fold of peritoneum that contains the left gastric vessels. Separate the stomach from the posterior wall right up to the roof of the lesser sac. Occasionally you will be surprised to find the scar of an unsuspected posterior gastric ulcer.

2 Pass the right index finger through the hole in the gastrocolic omentum and grasp the gastric antrum to draw it down, so stretching the lesser curve of the stomach. In all but the most obese patients the taut anterior nerve of Latarjet can be seen running parallel to the lesser curve, separating into branches which form a 'crow's foot' pattern as they cross the curvature at the angulus, accompanied by blood vessels from the descending branch of the left gastric artery (Fig. 13.12). The posterior nerve cannot usually be seen from the front but can be displayed by looking through the hole in the gastrocolic omentum after turning the stomach forwards and upwards.

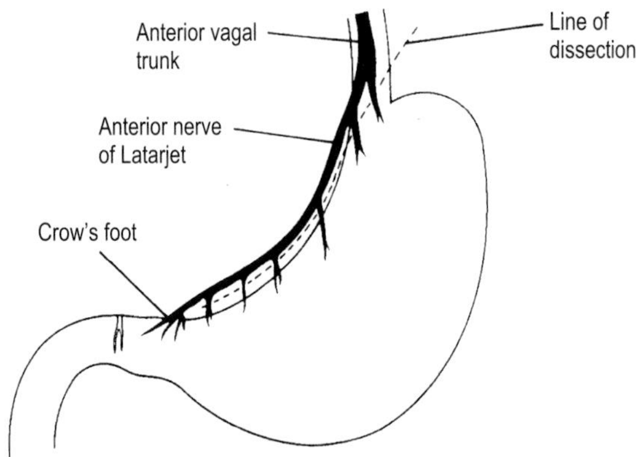

Fig. 13.12 Proximal gastric vagotomy. The anterior nerve of Latarjet, showing line of separation by dissection. The posterior nerve runs parallel to the anterior nerve.

3 Carefully make a hole through the lesser omentum close to the gastric wall, just to the left of the 'crow's foot' of nerves, while protecting the posterior structures from damage with the right index finger passed through the defect in the gastrocolic omentum. Pass one end of a tape through the hole in the lesser omentum, drawing it out through the hole in the gastrocolic omentum. The tape now encircles the stomach at the level of the angulus, marking the lower limit of dissection. Clip the ends of the tape together so they may be used to exert gentle downward traction on the stomach by an assistant to tauten and define the nerves of Latarjet.

4 Make a second, higher hole in the lesser curve close to the stomach just above the next visible vessels. Double-clamp, divide and ligate the vessels and accompanying nerve filaments.

KEY POINTS Take care!

- The length of tissue available for double-clamping between the nerve of Latarjet and the lesser curve is short.
- If you place the haemostats well apart you risk damaging the lesser curve, or the nerve of Latarjet or both.

5 A better method is to pass double ligatures with an aneurysm needle or with Lahey's fine curved forceps, tie them carefully and divide the tissue between them. It is possible to use haemostatic clips instead of ligatures, and one instrument applies two clips side by side and cuts between them; there is not usually sufficient length to use this here but it may be carefully used where the vessel and nerve length is adequate. If you do use haemostatic clips, take care that you do not inadvertently brush them off, thus tearing the delicate blood vessels.

6 Proceed upwards step by step, dividing the vessels and nerves that cross the lesser curve, carefully preserving the nerves of Latarjet as they are separated from the stomach. Higher up on the stomach, the vessels and nerves do not tend to penetrate at the lesser curve but cross it to enter on the posterior or anterior wall. Take advantage of this extra length by carrying the dissection onto the anterior and posterior walls. The separation of the anterior and posterior nerves of Latarjet from the stomach now proceeds independently onto the anterior and posterior gastric walls.

7 As the anterior and posterior layers of lesser omentum separate, slide non-toothed forceps under avascular sections and cut between the opened blades. Small vessels may be sealed with low-power diathermy applied for the minimum time through fine forceps applied well away from the main nerves and from the gastric musculature.

8 At the level of the main left gastric artery and vein quite large vessels must be ligated and divided on the anterior and posterior walls, together with their accompanying nerve filaments. Above these, the lowest portion of the oesophagus can be separated from the nerves of Latarjet without dividing any large vessels.

9 As the dissection reaches the cardia, the main trunks of the nerve are separated from the gullet, the nerves of Latarjet being the inferior prolongations of them. At this point temporarily stop the dissection.

10 Draw down the gastric fundus while an assistant retracts the left costal margin. Identify the angle of His between the fundus and the left edge of the lower gullet. Carefully incise the peritoneum in the angle, without damaging the stomach or oesophagus. Open up the hole gently with the right index finger and pass the right thumb through the upper part of the defect in the lesser omentum, behind the fundus of the stomach. Thumb and finger are prevented from meeting by the peritoneum of the roof of the lesser sac which can now be broken through.

11 At the level of the cardia separate, doubly ligate and divide the peritoneum, phreno-oesophageal ligament and nerve fibres across the anterior aspect of the lower oesophagus, leaving the muscle coat denuded but intact.

12 Divide loose tissue and nerve fibres around the posterior aspect of the lower oesophagus, rotating it to improve the view. A troublesome fragile vein is encountered running posteriorly from the cardia often in a crescentic peritoneal fold. Tie it, seal it with diathermy current or apply a haemostatic clip. Do not encroach more than 2 cm on the greater curve aspect of the gastric fundus or you will damage the short gastric vessels and the spleen.

? DIFFICULTY

1. *Bleeding into the lesser omentum?* A vessel retracts out of the ligature and continues to bleed between the layers of the omentum to form a large, spreading swelling. Do not try to grab it with large artery forceps. The ooze does not emerge directly from the vessel but trickles through the haematoma. Gently close the blades of a swab-holding forceps over the area and leave them for 5 minutes, timed by the clock. Remove the forceps. If bleeding does not recur during the remainder of the operation it is safe to leave the vessel. If oozing recurs or you are in doubt, gently dissect between the layers, identify the vessel and ligate it.
2. *Thick, fatty omentum?* Do not attempt to ligate it as a single layer. If you bunch it, subsequent traction on the stomach stretches the base of the bunch, and the ligature is forced off. If you are lucky, bleeding starts now. If you are unlucky, it will start later and you will miss it. Safeguard against this by picking up vessels with the minimum extraneous tissue. If necessary, perform the dissection in three separate layers, along the anterior leaf of lesser omentum, the lesser curve and the posterior leaf.
3. The operation can be difficult in an obese patient, in spite of taking steps to obtain a good view. Consider if truncal vagotomy would be easier, combined with a drainage operation. If you decide to proceed with proximal gastric vagotomy, concentrate on each step, not anticipating the difficulties of the next step. Remarkably, the dissection usually becomes easier as the stomach is mobilized.

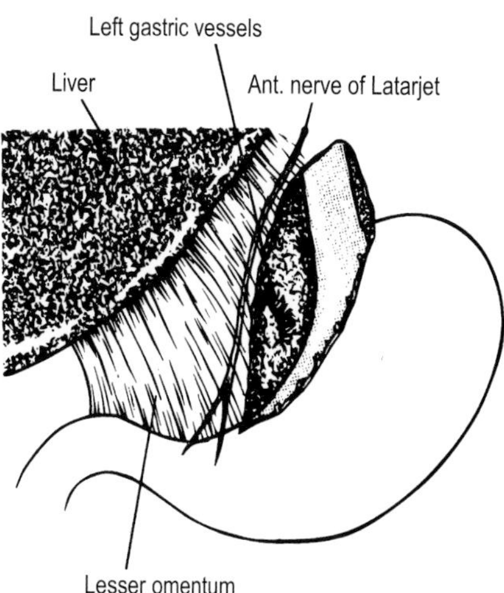

Fig. 13.13 Proximal gastric vagotomy. The nerves of Latarjet have been separated from the lesser curvature of the stomach.

13 Clear the whole circumference of the lower 5–7 cm of oesophagus of nerve fibres. Do not damage the longitudinal muscle coat. Catch any small veins that have retracted into the muscle coat using fine sutures if necessary (Fig. 13.13).

Checklist

1 Examine the lesser omentum, lesser curve of stomach, lower oesophagus and upper lesser sac for signs of damage or bleeding. Have the short gastric vessels or spleen been damaged?

2 Re-examine the lower oesophagus for the presence of persistent vagal fibres and for signs of damage to the muscular coat. Re-examine the incisura angularis, where vagal fibres to the parietal cell mass may also have escaped detection. Finally, look again at the gastric lesser curve to ensure there is no damage. Ensure that 5–6 cm of distal stomach remains innervated.

PYLOROPLASTY

Appraise

1 Re-formation of the pylorus has the effect of increasing the size of the lumen and also destroys the pyloric sphincteric metering function. It can be used to overcome stricture of the pylorus and also to improve gastric emptying following truncal vagotomy. Following proximal gastric vagotomy, the distal stomach or 'antral mill' remains innervated so that gastric emptying is not usually prejudiced and pyloroplasty is not required.

2 Pyloroplasty is simple to perform in most circumstances and has enjoyed great popularity as an adjunctive operation with truncal vagotomy for duodenal ulcer. It may be difficult to perform if the duodenum is very scarred and adherent to the pancreas and the structures in the free edge of the lesser omentum if the abdomen is obese and deep.

3 It is probable that many postvagotomy symptoms are attributable to the drainage procedure and not to the vagotomy. Many such patients are improved if the drainage procedure is reversed.

Although the pylorus can be anatomically restored to normal, the long-term results are not impressive.

4 Inevitably a number of methods of performing pyloroplasty have been described. The Heineke–Mikulicz method is the simplest, but some surgeons favour the Finney pyloroplasty.

5 The use of pyloroplasty or pyloromyotomy to facilitate gastric emptying following transection of the cardia for oesophagectomy is controversial. Some surgeons perform it only if there is evidence of stenosis (see Ch. 11). In the event of delayed gastric emptying they give cisapride 10 mg t.d.s. orally or metoclopramide 5–10 mg intravenously, and balloon dilatation of the pylorus under radiological control; they reserve re-operation for patients in whom these methods fail. The experience of other surgeons gives less cause for optimism so they routinely perform pyloroplasty or pyloromyotomy to circumvent gastric delay.

HEINEKE–MIKULICZ PYLOROPLASTY

Access

Gently mobilize the pyloroduodenal region by Kocher's manoeuvre and place a large pack behind the upper duodenal loop to bring it forwards in the wound.

Action

1 Make a longitudinal incision through all coats starting on the anterior wall of the duodenal bulb, carried through the pylorus and on to the anterior gastric antral wall (Fig. 13.14). Centre the incision, 4–5 cm long, on the narrowest part of the pyloroduodenal canal. If there is an active anterior ulcer, encircle it so that a lozenge-shaped segment of anterior pyloroduodenal wall is excised, containing the ulcer. This 'pylorectomy' was described by Judd.

2 Aspirate the contents and inspect the interior of the distal stomach and proximal duodenum. Sometimes there is a mucosal diaphragm with no evidence of ulcer in patients with typical features of pyloric stenosis in whom an endoscope would not pass. If a diaphragm is suspected, start the incision on the anterior antral wall 3–4 cm proximal to the pylorus and inspect the interior before cutting through the pyloric ring. Make sure there is not a second narrow duodenal segment distal to the pyloroplasty as may develop in postbulbar duodenal ulceration.

3 Gently apply tissue forceps to the middle of the upper and lower cut edges and draw them apart, allowing the proximal and distal limits of the incision to come together, transforming the longitudinal cut into a transverse slit.

4 Close the incision, starting from the upper tissue forceps and ending at the lower forceps. Three methods are possible. The traditional technique is to insert an invaginating continuous all-coats layer reinforced with a second seromuscular layer of sutures. The invaginated edges temporarily produce some hold-up and many surgeons insert a single layer of all-coats sutures placed closely together, uniting the walls edge-to-edge without invagination. In the last few years stapling devices have gained popularity. Place a single straight stapler along the edges as they are held in their new position, with the opposed edges everted. Close and activate the stapler. Cut off the excess tissue with a scalpel blade held in contact with the upper surface of the stapler, which is then removed. Insert a reinforcing layer of seromuscular stitches if desired.

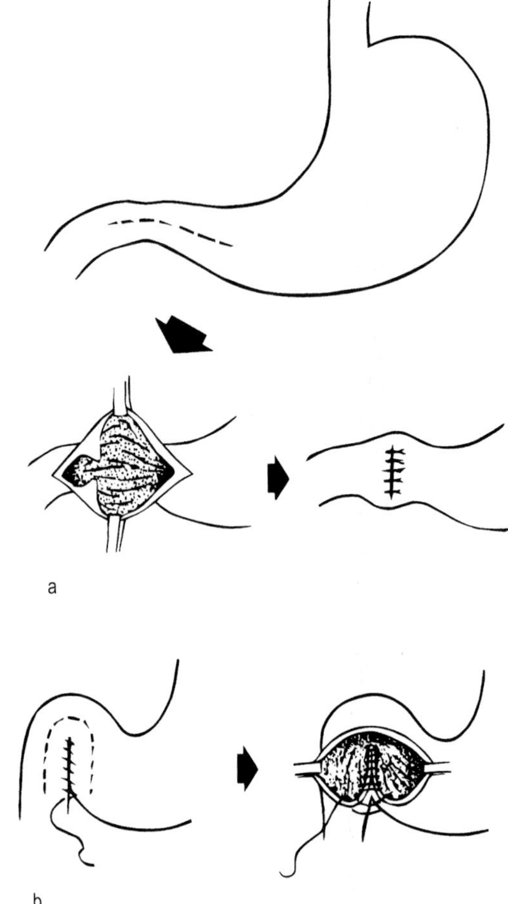

Fig. 13.14 Pyloroplasty: (a) Heineke–Mikulicz; (b) Finney.

FINNEY PYLOROPLASTY

Appraise

Advocates claim that this produces a wider lumen than the Heineke–Mikulicz pyloroplasty. Of course the lumen size depends to some extent on the length of the incision. The Finney technique merely represents a generously fashioned Heineke–Mikulicz pyloroplasty with the inferior 'dog ear' pushed in.

Action

1 Gently mobilize the duodenal loop by Kocher's manoeuvre so the descending duodenum can be laid alongside the greater curve part of the gastric antrum.

2 Unite the adjacent gastric and duodenal walls with a seromuscular stitch, from above downwards, closing the angle below the pylorus.

3 Incise the full thickness of the stomach, pylorus and duodenum along an inverted horseshoe-shaped line which runs from the gastric antrum 4–5 cm proximal to the pyloric ring, through the pylorus, curving through the duodenal bulb and down the descending duodenum.

4 Starting at the pylorus, unite with an all-coats stitch the adjacent walls of the stomach and duodenum. Continue the stitches round the lower limits of the incisions to unite the right duodenal cut edge to the left gastric cut edge, using an invaginating stitch.

5 Continue the seromuscular stitch to cover the anterior all-coats suture line.

DUODENOPLASTY

Appraise

1 The advent of proximal gastric vagotomy removed the need to perform an adjunctive drainage operation in the majority of patients with duodenal ulcer since in modern times most patients with incipient pyloric stenosis are operated upon before it becomes severe.

2 Even if pyloroplasty is necessary there are advantages in performing proximal gastric vagotomy. If truncal vagotomy is performed, gallbladder dilatation results and there is an increased risk of gallstones; loss of vagal supply to the pancreas reduces its exocrine secretion and there is a significantly increased risk of severe diarrhoea following truncal vagotomy. In some patients, stenosis is distal to the pylorus and can be overcome without damaging the sphincteric mechanism. This is particularly true when the patient has postbulbar duodenal ulceration. Proximal gastric vagotomy can then be justified.

Action

1 Mobilize the pyloroduodenal region by Kocher's manoeuvre and confirm that the pyloric ring itself is widely patent by invaginating the anterior antral wall through it on an index finger. The site of stenosis should have been determined before operation but this is not always easy to assess.

2 Make a longitudinal incision through the anterior duodenal wall, stopping short of the pyloric ring (Fig. 13.15). This needs to be only about 1.5–2 cm long. If the ulcer and stenosis are postbulbar remember that the distortion may draw the ampulla out of its normal place, exposing it to inadvertent damage.

3 Gently apply tissue forceps to the middle of each cut edge and separate them to produce a transverse slit.

4 Close the slit transversely. Insert a single layer of closely applied stitches, bringing the edges together without inversion.

GASTRODUODENOSTOMY

Appraise

- This resembles the Finney pyloroplasty but does not include division of the pyloric ring.

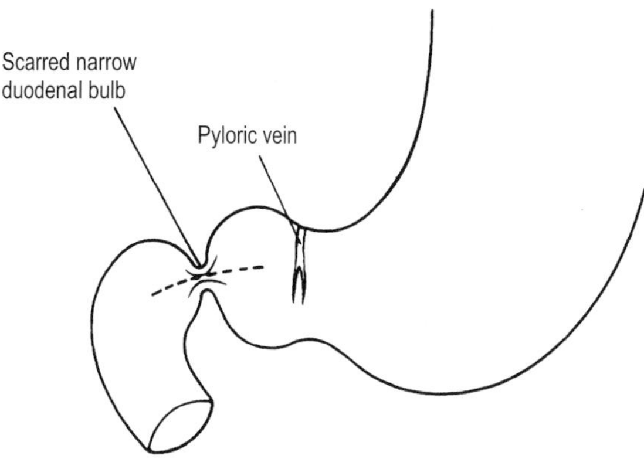

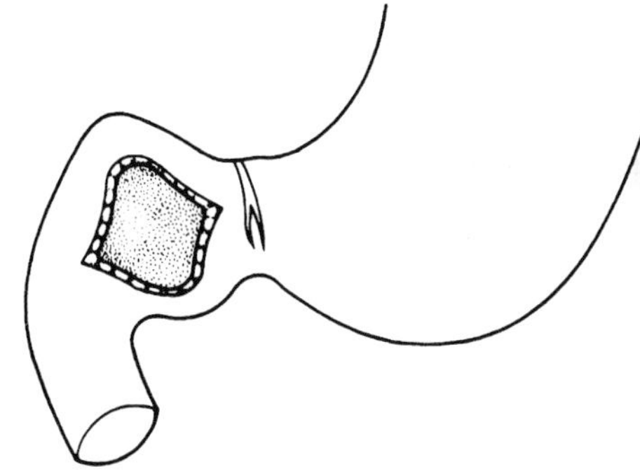

Fig. 13.15 Duodenoplasty.

- It is an alternative method to pyloroplasty or gastroenterostomy for overcoming pyloric obstruction and may be appropriate if the descending duodenum has been opened. It is seldom used.

Action

1 Mobilize the descending duodenum by Kocher's manoeuvre and join the descending duodenum to the anterior wall of the distal stomach with a running seromuscular stitch.

2 Incise the descending duodenum and anterior gastric walls for 5 cm, parallel and close to each side of the seromuscular stitch. Aspirate the contents and inspect the interior (Fig. 13.16).

3 Join the adjacent gastric and duodenal walls with a continuous all-coats stitch, carrying this round on to the anterior walls as an invaginating stitch to encircle the anastomosis.

4 Continue the seromuscular stitch onto the anterior wall to bury the all-coats stitch and complete the two-layer anastomosis.

5 The anastomosis can be accomplished using a stapling device that will insert four linear rows of staples and incise in the same line between the inner rows of staples. Bring the stomach and duodenum together with a posterior seromuscular stitch. Make a stab hole in the stomach and the duodenum at the lower limit of the intended anastomosis. Pass in the separated limbs of the stapler, one into each hole, with the points towards the pylorus. Lock the limbs together so they lie just anterior to the seromuscular stitch line with no extraneous tissues intervening. Actuate the stapler to insert the rows of staples and cut between the middle rows. Unlock the staples, withdraw the limbs,

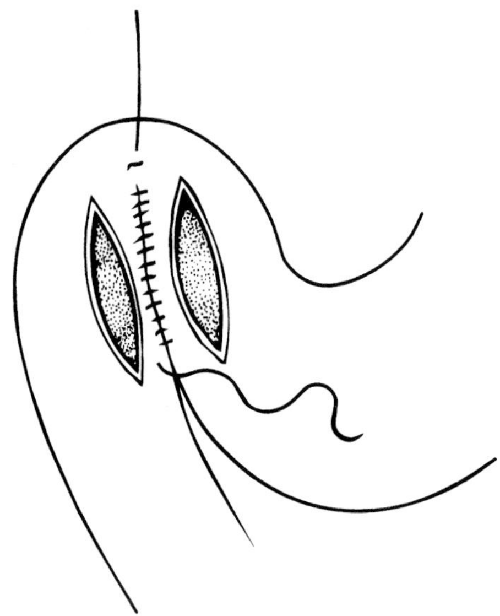

Fig. 13.16 Incisions for gastroduodenostomy.

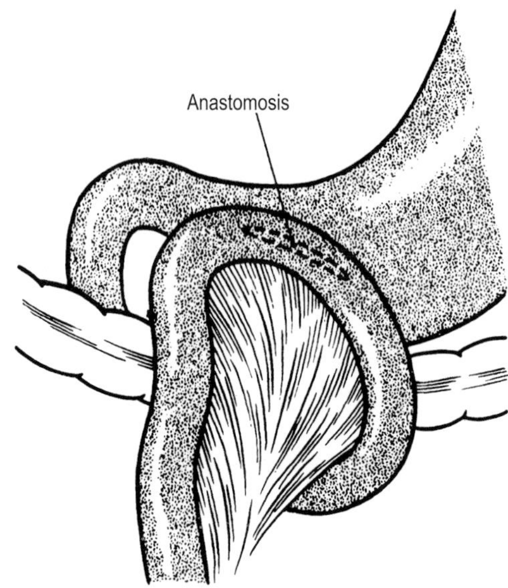

Fig. 13.17 Juxtapyloric anterior gastroenterostomy.

inspect the completeness of the union and pick up the extremities of the staple lines through the stab wounds, which are now united, with tissue forceps. Separate the tissue forceps to draw the defect into an everted slit. Close the defect with sutures or a linear stapler. Check the integrity of the anastomosis and if desired continue the seromuscular stitch from the posterior suture line to bury the anterior stapled line.

GASTROENTEROSTOMY

Appraise

1 Gastroenterostomy was originally applied to the relief of pyloric obstruction from distal gastric carcinoma. It offers an important method of relief when gastrectomy cannot be carried out because the growth is locally too extensive or has already metastasized. Always place the gastroenterostomy as high on the stomach as possible to guard against the stoma becoming obstructed by advancing growth. However, always prefer an exclusion gastrectomy if this is possible because high gastroenterostomy often fails to drain the stomach and may provoke bilious vomiting.

2 Gastroenterostomy was used for the relief of benign pyloric stenosis from duodenal ulceration, but in the absence of stenosis it diverts some of the acid away from the ulcer, which usually heals. A proportion of patients eventually develop an ulcer at the stoma although this may be delayed for many years. An advantage is that if the patient subsequently has postprandial symptoms from the drainage operation, it can be taken down quite simply provided that the pyloroduodenal canal is adequate. Gastroenterostomy for duodenal ulcer is placed as close to the pylorus as possible.

3 Gastroenterostomy may be used as a bypass in the presence of duodenal ileus or fistula. For many years surgeons argued about the merits of different techniques for gastroenterostomy. As a general rule surgeons now use only anterior juxtapyloric gastroenterostomy for benign disease (Fig. 13.17); this will be described in detail with a note on the previously very popular posterior gastroenterostomy.

Access

Use a right upper paramedian or midline incision 15 cm long.

Assess

1 Explore the abdomen.

2 If the patient proves to have extensive and inoperable carcinoma with no evidence of impending distal obstruction, carry out limited exploration only, but take a biopsy specimen.

Action

Suture technique

1 Pick up a longitudinal fold of anterior gastric wall and grasp it with one of Lane's twin clamps. Choose a fold as close to the pylorus as possible if this is for benign pyloric obstruction or accompanies vagotomy for ulcer. Choose a fold as high as possible if this is to bypass an unresectable distal gastric carcinoma.

2 Lift up the greater omentum and transverse colon to identify the duodenojejunal junction. Draw the first loop of jejunum up over the colon and greater omentum to the stomach, with the short but not taut afferent loop against the proximal part of the clamped gastric fold and the efferent loop against the distal end of the fold. Place the second twin clamp along the apposed bowel, avoiding the mesentery, to occlude the lumen but not the blood supply. Lock the clamps together.

3 Unite the adjacent gastric and jejunal walls with a running seromuscular stitch on an eyeless needle. Leave the ends long so that the stitch can be continued to encircle the anastomosis.

4 Open the stomach and jejunum parallel to the seromuscular stitch and 0.5 cm from it on each side, for 4–6 cm if this is for benign disease and for as long as possible if it is to bypass malignant obstruction.

5 Apply fresh drapes to isolate the area and keep separate instruments during the next part of the operation when the potentially infected interior of the bowel will be exposed.

6 Unite the adjacent gastric and jejunal walls with a running all-coats stitch. Carry the stitch round the corner on to the anterior wall to complete the anastomosis. As the anterior gastric and jejunal walls are brought together, invert the edges. A Connell mattress stitch may be used as an alternative to the simple over-and-over stitch but take care that the blood vessels are picked up and tied along the edges since the Connell stitch is not haemostatic.

7 Remove the twin clamps, discard and take sterile replacements for the soiled towels, instruments and gloves.

8 Carry the seromuscular stitch round the end on to the anterior wall and complete it to encircle the anastomosis, burying the all-coats stitch.

Checklist

1 Examine the anastomosis and make sure it is patent.

2 Make sure there is no tension on the loop of jejunum. Draw the transverse colon and greater omentum to the right so there is no weight of bowel to drag on the anastomosis.

? DIFFICULTY

1. The duodenum may be bound down in patients with severe duodenal ulcer. It is then difficult to make a juxtapyloric anastomosis. Make a more proximal, safe and easy anastomosis.
2. It may be difficult to draw down sufficient proximal stomach to make a high anastomosis as a palliative bypass operation for obstructing distal carcinoma. Do not hesitate to enlarge the incision and abandon clamps if they are difficult to apply.

Staple technique

1 The anastomosis can be fashioned using a linear-cutter stapling device. Draw the jejunum up to the stomach and attach it along the proposed line of the anastomosis with a seromuscular stitch at each end. Make stab wounds in the stomach and the jejunum close to the stitch uniting the afferent jejunal loop to the proximal stomach.

2 Insert a sucker to empty the gastric and jejunal contents.

3 Separate the two halves of the stapler and insert one blade into each of the stab wounds, pointing towards the distally placed stitch. Lock the blades together, taking care not to include extraneous tissue.

4 Actuate the device to insert four parallel rows of staples and cut between the central rows, forming an anastomosis between stomach and jejunum. Unlock the blades and withdraw them.

5 Inspect the anastomosis all round from within and without, inserting sutures to reinforce doubtful areas. Pick up the ends of the staple lines on each side of the defect and draw them apart to create a linear slit. Apply a linear stapling device along the everted edges of the defect, close the device and actuate it to seal the edges.

6 Remove the device and examine the anastomosis to ensure it is perfect, inserting further stitches if necessary.

7 Alternatively close the defect with sutures.

Checklist

1 Is the anastomosis intact and patent?

2 Ensure that there is no tension on the loop of jejunum. Draw the transverse colon and greater omentum to the right so there is no weight of bowel to drag on the anastomosis.

Technical points

- Suture material and stitches vary from surgeon to surgeon. I have described a sutured anastomosis using two layers of continuous absorbable stitches. A single all-coats stitch is also quite adequate. Many surgeons insert interrupted non-absorbable stitches such as silk on the outer, seromuscular layer. It is not the material or type of stitch but the care with which they are inserted that determines whether the patient will recover without complications.
- The use of non-crushing clamps is argued about by surgeons. Certainly many successful surgeons use them routinely when they can be conveniently applied to prevent the leakage of bowel content into the wound, and to hold the stomach and bowel perfectly apposed while the anastomosis is fashioned. If you use clamps, apply them to the bowel only and not across the mesentery. Apply them sufficiently firmly to occlude the arteries as well as the veins, otherwise the bowel becomes congested and oedematous.

POSTERIOR GASTROENTEROSTOMY

1 This method was used with success for many years. From time to time it offers a convenient way of fashioning the anastomosis for benign disease. It cannot be used conveniently for high gastroenterostomy to relieve malignant distal gastric obstruction.

2 Hold up the greater omentum and transverse colon in order to inspect the mesocolon. Identify the middle colic vessels and make a conveniently placed vertical hole through the mesocolon to one or other side of them, 5–7 cm long.

3 Identify the posterior wall of the stomach through the hole and draw it down. Select a dependent and distal part of the stomach.

4 Apply the twin clamps to the protruding part of the stomach and to the first loop of jejunum beyond the ligament of Treitz. Lock the clamps and carry out the anastomosis.

5 Suture the margins of the cut mesocolon to the stomach to prevent small bowel loops from slipping through into the lesser sac and becoming obstructed.

BILLROTH I PARTIAL GASTRECTOMY

Appraise

- Billroth I gastrectomy was originally used to resect distal gastric carcinoma in Frau Heller on 29 January 1881, by Theodore

Billroth (1829–1894) in Vienna. The size of the anastomosis between the proximal gastric stump and the duodenum is restricted to the diameter of the duodenal lumen and if the cancer recurs there is a risk of anastomotic obstruction. In the union of stomach to jejunum following gastrojejunostomy in the Billroth II or Polya gastrectomy the whole width of the cut end of the proximal gastric stump can be used and is at less risk of obstruction, so it has replaced the Billroth I operation.

- In its developed form the lesser curve of the proximal gastric stump is excised with closure to form a new lesser curve to match the duodenal lumen. It has an advantage that a proximal gastric ulcer can be included in the tongue of excised lesser curve. However, effective non-surgical treatment of gastric ulcers reduces the need for operation and, if it is needed, Polya gastrectomy is suitable.

POLYA PARTIAL GASTRECTOMY

Appraise

- At an emergency operation for bleeding peptic ulcer the most certain procedure is excision of the ulcer-bearing area. If the ulcer is duodenal then Polya gastrectomy with closure of the ulcer-bearing area duodenum gives good results if the main end-point is prevention of re-bleeding. However, the operative mortality is twice that following vagotomy with under-running of the bleeding vessel, and the side-effects and late sequelae may be more severe. Consequently, the most frequently performed procedure is vagotomy with pylorotomy following under-running the ulcer with non-absorbable stitches. Erosive bleeding rarely demands operation but multiple haemorrhages can be dealt with only by excision of the affected gastric wall by gastrectomy. Fortunately such bleeding is usually from the distal stomach.
- The most frequent indication for gastrectomy is distal gastric carcinoma. Polya gastrectomy allows the creation of a stoma the full width of the stomach and is thus unlikely to become obstructed if the tumour recurs. Since the duodenum is closed, this isolates it from distal spread as may occur if gastroduodenal anastomosis is used. The preferred method of resecting distal gastric carcinoma is by radical subtotal gastrectomy with Polya or Roux-en-Y reconstruction.

Access

Make a midline incision that skirts the umbilicus, extending downwards from the xiphoid process for 20 cm. Ligate and divide the ligamentum teres and divide the falciform ligament.

Assess

1 Explore the whole abdomen. If the operation is for carcinoma, start in the pelvis and lower abdomen, para-aortic region and root of the mesentery, proceeding to the liver before touching the stomach in order to avoid carrying malignant cells around the peritoneal cavity.

2 Carefully examine the stomach and duodenum to confirm the diagnosis and assess the strategy of the operation. If necessary, open the lesser omentum or gastrocolic omentum to examine the posterior wall of the stomach and contents of the lesser sac, including the glands around the coeliac axis and along the superior border of the pancreas.

Resect

Benign disease

1 Make a hole in an avascular area of the gastrocolic omentum to the left of the gastroepiploic vascular arch. Identify the posterior gastric wall and separate it from the pancreas and transverse mesocolon.

2 Clamp in sections, divide and ligate the gastrocolic omentum, extending on the left up to and including the main left gastroepiploic vessels and the first one or two short gastric vessels. Avoid damaging the spleen directly or by exerting heavy traction on the stomach. To the right, divide and ligate the main right gastroepiploic vessels as they lie near the inferior border of the pylorus. The separation of this vascular tissue can be accomplished rapidly using a stapling device which places two clips across the tissue and cuts between them in a single action.

KEY POINT Inadvertent vascular damage

- Identify to avoid damaging the middle colic vessels, which lie within 1 cm of the right gastroepiploic vessels.

3 Clamp, divide and ligate the right gastric vessels after identifying and isolating them as they run to the left in the lesser omentum just above the duodenal bulb and pylorus. Divide the lesser omentum proximally, if possible preserving an accessory hepatic artery if one is present.

4 Free the first 1–2 cm of duodenum after applying fine artery forceps on the small vessels posteriorly, dividing and ligating them with fine ligatures. Divide with a linear stapler or Payr's clamp across the duodenum just beyond the pylorus. Place a second clamp just proximal to this to occlude the stomach. If there is insufficient room for this, apply a non-crushing clamp across the distal stomach. Transect the duodenum just above the distal Payr clamp, ensuring that no gastric mucosa remains attached to the duodenum. Cover the cut distal stomach with a swab.

5 Dissect the duodenum free for 2–3 cm so that it can be safely closed, applying fine forceps and ligatures to the vessels, keeping close to the duodenal wall.

KEY POINTS Distorted anatomy?

- The common bile duct lies near the posterior and superior parts of the proximal duodenum and may be drawn out of its normal relationship by scar tissue.
- The gastroduodenal artery runs close to the medial wall of the duodenum.

6 Close the duodenal stump as a rule using a linear stapling device. This places a double row of staples across the duodenum. Apply

it just distal to the pylorus in place of the Payr's crushing clamp and place a proximal clamp across the distal stomach. Activate the stapling device to staple and seal the duodenum and transect this with a scalpel applied closely to the upper edge of the stapler. Alternatively, close the distal stomach and duodenal stump with GIA staplers. It is wise to invaginate or reinforce the everted staple line with a layer of sutures.

7 Alternatively close the duodenal stump with sutures. First use a running over-and-over spiral stitch that encircles the clamp and the enclosed crushed duodenum. Gently ease out the clamp, tightening the stitches seriatim as it is withdrawn. Tie the stitch. Insert a second invaginating seromuscular suture to cover the first stitch line or insert a purse-string suture and invaginate the first suture line as it is tightened and tied. If possible, insert a third stitch that picks up and draws together the ligated right gastric and right gastroepiploic vessel stumps, the anterior duodenal wall and the peritoneum over the head of the pancreas.

8 Exert a little tension on the left gastric vessels by elevating the pyloric end of the stomach. Identify the artery by feeling for the pulsations. Isolate the vessels from the lesser curve of the stomach, doubly clamp, divide and ligate them.

9 Select the line for the transection of the stomach (Fig. 13.18). When Polya gastrectomy was the standard operation for duodenal ulcer, a two-thirds gastrectomy was usually carried out.

10 Ask the anaesthetist to withdraw the nasogastric tube until the tip lies above the line of transection.

Malignant disease

1 Radical subtotal gastrectomy is described later, but non-radical partial gastrectomy is appropriate in frail patients and in those who have a resectable carcinoma but already have metastatic deposits in the liver or elsewhere which make radical resection impossible.

2 It may not be possible to be sure that the distal resection is clear of growth but always ensure that the proximal line of resection is well clear of growth. Aim at a minimum of 5 cm apparently tumour-free margin. If the resection line cuts through tumour, the anastomotic line may break down during recovery from the operation. If it does not do so, recurrent tumour at the anastomosis may soon obstruct the lumen.

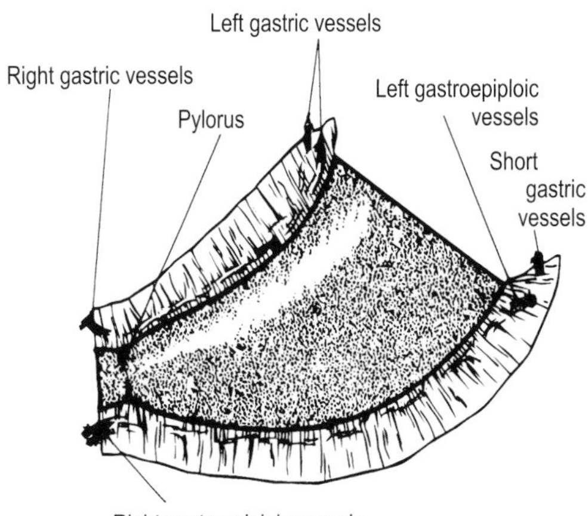

Fig. 13.18 Polya partial gastrectomy. The removed specimen.

3 It is useless to carry the line of resection widely beyond the stomach, so adopt the same technique as for resection for benign disease.

4 Plan to provide a full-width gastroenterostomy to guard against recurrent tumour causing obstruction.

Unite

Staples

1 The gastroenterostomy can be accomplished using stapling devices. Place and actuate a long straight stapling device across the stomach at the proposed line of section and cut off the distal gastric specimen with a scalpel run along the distal edge of the stapler. Remove the stapler.

2 Bring up a proximal loop of jejunum and suture it to the posterior wall of the stomach 5 cm above the staple line, placing a seromuscular stitch at each end, with the afferent loop to the lesser curve, the efferent loop to the greater curve. Make a stab wound in the greater curve aspect of the posterior wall of the stomach 2 cm proximal to the staple line and make a matching stab wound in the jejunum at the origin of the efferent loop.

3 Insert the two limbs of the stapler separately into the holes, with the tips pointing to the lesser curve. Ensure that there is no interposed tissue, lock the two limbs together and actuate the instrument. Four lines of staples will have united stomach to jejunum and the knife will have cut a stoma between the centre rows of staples. Unlock and withdraw the stapler.

4 Carefully check that the staple lines are perfect. Place tissue forceps at the ends of the inner and outer staple lines and separate the forceps to create an everted linear defect in the anastomosis. Place a short straight stapler across the everted lips of the defect, tighten and actuate it. Cut off the excess tissue, remove the stapler and check the line of closure carefully, if necessary reinforcing the whole anastomosis all round with sutures.

Sutured

1 Place one of the twin gastroenterostomy clamps across the stomach 2 cm above the proposed line of transection, from greater to lesser curve. Place a long non-crushing clamp across the stomach 3 cm distal to the twin clamp and parallel to it. The stomach will be transected just above this clamp.

2 Fold the distal part of the stomach upwards. Reach down and identify the duodenojejunal junction. Draw up to the stomach the first loop of jejunum, with afferent loop to lesser curve with no slack but not tight. The efferent loop is placed at the greater curve. Place the second of the twin clamps across this loop of bowel, occluding only the lumen and not the mesentery. Marry and lock the clamps together.

3 Run a continuous seromuscular stitch to unite the adjacent gastric and jejunal walls.

4 Incise the full width of the posterior gastric wall 0.5 cm above the clamp, taking care at this time to leave the anterior wall intact. Make a parallel incision in the jejunum, 0.5 cm from the seromuscular suture line. Join the adjacent gastric and jejunal edges with an all-coats stitch on an eyeless needle.

5 Now cut through the anterior wall of the stomach 1 cm distal to the clamp and remove the specimen of distal stomach.

Continue the all-coats stitch round on to the anterior wall and along it to completely encircle the anastomosis.

6 Remove the clamps, discard and take sterile replacements of the towels, gloves and instruments. Complete the seromuscular suture line onto the anterior wall to encircle the anastomosis.

Valved anastomosis

1 When performing gastrectomy for benign disease it is conventional to close the lesser curve half of the stomach and form a small stoma between the greater curve half of the stomach and the jejunum. This is referred to as a valved anastomosis (Fig. 13.19).

2 A different technique is used after uniting the stomach and jejunum in the twin clamps and with the posterior seromuscular stitch. Have the distal stomach held vertically and place halfway across it from the lesser curve, and 1 cm distal to the twin clamp, a short Payr's crushing clamp. Cut halfway across the stomach just distal to the Payr clamp, transecting the lesser curve half of the stomach. Oversew the clamp and contained crushed stomach edge with a running loose spiral stitch. Release and gently withdraw the clamp as the sutures are tightened seriatim. This manoeuvre leaves just the greater curve half of the stomach to be united to a matched hole made in the jejunum. The anastomosis is accomplished in a similar manner to the creation of a full-width stoma.

3 After the gloves, towels and instruments have been replaced, continue the posterior seromuscular stitch round and along the anterior wall to encircle the stoma and closed lesser curve.

Technical points

1 The inside of the stomach and bowel are infected with microorganisms. While fashioning anastomoses, isolate the interior of the bowel from the peritoneal cavity and wound edges by using separate towels, instruments and gloves. When the bowel is repaired, discard and replace them with sterile gloves, towels and instruments.

2 Retrocolic anastomosis may be fashioned following gastrectomy but it does not confer any benefits over the antecolic anastomosis.

3 Some surgeons avoid the use of clamps during the fashioning of gastric anastomoses. There is no evidence that clamps damage the bowel. However, every surgeon has firm ideas on techniques and should respect the convictions of others, especially when they are based on scientific evidence.

? DIFFICULTY 13.4

1. It may be difficult and hazardous to dissect out and close the duodenum in the presence of extensive scarring and distortion from chronic severe duodenal ulceration. There are alternative techniques available. If for some reason you are committed to closing the duodenum, then an alternative is to transect the gastric antrum, dissect out and excise the antral mucosa and close the cut edge of duodenal mucosa, leaving raw antral seromuscularis. Now close this using a series of internal purse-string sutures.
2. If you have committed yourself to dissecting out and closing the duodenum and now find yourself in difficulty, carefully stick close to the duodenal wall. If you encounter a large ulcer crater, this cannot be mobilized to help close the duodenum. There are three choices. The best choice is to carefully pinch off the duodenum just at the distal ulcer edge and carefully mobilize a sufficient cuff of duodenum beyond to close safely, leaving the ulcer crater undisturbed. The second choice is to leave the duodenum attached to the ulcer and mobilize the anterolateral duodenal wall so that it can be sewn down to the distal fibrotic edge of the ulcer crater, thus closing off the duodenum. If neither of these is possible or can be safely accomplished, then do not try to close the duodenum. Sew in a large tube and bring this to the surface of the abdomen. Leave it attached to a closed drainage system for 10 days and, if the patient is well, gradually withdraw it. The duodenal fistula will heal spontaneously provided there is no distal obstruction or adynamic ileus. Even if it does not to do so, the track is so well established that there will be no intra-abdominal complications of the manoeuvre.
3. *Is it difficult to mobilize the proximal stomach?* The spleen may be adherent to the diaphragm and the costal margin may be narrow in an obese patient. Make sure the stomach is not adherent posteriorly through adhesions or a previously unsuspected gastric ulcer; if it is, pinch off the ulcer and, if necessary, temporarily close the defect with sutures, and include the ulcer in the gastrectomy specimen.
4. In time of difficulty make sure that the light, the exposure and the assistance are all optimal.
5. *Bleeding?* Avoid panic measures. Control severe bleeding with local pressure while preparing to pick up the bleeding point accurately with artery forceps. Do not tie blood vessels together with large pieces of omentum or mesentery. The blood vessel may retract and quietly bleed into the closed mesentery. If the splenic capsule is torn, try to preserve the spleen by suture repair or packing with Surgicel. Splenectomy is undesirable because of the thrombotic, infective and immunological complications (but see Ch. 23).
6. *Damage to the common bile duct?* Correct it now, or call upon a more experienced person to do so. Ensure that you have available radiography to help in elucidating the damage. Repair the injured duct as you would at a routine biliary operation and plan to leave a 'T-tube' drain in the common duct to drain the biliary tract temporarily. Immediate and perfect repair of bile duct injuries ensures minimal disability. Missed or imperfectly repaired injuries seriously threaten the patient's life or well-being.

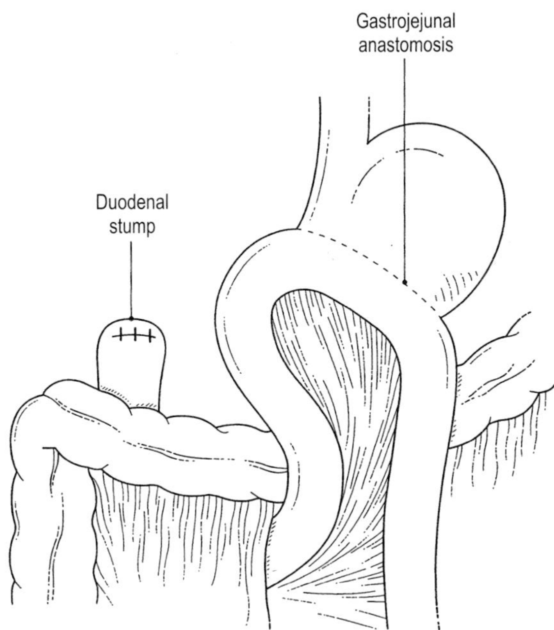

Fig. 13.19 Polya partial gastrectomy. The antecolic valved gastrojejunal anastomosis, with afferent loop joined to lesser curve, is complete. The duodenal stump is closed.

Checklist

1 Examine the anastomosis. See that it is perfectly fashioned and intact. If necessary insert extra sutures. Ensure that you can invaginate the gastric and jejunal walls through the stoma.

2 Check each of the main vascular ligatures. Re-tie them if they are insecure.

3 Check the spleen. Aspirate all the blood from under the left cupola of the diaphragm and re-check it just before closing the abdomen to ensure that there has been no further collection of blood.

4 Make sure the duodenal stump is safely closed. Should you leave a drain down to it? If so, does this replace careful technique and should you therefore re-close the duodenum or reinforce the closure?

5 Examine the colon to ensure there is no damage to it, or the mesocolon or middle colic vessels. Draw the greater omentum, transverse colon and mesocolon through to the right so there is no weight of colon resting on the anastomosis.

6 Aspirate any blood from under the right cupola of the diaphragm, from under the liver and in the right prerenal pouch. Finally, aspirate any blood that has collected in the pelvis.

GASTRODUODENAL BLEEDING

Appraise

1 Bleeding is the most life-threatening complication of peptic ulcer. Its management is best carried out by experienced clinicians, endoscopists and surgeons acting as a team. Dedicated units achieve much better survival than those undertaking it as part of a general service.

2 Erosive bleeding sometimes complicates bleeding elsewhere, sepsis, burns, head injury and major trauma. Drugs such as steroids and NSAIDs can cause erosive bleeding or be associated with ulcer bleeding. Alcohol causes acute gastritis with bleeding from this or, following retching, Mallory–Weiss tears around the cardia. For this reason take a careful history, asking specific questions about drugs.

3 Assess the patient's general condition so that you can carry out appropriate resuscitation. Check the blood haemoglobin and haematocrit, and exclude clotting deficiencies if suspected. In appropriate circumstances have blood cross-matched. Routinely give intravenous omeprazole or an equivalent proton-pump inhibitor.

4 Do not make a once-and-for-all assessment but carefully monitor the patient thereafter. Remember that mortality is highest among the over-60s, those with massive haemorrhage and shock, and those with serious associated disease.

KEY POINT Decision-making

- Remember that more than 80% of gastrointestinal bleeding stops spontaneously, but also remember that you do not know which 80%.

5 Carry out endoscopy as soon as possible to determine the cause, site, state and number of lesions. Look for continuing bleeding and the presence of visible vessels which indicate that the bleeding is likely to continue or recur. Even if you cannot identify the source you can usually exonerate particular areas, for example excluding oesophageal varices.

6 If you are expert in their use, have available instruments to control bleeding through the endoscope. These include the Nd-YAG laser, heater probes and diathermy together with needles for injecting adrenaline (epinephrine), ethanol or polidocanol through the biopsy channel. Other methods that are under trial include application or injection of cryoprecipitate or thrombin to induce clotting, the adhesive trifluoroisopropylcyanoacrylate to seal the vessel, and endoscopic clipping or suturing of vessels. Combinations of these methods are proving effective. Haemostatic substances can be injected in association with local application of heat. They should be the first line of treatment in most patients. They may be repeated if re-bleeding occurs.

7 For this reason, if you are inexperienced or do not have the equipment available, call in an expert or be willing to transfer the patient rather than operate precipitately. Surgery produces its own immediate and long-term complications. Inexpert and ineffective surgery is disastrous.

8 The origin of obscure recurrent upper gastrointestinal bleeding can sometimes be elucidated by injecting radioisotope-labelled red cells into the circulation with gamma-camera monitoring of leakage into the gut. Most surgeons would now opt for angiography carried out during bleeding episodes. In appropriate circumstances the radiologist may be able to embolize the feeding vessel.

9 Relative indications for operation when other methods of control have failed remain:

- Continuing bleeding which fails to respond to other measures.
- Bleeding that recurs.
- Patient more than 60 years old.
- Gastric ulcer bleeding.
- Cardiovascular disease patients, who do not withstand hypotension well. This makes it dangerous to defer operation if bleeding is serious and not controllable.

KEY POINTS Interoperative endoscopy

- Always have an endoscope available in the operating theatre, even when the diagnosis seems certain.
- When the patient is anaesthetized, be willing, in case of doubt, to perform endoscopy

10 Although exploratory laparotomy allows access to the abdomen, the exterior of the gut is exposed, not the interior, where the cause lies. Do not embark on surgery for upper gastrointestinal bleeding alone if there is someone more experienced available. Eschew the temptation to carry out 'blind' gastrectomy if you cannot identify the cause of bleeding. This merely confuses the problem while risking the possible complications.

Access

Make a generous upper abdominal paramedian or midline incision skirting the umbilicus, 20–25 cm long. Ligate and divide the ligamentum teres and incise the falciform ligament.

Assess

1 As the abdomen is opened, blood which appears bluish through the bowel wall may be seen in the small or large bowel. Dilated and congested veins on the viscera with a stiff cirrhotic liver make portal venous hypertension obvious. Scarring and oedema of the stomach or duodenum may indicate the site of bleeding.

KEY POINT Multiple sites

- Do not assume there is a single cause.

2 Remember that, in Britain, most upper gastrointestinal bleeds requiring emergency surgery are from peptic ulceration or erosions, but also remember that there are sometimes multiple causes and the detection of a possible site does not exclude the possibility of other causes. Therefore carry out a thorough check of the lower oesophagus, stomach and duodenum, remembering that there may be an unsuspected lesion in the small or large bowel.

3 If no cause is detected and there is no site of active bleeding, do not hesitate to repeat the endoscopy yourself or ask an experienced colleague to do so. It may be valuable first to have a large-bore gastric tube passed so that the stomach can be washed out if it contains blood or retained food.

4 Alternatively, but often less satisfactorily, perform gastrotomy or gastroduodenotomy. Make an incision through the anterior gastric wall midway between the greater and lesser curves in the distal stomach, carrying this through the pylorus into the anterior duodenal wall for 2–3 cm if necessary. Aspirate the gastric contents. Insert large-bladed retractors for your assistants, have the light adjusted to shine into the stomach and carefully examine the interior of the stomach and if necessary the duodenal bulb, seeking the cause of bleeding. Sometimes the gastric wall can be evaginated through the gastric wound to allow close inspection. If the pylorus has not been incised it is often possible to insert thin-bladed retractors through it to view the duodenal bulb, or a cystoscope may be passed, offering excellent views of the bulb.

5 Do not carry out a procedure unless the cause is found. 'Blind' gastrectomy was once recommended but this merely confuses the problem and adds to the patient's risk. Make a thorough examination of the whole gastrointestinal tract including structures that could produce bleeding into it, such as the biliary tract. If there is no active bleeding and no cause is found, close the abdomen and determine to repeat the endoscopy at the first sign of re-bleeding, followed if necessary by other methods of detection and isolation of bleeding sites.

Action

1 Bleeding duodenal ulcer is preferably treated at present by pyloroplasty or duodenotomy, and suture of the bleeding vessels. Vagotomy is now usually omitted in favour of postoperative medical treatment of the ulcer. Create a gastroduodenotomy of the size that would usually be made for a pyloroplasty. Aspirate blood and clot from the ulcer base and isolate the site of bleeding. This is usually from the gastroduodenal artery. Carefully insert stitches of 2/0 silk or other non-absorbable material on a round-bodied small curved eyeless needle placed transversely to pick up the artery (Fig. 13.20).

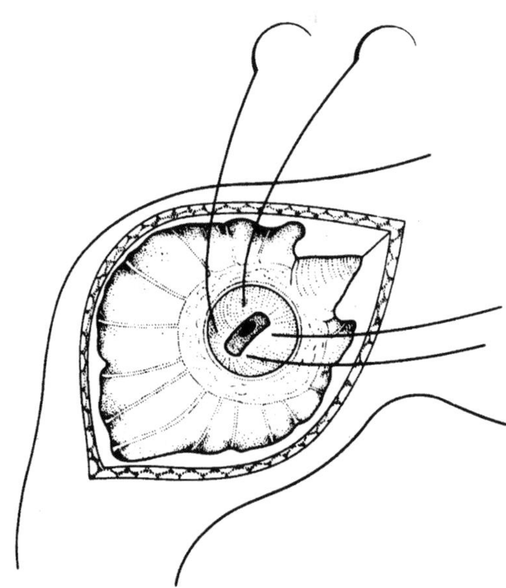

Fig. 13.20 Suture-ligature of gastroduodenal artery in the base of posterior duodenal ulcer, using 2/0 silk.

KEY POINTS Crucial aims

- Make sure you have completely controlled the bleeding.
- Insert the sutures carefully because the common bile duct lies close by.

2 Close the gastroduodenotomy either as a pyloroplasty or longitudinally as it was made.

3 The florid duodenal ulcers that were formerly seen are less common now but occasionally the duodenal ulcer is so large, the walls so thickened and distorted that pyloroplasty will not be successful. One possibility is to close the gastroduodenotomy longitudinally, and if necessary create a gastrojejunostomy. Alternatively, perform Polya gastrectomy, although this should rarely be necessary. The difficulty will be in freeing and closing the duodenum. If the duodenum has already been opened to perform pyloroplasty before the problem is appreciated, first control the bleeding with 2/0 silk sutures. Now decide whether to dissect the duodenum distal to the ulcer sufficiently to allow it to be closed. This is feasible only if the ulcer is close to the pylorus. If it lies distally, you will endanger the ampullary region. Nissen's manoeuvre may succeed: suture the anterior cut duodenal edge to the distal ulcer edge and, if there is sufficient free anterior duodenal wall, suture it over the ulcer to the proximal ulcer edge (see Fig. 13.21).

4 If the difficulty of performing pyloroplasty is appreciated early, perform Polya gastrectomy, preserving as much of the anterior duodenal wall as possible, provided the ulcer base can be exposed and the bleeding controlled with sutures. This allows the closure of the duodenum to be carried out securely.

5 Control of the bleeding may be difficult in the presence of a large ulcer and the base may be exposed most easily by 'pinching off' the duodenum from the ulcer edge to leave the base free. Control the bleeding. The problem of closing the duodenum can now be tackled calmly, either accomplishing it in the post-ulcer segment, or closing the hole created by the ulcer defect (see p. 188).

6 If all else fails, insert a large catheter into the duodenal defect and close the duodenum around it. Bring the catheter to the surface of the abdomen to create a controlled fistula. This can be removed after 10–14 days and always closes without complication unless there is distal obstruction.

7 The surgical treatment of erosive gastritis is often unsatisfactory and most surgeons are conservative whenever possible. If bleeding is uncontrollably severe, then perform high or even total gastrectomy. Roux-en-Y reconstruction is then usually appropriate.

8 Gastric carcinoma or sarcoma are rare causes of severe gastrointestinal bleeding and should have been diagnosed before surgery was contemplated. Ideally, the operation to be performed is the one that would be selected at an elective operation. However, as a life-saving operation, be prepared to carry out a limited resection. In suitable patients it is reasonable to plan re-operation after 2–3 weeks to carry out radical resection.

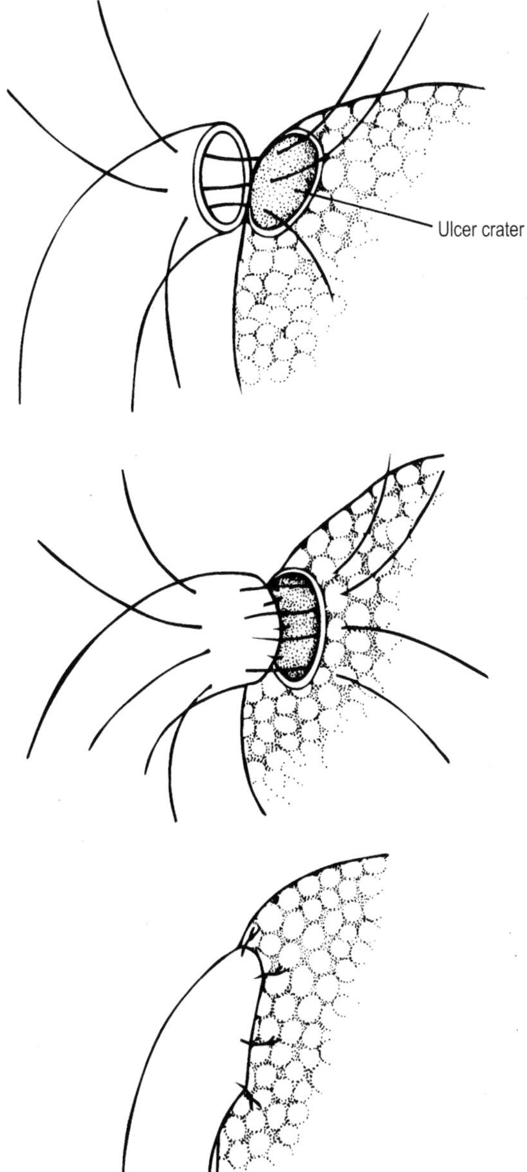

Fig. 13.21 Nissen's manoeuvre for closure of duodenal stump. The cut anterior duodenal edge is first sutured to the distal ulcer edge. The anterior duodenal wall is then sutured to the proximal ulcer edge.

RECURRENT PEPTIC ULCER

Appraise

1 The effectiveness of modern drugs has drastically reduced the indications for peptic ulcer surgery and therefore the risk of recurrent ulcer. In consequence, many surgeons are inexperienced in dealing with the challenging problems encountered in this field. Do not hesitate to refer patients with recurrent ulcer to someone who has specialized experience.

2 Test the basal, pentagastrin-stimulated and insulin-stimulated gastric acid secretion. High basal secretion suggests the possibility of a Zollinger–Ellison tumour. In all cases estimate the

serum gastrin level and exclude hyperparathyroidism (see Ch. 27). A positive insulin test may suggest incomplete vagotomy if that was the original operation.

3 An episode of recurrent ulcer does not necessarily demand re-operation. Try the effect of H_2-receptor-blocking drugs in high dosage or omeprazole, or omeprazole with antibiotics. The ulcer may heal and not recur.

3 If the recurrent ulcer is associated with high basal gastric acid output, carefully explore the pancreas and duodenum to exclude the presence of a Zollinger–Ellison tumour (see p. 206).

4 Recurrent gastric ulcer is rare following Billroth I gastrectomy but, if it does develop, carry out a higher gastrectomy, excising the ulcer. The anastomosis may once again be gastroduodenal, but Polya gastrectomy is highly effective in preventing recurrence. Recurrent ulcer following proximal gastric or truncal vagotomy with excision of the ulcer or a 'drainage procedure' is best treated by partial gastrectomy.

5 Recurrent ulcers may develop following conversion surgery to relieve dumping, bile vomiting or diarrhoea. Combine vagotomy and partial gastrectomy.

Action

1 Truncal vagotomy demands expert knowledge of the area. If the trunks were missed previously, search carefully not only around the lower oesophagus but also within the whole of the oesophageal hiatus. The posterior trunk may lie posteriorly on the right crus of the diaphragm. Remember that missed trunks may have been displaced at the first operation.

2 Partial gastrectomy is not necessarily more difficult than at a primary operation but great care is necessary to mobilize the stomach or remnant.

3 Do not leave a complicated anatomical result but prefer to take down anastomoses, leaving the anatomy simple. Blind and redundant loops of bowel endanger the patient's long-term well-being.

REVISIONARY SURGERY FOLLOWING PEPTIC ULCER SURGERY

Appraise

1 It is surprising how infrequently patients having gastric surgery for cancer develop disabling chronic symptoms compared with those having surgery for peptic ulcer.

2 If you are an inexperienced and occasional gastric surgeon do not embark on revisionary surgery for the relief of sequelae following operations for peptic ulcer. Resist the desire to 'do something'. Very few of the many papers written on revision operations are objective or have sufficient numbers, or sufficient follow-up. Many of the patients improve with time following reassurance, and almost all of them can be improved by adherence to simple rules such as avoiding large meals and food that they have learned is likely to be upsetting, by taking small meals separate from fluids and resting after meals, and by avoiding food and drinks containing excessive sugar. In any case, it is wise to wait at least 2 years from the primary operation before contemplating a revisionary operation.

2 Bilious vomiting following the creation of a gastroenterostomy stoma is most likely to respond to anatomical revision. Indeed, disabling bilious vomiting is the only symptom for which a mechanical conversion can be offered with reasonable confidence. It is thought that the afferent loop is functionally or mechanically obstructed and distends with bile, pancreatic juice and duodenal secretions discharging intermittently into the stomach. The gastric lining is irritated and the patient may vomit or regurgitate some of the bile-stained fluid. At endoscopy, the region of the stoma reveals florid gastritis. If bilious vomiting follows gastroenterostomy plus truncal vagotomy, the anastomosis can often be simply disconnected provided the pyloroduodenal canal has an adequate lumen. If it follows Polya gastrectomy, conversion to a Roux-en-Y anastomosis (see Fig. 13.22) with drainage of the duodenal loop into the efferent limb at least 50 cm from the stomach diverts bile away from the stomach.

3 An alternative is a Roux-19 conversion in which the afferent loop is divided and the ends are anastomosed into the efferent loop at least 50 cm apart; this procedure can be carried out without mobilizing the stomach. These operations increase the risk of stomal ulceration and, if the original operation was for duodenal ulcer, it is wise to perform truncal vagotomy.

4 Occasionally bilious vomiting complicates Billroth I gastrectomy. The anastomosis can be disconnected, the duodenum closed and the stomach connected to a Roux-Y loop of jejunum.

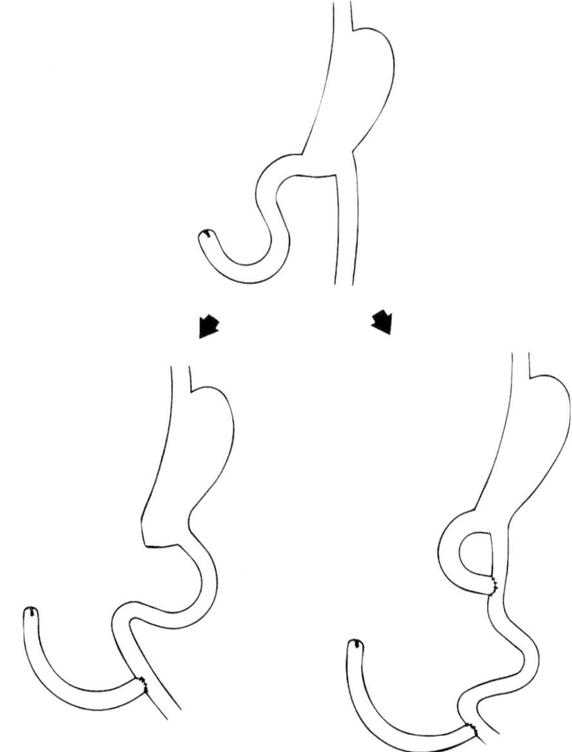

Fig. 13.22 Conversion surgery for relief of bile vomiting following Polya partial gastrectomy. Lower left is the Roux-Y operation. Lower right is the Tanner Roux-19 operation.

5 Dumping syndrome is named from the probability that it develops because of the destruction of pyloric metering of gastric contents into the small bowel. Thus food and fluid may be rapidly deposited into the jejunum, causing overdistension and discomfort usually within 30 minutes of the meal. This is called 'early dumping'. Rapid absorption of fluid may produce circulatory disturbances, while hyperosmolar solutions attract fluid into the lumen, depleting the circulating fluid volume and at the same time overfilling the jejunal lumen. Rapid absorption of sugars may evoke hyperglycaemia stimulating insulin release, followed by rapid fall in blood glucose and the symptoms of hypoglycaemia, usually 2–4 hours after meals. This is called 'late' dumping. Proximal gastric vagotomy without drainage for duodenal ulcer greatly reduces the incidence and severity of dumping, since the metering function of the antrum and pylorus is left intact.

6 Following Polya partial gastrectomy, dumping may be diminished by conversion to a Billroth I anastomosis or by conversion to a Roux-en-Y, adding truncal vagotomy if the first operation was for duodenal ulcer, to protect from recurrent ulceration. Neither of these procedures is totally satisfactory in every patient. Elaborations have been recommended, usually in the form of interposed antiperistaltic or isoperistaltic jejunal segments between the gastric remnant and the duodenum or efferent loop of small bowel. As a trainee surgeon, do not attempt to perform these complicated and often ineffective operations.

7 Severe dumping infrequently complicates Billroth I gastrectomy. It is sometimes improved by interposing an isolated isoperistaltic or antiperistaltic loop of jejunum between the gastric remnant and the duodenum.

8 Dumping following vagotomy is usual only when accompanied by an adjunctive procedure to improve gastric emptying. Gastroenterostomy can be taken down if the pyloroduodenal canal is adequate and the results are usually good. Pyloroplasty can be revised so that the pylorus is restored to anatomical normality but reports are varied on the success of the procedure. Probably it does little to improve the patient's symptoms in the long term.

9 Gastric retention produces postprandial bloating sensation and regurgitation or vomiting of gastric contents often with eructations. It was notorious in a proportion of patients treated by truncal vagotomy alone for the cure of duodenal ulcer and was relieved or prevented by the addition of gastrectomy, gastroenterostomy or pyloroplasty. As a rule, improvement occurs with time even when there is no drainage operation. Some patients appear to develop complete gastric atony following vagotomy, including proximal gastric vagotomy, whether or not a drainage operation has been added; this also tends to improve slowly with time. If a drainage operation was not used originally then perform gastroenterostomy.

10 Occasionally gastric retention develops from stomal obstruction associated with adhesions trapping the efferent bowel, intussusception of the afferent loop into the stomach or prolapse of hypertrophic gastric mucosal folds into the stoma, and from stenosis following recurrent ulcer. The diagnosis is made by contrast radiography and endoscopy. Treatment is surgical relief of the obstruction, or bypass. In the case of stenosis from recurrent ulcer, truncal vagotomy and gastrectomy are usually necessary.

11 In postgastrectomy patients who swallow indigestible food without first chewing it, the bolus of food may impact in the bowel, usually in the terminal ileum. Surgical relief is necessary: the bolus can usually be broken up without opening the bowel. If it cannot be broken up, 'milk' it proximally and open the bowel to extract the bolus. Then repair the incision in the bowel. Subsequently adjure the patient to avoid eating unchewed meat, fruit and other foods.

12 Diarrhoea may complicate peptic ulcer surgery. Make sure that the patient does not have some unrelated cause. An occult tendency to coeliac disease, colitis or irritable bowel disease may become manifest following peptic ulcer surgery. Dumping of food and fluid, especially hyperosmolar fluid, provokes intestinal hurry and diarrhoea as well as dumping syndrome and these symptoms can be controlled with simple dietary advice. Nearly all patients following gastrectomy have a tendency to steatorrhoea although this may not be clinically evident. In most patients diarrhoea can be controlled using codeine phosphate. A rare cause of diarrhoea is inadvertent gastroileostomy instead of gastrojejunostomy; this requires surgical correction.

13 A few patients have crippling, uncontrollable diarrhoea following truncal vagotomy and drainage for peptic ulcer. Diarrhoea is associated with dumping and can usually be alleviated by controlling the dumping. In the hope of controlling diarrhoea a 10–12-cm length of jejunum may be taken out of circuit, reversed and inserted 100 cm beyond the ligament of Treitz or alternatively an 8-cm loop of ileum 40 cm proximal to the ileocaecal valve. The results have been disappointing in the long term.

14 Surgery for peptic ulcer is thought to predispose to gastric carcinoma. The cause is probably excessive bile reflux onto the gastric mucosa following Polya gastrectomy or gastroenterostomy with vagotomy. The detergent bile breaks the protective mucosal barrier, which may provide access to the mucosa for ingested carcinogens. A diet poor in vitamins and antioxidants, together with hypoacidity in the stomach, may be other predisposing factors. Do not assume that all symptoms, especially those developing late or with a changed pattern from previous symptoms, are 'postpeptic ulcer surgery syndrome'. Carry out endoscopy and remove numerous biopsies, especially near the stoma. The reassurance that serious disease has been excluded often leads to an improvement in the symptoms. Successful resection is possible in some patients with stump carcinoma.

GASTRIC CARCINOMA

Appraise

1 At present, the best hope of cure is radical resection. Gastric carcinoma is usually resistant to radiation therapy, but responses to chemotherapy are improving.

2 Unfortunately most tumours present late. In Japan a high proportion of early cancers are detected by screening or open-access

endoscopy and are successfully treated by surgery. Early gastric cancer is defined as a cancer that is confined to the mucosa or submucosa, with or without spread to the lymph nodes. In the UK, not even those at higher than normal risk are routinely and regularly screened. They include those with a family history of the disease, pernicious anaemia and gastric atrophy, hypergammaglobulinaemia, atrophic gastritis, intestinal metaplasia, dysplasia, polyps and previous gastric surgery. Blood group A confers a higher than normal risk. Early gastric cancer is often asymptomatic, yet even patients presenting with dyspepsia are not routinely endoscoped.

2 Lauren of Finland described in 1965 two types of gastric carcinoma. The first is intestinal in type, developing in areas of intestinal metaplasia and tending to be localized. The reduction in gastric cancer that is seen in many Western countries stems from a reduced incidence of this type. The second type is infiltrating and it tends to spread rapidly within the stomach, often in the submucosa, causing the rigidity that gives it the name 'linitis plastica'. It also spreads widely outside the stomach and carries a gloomy prognosis. Nevertheless, gastric cancer should be primarily regarded as a locoregional disease which is potentially curable by classical oncological surgery that removes the primary tumour and its draining lymph nodes.

3 Although most gastric carcinomas are sited distally, a tendency for a higher proportion to develop proximally has been noticed in recent years; the reason is unknown.

4 Endoscopy with cytology and biopsy is the best method of screening and diagnosis. It is valuable in detecting early gastric cancer (Fig. 13.23).

5 Improvements in imaging have facilitated preoperative staging. Barium meal X-ray is often now deprecated if endoscopic diagnosis has been made, but in expert hands it can sometimes give valuable information. For example, gastric rigidity and lack of peristalsis suggest extensive submucosal spread. Chest X-ray may reveal enlarged mediastinal nodes or pulmonary metastases. Conventional ultrasound and CT scanning show up spread into adjacent organs, the liver and lymph nodes but do not pick up very early lesions. Endoluminal ultrasound is a valuable means of assessing infiltration and local nodal involvement. Laparoscopy, for so long ignored by general surgeons, is useful for determining tumour spread in the peritoneal cavity.

6 The ability to determine the extent of the tumour before operation saves many patients from fruitless exploratory laparotomy, although the preoperative, perioperative and postoperative staging may prove to be different. The combined TNM (tumour, nodes, metastases) staging of the International Union against (*contre*) Cancer (IUCC) in 1987 modified the staging to reflect the realization that the depth of invasion is more important than the topographical distribution.

7 Careful studies, carried out mainly in Japan, have demonstrated the sequential spread of cancer from various sites in the stomach to the lymph nodes. Local nodes within 3 cm of the primary tumour are designated N_1, the next nodes to be affected are N_2, the third tier is N_3 and distant spread is N_4 (Fig. 13.24, Table 13.1). If the tumour has not spread into unresectable local structures, or metastasized by the blood stream, curative resection can be attempted. En bloc resection of the tumour with the

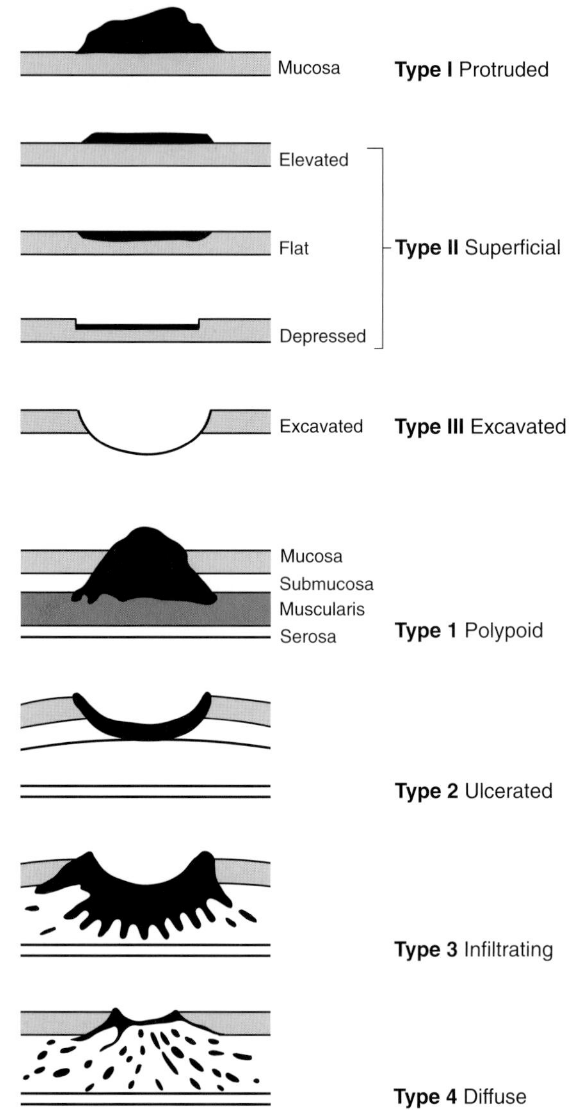

Fig. 13.23 Early and invasive gastric cancer. The upper types I–III are superficial carcinoma confined to the mucosa, described by the Japanese Society of Gastroenterological Endoscopy. The lower types 1–4 show advanced carcinoma described by Borrmann.

N_1 nodes is designated a D_1 resection, with the N_1 and N_2 nodes a D_2 resection. D_2 resection is the standard procedure. On occasion a D_3 resection may be performed, incorporating the N_3 nodes.

8 Other structures may be removed in continuity with the stomach including the parietes, a portion of the liver, small bowel, colon or pancreas. The aim is to achieve circumferential resection margins that are clear of tumour, just as in rectal surgery. If you succeed in this endeavour, there is a 20–90% chance of cure, depending on the stage (90% in early gastric cancer, 20% in stage IIIb). Overall 5-year survival is now about 40% after potentially curative D_2 resection in Britain.

9 Radical subtotal gastrectomy carried out through the abdomen is the standard operation for localized distal tumours. For diffuse distal growths and those in the body of the stomach a radical total gastrectomy is required. This is sometimes per-

TABLE 13.1 The successive tiers of lymph nodes affected by adenocarcinoma at different sites within the stomach

	N_1	N_2	N_3	N_4
Distal primary carcinoma	Lesser curve Greater curve Suprapyloric Subpyloric	Right paracardial Left gastric Common hepatic Coeliac axis	Hepatoduodenal ligament	Middle colic artery
Middle third carcinoma	Right paracardial	Splenic artery	Posterior aspect of pancreas	Para-aortic
	Lesser curve Greater curve Suprapyloric	Splenic hilum Left paracardial Left gastric		
Subpyloric	Common hepatic	Para-oesophageal Coeliac axis		
Upper-third carcinoma	Left paracardial	Suprapyloric		
	Right paracardial Lesser curve Greater curve	Subpyloric Common hepatic Left gastric Splenic artery Splenic hilum Coeliac axis	Diaphragmatic Root of mesentery	

formed through a left thoracoabdominal incision but can often be performed satisfactorily through the abdomen. For lesions at the cardia, a radical oesophagogastrectomy is required and this must be performed through a left or right thoracoabdominal approach.

10 Removal of the primary tumour is valuable even when the growth has spread beyond the limits of radical resection. Palliative distal gastrectomy is suitable for distal growths. Palliative total gastrectomy is appropriate for proximal growths. Upper partial gastrectomy should seldom be employed. Try not to leave tumour at the resection lines; wherever possible, excise 4–5 cm of apparently normal stomach or duodenum or oesophagus beyond detectable growth.

11 When resection is impracticable, try to relieve existing or impending obstruction. Distal obstruction can usually be bypassed using a proximal gastrojejunostomy. Proximal obstruction may demand anastomosis of bowel to the oesophagus in the chest or neck. When surgical bypass is impossible or unjustified, consider dilating a stricture with bougies or inflatable balloons followed by the insertion of a splinting tube. If a large tumour bulges into and blocks the lumen, reduce it using radiotherapy or endoscopically delivered Nd-YAG laser beam vaporization.

D_2 RADICAL ABDOMINAL SUBTOTAL AND TOTAL GASTRECTOMY

RADICAL SUBTOTAL GASTRECTOMY

Appraise

- Radical resection for localized carcinoma of the distal stomach will be described. It resembles radical total gastrectomy except that a fringe of proximal stomach is retained, its size determined by the extent of proximal spread of the tumour since the resection margin should be 5 cm clear of detectable tumour. Preservation of the proximal stomach allows gastrojejunostomy to be accomplished through the abdomen. It is carried out on patients who have no evident involvement of the peritoneum distant from the tumour or of N_3 and N_4 nodes. Any local invasion of contiguous structures must be resectable with the stomach, such as proximal duodenum, a segment of small bowel, transverse colon, pancreas, liver lobe or parietal wall.
- If radical resection cannot encompass all the detectable growth, carry out a more modest palliative resection if possible. Ensure that the resection margin is well clear of growth, because a resection that does not protect the patient against stomal recurrence and obstruction is not worth carrying out. If there are extensive metastases, even palliative resection is probably inappropriate. Bypass existing or impending pyloric obstruction with proximal gastroenterostomy.

Access

1 Make a long vertical midline incision skirting the umbilicus, or a paramedian incision.

2 If necessary excise the xiphoid process. Be prepared to mobilize the left lobe of liver and fold it to the right.

Assess

1 Do not immediately palpate the stomach. Note any ascites and peritoneal deposits. Start your complete exploration from the pelvis and work towards the stomach in order not to disperse malignant cells. Exclude pelvic deposits and, in the female, ovarian seedlings. Examine the greater omentum for deposits and then raise it to feel the para-aortic nodes and those around the root of the mesentery, and the right colic and middle colic arteries. Examine the full length of the small and then large intestine, seeking peritoneal deposits on the bowel wall, the mesentery and the parietal peritoneum. Look for incidental

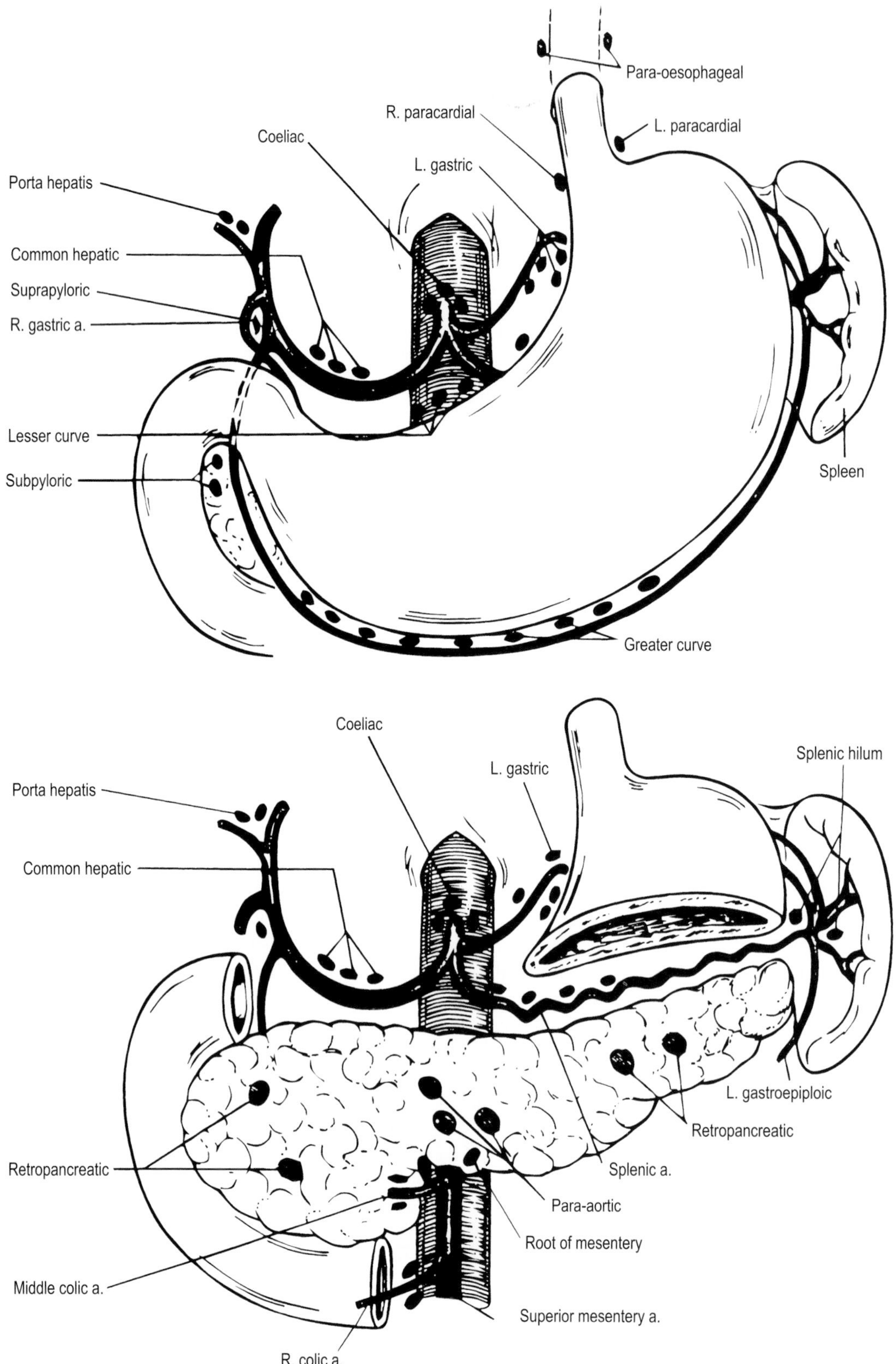

Fig. 13.24 The lymph nodes likely to be involved by gastric carcinoma. In the lower diagram the body of the stomach has been removed to display the deeply placed nodes.

disease. Throughout the examination confirm the pulsations in the arteries, noting atheromatous rigidity, aneurysms and venous or lymphatic obstruction.

2 Now draw the omentum caudally to examine the upper compartment. Feel both lobes of the liver and adjacent diaphragm, gallbladder and free edge of the lesser omentum, the spleen, kidneys and adrenal glands. Starting at the oesophageal hiatus and working distally, look and feel for tumour involvement, fixity, glands and also incidental disease. Systematically move distally, avoiding handling or squeezing the tumour if possible.

3 Palpate the duodenum and initially split the floor of the aditus to the lesser sac to feel the head of the pancreas between finger and thumb. Now palpate the body and tail of the pancreas through the lesser omentum and transverse mesocolon, then the region of the coeliac axis just above the neck of the pancreas. This part of the examination cannot be exact and must be repeated as the dissection allows. If you are seriously in doubt whether to proceed, incise the lesser omentum in an avascular area near the liver and examine the coeliac axis and emerging arteries and assess the spread across the lesser sac. To assess the left part of the lesser sac and body and tail of the pancreas, carefully make a hole in the base of the transverse mesocolon to the left of the middle colic vessels. If you are doubtful about involvement of the head of the pancreas, perform Kocher's manoeuvre in order to palpate it adequately. None of these manoeuvres commits you to proceed with radical resection if you discover unsuspected spread.

KEY POINTS Avoid too early commitment to resection

- If you are still in doubt, plan to mobilize the stomach without dividing any vital structures until you have ensured that resection is appropriate and achievable.
- This may entail a change in the order of the procedure, approaching the suspect area from different aspects.

Resect

1 Lift the great omentum and dissect it from the transverse colon. There is a bloodless plane of fusion between the folded omentum, which was part of the dorsal mesogastrium, and the anterior leaf of mesocolon. Gently peel off the omentum, taking care not to damage the anterior leaf of mesocolon or the middle colic and marginal vessels. Continue on to the pancreas until you reach its upper border. Take care to avoid damaging the pancreas or its blood vessels.

2 At the left extremity of the greater omentum the left gastroepiploic vessels pass forwards in the gastrosplenic omentum from the hilum of the spleen. Carefully dissect out the lymph nodes at the origin of the left gastroepiploic artery, then doubly ligate and divide the artery and vein.

3 At the right extremity of the greater omentum the right gastroepiploic vessels pass forwards from the gastroduodenal vessels. Carefully isolate them and the subpyloric lymph nodes before doubly ligating and dividing them at their origins.

4 Now draw the distal stomach caudally to put on stretch the free edge of the lesser omentum. Carefully make a transverse incision in the anterior leaf above the pylorus to reveal the right gastric vessels and the suprapyloric lymph nodes. Dissect the nodes and doubly ligate and divide the right gastric blood vessels.

5 Gently burst through an avascular area of the lesser omentum close to the liver and extend this towards the cardia, keeping close to the liver. Look for and divide between ligatures the accessory hepatic artery crossing from the left gastric artery.

6 Perform Kocher's mobilization of the duodenum so that the first part can be dissected from the head of the pancreas. The blood vessels are short and fragile. In order to avoid damaging the pancreas, apply fine haemostasis forceps on the vessels a few millimetres from the duodenal wall, divide the vessels between the tips of the forceps and the duodenal wall, then pick up the short duodenal cut ends to ligate them.

7 Mobilize 5–6 cm of duodenum beyond the pylorus.

KEY POINT Keep in the correct tissue plane

- Do not wander from the duodenal wall; you risk damaging the bile duct and pancreas.

8 Use a GIA or similar mechanical stapler to transect the duodenum.

9 From the site of ligature of the right gastric artery, strip the peritoneum, connective tissue and lymph nodes from the hepatic artery, proximally along the upper border of the pancreas, to the coeliac artery.

10 Have the distal stomach elevated by an assistant, to tauten the left gastric vessels in their peritoneal fold. In the free edge of the fold lies the left gastric vein; identify, doubly ligate and divide this first. Now extend the dissection of the hepatic artery to the coeliac artery, in order to dissect all the glands from this area, including those around the origin of the splenic artery. Elevate the gland mass into the column of tissue around the now cleaned origin of the left gastric artery. Doubly ligate and divide the left gastric artery. We always place two ties on the proximal cut stump or transfix it with an arterial suture.

11 Have the stomach drawn caudally and to the patient's left, to place the cardia on stretch. Complete the division of the lesser omentum until the right side of the cardia is reached; now gently clean the upper lesser omentum, connective tissue and right cardiac lymph nodes from the gastric lesser curve down to the selected site of transection. The nerves of Latarjet will be transected during this manoeuvre.

12 Turn the distal stomach cranially again, to examine the upper posterior wall, ensuring that it is free of adhesions; there is often a vein, arching backwards in a peritoneal fold from the posterior gastric fundus, which bleeds annoyingly if it is torn.

13 Transect the stomach with a mechanical stapling device. When the stomach is transected it appears as in Fig. 13.25.

Technical

1 Remember that the more extensive the operation the greater the morbidity and mortality. Do not deprive a fit patient of the

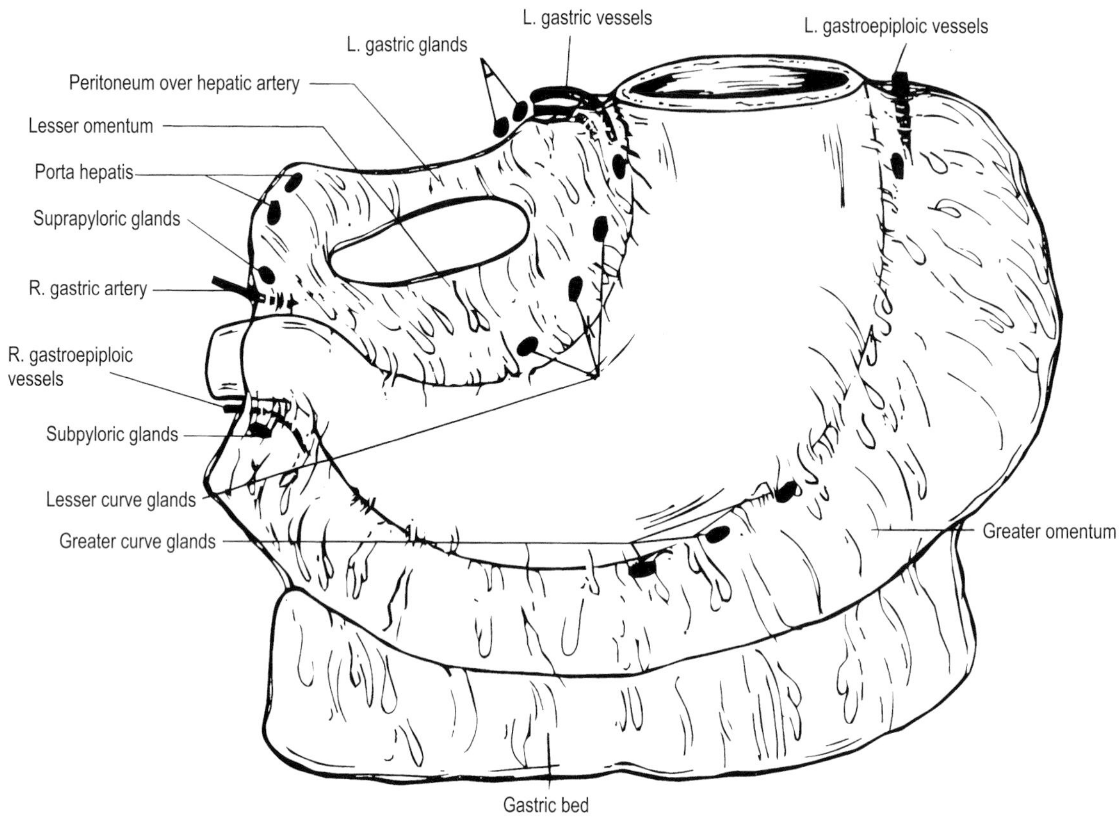

Fig. 13.25 Radical subtotal gastrectomy; the removed specimen.

chance for cure by being too conservative. However, do not place a patient at risk unnecessarily with a radical resection if the N_3 nodes (porta hepatis, root of mesentery, para-oesophageal and retropancreatic) and N_4 nodes (middle colic and para-aortic) are already involved. If in doubt, take biopsies of these nodes and obtain frozen-section histology by an expert.

2 Remember the principles of cancer surgery enunciated by the great surgeons, William Halsted and Keiichi Maruyama: whenever possible, dissect the lymph nodes en bloc with the primary tumour so that you do not transect the intervening lymphatics, and obtain clear circumferential resection margins.

3 An argument could be made for less extensive nodal dissection for early gastric cancer. However, in a fit patient, perform D_2 resection, because 10–30% of UK patients with early gastric cancer have nodal metastases.

4 The D_2 resection may be selectively extended to encompass N_3 nodes (a $D_{2/3}$ resection):

- Tumour cells may travel retrogradely towards the hilum of the liver. Routinely remove these nodes when radically excising distal gastric carcinoma, in continuity with the dissection of the common hepatic artery. Make a careful incision across the upper free edge of the lesser omentum over the hepatic arteries, which can be found by palpation between a finger placed in the upper aditus to the lesser sac, and a thumb placed anteriorly. Carefully strip down the connective tissue and glands from the hilum of the liver to the point of right gastric artery ligation and beyond, along the common hepatic artery to the coeliac axis. Take care not to damage the common bile duct; the portal vein is less at risk since it lies posteriorly.
- After Kocher's manoeuvre has been performed to dissect off the duodenal bulb, carefully seek and excise retropancreatic (N_3) nodes from the posterior aspect of the pancreatic head. Of course these cannot be removed in continuity with the main specimen. During this manoeuvre also look for and remove nodes at the root of the mesentery (N_3 nodes) and close to the aorta (N_4 nodes). Always have isolated nodes placed separately in labelled pots for histology and prognostication.
- If the distal carcinoma extends proximally into the body of the stomach it is wise to excise the nodes along the upper and lower borders of the pancreas (N_2 nodes for carcinoma in the body of the stomach). When the omentum has been stripped as far as the pancreas, gently dissect the mesocolon caudally to display the lower border of pancreas. Seek and remove any glands that lie around the emerging superior mesenteric vessels and the inferior mesenteric vein.
- Having stripped the greater omentum as far as the pancreas, peel the continuation of posterior parietal peritoneum in a cephalad direction, from the upper part of the body and tail of the pancreas to reveal the serpentine splenic artery. Carefully dissect from it the connective tissue and lymph nodes proximally along its whole length from its origin at the coeliac artery.
- Some surgeons remove the spleen and body and tail of the pancreas in order to remove the supra- and infrapancreatic nodes together with retropancreatic nodes around the

splenic vein (see p. 202). To achieve this, draw the spleen forwards and to the right to display and divide the left leaf of the lienorenal ligament. Gently mobilize the spleen and tail and body of pancreas forwards with the splenic artery and vein. Doubly ligate and divide the splenic vein just distal to the entry of the inferior mesenteric vein. Carefully dissect the lymph nodes from the splenic artery, starting at the coeliac artery and working distally until you reach the level at which the splenic vein was divided. Now doubly ligate and divide the splenic artery, leaving the dissected nodes attached to the distal segment. Transect the body of the pancreas, carefully preserving the inferior mesenteric vein junction with the splenic vein. If possible, isolate and separately ligate the cut pancreatic duct. Oversew the proximal cut end of the pancreas with fine non-absorbable sutures. Since the splenic artery no longer supplies the proximal stomach through the short gastric vessels, the proximal stomach will receive its blood supply only from the oesophagus, so perform a near-total gastrectomy, leaving but a fringe of stomach.

KEY POINTS Cost/benefit decision

- Addition of splenopancreatectomy to D_2 subtotal gastrectomy doubles or triples the operative mortality, from approximately 4% to 10–15%. Spleen and pancreas so removed are usually uninvolved.
- Do not, therefore, routinely perform splenectomy or pancreatectomy in standard D_2 subtotal gastrectomy but assiduously try to clear suprapancreatic lymph nodes.
- However, direct posterior invasion of the pancreas may force you to carry out splenopancreatectomy en bloc with stomach.

Unite

1 Draw up a loop of proximal jejunum in exactly the same manner as following Polya gastrectomy for benign disease.

2 The anastomosis can be made using a combined linear stapling and cutting device. In this case transect the stomach with a double line of staples applied with a long linear stapler and transect it below the line of staples. Bring up the selected jejunal loop and suture it at each end to the posterior wall of the stomach. Make stab wounds through the gastric and jejunal walls close to the uniting stitch at the greater curve end of the proposed anastomosis and pass in the separate blades of the combined linear stapler and cutter, one into the stomach, one into the jejunum, lying parallel to each other and pointing to the gastric lesser curve.

3 Lock the two blades together after ensuring that there is no intervening tissue. Actuate the stapler to insert four parallel rows of staples uniting the stomach and jejunum and cutting between the middle rows to form a stoma. Unlock and remove the stapler. Inspect the interior to ensure the anastomosis is perfect.

4 Pick up the incomplete ends of the staple lines with tissue forceps and separate them to leave a longitudinal defect. Close this with a short straight stapling device.

5 Alternatively, use a Roux-en-Y method of reconstruction, which spares some patients the discomfort of bilious vomiting.

ABDOMINAL TOTAL GASTRECTOMY

Resect

1 Complete the gastric mobilization by dividing the lesser omentum right up to the diaphragm and dividing the gastrophrenic ligament close to the diaphragm. Posteriorly, there is a vein arching backwards from the upper stomach that must be ligated or occluded with haemostatic clips and divided. Splenectomy and distal pancreatectomy are not always necessary.

2 The stomach is now attached only to the oesophagus. Gently free this in the hiatus. Transect the anterior and posterior vagal trunks and decide on the level of transection. Do not divide the oesophagus until either the posterior oesophagojejunal outer Lembert suture line is in place after turning the specimen upwards over the patient's chest to prevent the oesophagus from retracting out of sight, or until most of the purse-string suture has been inserted for use with a circular stapling device. Prevent retraction of the oesophagus into the chest by application of a Crafoord or Satinsky clamp, and slow intravenous injection of up to 20 mg of hyoscine butylbromide (Buscopan).

3 If a nasojejunal tube is to be used, have it drawn up into the lower oesophagus. It can be pulled down when making a sutured anastomosis when the posterior all-coats suture is in place and pushed on into the jejunum. If a stapled anastomosis is made, have the anaesthetist push it on with a twisting motion when the stapler is withdrawn.

Unite

1 Oesophagojejunostomy is preferably performed using a Roux-en-Y jejunal loop (see Ch. 11). Transect the jejunum close to the ligament of Treitz and divide sufficient primary vascular arcades to allow the distal portion to be taken up to the oesophagus. Transect the bowel beyond the duodenojejunal junction and join the cut proximal end into the side of the Roux loop 50 cm downstream. If a sutured oesophagojejunal anastomosis is used, close the end of the jejunum in two layers, or staple it. The loop should be led up to the oesophagus posterior to the transverse mesocolon. Make sure it lies without tension or twisting. Insert a posterior running suture line of Lembert stitches joining the posterior wall of the oesophagus to the posterior wall of the Roux loop about 5 cm from the closed end. Now transect the oesophagus below the suture line and remove the specimen.

2 Create a hole in the antimesenteric border of the jejunum exactly matching the oesophageal lumen. Insert a stitch through all coats of the oesophagus and jejunum at each end so they can be slightly stretched. Carefully insert a circular all coats stitch to produce perfect union (see p. 171). Now carry the posterior Lembert stitch onto the anterior wall to encircle the anastomosis, trying to draw up the jejunal wall to cover the inner all-coats stitch.

3 Discard and replace the soiled towels, instruments and gloves.

4 End-to-end Roux loop anastomosis is rarely possible if the oesophagus is sufficiently dilated so that its lumen matches that of the cut end of the jejunum and if the jejunum can be laid straight with not too much tendency to curve at its free end. A two-layer anastomosis is usually fashioned, but one-layer anastomosis is probably equally satisfactory.

5 The oesophagojejunal anastomosis may be accomplished using one of the circular stapling devices. Before the oesophagus is completely transected, most of an encircling all-coats purse-string suture is inserted and the specimen is then resected below it and removed. Introduce a size-testing head so that the correct size of stapler can be used. An end-to-side Roux anastomosis does not require a separate stab since the instrument, without the anvil, can be passed in through the cut end of bowel which will be closed in two layers after it is withdrawn. In an end-to-end anastomosis the anvil remains in place but well separated from the staple cartridge, and a purse-string suture is used to draw in the jejunal end over the cartridge.

6 Now feed the anvil head into the cut end of oesophagus, tighten and tie the purse-string suture and close the anvil head onto the cartridge after ensuring there is no extraneous tissue trapped and that the oesophagus and jejunum lie without tension or twist. Release the safety catch and actuate the gun. Open it, remove it, check the intactness of the anastomosis and of the doughnut-shaped rings on the spindle. Close the portal of entry of the device in two layers. If the oesophageal wall is very thick, dissect back a cuff of muscularis so that it is not included in the stapler. After uniting the oesophagus to jejunum, insert a layer of stitches drawing the muscle coat onto the jejunum around the stapled anastomosis.

7 Anastomosis has been made easier by the development of improved circular stapling devices in which the anvil head and the spindle can be detached together. A temporary pointed trocar can be fitted to the main instrument and pushed through the wall of the bowel, then removed. Introduce the anvil on its spindle into the lower oesophagus and tighten and tie the previously inserted purse-string suture. Attach the anvil on its spindle to the instrument and bring together the jejunum and oesophagus by closing the anvil down onto the cartridge. Actuate the stapler. Always, before loosening the stapler, feel again around the anastomosis to ensure that nothing is interposed, nothing is protruding. In case of doubt about the integrity of the anastomosis, retain the closed stapler and use it to rotate the anastomosis while inserting reinforcing sutures around the circumference of the stoma. Only now release and remove the stapler.

Check

1 Stop all bleeding.

2 Ensure that the anastomoses are perfect, the bowel is a good colour, untwisted and not stretched and the mesentery lies free.

3 Check all the other structures that have been disturbed. The hiatus does not need to be repaired if total gastrectomy has been carried out. The liver must be replaced if the left lobe was folded to the right. Repair the transverse mesocolon if there is a hole through which small bowel may prolapse.

Closure

1 Drain the cut end of the pancreas and leave the drain in situ for 6–10 days to form a track. Pancreatic fistula is common and very dangerous if it cannot freely drain externally.

2 Close the abdomen in routine fashion.

Postoperative

1 Manage a patient following subtotal gastrectomy in the same manner as following gastrectomy for benign disease.

2 Following transabdominal total gastrectomy manage the patient in a similar manner to one who has had thoracoabdominal total gastrectomy (see p. 204).

RADICAL THORACOABDOMINAL TOTAL GASTRECTOMY

Appraise

1 Never embark upon this operation without first obtaining a tissue diagnosis with endoscopic biopsy or cytology or frozen-section histology at operation. Never embark upon it without making every effort by preoperative and operative assessment to exclude metastatic tumour.

2 As a rule, this is a radical operation undertaken for carcinoma of the proximal stomach or cardia which can apparently be totally encompassed by this major resection of the stomach, lower oesophagus, omenta, spleen, body and tail of the pancreas, with all the primary lymph nodes and the next tier, completing a D_2 resection.

3 Accomplish it through a left thoracoabdominal incision. It can be carried out through an upper midline abdominal incision only if the upper stomach is free of growth and in that case it is merely an extension of radical partial gastrectomy to include the upper fringe of stomach in the resection. Transabdominal total gastrectomy is usually contraindicated, except in very thin patients, if the growth extends proximally to within 2–3 cm of the gastro-oesophageal junction since at least a 3-cm segment of apparently uninvolved lower oesophagus should be resected. Do not attempt it in an obese patient with a narrow costal margin.

3 Total gastrectomy is justifiable as a palliative procedure in the presence of metastases provided the patient is expected to survive for a reasonable period. In this case the resection is as extensive longitudinally as a radical gastrectomy, but is not carried widely from the stomach.

KEY POINTS Insure against anastomotic recurrence

- Do not compromise on the longitudinal proximal clearance in a palliative total gastrectomy.
- It is tragic for the patient to undergo a major resection only to rapidly develop malignant stenosis at the anastomosis.

4 Lymphoma and sarcoma of the stomach are best treated by radical gastrectomy but even if they extend beyond the scope of the operation total gastrectomy may be justified to reduce the bulk of the tumour. Radiotherapy and chemotherapy may then be more effective, with a reduced risk of hollow viscus perforation.

5 Non-radical total gastrectomy through the abdomen was conventionally carried out on patients with Zollinger–Ellison syndrome, whether or not a gastrin-secreting tumour had been totally excised. It is now reserved for the minority of patients whose ulcer cannot be controlled medically or by extirpation of the tumour (see p. 206).

6 This major resection must sometimes be offered to patients who are elderly, have other conditions that prejudice recovery and are also malnourished. Ensure that the nutritional state is restored by oral feeding with high-calorie, high-protein and vitamin-rich diet, nasoenteric feeding or, if necessary, intravenous feeding through a centrally placed venous catheter. Organize preoperative chest physiotherapy and check all other body systems to anticipate and prevent complications. Make sure that the patient has an indwelling urinary catheter in place during and after the operation to allow the urinary output to be monitored.

Access

1 The anaesthetized, intubated patient lies on the right side (Fig. 13.26), tilted backwards 30°, right hip and knee flexed, left leg straight and separated from the right leg by a pillow. The pelvis is fixed by a wide strip of adhesive tape to prevent it from rolling backwards; a fixed post, covered with sponge, supports the left scapula posteriorly to maintain its position. The arms are brought in front of the face in the 'hornpipe' position.

2 Stand at the patient's back.

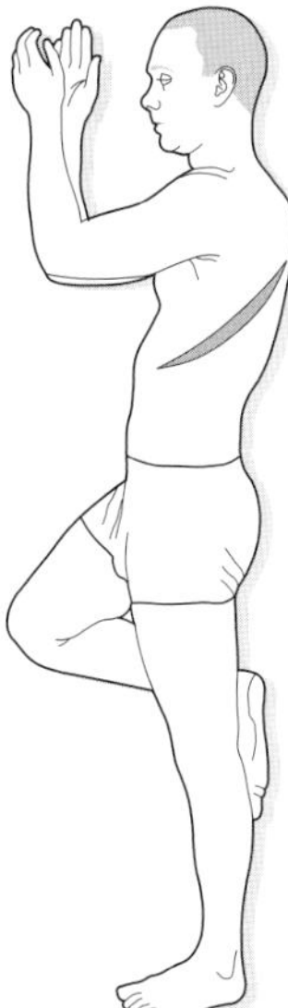

Fig. 13.26 Left thoracoabdominal approach to total gastrectomy, as seen from above the patient. The shaded section shows the extent of the incision.

3 Open the abdomen obliquely from the midline to the costal margin in the line of the left seventh or eighth rib.

Assess

1 Note any free fluid. Feel the pelvic peritoneum for deposits, then the para-aortic and middle colic nodes, then the liver.

2 Examine the stomach and its related nodes, in particular the coeliac nodes by making a hole in an avascular part of the lesser omentum near the liver. Note if the tumour is fixed to adjacent structures such as the liver, pancreas, colon or abdominal wall and if partial resection of these allows radical resection to be accomplished. Decide if radical resection is feasible.

Resect

1 Extend the incision along the seventh or eighth rib as far as the lateral border of the sacrospinalis muscle. Open the chest either by resecting the rib or along the upper border of the rib. If the rib remains, remove a 2-cm length posteriorly and cut a similar piece from the next rib above. Isolate and divide the intercostal nerve posteriorly to prevent postoperative girdle pain.

2 Incise the diaphragm radially down towards, but not into, the hiatus. It may be necessary to resect the crural part en bloc with the growth.

3 Mobilize the spleen forwards (Fig. 13.27) after incising the lienorenal ligament, lifting up the tail and body of the pancreas. When the inferior mesenteric vein is encountered, doubly ligate and divide the splenic vein distal to it and separate the proximal pancreas from the right part of the splenic vein, ligating any small vessels joining the two structures.

4 Lift up the greater omentum and separate its whole length from the transverse colon in the bloodless plane just above the colon, so that the omentum can be stripped upwards as an intact leaf from the mesocolon. Avoid damaging the mesocolon or its contained blood vessels.

5 Carry out Kocher's manoeuvre of duodenal mobilization. Carefully identify and dissect out the lymph nodes on the posterior surface of the pancreatic head, para-aortic area, origin of the superior mesenteric artery, and also the origins of the middle colic and right colic arteries. Separately pot these in formalin for histology.

6 Rotate the spleen, tail of pancreas, omentum and greater curve of stomach over to the right. At the pyloric end the right gastroepiploic vessels are taut and at the cardiac end of the stomach the left gastric vessels are tensed. Dissect out the right gastroepiploic vein on the pancreas and doubly clamp, divide and ligate it. Dissect out the origin of the right gastroepiploic artery. Doubly clamp, divide and ligate it, dissecting out the lymph nodes with the vessels. Above the pylorus, identify the right gastric vessels, trace the arteries up to their origin from the hepatic artery and doubly clamp, divide and ligate them, dissecting out the lymph nodes with the vessels. Mobilize the duodenum for at least 5–7 cm beyond the pylorus. There are small vessels connecting it to the pancreas; clamp these close to the duodenum, divide them between the clamps and the duodenum, pick up the vessels on the duodenal wall and ligate them.

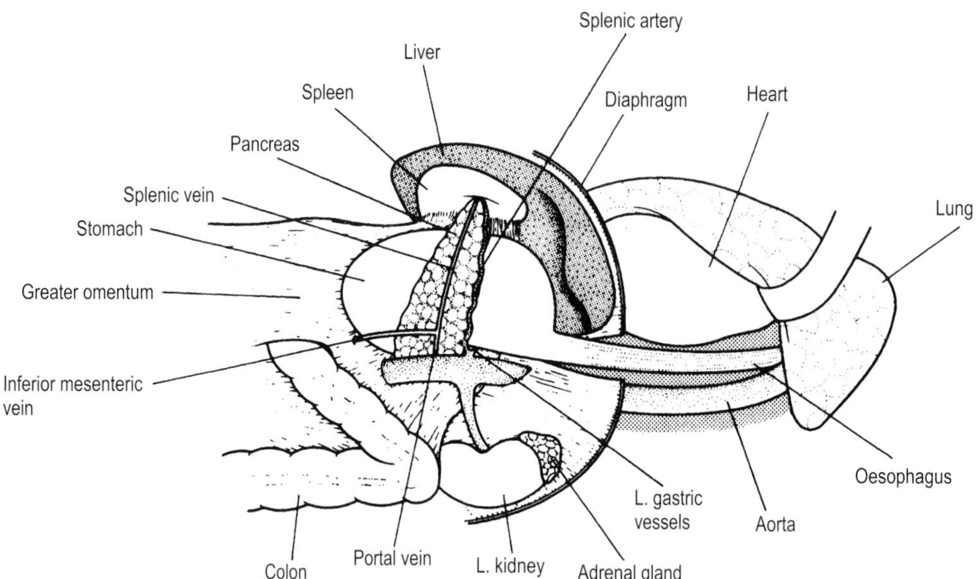

Fig. 13.27 Through a left thoracoabdominal incision the diaphragm has been incised. The spleen, splenic vessels and body and tail of the pancreas have been elevated, together with the greater curve of the stomach.

7 Isolate the area with distinctive coloured towels. Transect the duodenum 3–5 cm beyond the pylorus between thin crushing clamps such as Lang Stevenson's. Close the distal cut end with a loose running over-and-over absorbable stitch on an eyeless needle, including the clamp. Withdraw the clamp and tighten the sutures seriatim. Insert a second layer of invaginating stitches to bury the first layer. Alternatively, close the duodenum with a straight stapling device, with or without a row of reinforcing invaginating stitches.

8 Fold the distal stomach to the left. Expose the porta hepatis and incise the peritoneum over the hepatic artery, recognized by palpation. Strip the peritoneum, connective tissue and lymph nodes from the hepatic artery back to the coeliac artery. Continue the peritoneal incision in the porta hepatis to the left, keeping close to the liver, to detach the lesser omentum up to the diaphragm.

9 Have the distal stomach drawn upwards to place the left gastric vessels on stretch within their peritoneal fold. Continue the dissection of peritoneum, connective tissue and nodes along the hepatic artery to clear the coeliac axis and origins of the splenic and left gastric arteries. Dissect in continuity any glands from the aorta above the coeliac axis. Isolate, doubly clamp, divide and ligate the left gastric vein on the posterior abdominal wall. Doubly clamp, divide and ligate the left gastric artery at its origin.

10 Just below and to the right of the coeliac axis gently separate the neck of the pancreas from the splenic vein lying behind it and transect the pancreas here, picking up and ligating the small vessels above and below. Identify the main duct and separately ligate it. Close the raw proximal cut end of the pancreas with a running absorbable stitch or with interrupted sutures.

11 The coeliac axis has been cleared of connective tissue and nodes. Now sweep off the tissue on the left-hand side to reveal the cleaned origin of the splenic artery. Doubly clamp, divide and ligate the splenic artery at its origin. Separate the splenic vein from the posterior surface of the pancreas as far as the ligature placed distal to the entrance of the inferior mesenteric vein. The distal splenic artery with its associated glands is now freed together with the body and tail of the pancreas and spleen.

12 The distal stomach is free. Decide whether or not to excise a cuff of diaphragmatic crura in continuity with the upper stomach and lower oesophagus. In any case, continue up the dissection of the upper stomach and lower oesophagus keeping well away from them so the loose connective tissue, paracardial glands and lymphatics will be incorporated in the specimen.

13 Have the left lower lung held forwards with a lung retractor. Incise the pleura over the lower oesophagus. Mobilize the oesophagus above the diaphragm and dissect downwards stripping all the surrounding connective tissue, lymphatics and lymph nodes with it and from the aorta lying posteriorly.

14 Extend the radial cut in the diaphragm to the crura. Now preferably dissect on either side to leave a cuff of crus still attached to the free oesophagus. If the tumour is well away, it is permissible to split through the crus and dissect out all the loose tissue with the oesophagus.

15 The specimen is now attached only by the oesophagus and vagal trunks. Divide the vagi. Decide the level of oesophageal transection to be 5–10 cm clear of detectable tumour. In case of doubt, obtain frozen-section histological confirmation that the resection margin is free from tumour. Reconstruction will be easy if the oesophagus is cut across midway between the aortic arch and the diaphragm since the upper end will retract up to just below the arch. Do not stint on the resection, however. It is tragic to succeed in extirpating all the peripheral growth only to have the patient develop recurrence at the stoma. If necessary, the oesophagus can be freed and united on the outside of

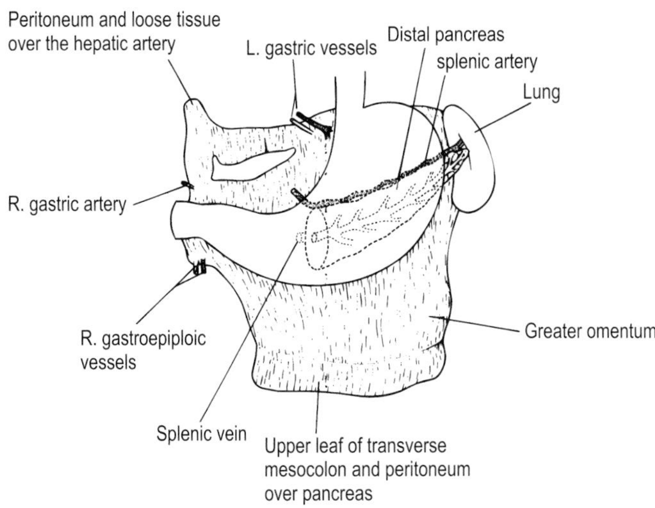

Fig. 13.28 Radical total gastrectomy. The resected specimen.

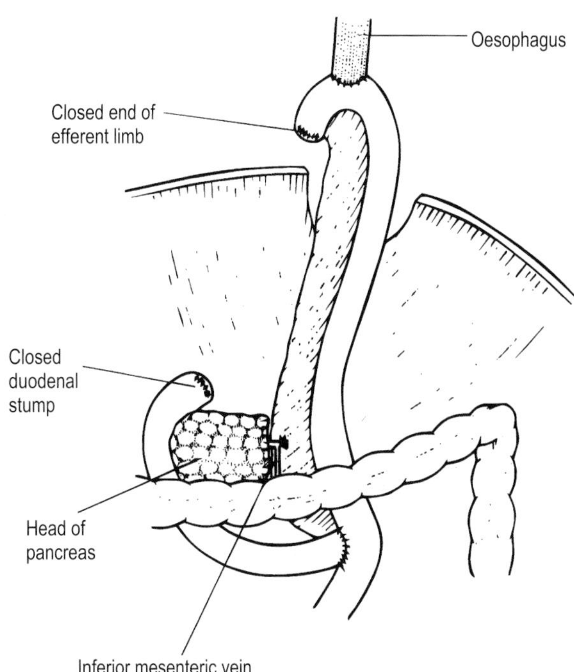

Fig. 13.29 Radical total gastrectomy. The oesophagojejunal anastomosis is complete, using a Roux loop of jejunum taken behind the mesocolon. The duodenal bulb is closed, and duodenal loop is joined end-to-side to the jejunum.

the arch, or freed up to the neck and united to a conduit there. Transect the oesophagus cleanly (Fig. 13.28). If a nasogastric tube was in place have it first withdrawn to just above the line of transection.

16 Scrupulously ensure total haemostasis now. It will be impossible to examine the area when the reconstructive conduit is in place.

Unite

1 Pick up the proximal jejunum. Carefully examine the vascular pattern. Hold up the loops and view them against a light. Create a Roux loop that will easily reach the retracted oesophagus (p. 220). Draw the loop through a hole in an avascular portion of the posterior part of the mesocolon, subsequently suturing the margins of the mesocolon carefully to the loop and its mesentery to prevent other loops of bowel from herniating through.

2 The anastomosis may be end-to-end but the jejunum usually sits most comfortably with the oesophagus joined end-to-side. If this is a sutured anastomosis, close the end of the jejunum with a purse-string suture reinforced with an invaginating seromuscular stitch. Make a hole in the antimesenteric border of the jejunum to match the lumen of the oesophagus. Place stay sutures through all coats of oesophagus and jejunum at each end and have these drawn apart to slightly stretch the anastomotic lines. Now carefully insert an all-coats stitch uniting the adjacent oesophageal and jejunum walls, placing the sutures 2 mm apart, with 2–3-mm bites. The stitches may be continuous or interrupted, absorbable, silk or monofilament plastic thread. The material and method are less important than the perfection of every stitch (Fig. 13.29).

4 Many surgeons employ a single suture layer. Alternatively, a second layer may be inserted of continuous or interrupted stitches which pick up the muscularis and submucosa of the oesophagus close to the anastomosis and the seromuscularis of the jejunum 5 mm below the anastomosis so that as it is gently tightened it draws a cuff of bowel up and over the all-coats suture line. The anastomosis can be rotated to allow the stitch to be inserted around the whole circumference.

5 Now discard and replace the soiled towels, instruments and gloves.

6 The anastomosis can be fashioned using circular staplers. Choose a suitable cartridge size by inserting a test head into the oesophagus. Do not unite the jejunal end. When turned over the cartridge head with a purse-string suture, it would prove too bulky in conjunction with the thick-walled oesophageal end also drawn into the gap between anvil and cartridge by a purse-string suture.

7 Apply the stapler safety catch and remove the anvil from the spindle. Introduce the spindle and cartridge through the open end of the jejunum, cut down upon the spindle end 5–7 cm from the jejunal end, on the antimesenteric border, and advance the spike through the jejunum. Replace the anvil. Introduce a purse-string suture of monofilament plastic suture around the cut oesophageal end. Introduce the anvil into the oesophagus and tighten the purse-string suture, cutting off the spare thread. Close the anvil onto the cartridge with the intact purse-stringed oesophagus and jejunal wall separating them and with no extraneous tissue caught. Release the safety catch and actuate the stapler. Separate the anvil from the cartridge and gently withdraw the instrument.

8 Confirm that there are two intact toroidal fragments ('doughnuts') of oesophagus and jejunum on the spindle. Check the suture line. If necessary reinforce it partially or completely with sutures.

9 Now close the cut jejunal end with two purse-string sutures or use a short straight stapler. If the oesophagus is very thick, dissect back the muscular coat as a cuff which is not included in the stapler. After 'firing' and withdrawing the stapler, unite the oesophageal muscle to the jejunum with a continuous ring of sutures. The technique is simplified using the stapling device in which the anvil, together with the spindle, can be separated from the cartridge.

10 Manoeuvre the nasogastric tube through the anastomosis and if possible down to or beyond the duodenojejunal anastomosis if it is intended to use it for feeding.

Technical points

1 Radical and potentially curative resection may be accomplished if the tumour has invaded the abdominal wall or diaphragm provided it is possible to excise part of these en bloc with the tumour. If the body or tail of the pancreas is invaded posteriorly, this part of the gland will have been removed as a routine together with the spleen. The transverse colon can be resected en bloc with the stomach, and the left lobe of the liver may also be resected. If the tumour spreads distally into the duodenum or into the head of the pancreas then pancreatoduodenectomy would be necessary and this is very rarely feasible.

2 It is important to stretch the anastomosis slightly when uniting it with sutures, since the oesophagus contracts down to a narrow tube and sutures placed close together become widely separated when a bolus of food stretches it, allowing leakage to occur.

3 If the oesophagus retracts under the aortic arch gently free it until it can be brought onto the outside of the arch and complete the anastomosis there. With care this can be accomplished perfectly but occasionally it is worth creating a second, higher thoracotomy. If anastomosis cannot be safely performed, do not persist. Dissect up the oesophagus to the neck and complete it safely there, using a suitable conduit such as a segment of colon.

4 A jejunostomy may be created (see Ch. 14) to allow early feeding if the patient was severely undernourished or if slow recovery is possible. Alternatively the nasal tube may be passed into the upper jejunum for feeding purposes. In patients who find the tube intolerable, the upper end can be brought out in the neck as a pharyngostomy.

Checklist

1 Check that you have completed the D_2 glandular clearance (see Table 13.1).

2 In the chest make sure the anastomosis is perfectly executed, that it lies without tension and is not twisted. Ensure that the lung is undamaged and that it can be re-expanded by the anaesthetist if he has deliberately collapsed it.

3 Check all the main ligatures. Re-examine the closed neck of pancreas and duodenal stump closure. Check that there is no continuing oozing from the raw surfaces.

4 Check the duodenojejunal anastomosis, ensure that the Roux loop passes upwards without twisting, and that its blood supply is not prejudiced. Re-examine the passage of the jejunum through the mesocolon and ensure that the blood supply to the colon is not damaged.

Closure

1 Insert a left basal chest drain and connect it to an underwater seal. Insert an abdominal drain to the distal cut pancreas.

2 Close the cut diaphragm using mattress sutures of non-absorbable material. Even if a cuff of crura has been removed it will close without tension. Do not tighten the new hiatus to constrict the jejunal loop. Do not suture the bowel to the diaphragm but allow it to lie freely.

3 Close the chest in layers.

4 Close the abdomen.

Postoperative

1 Nurse the patient in the intensive therapy unit for the first 24 hours.

2 Institute physiotherapy for the chest. Remove the drain to the pancreas and the underwater drain after 48 hours and the drain to the pancreas after 6–10 days. Order daily chest X-rays until the chest is clear. If fluid collects in the base of the left pleural cavity, aspirate it.

3 Give jejunostomy feeds or parenteral feeds. After 4–5 days examine the anastomosis radiologically after the patient has swallowed water-soluble radio-opaque medium. If leakage is excluded remove the nasogastric tube and start oral fluids proceeding to food.

PALLIATIVE OPERATIONS FOR GASTRIC CARCINOMA

Appraise

- Palliative resection for carcinoma should be interpreted to mean apparently complete removal of the primary tumour, even though there is metastatic growth outside the scope of a radical resection. If growth is cut across in the stomach then the anastomosis may not heal so that the patient develops leakage and peritonitis, or soon develops stomal obstruction from recurrent tumour, or the growth is spread widely during the procedure. This view may need to be modified as cytotoxic chemotherapy improves since some of the agents are more effective if the tumour bulk is reduced.
- If palliative resection is precluded, the patient can be relieved of impending or existing obstruction in many cases.

PALLIATIVE TOTAL GASTRECTOMY

Appraise

- Fit patients with carcinoma of mid-stomach or proximal stomach may be given dramatic and often long-term palliation by total gastrectomy. Occasionally what appeared to be metastatic tumour proves to be reactive changes producing enlarged lymph nodes, and the patient survives indefinitely.
- Abdominal total gastrectomy is appropriate for carcinoma of the mid-stomach and many cases of upper-third carcinoma. If palliative total gastrectomy is planned for upper gastric

carcinoma, the thoracoabdominal route may be required to avoid cutting through tumour or prejudicing the anastomosis of oesophagus in the abdomen in an obese patient with a narrow costal margin.

- Try to preserve the spleen and pancreas in most cases.

Action

1 Whether the abdominal or abdominothoracic route is used, proceed as for partial gastrectomy for peptic ulcer (p. 186), dividing the gastrocolic omentum but continuing higher so that all the short gastric vessels are doubly clamped, divided and ligated, leaving the spleen intact.

2 Distally, doubly clamp, divide and ligate the right gastroepiploic and right gastric vessels and divide the duodenum. A wide, clear margin is not so essential here if the duodenum is to be closed. Close the distal cut end of duodenum.

3 Elevate the stomach to display the left gastric vessels and isolate, doubly clamp, divide and ligate them.

4 Gently mobilize the upper stomach and lower oesophagus and select a point of transection that is at least 5–7 cm clear of detectable growth. Cut across the gullet and vagal trunks.

5 In a small number of patients an uninvolved duodenum can be brought up to the lower oesophagus after fully mobilizing it by Kocher's manoeuvre and it can then be anastomosed end-to-end. As a rule it is necessary to bring up jejunum to the oesophagus. This may be a Roux loop (see Ch. 14), or occasionally an intact proximal loop. The intact loop has the disadvantage that bile reflux into the oesophagus may be troublesome. Such bile reflux is not always prevented by creating an anastomosis between the afferent and efferent loops in the hope of diverting bile away from the oesophageal stoma. These patients have a limited outlook so prefer the simplest operation.

PALLIATIVE PARTIAL GASTRECTOMY

Appraise

For distal gastric carcinomas associated with metastases outside the scope of radical surgery, distal gastrectomy may still offer good palliation. However, the proximal cut edge should be well clear of growth or the stoma will either leak or subsequently obstruct from recurrent growth.

If the growth is very extensive in the stomach, however, it may be more damaging to perform gastrectomy than to leave the patient alone.

Action

1 Perform the gastrectomy in the same manner as for benign disease (see p. 186). Make sure that the line of proximal section is at least 5–7 cm above detectable disease.

2 Close the duodenal stump and bring up a proximal loop of jejunum and create a full-width stoma to guard as far as possible against stomal obstruction if the carcinoma recurs here. Alternatively use a Roux-en-Y reconstruction.

PALLIATIVE UPPER PARTIAL GASTRECTOMY

Appraise

- This procedure may be carried out through the abdomen but is better performed through a left thoracoabdominal incision. It may be useful to palliate proximal gastric carcinoma but it is essential to transect the lower oesophagus sufficiently high to insure against local recurrence and this usually means that the transection and anastomosis must be performed in the chest.
- Its main advantage over palliative total gastrectomy is that, if the distal stomach is free of tumour, it provides a convenient conduit to unite to the gullet.

Action

1 Open the gastrocolic omentum and divide the vessels upwards including the left gastroepiploics and the short gastrics. Alternatively, remove the spleen.

2 Distally preserve the right gastroepiploic and right gastric vessels but mobilize the duodenal loop by Kocher's manoeuvre until the pylorus can be drawn up to the oesophageal hiatus. Ensure that there is no pyloric obstruction by invaginating the anterior gastric antral wall through the pylorus on an index finger.

3 Incise the lesser omentum proximal to its free edge to gain access to the lesser sac to the right of the stomach. Identify, isolate, doubly clamp, divide and ligate the left gastric vessels.

4 Decide the upper and lower limits of the resection. Both of them should be 5–7 cm clear of detectable growth. Transect the oesophagus and vagal trunks. Transect the stomach, and remove the specimen.

5 The cut edge of the stomach may be partially closed from the lesser curve aspect to leave a hole equal in size to the oesophagus so that an end-to-end anastomosis can be made between the oesophagus and the greater curve part of the cut stomach. Alternatively the cut proximal edge of the stomach may be closed using a stitch or a straight stapling device. An anastomosis can now be created between the oesophagus and the anterior or posterior wall of the greater curve portion of stomach at least 2 cm proximal to the line of closure (Fig. 13.30). This again may be sutured or created with a stapling device. To staple the anastomosis make a hole in the middle of the anterior wall of the gastric remnant and pass through it the spindle of the circular stapling device after removing the anvil. Press the spindle end against the posterior wall of the stomach near the greater curvature at least 2 cm proximal to the closed end. Make a small cut to enable the spindle to emerge and replace the anvil. Place a purse-string suture around the cut end of the oesophagus, insert the anvil of the stapler into the oesophagus and tighten and tie the purse-string, cutting off the loose ends. Close the anvil down onto the cartridge and actuate the stapler. Open the device, gently withdraw it, and check that there are two intact toroids of excised oesophagus and stomach. Check the anastomosis and insert reinforcing stitches if necessary.

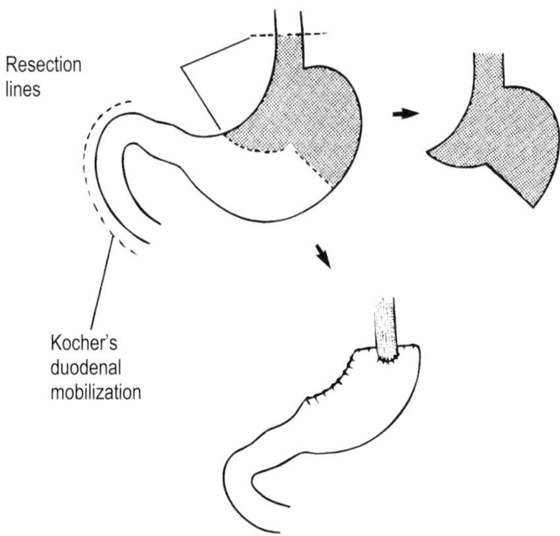

Fig. 13.30 Upper partial gastrectomy.

GASTROENTEROSTOMY

Appraise

- If a distal growth is extensive and cannot be resected or if there are gross metastases, relieve the existing or impending obstruction in the pyloric region by creating a proximal gastroenterostomy.
- Bypass may offer as good palliation and disturb the patient less than resection that cuts through tumour.

Action

1 Reach below the transverse mesocolon and draw up the proximal jejunum, selecting the first loop that will reach easily to the upper stomach.

2 Create a high, wide stoma between the upper anterior gastric wall and the jejunum. Use twin gastroenterostomy clamps only if they facilitate the procedure.

CARDIAC OBSTRUCTION

Appraise

1 An inoperable proximal carcinoma that obstructs the cardia offers a challenge. If nothing is done the patient will starve to death.

2 Rarely it is reasonable to draw a loop of intestine or colon into the chest or neck to bypass the obstruction (see Ch. 11).

3 Either a Mousseau–Barbin, Celestin or Atkinson type of tube may be passed after dilating the malignant stricture. This can be achieved using a balloon or the pulsion technique from above. If the abdomen is open, make a small high gastrotomy and dilate the cuff of tumour from below. Pass up a bougie and ask the anaesthetist to attach the leader of a Mousseau–Barbin or Celestin tube to it and draw it down until the tube is impacted in the malignant stricture. Cut off the excess tube and close the gastrotomy. Alternatively, the stent may be introduced under radiological control.

4 Occasionally, it is valuable to insinuate a nasogastric tube through into the stomach for feeding purposes before trying the effect of radiation therapy. In some patients, the effect is dramatic in shrinking the tumour and relieving the obstruction.

5 Many surgeons deprecate use of a gastrostomy in patients with terminal disease and attitudes are determined by one's philosophy.

GASTRIC LYMPHOMA

- Most lymphomas are generalized, nodal, affecting the stomach secondarily. Primary gastric lymphoma does occur. It is a non-Hodgkin's B-cell lymphoma. It is characterized by the absence of peripheral node enlargement, mediastinal gland enlargement on chest X-ray, or liver and spleen enlargement. In addition, there is no bone marrow evidence of leukaemia. Some tumours that appear to be neoplastic run a benign course and are labelled pseudolymphomas. They may represent reactive hyperplasia.
- Both symptomatically and at endoscopy it often resembles adenocarcinoma. There may be a mass, a plaque, sessile or pedunculated polyps, or infiltration resembling linitis plastica. Ulcers are irregular and dendritic, sometimes with raised edges, sometimes multiple. The rugae tend to be hypertrophic. The condition can be multicentric. Since the lesions are essentially in the submucosa, the best diagnostic method is deep biopsy.
- There are a number of classifications.
- Staging is by clinical, endoscopic, ultrasound and CT scanning.
- The best method of treatment is by radical surgery. Perform a D_2 resection if possible; if not, carry out a palliative resection. Mark residual diseased areas with metal clips to aid the planning of postoperative radiotherapy. Adjuvant chemotherapy improves survival, which is, overall, better than for adenocarcinoma.

BENIGN AND NON-EPITHELIAL TUMOURS

- Polyps may be regenerative hyperplastic or adenomatous. Employ endoscopic biopsy, snare and diathermy to establish the diagnosis.
- Leiomyomas and leiomyosarcomas are difficult to distinguish histologically. Excise lesions with a clear margin of healthy gastric wall. For larger and doubtful lesions carry out an appropriate gastric resection.
- Fibrosarcoma, angiosarcoma, Kaposi's sarcoma and haemangiopericytoma are rare in the stomach.

ZOLLINGER–ELLISON SYNDROME

Appraise

1 The classic syndrome consists of severe and sometimes intractable peptic ulcer developing as a rule in expected sites but

sometimes distally in the duodenum and proximal jejunum, associated with gastric acid hypersecretion of marked degree.

2 Exclude it in all patients developing recurrence following surgical treatment of duodenal ulcer. The ulcers may be multiple. There may be diarrhoea, usually attributed to irritability of the bowel from contact with its high acid content. The syndrome is caused by a gastrin-secreting tumour of the pancreatic islets which may be benign or malignant, or there may be hyperplasia without tumour formation (see Ch. 21). The serum gastrin is raised and appears to act as a trophic hormone acting on gastric parietal cells which undergo hyperplasia. The gastric fundic mucosa appears hypertrophied and extends almost to the pylorus, hypersecreting acid in response to the hypergastrinaemia at basal rates approaching maximal acid output. Zollinger–Ellison syndrome is part of a multiple endocrine neoplastic (MEN) syndrome in a quarter of cases, the parathyroid glands being particularly frequently involved. The features of hypergastrinaemia are reproduced in the absence of a pancreatic tumour when the antrum is congenitally duplicated and when it is sequestered in an alkaline medium.

3 Suspect the diagnosis when duodenal ulcer does not respond as expected to medical treatment; or is multiple; or ulcers occur in the stomach, distal duodenum and upper jejunum or in unexpected areas of the stomach such as the greater curvature. The suspicion is confirmed when very high basal levels of acid output are measured and maximal pentagastrin stimulation has little or no added effect. Serum gastrin is raised. In case of doubt, carry out calcium stimulation (5 mg/kg/hour infused for 3 hours) or a secretin challenge (4 units/kg intravenously). These cause a sharp release of gastrin from tumours. Search for other endocrine abnormalities, particularly of the parathyroid glands.

4 Total gastrectomy was previously advocated but should now be reserved only for those who fail to respond to adequate treatment with H_2-receptor-blocking drugs, omeprazole or somatostatin analogue.

5 After employing scanning techniques to exclude metastases, and angiography to try to localize the tumour, plan to explore the abdomen and carefully examine the pancreas, duodenum, stomach, liver and remainder of the abdomen, searching for single or multiple tumours and metastasis. Debulking of metastases is worthwhile. If a solitary tumour is found in the head of the pancreas in the absence of metastases, enucleate it. If a tumour is found in the body or tail of the pancreas, excise the body and tail. If no tumour is found in the pancreas, duodenum or elsewhere, excise the body and tail of the pancreas for histological exclusion of hyperplasia.

GASTRIC OPERATIONS FOR MORBID OBESITY

Appraise

- Patients with morbid obesity (i.e. a body mass index (BMI) greater than 40) have a seriously reduced life-expectancy for a number of reasons. Some have an underlying metabolic disorder such as Cushing's disease, others over-eat for psychological reasons. When dietary management has failed, and attempts to restrict food intake using teeth wiring have failed to produce a long-term weight reduction, surgery is sometimes advocated on the ground that weight loss, however achieved, is just as much a life-saving procedure as cancer surgery. Type 2 diabetes often disappears and coronary artery risk is reduced.
- There are certain ethical considerations. In the first place it can argued that in circumstances of starvation or near starvation, such as the Nazi concentration camps, morbid obesity did not occur, so that voluntary restriction of food intake by the patient will overcome even the most stubborn metabolically generated obesity. Morbid obesity is seen with greatest frequency in prosperous countries, especially the USA, but is now epidemic in the Western world.
- All surgeons agree that, if operations for morbid obesity can be justified, they must be performed by surgeons working in conjunction with specialist colleagues so that the indications for surgery and the results can be monitored. Therefore, do not embark upon such surgery if you are in training or working in isolation.
- The gastric operations in vogue are designed to place a restriction on the passage of food into the gastrointestinal tract. The first convenient region for this restriction beyond the teeth is the upper stomach. Most of the operations utilize the convenient long straight stapling device that places a double row of staples through the full thickness of the gastric wall. After mobilizing the stomach, two double rows of staples are placed across the upper stomach to form a small loculus. A Roux-en-Y loop of jejunum may be brought up for anastomosis to the upper loculus (Fig. 13.31).
- Many other techniques have been devised to overcome the tendency of the small passage to stretch and become ineffective. The operations currently favoured are vertical banding or vertical plastic ring gastroplasty, forming a 20-ml reservoir above the restriction (Fig. 13.32). Laparoscopic banding, 2 cm below the cardia, is gaining popularity and seems to be effective, safe in expert hands, and permits early (2–5 days) discharge from hospital.

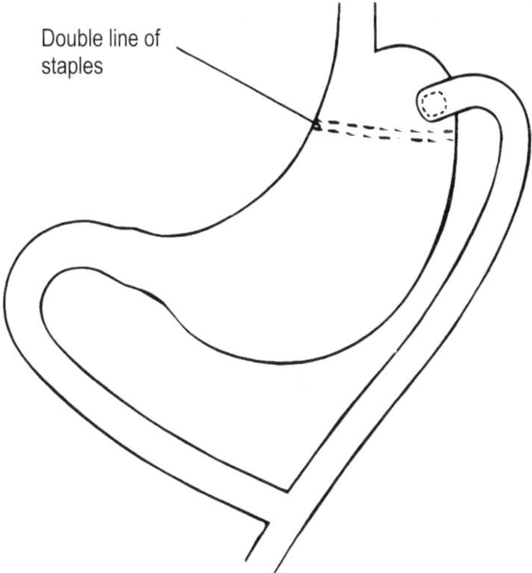

Fig. 13.31 Roux-Y gastric bypass. The gastric staple line is now usually made vertically. The proximal pouch is very small (about 10–20 ml).

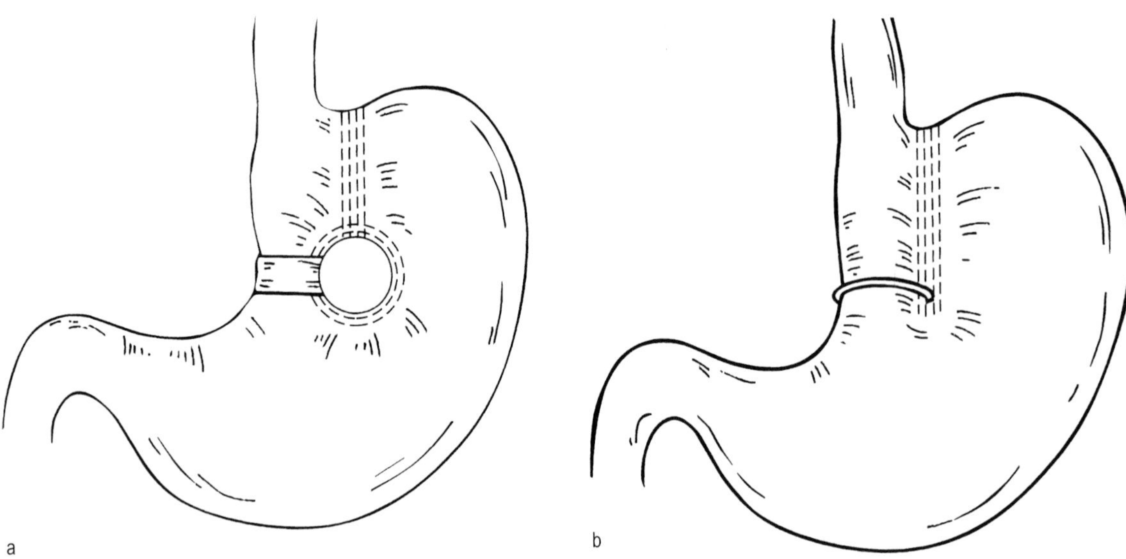

Fig. 13.32 Vertical banded gastroplasty (a) and vertical plastic ring gastroplasty (b).

- The gastric operations are not the sole method of surgically controlling morbid obesity. The majority of the small bowel may be bypassed but the risks of sequelae are greater.

FURTHER READING

Akiyama H 1979 Thoracoabdominal approach for carcinoma of the cardia of the stomach. American Journal of Surgery 137:345–349

Allum WH, Griffin SM, Watson A et al on behalf of the Association of Upper Gastrointestinal Surgeons of Great Britain and Ireland, the British Society of Gastroenterology, and the British Association of Surgical Oncology 2002 Guidelines for the management of oesophageal and gastric cancer. Gut 50(Suppl V):v1–v23

Barkun A 2001 *Helicobacter pylori* eradication prevents ulcer recurrence after simple closure of duodenal ulcer perforation. Evidence-Based Gastroenterology 2:6–8

Bell GD, McCloy RF, Charlton JE et al 1991 Recommendations for standards of sedation and patient monitoring during gastrointestinal endoscopy. Gut 32:823–827

Higham J, Kang J-Y, Majeed A 2002 Recent trends in admissions and mortality due to peptic ulcer in England: increasing frequency of haemorrhage among older subjects. Gut 50:460–464

Rabine JC, Barnett JL 2001 Management of the patient with gastroparesis. Journal of Clinical Gastroenterology 32:11–18

Sasako M 2003 Principles of treatment of curable gastric cancer. Journal of Clinical Oncology 21:(23 Suppl):2745–2755

So JBY, Yam A, Cheah WK et al 2000 Risk factors related to operative mortality and morbidity in patients undergoing emergency gastrectomy. British Journal of Surgery 87:1702–1707

Thorban S, Bottcher K, Etter M et al 2000 Prognostic factors in stump carcinoma. Annals of Surgery 231:188–194

14

Small bowel

R.C.N. Williamson, L.R. Jiao

CONTENTS

EXAMINATION OF THE SMALL BOWEL

Normal appearance

1 The duodenum [Latin: =twelve. Originally Greek: *duodekadaktulon*=12 fingers (breadth)] is 25 cm long. Apart from the proximal 2–3 cm, it is retroperitoneal. The remaining small bowel, which has a mesentery, is variable in total length (about 3–5 m) and difficult to measure with accuracy in vivo. It is arbitrarily divided into a proximal 40%, the jejunum (Latin: *jejunus*=hungry, empty), and a distal 60%, the ileum (Greek: *eilios*=twisted; used by Galen only in a pathological sense). On palpation the jejunal wall is thicker than that of the ileum, so that the examining fingers gain the impression of a double layer, rather like feeling a shirt through the sleeve of a jacket.

2 Examine the duodenal loop. Locate the duodenojejunal flexure by displacing the transverse colon upwards and tracing the coils of jejunum proximally to the ligament of Treitz. Pick up the small bowel at the duodenojejunal flexure and feed it through your fingers down to the ileocaecal valve. Note the diameter and contents of the bowel and the thickness and colour of its wall. In a thin person lacteals may appear as white lines crossing the jejunum and its mesentery.

3 Examine the small-bowel mesentery throughout. Its thickness varies with the patient's adiposity. In a thin patient mesenteric lymph nodes can often be seen. Determine whether the nodes are enlarged or inflamed and whether the mesenteric blood vessels are normal.

> **KEY POINTS What is normal?**
>
> - Take every opportunity to see and feel normal bowel.
> - You can determine what is abnormal only by knowing the limits of normality.
> - You can determine the limits of normality by taking every opportunity to examine normal bowel.

Abnormalities

- *Diverticula*. These are quite common. Meckel's diverticulum, which arises from the distal ileum, is considered below. Acquired diverticula may affect the duodenum, jejunum and to a lesser extent the ileum, and are frequently multiple. Do not remove incidental diverticula, but excise localized groups if they are causing symptoms, such as pain or bleeding.
- *Inflammation*. Crohn's disease may affect any part of the alimentary canal but especially the terminal ileum. Affected segments of bowel are inflamed, thickened, narrowed and often covered with fibrinous exudate. The mesentery is thickened and encroaches on a greater proportion of the circumference of the bowel; adjacent lymph nodes are enlarged. Look for evidence of disease elsewhere in the small and large bowel. Segmental resection is usually indicated for chronic Crohn's enteritis (see below). Tuberculous and yersinial infection can produce similar changes of ileitis; if in doubt remove a gland for bacteriological and histological examination. Coeliac disease particularly affects the jejunum. The diagnosis is indicated by dilatation of subserous and mesenteric lymphatics, thinning and pigmentation of the bowel wall and splenic atrophy, and it is confirmed by full-thickness biopsy (see below). Small-bowel ulcers and strictures may occur spontaneously or follow either radiotherapy, transient strangulation in an external hernia or the ingestion of potassium tablets.
- *Infarction*. The viability of the small bowel must be carefully checked after reduction of a strangulated hernia or untwisting of a volvulus in adhesion obstruction. Any frankly necrotic or perforated loops should be excised. If you are in doubt about the viability of a dusky segment, return it to the abdomen and wait for 5 minutes (timed by the clock). The return of a shiny, pink appearance, pulsation of the mesenteric vessels (or bleeding if pricked) and peristalsis across the affected segment indicate viability. If you are still in doubt, resect. Clinical judgement will usually determine intestinal viability, but possible adjuncts are the use of a small Doppler ultrasound probe and injection of fluorescein with

examination under ultraviolet light. Constriction rings may be carefully invaginated, using interrupted seromuscular sutures.

- *Tumours*. Serosal deposits occur in carcinomatosis peritonei and may cause kinking and obstruction of the small bowel, requiring side-to-side bypass (see later). Primary neoplasms are less common. Benign tumours include adenoma, leiomyoma, lipoma and Peutz–Jeghers hamartomas; they can cause intussusception. Carcinoid tumours favour the ileum, but may be multiple and metastasizing; they are hard with a yellowish cut surface. Malignant tumours comprise adenocarcinoma, lymphoma and leiomyosarcoma in that order of prevalence. Primary neoplasms should be excised or, if irresectable, bypassed and biopsied.

Biopsy

- Duodenal lesions can be biopsied endoscopically under direct vision, and the increasing availability of flexible enteroscopy has extended this possibility to further down the small intestine. Multiple 'blind' biopsies of duodenal and jejunal mucosa can safely be obtained by the per-oral route; the patient swallows an appropriate, retrievable capsule.
- Small intestine endoscopy (enteroscopy) is now feasible, formerly being both time-consuming and incomplete. Increasingly, push enteroscopy has superseded Sonde enteroscopy (which relies on peristalsis to carry the instrument distally), principally because of its ability to provide therapy as well as diagnosis. A stiff overtube limits looping of the instrument within the stomach and permits deeper jejunal insertion. A separate working channel allows for therapeutic intervention. Capsule endoscopy has now been widely used clinically, replacing other enteroscopic techniques.[1] It consists of a capsule endoscope, an external receiving antenna with attached portable hard drive, and a personal computer workstation for review and interpretation of images. The technique is increasingly used for the diagnosis and treatment of small intestinal disorders, particularly obscure gastro-intestinal haemorrhage, iron-deficiency anaemia or Crohn's disease.[1,2]
- Operative biopsy of the small intestine is seldom indicated. It is usually possible to excise the segment of bowel in question, and intestinal biopsy should be avoided in Crohn's disease. If a full-thickness biopsy is required, however, the incision should be closed in two layers just like an intestinal anastomosis.
- Mesenteric lymph nodes can be biopsied with relative impunity. Where possible, select a node close to the bowel wall and avoid dissecting deep in the root of the mesentery. Carefully incise the peritoneum and dissect out the entire node, using diathermy to coagulate its small blood vessels.

REFERENCES

1. Hartmann D, Schilling D, Bolz G et al 2004 Capsule endoscopy, technical impact, benefits and limitations. Langenbeck's Archives of Surgery 389:225–233
2. Maieron A, Hubner D, Blaha B et al 2004 Multicenter retrospective evaluation of capsule endoscopy in clinical routine. Endoscopy 36:864–868

INTESTINAL ANASTOMOSIS

General principles

1 Several hundred intestinal anastomoses are carried out each week in Britain, and the vast majority heal rapidly by primary intention. It is fortunate that the small bowel does heal so satisfactorily, since discharge of intestinal contents into the abdominal cavity is potentially lethal and inability to use the gut within a few days of operation makes adequate nutrition much more difficult. Healthy large intestine heals almost as well as small intestine, with the exception of anastomoses situated in its last few centimetres, which do not enjoy serosal cover.

2 Remember that most of the intestinal canal is contaminated with bacteria, disproportionately so towards the distal end. Elaborate techniques were devised in the past to avoid exposing open bowel, but it is now accepted that a secure anastomosis is more easily achieved by opening the bowel. Take appropriate precautions against disseminating faecal organisms (Ch. 4) before dividing and re-suturing the bowel; clamps are usually indicated to prevent faecal spillage. Postoperative abscess formation is likely to impair anastomotic healing.

3 Ensure that the bowel ends are pink and bleeding freely, and leave the mesentery attached to the bowel right up to the point of intestinal transection. If either cut end is bruised or dusky, it is usually sensible to sacrifice a few more centimetres of intestine, even if, in the case of the large bowel, this requires further mobilization.

4 Tension puts the mesenteric vessels on stretch and tends to distract the bowel ends. It usually results from inadequate mobilization, especially of the colon. Though readily avoidable, twisting of the mesentery can also render an anastomosis ischaemic. As a rule repair mesenteric/mesocolic defects after completing an intestinal anastomosis to prevent postoperative internal herniation, but take care in so doing not to compromise the vessels supplying the bowel ends.

5 Distended loops of bowel are heavy and difficult to handle. Moreover, healing is impaired, probably because the bowel wall is thinner and somewhat ischaemic. Distended small bowel may be decompressed by milking contents upwards into the reach of the nasogastric tube or by enterotomy and insertion of a sucker (see later). Gaseous distension of the large bowel can be relieved by introducing a needle obliquely through its wall. Try to avoid leaving hard faecal lumps proximal to a colonic anastomosis. If possible, milk them beyond the site of intended colonic transection.

KEY POINT A safe small-bowel anastomosis

- The key to a successful anastomosis is the accurate union of two viable bowel ends with complete avoidance of tension.

Hand-suturing techniques

1 Traditionally, bowel is united in two layers, using absorbable suture material such as polyglactin 910 for the inner, all-coats layers and an outer stitch, named after its inventor in 1826, the Parisian surgeon Antoine Lembert (1802–1851), to join the seromuscular layers. In certain sites only a one-layered anastomosis can sometimes be achieved, such as colorectal and biliary–enteric anastomoses and oesophagojejunostomy.

2 Surgeons have long disputed the best suture material, the best type of stitch and the best methods of fashioning a suture line. We believe that these technical points are less important than the principle stated above: to achieve accurate and tension-free coaptation of two healthy mucosal surfaces. Nevertheless, each surgeon develops his own variations of technique, which he believes to be the most appropriate. As an assistant, therefore, follow the method of your present chief and hope to experience a number of methods before you have to select one for yourself.

3 Surgical trainees are often uncertain whether to use continuous or interrupted sutures in a given situation. A continuous (running) stitch is undoubtedly quicker and it achieves good haemostasis. It is therefore appropriate for straightforward gastric, enteric and colonic anastomoses. Be careful to maintain the tension on the previous stitch when inserting and pulling through its successor. The assistant should keep the suture material taut until you are ready to pull up the next stitch.

4 Interrupted sutures allow slightly greater precision and may be more convenient than a continuous stitch when there is marked disparity in the size of the bowel ends to be united or the anastomosis is technically difficult. In inaccessible situations such as a colorectal anastomosis deep in the pelvis, or hepaticojejunostomy, it may be wise to insert the entire posterior row of interrupted sutures before trying any individual stitch.

5 Many surgeons routinely use two layers of continuous absorbable sutures for gastric and intestinal anastomoses. If impaired healing is anticipated, as in Crohn's disease, consider whether an inner layer of continuous polyglactin 910 (Vicryl) and an outer layer of interrupted silk would provide added security. Non-absorbable sutures are usually indicated when joining small bowel or colon to the oesophagus, pancreas or rectum; suitable materials include silk (2/0 or 3/0), polypropylene (Prolene), monofilament nylon and stainless-steel wire.

6 Whichever type of suture and suture material you employ, take care to achieve the correct degree of tension when pulling through and tying the stitch. Insert each stitch separately and invert the bowel edges as the suture is tightened. Once the bowel edge is inverted, prevent the suture material from slipping by getting your assistant to follow up. Alternatively, follow up yourself, using the taut suture as a means of steadying the bowel against the thrust of the needle. The objective is a snug, watertight anastomosis. Excessive tension risks strangulating the bowel incorporated in the stitch and perhaps causing subsequent leakage.

7 Do not place the sutures so close to the edge of the bowel that they might tear out or so deep that they turn in an enormous cuff of tissue and narrow the bowel; usually 3–5 mm is about the correct depth of 'bite'. Be sure that the all-coats suture does in fact incorporate all coats of the bowel wall. The muscularis tends to retract and may escape being sutured, especially posteriorly. The best way to master these important technical points is to assist at, and then perform under supervision, a number of intestinal anastomoses.

8 The seromuscular stitch unites the adjacent bowel walls outside the all-coats stitch. Sometimes the posterior seromuscular layer is inserted before opening the gut, as in side-to-side anastomoses (Fig. 14.1). After the all-coats stitches have been inserted, carry the seromuscular sutures round the ends of the anastomosis and across the front wall, ultimately encircling the anastomosis so that the all-coats stitches can no longer be seen. For end-to-end anastomoses in small and large intestine it may be simpler to complete the all-coats layer before placing any Lembert sutures. Thereafter, the seromuscular layer can be inserted all the way round by rotating the bowel.

9 The all-coats stitch is accepted as the paramount stitch for holding bowel edges, since it catches the strong submucosa. There are many ways of inserting these stitches; three popular methods are described here:

- *Continuous over-and-over suture*. Approximate the two edges of cut bowel. Starting at one end, insert a corner stitch from outside to in, then over the adjacent edges of bowel and out through the other corner. Tie the suture and clip the short end. Pass the stitch back through the nearest bowel wall, over the contiguous cut edges and back through the full thickness of both walls. Continue over-and-over stitches to the opposite corner (Fig. 14.2a). After the last stitch is inserted right into the corner, take it back through the nearest corner leaving a loop on the mucosa so that the stitch emerges from the outer wall of the bowel (Fig. 14.2b). Now sew the front walls together by passing the stitch over and over, from out to in and then from in to out (Fig. 14.2c). Continue until the anastomosis has been encircled and the edges inverted, then tie off the ends of suture material. This over-and-over stitch is haemostatic.

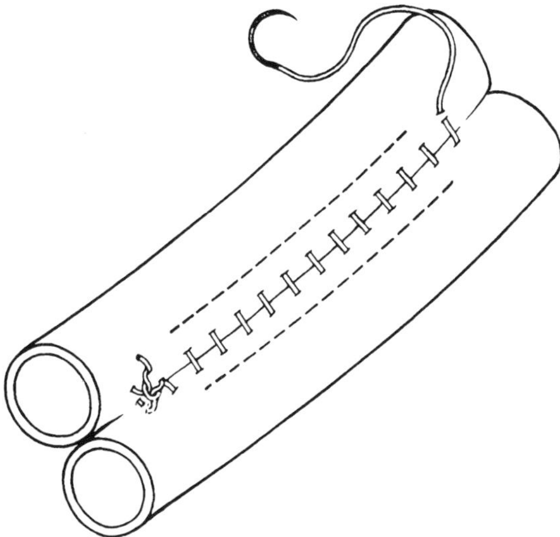

Fig. 14.1 A continuous layer of posterior seromuscular sutures has been inserted before fashioning a side-to-side anastomosis. The dotted lines indicate the lines of incision of the bowel.

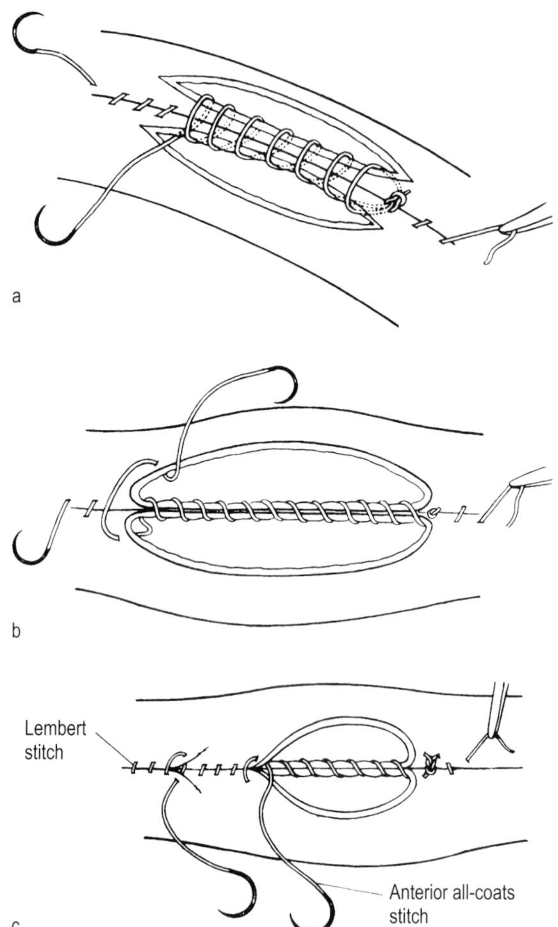

Fig. 14.2 Continuous over-and-over stitch. (a) The all-coats stitch is being inserted in a continuous over-and-over fashion. Care is taken to include mucosa and muscularis in each bite. (b) The all-coats stitch is continued round the corner. A single loop-on-the-mucosa stitch starts the return over-and-over stitch. (c) The anterior all-coats stitch is continued, then the anterior seromuscular stitch completes the anastomosis.

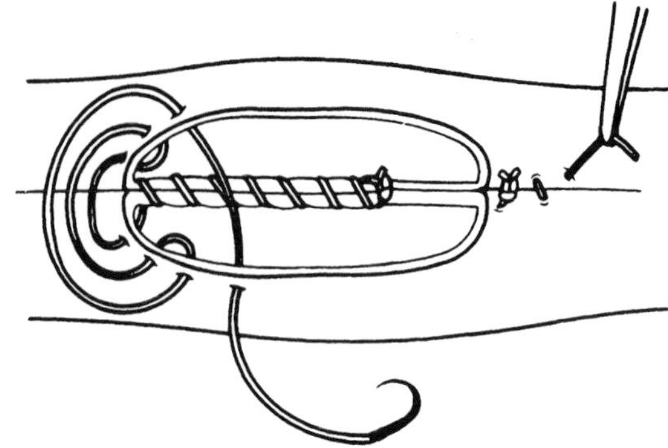

Fig. 14.3 Starting from the middle of the back wall, an over-and-over stitch has been inserted as far as the corner. Two or three Connell stitches are placed to turn the corner, followed by an anterior over-and-over stitch. A separate suture is used to fashion the other half of the anastomosis.

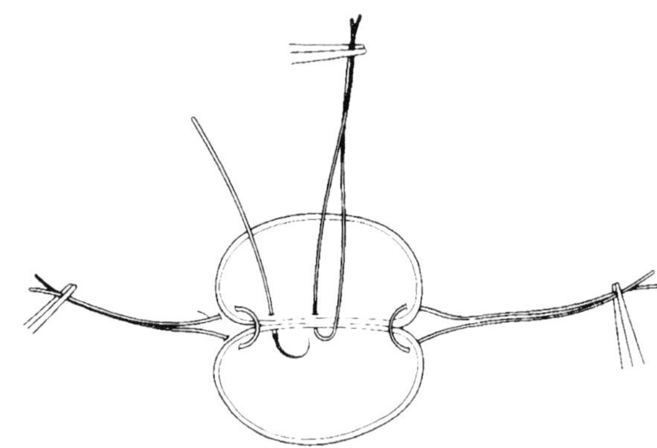

Fig. 14.4 End-to-end anastomosis using interrupted sutures. The two corner stitches are tied with the knots on the outside, but for the remainder of the posterior wall the knots are placed on the inside. If access is restricted, each suture is inserted and held in a clip before any one is tied (as shown).

- *Continuous over-and-over plus Connell suture.* Commence in the middle of the posterior wall by placing a stitch between the adjacent cut edges of bowel and tying it on the luminal surface. Now continue towards one corner with over-and-over stitches. At the corner the needle passes from in to out on the nearside cut surface, then crosses to the far edge and is passed in and out to leave a loop on the mucosa (Fig. 14.3). The needle returns to the near edge and another loop-on-the-mucosa stitch (named after the American surgeon Gregory Connell born 1875, who popularized it) is inserted. These Connell stitches turn the corner neatly. Once you are round the corner, leave this stitch and return to the middle of the posterior wall. Use a new length of suture material, unless there is a needle at each end of the original length. Insert and tie a stitch close to the site of the original ligature, tie the two short ends of suture material and proceed towards the opposite corner, using Connell sutures to negotiate the corner again. Either continue with Connell stitches along the anterior wall from each end or return to over-and-over stitches once you are round the corners. Tie off the ends of suture material in the middle of the anterior wall. The Connell stitch is not fully haemostatic, so secure all bleeding points.
- *Interrupted suture.* Insert a stitch from out to in and in to out at each corner. If the anastomosis is easily accessible, tie each stitch at this stage. Clip the ends of suture material and get your assistant to hold the clips to exert traction on the posterior cut edges of bowel (Fig. 14.4). Insert a row of posterior sutures 2–3 mm apart, tying the knots on the luminal surface. If the anastomosis is relatively inaccessible, avoid tying any sutures until the entire posterior row has been inserted. Then approximate the bowel ends and tie the sutures snugly and in order, proceeding from one corner to the next. Now place an anterior row of interrupted sutures. It is easier to tie the knots on the outside at this stage, and inversion does not appear to be essential. Indeed, some surgeons practise edge-to-edge or eversion techniques routinely for intestinal anastomosis, preferring not to turn in a ridge of tissue that might obstruct the lumen.

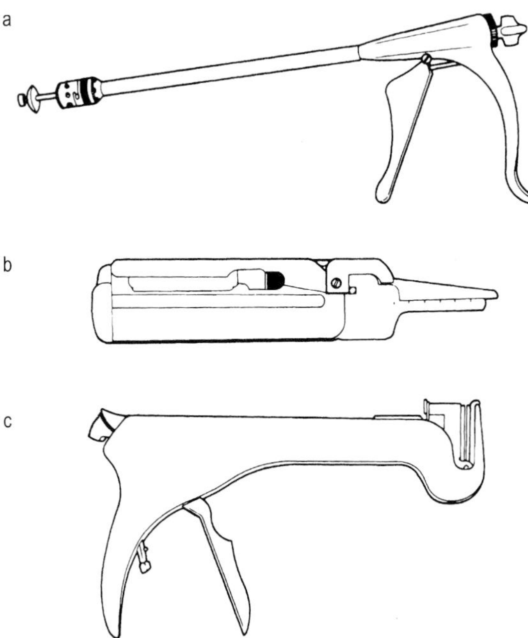

Fig. 14.5 Auto Suture instruments used for gastrointestinal anastomosis: (a) model EEA is for end-to-side anastomosis; (b) model GIA is for side-to-side anastomosis; (c) model TA30 is for closing off the end of the bowel.

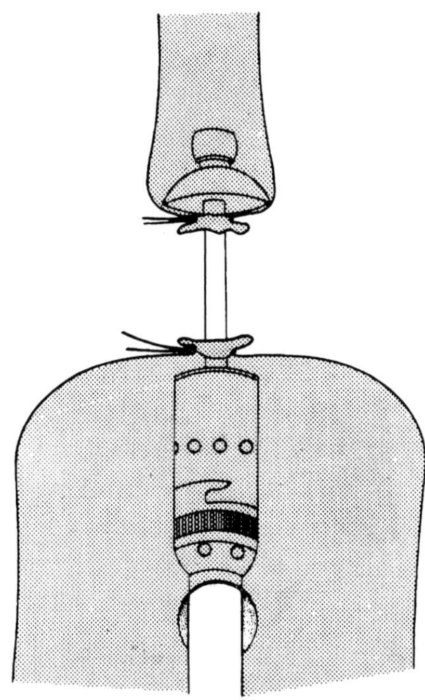

Fig. 14.6 Oesophagogastric anastomosis, using the EEA stapling gun inserted through a small gastrotomy. After tying each purse-string suture around the central rod, the anvil is approximated to the cartridge and the staples are discharged.

Mechanical stapling techniques

- Stapling machines are now available to carry out most types of gastrointestinal anastamosis.[1] Disposable and angled instruments are available for use in particular circumstances, and the metal staples come in different lengths to accommodate the different tissue thicknesses encountered. For end-to-end anastomosis (e.g. colorectal, oesophagojejunal) the stapling gun (Fig. 14.5a) is introduced into the intestinal lumen downstream, brought out through the distal cut end of bowel and then insinuated into the proximal cut end.

  Choose the largest anvil that will fit comfortably into the proximal lumen. Tightly snug the proximal and distal gut around the central rod using purse-string sutures, and then approximate the anvil to the cartridge by closing the instrument. When the gun is fired, a circular double row of stainless-steel staples is inserted and at the same time a complete 5-mm rim of each bowel end (the 'doughnut') is resected. Withdraw the machine and check the 'doughnuts' to confirm that they are complete and that the anastomosis is perfect.
- For side-to-side anastomosis use a different instrument, resembling a pair of scissors (Fig. 14.5b). One 'blade' is inserted into each of the two intestinal segments to be united, and the blades are closed. Firing the gun advances a knife, which divides the adjacent surfaces of bowel between two parallel rows of staples.
- Yet another set of instruments has been designed to place a double row of staples across the end of a segment of intestine or stomach (Fig. 14.5c). The staple line can be 30, 55 or 90 mm long. After firing the staples, leave the instrument attached and use it as an anvil on which to transect the gut. Some surgeons prefer to bury the staple line with a continuous Lembert suture.

KEY POINTS Stapled anastomosis

- Using a mechanical stapler does not guarantee a perfect result. It is just as important to prepare healthy bowel ends and avoid tension as it is in hand-sewn anastomoses, and a different set of technical details has to be learnt.
- Sutures are more versatile than staples. As a trainee, take every opportunity to practice perfect stitching.

- Stapling machines reduce the time involved in fashioning an anastomosis and facilitate certain operations that can be difficult to complete by hand, such as oesophageal transection, oesophagogastrectomy (Fig. 14.6) or low anterior resection of the rectum. The introduction of disposable stapling guns obviates the need for careful maintenance of the reusable instrument and may reduce the substantial costs involved in mechanical stapling. On the other hand, there are many situations where the stapler is inappropriate such as choledochojejunostomy, or unnecessary as in most small-bowel anastomoses.

Types of anastomosis

End-to-end anastomosis

1 This is the simplest way of restoring intestinal continuity after partial enterectomy and/or colectomy. After removal of the resected specimen, clean and approximate the bowel ends. The anastomosis is usually created in two layers, using a continuous absorbable suture (e.g. 2/0 or 3/0 Vicryl) swaged on to an eyeless needle (Fig. 14.7).

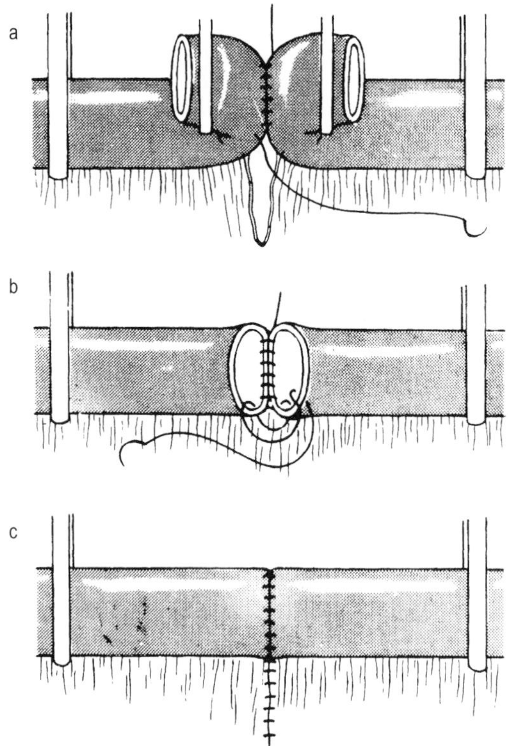

Fig. 14.7 End-to-end intestinal anastomosis: (a) and (b) two layers of stitches being inserted; (c) the completed anastomosis with the mesentery repaired.

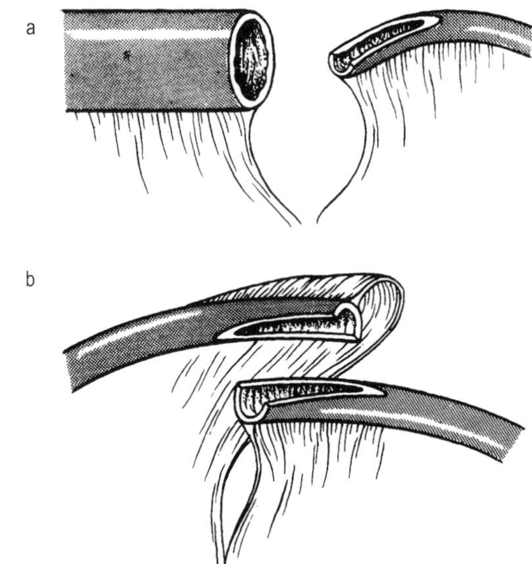

Fig. 14.8 Oblique anastomoses: (a) end-to-back anastomosis; the narrow bowel has been opened along its antimesenteric border so that its lumen matches the end of the wider bowel; (b) back-to-back anastomosis; two narrow segments of bowel have been opened along their antimesenteric borders to create a wide anastomosis.

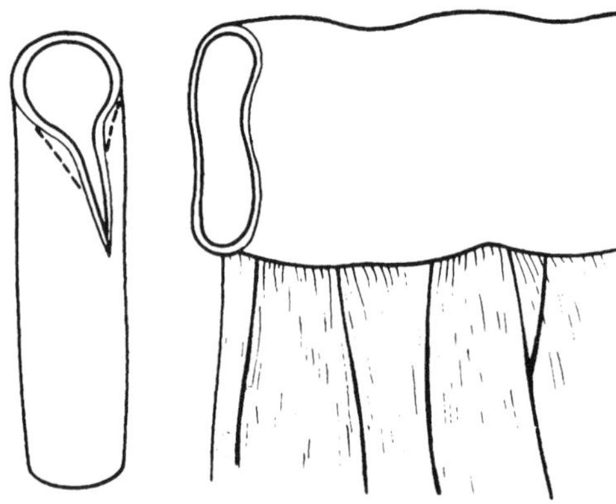

Fig. 14.9 End-to-lateral anastomosis. Poth's variation of the oblique anastomosis may be used to unite ileum to colon. The comers on the ileal segment are trimmed along the dotted lines.

2 Insert the all-coats stitch, using one of the techniques described above or a variant that you have been shown. Remove the intestinal clamps and check that the anastomosis is airtight and watertight by gently squeezing intestinal contents across it. Now insert the circumferential seromuscular stitch, taking care not to turn in too thick a cuff of tissue. Make sure the thumb and forefinger can invaginate bowel wall on each side through the anastomosis. Some surgeons prefer to unite the bowel ends with a posterior layer of Lembert sutures before embarking on the all-coats stitch, but we resort to this manoeuvre with end-to-end anastomosis only if we anticipate subsequent difficulty in placing the posterior seromuscular layer. Lastly, unite the cut edges of mesentery and/or mesocolon on each aspect with interrupted Vicryl sutures, taking care to avoid damaging the vessels.

Oblique anastomosis

1 When the ends of bowel are disproportionate in size, they may be matched by incising the antimesenteric border of the narrow bowel longitudinally (Fig. 14.8a).

2 This manoeuvre is useful in joining obstructed bowel to collapsed bowel or ileum to colon. In neonates with congenital intestinal atresia, the lumen of the distal bowel is particularly narrow and this type of 'end-to-back' anastomosis is necessitated. The mesentery of the proximal bowel is also disproportionately big and should be shortened with a few gathering stitches before being united to the distal cut edge of mesentery. When two segments of narrow intestine must be united, they may both be opened along their antimesenteric borders, which are then joined back-to-back (Fig. 14.8b). The mesenteries are now on opposite sides of the anastomosis and cannot always be neatly approximated. Poth has described an elegant variant of this technique, in which the end of the larger segment is sutured to the end-to-lateral aspect of the smaller segment of bowel (Fig. 14.9).

End-to-side anastomosis

1 This is most commonly used when creating a Roux-en-Y anastomosis. Approximate the cut end to the side of bowel to which it will be joined and insert a posterior seromuscular suture (Fig. 14.10).

2 Incise the antimesenteric border of the side of bowel to accommodate the cut end. Insert the all-coats stitch as before, remove the clamps and complete the seromuscular stitch. Lastly,

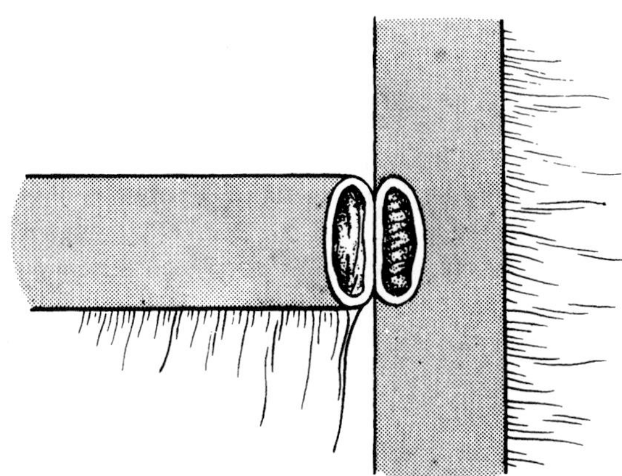

Fig. 14.10 End-to-side anastomosis.

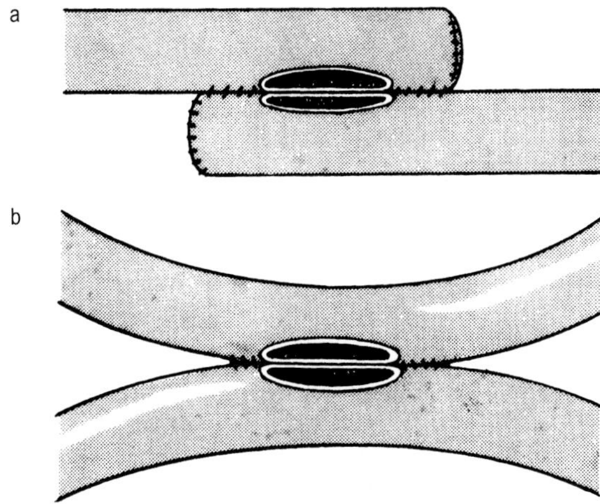

Fig. 14.11 Side-to-side anastomoses: (a) after transection of the bowel, with closure of each end; (b) two segments are joined without dividing the bowel.

join the cut edge of mesentery to the side of the intact mesentery.

Side-to-side anastomosis

1 This can be used to joint two loops of bowel without resection, or to unite intestine to stomach, bile duct, etc. (Fig. 14.11).

2 It may also be employed as an alternative to end-to-end anastomosis after intestinal resection, in which case the cut ends of bowel should first be closed and invaginated. The advantages of the side-to-side anastomosis are that the segments of bowel to be united have no interruption to their blood supply at all and that the incisions can be made exactly congruous. The disadvantages are that there are more suture lines involved and that there may be some degree of stasis and bacterial overgrowth; Poth's adaptation of the side-to-side anastomosis may overcome these objections (Fig. 14.12).[2]

3 Lay the segments to be joined side by side in contact for 8–10 cm and insert a posterior seromuscular stitch. Incise the antimesenteric borders for about 5 cm and insert an all-coats stitch. Remove the clamps and complete the anterior seromuscular layer of stitches. When side-to-side anastomosis follows bowel resection, suture the cut edge of mesentery to the adjacent intact mesentery on each side of the anastomosis.

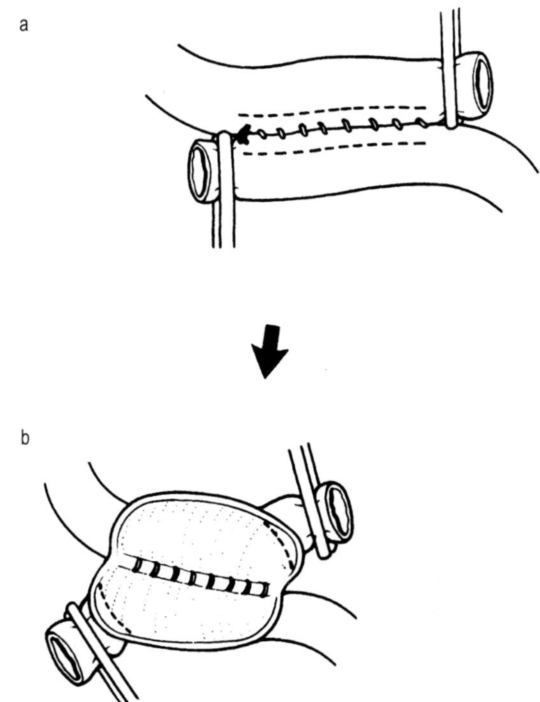

Fig. 14.12 Poth's modification of the side-to-side anastomosis: (a) the posterior seromuscular stitch has been inserted; each segment is opened along the dotted line; (b) the posterior all-coats stitch has been placed; the corners are trimmed along the dotted lines.

REFERENCES

1. Steichen FM, Ravitch MM 1987 Mechanical sutures in operations on the small intestine. In: Nelson RL, Nyhus LM (eds) Surgery of the small intestine. Appleton & Lange, Norwalk, pp 375–399
2. Poth EJ 1950 A technique for suturing bowel. Surgery, Gynecology and Obstetrics 91:656–659

ENTERECTOMY (SMALL-BOWEL RESECTION)

Appraise

- Resection is often indicated for congenital lesions of the small bowel such as atresia and duplication; traumatic perforation; critical ischaemia from mesenteric trauma, strangulation or arteriosclerosis; Crohn's disease or other cause of stricture; tumours of the bowel or its mesentery. Resection is sometimes indicated for fistula, diverticulitis, intussusception and a symptomatic blind loop. Small portions of the duodenum and ileum are removed during partial gastrectomy and right hemicolectomy respectively.
- There are several reasons for being conservative in the management of *Crohn's disease*: the indolent nature of the disease, its relapsing course and its strong tendency (>50%) to recur anywhere in the intestinal tract, but especially at and just proximal to the anastomosis. Despite many advances in the treatment of Crohn's disease, the course of the disease in any given patient remains unpredictable. There is little agreement as to which factors predispose a patient to recurrence. A multivariate analysis has shown that the only independent predictors of earlier

postoperative recurrence after initial operation are an initial presentation with peritonitis, secondary to perforation, and a longer preoperative disease duration.[1]

KEY POINT Avoid unnecessary intestinal resection in Crohn's disease

- Do not resect for Crohn's ileitis discovered incidentally during laparotomy for suspected appendicitis.

- On the other hand, most patients with chronic Crohn's enteritis eventually require resection of the affected segment because of subacute obstruction, fistula or abscess. Bypass is obsolete: the defunctioned segment is unlikely to heal, bacterial overgrowth of the blind loop may aggravate diarrhoea and there is a long-term risk of carcinoma. For 'burnt-out' stenotic areas of bowel, strictureplasty (see later) is an alternative to resection.
- When operating for *radiation enteropathy* certain principles should be observed. Establish the extent both of the original cancer and of the radiation damage. Where possible, avoid bypass or exclusion procedures: the leakage rate is probably no lower than after resection and anastomosis, and the defunctioned bowel may still give rise to problems such as bleeding and fistula. Wide resection is the optimal approach, ensuring that at least one side of the subsequent anastomosis employs healthy, non-irradiated, bowel.

Prepare

1 In the presence of an obstructing lesion, ensure that the patient is adequately resuscitated before operation with nasogastric intubation and intravenous rehydration. In non-obstructed patients undergoing small-bowel operations, a nasogastric tube should be passed after induction of anaesthesia.

2 Healthy ileum has a resident bacterial flora, and in the presence of obstruction the entire small bowel may be colonized. It is sensible to cover all operations likely to involve intestinal resection with appropriate prophylactic antibiotics, such as a cephalosporin plus metronidazole given preoperatively in a single intravenous injection.

3 Nutritional status may be impaired in some patients requiring small-bowel resection, for example those with Crohn's disease, cancer, radiation enteropathy or enterocutaneous fistula. In the absence or obstruction on fistula, supplemental enteric feeds may reverse the nutritional defect, but some patients require a period of preoperative parenteral nutrition.

Access

1 Adequate exposure of the entire small bowel can be provided by a number of different incisions. We usually employ a midline incision that skirts the umbilicus and can be extended in either direction as necessary.

2 Remember that the small bowel quite often adheres to the back of a previous laparotomy incision, and take particular care during abdominal re-entry. The chances are that an accidental perforation will not be located in a segment of bowel that you would in any case have intended to remove.

Assess

1 Expose and examine the entire small bowel. Continue by examining the stomach, large bowel and remaining abdominal viscera (Ch. 4).

2 If a loop of small bowel has been strangulated in an external hernia, for example, release the obstruction and check the viability of the bowel after allowing a minimum period of 5 minutes for possible recovery in doubtful cases (Ch. 6).

3 Healthy small intestine possesses both a considerable functional reserve and the capacity to adapt to partial tissue loss by compensatory villous hyperplasia of the portions that remain. Nevertheless, do not gratuitously sacrifice healthy bowel, particularly terminal ileum, which has specialized transport functions. Except when operating for primary malignant tumours it is quite unnecessary to excise a deep wedge of mesentery, which might increase the extent of small bowel requiring removal. In Crohn's disease do not remove more than a few centimetres of gut on either side of the affected segment, but include any fistulas or sinuses. It is more than likely that further resection will be required in future, and microscopic inflammation of the bowel at the resection margin does not appear to increase subsequent anastomotic recurrence. Conventional right hemicolectomy is unnecessary for small-bowel Crohn's disease; undertake conservative ileocaecal resection.

4 Sometimes a partial resection of small bowel can be performed, leaving the mesentery intact. Appropriate conditions include Richter's hernia, Meckel's diverticulum and small tumours arising on the antimesenteric border.

Action

1 Isolate the diseased loop of bowel from the other abdominal contents by means of large, moist packs or a special towel.

2 Hold up the bowel and examine the mesentery against the light. Note the vascular pattern.

Standard resection

1 Determine the proximal and distal sites for dividing the bowel, and select the line of vascular section in between; keep fairly close to the bowel wall (Fig. 14.13), except when resecting a neoplasm (Fig. 14.14). Incise the peritoneum along this line on each aspect of the mesentery. This manoeuvre is most easily accomplished by inserting one blade of a pair of fine, curved

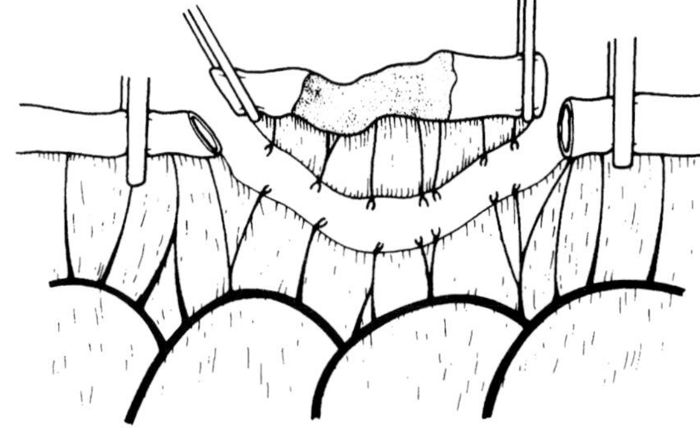

Fig. 14.13 Resection of an ischaemic segment of small bowel including a shallow wedge of mesentery. The narrower bowel end has been cut obliquely to match the wider end.

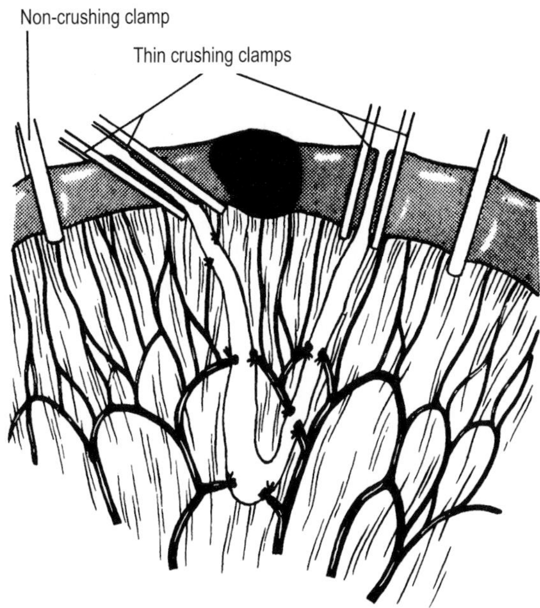

Fig. 14.14 Resection of a small-bowel tumour. A deeper wedge of mesentery is included than in operations for benign disease (see Fig. 14.13). As before, the narrower segment of bowel (on the left) is transected obliquely, removing more of the mesenteric border with the specimen.

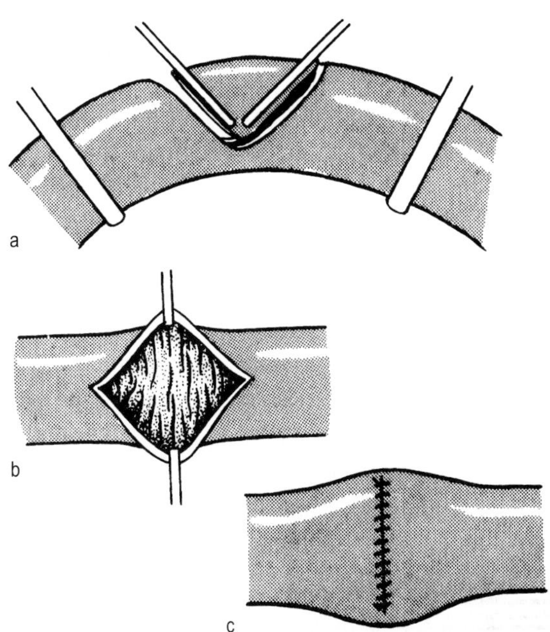

Fig. 14.15 Partial resection of small bowel: (a) a wedge of antimesenteric bowel is removed; (b) the defect is opened out transversely; (c) closure across the long axis of the bowel prevents narrowing.

scissors beneath the peritoneum and cutting superficially to expose the mesenteric vessels.

2 Using small artery forceps, create a small mesenteric window right next to the bowel wall at each point chosen for intestinal transection. Starting at one end, insinuate a curved artery forceps through this window and back through the mesentery, denuded of peritoneum, 1–2 cm away, thus isolating a small leash of mesentery with its contained vessels. Either doubly ligate this leash in continuity and divide between ligatures, or divide between artery forceps, ligating the mesentery beneath each pair of forceps. Proceeding in this manner, divide the mesentery right up to the bowel wall at the further end of the line of peritoneal incision. Take care in placing and tying each ligature; if the knot slips, there can be troublesome haemorrhage. We use polyglactin 910 (Vicryl) or silk ties, 2/0 or 3/0 according to the thickness of the mesentery.

3 Apply four intestinal clamps (Fig. 14.13). The first two clamps are crushing clamps (Payr's, Lang Stevenson's or Pringle's). They should be applied obliquely at the points of intended intestinal transection, so that slightly more of the antimesenteric border is resected than of the mesenteric border; the obliquity reduces the risk of a tight anastomosis. Now apply a non-crushing clamp about 5 cm outside each crushing clamp, having milked the intervening bowel free of contents.

4 Place a clean gauze swab beneath the clamps at each end to catch spills, and divide the bowel with a knife flush against the outer aspect of each crushing clamp. Place the specimen and the soiled knife in a separate dish, which is then removed.

5 Cleanse each bowel end, using small swabs or pledgets of gauze soaked in cetrimide. Then remove the protective gauze swab and proceed to intestinal anastomosis. In an attempt to limit contamination, some surgeons divide the intestine between two pairs of light crushing clamps (i.e. six clamps in all) and insert the posterior seromuscular layer of sutures before removing the outer clamps and excising the narrow rim of crushed tissue (Fig. 14.14).

6 Perform a two-layer, end-to-end anastomosis, as described in the previous section.

Partial resection

1 A diverticulum on the antimesenteric border may be locally excised. Clamp and cut it off at the neck, then close the defect in two layers as a transverse linear slit. Try to avoid narrowing the intestinal lumen during this procedure.

2 A diamond-shaped area of the antimesenteric border may be included in the resection of a localized tumour or wide-mouthed Meckel's diverticulum. Apply two light crushing clamps (Lang Stevenson's or Pringle's) across the antimesenteric border, meeting in a 'V' (Fig. 14.15). Incise the bowel flush with the outer aspect of each clamp, and close the wall in two layers, leaving a transverse suture line.

3 A similar defect results if the antimesenteric lesion is excised through a longitudinal ellipse. Approximate the ends of the ellipse, pull apart the sides and close transversely as before.

Checklist

1 Take a last look at the anastomosis. Check that the bowel is pink, that haemostasis is secure and that all mesenteric defects are closed.

KEY POINTS Swabs

- It is easy to lose a swab among the coils of small intestine.
- Check the entire abdominal cavity and make sure that the swab count is correct.

2 Remove any ends of suture material that might provoke subsequent adhesions.

3 Replace the intestine and the greater omentum in their normal anatomical position.

4 Suck out the peritoneal cavity. Place a fine-bore suction drain to the region of the anastomosis.

? DIFFICULTY

1. *Is the bowel obstructed?* Decompress obstructed jejunum by milking its contents upwards until they can be aspirated through the nasogastric tube. Decompress obstructed ileum by inserting a sucker tube, either into the end of the proximal bowel after releasing the clamps or via a separate enterotomy. Do this without allowing bowel contents to spill.
2. In the presence of obstruction there may be marked disparity between the diameters of the bowel ends. In practice, moderate incongruities can be overcome by adjusting the size of bite, while suturing proximal to distal bowel. The diameter of the distal bowel can be increased by transecting it more obliquely, sparing the mesenteric border, and by opening it along the antimesenteric border. If there is gross disparity, consider oblique or side-to-side anastomosis.
3. Resection and anastomosis can usually be completed outside the abdomen. Sometimes this is not possible, in which case you may not be able to apply all the clamps described above. Try and retain the non-crushing clamps placed at a distance from the anastomosis, if possible. In difficult circumstances, concentrate on completing the all-coats suture without defect, if necessary using interrupted sutures. You may subsequently be able to insert seromuscular sutures around all or most of the circumference.
4. *A haematoma develops in the mesentery or in the submucosa at the point of intestinal transection.* Compression of the area with a swab usually stops the bleeding. Alternatively, gently close swab-holding forceps or non-crushing clamps across the bleeding point and wait for a few minutes. If the bleeding is not fully controlled, incise the peritoneum, find the bleeding point, pick it up with fine artery forceps and ligate it. Check the colour of the bowel to confirm that the blood supply is not prejudiced.
5. *One or other intestinal end becomes dusky during the anastomosis.* Allow time to declare the issue. Non-viable bowel will not heal, so if you are in any doubt excise a few more centimetres and make a fresh start. Leave the mesentery attached to the bowel as close as possible to the point of transection, and check for visible pulsations in the edge of the mesentery.

Aftercare

1 Anticipate a period of postoperative paralytic ileus during which maintain the patient on intravenous fluids. Leave the nasogastric tube on open drainage, aspirated regularly for the first 24–48 hours. Allow water 30 ml/hour by mouth. The tube can usually be removed when bowel sounds return, the volume of aspirate drops below the volume of fluid taken by mouth and there is passage of flatus. Peristalsis returns to the small bowel before the stomach and colon regain their motility.

2 Remove the drain when the fluid loss diminishes, generally at 2–3 days.

3 If restoration of oral feeding is very delayed, consider instituting a period of parenteral nutrition.

Complications

1 Wound infection is a potential risk of any procedure involving an intestinal anastomosis. Good surgical technique in limiting contamination from bowel contents certainly reduces the incidence. If wound sepsis develops, remove sufficient sutures to allow the pus to drain, irrigate the wound, obtain bacteriological cultures and, in severe cases, institute appropriate antibiotic therapy. Once the infection is controlled, the wound usually heals without the need for secondary suture. Wound dehiscence is considered in Chapter 4.

2 As with any abdominal operation there is a risk of chest infection resulting from atelectasis. Institute vigorous physiotherapy to avert the need for antibiotics.

3 Occasionally a collection of infected material develops within the abdominal cavity. Abscess sites may be subphrenic, subhepatic, pelvic or adjacent to the anastomosis. The patient develops fever and leucocytosis. Ultrasound scan localizes the collection and allows percutaneous drainage in many cases (Ch. 8).

4 A leaking anastomosis often presents with pain, fever, tachycardia and erythema of the wound or drain site before intestinal contents begin to discharge. The management of an established small-bowel fistula is described at the end of this chapter.

5 It is occasionally necessary to undertake massive resection of the small bowel, for example when volvulus complicates an obstruction.[2] Repeated enterectomies in Crohn's disease can similarly remove a substantial percentage of the small intestine. Increased frequency of bowel actions may follow loss of a third to a half of the small bowel, and more extensive resections produce short-bowel syndrome.[3] During the initial phase of recovery and adaptation, anticipate and replace losses of fluid and electrolytes, notably potassium. Give codeine or loperamide to control diarrhoea. The body compensates better for proximal than distal enterectomy. After an extensive ileal resection regular injections of vitamin B_{12} may be needed indefinitely; colestyramine may diminish the irritative diarrhoea that results from bile-acid malabsorption. Consider nutritional support by the enteral or parenteral routes in severe short-bowel syndrome. Cimetidine or, rarely, vagotomy may be needed for gastric acid hypersecretion.

REFERENCES

1. Bernell O, Lapidus A, Hellers G 2000 Risk factors for surgery and postoperative recurrence in Crohn's disease. Annals of Surgery 231:38–45
2. Hill GL 1985 Massive enterectomy: indications and management. World Journal of Surgery 9:833–841
3. Bristol JB, Williamson RCN 1985 Postoperative adaptation of the small intestine. World Journal of Surgery 9:825–832

ENTERIC BYPASS

Appraise

- Small-bowel loops may become obstructed as a result of carcinomatosis peritonei or a particularly dense set of adhesions, sometimes deep in the pelvis. Irradiated small bowel may fistulate into other organs, such as the bladder or vagina. In these unfavourable circumstances it is often better just to bypass the affected segment of intestine (Fig. 14.16) rather than embark on a difficult and hazardous disentanglement. In radiation enteritis choose overtly normal bowel for the anastomosis, since healing is likely to be impaired.
- Resection is almost always a better option than simple defunction in Crohn's disease of the small bowel. For irresectable carcinoma of the caecum, however, side-to-side bypass is indicated between the terminal ileum and the transverse colon—ileotransversostomy.
- Subtotal jejunoileal bypass has been recommended for intractable morbid obesity (Fig. 14.17). Patients lose weight because of malabsorption, diarrhoea and impaired appetite. The operation provides a metabolic insult to the body, and there are many potential long-term complications. The alternative procedure of gastric reduction causes fewer metabolic upsets and is generally preferred nowadays.

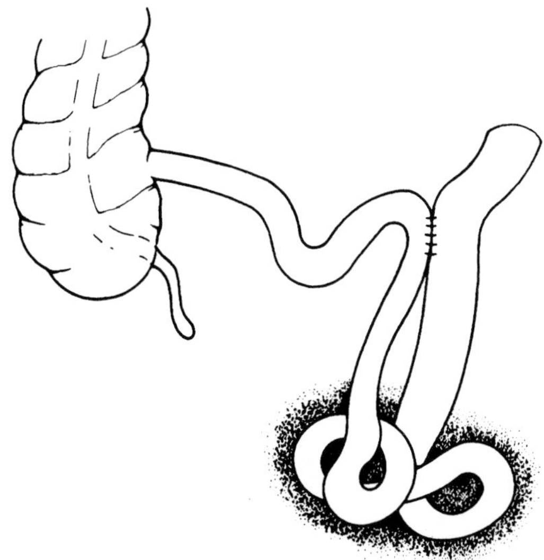

Fig. 14.16 Bypass procedure for small-bowel obstruction resulting from irresectable pelvic cancer. A side-to-side anastomosis is fashioned between a (proximal) distended loop of bowel and a (distal) collapsed loop.

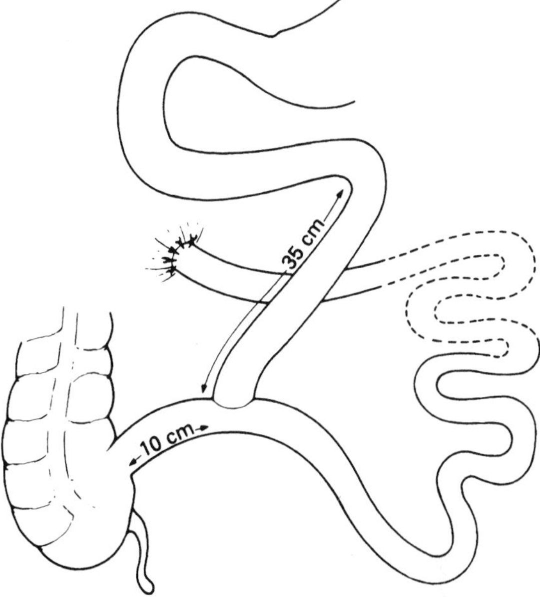

Fig. 14.17 Subtotal jejunoileal bypass for morbid obesity. An end-to-side anastomosis is fashioned between 35 cm of functioning jejunum and 10 cm of functioning ileum. The top end of the blind loop is closed and invaginated and tacked to the posterior abdominal wall to prevent intussusception.

- Bypass of the distal one-third of the small intestine is rarely indicated for certain types of hyperlipidaemia. The ileum is divided, the distal end is closed and the proximal end is reimplanted into the caecum. The operation reduces the levels of cholesterol and triglyceride in the blood.

Action

Bypass of an irresectable lesion

1. A midline incision is usually appropriate. Aim to anastomose healthy bowel on either side of the diseased segment. Side-to-side anastomosis avoids the risk of closed-loop obstruction developing in a sequestered loop of bowel.
2. Occasionally if there are multiple sites of actual or imminent obstruction, two or more side-to-side anastomoses between adjacent loops may cause less of a short circuit than one enormous bypass.
3. Approximate a distended loop of proximal intestine to a collapsed loop of distal small bowel (Fig. 14.16) or transverse colon. Pack off the remaining viscera. Consider decompression of the obstructed loops.
4. Carry out a two-layer, side-to-side anastomosis, as previously described. Take care with the anastomosis and subsequent wound closure, since healing may be impaired, but do not prolong the operation unnecessarily if the patient has advanced disease.

Aftercare and complications

The principles of management are as for enterectomy. Short-bowel syndrome is inevitable after subtotal (about 90%) jejunoileal bypass, although adaptation can still be anticipated.

STRICTUREPLASTY

Appraise

- This technique is virtually confined to patients with Crohn's disease causing a single or a few strictures in the small intestine.[1] It can avoid the need for resection and may therefore be appropriate for patients with disease at several sites or those with recurrent disease and a limited length of residual small bowel.
- Florid inflammatory change or bowel containing several strictures within a relatively short segment is better treated by local resection. Sometimes you may combine one or more strictureplasties with resection to reduce the total length of bowel excised.

Assess

The tightness of the stricture(s) can be assessed by making a small enterotomy and passing a balloon catheter. Moderate strictures of 20–25 mm diameter may be treated by balloon dilatation, but tight strictures of less than 20 mm diameter require either strictureplasty or resection.

Action

1. Carry a longitudinal full-thickness incision across the stenotic area and for 1 cm into the 'normal' bowel on either side.
2. Close the bowel transversely, using either one or two layers of 3/0 Vicryl sutures. Test that the anastomosis is airtight and watertight.
3. This modification of the Heineke–Mikulicz pyloroplasty is suitable for short stenoses. For long stenoses, a modification of the Finney pyloroplasty (Ch. 13) can be performed, but local resection may be a simpler alternative.

Complications

- Wound infections are uncommon.
- Anastomotic leakage may occur, particularly if tight strictures distal to the strictureplasty are not treated.
- As strictureplasty is a relatively recent innovation, long-term follow-up is limited. Several studies have reported excellent symptomatic improvement following operation, however. Moreover, perioperative complication rates are comparable to standard surgical treatment, with low rates of recurrent stricture. Recurrent stricture can sometimes occur at a later date.
- It is of concern that small bowel adenocarcinoma has been reported at the site of a previous strictureplasty, so bear this possibility in mind if there is a sudden clinical deterioration.[2]

REFERENCES

1. Andrews HA, Keighley MRB, Alexander-Williams J et al 1991 Strategy for management of distal ileal Crohn's disease. British Journal of Surgery 78:679–682
2. Jaskowiak NT, Michelassi F 2001 Adenocarcinoma at a strictureplasty site in Crohn's disease: report of a case. Diseases of the Colon and Rectum 44:284–287

THE ROUX LOOP

Appraise

- A defunctioned segment of jejunum provides a convenient conduit for connecting various upper abdominal organs to the remaining small bowel. The technique was originally described by the Swiss surgeon César Roux in 1907 for oesophageal bypass.

> **KEY POINT The versatile Roux loop**
>
> - The method has proved invaluable in gastric, biliary and pancreatic surgery.[1] It can be used to bypass or replace the stomach, the distal bile duct and to drain the pancreatic duct or pseudocyst.

- Roux-en-Y anastomosis has two advantages over an intact loop: it can stretch further and it is empty of intestinal contents, thus preventing contamination of the organ to be drained such as the bile duct. Active peristalsis down the loop encourages this drainage.[2]
- Probably the commonest indications for Roux-en-Y anastomosis are biliary drainage in irresectable carcinoma of the pancreatic head and reconstruction after total gastrectomy (Fig. 14.18) or oesophagogastrectomy. Conversion to a Roux loop may cure duodenogastric reflux after partial gastrectomy, provided the loop is 40–50 cm long. Allison has shown that with meticulous attention to technique it is possible to bring a Roux loop up to the neck to replace the oesophagus.[1]

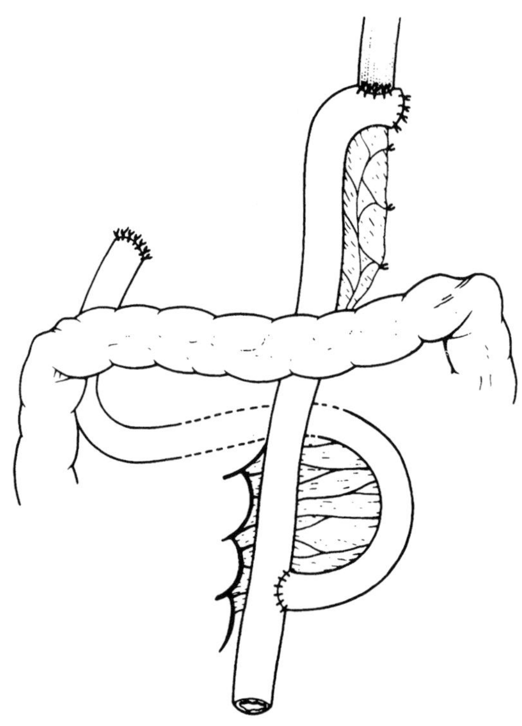

Fig. 14.18 One indication for a Roux loop: Roux-en-Y anastomosis between the oesophagus and jejunum after total gastrectomy.

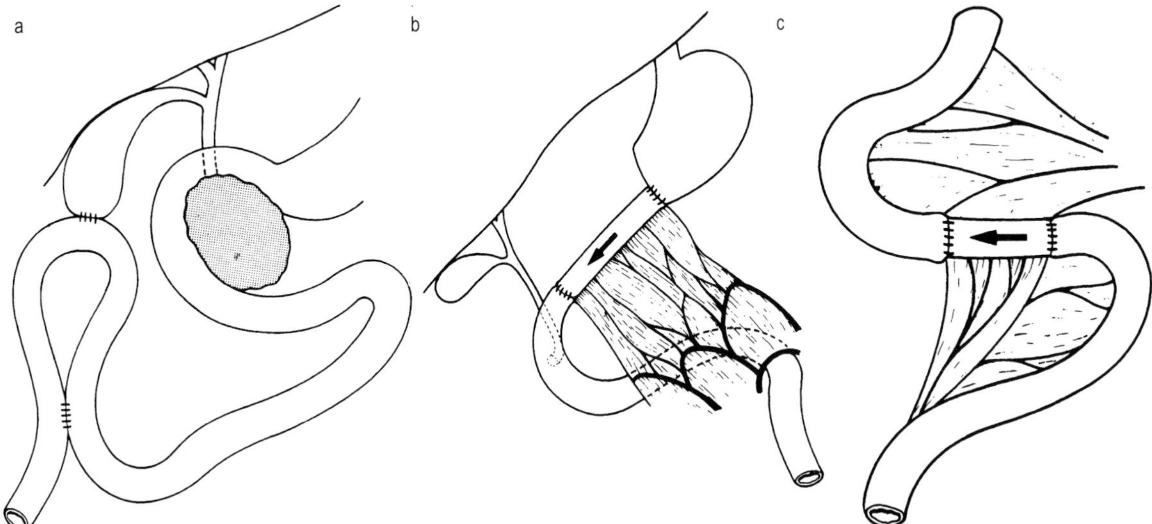

Fig. 14.19 Other types of enteric loop: (a) intact loop used to drain the distended gallbladder in a case of irresectable pancreatic cancer; side-to-side anastomosis below the cholecystojejunostomy may divert food away from the biliary tree; (b) isoperistaltic 20-cm jejunal loop interposed between the stomach remnant and the duodenum to treat reflux alkaline gastritis after partial gastrectomy; (c) reversed 10-cm loop inserted 1 m distal to the ligament of Treitz to treat severe postoperative diarrhoea.

- Although Roux-en-Y anastomosis is the most versatile technique, other types of jejunal loop are sometimes indicated (Fig. 14.19). Intact loops are used for cholecystoenterostomy, gastroenterostomy and Polya (Billroth II) reconstruction after partial gastrectomy. Isolated loops may be interposed between the stomach and duodenum in an isoperistaltic or antiperistaltic direction for different facets of the postgastrectomy syndrome. A reversed loop can be used further downstream in certain cases of intractable diarrhoea. These alternatives are further discussed in Chapter 13.

Action

1 Select a loop of proximal small bowel, beginning 10–15 cm distal to the ligament of Treitz. Hold up the jejunum and transilluminate its mesentery to display the precise blood supply, which varies from patient to patient. The number of vessels requiring division depends on the length of conduit required.

2 Starting at the point chosen for intestinal transection, incise the peritoneal leaves of the mesentery in a vertical direction (Fig. 14.20). Divide at least one vascular arcade and the smaller branches that lie between the arcade vessels and the bowel. Ligate these vessels neatly in continuity and avoid using artery forceps, which can bunch up the tissues and prevent mobilization of the loop. Now divide the bowel between clamps.

3 If a longer loop is required, sacrifice two or three main jejunal vessels, preserving an intact blood supply to the extremity of the bowel via the arcades (Fig. 14.20). The peritoneum may require further incision to facilitate elongation of the loop without tension. Individual ligation of the arteries and veins is recommended, using fine silk sutures. Check the viability of the bowel at the tip of the loop, and sacrifice the end if it is dusky.

4 Straighten out the efferent limb and take it up by the shortest route for anastomosis to the oesophagus, stomach, bile duct, common hepatic duct or pancreatic duct. It is often easier to close the end of the limb and fashion a new subterminal opening of the correct diameter. Make a window in the base of the transverse mesocolon, to the right of the duodenojejunal flexure, for passage of the Roux loop. At the end of the operation suture the margins of this defect to the Roux loop to prevent internal herniation.

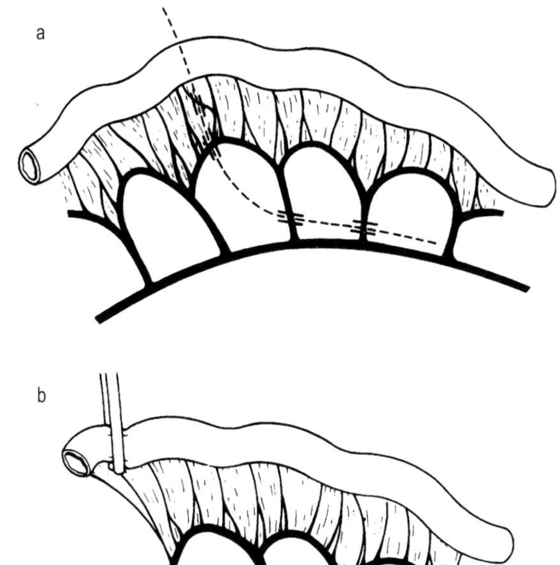

Fig. 14.20 Creation of a long Roux loop: (a) three arcade vessels have been divided; (b) the bowel is transected at a point previously selected and the loop is mobilized.

5 Restore intestinal continuity by uniting the short afferent limb to the base of the long efferent limb, using an end-to-side anastomosis. Ensure that the efferent limb is at least 30 cm long and that the afferent loop is joined to its left-hand side.

REFERENCES

1. Allison PR, da Silva LT 1953 The Roux loop. British Journal of Surgery 41:173–180
2. Kirk RM 1985 Roux-en-Y. World Journal of Surgery 9:938–944

ENTEROTOMY

Appraise

- Probably the commonest reason for making an incision into the lumen of the small bowel is to decompress the intestine proximal to the site of an obstruction. The enterotomy should be made halfway between the ligament of Treitz and the site of obstruction, so that the sucker can be inserted both proximally and distally to reach all the distended loops. It is usually possible to avoid enterotomy in a high obstruction by advancing the nasogastric tube through the duodenum and squeezing luminal contents upwards until they can be aspirated. In other circumstances the decompressing sucker can be inserted through the proximal cut end of bowel, if enterectomy is planned, or through the caecum and ileocaecal valve after appendicectomy.
- Sometimes enterotomy is needed to extract a foreign body, for example in gallstone ileus or bolus obstruction. After partial gastrectomy, the absence of the antropyloric mill means that whole orange segments or pith, for example, are inadequately broken up and may impact further down the gut. Benign mucosal or submucosal tumours may be explored and removed through an enterotomy incision.
- Traumatic enterotomy can result from blunt or penetrating abdominal injuries. After a closed injury there is typically a rosette of exposed mucosa on the antimesenteric border of the upper jejunum. After knife or gunshot injuries, look for entry and exit wounds; holes in the small bowel nearly always come in multiples of two.
- Occasionally, operative enteroscopy may be indicated for unexplained bleeding localized to the small bowel. A flexible colonoscope can be introduced through a mid-enterotomy and threaded up and down the gut.

Action

Decompression enterotomy

1 The objective is to empty the small bowel without contaminating the peritoneal cavity. Pack off the area and apply non-crushing clamps on either side of the site chosen for enterotomy. Insert an absorbable purse-string stitch, make a small nick through the wall of the bowel and introduce a Savage decompressor, which consists of a long trocar and cannula connected to the sucker tubing (Fig. 14.21).

2 Pass the sucker up and down the bowel, removing first one clamp and then the other. The assistant feeds the distended loops of gut over the end of the sucker, while you control the force of suction by placing a finger over a side-port on the decompressing cannula. Sometimes the bowel appears to be only partly deflated, because of interstitial oedema.

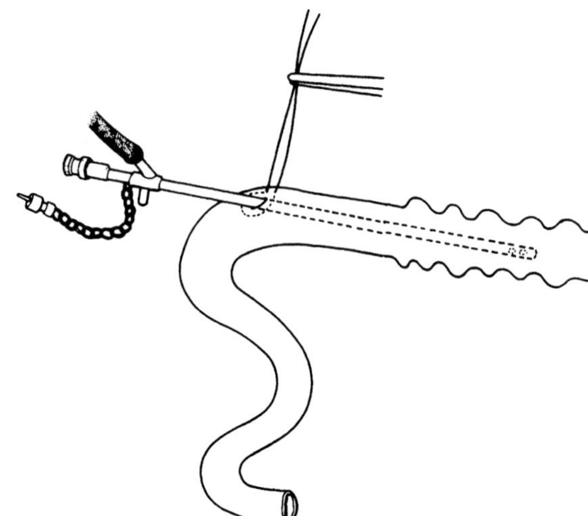

Fig. 14.21 Decompression enterotomy. After insertion of the Savage decompressor, the trocar is withdrawn and the cannula is gently passed along the distended loops of bowel in either direction. Suction tubing is attached to the side-arm of the decompressor.

3 After emptying the bowel, remove the sucker, tighten and tie the purse-string and discard the contaminated packs. Place a second purse-string suture or Lembert sutures to bury the wound.

Extraction enterotomy

1 It may be possible to knead a foreign body, especially a bolus of food, onwards into the caecum. If so, it will pass spontaneously per rectum. Do not persist with this manoeuvre if it is difficult.

2 Before opening the bowel, pack off the area carefully. Try and manipulate an impacted foreign body upwards for a few centimetres, away from the inflamed segment in which it was lodged.

3 Apply non-crushing clamps across the intestine on either side of the enterotomy site. Open the bowel longitudinally over the foreign body or tumour and gently extract or resect the lesion. Close the bowel transversely in two layers to prevent stenosis.

4 In gallstone ileus examine the right upper quadrant of the abdomen. Consider whether it is appropriate to proceed to cholecystectomy, choledochotomy and possible closure of the biliary–enteric fistula. Since the patient is often elderly and unfit, concentrate on relieving the intestinal obstruction. Examine the rest of the small bowel to exclude a second gallstone.

Traumatic enterotomy

1 Excise devitalized tissue and close the intestinal wound(s) in two layers. Explore an associated haematoma in the mesentery and ligate any bleeding points. Check the viability of the bowel thereafter, and if in doubt resect the damaged segment with end-to-end anastomosis.

2 Examine the other abdominal viscera for concomitant injuries (see Ch. 4).

ENTEROSTOMY

Appraise

- A feeding jejunostomy permits enteral nutrition in patients who are unable to take sufficient food by mouth.[1] The development of parenteral nutrition has limited its use to certain circumstances, for example the preoperative hyperalimentation of malnourished patients with cancer of the stomach or oesophagus. Better still, it may be possible to pass a fine transnasal feeding tube through the malignant stricture under endoscopic control.
- A feeding tube should always be placed as high as possible in the jejunum. Nevertheless it can be difficult to introduce enough calories and nitrogen by this route without causing troublesome diarrhoea. Some surgeons use feeding jejunostomy routinely after major oesophagogastric resections. Others reserve it for postoperative complications such as fistula, or serious upper gastrointestinal conditions such as corrosive oesophagogastritis or pancreatic abscess.
- The ideal feeding jejunostomy is easily inserted, if necessary under local anaesthesia, and seals off immediately it is removed. It neither obstructs the bowel nor permits the escape of intestinal contents. We favour the use of a T-tube for this purpose.
- A feeding jejunostomy tube can be placed at laparotomy either transnasally or via an enterostomy. Insert a fine-bore nasojejunal tube peroperatively and milk it down into jejunum. The sophisticated Frecka tube contains three separate lumens—to allow gastric aspiration, pressure measurement, and jejunal feeding; it includes a clever device for insertion. It is sometimes possible to avoid laparotomy for insertion of a feeding jejunostomy by radiological puncture of the jejunum and initial placement of a guidewire, using a Seldinger technique similar to that for Hickman line insertion.
- A terminal ileostomy replaces the anus after total colectomy for multiple neoplasia, ulcerative proctocolitis or Crohn's colitis. The ileostomy may be temporary, if subsequent ileorectal anastomosis is planned, or permanent after panproctocolectomy. Improvements in stoma care make ileostomy less of a burden to patients, many of whom are young. It is desirable and usually possible to select and mark the site for ileostomy preoperatively. Choose a point just below waist level and 5 cm to the right of the midline, unless there is a previous scar in this region. It is important to create a spout that will discharge its irritative contents well clear of the skin.
- Other types of ileostomy are sometimes fashioned. Increasingly, defunctioning loop ileostomies are being used as forms of faecal diversion. Historically this stoma was used to defunction distal bowel affected by inflammatory bowel disease or to cover a precarious anastomosis in the right colon. With the advent of ultralow anterior resection, however, its use has spread. In comparison with transverse colostomy, it produces predictable volumes of relatively inoffensive faecal effluent and it is a truly defunctioning stoma to which an appliance can easily be attached. For these reasons, it has become the temporary stoma of choice. Split ileostomy, with separated stomas, completely defunction the distal bowel and has been advocated in selected cases of colitis. Split enterostomy has also been advocated to protect a lower enteric anastomosis created in the presence of peritonitis. The distal cut end is either exteriorized as a mucous fistula or oversewn and fixed to the parietal peritoneum to facilitate later retrieval. Kock's continent ileostomy consists of an ileal reservoir discharging by a short conduit to a flush stoma; a nipple valve is created to preserve continence, and the patient empties the reservoir regularly with a soft catheter. Lastly, a 'wet' ileostomy together with an ileal conduit provides one of the commoner methods for achieving urinary diversion.

Action

Feeding jejunostomy

1 Expose the upper jejunum through a small left upper paramedian or transverse incision. Trace the bowel proximally to the duodenojejunal flexure. Select a loop a few centimetres distal to this point, so that it will easily reach the anterior abdominal wall.

2 Insert a Vicryl purse-string suture on the antimesenteric border of the bowel. Make a tiny enterotomy in the centre of the purse-string and introduce a T-tube (14F) into the lumen of the bowel (Fig. 14.22). Tighten the purse-string snugly around the tube.

3 An alternative method employs a Foley catheter subsequently inflated with 5–10 ml of water. After tightening the purse-string, the catheter and its point of entry into the bowel are buried with Lembert sutures. This is a Witzel jejunostomy.

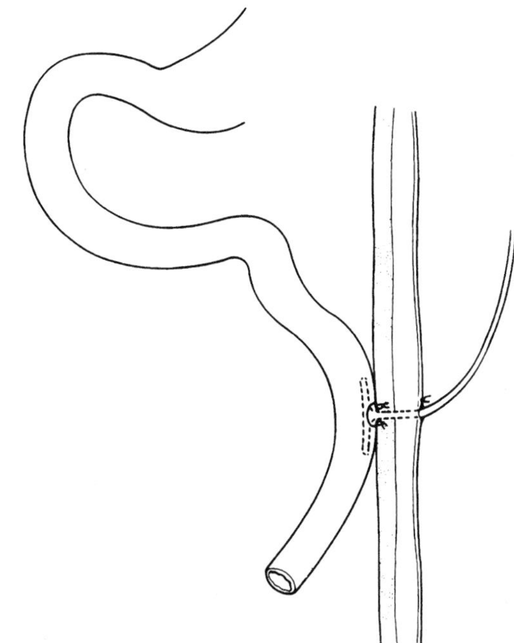

Fig. 14.22 Feeding jejunostomy. The T-tube is brought out through the abdominal wall, and the jejunum is stitched to the peritoneum around the margins of the stab incision.

4 Whichever tube is used, introduce it first through a stab incision in the abdominal wall and then into the jejunum. Traction on the tube approximates the intestine to the underside of the abdominal wall. Suture the bowel to the parietal peritoneum.

Terminal ileostomy

KEY POINT A durable ileostomy

- Permanent ileostomies are prone to complications such as retraction, prolapse, parastomal hernia, that require operative correction. Take extra care when fashioning an ileostomy to reduce the incidence of these problems

1 Excise a circular disc of skin and subcutaneous fat, 3 cm in diameter, at the site chosen and marked preoperatively. Make a cruciate incision in the exposed anterior rectus sheath, split the fibres of the rectus muscle and open the posterior sheath and peritoneum. The defect should comfortably accommodate two fingers.

2 The terminal ileum will previously have been clamped and transected. Now exteriorize 6–8 cm of bowel with its mesentery intact, through the circular opening in the abdominal wall, leaving its end securely clamped. Make sure that the mesentery is neither twisted nor tight and that the tip of the ileum remains pink.

3 Some surgeons close the lateral space between the ileostomy and the abdominal wall, using a running Vicryl suture (Fig. 14.23). Others tunnel the ileum extraperitoneally. We prefer transperitoneal ileostomy, leaving the lateral space widely open. In this case, however, it is important to suture the seromuscular layer of the bowel to the margins of the defect at peritoneal level. Take great care not to enter the lumen of the ileum when inserting these stitches.

4 After closing the main abdominal incision, remove the clamp and trim the crushed portion of ileum. Now suture the edge of the ileum directly to the skin, using Vicryl mounted on an atraumatic taper-pointed needle. After inserting three or four evenly spaced sutures, the bowel begins to evert spontaneously; if not, use Babcock's forceps to encourage eversion. Complete the circumferential sutures, producing a spout, which should project about 3 cm from the abdominal wall.

5 Carefully clean and dry the skin around the ileostomy and apply an ileostomy bag at once.

Loop ileostomy

1 Excise a disc of skin and fat and deliver a loop of ileum on to the abdominal wall.

2 Open the bowel, not at the apex of the loop as for a loop colostomy (Ch. 16), but close to skin level.

3 Suture the mucosa of the distal bowel to the skin. Use Babcock's forceps to evert the mucosa of the proximal bowel before suture.

4 The completed loop ileostomy looks very like a standard end ileostomy. As for loop colostomy, insert a plastic rod to prevent the bowel slipping back in, and fit a suitable appliance, with flange and clip-on bag, to the skin over the stoma.

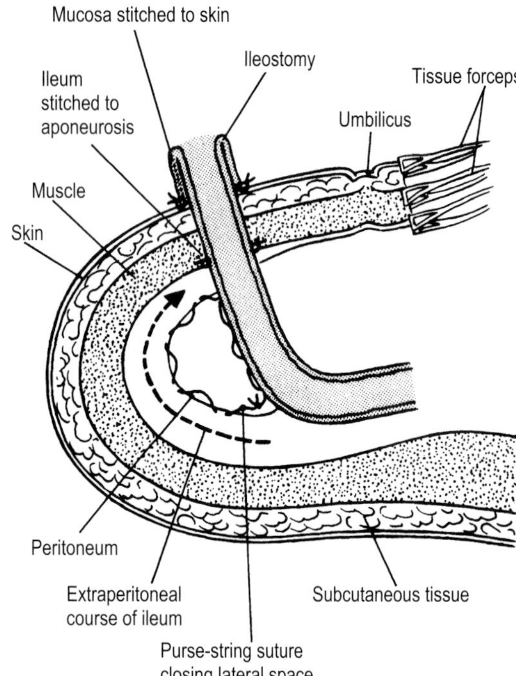

Fig. 14.23 Terminal ileostomy. Two methods of closing the lateral space are shown: a purse-string suture or taking the ileum along an extraperitoneal track. Alternatively, the lateral space can be left widely open. Tissue forceps on each layer of the wound edge prevent retraction of the layers while the ileostomy is being fashioned.

Aftercare

- *Feeding jejunostomy*. Keep the tube patent by introducing 5–10 ml of sterile water hourly. When bowel sounds return, increase the amount of water before switching to half-strength and then full-strength liquid feed. Consult the dietitian about the patient's individual nutritional needs. Give codeine or loperamide to control diarrhoea. When oral feeding is resumed, spigot the tube for 24–48 hours before removal.
- *Ileostomy*. Increase oral fluids when the stoma commences to discharge. The effluent will be very loose at first but will gradually thicken as the ileum adapts. Give bulking agents or antidiarrhoeal drugs as needed. Consult the stomatherapist directly, if he has not already seen the patient before operation. Make sure that the patient is competent and confident at managing the stoma before he leaves hospital.

REFERENCE

1. Hesp WLEM, Lubbers EJC, de Boer HHM et al 1988 Hendriks T enterostomy as an adjunct to treatment of intra-abdominal sepsis. British Journal of Surgery 75:693–696

MISCELLANEOUS CONDITIONS

MECKEL'S DIVERTICULUM

- Potential complications include bleeding, infection, peptic ulceration, perforation, intestinal obstruction or fistulation to the umbilicus. Usually this remnant of the allantois gives no trouble at all, however, throughout the patient's life.

- Incidental Meckelian diverticulectomy has been advocated by some surgeons because of the supposed lower morbidity and mortality rates before complications arise. Others have argued that the low risk of complications arising from a Meckel's diverticulum does not justify prophylactic resection. A retrospective analysis[1] found that the conditional probabilities of producing surgical morbidity and mortality in the adult population were far higher when resecting incidental diverticula.

KEY POINT Removal of Meckel's diverticulum

- Do not carry out incidental Meckelian diverticulectomy in adults.

- The first step in Meckelian diverticulectomy is to divide the small vessel that crosses the ileum to supply it. Depending on the size of its mouth, the diverticulum can simply be transected across the neck using a linear stapler or excised with a portion of the antimesenteric border of the bowel. Local resection of the ileum with end-to-end anastomosis may be preferable in a complicated case.

INTUSSUSCEPTION

In infants

1 Ileocolic intussusception usually presents in a child of a few months old with abdominal colic and rectal passage of blood and mucus. Besides confirming the diagnosis, barium enema may reduce the intussusception totally or subtotally. On examination under anaesthetic, if not before, a mass can be felt in the central or upper abdomen with an 'empty' right iliac fossa.

2 Open the abdomen through a right Lanz incision and find the sausage-shaped mass. Starting at the apex, squeeze the intussusceptum back along the intussuscipiens as though extracting toothpaste from the bottom of the tube. Do not remove the bowel from the abdominal cavity during this manoeuvre.

3 The final portion of the intussusception is the most difficult to reduce. Deliver the affected segment from the abdomen and gently compress it with a moist swab, before resuming the squeeze. Make certain that reduction is complete before replacing the bowel. No fixation is required, except in the rare event of a recurrent intussusception.

4 If the bowel is clearly gangrenous or the intussusception cannot be reduced, proceed to resection. Usually an end-to-end ileoileostomy can be performed.

In adults

1 Intussusception is rare and is nearly always associated with an underlying lesion in the bowel wall such as a benign tumour or Meckel's diverticulum.

2 Reduce the intussusception as far as possible, then proceed to local resection of the affected segment of bowel with end-to-end anastomosis.

INTESTINAL ISCHAEMIA

1 The small intestine is supplied by the superior mesenteric, midgut, vessels. Thrombosis may occur on arteriosclerotic plaques at the origin of the superior mesenteric artery, especially if the patient is shocked. The superior mesenteric artery is an uncommon site for peripheral embolism in patients with cardiac arrhythmia or a recent myocardial infarction. Venous gangrene may result if the superior mesenteric or portal veins suddenly undergo thrombosis, for example in extreme dehydration or disseminated intravascular coagulation. Lastly, non-occlusive mesenteric infarction may occur secondary to microcirculatory damage in critically ill patients. With the advent of ever-improving intensive care units, a greater proportion of patients have mesenteric ischaemia secondary to this cause. Although the diagnosis may be difficult to make, suspect it if unexplained acidosis develops in a postoperative or critically ill patient.

2 Patients with severe mesenteric vascular insufficiency are extremely ill with evidence of peritonitis and shock. Early operation is needed to prevent death.[2] At laparotomy, the bowel appears ischaemic or frankly infarcted without evidence of strangulation.

3 Examine the whole intestinal tract and feel for pulsation in all accessible gut arteries. Examine the aorta and its main divisions to determine the extent of atherosclerosis. If the main intestinal vessels and their arcades are patent, the circulation is probably occluded at capillary level.

4 Resect obviously necrotic bowel. Recovery is unlikely if the entire midgut is infarcted following occlusion of the main superior mesenteric vessels. If an extensive segment is affected, be as conservative as possible to avoid severe short-bowel syndrome. Multiple patches of ischaemia can be oversewn or locally resected.

5 Early cases of arterial embolus or acute in-situ thrombosis may be amenable to revascularization. It is much easier to mobilize the caecum and identify the ileocolic artery than to expose the origin of the superior mesenteric artery itself. Control the vessel with tapes and perform a longitudinal arteriotomy. Pass a Fogarty catheter proximally into the superior mesenteric artery and aorta to dislodge the clot, and try to establish free flow. Rapid injection of heparin saline up the vessel may achieve the same effect. If the bowel regains its normal colour, close the arteriotomy with a venous patch. Otherwise consider side-to-side anastomosis between the ileocolic and right common iliac arteries.

6 Following direct arterial surgery, or in any case in which bowel of doubtful viability has been left in the abdomen, plan to repeat the laparotomy after 24 hours. Further resection of bowel may be clearly indicated at this time.

KEY POINT Mesenteric ischaemia: urgency of management

- Regardless of aetiology, the prognosis of patients with mesenteric ischaemia is dependent upon rapid diagnosis and institution of treatment. Conservative management may be sufficient in selected cases; more often laparotomy is required and can be life-saving.

SMALL-BOWEL FISTULA

1 The spontaneous discharge of bowel contents on to the abdominal wall is a rare event. The vast majority of external fistulas arise either from a leaking anastomosis or from operative injury to the intestine. Besides impaired healing, radiation enteritis, multiple adhesions, diffuse carcinoma and Crohn's disease predispose to fistula formation.[3]

2 Do not rush to re-operate once there is an established small-bowel fistula. Correct fluid and electrolyte depletion. Switch to total parenteral nutrition both to maintain health and to reduce the amount of intestinal contents discharged. Consult a stomatherapist on how best to protect the wound and abdominal wall from the effluent, using adhesive seals and collecting bags as appropriate. Consider constant suction through a catheter placed in the fistula if the discharge is particularly profuse.

3 Obtain an early fistulogram to delineate the leak. A side hole may well close if there is no distal obstruction, but a complete anastomotic dehiscence is almost certain to require re-operation once the patient's general condition allows.

4 If the patient is toxic, early drainage of an associated abscess may improve the patient's general health and sometimes allow the fistula to heal. If you encounter a complete dehiscence at this time, it is probably better to exteriorize the bowel ends rather than attempt a repeat anastomosis under unpromising circumstances. This counsel may not be appropriate for a high jejunal fistula, however.

5 Do not ordinarily undertake a definitive operation to close a small-bowel fistula if you are an inexperienced surgeon. As a rule resect the damaged portion of bowel. Take care to divide any adhesions that could partially obstruct the distal gut and lead to recurrence of the fistula. Continue nutritional support during the postoperative healing phase.

REFERENCES

1. Peoples J 1995 Incidental Meckel's diverticulectomy in adults. Surgery 118:649–652
2. Bradbury A 1995 Mesenteric ischaemia: a multidisciplinary approach. British Journal of Surgery 82:1446–1459
3. Frileux P, Parc Y 1999 External fistulas of the small bowel. In: Taylor TV, Watson A, Williamson RCN (eds) Upper digestive surgery. Oesophagus, stomach and small intestine. Saunders, London, pp 741–763

LAPAROSCOPIC APPROACH TO THE SMALL BOWEL

Appraise

1 Diagnostic laparoscopy can be performed with little morbidity and can obviate additional complications arising from laparotomy. In addition to this diagnostic role, laparoscopic surgical techniques can now be applied to a variety of therapeutic procedures that traditionally were performed in an open fashion.

> **KEY POINT Laparoscopy: risk of small-bowel injury**
>
> - In patients in whom previous laparotomy has been carried out and in those with distended loops of bowel, prefer the open method of trocar placement to avoid inadvertent puncture of the small bowel.

2 With regard to diagnosis, laparoscopy is useful in patients with peritonitis or possible small-bowel ischaemia, any therapeutic procedures being carried out either laparoscopically or via the open route. The small bowel can be examined in detail via the laparoscope. Use a standard infra-umbilical port and a 30°-angled endoscope. Identify the ligament of Treitz initially. Thereafter, by alternately using two atraumatic graspers, expose the entire length of the small bowel to the caecum, dividing any intervening adhesions with scissors. Inspect both the serosal surface and the mesentery.

3 The clinical diagnosis of small-bowel ischaemia is notoriously difficult to make. Laparoscopic examination of the bowel is helpful, therefore, and other diagnostic aids such as fluorescein and Doppler examinations, which assess perfusion and viability of the bowel, can be adapted for use via the laparoscope. If you are in doubt about the viability of the bowel, make a small incision in order to deliver the suspect segment for closer inspection. Diagnostic laparoscopy is safe and can be performed with minimal risk and a negligible mortality rate. It is perhaps most useful in critically ill patients in whom you wish to avoid unnecessary laparotomy.

4 Small-bowel resection can be performed entirely laparoscopically or with laparoscopic assistance (Ch. 5). Determine the segment for resection, dissect the mesentery and devascularize it using clips, sutures or linear cutting staplers that have been designed to fit through a laparoscopic port. Perform subsequent anastomosis intraperitoneally or, as is more conventional, by standard extracorporeal anastomosis after delivering the bowel to the exterior through a small abdominal incision. Intraperitoneal resection and anastomosis is possible, using either stapling devices or laparoscopic suturing.

5 The placement of a feeding jejunostomy can be achieved via the percutaneous route using a laparoscope to anchor the bowel to the anterior abdominal wall. Sutures, clips or T-fasteners, with a metal bar attached to a nylon suture, can be used to secure the bowel. Once attached, the bowel is cannulated using an 18G needle and a guidewire. When performed by experienced laparoscopic surgeons, this technique is safe, effective and perhaps superior to open jejunostomy. Complications can still arise, however, and as with open jejunostomy catheters may become dislodged. Leaks seldom occur as the bowel is flush to the abdominal wall, and catheter replacement can usually be carried out without resorting to laparotomy.

6 Laparoscopic creation of stomas for faecal diversion can be performed using a variety of organs as conduits; loop ileostomy, loop sigmoid colostomy and end colostomy have all been described. Studies have reported a high success rate, in excess of 95%, and a low morbidity rate.

7 Laparoscopic management of acute small-bowel obstruction is theoretically attractive, but experience is limited.[1] Adhesions

and distended loops of bowel make trocar placement more hazardous, therefore prefer open trocar placement. If obstruction is due to a single adhesion, as is often the case, this can easily be identified and divided. If adhesions are more extensive, adhesiolysis and relief of obstruction are more difficult. The procedure demands painstaking care, whether performed by the open or the laparoscopic route. Several studies have shown that laparoscopy is both effective and safe in patients with small-bowel obstruction. One study in particular[2] reported that laparoscopy was effective in a high proportion of patients and that hospital stay was reduced; early unplanned re-operation was increased in patients managed laparoscopically, reinforcing the fact that experience is limited in this field.

REFERENCES

1. Navez B 1998 Laparoscopic approach in acute small bowel obstruction. A review of 68 patients. Hepatogastroenterology 45:2146–2150
2. Wullstein C, Gross E 2003 Laparoscopic compared with conventional treatment of acute adhesive small bowel obstruction. British Journal of Surgery 90:1147–1151

SMALL-BOWEL OBSTRUCTION

See Chapter 4.

FURTHER READING

Duh Q 1993 Laparoscopic procedures for small bowel disease. Baillière's Clinical Gastroenterology 7:833–850

Durdey P 1996 Small intestine. In: Keen G, Farndon J (eds) Operative surgery and management, 3rd edn. Butterworth-Heinemann, London, pp 210–225

Galland RB, Spencer J 1990 Radiation enteritis. Edward Arnold, London

Hyman NH, Fazio VW 1991 Crohn's disease of the small bowel. Comprehensive Therapy 17:38–42

Irwin ST, Krukowski ZH, Matheson NA 1990 Single layer anastomosis in the upper gastrointestinal tract. British Journal of Surgery 77:643–644

Mackey WC, Dineen P 1983 A fifty year experience with Meckel's diverticulum. Surgery, Gynecology and Obstetrics 156:56–64

Marston JAP 1986 Vascular disease of the gut: pathophysiology, recognition and management. Edward Arnold, London

McConnell DB, Turkey DD 1999. Injuries to the small intestine. In: Taylor TV, Watson A, Williamson RCN (eds) Upper digestive surgery. Oesophagus, stomach and small intestine. Saunders, London, pp 732–740

Michelassi F 1998 Strictureplasty for Crohn's disease: techniques and long-term results. World Journal of Surgery 22:359–363

Murray J 1998 Controversies in Crohn's disease. Baillière's Clinical Gastroenterology 12:133–155

Newman T 1998 The changing face of mesenteric infarction. American Surgeon 64:611–616

O'Toole G 1999 Defunctioning loop ileostomy: a prospective audit. Journal of the American College of Surgeons 188:6–9

Ottinger L 1990 Mesenteric ischaemia. In: Williamson RCN, Cooper MJ (eds) Emergency abdominal surgery. Churchill Livingstone, Edinburgh, pp 242–257

Richelsen B 1998 Long term follow up of patients who underwent jejunoileal bypass for morbid obesity. European Journal of Surgery 164:281–286

Studley JGN, Williamson RCN 1999 Malignant tumours of the small bowel. In: Taylor TV, Watson A, Williamson RCN (eds) Upper digestive surgery. Oesophagus, stomach and small intestine. Saunders, London, pp 949–962

Thodiyil PA, El-Masry NS, Peake H et al 2004 T-tube jejunostomy feeding after pancreatic surgery: a safe adjunct. Asian Journal of Surgery 27:80–84

Thomas WEG 1990 Complications of small bowel diverticula. In: Williamson RCN, Cooper MJ (eds) Emergency abdominal surgery. Churchill Livingstone, Edinburgh, pp 191–208

Williams JG, Wong WD, Rothenberger DA et al 1991 Recurrence of Crohn's disease after resection. British Journal of Surgery 78: 10–19

Williams NS, Nasmyth DG, Jones D et al 1986 De-functioning stomas: a prospective controlled trial comparing loop ileostomy with loop transverse colostomy. British Journal of Surgery 73:566–570

Williamson RCN 1991 Small intestine. In: O'Higgins NJ, Chisholm GD, Williamson RCN (eds) Surgical management, 2nd edn. Butterworth-Heinemann, Oxford, pp 562–593

15

Colonoscopy

R.J. Leicester

DESCRIPTION OF OPERATION

Appraise

1 Colonoscopy has revolutionized the diagnosis and treatment of colonic disease, allowing accurate mucosal visualization, biopsy and therapeutic polypectomy. Technological advances in instrumentation allow rapid and safe examination of the whole colon, provided the endoscopist has been adequately trained in the technique.

2 Use diagnostic colonoscopy to evaluate an abnormal or equivocal barium enema, particularly where diverticular disease or colonic spasm may often obscure a small mucosal lesion. In elderly patients, who often tolerate barium enema badly, colonoscopy should be the first-line investigation for unexplained rectal bleeding or anaemia and is the investigation of choice for all patients with a positive faecal occult blood test. Colonoscopy is the most accurate diagnostic tool for differential diagnosis and assessment of extent in inflammatory bowel disease, but should be avoided in acute disease, where technetium-labelled white cell scanning is a safer alternative.

3 Therapeutic colonoscopy has changed the surgical management of colorectal polyps, facilitating removal of all pedunculated and most sessile adenomatous lesions, thus providing an opportunity for colorectal cancer prevention. Diathermy coagulation or laser therapy of vascular abnormalities such as angiodysplasia may pre-empt laparotomy in acute colonic haemorrhage or cure anaemia due to chronic blood loss.

4 Relief of obstruction in colorectal cancer, either as an initial procedure prior to surgical resection or as long-term palliation, may be achieved using either laser vaporization or stent insertion.

5 Perform surveillance colonoscopy with multiple biopsies at least biennially in all patients with total ulcerative colitis, for more than 8 years, thus avoiding colectomy in over 80% of cases. Surgery is indicated only in those with definite dysplasia or carcinoma.

6 Following polypectomy or curative resection for colorectal cancer, carry out regular follow-up colonoscopy, initially after 3 years and thereafter 5-yearly if no new polyps are detected.

7 Commence screening of high-risk groups (e.g. polyposis coli) from age 15 years (if gene-positive) and continue approximately 2-yearly until the age of 40 years. Hereditary non-polyposis coli families should undergo 1–2-yearly surveillance, commencing at least 10 years younger than the index case. If facilities exist, then screen subjects with a strong family history of colorectal cancer (i.e. one first-degree relative with onset before 40 years of age, or more than one first-degree relative of any age) in the hope of reducing the incidence of colorectal cancer by removing adenomatous lesions.

8 Carry out emergency colonoscopy in cases of acute, severe rectal bleeding after anorectal and upper gastrointestinal causes have been excluded by rigid proctosigmoidoscopy and gastroscopy. Bleeding usually ceases in up to 80% of patients, allowing colonoscopy within 24–48 hours, after bowel preparation. Even in the presence of active bleeding, while small mucosal lesions may be overlooked, you can obtain valuable clues as to the segment of colon from which the haemorrhage is arising, or note blood emerging through the ileocaecal valve, indicating a small-bowel lesion. When a diagnosis has not been reached and emergency laparotomy becomes necessary, you may perform colonoscopy under general anaesthetic with the peritoneal cavity exposed, following on-table lavage with saline or water introduced via a Foley catheter through a caecostomy.

Prepare

1 Accurate, rapid examination depends upon effective bowel preparation. Advise patients to discontinue any iron preparation or stool-bulking agents 1 week prior to endoscopy, and change to a low-residue diet. 24 hours before examination restrict oral intake to clear fluids such as coffee or tea without milk, concentrated meat extract and glucose drinks. Give a purgative such as sodium picosulfate 12–18 hours before colonoscopy and repeat it 4 hours before examination. Alternatively, give balanced electrolyte solutions combined with polyethylene glycol, which have been shown to produce rapid preparation without the need for dietary restriction. Give oral metoclopramide 10 mg prior to ingestion of the 3–4 litres of solution, which enhances gastric emptying and reduces nausea and vomiting.

2 Obtain from all patients written, informed consent for the procedure. Give reassurance about the examination to allay fears, allowing minimal levels of sedation to be used.

3 Colonoscopy is usually performed under intravenous sedation with the addition of an analgesic. Do not give excessive sedation or analgesia, to avoid circulatory or respiratory depression. Additionally, it will dull appreciation of severe pain, which should occur only when a poor technique is used, causing dangerous overstretching of the bowel. For similar reasons do not perform colonoscopy under general anaesthesia, apart from as an intraoperative procedure in cases of acute colonic haemorrhage. Elderly patients in particular can suffer significant hypotension following pethidine, and this, combined with the synergistic effect of opiates and benzodiazepines, can also cause significant falls in oxygen saturation. In order to avoid these complications, use only small doses of analgesic and hypnotic

such as intravenous pethidine 50 mg or pentazocine 30 mg plus midazolam 2.5–5 mg. Monitor all patients by pulse oximetry, during and after the procedure, and give added inspired oxygen as appropriate. Always have available antidotes to benzodiazepines (flumazenil) and opiates (naloxone), together with full cardiorespiratory resuscitation equipment and trained staff to use it in case of emergency. Occasionally an antispasmodic, either intravenous hyoscine butylbromide (Buscopan) or intraluminal peppermint oil suspension, may be employed.

4 As a rule, examine the patient in the left lateral position or, alternatively, supine. Use a tipping trolley in case of cardiorespiratory problems. Have available at least two trained assistants: one to observe the patient's vital signs and the other to assist with the accessories for biopsy or snare polypectomy. Videoendoscopes are an essential tool to ensure accurate and safe polypectomy and also to maintain the interest of the assistants.

5 Check all equipment prior to intubation. The colonoscope must have been adequately cleaned and disinfected. The light source, endoscope angulation controls, air–water insufflation and suction facilities must be in full working order. Check the diathermy equipment for correct, safe operation. Ensure that all accessories such as biopsy forceps and polypectomy snares operate correctly.

Access

1 Modern colonoscopes are sophisticated precision instruments designed to enhance intubation of the colon in the most efficient manner. As well as a wide-angled lens to allow a greater field of vision, a graduated torque characteristic assists variability in the stiffness of the instrument.

2 During intubation, the instrument may be pushed forward or pulled back. Change of direction may be achieved by angulation of the distal end, up/down or left/right. Change of direction may also be achieved by up/down deflection, combined with rotation. Keeping the distal section of the instrument as straight as possible, restoring this to a neutral position as soon as possible after angulation around an acute bend helps to prevent loop formation. Avoid maximum up/down and left/right angulation, as this results in a J-shape and rotation of the end of the instrument rather than change of direction. Advancement may also be achieved by the straightening of a loop using torque and withdrawal or by suction causing a concertina effect of the bowel over the endoscope.

3 Colonoscopy is made easier if the anatomy of the colon is properly understood. The rectum is fixed in a retroperitoneal position and consists of alternating mucosal folds forming the valves of Houston. The sigmoid colon is freely mobile on its mesentery and of variable length and configuration. The descending colon and splenic flexure are relatively fixed by their peritoneal attachments. At the splenic flexure, the direction of the colon is forwards and downwards to the transverse colon which, like the sigmoid, is of variable length and freely mobile on the transverse mesocolon. The bowel becomes fixed again at the hepatic flexure and the direction passes forwards and downwards into the ascending colon and caecum, which are usually fixed by peritoneal attachments, though less consistently than the descending colon. It is the mobile and variable-length sigmoid and transverse colon that cause the most difficulty through looping of the instrument.

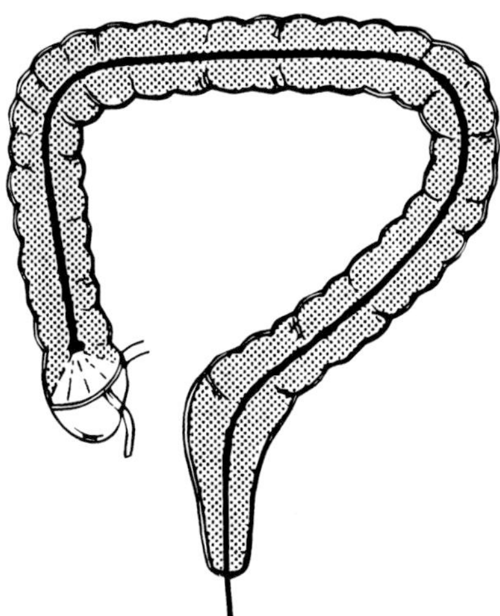

Fig. 15.1 Colonoscope inserted to the caecal pole.

4 The aim of colonoscopy is to achieve intubation from the anus to caecum with the minimum possible length of instrument. Characteristically, the colonoscope, when straight and without loop formation, should be in a roughly U-shaped configuration with 70–80 cm of instrument inserted to the caecal pole (Fig. 15.1). Significantly greater insertion length indicates the presence of a loop.

KEY POINTS Achieving successful colonoscopy

- To achieve the optimum insertion length, aim to straighten out the natural loops of the bowel and concertina the colon on to the instrument. This is achieved by a combination of advancement, withdrawal, distal end angulation and rotation, applying torque to the instrument and finally suction to draw the colon over the end of the instrument.
- Successful colonoscopy depends on the rapid application of any one or more of these techniques as visual appearances and feedback of longitudinal and rotational forces on the colonoscope are detected by you via the instrument shaft and control wheels. By using a tactile approach, assessing the forces on the instrument, you can often prevent unnecessary looping before it occurs.

5 Liberally lubricate the anus and perianal area with lubricating gel. Carry out a thorough digital examination, then introduce the instrument along the forefinger of the right hand. Repeated lubrication is required to prevent friction at the anus, one of the commonest causes of failure to advance the endoscope. Control of the instrument is best achieved by rotation of the up/down wheel, using your left thumb. Place your index finger to allow it to operate the air/water and suction valves. Manipulation of the colonoscope shaft is performed with the right hand (Fig. 15.2), this hand leaving the shaft only for short periods, to make minor adjustments to the left/right wheel.

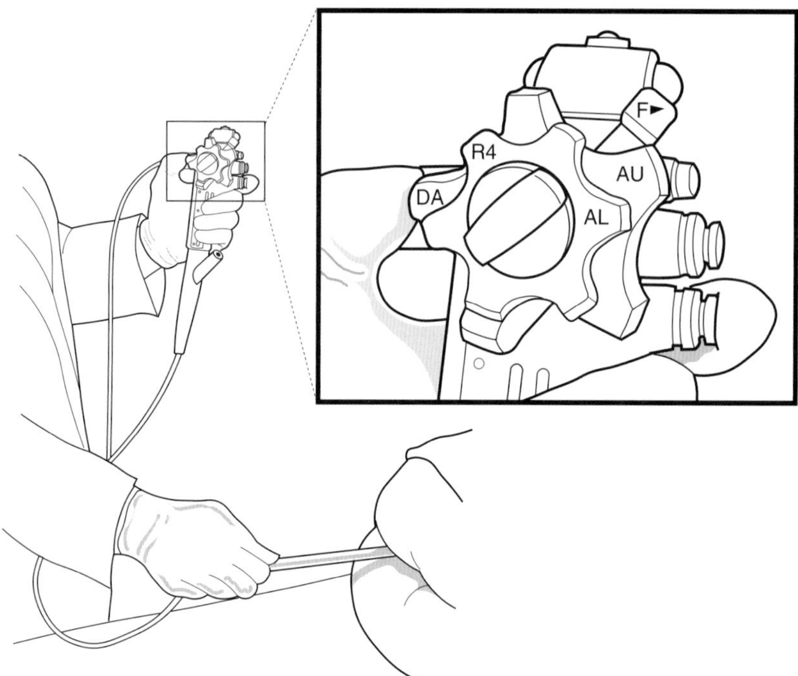

Fig. 15.2 The right hand, which should be gloved, manipulates the colonoscope shaft.

6 On entering the rectum, aspirate excess fluid and adjust the tip of the instrument until it is in the centre of the lumen. During intubation, insufflate only the minimum amount of air to allow adequate visualization of the lumen. Excessive air leads to distal distension and accentuation of angles in the bowel. At the rectosigmoid junction the lumen passes upwards and to the right. Intubation at this point can be achieved by upward deflection of the tip and clockwise rotation of the shaft. In patients with a relatively short sigmoid colon, continuation of the clockwise rotation with advancement often leads to passage as far as the descending sigmoid junction. However, in many patients, particularly those with diverticular disease or those who have undergone pelvic surgery, the configuration is variable and there may be a number of acute angles. In these cases, achieve advancement by a combination of rotation and adjustments to the left/right wheel. Aim to take the shortest possible route through the bowel, keeping the instrument tip in the centre of the lumen and keeping to the inside of each bend.

? DIFFICULTY

1. If at any time the luminal view is lost, withdraw the instrument until the view is regained.
2. Pushing against the colon wall tends to create loops and may also lead to perforation. This precaution is particularly important in patients with diverticular disease, as advancement of the instrument into a diverticulum is potentially hazardous.
3. Clues as to the position of the lumen can be obtained from the arcuate folds and the light reflex caused by the instrument. As a general rule, steer towards the concavity of the folds and away from the bright light reflex (Fig. 15.3).

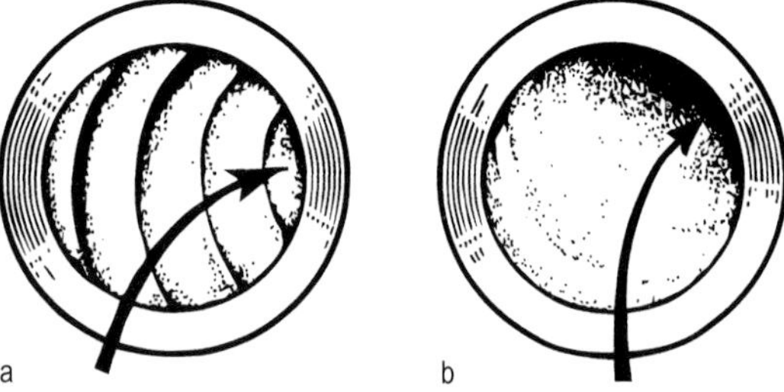

Fig. 15.3 Steer towards the concavity of the folds (a) and away from the bright light reflex (b).

7 Looping of the colonoscope may occur in the sigmoid colon, indicated by a lack of one-to-one advancement of the instrument tip compared with the shaft, which may cause the patient some discomfort. Straighten the loop by applying rotational torque to the shaft, in the direction that produces the least resistance, while at the same time withdrawing the instrument. Once one-to-one withdrawal has been achieved, re-advance the instrument while maintaining the same torque, preventing re-formation of the loop. In the sigmoid colon, the torque usually needs to be applied in a clockwise direction. The effect of this is to fold the sigmoid loop over and achieve a relatively straight sigmoid colon (Fig. 15.4).

On reaching the descending colon, often recognizable by its long, straight appearance, straighten the tip of the instrument and advance it by insertion, maintaining the torque applied to keep the sigmoid colon in a straight configuration. The splenic flexure may be recognized by a bluish discoloration produced by the spleen adjacent to the colon wall, or a gate-like appearance at the entrance to the transverse colon.

8 Although there are variations between patients, the transverse colon is usually found by angling the tip to the left and downwards. Once the characteristic triangular lumen of the transverse

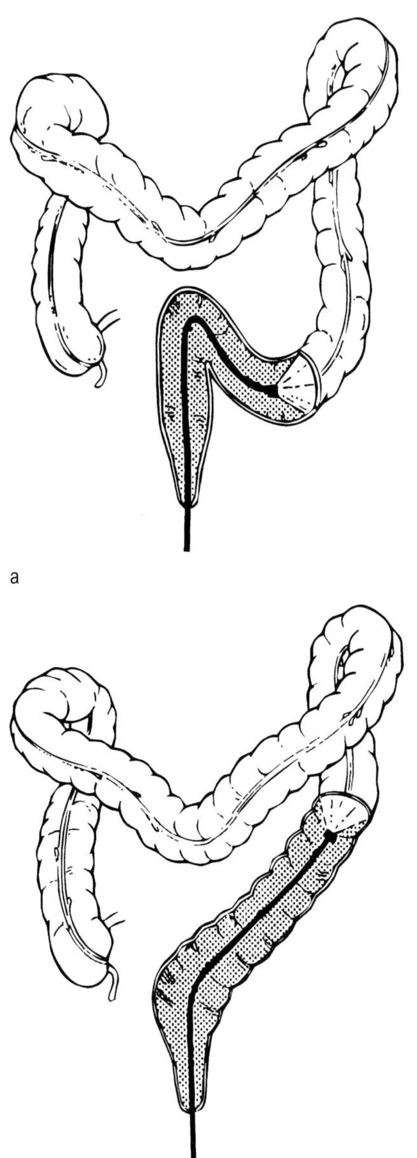

Fig. 15.4 Apply torque in the direction that produces the least resistance while withdrawing the instrument, to straighten the sigmoid colon so that the colonoscope can advance into the descending colon.

colon is recognized, straighten the tip of the instrument and advance the instrument with a combination of intermittent suction and insertion. This has the effect of making the bowel concertina over the colonoscope and shortening the effective length. The transverse colon usually has at least one acute angle at its centre point, but may have more, particularly if postoperative adhesions are present. On reaching such an angle, angle the tip around the bend and, while maintaining a luminal view, apply torque and withdrawal as for the sigmoid loop, again in the direction of least resistance. In order to prevent possible trauma to the colon, always maintain a luminal view and do not hook the end of the instrument into the bowel wall. The effect of this manoeuvre is to straighten the transverse colon (Fig. 15.5).

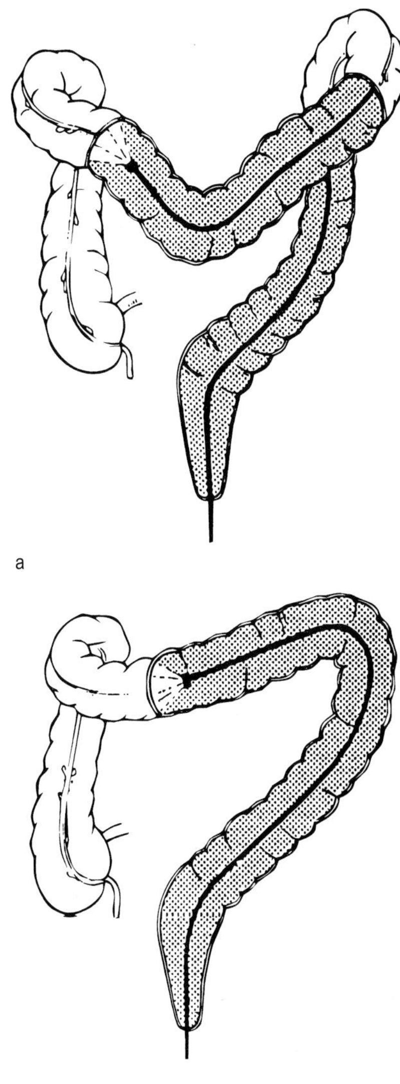

Fig. 15.5 Negotiating the transverse colon. Always maintain a luminal view.

As soon as one-to-one advancement is achieved, straighten the tip and advance the instrument, again using intermittent suction. The tip of the instrument should then pass rapidly to the hepatic flexure, which may be recognizable by a bluish hue of the right lobe of the liver visible through the colonic wall. However, this is an unreliable landmark as the left lobe of the liver can give the same appearance in the mid-transverse colon. Occasionally, during the process of straightening the transverse colon, the sigmoid loop may re-form. It is useful at this stage, having re-straightened the sigmoid loop, to employ an assistant to hold the sigmoid or transverse loop in its straightened configuration. In the case of the sigmoid colon, this is performed using the flat of the hand to exert pressure downwards and towards the left iliac crest (Fig. 15.6a). For recurrent transverse looping, the colon is splinted by the assistant's hand pushing upwards from just above the umbilicus (Fig. 15.6b).

9 At the hepatic flexure, entrance to the caecum is usually found by angulation down and to the left. The caecum often has a pool

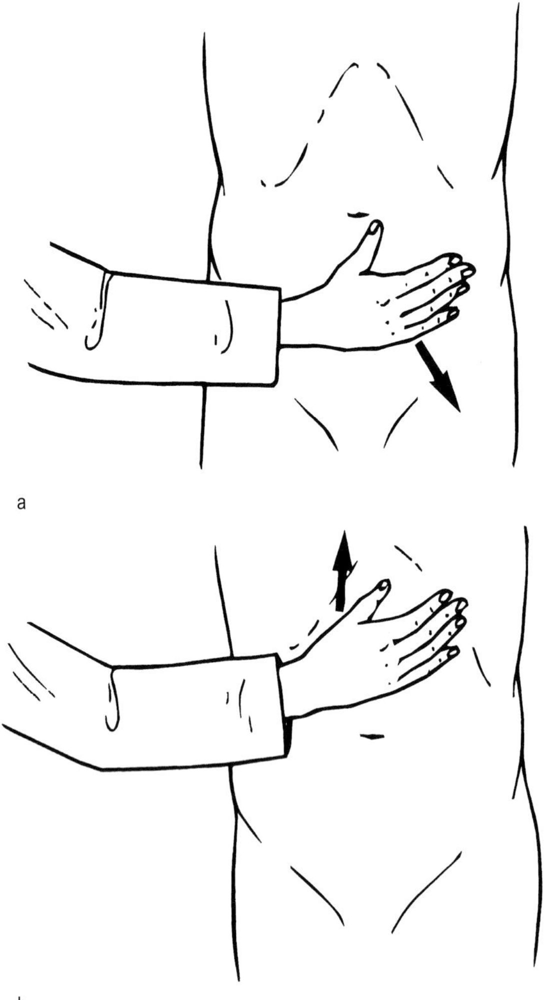

Fig. 15.6 (a) Have the colon held in the straightened configuration by an assistant's hand placed on the abdominal wall. (b) For recurrent transverse colon looping, have the assistant's hand push upwards from just below the umbilicus.

of fluid at its pole and the ileocaecal valve is visible as a shelf-like protrusion, with a lip-like centre. Advancement to the caecal pole can usually be achieved by a combination of suction and gentle advancement. If a transverse loop has re-formed, then straighten the loop and re-advance, using assistant compression, or, providing the patient does not experience excessive discomfort and there is no resistance to intubation, a transverse loop can be deliberately formed and then, following angulation of the tip into the upper ascending colon, straightening of the scope by withdrawal combined with torque achieves advancement to the caecal pole. An alternative solution to difficulties with transverse colon looping is to alter the position of the patient, either prone or supine, which will often result in a less-acute angle to be negotiated.

10 The only reliable landmarks in colonoscopy are seen on entering the caecum. Typically, there is a triradiate fold at the caecal pole, representing the convergence of the taenia coli, at the centre of which may be seen the base of the appendix. Palpation of the abdomen, laterally in the right iliac fossa, produces indentation of the caecal wall, and the light of the colonoscope may also be visible through the abdominal wall. However, all of these appearances can be present in a deep transverse loop and the ileocaecal valve is the only reliable sign that the caecum has been reached. Its appearance may vary, but its usual appearance is of a lip-like structure. Intubation of the valve shows an obvious change in the mucosal pattern, from the shiny mucosa of the colon with visible blood vessels to the rather granular appearance of the distal ileum, often with visible lymphoid patches, and a characteristic advancing peristaltic movement.

? DIFFICULTY

If you experience difficulty with loop formation, carry out the following in sequence:

1. If no resistance to intubation and no patient pain, try 'pushing through' the loop.
2. Try withdrawal with clockwise torque.
3. Try withdrawal with anticlockwise torque.
4. Try changing patient position, supine in the first instance.

Assess

1 While much of the examination is carried out during intubation, perform a thorough inspection of the colon during withdrawal of the instrument. By using a combination of up/down deflection and rotation to create a figure-of-eight motion, it is possible to examine the colonic mucosa completely, particularly behind the circular muscle folds.

2 Keep your right hand on the shaft of the colonoscope, approximately 15–20 cm from the anus, since straightening of a loop often leads to rapid distal progression of the instrument. This requires rapid re-insertion to avoid overlooking any area of the mucosa. During extubation, insufflate more air in order to straighten the haustral folds. As each segment of colon is examined, suck out the air in order to prevent undue discomfort and possible vasovagal attacks due to overdistension. At this stage, if spasm becomes a problem, then inject intravenous hyoscine butylbromide or instil peppermint oil suspension into the colon via the biopsy channel to relieve the spasm and allow adequate visualization.

3 The normal appearance of the colon is a shiny mucosal surface, with a clearly visible vascular pattern. Loss of vascular pattern is the earliest sign of inflammatory bowel disease, followed by granular, friable mucosa and frank ulceration as the disease intensifies. Chronic disease may be manifest by pseudopolyps and stricture formation. The presence of areas of normal mucosa, aphthous ulceration and fistulas is characteristic of Crohn's disease. The commonest types of polyp to be encountered are either adenomatous or hyperplastic; remove all of these for histological assessment, as visual appearances are not reliable. Biopsy polypoid or plaque-like areas in cases of established ulcerative colitis to exclude dysplastic or neoplastic change.

Action

1 During colonoscopy, take biopsies or perform polypectomy. Introduce endoscopic accessories only when there is a clear

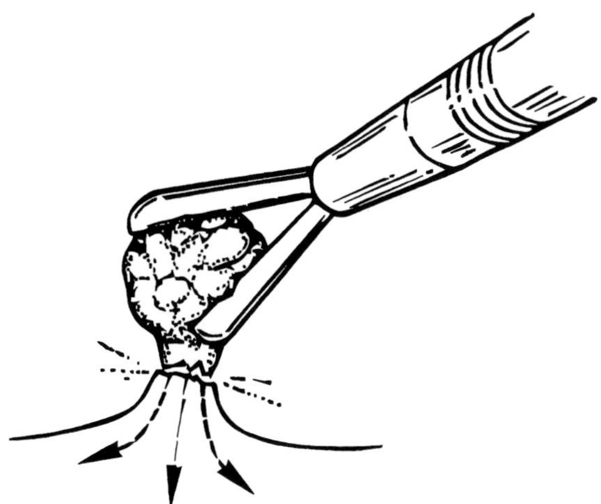

Fig. 15.7 Draw a polyp away from the colonic wall while applying diathermy current to avoid overheating the colonic wall.

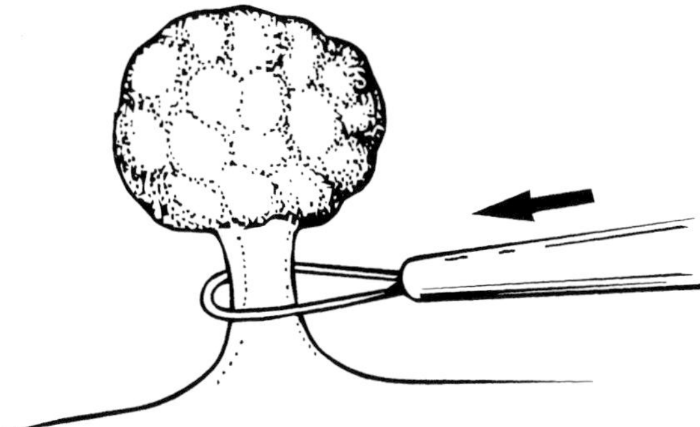

Fig. 15.8 When snaring a polyp, gradually close the snare while advancing the covering tube up to the stalk.

luminal view, to avoid the risk of perforation. The most convenient biopsy forceps are those of the spiked variety, which remove adequate-sized samples of tissue and will not slide off the mucosa when attempting biopsy at a tangent. Mount biopsy specimens carefully according to the preference of the histopathologist. Clearly label containers. Use a diagram of the colon on the histology request form, with specimens appropriately labelled to allow accurate identification of biopsy sites. In the case of strictures, use brush cytology when adequate biopsies cannot be obtained.

2 Hot biopsy forceps allow tissue sampling and simultaneous fulguration of small sessile polyps, or the coagulation of areas of vascular abnormality such as angiodysplasia. In the case of polyps, grasp the lesion and then tent it away from the colonic wall, to avoid excessive heat from the diathermy being dissipated to the colonic wall (Fig. 15.7). Apply short bursts of coagulating current until a white appearance is produced around the polyp. Withdraw the forceps and recover the tissue sample. The base of the polyp will slough in due course. Because of the risk of perforation in the relatively thin-walled caecum, this technique should be reserved for small, left-sided polyps.

3 Perform coagulation of areas of angiodysplasia using hot biopsy forceps, picking up the edge of the lesion, tenting it away from the colonic wall and drawing it over the centre of the lesion before applying the current. Alternatively use argon plasma coagulation or laser vaporization.

4 Videoendoscopes facilitate snare polypectomy, allowing the assistant to view the procedure. After introducing the snare, open it and manoeuvre it over the polyp. Adjust its position around the polyp stalk. Gradually close the snare while advancing the covering tube up to the stalk (Fig. 15.8). When it is closed snugly a feeling of resistance is felt by the assistant. Avoid over-enthusiastic tightening at this stage or 'cheese-wiring' of the polyp results, with the risk of subsequent haemorrhage. As a helpful guide, mark the snare handle at the point of full closure, allowing the assistant to assess the degree of closure of the snare loop. Do not apply diathermy current until the snare is closed tightly around the polyp stalk, or the colonic wall beyond the polyp could be burned. Apply coagulation diathermy in short bursts while the assistant slowly tightens the snare.

KEY POINT Take care with diathermy coagulation

- For safe diathermy coagulation of a polyp, look for blanching of the stalk; as this occurs, gradually draw the wire through.

On separation of the polyp head, observe the remaining stalk for bleeding. If haemorrhage does occur, replace the snare over the stalk, tighten it and leave it in place for 2–3 minutes. Do not apply further diathermy, but if necessary inject the stalk with a 1:10 000 adrenaline (epinephrine) solution, using an endoscopic injection needle.

5 Retrieve polyps for histological examination by either lassoing them with the snare or grasping them with tripod forceps. Alternatively, they may be sucked on to the end of the endoscope and withdrawn en masse by extubation, or small polyps (5 mm) may be sucked through the biopsy channel and retrieved into a polyp trap inserted into the suction line. Snares may be used not only for pedunculated polyps but also for piecemeal polypectomy of large sessile lesions when the patient is unfit for an operative procedure. Such lesions may require several sessions to achieve complete eradication. Large sessile polyps may also be removed by endoscopic mucosal resection, using either a snare or diathermy needle, following submucosal injection of saline to raise the polyp from the muscularis mucosae. If the polyp does not completely rise after the injection and there is central tethering, malignancy should be suspected and biopsy taken.

Aftercare

1 Have the patient observed by a trained nurse during recovery from sedation and ensure continuation of pulse oximetry monitoring until the patient is fully awake. Excessive insufflation of air during intubation may lead to nausea and vomiting, which is potentially dangerous in the sedated patient. Once fully awake, allow patients to go home, provided they are accompanied by a responsible adult. Advise patients against driving or operating machinery for a period of 24 hours after sedation.

2 Ensure that the colonoscope is cleaned and disinfected following the procedure, and all equipment is checked for correct operation. Non-disposable endoscopic accessories should be cleaned in an ultrasonic cleanser and then sterilized by autoclaving.

Complications

1 Apart from the effects of sedation, complications of diagnostic colonoscopy include perforation and haemorrhage, occurring in 0.17% and 0.03% of cases respectively, with approximately 10 times this rate following polypectomy. However, these rates are quoted from a number of colonoscopic series, some very early in the history of colonoscopy, when instrument design was less advanced and endoscopists were learning the techniques. Nevertheless, complications still occur, particularly when the colonoscopist is inexperienced, so remember that patient pain is an important warning sign of dangerous overstretching of the bowel. This must not be masked by heavy sedation or analgesia. Similarly, never perform routine colonoscopy under general anaesthesia.

2 Many of the reported cases of postpolypectomy perforation and haemorrhage occur late (up to 72 hours post-procedure), usually because excessive diathermy current has been used, causing transmural burns or secondary haemorrhage. Advise patients to be seen by an experienced clinician if pain or bleeding occur at any time following the procedure.

FURTHER READING

American Society for Gastrointestinal Endoscopy 1998 The role of endoscopy in the patient with lower gastrointestinal bleeding. Gastrointestinal Endoscopy 48:685–688

Bell GD, McCloy RF, Charlton JE et al 1991 Recommendations for standards of sedation and patient monitoring during gastrointestinal endoscopy. Gut 32:823–827

Bond JH 1999 Colorectal surveillance for neoplasia: an overview. Gastrointestinal Endoscopy 49(3 Pt 2):S35–S40

BSG Endoscopy Committee Working Party 1998 Cleaning and disinfection of equipment for gastrointestinal endoscopy. Report of a Working Party of the British Society of Gastroenterology Endoscopy Committee. Gut 42:585–593

Cotton PB, Williams CB 1996 Practical gastrointestinal endoscopy, 4th edn. Blackwell Science, Oxford

Habr-Gama A, Waye JD 1989 Complications and hazards of gastrointestinal endoscopy. World Journal of Surgery 13:193–201

Hunt RH, Waye JD 1981 Colonoscopy techniques, clinical practice and colour atlas. Chapman & Hall, London

Macrae FA, Bhathal PS 1997 Colonoscopy and biopsy. Baillière's Clinical Gastroenterology 11:65–82

Rex DK 1995 Colonoscopy: a review of its yield for cancers and adenomas by indication. American Journal of Gastroenterology 90:353–365

Waye JD 1997 New methods of polypectomy. Gastrointestinal Endoscopy Clinics of North America 7:413–422

Webb WA 1991 Colonoscoping the 'difficult' colon. American Surgeon 3:178–182

Zauber AG 1997 Initial management and follow-up surveillance of patients with colorectal adenomas. Gastroenterology Clinics of North America 26:85–101

16

Colon

C.R.G. Cohen, C.J. Vaizey

CONTENTS

EXAMINATION OF THE LARGE BOWEL

Preoperative assessment

1 Obtain a full history and carry out a complete examination before any surgical procedure. Examine the abdomen, anus and rectum in every patient before undertaking surgery of the large bowel. This implies a thorough digital examination of the rectum and the passage of a rigid sigmoidoscope, which is an outpatient or bedside procedure. Carry out further investigations as necessary.

- *Fibreoptic sigmoidoscopy.* This is a simple outpatient procedure undertaken after one or two phosphate enemas. It reveals polyps or a carcinoma in the proximal sigmoid or descending colon.
- *Colonoscopy* (see Ch. 15). This is currently the investigation of choice for the large bowel although it is not without risks, especially in the elderly or if polyp removal is carried out. The risk of perforation is approximately 1:500 but this is obviously dependent on the age of the patient, their co-morbidity, especially diverticular disease, and on the associated procedures to be performed via the scope. Removal of large polyps also carries a significant risk of bleeding although this can usually be controlled endoscopically. Biopsies can be obtained from tumours and inflammatory bowel disease in the proximal colon. Pedunculated polyps can be removed by colonoscopic snaring and more advanced procedures such as endoscopic mucosal resection and stenting are now available in many centres. Colonoscopy is often useful in cases of gastrointestinal bleeding and can be safely carried out at the acute admission.
- *CT colography and virtual colonoscopy.* With the advent of spiral computed tomography (CT), the technique of CT colography or virtual colonoscopy has become a sensitive alternative to colonoscopy. The obvious advantages over colonoscopy are the reduced risk of perforation, the ability to image the bowel proximal to a tight stricture and the visualization of other intra-abdominal and pelvic organs. There is increasing interest in the technique of barium subtraction CT colography which can be used to image the bowel without conventional bowel preparation. Oral barium taken on a couple of consecutive days prior to the examination coats the stools and these can then be removed from the images on the computer.
- *Barium enema.* Double-contrast barium enema is less sensitive than colonoscopy but does still have a place in some hospitals where access to superior tests is limited. It can also play a complementary role to flexible sigmoidoscopy. Instant barium enema, with barium introduced into the rectum without any preparation, is still favoured by some colorectal surgeons. This can be useful in inflammatory bowel disease to demonstrate the upper limit of disease during the outpatient visit. It can also differentiate mechanical obstruction from pseudo-obstruction.
- *Other examinations.* These include: mucosal biopsy in inflammatory bowel disease to help in the differentiation of ulcerative colitis, Crohn's disease and infective colitis; stool microscopy and culture to differentiate bacterial and parasitic infection from inflammatory bowel disease; straight X-ray of the abdomen in suspected large-bowel obstruction or perforation. Serial abdominal films are important in evaluating the progress of acute colitis and the onset of toxic megacolon. Imaging scans are of value in elucidating abdominal masses, abscesses and possible metastases. Ultrasonography is more readily available than CT scanning, but diagnostic accuracy is operator-dependent. Angiography can help in the evaluation of severe gastrointestinal haemorrhage and localizes haemangiomatous malformations.

KEY POINTS Preoperative diagnosis

- Avoid elective operations to establish colonic or rectal disease.
- Diagnostic laparotomy allows access to the exterior of the bowel; disease is mainly confined to the interior.
- Skilled endoscopy usually provides the diagnosis of intraluminal disease.

ELECTIVE OPERATIONS

CARCINOMA

KEY POINTS Precautions

- Plan elective surgery carefully.
- Always get informed consent for removal of any adjacent organs that may be affected by the disease process.
- Always have X-ray films and results of other investigations available for study in the operating theatre.
- Ensure you have the right equipment and assistance available.
- Should you have an endoscope available to re-examine the bowel lumen if necessary during the procedure?
- Re-examine the abdomen and rectum when the patient is asleep and relaxed.

Assess

1 Examine the contents of the whole abdomen.

2 Examine the whole of the colon from the appendix to the anus. Small adenomatous polyps cannot be felt.

3 Synchronous carcinomas occur in 4% of patients. Avoid handling the carcinoma; cover it with a swab soaked in dilute aqueous povidone–iodine (Betadine) solution.

4 Feel for enlarged lymph nodes in the mesentery and in the para-aortic regions. Look and feel for liver metastases. Look for peritoneal metastases.

Appraise

1 Estimate the resectability and curability of the tumour.

2 Palpate and visualize the liver to exclude metastases or biopsy them to confirm the diagnosis.

? DIFFICULTY

1. If a tumour is locally resectable but fixed to other organs such as bladder, uterus, another piece of large or small intestine, the duodenum, stomach, gallbladder, liver or kidney, or to the abdominal wall, it may still be curable, so be prepared to resect it en bloc with part or all of the adjacent organ or abdominal wall.
2. If the carcinoma is resectable but metastases are present, be willing to modify surgical treatment, but tumour resection provides better palliation than a bypass procedure.

3 Subsequent investigation allows you to make an accurate assessment. You may then plan to perform partial hepatectomy or an ablation technique in 3–4 months' time.

4 Treat potentially curable carcinoma of the right colon by one-stage right hemicolectomy, taking the ileocolic and middle colic vessels at their origin from the superior mesenteric vessels. If metastases are present perform a less-extensive resection without wide mesenteric clearance.

5 Treat carcinoma of the transverse colon by extended right hemicolectomy or transverse colectomy, taking the hepatic and/or splenic flexure if the lesion is situated proximally or distally in the transverse colon. With a lesion at the splenic flexure and distal diverticular disease, you may need to perform an extended left hemicolectomy; swing the right colon down on the right side of the abdomen and perform an anastomosis to the rectum (Fig. 16.1). Alternatively, perform an extended colectomy and ileosigmoid anastomosis.

6 Treat carcinoma of the descending and sigmoid colon by left hemicolectomy, taking the inferior mesenteric artery at its origin from the aorta and the inferior mesenteric vein at the same level.

7 Surgical management of rectal carcinoma has evolved rapidly in the last 5 years. Treat most cases of carcinoma of the rectum by anterior resection using either a sutured, stapled or per-anal anastomosis. Abdominoperineal excision of the rectum is required in only 15–20% of cases when it is impossible to obtain a 2–5-cm distal clearance of the tumour. Dissection in the pelvis is essential to ensure removal of the lymphovascular bundle (mesorectum) without breaching the fascial plane in which it is contained. Identify and preserve the hypogastric nerve plexus, if it is uninvolved with tumour. This avoids ejaculatory, erectile and urinary complications. A discussion of the merits and problems with so-called 'total mesorectal excision' is beyond the scope of this chapter; suffice to say that in expert hands it provides very low local recurrence rates with an acceptable incidence of complications.

8 For rectal carcinoma with metastases, carry out anterior resection if you can perform this safely without the need to perform a defunctioning colostomy, since many of these patients deteriorate and never have the colostomy closed. For low rectal carcinoma with local extension to the side walls of the pelvis or involved internal iliac nodes, select a palliative abdominoperineal excision of the rectum or a Hartmann's operation.

DIVERTICULAR DISEASE

1 Diverticular disease is very common and most elderly patients having operations for other abdominal conditions are found to have diverticula, mainly in the sigmoid colon. Although diverticular disease may be widespread in the colon, symptomatic disease is usually produced by muscle hypertrophy, thickening and shortening of the sigmoid colon.

2 Even in elective resection, the disease may be associated with marked pericolic inflammation and oedema with pericolic abscess formation in the mesentery.

3 Indications for elective resection are not always definite and fewer operations are now undertaken than formerly. However,

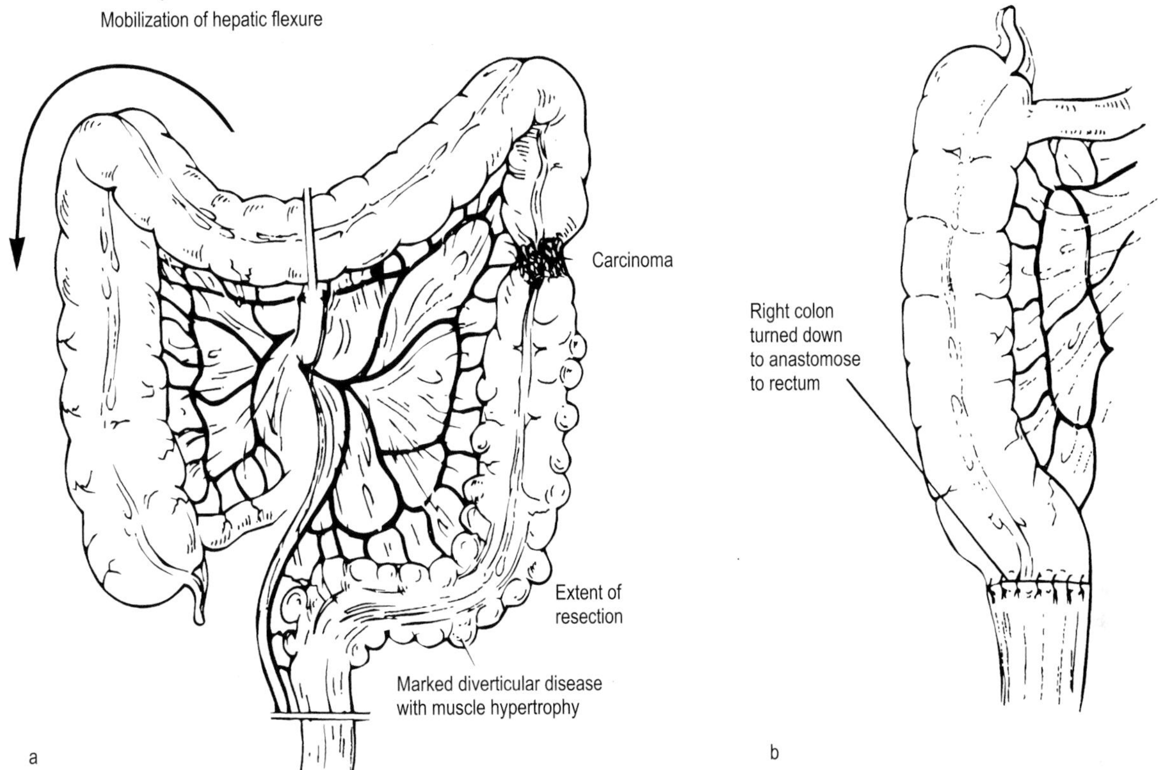

Fig. 16.1 Management of carcinoma of the splenic flexure or distal transverse colon with significant diverticular disease. This is better than an ileorectal anastomosis in patients with a compromised sphincter.

offer operation to patients in good general health who have severe attacks of lower left-sided and suprapubic pain with marked diverticular disease on a barium enema X-ray, with muscle hypertrophy and narrowing of the colonic lumen unresponsive to dietary change and antispasmodic drugs. The barium enema findings and pathology do not always correlate, and patients often wait too long before being offered surgical treatment. Definite indications for surgical treatment include:

- Male patients under the age of 50 years with symptomatic disease, since statistically over 80% eventually come to surgery, many with complications.
- Patients with urinary infection associated with their attacks, indicating adhesion to the bladder or ureter and an impending fistula, and indeed those with an established colovesical fistula.
- Patients fit for operation with recurrent attacks of acute diverticular disease within a short period of time, associated with a fever, mass and radiological signs of a pericolic abscess.
- Patients fit for operation with recurrent bleeding. A single episode does not make surgery mandatory.

KEY POINT Avoid operation

- Avoid operation in patients with irritable bowel syndrome and few diverticula; their symptoms will persist.

4 It is unnecessary to remove all the proximal diverticula. Resect all hypertrophied sections of bowel, usually including the whole of the sigmoid colon, with anastomosis between the middle or upper descending colon and the upper third of the rectum below the sacral promontory.

5 Operative treatment is always by resection and anastomosis. If there is acute on chronic inflammation at the time of surgery or the anastomosis is difficult, then be prepared to perform a defunctioning ileostomy as a temporary measure.

ULCERATIVE COLITIS

1 Offer elective operation to patients with persistent or recurrent attacks of diarrhoea with the passage of blood, anaemia, weight loss and general ill-health who do not respond to treatment with corticosteroids and salazines. The majority of these patients have total or extensive colitis. Patients with purely distal disease, such as sigmoid or left-colon, do not usually require operation. Try to operate on patients who have several severe attacks of acute colitis during remission.

2 Total colitis of 10 or more years' duration may result in dysplastic epithelial changes and eventual carcinoma, even in the absence of any symptoms. Carefully monitor them with colonoscopy and mucosal biopsy. Operate if they develop moderate or severe dysplasia. Operate on patients with total colitis and strictures or filling defects on barium enema X-ray or colonoscopy. Steroid therapy does not contraindicate surgery as

it makes no difference to the outcome, but administer steroid cover during and after the operation.

3 In quiescent total colitis, the colon is slightly thickened, shortened and greyish white in colour. Even at elective operation, part of the colon may appear much more actively inflamed with thickening, oedema and marked hyperaemia. The paracolic and mesenteric nodes may be considerably enlarged.

4 The most straightforward procedure is a proctocolectomy with a conventional Brooke ileostomy.

5 Consider alternative procedures:
- If operation is performed early in the course of the disease when the rectum is still distensible and there is no dysplasia in rectal biopsies, consider performing a colectomy and ileorectal anastomosis.
- To spare patients from permanent conventional ileostomy, perform a conservative proctocolectomy leaving the anal sphincters and create an ileoanal reservoir.
- If the patient is incontinent as a result of previous sphincter damage, you may construct a Kock reservoir ileostomy to avoid the patient having to wear an appliance.

6 If you are inexperienced in these operations, carry out a colectomy and ileostomy, retaining the whole rectum.

CROHN'S DISEASE

1 This can develop anywhere within the gastrointestinal tract and is primarily treated medically.

2 Undertake surgical treatment if medical treatment fails to control the disease, or for complications such as stenosis causing obstructive symptoms, abscesses or internal or external fistula formation.

> **KEY POINT Operate on clinical grounds, not merely on investigation results**
>
> - Surgery is not curative, so make sure you treat the patients and their symptoms, not appearances on radiological imaging.

3 The whole or part of the colon may be involved in Crohn's disease. Carefully exclude disease in the stomach, duodenum and the whole of the small bowel. Measure and record the length of the small bowel and the sites and extent of the disease. These patients often require multiple operations and may end up with 'short-bowel syndrome' unless surgery is carefully planned.

4 When the disease affects the terminal ileum and/or caecum and ascending colon, carry out ileal resection with removal of the caecum or right colon as necessary. In a primary operation, remove 5–10 cm of macroscopically normal ileum proximal to the lesion. If there is a chronic abscess cavity in the right iliac fossa, extend the right hemicolectomy so that the anastomosis lies in the upper abdomen away from the abscess cavity.

5 If the whole colon is severely involved and requires resection, perform a colectomy and ileorectal anastomosis or a total proctocolectomy and conventional ileostomy. Distal disease involving only the rectum may require an abdominoperineal excision with an end colostomy.

6 Segmental colonic resection is rarely required because segmental involvement of the colon is unusual.

POLYPS AND POLYPOSIS

1 When you discover rectal polyps on routine sigmoidoscopy, remove one or more for histology. If the polyp proves to be an adenoma, carry out a colonoscopy to search for and treat proximal polyps. Sessile villous adenomas usually occur in the rectum and can be removed by endoanal local excision. Transanal endoscopic microsurgery is available in specialist centres.

2 If several large polyps are present in a patient with carcinoma, extend the resection to include these. In a patient with one or more carcinomas and several large polyps, consider colectomy and ileorectal anastomosis.

3 Perform anterior resection with coloanal anastomosis or a modified Soave procedure on circumferential villous tumours extending above 10 cm from the anal vent.

4 Familial adenomatous polyposis demands operation to avoid inevitable malignant change. Options include colectomy and ileorectal anastomosis, or proctocolectomy and ileoanal pouch reconstruction. Following ileorectal anastomosis the rectum still carries the potential for malignant change, so plan to perform follow-up sigmoidoscopy every 6 months. Fulgurate rectal polyps if they are over 5 mm in diameter.

URGENT OPERATIONS

1 Urgent operations on the colon or rectum are carried out for obstruction, perforation, acute fulminating inflammatory bowel disease and acute haemorrhage.

2 Improve the patient's condition before operation by replacing blood, fluid and electrolyte loss. Counteract major sepsis with antibiotics such as a cephalosporin, together with metronidazole.

3 Decide on the best time for operation:
- Severe bleeding, major abdominal sepsis or perforation demand operation as soon as the patient's condition allows.
- Large-bowel obstruction and inflammatory bowel disease rarely require emergency surgery.

> **KEY POINT Operate under the best conditions**
>
> - Whenever possible avoid operating in haste at night, when you are tired, the patient is ill-prepared and your assistance and equipment are inadequate.

OBSTRUCTION

1 Define the level of obstruction with a CT scan or water-soluble contrast enema.

2 If the patient is medically unfit for operative surgery, the stenosing tumour may be suitable for radiological insertion of a stent to open up the lumen. This may allow the patient to be optimized for elective surgery.

3 If you need to carry out an urgent resection, make sure it is as radical as would be achieved at an elective operation at the same site, provided cure is possible. If there are metastases, carry out palliative resection. It is rare to find a proximal tumour that is not resectable. Avoid the alternative procedure of a bypass operation if possible as this may relieve the obstruction but it will not stop bleeding from the tumour and consequent anaemia nor will it stop the pain or complications from the mass invading other structures. If a left-sided tumour is unresectable, create a proximal defunctioning colostomy.

KEY POINTS Do not lose sight of your objective

- You are operating in an emergency to achieve a specific, urgent goal.
- Do not lightly undertake procedures that prejudice the patient's recovery.

4 Perform a right hemicolectomy for carcinoma of the right colon causing acute intestinal obstruction.

5 In the past, left-sided obstruction was treated by a staged procedure. Initially a proximal defunctioning stoma was created to relieve the obstruction; subsequently the tumour was resected and, when it was safely healed, the stoma was closed. More commonly, carcinoma of the sigmoid or descending colon is resected by a one-stage colectomy with ileosigmoid or ileorectal anastomosis (Fig. 16.2).

6 Treat carcinoma of the rectosigmoid junction or rectum by resection, peroperative irrigation of the obstructed colon and primary anastomosis with or without a defunctioning ileostomy (Fig. 16.3). Alternatively, perform a Hartmann's procedure (see later).

7 Acute obstructive diverticular disease is rare but is often complicated by paracolic abscess formation. The most commonly performed operation is immediate resection with a Hartmann's procedure. However, if the infection is localized and would be completely removed by resection, it should be safe to carry out a resection and anastomosis with or without a defunctioning ileostomy.

PERFORATION

1 Perforation of a carcinoma or diverticular disease demands resection and anastomosis with a covering colostomy or, in the presence of major faecal contamination, a Hartmann's procedure.

2 If you detect a significant abscess using CT, drain it percutaneously.

3 If initially localized abdominal signs become more generalized, or if the infection fails to settle despite adequate conservative therapy, operate. A minority of patients operated on for localized diverticulitis are amenable to primary resection and primary anastomosis. Generalized peritonitis secondary to a free perforation is more commonly associated with purulent peritonitis than with faecal peritonitis. Resection and primary anastomosis is possible in the majority of cases without faecal contamination but do not carry this out in the presence of faecal peritonitis.

4 Primary anastomosis is popular because:

- Patients require one operation rather than two.
- Following a Hartmann's operation many patients are left with a permanent stoma, either because of unwillingness or unfitness to have further surgery.
- Reversal operation after Hartmann's resection can be very difficult.

5 If possible, aim to resect the perforated segment, even in the acutely ill patient, because it minimizes the risk of continued contamination. An additional reason for advocating primary resection is because it is difficult, at operation, to decide whether the lesion is a perforated carcinoma or an area of diverticulitis. As many as 25% of patients with a preoperative diagnosis of perforated diverticulitis may have a perforated carcinoma. If there is reasonable suspicion of carcinoma, perform a radical resection of the lesion, together with the colonic mesentery. Examine the resected specimen in the theatre as an aid to further decision-making.

ACUTE INFLAMMATORY OR ISCHAEMIC BOWEL DISEASE

1 Treat acute fulminating colitis, with or without toxic megacolon, by colectomy and ileostomy with a mucous fistula. Do not excise the rectum. It is much safer to make a mucous fistula than to close the rectal stump. In order to avoid creating a second stoma, close the stump directly under the wound so that if it breaks down it will not contaminate the peritoneal cavity.

2 Excise a segment of acute ischaemic colitis and create a proximal and distal colostomy. Always leave the rectum and sigmoid colon as these usually recover sufficiently for an anastomosis to be carried out later.

ACUTE MASSIVE HAEMORRHAGE

1 Determine if possible the site of bleeding by sigmoidoscopy, colonoscopy, upper gastrointestinal endoscopy and angiography. Remember that 50% of patients with episodes of haemorrhage and diverticular disease have another cause for the bleeding.

2 If the site can be accurately determined it may be possible to stop the bleeding by interventional radiologically controlled embolization. If you cannot determine the site and origin of colonic bleeding preoperatively, organize on-table colonoscopy and possible enteroscopy.

SURGERY OF THE LARGE BOWEL

Appraise

1 Morbidity and mortality following colonic surgery is higher than following resections of the small bowel.

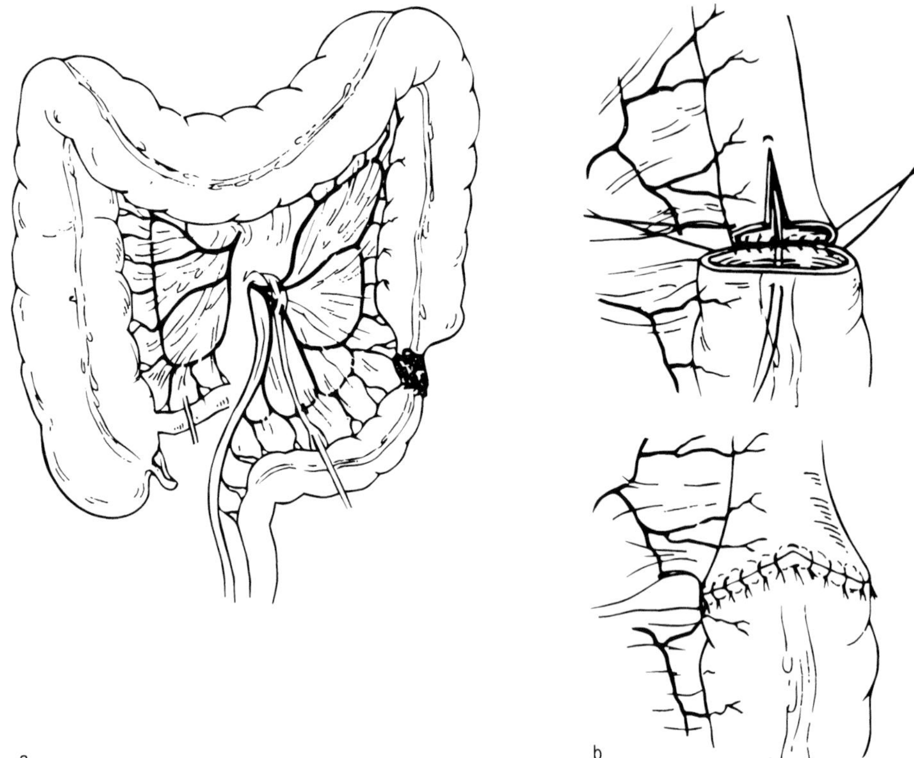

Fig. 16.2 (a) Obstructing carcinoma of the sigmoid colon: colectomy and ileorectal or ileosigmoid anastomosis. (b) Cheatle slit on antimesenteric aspect of the ileum to accommodate the discrepancy in size.

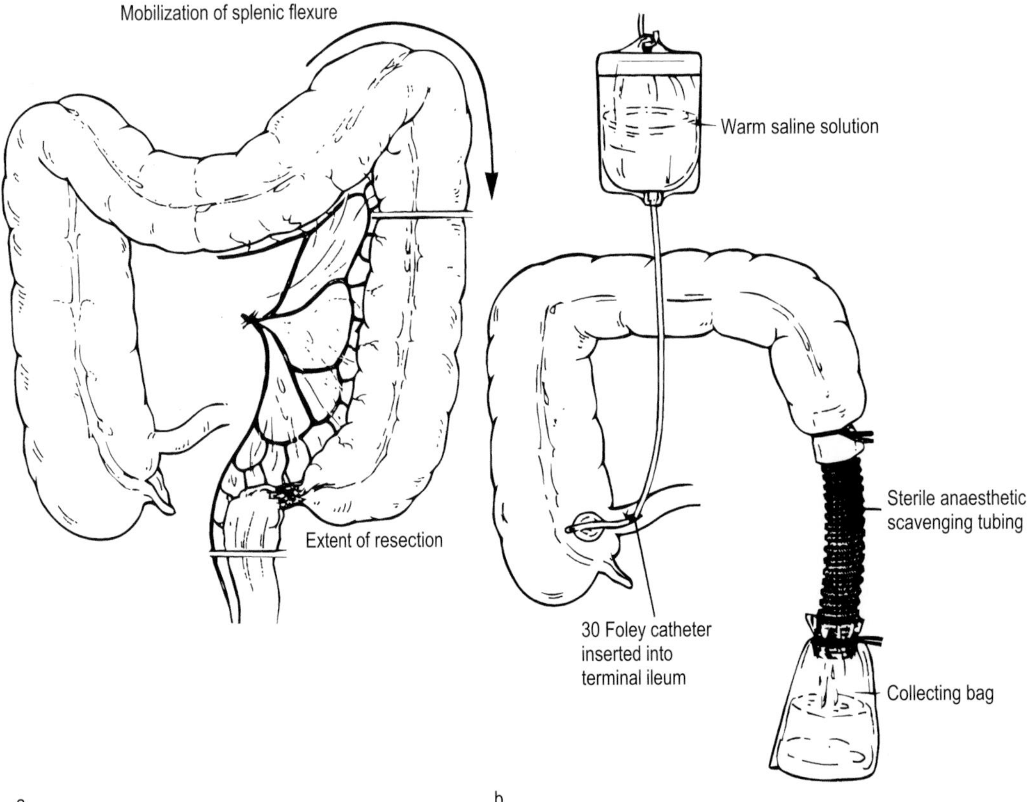

Fig. 16.3 (a) Obstructing carcinoma of the rectosigmoid or lower sigmoid colon. (b) Closed orthograde irrigation of the obstructed colon after primary resection. Four or more litres of warm saline are necessary to completely clean the colon.

2 The colonic blood supply is more tenuous and easily damaged. Tissue perfusion is often decreased postoperatively, resulting in a degree of ischaemic colitis.

3 Infection is more common, resulting in abscess formation with potentiation of collagenase activity. Collagen undergoes lysis and may result in anastomotic dehiscence.

Prepare

1 Ensure that imaging results are available at operation.

2 Most surgeons use bowel preparation before elective operations although there is no clear-cut evidence to support it. Certainly there is no need to clear the colon for a right hemicolectomy. Sodium picosulfate and magnesium citrate provide a stimulant preparation, polyethylene glycol is a mechanical preparation. Give adequate fluids for 24 hours preoperatively. Intravenous fluids may be required in elderly patients. If necessary order enemas in the absence of a bowel preparation to reduce the presence of hard stools distal to the anastomosis.

3 Preoperative oral antibiotics are of little value. Give peroperative prophylactic antibiotics at induction of anaesthesia. A cephalosporin and metronidazole or beta-lactamase inhibitor/broad-spectrum penicillin (Augmentin) are popular. Give a further dose of antibiotics if the operation is prolonged more than 2 hours, or if there is significant intraoperative contamination. There is no evidence that routine use of more than one dose of prophylactic antibiotics reduces the risk of infection although gross faecal contamination may lead you to continue therapeutic antibiotics for several days postoperation.

4 Catheterize the patient after induction of anaesthesia and monitor urinary output during and after surgery.

KEY POINTS Are you well prepared?

- Are the barium enema films and other imaging results available?
- Do you have adequate assistance and the necessary equipment?
- Is this the right patient, accompanied by the completed consent form?

Action

1 Clamp the bowel to be resected with Parker–Kerr clamps or use a cross-stapling technique. Place no clamps on the ends to be sutured but use non-crushing clamps away from the bowel ends to avoid contamination.

2 Clean the ends of the bowel to be sutured with moistened swabs wetted in 1:2000 aqueous chlorhexidine solution on aqueous 10% povidone–iodine (Betadine) solution.

3 Divide the colon at right-angles to the mesentery. If there is disparity in size between the ends, particularly when carrying out a right hemicolectomy or an ileorectal anastomosis, slit up the antimesenteric border of the ileum or narrower colon until the two ends approximate in size. Alternatively carry out an end-to-side or side-to-side anastomosis. When a long length of mobilized colon is to be anastomosed to the rectum make certain there is not a 360° twist.

4 Suture the bowel in a one-layer seromuscular fashion with an appropriate suture such as 3/0 PDS (polydioxanone), or 4/0 Ethibond (polybutylate-coated polyester). Use either an interrupted or continuous stitch. Invert the edges but not so much as to produce a cuff that will create an obstructive anastomosis. Ensure that the mucosa does not protrude from the suture line. Alternatively, there are a number of methods for carrying out a stapled anastomosis; apart from speed they add little to the more traditional approach and are significantly more expensive. Undertake rectal anastomosis using a circular stapling device such as the EEA stapler, using a 28- or 31-mm diameter device, particularly when forming an anastomosis low in the pelvis, when suturing is technically difficult.

5 Avoid contamination during the operation. If the colon is loaded, place a non-crushing clamp across the bowel 10 cm from the end before this is swabbed out and cleaned. If possible, screen the anastomosis from the peritoneal cavity and contents while it is being constructed. When it is complete, discard and replace the towels, gloves and instruments before closing the abdomen.

6 It is traditional for British surgeons to drain any colonic anastomosis. This is probably unnecessary in most cases. You may wish to drain a very low pelvic anastomosis.

RIGHT HEMICOLECTOMY

Appraise

1 Perform this operation for carcinoma of the caecum and ascending colon and for the occasional benign tumour of the right colon. Undertake it for a perforated caecal diverticulum, so-called solitary ulcer of the caecum and carry out a limited resection for carcinoma of the appendix or a carcinoid tumour at the base of the appendix. If possible avoid performing an ileocolic bypass even for an extensive carcinoma; a palliative resection gives better results.

2 Treat benign disease of the terminal ileum, particularly Crohn's disease, by resecting an appropriate amount of ileum together with the caecum and 2–3 cm of the right colon. When Crohn's disease is associated with abscess formation in the right iliac fossa, extend the operation so that the anastomosis lies in the upper abdomen away from the abscess with the intention of protecting it from postoperative fistula formation.

3 Never make a small-bowel anastomosis close to the ileocaecal valve. Preferably remove the caecum and a small part of the ascending colon, and carry out an ileocolic anastomosis.

4 In the presence of obstructing lesions of the colon the caecum may be ischaemic. You must include the region in any resection, either in the form of an extended right hemicolectomy or even a colectomy with ileorectal anastomosis.

Action (Fig. 16.4)

Resect

1 Handle the tumour as little as possible. If the serosa and surrounding fat are infiltrated by carcinoma, cover it with a swab soaked in aqueous 10% povidone–iodine solution.

2 Leave the omentum adherent to the right colon.

3 Draw the caecum and ascending colon medially. Cut through the parietal peritoneum lateral to the colon from the caecum to the hepatic flexure. If the carcinoma infiltrates the lateral abdominal wall, excise a large disc of peritoneum and underlying muscle with the specimen.

4 Dissect the right colon from the posterior abdominal wall. Identify and preserve the right ureter, gonadal vessels and duodenum.

5 Mobilize the hepatic flexure and divide any ileal bands so that the whole of the right colon can be lifted from the abdomen.

KEY POINTS Anatomy

- You are elevating the bowel on its embryological mesentery, containing its blood vessels, lymphatics, nerves and contained fat.
- Keep meticulously in the correct plane between the mesentery and posterior wall peritoneum.

6 Transilluminate the mesentery to identify the vessels. Clamp and divide the ileocolic artery and vein close to the superior mesenteric vessels. Divide the right colic vessels and the right branch of the middle colic vessels close to their origin.

7 The extent of the resection depends to some degree on the size and site of the tumour but normally includes approximately 25 cm of terminal ileum to the middle third of the transverse colon.

8 Remove the right half of the greater omentum with the specimen. If the tumour is situated near the hepatic flexure remove the right side of the gastroepiploic arch of vessels to obtain a wider clearance.

9 Place a Parker–Kerr clamp or cross-staples across the ileum and transverse colon at the site of division. If the patient is obstructed or the colon is unprepared, place towels around the bowel at the time of division.

10 Divide the bowel and remove the specimen.

11 Hold the ends of the ileum and colon to be anastomosed in Babcock's forceps and clean them with mounted swabs wetted with aqueous 10% povidone–iodine solution.

Unite

1 Anastomose the terminal ileum end-to-end to the transverse colon, if necessary widening the ileum with an antimesenteric slit (described by the English surgeon Sir George Cheatle, 1865–1951). Mark the anastomosis with haemostatic clips if

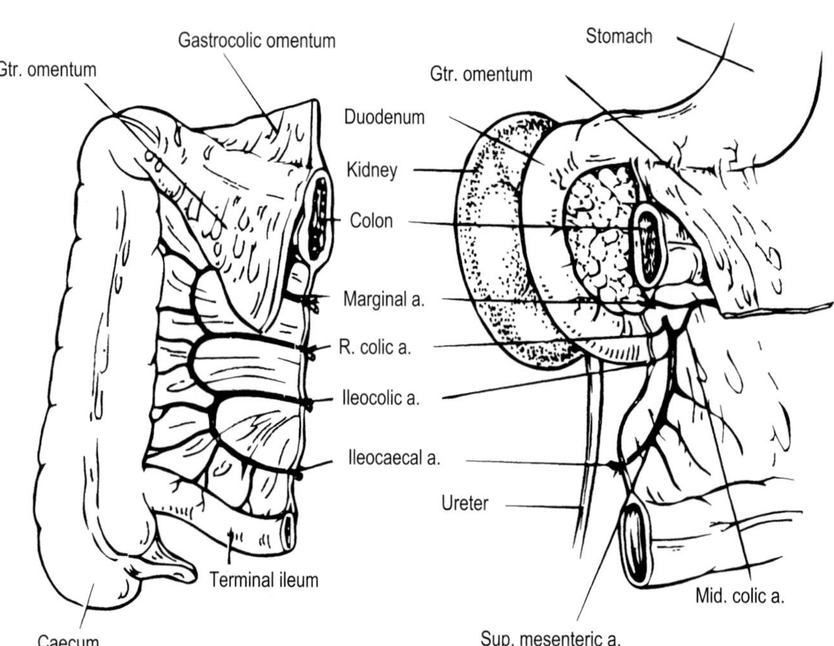

Fig. 16.4 Radical right hemicolectomy. The resected specimen is on the left and comprises the right half of the colon, the terminal ileum and the mesentery with vessels and nodes. Also included are the right halves of the gastrocolic and greater omenta. The ileocolic artery and vein are divided at their origins from the superior mesenteric vessels. The right branch of the middle colic artery is divided. The duodenum, pancreas and right kidney and ureter have been identified and protected from damage.

desired. Alternatively, divide the colon using a linear cutter stapling device and perform an end-to-side anastomosis, or construct a functional end-to-end anastomosis using the same linear cutter stapling device.

2 Suture the cut edges of the mesentery with a polyglactin 910 (Vicryl) suture.

3 Cover the anastomosis with the remaining omentum.

Technical points

1 If the resection is for a benign condition such as Crohn's disease or a caecal diverticulum, it need not be extensive. The vessels can be divided in the middle of the mesentery rather than at their origin.

2 If the carcinoma is locally invasive but can be excised radically, widen the scope of the operation to include abdominal wall or part of the involved organs.

3 If the carcinoma is situated at the hepatic flexure or in the right side of the transverse colon, mobilize the splenic flexure as well. Divide the middle colic vessels close to their origin and anastomose the terminal ileum to the descending or sigmoid colon. If there are multiple metastases carry out a limited segmental resection rather than a bypass procedure.

Checklist

1 Make sure the bowel on each side of the anastomosis is viable and check that the anastomosis lies freely without twist or tension.

2 Examine the raw surfaces, particularly in the right flank, and stop any bleeding. Remove any blood collected above the right lobe of the liver and in the pelvis.

LEFT HEMICOLECTOMY

Appraise

1 Undertake left hemicolectomy for carcinoma of the left and sigmoid colon, and for diverticular disease.

2 If the operation is for an obstructed neoplasm, carry out an extended colectomy with an ileosigmoid or ileorectal anastomosis. Alternatively, carry out a resection with on-table irrigation of the obstructed proximal colon and create a primary anastomosis. Try to avoid a Hartmann's operation as patients are frequently left with their stoma and reversal can be a major undertaking.

3 In diverticular disease, resect the sigmoid colon and as much of the ascending colon as is necessary. Leave isolated diverticula in the upper descending and transverse colon, providing the bowel wall is not thickened. Anastomose the proximal bowel to the upper third of the rectum below the sacral promontory and not to the sigmoid colon.

4 In any left hemicolectomy, the splenic flexure and the left half of the transverse colon must be mobilized.

Prepare

1 Place the patient in the lithotomy Trendelenburg (Lloyd-Davies) position (Fig. 16.5).

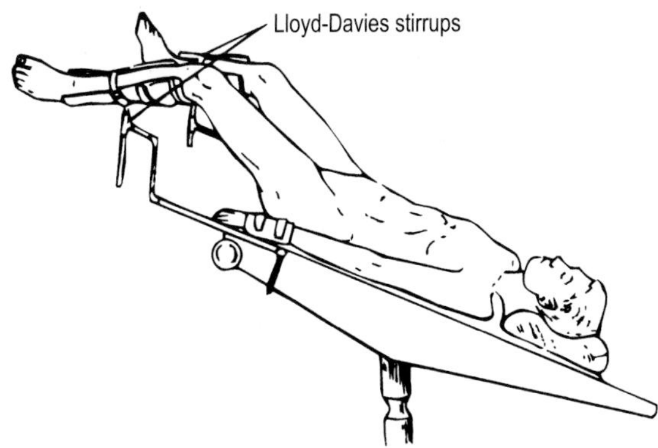

Fig. 16.5 Place the patient in the lithotomy Trendelenburg (Lloyd-Davies) position for any operation on, or involving, the left side of the colon or the rectum. This allows simultaneous approaches to be made to the perineum or rectum and the abdomen without altering the patient's position.

2 Pass a catheter to empty the bladder and to monitor the urine flow during and after the operation.

Access

1 Stand on the patient's right side.

2 Make a long midline incision. You require access to the spleen when you mobilize the splenic flexure of colon, and in the pelvis when you construct the anastomosis.

Assess

1 If the operation is for a carcinoma, carefully palpate the liver bimanually, examine the colon and the whole of the small bowel, palpate the mesenteric and para-aortic nodes and the whole of the peritoneal cavity and pelvis.

2 Gently palpate the carcinoma to assess its mobility but touch it as little as possible. If the serosal surface is involved, cover it with a swab soaked in 10% aqueous povidone–iodine solution.

3 If you are performing partial colectomy for a benign condition, assess the diseased and normal colon to decide the extent of resection.

KEY POINTS Decisions

- Carry out a radical resection of a carcinoma if possible. Tie the inferior mesenteric artery at its origin from the aorta and the inferior mesenteric vein below the inferior border of the pancreas.
- If the patient is very elderly and clearly unfit, and the blood supply to the colon is tenuous because of severe atheroma, undertake a less-radical procedure, retaining the origin of the inferior mesenteric artery, and ligate the left colonic artery and sigmoid branches as appropriate.
- If the resection is for a benign condition, or a palliative resection for carcinoma, then the bowel resection need not be so wide and you may ligate and divide the vessels close to the bowel wall.

RADICAL RESECTION OF THE LEFT COLON

Action (Fig. 16.6)

1 Exteriorize the small bowel to the right side and cover it with a moist pack. Never pack the small bowel into the wound as it severely restricts access.

2 Divide the congenital adhesions that bind the sigmoid colon to the abdominal wall in the left iliac fossa and then divide the adhesions between the descending colon and the lateral peritoneum. This is most efficiently achieved by following the plane of zygosis (Greek: *zygon*=yoke; true conjunction of posterior peritoneum and visceral peritoneum) or white line. Do not divide the peritoneum but stay on the mesenteric side of the white line to ensure that you remain in the correct plane.

3 Rotate the patient to the right side and then mobilize the splenic flexure by dividing the phrenocolic ligament. Ligate the few vessels in it. Avoid damaging the spleen and the tail of the pancreas. If the carcinoma is distal you may preserve the greater omentum by dividing the adhesions between the omentum and the colon as far proximally as the middle of the transverse colon and dividing the peritoneum along the end of the lesser sac. If the tumour is situated near the flexure, excise the left half of the greater omentum with the tumour by dividing the left side of the gastroepiploic arch and removing the lesser and greater omentum with the specimen.

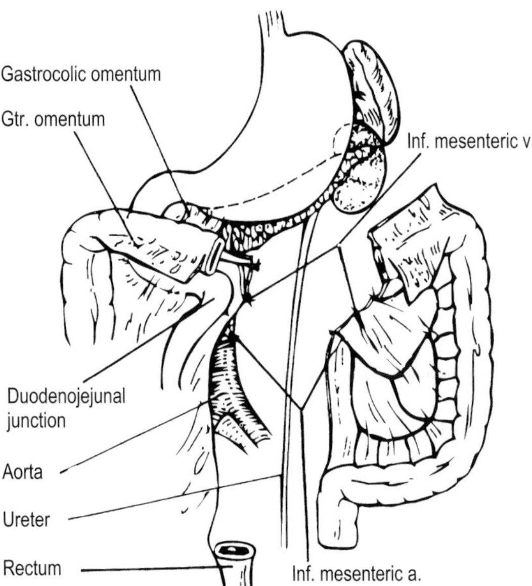

Fig. 16.6 Radical left hemicolectomy. The resected specimen is on the right and comprises the left half of colon, the mesocolon and the left halves of the gastrocolic and greater omenta. The left division of the middle colic artery and the origin of the inferior mesenteric artery have been ligated and divided. The duodenojejunal junction, left ureter and kidney, pancreas and spleen have been protected from damage.

4 Elevate the left colon on its mesentery and dissect it free from the duodenojejunal flexure, the left ureter and gonadal vessels.

5 Incise the peritoneum overlying the aorta and mobilize the inferior mesenteric artery to its origin. Ligate and divide the artery and then identify the inferior mesenteric vein lying laterally and clamp, ligate and divide it a little below the lower border of the pancreas.

6 Mobilize the sigmoid colon if the anastomosis is to be made to the upper third of the rectum. Do not divide the sigmoid higher than about 10 cm above the rectum or you will endanger its blood supply.

7 Divide the mesentery and marginal vessels to the edge of the colon at the site chosen for resection in the transverse colon and rectum or sigmoid colon.

8 Place a non-crushing right-angled clamp across the rectum at the site of resection. Then irrigate the rectum by means of a catheter passed through the anus with povidone–iodine solution or a 1:2000 aqueous chlorhexidine solution, until it is perfectly clean.

? DIFFICULTY

1. If the abdominal wall is involved with carcinoma, excise part of the wall with the tumour and repair the defect at the end of the procedure. If small bowel is involved, be prepared to resect one loop or more as necessary and anastomose the cut ends. Be willing to excise a portion of the bladder fundus. If other organs are involved, such as the left ureter or uterus, deal with them appropriately.
2. Do not hesitate to involve another specialist if you are not experienced enough to deal with unfamiliar techniques.
3. If the tumour is situated in the left half of the transverse colon or at the splenic flexure, excise most of the transverse colon and unite the hepatic flexure or ascending colon to the lower descending or sigmoid colon. Alternatively, perform an extended right hemicolectomy with an ileo-descending anastomosis.

9 While the rectal irrigation is being carried out, prepare the proximal colon for division. Place a non-crushing clamp across the bowel well proximal to the intended site of division. Cross-staple or use a Parker–Kerr clamp just distal to the intended site of division. Divide the colon, hold the proximal end in Babcock's forceps and swab the bowel out with Betadine solution or 1:2000 aqueous chlorhexidine solution.

10 Divide the rectum or sigmoid colon below the right-angled clamp and remove the specimen consisting of the left half of the colon, the inferior mesenteric artery and vein and the whole of the mesentery.

11 If you need to mobilize the transverse colon or hepatic flexure to ensure a tension-free anastomosis, do this before dividing the colon.

Unite

1 Unite the bowel ends with one layer of seromuscular-inverting sutures according to your preferred technique.

KEY POINT Stapling care

- Beware of using the EEA stapler at the top of the rectum. Introducing it around the rectal valves may tear the rectum. If you employ this technique, either resect more of the rectum or anastomose the colon end-to-side to the rectum.

2 Suture the cut edge of the transverse mesocolon to the cut edge of the peritoneum overlying the aorta.

CARCINOMA OF THE RECTUM

Appraise

1 Assess all patients before operation by sigmoidoscopy, rectal biopsy and a colonoscopy or CT colography to evaluate the proximal colon.

2 Assess low tumours and those placed anteriorly, with magnetic resonance imaging, to assess tumour stage.

3 Consider preoperative radiotherapy particularly for T_3 and T_4 lesions.

4 A few patients with small early carcinomas (assessed by transrectal ultrasound) are suitable for a per-anal local excision.

ANTERIOR RESECTION OF THE RECTUM

Prepare

1 Place the anaesthetized patient in the lithotomy Trendelenburg (Lloyd-Davies) position.

2 Insert an indwelling Foley catheter.

3 Carry out an examination under anaesthetic to assess the fixity of low tumours (below the peritoneal reflection).

Access

1 Stand on the patient's right.

2 Make a long midline incision, as the splenic flexure will require mobilization and the rectal anastomosis may be deep within the pelvis.

Assess

1 Palpate and visualize the liver to establish if there are metastases.

2 Note any local or distant peritoneal metastases. Examine the omentum.

3 Palpate any nodes in the mesentery and note any para-aortic nodes.

4 Finally, palpate the tumour, note its size and position above or below the peritoneal reflection and decide whether it is mobile, adherent to other organs or fixed within the pelvis.

? DIFFICULTY

1. Do not be daunted to discover that a large rectal carcinoma lies in a small male pelvis.
2. Determine not to compromise on the standard of radical resection by breaching the planes of dissection. Take time and proceed in an ever-deepening circumferential manner. As you mobilize the rectum, dissection becomes progressively easier.

Action (Fig. 16.7)

1 Mobilize the left side of the colon from the peritoneum by dividing the congenital adhesions from the sigmoid colon to the splenic flexure.

2 Fully mobilize the splenic flexure and the left half of the transverse colon, preserving the omentum unless there are metastases present in it. Avoid damage to the spleen.

3 Mobilize the left colon, pull it to the right on its mesentery and separate and preserve the left ureter and gonadal vessels. Take care not to damage the duodenojejunal flexure or the tail of the pancreas.

KEY POINTS Anatomy

- You are mobilizing the left colon onto its embryological mesentery.
- Make sure you do not wander from the correct tissue plane.

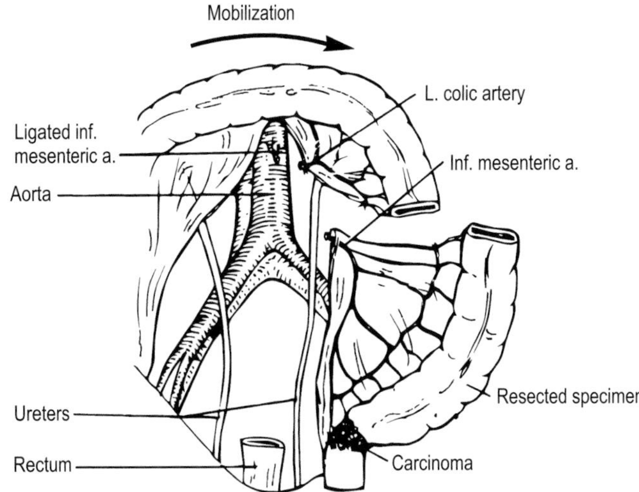

Fig. 16.7 Anterior resection of the rectum: the resected specimen is on the right and consists of the upper rectum, the sigmoid and part of the descending colon, together with the sigmoid mesocolon. The inferior mesenteric artery has been ligated and divided on the aorta and the inferior mesenteric vein at the upper border of the pancreas. The splenic flexure has been mobilized. Both ureters have been identified and preserved.

4 To enter the 'mesorectal plane' lift the sigmoid loop vertically. Observe the arc of the inferior mesenteric artery as it leaves the aorta and enters the mesorectum. Divide the peritoneum on the right side just beneath the arc of the artery, follow it back up to its origin and down into the loose areolar tissue that denotes the beginning of the mesorectal plane. Push away the tissue deep to this arcing peritoneal incision, which contains the pelvic nerve plexus. Both branches of this plexus should be apparent as they divide around the rectum at the level of the sacral promontory.

5 Make a similar incision in the peritoneum of the left side to produce a window with artery above and nerves below from the origin of the inferior artery to the start of the mesorectal plane. Clamp, divide and ligate the inferior mesenteric artery at its origin from the aorta, but if the patient is old and arteriosclerotic, preserve the left colic artery. Divide the inferior mesenteric vein at a slightly higher level, close to the lower border of the pancreas. Select a suitable area to transect the descending colon and divide the mesentery up to this point. Bowel transection at this stage facilitates the rectal dissection because the specimen can be pulled anteriorly while leaving the descending colon and small bowel packed up and out of the way in the upper abdomen.

6 The extent of rectal mobilization depends upon the level of the tumour. If it is retroperitoneal, you must completely mobilize the rectum and its mesorectum.

7 Move to the left of the patient. Pull the rectum forwards and dissect anteriorly to the sacral promontory and presacral fascia, as far down as the tip of the coccyx and the pelvic floor muscles. This is best done by holding a St Mark's lipped retractor in your left hand to pull the rectum forwards while carrying out sharp dissection with scissors or diathermy. Take care to visualize and preserve the presacral nerves.

8 As the posterior dissection deepens, divide the peritoneum over each side of the pelvis, close to the lateral wall. Eventually join the incisions anteriorly in the midline. The ideal site for this anterior division is about 1 cm above the most dependent part of the peritoneum. This usually corresponds to the bulge in the peritoneum overlying the seminal vesicles.

9 Hold the seminal vesicles forwards with a St Mark's lipped retractor and dissect between the vesicles and the rectum to uncover the rectovesical fascia described by the Parisian anatomist and surgeon Charles Denonvilliers (1808–1872). Incise this transversely and dissect down between the fascia and the rectum as far distally as necessary, and down behind the prostate to the pelvic floor. In a female, dissect distally between the rectum and vagina as far down as necessary, even to the pelvic floor.

10 By traction on the rectum to one side and then the other side of the pelvis, identify the tissue described as the 'lateral ligaments'. This can be cauterized and divided without the need for formal clipping and dividing. Avoid tenting up and damaging the third sacral nerve root at this point.

11 Straighten out the rectum and draw the tumour upwards. Choose a suitable site for division of the rectum. If possible allow a 5-cm clearance below the lower edge of the carcinoma. If the tumour is low down, this degree of clearance may be impossible to achieve in a restorative procedure. Be willing to compromise but without jeopardizing a curative procedure. Obtain at least a 2-cm clearance. For lesions of the upper rectum, the mesorectum is present at the site selected for division of the rectum. Divide this perpendicularly to the rectal wall, taking care not to 'cone down' on to the rectum, getting so close that you risk leaving mesorectum containing tumour deposits. Apply a transverse stapler or right-angled clamp to the rectum at the site selected for division. Remember, if you intend using a stapled anastomosis, that the stapler removes an extra 8 mm of rectum.

12 Irrigate the rectum through the anus with povidone–iodine solution or 1:2000 aqueous chlorhexidine solution. If only a small cuff of sphincter and rectum remains, simply swab it out.

13 If you have not already divided it, select the site for division of the descending colon, place a Parker–Kerr clamp at right-angles across the bowel and transect above it, holding the upper end of the colon with Babcock forceps so that it can be swabbed out.

14 Divide the rectum below the stapler or clamp with a long-handled knife. Remove the specimen containing the rectal carcinoma, the complete mesentery and nodes up to the origin of the inferior mesenteric artery.

Unite

The anastomosis can be carried out in one of two ways, depending upon the level of anastomosis, the ease of access to the pelvis and the obesity of the patient.

Sutured anastomosis (Fig. 16.8)

1 Suture the bowel in one layer to produce an end-to-end inverted anastomosis.

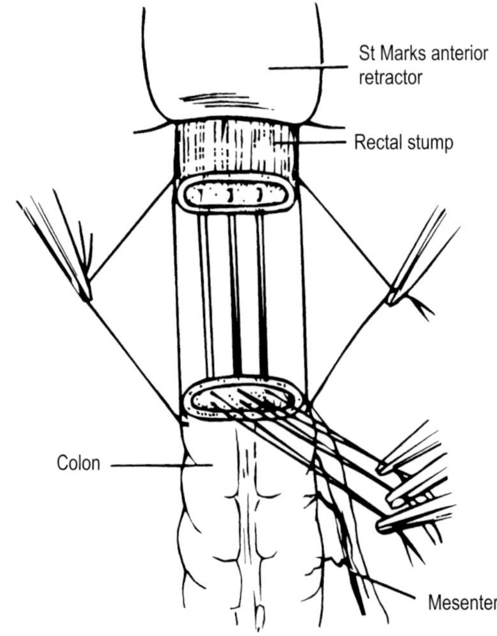

Fig. 16.8 Anterior resection of the rectum with sutured anastomosis. One-layer anastomosis, showing the insertion of sutures in preparation for the descending colon to be 'railroaded' down to the rectum.

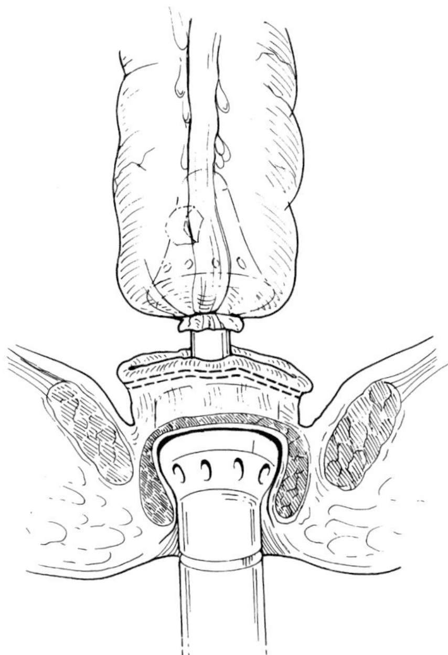

Fig. 16.9 Anterior resection of the rectum with stapled anastomosis, showing insertion of the circular stapling device through the anus with stapled rectal stump with the descending colon tied over the anvil.

2 Insert vertical mattress sutures into the posterior layer and hold each suture with artery forceps until they have all been inserted.

3 Now 'rail-road' the descending colon down to the rectum. The sutures are all held taut while the descending colon is pushed down until its posterior edge is in contact with the rectum, sometimes also called the 'parachute' technique. Tie the sutures with the knots within the lumen. Hold the two most lateral sutures and cut the others. Suture the anterior layer using interrupted seromuscular-inverting stitches, inserting them all before they are tied.

4 Place a haemostatic clip on each side of the anastomosis to mark it radiologically.

Stapled anastomosis (Fig. 16.9)

1 If the anastomosis is too low to suture conventionally or if you prefer the technique, unite the bowel with the EEA circular stapling device. Carry out the operation exactly as described until the ends of the bowel have been prepared for anastomosis. Now insert the sizing heads into the colon to see if the stapling gun should be 25, 28 or 31 mm in diameter. For the colon it is best to select a 28- or 31-mm gun. Remember that the stapler removes an extra 8 mm of rectum and this can be taken into account when estimating the distal clearance below the tumour.

2 Introduce the EEA gun through the anus and open it. Allow the spike of the gun to pass through the posterior aspect of the stapled rectal stump in the middle and just behind the staple line. Insert a purse-string suture into the end of the descending colon. Manipulate the end of the descending colon over the top of the anvil and tie the purse-string suture as tightly as possible. Connect the anvil and secured descending colon into the cartridge.

3 Have the assistant operating the gun approximate the anvil to the cartridge while you make sure that the gun is pushed firmly upwards and that the descending colon is pulled up tightly over the anvil. Ensure that no appendices epiploicae and no part of the vagina are trapped between the ends of the bowel to be stapled. Rotate the descending colon 90° to the left so that the mesentery lies to the right side. Fire the staple gun to construct the anastomosis. Open the gun to separate the anvil from the cartridge, twist it to make sure the anastomosis is lying free, and then gently rock it and pull it free from the anus.

4 Check the integrity of the stapled anastomosis:
- Examine the 'doughnuts' of colon and rectum removed from the gun. They should be complete. Identify the distal doughnut and send it for histological examination.
- Feel the anastomosis digitally with a finger through the anus.
- Pass a 1-cm sigmoidoscope to examine the anastomosis.
- Place fluid in the pelvis and gently blow air into the colon through the sigmoidoscope. If no bubbles appear and the doughnuts are complete, the anastomosis is satisfactory.

Checklist

1 Make certain that there is no bleeding, particularly in the region of the splenic flexure and spleen.

2 Check that the anastomosis is under no tension and that the descending colon lies in the sacral hollow.

3 Ensure that the descending colon is viable.

4 Following a low anastomosis, do not close the mesentery.

5 Drain the pelvis, preferably using a sump suction drain inserted through a stab wound in the left iliac fossa.

6 Replace and arrange the small bowel and cover it with omentum before closing the abdomen.

HARTMANN'S OPERATION

Appraise

1 This was described by the Berlin anatomist Robert Hartmann (1831–1893).

2 After carrying out an anterior resection of the rectum or rectosigmoid it may be inadvisable to proceed with an anastomosis if:
- The procedure is palliative and the anastomosis would demand the addition of a defunctioning colostomy.
- There is residual carcinoma in the lateral pelvic wall or internal iliac nodes.

Action

1 Close the distal rectum. If the rectum is cut off low down and the end is difficult to suture, leave it open and insert a drain through the anus into the pelvis.

2 Close the peritoneum over the rectal stump if possible. Bring out an end colostomy as described later (following abdominoperineal excision of the rectum).

ABDOMINOPERINEAL EXCISION OF THE RECTUM

Prepare

1 Involve the stoma care team to mark on the skin of the left iliac fossa the site of the colostomy.

2 This operation may be carried out by one surgical team carrying out the abdominal part of the operation and then the perineal part, or by a synchronous combined approach with two teams.

3 Place the patient in the lithotomy Trendelenburg position.

4 Rest the sacrum on a pad to allow the coccyx to overhang the end of the table.

5 Insert a urinary catheter.

6 Suture or strap up the scrotum clear of the perineal operation field.

7 Assess the carcinoma digitally to ascertain that the tumour is technically operable. If the tumour is too low for an anastomosis to be constructed, excision of the anus and rectum is the preferred procedure.

8 Close the anus with a strong purse-string suture.

ABDOMINAL OPERATOR

Access

1 Stand on the patient's right side.

2 Construct a trephine in the left iliac fossa at the previously marked site for the colostomy. Remove a disc of skin 2 cm in diameter together with a minimum of subcutaneous fat. Divide the aponeurosis of rectus abdominis in a cruciate manner. Separate the underlying muscle fibres rather than cut across them. Leave the cruciate incision in the peritoneum until you have opened the abdomen.

3 Open the abdomen through a lower midline incision extending above the umbilicus.

Assess

1 Palpate the liver for metastases.

2 Examine the whole of the colon and then the small intestine.

3 Examine the mesentery and para-aortic region for enlarged lymph nodes.

4 Examine the peritoneal cavity, particularly in the rectovesical pouch, for peritoneal metastases.

5 Finally, palpate the tumour which is retroperitoneal.

Action (Fig. 16.10)

1 Cover the wound edges with damp packs and suture the lower cut edge of the peritoneum to the skin.

2 Place the small bowel to the right side of the incision so that it is lying outside the wound if possible, and cover it with a pack.

3 Divide the lateral adhesions from the sigmoid colon and along the lateral aspect of the descending colon.

4 Lift the colon upwards and to the right and identify the left ureter and gonadal vessels and sweep them away from the vascular pedicle.

5 Enter the mesorectal plane and preserve the pelvic nerve plexus in the same manner as for anterior resection of the rectum. Divide the inferior mesorectal artery at its origin from the aorta, and the inferior mesenteric vein at the same level, or a little higher.

6 Select a suitable site in the sigmoid colon for transection of the bowel. Pull the colon down until it easily reaches the symphysis pubis and this will be found to leave approximately the correct length of colon for construction of the colostomy. Cut the mesocolon, ligating and dividing the marginal vessels to this point. Divide the colon using a Parker–Kerr clamp on the rectal side and non-crushing clamp on the colonic side, or alternatively divide the colon with a linear cutting stapler. This maintains sterility and the staple line can be excised from the colonic end when the wound is closed and the colostomy is about to be constructed.

7 Move to the patient's left side and continue the mesorectal dissection posteriorly, laterally and anteriorly as for anterior resection of the rectum. Continue the dissection as far as possible down to the pelvic floor but at least to the tip of the coccyx posteriorly.

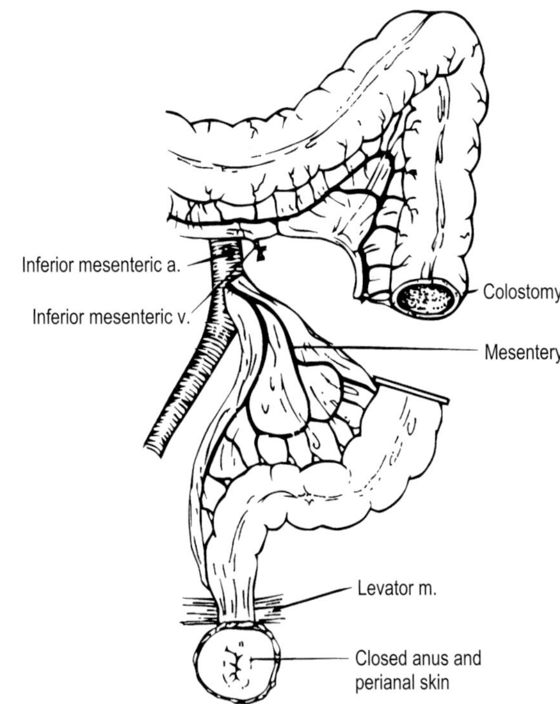

Fig. 16.10 Abdominoperineal excision of the rectum. The excised specimen consists of the rectum, anus, perianal skin and sigmoid colon and mesocolon. The inferior mesenteric artery is divided at its origin from the aorta and the inferior mesenteric vein is divided at a similar level.

> **KEY POINTS Anatomy**
>
> - Take care as you approach the tumour low down, to stay outside the mesorectum.
> - If you stray into the mesorectum you risk spilling cancer cells.
> - Identify and preserve the presacral sympathetic nerves.

8 At this stage the abdominal and perineal operators meet behind the mesorectum. Define the course of both ureters in the pelvis and carefully preserve them.

9 When the perineal dissection is completed have the excised colon and rectum withdrawn through the perineum.

10 Irrigate the pelvic cavity with 500 ml of povidone–iodine solution.

11 Pass the end of the colon through the colostomy trephine hole.

12 Before you close the pelvic peritoneal floor, both you and the pelvic operator must be certain that you have achieved complete haemostasis.

13 Gently mobilize the peritoneum from the lateral walls of the pelvis and the iliac fossae with your fingers and suture the edges together over the empty pelvis with a continuous polyglactin 910 suture.

14 Close the abdominal wound.

15 Trim the staple line from the colostomy to leave 1 cm projecting above the skin. Suture the edge of the colon to the edge of the skin wound with a polyglactin 910 suture on a cutting needle.

PERINEAL OPERATOR

Start the perineal operation when the abdominal operator has opened the abdomen, carried out a full laparotomy, and ligated and divided the inferior mesenteric artery and vein.

In the male (Fig. 16.11a)

1 Make an elliptical incision around the closed anal canal from a point midway between the anus and the bulb of the urethra anteriorly, extending backwards to the sacrococcygeal articulation. Deepen the incision to expose the lobulated fat of the ischiorectal fossae and the coccyx. Pick up the skin edges and the anal skin with tissue forceps.

2 In a male with a small pelvis and a large posterior tumour low in the rectum, remove the coccyx. Flex the coccyx to open a coccygeal joint and divide across it with a scalpel to separate the distal portion of the coccyx. Coagulate the middle sacral vessels.

3 Make small incisions on either side of the coccyx through the fibrous attachment at the coccygeal raphe and with a finger separate the levator muscles from the underlying rectal fascia described in 1899 by Heinrich Waldeyer-Hartz (1836–1921), pathological anatomist in Breslau and Berlin.

4 Divide the levator muscles well out on the lateral wall of the pelvis and ligate or coagulate the inferior haemorrhoidal vessels.

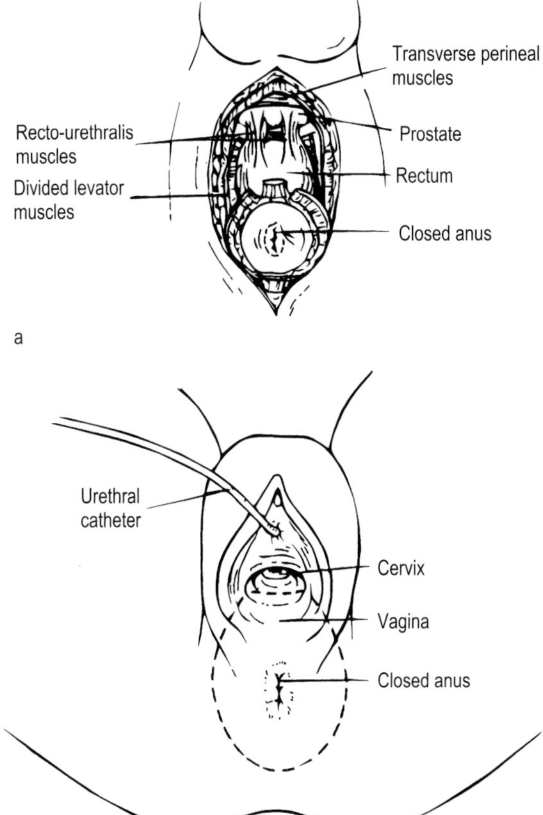

Fig. 16.11 Perineal approach to abdominoperineal excision of the rectum: (a) the male pelvis; (b) the female pelvis. The broken lines indicate the extent of the excision. In the female the posterior vaginal wall is removed up to the posterior fornix. In the male the initial plane is posterior to the transverse perineal muscles.

5 Insert a St Mark's pattern self-retaining perineal retractor. Clearly identify Waldeyer's fascia and cut it across, just in front of the divided coccyx. Extend the incision laterally to expose the mesorectum.

6 Separate the mesorectum from the anterior aspect of the presacral fascia and join up with the abdominal operator.

7 Retract the rectum posteriorly and make a transverse incision anteriorly, to expose the superficial and the deep transverse perineal muscles.

> **KEY POINT Anatomy**
>
> - Keep the plane of dissection behind the transverse perineal muscles to avoid injuring the urethra.

8 Divide the broad, strap-like pubococcygeus muscle on either side of the rectum. Then divide the underlying fascia, which is the lateral continuation of the fascia of Denonvilliers and Waldeyer, to expose the rectal wall. Palpate the prostate gland anteriorly and define the plane between the rectum and prostate.

9 Insert an artery forceps anteriorly between the rectum and the prostate to separate the recto-urethralis muscle fibres. Divide these fibres to expose the prostatic capsule. Cut the visceral pelvic fascia, which is condensed anteriorly to the lateral aspect of the prostate, to expose the whole of the prostate and the seminal vesicles above. Anteriorly, your dissection now meets that of the abdominal operator.

10 Divide the lower parts of the lateral ligaments and then draw the rectum and sigmoid colon through the perineal incision.

11 Flatten the operating table and secure pelvic haemostasis.

12 If haemostasis is perfect and there is no significant sepsis, place a suction drain into the pelvis through a lateral stab wound on the anterior abdominal wall and secure it to the skin. Do not drain the pelvis through the buttocks.

13 Close the incision with subcutaneous and skin sutures of 3/0 interrupted polyglactin 910. If the wound is unsuitable for primary closure leave the centre open to take three fingers and insert a corrugated drain into the pelvis.

In the female (Fig. 16.11b)

1 Unless the tumour is small and situated in the midline posteriorly, always remove the posterior vaginal wall. Make an incision from the posterior lateral aspects of the labia around the anus to the coccyx.

2 The posterior part of the dissection is as in the male until you reach the anterior part of the dissection. Carry the anterior incision upwards through the lateral aspect of the vagina as far as the posterior fornix. Make a transverse incision to join the two lateral incisions and deepen it to expose the rectal wall and so to meet the abdominal operator.

3 Make no attempt to reconstruct the vagina. Obtain haemostasis by oversewing the cut edge of the vagina with a continuous 2/0 synthetic absorbable suture.

4 Close the subcutaneous tissue and skin with interrupted mattress sutures of polyglactin 910.

5 Drain the pelvis by placing a corrugated or sump suction drain through the re-formed vaginal orifice.

? DIFFICULTY

1. In the male or female, it may be impossible to close the peritoneal floor to prevent small-bowel herniation to the skin incision or out through the vagina. In these circumstances, place a plastic (Aldon) bag into the pelvis from below. Fill it with gauze roll to pack the bag and keep the small intestine in the abdominal cavity. Loosely close the skin of the perineal wound to keep the bag in place. Remove the gauze and bag after 3–5 days.
2. If pelvic haemorrhage cannot be controlled, pack the pelvis with gauze directly. Leave the packs for 72 hours and gently remove them under an anaesthetic so that you can inspect the pelvis.

TRANSVERSE COLOSTOMY

Appraise

▶ KEY POINT Carefully assess the options

- Transverse colostomy is a particularly unpleasant stoma so try to avoid it if at all possible.

1 Carry out a transverse colostomy in the rare cases of distal obstruction in patients unfit to have an urgent resection carried out, or if you are too inexperienced to do this. It can be performed under a local anaesthetic in a severely ill patient.

2 Site the stoma in the right upper quadrant of the abdomen, midway between the umbilicus and the costal margin.

3 Place the colostomy as far to the right in the transverse colon as possible to minimize the risk of prolapse. The next stage of the operation may require you to take down the splenic flexure and mobilize the distal transverse colon.

Access

1 Make a transverse incision 5 cm long centred on the upper right rectus muscle between the umbilicus and the costal margin so that an appliance can be fitted without encroaching upon either. Divide the anterior and posterior rectus sheath, and split the rectus muscle. Through this locate the transverse colon, which you can recognize by the presence of omentum, and the lack of appendices epiploicae.

2 The abdomen may be already open when you make a decision to perform a colostomy. When a midline or left paramedian incision has been used, make a transverse incision as described above but only 6–7 cm long. If a right upper paramedian incision was used, bring the colostomy through the upper end of the incision, provided it is clear of the costal margin.

Assess

1 If the operation is undertaken through a laparotomy to relieve a distal obstruction, examine the relevant structures and feel the obstructing mass in the distal colon. It may be impossible to determine if this is due to carcinoma or diverticular disease.

2 Palpate the liver for metastases.

3 Palpate the rest of the colon and the peritoneal cavity to determine if there are other metastases.

Action (Fig. 16.12a)

1 Draw the right side of the transverse colon and omentum out of the wound. Manipulate it so that a loop of proximal transverse colon lies in the wound without tension.

2 Separate the omentum from the colon and turn it upwards to expose the mesentery.

3 Pull the loop upwards through the incision and make a hole through the mesentery close to the bowel wall at the apex of the

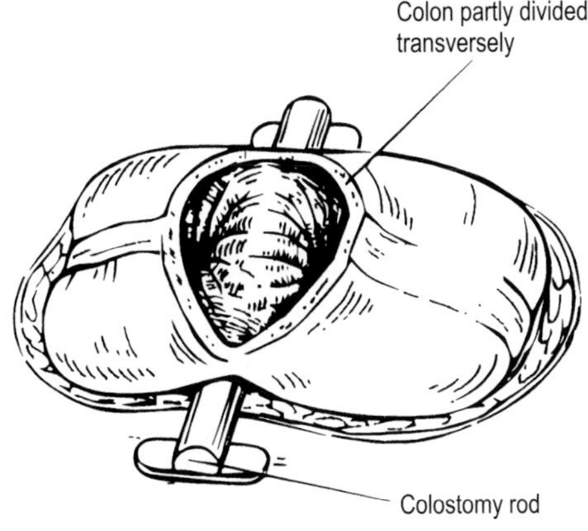

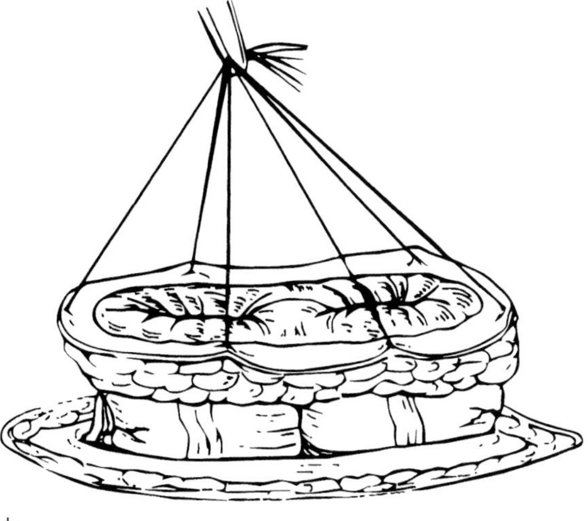

Fig. 16.12 (a) Transverse colostomy: bring a loop of colon through the wound and keep it in place with a colostomy device or simple glass rod. Open the colostomy by a transverse incision. (b) Closure of colostomy: insert stay sutures to help mobilization.

loop with a pair of long artery forceps, taking care not to damage the blood supply.

4 Pass a piece of narrow rubber tubing or a catheter under the mesentery. Pull the loop right out through the incision with the rubber tubing, making certain that the loop is not twisted and that the proximal opening is to the right and the distal opening to the left.

5 Pass a plastic colostomy device through the mesentery to form a bridge for the colostomy. Open the end of the colostomy device to keep it in place.

6 Do not insert any internal sutures.

7 If the colostomy is made to relieve obstruction, open it immediately by cutting across the apex of the bowel through half the circumference.

8 Turn back the edges of the opened colon and suture the whole thickness of the colon to the edge of the skin incision with interrupted 2/0 Vicryl sutures mounted on a cutting needle.

9 Insert a finger into each loop of the colostomy to make sure it is not too narrow and that the finger passes straight into the underlying colon.

10 Fix a suitable disposable appliance over the loop colostomy rod.

Aftercare

1 A transverse colostomy is a temporary defunctioning stoma made with a view to closure. Closure should be as easy as possible and not require excision of the colon and re-anastomosis.

2 Remove the colostomy device forming the bridge in about 7 days, depending on the obesity of the patient and the difficulty in bringing up the loop of colon.

Closure

1 Do not close the colostomy until at least 6 weeks after it has been formed. This allows the oedema to settle down and makes the operation safer and easier.

2 Before closure ensure that any distal anastomosis is satisfactory following the definitive operation, as shown on sigmoidoscopy and/or Gastrografin enema X-ray. Prepare the proximal bowel as for colonic resection and anastomosis.

3 Make an incision in the skin close to the mucocutaneous junction.

4 Insert six 2/0 silk stay sutures into the mucocutaneous junction, each held in an artery forceps so that traction may be applied while dissecting (Fig. 16.12b).

5 Deepen the incision to reveal the colon and the external rectus sheath. Dissect the colonic loops from the abdominal wall until the whole of the loop is freed and can easily be drawn out from the abdominal cavity.

6 Excise the mucocutaneous junction.

7 Close the colostomy transversely using a single layer of seromuscular sutures.

8 Replace the re-sutured colostomy in the peritoneal cavity, place the omentum over it and manipulate it so that it lies away from the abdominal incision.

9 Close the abdominal wound in one layer with a continuous or interrupted nylon suture. If the patient is obese, drain the subcutaneous space with a slip of corrugated latex sheet brought out through the end of the wound, or through a separate stab wound. Close the skin.

SIGMOID END COLOSTOMY

Appraise

1 Use this when you require to fashion a permanent colostomy because of sphincter damage, in some cases of constipation, prolapse and solitary ulcer when no other definitive operation is possible. If no previous surgery has been undertaken, you do not need to perform a laparotomy.

2 Consider performing the operation using the laparoscope.

Action (Fig. 16.13)

1 Place the patient in the lithotomy Trendelenburg (Lloyd-Davies) position.

2 Make a trephine hole in the left iliac fossa at the site marked for the colostomy.

3 Find the sigmoid colon and make sure the mesentery is not twisted. Identify it by the lack of omentum and the presence of appendices epiploicae.

4 Locate the lateral peritoneal attachments (white line). This allows you to identify the correct orientation of the colon and to ensure that the proximal end is delivered as the stoma. Place a sigmoidoscope or Foley catheter with bellows attached into the rectum and inflate it with air. Once the stoma has been secured, ensure that an examining finger is directed up and to the left.

5 Divide the loop of sigmoid across, together with 5–6 cm of mesentery. Close the distal end with polyglactin 910 or polypropylene sutures and push it back into the peritoneal cavity. Fashion a colostomy from the divided proximal colon by suturing the colon to the skin edge with interrupted 2/0 Vicryl sutures.

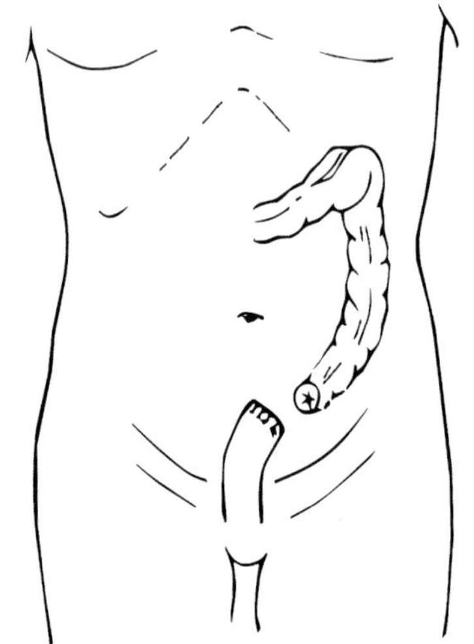

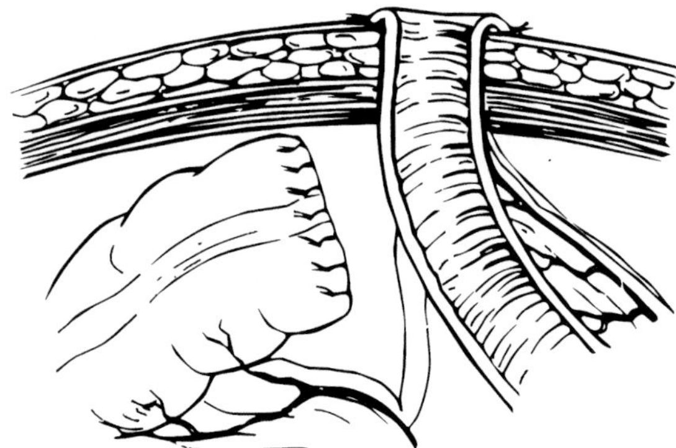

Fig. 16.13 Trephine end sigmoid colostomy.

6 Alternatively, divide the bowel with a linear cutting stapler. Trim the proximal end to secure the colostomy as above.

7 The stoma can be constructed laparoscopically. This allows excellent vision and ensures that the correct end of the bowel is delivered as a stoma.

KEY POINTS Anatomy

- It is possible, and may be disastrous, to bring out the wrong end of the bowel.
- If in doubt create a loop sigmoid colostomy.
- Laparoscopy-assisted colostomy allows you to confirm which is the correct end.
- Have air insufflated via the rectum; the distal limb should distend.
- Perform a flexible sigmoidoscopy on table.
- Formal laparotomy also allows you to select the correct end to form the colostomy.

COLECTOMY FOR INFLAMMATORY BOWEL DISEASE

Appraise

1 Acute fulminating colitis, with or without toxic megacolon, usually occurs in idiopathic ulcerative colitis but may occur in Crohn's colitis.

2 The operation of choice is colectomy and ileostomy. Emergency proctocolectomy carries a higher mortality and morbidity, and there is no opportunity to carry out a secondary ileorectal anastomosis.

3 Manage these patients jointly with a senior gastroenterologist.

4 Surgical treatment is usually indicated if:
- The patient's condition does not improve within 72 hours.
- The patient does not improve in 24 hours and still has more than six bowel actions containing blood each day.
- There is a fever of more than 38 °C and a tachycardia over 100 beats/min.

5 Carry out daily plain X-ray of the abdomen to see if toxic dilatation develops.

6 If there is toxic dilatation or evidence of perforation, carry out an emergency operation.

7 Beware of being lulled into a false sense of security, as the patient's condition is more critical than may be apparent.

Prepare

1 Continue steroid therapy with 100 mg of hydrocortisone 6-hourly. Commence full antibiotic cover with gentamicin or a cephalosporin and metronidazole.

2 Mark the site of ileostomy if the patient is fit enough.

3 Place the patient in the Lloyd-Davies position. If there is any degree of toxic dilatation, gently insert a sigmoidoscope and suck gas from the rectum and colon.

4 Catheterize the patient.

Access

1 Make an ileostomy trephine 2 cm in diameter at the previously marked site. If the patient is very sick and this has not been done, make it in the right iliac fossa over the infra-umbilical fat pad. Employ the trephine in the same way as in the construction of a colostomy (see above).

2 Open the abdomen through a long midline incision.

Assess

1 The colon is hyperaemic, thickened and oedematous. Do not handle it excessively and do not pull away adherent omentum or lateral pelvic wall adhesions as these may be the site of sealed perforations.

2 Note any free gas, denoting that perforation has occurred. If there is a perforation, try and close it with a purse-string suture then place omentum over it before proceeding. Note any free fluid and obtain a swab for culture and antibiotic sensitivity.

3 Examine the liver to note the presence of cirrhosis, and the small bowel to see if the diagnosis could be Crohn's disease. Examine the mesentery for enlarged lymph nodes.

Action (Fig. 16.14)

1 Ensure that there is good access. Gently dissect the omentum from the lateral walls starting at the caecum and mobilize the colon completely down to the rectum, taking care to avoid too much traction. In a severe case, remove the omentum with the colon as any attempt to dissect it away may lead to a perforation. If the colon is fixed to the lateral abdominal wall, remove a disc of peritoneum with the colon rather than risk opening a sealed perforation.

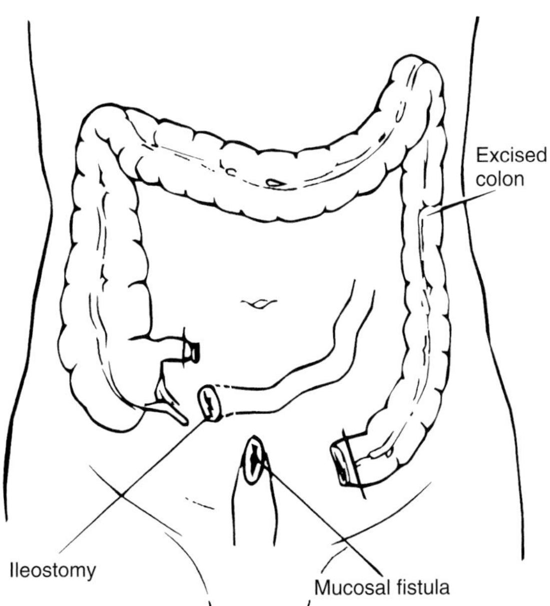

Fig. 16.14 Colectomy for acute colitis. The colon is resected to the mid-sigmoid colon, which is brought out as a mucous fistula through the lower part of the midline incision. An end ileostomy is constructed in the right iliac fossa.

2 Transilluminate the mesentery and divide the vessels at a suitable place in the centre of the mesentery.

3 Mobilize the terminal ileum and transect it using a linear cutting stapler 1–2 cm proximal to the ileocaecal valve.

4 Divide the sigmoid colon between Parker–Kerr clamps so that the distal bowel can be brought out as a mucous fistula, without tension. Do not divide the colon close to the sacral promontory in the mistaken belief that all the colon must be resected.

5 Bring the ileum through the ileostomy trephine hole and trim the staple line prior to suturing it with polyglactin 910, and close the lateral space with a continuous purse-string suture (see earlier). It is not necessary to suture the mesentery to the abdominal wall.

6 Secure haemostasis and close the abdomen with the sigmoid colon brought out through the lower end of the wound.

7 Construct the ileostomy (see above).

8 Bring the mucous fistula into the lower aspect of the abdominal wound and suture it to the skin with polyglactin 910. Alternatively, close the colon with sutures or staples and leave it under the closed skin incision.

Technical

If you are carrying out elective colectomy and ileostomy, you can oversew the sigmoid colon and replace it in the peritoneal cavity.

KEY POINTS Anticipate

- In any operation for inflammatory bowel disease or familial adenomatous polyposis, never carry out a proctocolectomy without considering whether a sphincter-saving operation would eventually be more appropriate.
- If there is any doubt in your mind, leave the rectum intact.

ELECTIVE COLECTOMY AND ILEORECTAL ANASTOMOSIS

Appraise

1 Elective colectomy and ileorectal anastomosis may be indicated for ulcerative colitis, Crohn's disease or familial adenomatous polyposis.

2 In ulcerative colitis there must be no carcinoma or severe dysplasia associated with colitis. The rectum must be distensible to act as a reservoir and the anal sphincter function normal.

3 In Crohn's disease the rectum must be relatively free of disease and the sphincter function normal with no evidence of severe perianal disease such as fistulas.

4 In familial adenomatous polyposis there must be no carcinoma in the rectum. If the rectum contains confluent polyps, it is not suitable for an ileorectal anastomosis; prefer proctocolectomy, possibly with an ileoanal reservoir.

5 Never assume a patient with multiple polyps has familial adenomatous polyposis until several have been biopsied and proved to be adenomas. 20% of patients have no family history: the condition has arisen as a new genetic mutation.

Access

1 Place the patient in the lithotomy Trendelenburg position with the legs supported on Lloyd-Davies stirrups. Insert a Foley catheter into the bladder for continuous drainage.

2 Open the abdomen through a long midline incision.

Assess

1 Palpate and visualize the liver.

2 Examine the whole of the gastrointestinal tract, the stomach, the duodenum, the whole of the small bowel and the colon.

3 In a patient with familial adenomatous polyposis examine the duodenum carefully for possible adenomas. If you feel any abnormality make certain the patient has upper gastrointestinal endoscopy carried out. Examine the colon and rectum carefully to make sure there is no carcinoma. If it is, carry out a radical operation as for carcinoma. An ileorectal anastomosis is still possible provided the carcinoma is not in the rectum. In Crohn's disease examine particularly the small bowel. Measure its length and look for skip lesions.

Action

1 Mobilize the colon completely as previously described, starting at the caecum. Work around to the rectosigmoid junction. Preserve the omentum by separating the congenital adhesions from the transverse colon.

2 Divide the mesenteric vessels at a suitable place in the mid-part of the mesocolon. Preserve the superior rectal artery and vein and avoid damaging the presacral nerves. In ulcerative colitis or Crohn's disease, ligate the superior rectal artery in continuity to decrease the vascularity of the rectum. This is claimed to decrease the chances of exacerbation of inflammation in the rectum.

3 Place a Lloyd-Davies right-angled clamp across the rectosigmoid junction and irrigate the rectum through the anus with 1:2000 aqueous chlorhexidine solution.

4 Divide the terminal ileum. Place a Parker–Kerr clamp at right-angles across the terminal ileum close to the ileocaecal valve. Wrap a gauze swab soaked in 1:2000 aqueous chlorhexidine around the ileum at the site of division and hold it between the forefinger and thumb of the left hand. After protecting the abdominal contents with packs, divide the ileum close to the proximal side of the clamp.

5 Pick up the divided ileum with Babcock's forceps, which also grasps the surrounding swab, holding it in place. Swab out the lumen with chlorhexidine solution.

6 Divide the rectum below the Lloyd-Davies clamp with scissors and remove the specimen. Hold up the rectum with Babcock's forceps.

7 The ileal lumen is usually narrower than that of the rectum. Widen the ileum with a longitudinal cut along the antimesenteric border; this matches the ileum and colon for size ready for anastomosis.

8 Construct an anastomosis with a single layer of interrupted seromuscular sutures. Alternatively, staple the rectum with a transverse stapler and construct the anastomosis with an EEA stapler. Do not force the stapling gun to get it high in the rectum or it may tear and perforate it.

9 Arrange the terminal ileum so that the terminal loop lies in the left iliac fossa. This prevents acute kinking of the anastomosis. Arrange the remaining loops of bowel anatomically and cover them with the omentum. Do not drain the anastomosis.

10 Close the abdomen.

Technical

If the colectomy and ileorectal anastomosis is carried out for polyposis, excise or destroy with diathermy any polyps that are going to impinge on the anastomosis, through the cut end of the rectum, before constructing the anastomosis.

ELECTIVE TOTAL PROCTOCOLECTOMY

Appraise

1 Either excise the rectum conservatively using a close rectal dissection to conserve the pelvic floor and protect the pelvic autonomic nerves, or ensure that similar care is taken as for 'mesorectal excision' of the rectum for cancer to ensure these structures are preserved.

2 Excise the rectum as part of the proctocolectomy, or following previous colectomy and ileostomy, with a mucous fistula.

3 Mark the ileostomy preoperatively. Place it in the right iliac fossa in the infra-umbilical fat pad through right rectus muscle.

Access

1 Place the patient in the lithotomy Trendelenburg position.

2 Catheterize the bladder for continuous drainage.

3 Open the abdomen through a long midline incision.

Action (Fig. 16.15)

1 Carry out the colectomy and ileostomy as previously described. If the patient has previously had a colectomy and a mucous fistula, mobilize the mucous fistula when the wound is re-opened and oversew the sigmoid colon.

2 Mobilize the rectum with peritoneal incisions on both sides of the rectum close to the rectal wall joined anteriorly just above the lowest part of the peritoneal floor. Preserve the superior rectal artery together with the presacral fat and nerves. Clamp, divide and ligate the individual sigmoid and rectal arteries close to the rectal wall with fine ligatures. Alternatively, excise the

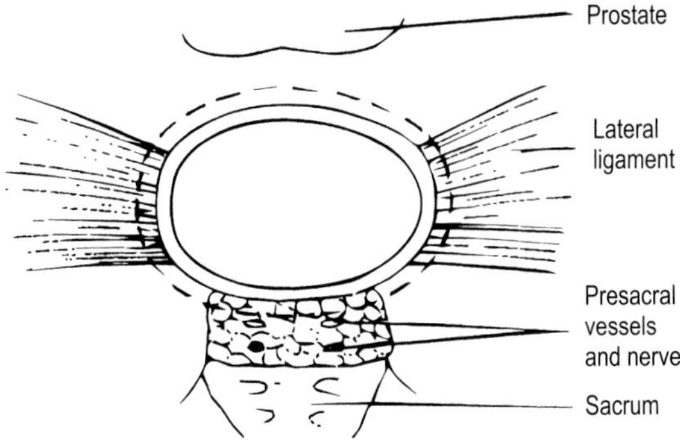

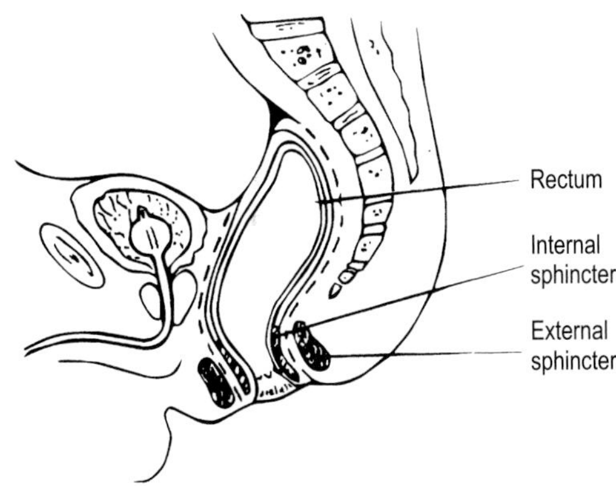

Fig. 16.15 Proctocolectomy for inflammatory bowel disease. The rectal excision is not the same as for malignant disease. The abdominal operator, standing on the left of the patient, preserves the superior rectal vessels, presacral fat and nerves. The perineal excision below is in the plane between the internal and external sphincters.

mesorectum as for anterior resection of the rectum for cancer but do not breach the presacral fascia or damage the presacral nerves.

3 Dissect posteriorly as far as the coccyx to meet the upward dissection of the perineal operator.

4 Dissect anteriorly between the rectum and the vagina in the female. In the male, hold up the seminal vesicles with a St Mark's lip retractor. Divide the fascia of Denonvilliers transversely and dissect downwards between the rectum and the prostate gland.

5 Approach the lateral dissection as for anterior resection, dividing this tissue using diathermy and sharp dissection. It is not necessary to formally clip and divide the so-called lateral ligaments.

6 If the operation is being carried out as a synchronous combined procedure, the perineal operator will have completed the rectal excision and the specimen can be removed through the perineal wound.

7 Close the pelvic peritoneum with continuous synthetic absorbable sutures.

Perineal operation

1 Place a strong purse-string suture around the anus close to the anal margin, since a minimum of skin will be removed.

2 Make a circumferential incision over the intersphincteric groove and deepen it to expose the intersphincteric plane between the pale fibres of the internal sphincter and the dark red fibres of the voluntary muscle of the external sphincter. The lone-star retractor is extremely useful for this dissection.

3 Divide the longitudinal fibres crossing the internal sphincter to fix the mucosa at the dentate line. Separate the internal sphincter from the puborectalis and levator muscles, easily establishing a plane into the pelvis. Carry out a similar dissection on the other side of the anus and then dissect the posterior part of the external sphincter to the puborectalis muscle.

4 Deepen the anterior part of the dissection behind the superficial and deep transverse perineal muscles and then continue the dissection upwards in the female between the vagina and the rectal wall. The wound is small and a self-retaining retractor cannot be inserted. Improve the exposure using a Langenbeck retractor, or a pelvic lateral wall retractor of the Lockhart–Mummery type. In the male, the external sphincter decussates in the midline and becomes attached to the fibres of the rectourethralis muscle. Cut the strap-like parts of the rectourethralis muscle to expose the posterior aspect of the prostate gland. Divide the visceral pelvic fascia laterally on each side where it is condensed on to the lateral lobes of the prostate. The seminal vesicles are then apparent in the upper part of the wound.

5 Divide Waldeyer's fascia posteriorly and meet the abdominal surgeon. Divide the lower parts of the lateral ligament and then remove the specimen through the perineal wound. This excision leaves a small wound with the external sphincter and the whole of the levator muscles intact.

Closure

1 Drain the pelvis with a suction drain inserted through a lateral stab wound on the anterior abdominal wall. Do not drain the pelvis through the buttocks.

2 Approximate the puborectalis and levator muscles with polyglactin 910 sutures. Approximate the subcutaneous fat and close the skin with interrupted mattress sutures, also of polyglactin 910.

3 Start continuous suction drainage immediately.

Technical

In patients with ulcerative colitis or familial adenomatous polyposis who wish to avoid a permanent conventional ileostomy but are not suitable for an ileorectal anastomosis, two alternative procedures can be carried out.

Restorative proctocolectomy

1 The rectum is divided across at the level of the puborectalis and the internal and external sphincter muscles are preserved.

2 A pelvic reservoir can then be constructed and anastomosed to the anal canal. The configuration of this reservoir can be of the 'S', 'J', 'W' or 'K' type and the function depends on its capacity and compliance rather than its shape. The reservoir can be constructed with sutures or staples but the ileoanal anastomosis is now commonly stapled to the anal canal 1–2 cm above the dentate line.

3 These procedures are normally covered by a defunctioning ileostomy (Fig. 16.16).

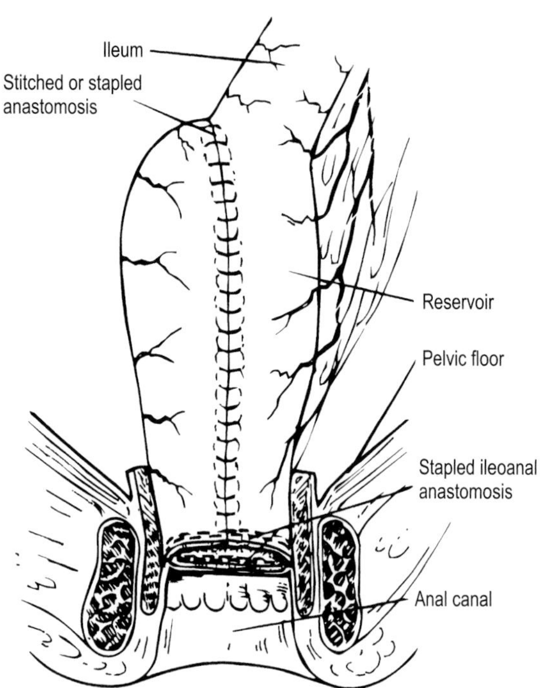

Fig. 16.16 Ileoanal reservoir. Depicted is a 'J' configuration reservoir, stapled to the anal canal 1–2 cm above the dentate line.

Kock reservoir ileostomy

1 This consists of a reservoir constructed from 45 cm of terminal ileum with an intussuscepted nipple valve in the efferent ileum. The reservoir is continent and emptied by catheterization, so no external appliance is necessary.

2 This procedure still has a place when the patient wishes to avoid a conventional Brooke ileostomy but is not suitable for an ileoanal reservoir as the sphincters have previously been removed or damaged.

DUHAMEL OPERATION

Appraise

1 Described by the Parisian surgeon Bernard Duhamel in 1956, this is the most satisfactory procedure for treating adult Hirschsprung's disease, described in 1888 by the Copenhagen paediatrician. A variety of operations are carried out for this condition in children but will not be considered here (see Ch. 40).

2 Confirm the diagnosis of Hirschsprung's disease by anorectal manometry to show the absence of the rectosphincteric reflex. Remove a full-thickness biopsy to show the absence of ganglia and abnormal autonomic nerve plexuses within the bowel wall.

3 Adults with Hirschsprung's disease do not always have short-segment disease.

Prepare

1 It is unnecessary to carry out a preliminary colostomy in these patients.

2 Place the patient in the lithotomy Trendelenburg position.

3 Insert an indwelling catheter.

4 Open the abdomen through a long midline incision.

Assess

1 After carrying out a general laparotomy examine the colon carefully. The narrow segment may be quite short.

2 The bowel proximal to the narrow segment is dilated and thickened and then gradually becomes of normal diameter.

3 Plan to excise the thickened dilated bowel.

Action (Fig. 16.17)

Abdominal operation

1 Mobilize the colon. The splenic flexure will probably need to be taken down so mobilize it initially as previously described.

2 Mobilize the rectum to its upper third.

3 Place a right-angled clamp across the middle third of the rectum at the site of division to leave a rectal stump of approximately

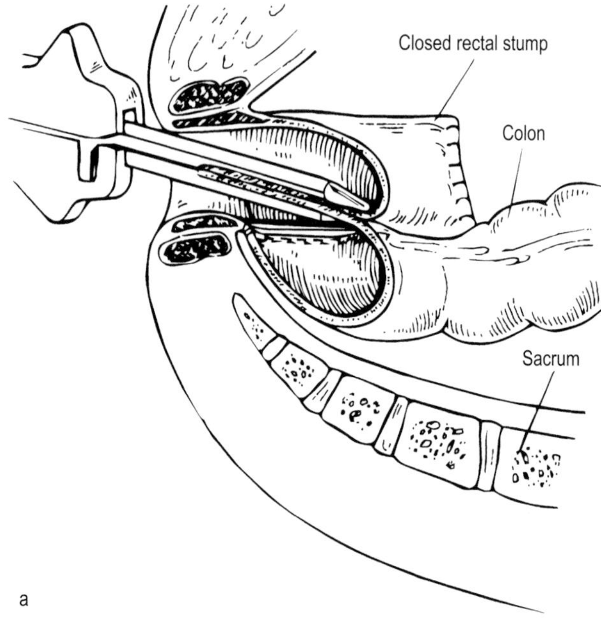

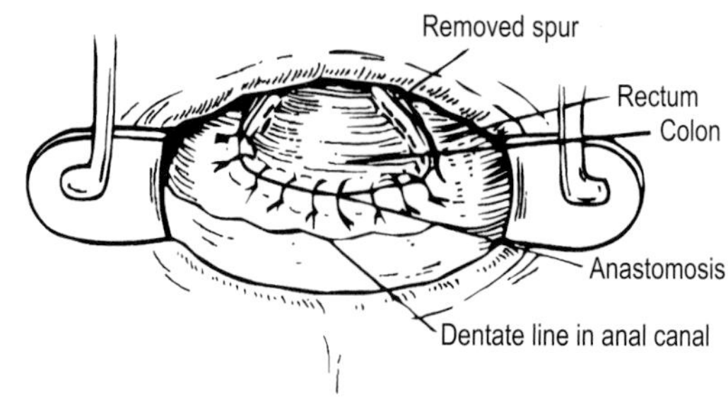

Fig. 16.17 Duhamel operation. (a) The retained rectum with the colon anastomosed to the posterior wall at the level of the puborectalis. (b) The septum between the rectum and colon is removed with two GIA staplers.

10 cm. Have the rectum below the clamp carefully washed out through the anus with 1:2000 aqueous chlorhexidine solution.

4 Dissect behind the rectum down to the tip of the coccyx.

5 Transect the rectum below the clamp and close the divided rectum with polyglactin 910 sutures in two layers. The rectum is usually too thickened to allow closure by stapling.

6 Divide the colon at an appropriate place above the dilated hypertrophied segment in the descending or sigmoid colon.

7 Remove the specimen. Arrange for frozen sections to be carried out on the upper end of the specimen to make sure ganglia are present. Swab out the colon with 1:2000 aqueous chlorhexidine solution.

Per-anal operation

1 Insert a self-retaining anal retractor and make a transverse incision through the posterior half of the rectal wall at the level of the puborectalis muscle.

2 Deepen the wound until you enter the space that has been dissected behind the rectum.

3 Bring down the mobilized colon to the upper anal canal with stay sutures.

4 Suture the lower edge of the anal incision to the posterior edge of the colon with interrupted sutures of polyglactin 910. Similarly, suture the anterior wall of the rectum to the upper end of the anal incision.

5 Resect the spur between the rectum and colon by placing two linear cutting staple lines from the lateral aspects of the anastomosis to meet at the top of the rectal stump. The intervening piece of the rectal and colonic wall will be removed. It is usually necessary to suture the top end of the rectum and colon between the lines of staples.

6 Drain the pelvis and close the abdominal wound.

SOAVE OPERATION

Appraise

1 This operation was devised by the Italian surgeon F. Soave in 1964, initially for the treatment of Hirschsprung's disease, but is rarely used for this in adults. It is a useful procedure in patients undergoing revision of a failed pelvic anastomosis.

2 A modified Soave operation is very useful for the treatment of large villous tumours, irradiation proctitis, rectovaginal and rectoprostatic fistulas and haemangiomas of the rectum.

Access

1 Place the patient in the lithotomy Trendelenburg position. Drain the bladder with an indwelling catheter.

2 Open the abdomen through a long midline incision.

3 Assess the nature and extent of the pelvic disease. Carry out a general exploration of the abdomen.

Action (Fig. 16.18)

1 Mobilize the sigmoid, descending colon and splenic flexure. Transect the rectum to leave 10 cm.

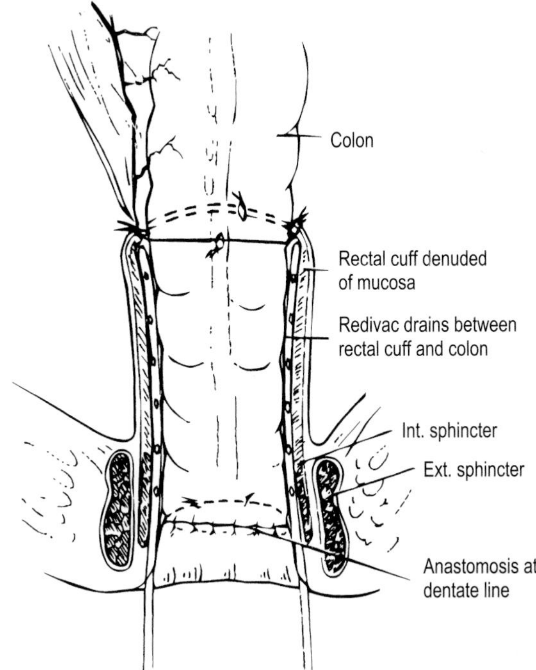

Fig. 16.18 Soave operation. The mobilized left colon is drawn through the retained rectum which has been denuded of mucosa, and sutured to the dentate line. Fine suction drainage tubes are inserted through the perianal skin to drain the potential space between the rectum and colon.

2 Resect any diseased bowel above this.

3 Working from above and through the anus with a self-retaining retractor, inject a solution of 1:300 000 adrenaline (epinephrine) in saline under the mucosa to lift it clear of the underlying circular muscle.

4 Remove the mucosa from the whole of the rectum down to the dentate line.

5 Bring down normal colon through this muscular tube and suture it with polyglactin 910 sutures to the dentate line, making certain that the anal sutures include part of the internal sphincter muscle. Three or four sutures approximate the upper end of the rectal cuff of the descending colon.

6 Close the abdomen without drainage.

7 Place Redivac drains close to the anus, led up through the intersphincteric plane to drain the space between the colon and the rectal cuff.

FURTHER READING

Dudley HAF 1983 Operative surgery: alimentary tract and abdominal wall, 4th edn. Butterworths, London

Goligher JC 1984 Surgery of the anus, rectum and colon, 5th edn. Baillière Tindall, London

Keighley MRB, Williams NS 1999 Surgery of the anus, rectum and colon, 2nd edn. Saunders, London

Nicholls RJ, Dozois RR 1997 Surgery of the colon and rectum. Churchill Livingstone, Edinburgh

Phillips RKS 1998 Colorectal surgery: a companion to specialist surgical practice. Saunders, London

Schwartz SI, Ellis H 1985 Maingot's abdominal operations, Vol 2, 8th edn. Butterworths, London

17

Laparoscopic colorectal surgery

A. Darzi, T. Rockall, P.A. Paraskeva

CONTENTS

PREOPERATIVE CONSIDERATIONS

Appraise

1 Advocates cite numerous potential advantages: less pain, faster patient recovery with less postoperative disability, shorter hospitalization, earlier return to work, better quality of life, with better cosmetic results. Technical capability is comparable to that of the open technique.

2 Laparoscopic colectomy is technically demanding and may be difficult. Learning the technique is challenging and may be prolonged. Analysis of total operative time as an indication of learning shows that it requires approximately 10–15 completed laparoscopic-assisted colectomies to achieve competence.

3 It has not yet been demonstrated how laparoscopic colectomy compares with open operation in terms of recurrence and survival.

4 Because the internal organs cannot be palpated during laparoscopy, preoperative colonoscopy is necessary to inspect the bowel mucosa and computed tomography (CT) scans to evaluate the liver and other structures such as enlarged lymph nodes.

5 Potential advantages are claimed for sigmoid resection, abdominoperineal resection, Hartmann's procedure, and assisted right hemicolectomy. Restorative proctocolectomy and completely intracorporeal right hemicolectomy require advanced technical skill.

6 Conditions amenable to a laparoscopic approach (Table 17.1) include:

- *Carcinoma*. Technological innovations facilitate the resection of colorectal malignant conditions but the propriety of performing such operations is questionable except in the context of randomized controlled trials.
- *Benign neoplasms* such as adenomas or lipomas can be removed, through either a colotomy or resection.
- *Diverticular disease*. Some but not all patients with diverticulitis are suitable for laparoscopic colectomy. Open resection is safer for large masses or in the presence of dense adhesions. Colovesical or colovaginal fistulas are not absolute contraindications, but may require intracorporeal suturing. Reversal of Hartmann's procedure offers training to acquire laparoscopic expertise, since there is no resection and little mesenteric dissection. In the absence of malignancy, oncological considerations can be ignored.
- *Inflammatory bowel disease*. Crohn's disease affecting the ileocaecal region is frequently amenable to a laparoscopic approach. Segments of the colon are also approachable laparoscopically.
- *Rectal prolapse*. From the available procedures those applied laparoscopically include anterior resection, rectopexy and sacral fixation with and without a mesh.
- *Idiopathic constipation* from colonic inertia can be treated laparoscopically by total abdominal colectomy and ileorectal anastomosis.
- *Volvulus* of the sigmoid or caecum can be resected laparoscopically.
- Intestinal stomas for diversion include colostomy for *anal incontinence, distal obstruction* and *complex pelvic and perianal sepsis*.

Prepare

1 Discuss with the patient the reasonable expectation for the pathological condition and warn that intraoperative circumstances may require conversion to open operation. Some patients decline the option of a laparoscopic approach. Until the laparoscopic approach is demonstrably acceptable, recruit patients within the context of trials.

2 Prepare the colon mechanically and with antibiotics as for laparotomy. Order compression stockings and deep vein thrombosis prophylaxis.

3 The table must be equipped to hold the patient in place, even when it is markedly tilted. A bean-bag torso holder and shoulder braces work well. Have the patient supine, legs in stirrups. Place the perineum just beyond the inferior end of the table, allowing access for intraoperative colonoscopy and facilitating stapled anastomosis if necessary. Position the patient's legs to allow you, or your assistant, to stand between them. Flex hips and knees less than usual to avoid impeding your arm movements and to keep the patient's thighs from obstructing the movements of instruments (Fig. 17.1).

4 Insert a nasogastric tube and a urinary catheter.

TABLE 17.1 Conditions amenable to a laparoscopic approach

Conditions
Colorectal carcinoma
Colonic polyps
Diverticular disease
Inflammatory bowel disease
Rectal prolapse
Idiopathic constipation
Volvulus
Stoma formation and closure

5 If the operation is for rectal disease, wash out the rectum.

6 Wash, prepare and drape the abdomen as for a laparotomy.

7 The arrangement of the operating team varies, depending on the site of the pathology. As a rule you and the camera controller stand next to each other on the side opposite to the lesion, your first assistant facing you, on the same side as the lesion. Site monitors so that the eyes and hands of you and your first assistant are aligned to view them directly without the need to turn your heads. Assistants and monitors change whenever you need to alter your position.

KEY POINTS Identifying the pathology

- It is frustrating if you cannot identify the pathology at the time of laparoscopic colectomy.
- Recognition may be difficult or impossible when there is no serosal involvement, unless a hand-assisted device is used (see later).
- Accurate delineation of the lesion is aided by preoperative injection of carbon particles into the normal colonic wall around the lesion; this avoids time-consuming intraoperative colonoscopy.

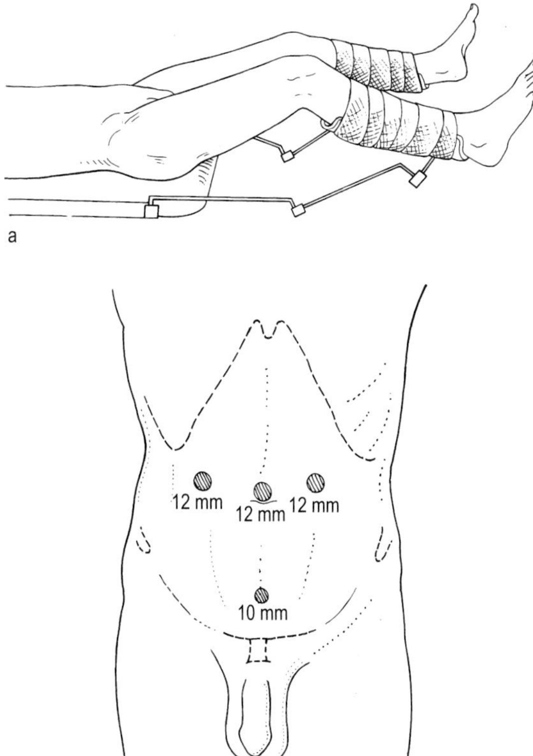

Fig. 17.1 Position of legs (a) and port sites (b) for colonic laparoscopic surgery.

KEY POINTS Principles of laparoscopic colonic resection

- Identification of lesion.
- Assess resectability/convert to open.
- Mobilization.
- Pedicle division.
- Resection.
- Restore continuity.

RIGHT-SIDED COLECTOMY

Access

1 Access apart, the operation resembles the open procedure.

2 Stand on the left side facing the right upper quadrant but, if necessary, stand between the patient's legs. Your monitor is placed facing the patient's right shoulder (Fig. 17.2a).

3 Achieve a pneumoperitoneum with either the Veress needle or open technique.

4 A variety of trocar positions have been described according to individual preference or because previous operation scars need to be avoided. A trocar is usually placed at the infra-umbilical site, with the patient in a head-down position. Place further ports in a semicircle centred on the lesion in the right colon (Fig. 17.2b).

5 Place the patient in steep head-down position and rolled to the left so that the small bowel falls away from the caecum and terminal ileum. Re-position the patient into the head-up position as the operation field moves up to the hepatic flexure and transverse colon.

Action

1 Begin the dissection in the right lower quadrant to free up the terminal ileum and appendix, moving cranially along the white line, mobilizing the colon medially. As you lift the caecum, identify and avoid the ureter and gonadal vessels. As you approach the hepatic flexure, have the table tilted to the head-up position, so helping to keep the small bowel dependent towards the pelvis. As you mobilize the transverse colon by dividing the gastrocolic ligament, the duodenum is revealed posteriorly. Use electrosurgical scissors or harmonic scalpel for the dissection, and graspers to reflect and hold the bowel.

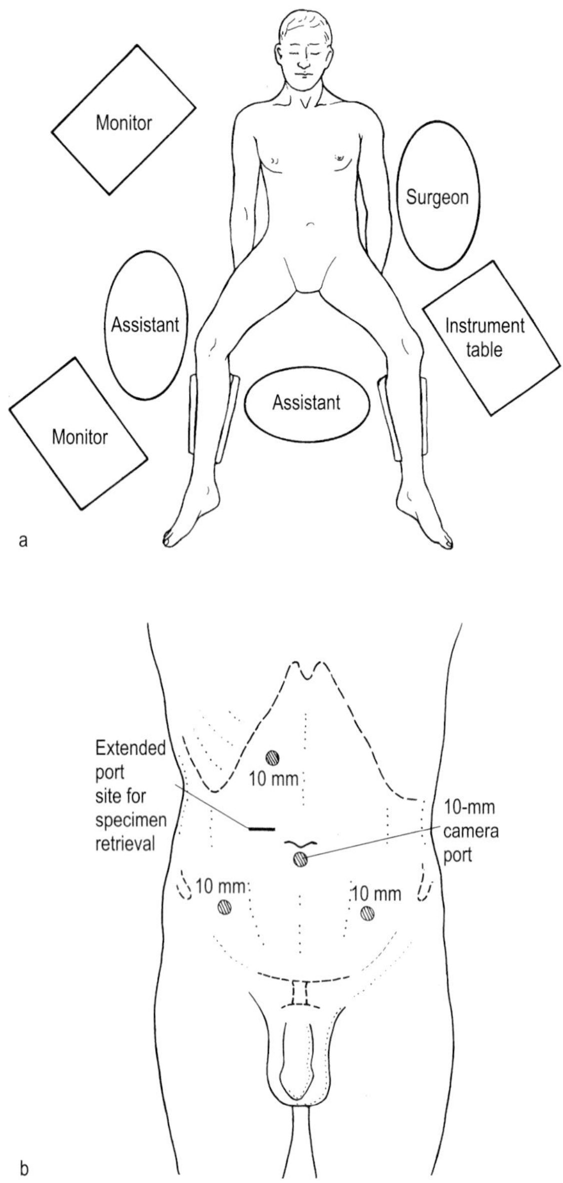

Fig. 17.2 Set-up (a) and port sites (b) for right hemicolectomy.

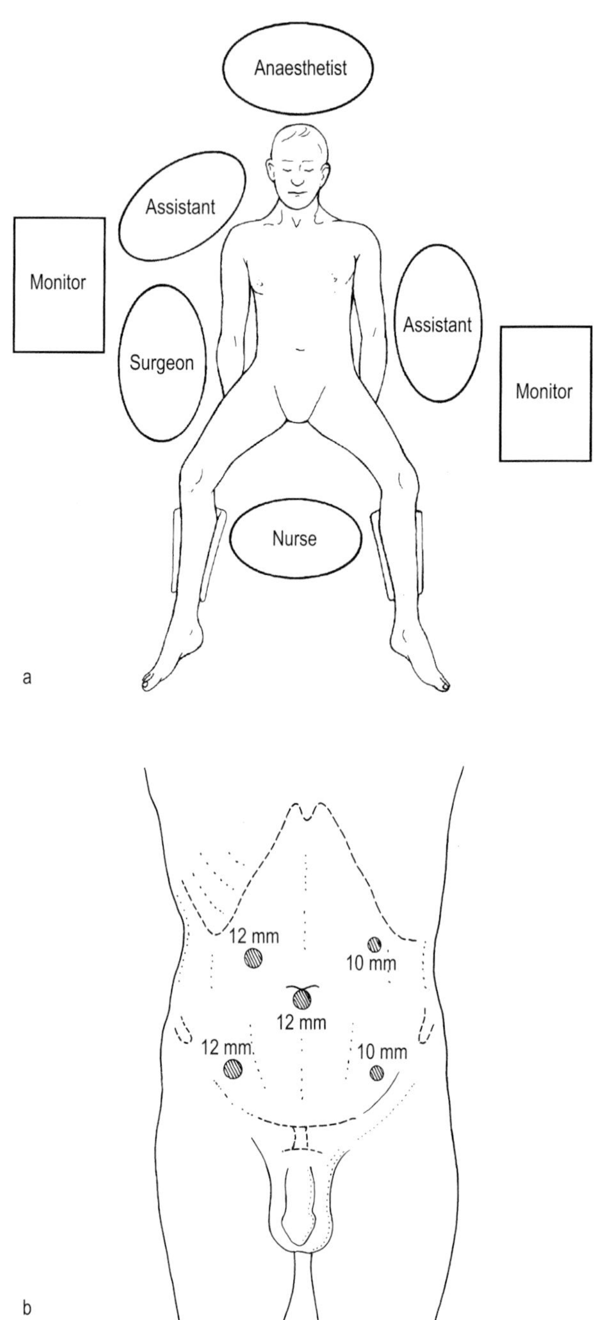

Fig. 17.3 Set-up (a) and port sites (b) for left hemicolectomy.

2 When the mobilization is complete, the colon is suspended by the mesentery containing the three named vessels: ileocolic, right colic and the right branch of the middle colic. Individually free, clip, ligate or staple these vessels, then divide the remaining vessels and mesentery.

3 The colectomy can be performed with a laparoscopic-assisted technique by making a small incision to allow the bowel to be delivered to the surface of the mid-abdominal wall. If the procedure is performed for carcinoma, shield the incision with a wound protector to avoid contamination by malignant cells. Transect the bowel, usually with staples, and perform the anastomosis, either by functional end-to-end anastomosis using a stapling device or by suturing.

LEFT COLECTOMY

Access

1 Stand on the right side of the patient with your hands and eyes aligned facing a monitor. A second monitor is positioned as needed for the assistant (Fig. 17.3a).

2 Place the ports as shown in Figure 17.3b, in a semicircle around the infra-umbilical port, which usually transmits the camera.

3 Have the patient placed in a steep head-down position with the table rotated to the right, so that the small bowel falls away from

the left lower quadrant. Depending upon whether the sigmoid colon alone or the descending colon or the rectum are also to be resected, modify the length of the mobilization and port placement.

Action

1 Retract the sigmoid colon medially, exposing the left lateral attachment of the descending colon and sigmoid colon. Usually, employ diathermy scissors to incise the white line. After the left lateral attachments are freed to the rectum, have the sigmoid colon retracted laterally, exposing the vessels, which can be put under tension.

2 The left ureter is more difficult to find than the right but, as mobilization proceeds, identify and separate the gonadal vessels and ureter from the specimen.

3 Score the mesentery across the base near the aorta and carry the incision down along the rectum on the right. Skeletonize, ligate, clip or staple the vessels with a vascular stapler.

4 If you are performing an anterior resection or a left colon resection, you must mobilize the splenic flexure. This requires a shift of team and realignment of monitors.

5 Prefer dissection into the pelvis under direct vision, using diathermy for cutting and coagulation. Identify and preserve the autonomic nerves of the pelvis.

6 If the rectum must be mobilized, incise its lateral attachments to the pelvic floor. Pull the rectum anteriorly so that the presacral space can be entered over the sacral prominence. Separate the rectum from the presacral fascia down to the coccyx. Cut the lateral stalks, carefully coagulating the middle rectal vessels, if present. Anteriorly, carry the dissection down to the rectovaginal septum in females or to below the seminal vesicles in males. This dissection is the same as that in open procedures.

7 When you have decided upon the two sites for bowel transection, dissect off the mesenteric fat in preparation for an anastomosis. Transect the bowel with a 30- or 60-mm linear stapler.

8 The specimen can be removed. Perform an intracorporeal stapled anastomosis via the anus using a triple-staple technique.

9 Alternatively, use the laparoscopically assisted colectomy techniques. Make the planned incision for specimen removal and draw the mobilized colon into the wound. Isolate, ligate and divide the vessels. Dissect the transection sites clean of fat and accomplish standard stapler transection. Anastomosis can be performed intraperitoneally, but it is easier to use a double-stapling technique.

RECTOPEXY

Assess

Laparoscopic surgery can be especially effective in benign disease such as rectal prolapse.

Access

Port placement is similar to that for an anterior resection (Fig. 17.4), as is the conduct of the operation.

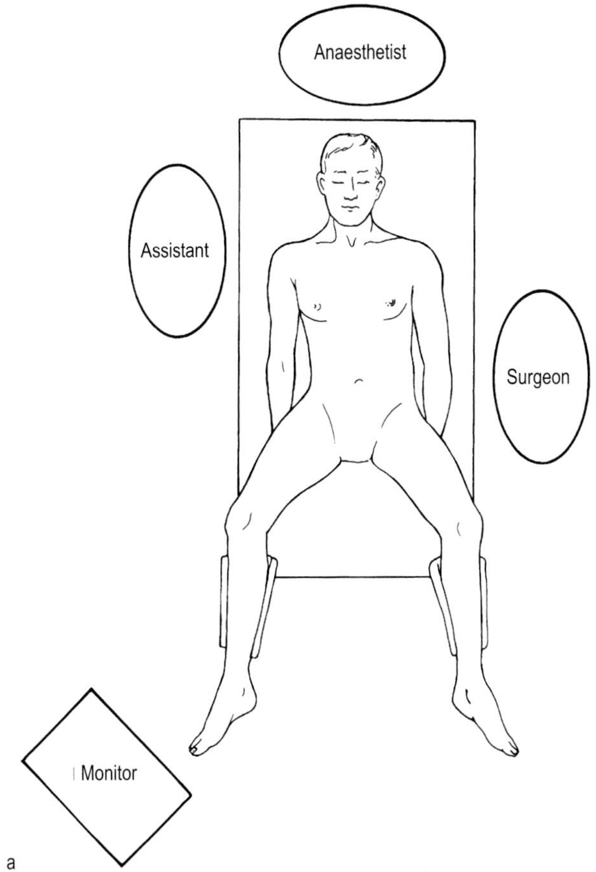

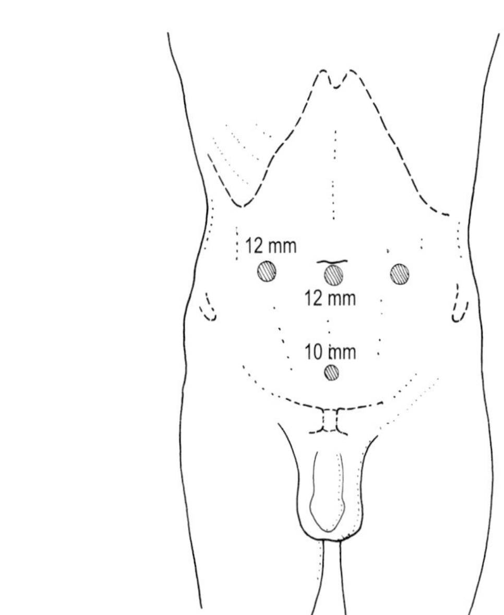

Fig. 17.4 Set-up (a) and port sites (b) for anterior resection or rectopexy.

Action

1 Mobilize the rectum while identifying the ureters and preserving the lateral stalks. Clear the sacrum of overlying tissues on the sacral promontory. Sew the lateral stalks to the clean site on

the sacrum; this pulls and holds the rectum up in the pelvis. Insert two sutures as a rule through each lateral stalk. In time, the rectum will adhere, preventing further prolapse.

2 If the patient has significant constipation, you may include a laparoscopically assisted colectomy. The technique resembles left colon resection.

3 Some authors use a mesh to fix the rectum to the sacrum. First attach the mesh to the sacrum. A device is available for applying tacks to hold the mesh to the sacrum. Wrap the mesh around, and sew it to the posterior half of the rectum, leaving the anterior half of the rectum unwrapped. Scar tissue will form between the rectum and sacrum, fixing it and preventing further prolapse.

HAND-ASSISTED LAPAROSCOPIC COLORECTAL SURGERY

Appraise

1 This is a newly developed technique involving the insertion of a hand or forearm through a mini-laparotomy incision, while maintaining pneumoperitoneum. Its advantages are summarized in Table 17.2. The hand can then be used as in an open procedure to palpate organs or tumour, reflect organs atraumatically, retract structures, identify vessels, dissect bluntly along a tissue plane and provide finger pressure to bleeding points while proximal control is achieved.

2 Make a transverse incision at a convenient place in the anterior abdominal wall with a length in centimetres equivalent to your glove size (e.g. $7\frac{1}{2}$). Site the incision away from bony prominences. Insert a special port in the wound and inflate the cuff, resulting in a stable port through which your hand can enter. An airtight flange is attached to your arm (usually the non-dominant one) and your hand is well lubricated. Pass the hand through the port and connect the flange in order to maintain a pneumoperitoneum. The presence of the hand in the abdomen allows for excellent controlled manipulation with tactile feedback. The port is then also available for specimen retrieval and extracorporeal anastomosis, and acts as a convenient wound protector.

3 This technique is more economical than a total laparoscopic approach, reducing both the number of laparoscopic ports and the number of instruments required. Some advocates claim that it is also easier to learn and perform than a total laparoscopic approach, and may increase patient safety.

TABLE 17.2 Advantages of the hand-assisted approach
Gives tactile feedback
Allows retraction for identification of tissue planes
Hand-device incision allows anastomosis and extraction of specimen
Useful in difficult cases
Useful in initial parts of operative learning curve

Postoperative care

1 Remove the nasogastric tube after completing the procedure.

2 Postoperative feeding has been initiated as early as the night of the operation, but it is usually more sensible to start oral intake on the first or second postoperative day if there is no evidence of nausea or abdominal distension. Progress with diet as it is tolerated.

3 Institute pain control as that after an open technique, with patient-controlled analgesia or systemic medication, but less analgesic medication is usually required.

Complications

1 Complications inevitably rise as the techniques increase in popularity, and this is certainly true of colonic operations. Any structure may be injured during trocar insertion. Minimize this by using open insertion of the first cannula and subsequent cannula insertion under vision. The viscera and small bowel, including the duodenum, may be damaged by grasping or cauterizing instruments. Avoid splenic injury by exercising caution during retraction in the left upper quadrant to expose the splenic flexure of the colon.

2 Avoid injury to the mesenteric, iliac, epigastric and innominate vessels by initial open cannulation and subsequent cannula insertion with direct laparoscopic viewing of the undersurface of the abdominal wall.

3 The ureter is at risk of surgical transection or diathermy burn during colectomy. Some authors suggest inserting illuminated ureteral catheters preoperatively to provide visualization of the ureter in its entirety.

4 Bleeding, either intra-operatively or postoperatively, is not unique to laparoscopic procedures. It may be mesenteric or originate in other locations.

Abdominal wall recurrence

1 One of the concerns about adopting a laparoscopically assisted approach to colorectal malignancy is the reported development of recurrence at a port site and not necessarily the one through which the specimen was retrieved or even one created during the operation in question. Reported incidences vary from 1.5% to 21%. Although most authors report laparoscopic colectomies for carcinoma without any evidence of port-site implantation, at least three port-site recurrences have been described. The number of procedures performed is unknown and hence the exact incidence of this complication is unknown.

2 The exact reasons for these abdominal wall metastases have not been elucidated. Possible explanations include seeding of malignant cells from intraoperative manipulation and instrument contamination. Gas flow generated during the pneumoperitoneum may also spread malignant cells, and gas leaking around a port may lead to implantation of malignant cells into the wounds. Experimentally, a pneumoperitoneum with carbon dioxide stimulates the growth of malignant cells.

3 Hopefully the trials sponsored by the MRC, the COLOR trial in Europe and large American trials to compare laparoscopic-assisted colectomy with open colectomy for colon carcinoma

will answer the issue of whether the disease-free survival rates and overall survival rates are equivalent, whether laparoscopic-assisted colectomy is safe compared with open colectomy and whether laparoscopic-assisted colectomy is a cost-effective alternative to open colectomy and results in superior quality of life.

FURTHER READING

Darzi A, Lewis C, Menzies-Gow N et al 1995 Laparoscopic abdominal perineal excision of the rectum. Surgical Endoscopy 9:414–417

Guillou PJ, Darzi A, Monson JRT 1993 Laparoscopic assisted colectomy for colorectal cancer. Surgical Oncology 2:43–49

Monson JRT, Darzi A, Carey PD et al 1992 Prospective evaluation of laparoscopic assisted colectomy in an unselected group of patients. Lancet 340:831–833

Monson JRT, Hill ADK, Darzi A 1995 laparoscopic colonic surgery. British Journal of Surgery 82:150–157

Paraskeva PA, Purkayastha S, Darzi A 2004 Laparoscopy for malignancy. Current status. Seminars in Laparoscopic Surgery 11:27

Puttick M, Gould SW, Darzi A 1999 Early experience with a new device for hand assisted laparoscopic colorectal surgery. British Journal of Surgery 86 (Suppl 1): 94 (abstract)

Scott HJ, Darzi A 1997 Tactile feedback in laparoscopic colonic surgery. British Journal of Surgery 84:1005

Wing Tai Siu, Michael Ka Wah Li 2004 Laparoscopy for malignancy: the role of handoscopy. Seminars in Laparoscopic Surgery 11:53–60

18

Anorectum

C.R.G. Cohen, C.J. Vaizey

CONTENTS

INTRODUCTION

You require meticulous attention to detail and carefully supervised postoperative care for successful results. You must have a sound understanding of the anatomy of the area in order to make a precise diagnosis and perform effective treatment.

Invariably perform a full rectal examination, including inspection, palpation, sigmoidoscopy and proctoscopy, before carrying out any procedure. In appropriate circumstances exclude serious diseases, such as neoplastic or inflammatory bowel disease with colonoscopy or computed tomography (CT) colography.

Most operations can be performed with the patient in the lithotomy position. The prone (Latin: *pronus*=bent forward) jack-knife position has the advantage of superior visibility and access for your assistant.

ANATOMY

The anal canal extends from the anorectal junction superiorly to the anus below and is approximately 3–4 cm long in men and 2–3 cm long in women. The lining epithelium is characterized by the anal valves midway along the anal canal. This line of the anal valves is often loosely referred to as the 'dentate line' (Fig. 18.1).

It does not represent the point of fusion between the embryonic hindgut and the proctoderm, which occurs at a higher level, between the anal valves and the anorectal junction. In this zone, sometimes called the transitional zone, there is a mixture of columnar and squamous epithelium.

Sphincters

The anal canal is surrounded by two sphincter muscles. The internal sphincter is the expanded distal portion of the circular muscle of the large intestine. It is only about 2 mm thick, composed of smooth muscle and is grey/white in colour. The external sphincter lies outside the internal sphincter with a palpable gutter between them. It is usually nearly a centimetre thick, composed of striated muscle and is brown in colour.

There is usually a pigment change in the skin over the outer margin of the external anal sphincter muscle with lighter skin outside and darker skin over the muscle and towards the anal canal. This demarcation is useful when siting the skin incision to operate on the external anal sphincter.

? DIFFICULTY

1. Identification and differentiation of the internal and external sphincters can be difficult. Electrical stimulation, using an electrical stimulator or electrocautery, causes twitching of the external sphincter but the internal sphincter does not respond in this way. Superiorly it is contiguous with the puborectalis and levator ani muscles, forming one continuous striated muscle sheet (Fig. 18.1). The external sphincter is supplied by the pudendal nerve entering the muscle from its outer aspect posterolaterally, and the levator ani from branches of the fourth sacral nerve on its superior aspect.
2. The levator ani and puborectalis muscles are responsible for holding the anal canal in its correct position in relationship to the bony pelvis; this is with the top of the anal canal on the line joining the tip of the coccyx to the inferior aspect of the symphysis pubis. They also maintain the correct angle between the rectum and anal canal at less than 90° (Fig. 18.2).

Spaces

There are three important spaces around the anal canal: the intersphincteric space, the ischiorectal fossa and the supralevator space (Fig. 18.1). These spaces are important in the spread of sepsis and in certain operations.

- The *intersphincteric space* lies between the two sphincters and contains the terminal fibres of the longitudinal muscle of the large intestine. It also contains the anal intermuscular glands, approximately 12 in number, arranged around the anal canal. The ducts of these glands pass through the internal sphincter and open into the anal crypts.

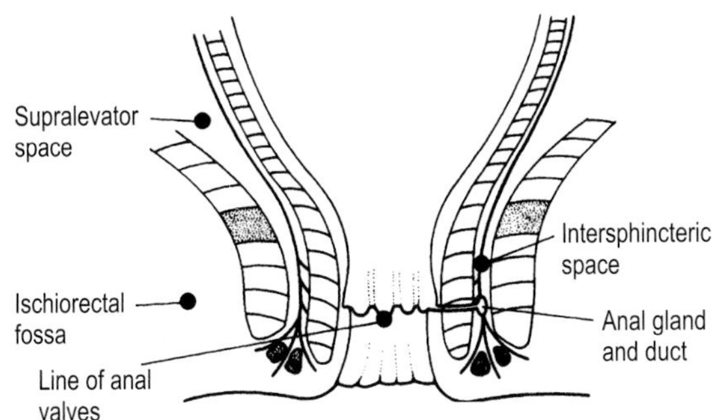

Fig. 18.1 Diagram to show the essential anatomy of the anal canal.

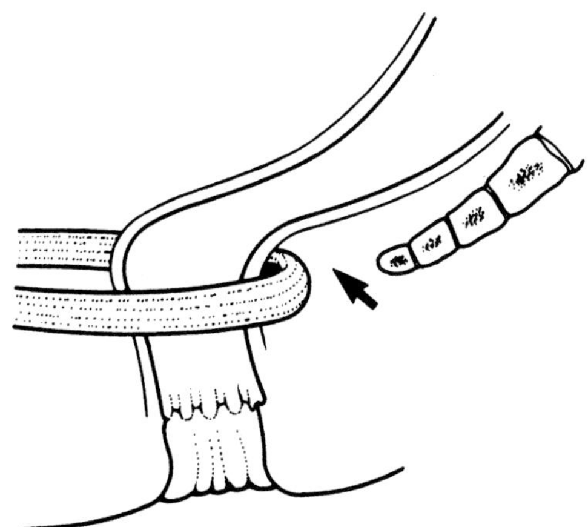

Fig. 18.2 Sagittal diagram to show the relationship of the distal rectum to the anal canal. The anorectal angle is just less than a right-angle in most people.

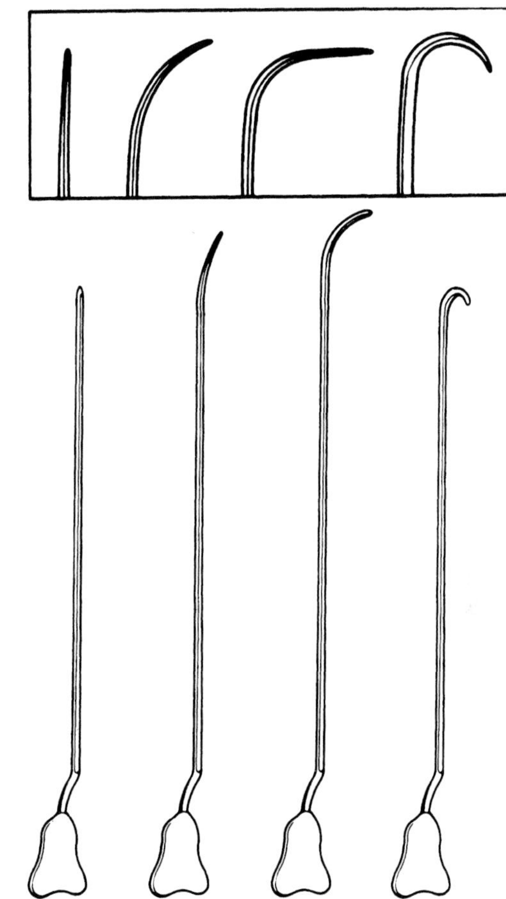

Fig. 18.3 A set of four Lockhart–Mummery fistula probes.

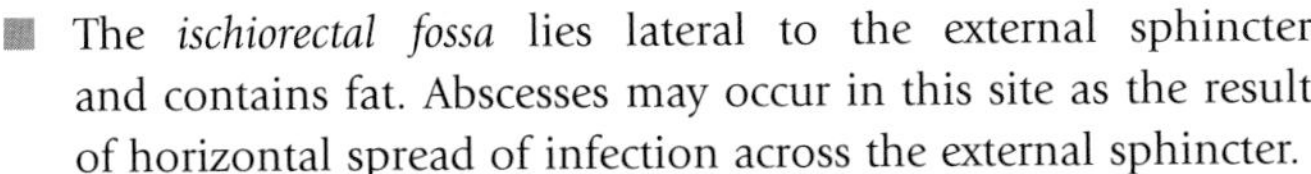

- The *ischiorectal fossa* lies lateral to the external sphincter and contains fat. Abscesses may occur in this site as the result of horizontal spread of infection across the external sphincter.

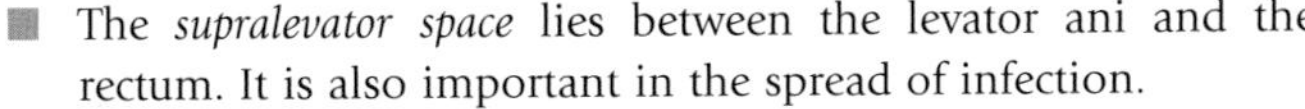

- The *supralevator space* lies between the levator ani and the rectum. It is also important in the spread of infection.

Prepare

- Familiarize yourself with the small range of essential instruments for examination of the patient, such as the proctoscope and the rigid sigmoidoscope. In awake patients with anal sphincter spasm, use a small paediatric sigmoidoscope.
- Operating proctoscopes of the Eisenhammer, Parks and Sims type are essential for operations on and within the anal canal.
- Use a pair of fine scissors, fine forceps (toothed and non-toothed), a light needle-holder, Emett's forceps and a small no. 15 scalpel blade for intra-anal work. Alternatively, diathermy dissection creates a virtually bloodless field.
- For fistula surgery have a set of Lockhart–Mummery fistula probes (Fig. 18.3), together with a set of Anel's lacrimal probes.
- Most patients require no preparation, or two glycerine suppositories, to ensure that the rectum is empty before anal surgery. If for any reason the bowels need to be confined postoperatively, then carry out a full bowel preparation to empty the whole large intestine.

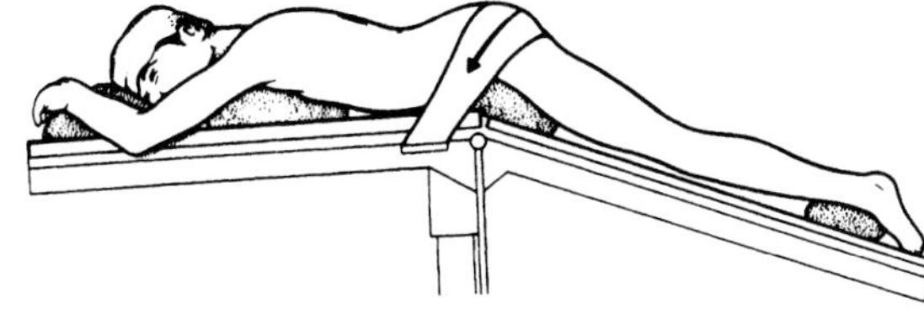

Fig. 18.4 The jack-knife position.

- Minor operations can be performed under local infiltration anaesthesia; larger procedures demand regional or general anaesthesia.
- For outpatient procedures use the left lateral position, or alternatively the knee–elbow position. For anal operations most British surgeons favour the lithotomy position, although the prone jack-knife position (Fig. 18.4) can also be used.
- If you prefer to shave the area before starting an anal operation, carry it out in the operating theatre immediately beforehand, where there is good illumination.

HAEMORRHOIDS

Appraise

KEY POINT Primary, secondary or incidental?

- Have you excluded pelvic tumours, large-bowel carcinoma and inflammatory bowel disease?

1 Haemorrhoids do not always need treatment if the symptoms are minimal and you have excluded a primary cause.

2 Small internal haemorrhoids can be treated by injection sclerotherapy. Prolapsing haemorrhoids may be ligated with rubber-bands. Large prolapsing haemorrhoids, which are usually accompanied by a significant external component, are best treated by haemorrhoidectomy. With the advent of day-case diathermy haemorrhoidectomy, which gives a satisfactory result, we are willing to offer surgical treatment more readily than in the past.

3 As a rule avoid treating haemorrhoids if the patient also has Crohn's disease.

INJECTION SCLEROTHERAPY

This is an outpatient procedure and does not require any anaesthesia. It is most conveniently carried out following a full rectal examination if no further investigation is required. Leave the patient in the left lateral position.

Action

1 Pass the full-length proctoscope and withdraw it slowly to identify the anorectal junction—the area where the anal canal begins to close around the instrument.

2 Place a ball of cotton wool into the lower rectum with Emett's forceps to keep the walls apart. Since you will not usually remove it, warn the patient that it will pass out with the next motion.

3 Identify the position of the right anterior, left lateral and right posterior haemorrhoids.

4 Fill a 10-ml Gabriel pattern syringe with 5% phenol in arachis oil with 0.5% menthol (oily phenol BP).

5 Through the full-length proctoscope, insert the needle into the submucosa at the anorectal junction at the identified positions of the haemorrhoids in turn. Inject 3–5 ml of 5% phenol in arachis oil into the submucosa at each site, to produce a swelling with a pearly appearance of the mucosa in which the vessels are clearly seen. Move the needle slightly during injection to avoid giving an intravascular injection.

6 Delay removing the needle for a few seconds following the injection, to lessen the escape of the solution. If necessary, press on the injection site with cotton wool to minimize leakage.

7 Warn the patient to avoid attempts at defecation for 24 hours.

KEY POINTS Injection sclerotherapy caution

- Avoid injecting the solution too superficially. This produces a watery bleb, which may ulcerate and subsequently cause haemorrhage.
- Avoid injecting the solution too deeply. This produces an oleogranuloma with subsequent features of an extrarectal swelling. Too deep anterior injection in male patients causes perineal pain and sometimes haematuria from prostatitis. This is a serious problem. Halt the injection immediately.
- If you suspect that the needle has entered the urinary tract, administer antibiotics. Do not hesitate to admit the patient, since septicaemia is common and may be severe.

RUBBER-BAND LIGATION

1 This is also an outpatient procedure and does not require anaesthesia.

2 There are several different designs of band applicator; the simplest is illustrated in Figure 18.5. The suction bander is relatively expensive but is convenient and easy to use.

3 Have available a pair of grasping forceps such as Patterson's biopsy forceps.

4 There are two conceptually different strategies:
- Band, or inject, above the haemorrhoid in order to 'hitch' it back into its normal place. Grasp the redundant mucosa proximal to the haemorrhoid and band that.
- Try to destroy the haemorrhoid itself. This method will be described.

Action

1 Load two elastic bands on to the band applicator.

2 Pass the full-length proctoscope and withdraw it slowly to identify the anorectal junction. Position the end of the proctoscope midway between the anorectal junction and the dentate line.

3 Pass the tips of the grasping forceps through the ring of the band applicator, within the lumen of the proctoscope, and take hold of the selected haemorrhoid, or above it if you are employing the 'hitch-up' approach.

4 Pull the haemorrhoid through the ring of the band applicator while pushing the band applicator upwards. If the patient experiences little additional discomfort when asked, 'fire' the band on to the haemorrhoid. If the manoeuvre causes increased discomfort, reposition the grip on the haemorrhoid slightly higher and retest before applying the band.

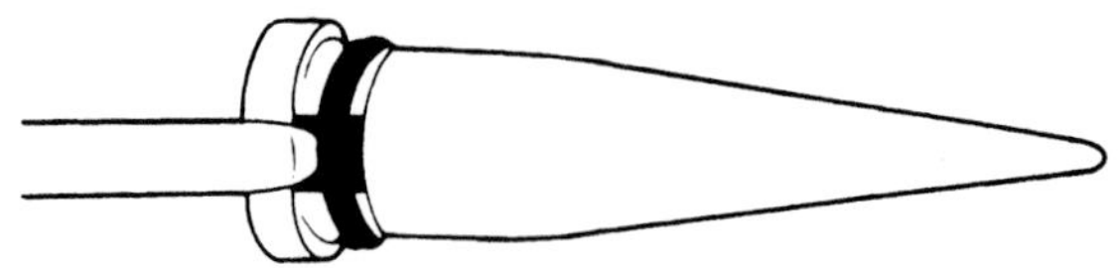

Fig. 18.5 A simple instrument with which to perform elastic-band ligation of haemorrhoids.

5 Any number of haemorrhoids can be banded on each occasion. Repeat banding when necessary but delay it for 6–8 weeks.

Aftercare

1 Warn the patient to avoid attempts at defecation for 24 hours.

2 Advise the patient to take a mild analgesic if the procedure causes discomfort.

? DIFFICULTY

1. If the procedure produces severe pain it may be because you applied the band too low on to sensitive epithelium.
2. Try the effect of analgesics.
3. If they do not control the pain, remove the bands in the operating theatre under general anaesthesia, using an operating proctoscope.

3 Pain developing slowly in 1–2 days may be from ischaemia. Analgesics relieve the pain. Give metronidazole tablets 200 mg three times daily, which may help reduce inflammation.

4 Advise the patient that the haemorrhoid and the band should drop off after 5–10 days and may be accompanied by a small amount of bleeding.

5 Warn the patient that secondary haemorrhage occurs in approximately 2% any time up to 3 weeks after the application. Tell the patient to report to hospital if this is severe, since it may require transfusion and operative control of the bleeding.

▶ KEY POINT Monitor temperature

- If the patient develops severe fever, suspect HIV infection. Admit the patient for treatment with intravenous antibiotics.

HAEMORRHOIDECTOMY

Appraise

1 There are several methods of performing a haemorrhoidectomy. We shall describe the diathermy technique, which has evolved out of the ligation and excision technique of Milligan and Morgan.

2 Haemorrhoidectomy should be a curative procedure. Perform it carefully and thoroughly.

Prepare

1 Start lactulose, a non-absorbed disaccharide which produces an osmotic bowel action, 30 ml twice daily 2 days preoperatively. This reduces postoperative pain.

2 Give oral metronidazole 400 mg t.d.s. for 5 days, which also significantly reduces postoperative pain.

3 Place the anaesthetized patient in the lithotomy position with some head-down tilt. Avoid caudal anaesthetic as it may provoke retention of urine.

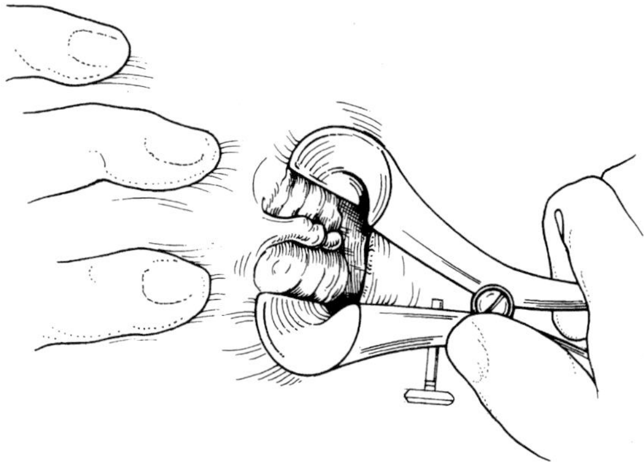

Fig. 18.6 Plan the operation by inserting the Eisenhammer retractor, establish the site and size of the haemorrhoids and identify the skin bridges to preserve them.

Assess

1 Plan the operation by inserting the Eisenhammer retractor and establish which haemorrhoids need to be removed; also estimate the state and size of the skin bridges (Fig. 18.6).

2 Determine whether:
- A three-quadrant haemorrhoidectomy will be sufficient.
- There is one additional haemorrhoid that needs removal, or the situation is more complex than this.

3 If there is one additional haemorrhoid you may:
- Leave it and be prepared to return on another occasion if it proves troublesome.
- Fillet it out by undermining the skin bridge.
- Another technique is to divide the skin bridge above the dentate line, reflect it out of the anus, and trim the haemorrhoid with the back of a pair of scissors. Now excise any redundant mucosa and stitch the trimmed flap back into position with 2/0 synthetic absorbable sutures of Vicryl (Fig. 18.7).

4 The haemorrhoids may be even more extensive and may be circumferential:
- One possibility is to perform a standard three-quadrant haemorrhoidectomy and return on another occasion to deal with any residual haemorrhoids.
- If you are experienced in the technique, consider performing the circumferential Whitehead haemorrhoidectomy described in 1882 by the English surgeon Walter Whitehead (1840–1914). He described the excision of a tubular segment of the anal canal, with mucosal–cutaneous re-anastomosis. Use polyglactin 910 (Vicryl). Beware of the difficulty, avoiding Whitehead deformity—mucosal ectropion (Greek: *ek*=out+*trepein*=to turn)—and later stenosis.

Action

1 Inject bupivacaine (Marcaine) 0.25% with adrenaline (epinephrine) 1:200 000 into each skin bridge and into the external component of each haemorrhoid to be excised.

2 Wait, and gently massage away excess fluid from the injection with a moistened gauze.

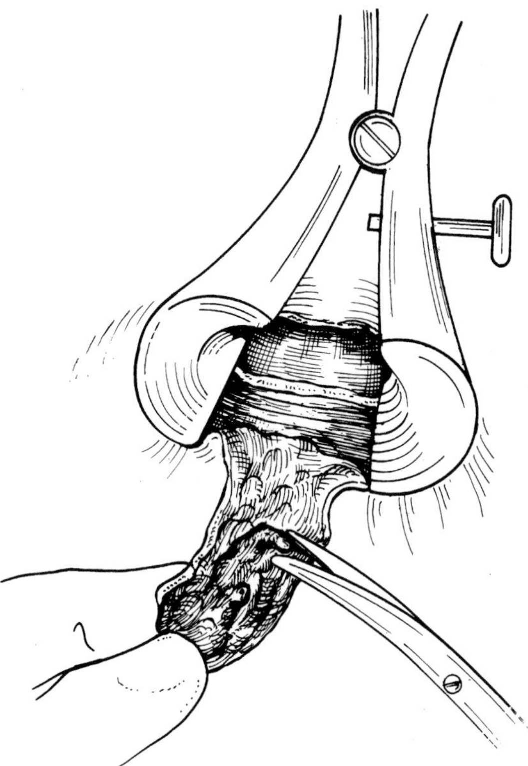

Fig. 18.7 In the event that there is an additional haemorrhoid, over and above the usual three, divide the skin bridge above the dentate line, reflect it out of the anus, trim the haemorrhoid with the back of a pair of scissors, excise redundant mucosa and stitch the trimmed flap back into position with 2/0 Vicryl.

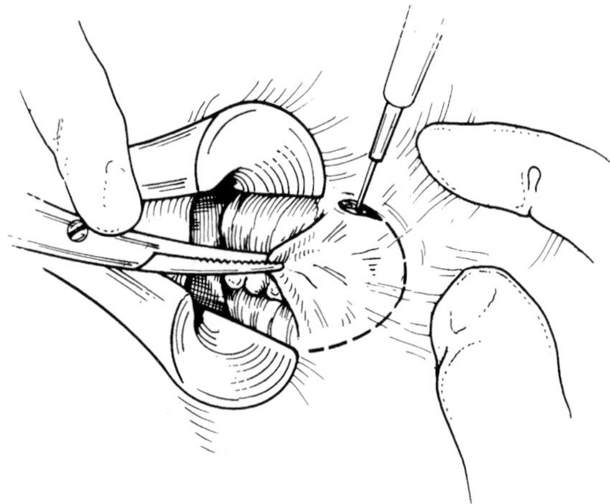

Fig. 18.8 Commence with the left lateral haemorrhoid. With the Eisenhammer in the anal canal the internal sphincter is put on stretch allowing easy identification.

3 Commence with the left lateral haemorrhoid. Place the Eisenhammer retractor in the anal canal and open it sufficiently to put the internal sphincter under tension. This demonstrates the plane of the dissection (Fig. 18.8).

4 Group the external component and excise it with electrocautery, using cutting diathermy on skin and coagulating diathermy for all other dissection (Fig. 18.9).

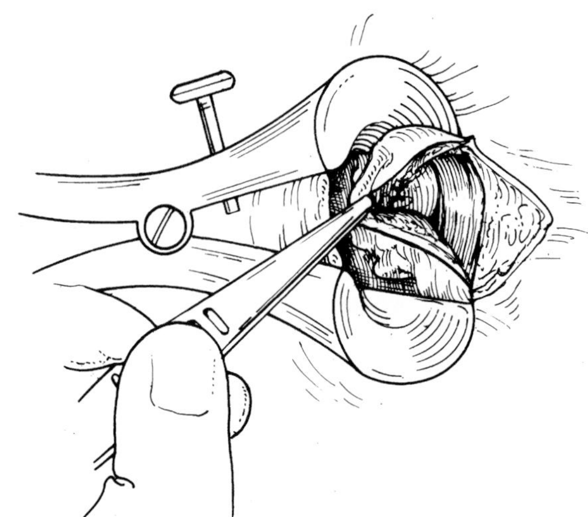

Fig. 18.9 Using electrocautery dissection, excise the external skin component and then continue the dissection up the anal canal separating haemorrhoid from anal sphincter.

KEY POINT Avoid diathermy burns

- When using cutting diathermy on skin, do not linger in one area or the skin develops indolent burn marks.

5 Now extend the haemorrhoidal dissection up the anal canal, separating the haemorrhoid from the underlying internal sphincter.

6 Narrow the pedicle as you dissect up towards the apex, otherwise you risk encroaching on the skin bridge.

7 When you have encompassed the internal component of the haemorrhoid, simply transect the pedicle with diathermy.

8 Repeat the procedure on the right anterior haemorrhoid and then the right posterior haemorrhoid.

9 Ensure complete haemostasis and check each wound and apex.

KEY POINT Haemostasis

- Remember that bleeding comes from what remains inside the patient, not from what has been removed.

10 Inspect the skin bridges and perform any further procedure as necessary and as earlier decided in the 'Assess' section (Fig. 18.10).

11 Do not apply any anal canal dressing.

12 Insert a diclofenac (Voltarol) suppository into the anus.

Aftercare

1 Allow the patient home after recovery from the anaesthetic.

2 Warn that there is likely to be an early increase in pain days 3–5 postoperatively.

3 Pain can usually be satisfactorily controlled with non-steroidal anti-inflammatory drugs (NSAIDs).

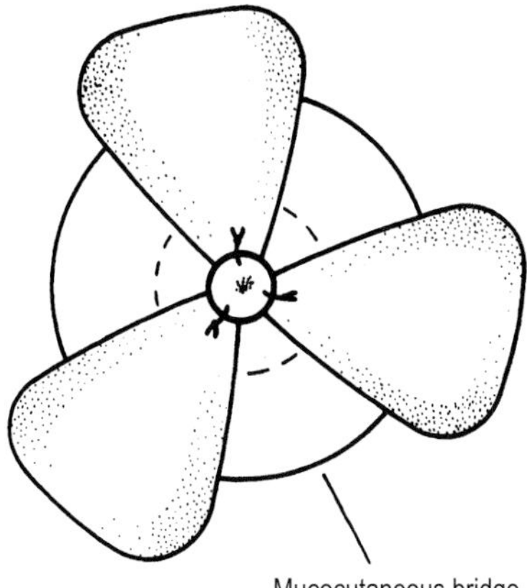

Fig. 18.10 Haemorrhoidectomy: it is essential to preserve three mucocutaneous bridges.

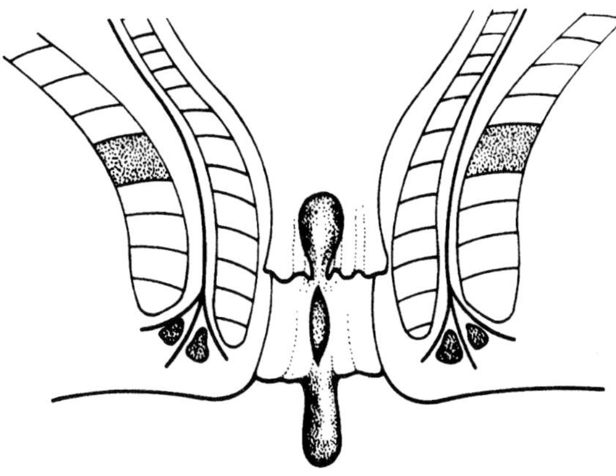

Fig. 18.11 A fissure with a sentinel skin tag, an anal polyp and undermining of the edges of the ulcer.

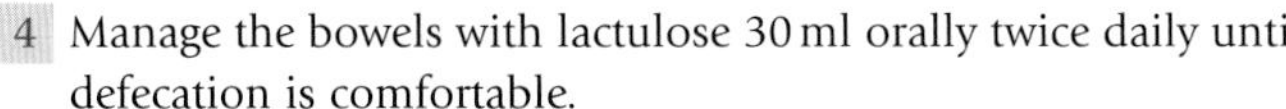

4 Manage the bowels with lactulose 30 ml orally twice daily until defecation is comfortable.

5 Try the effect of creating a reversible chemical sphincterotomy with locally applied 0.2% glyceryl trinitrate (GTN) applied three times daily.

6 Review the patient in the outpatient clinic within 10–12 days.

OTHER PROCEDURES

Closed haemorrhoidectomy

The principle is a limited removal of anoderm with immediate suturing. Randomized trials have failed to show any advantage.

Stapled haemorrhoidectomy

Linear staples impinging on skin or the rectum are painful. Circular stapling above the dentate line has been advocated by Longo but has yet to be evaluated adequately by others.

FISSURE

Appraise

1 Most ulcers at the anal margin are simple fissures in ano, possibly associated with a sentinel skin tag and/or hypertrophied anal papilla or anal polyp.

2 Exclude excoriation in association with pruritus ani, Crohn's disease, primary chancre of syphilis, herpes simplex, leukaemia and tumours.

3 Treat superficial fissures with 0.2% GTN (glyceryl trinitrate) cream twice a day or 2% diltiazem ointment, a calcium-channel-blocking drug, also twice daily. GTN can cause headaches; occasionally diltiazem causes local irritation.

4 Botulinum toxin injection is an alternative therapy, especially useful in patients who are non-compliant in regularly applying creams. Doses of botulinum toxin type A (Botox) may range from 2.5 to 50 units and reports have included injections into the internal and external anal sphincter either directly into the fissure or at sites removed from it. Dysport is an alternative preparation which requires roughly three times the number of units used with Botox. However, studies suggest that the two formulations are not bioequivalent, whatever the dose relationship.

5 Reserve operation for failures, which are more common when there is a sentinel tag, an anal polyp, exposure of the internal sphincter or undermining of the edges (Fig. 18.11).

6 Anal dilatation is no longer an acceptable treatment as it causes unpredictable stretching of the internal and external sphincters, and lower rectum, producing an unacceptable risk of incontinence.

7 The standard procedure is a lateral (partial internal) sphincterotomy.

LATERAL SPHINCTEROTOMY

Appraise

1 This is very successful, curing more than 95% of patients. It was introduced by Eisenhammer in 1951.

2 To avoid exacerbating the pain, avoid preoperative preparation.

3 The operation can be carried out as a 'day-case' procedure.

4 Warn the patient of a 1 in 20 chance of permanent flatus incontinence and a 1 in 200 chance of faecal leakage.

Action

1 Place the patient in the lithotomy position, with general or regional anaesthesia.

2 Pass an Eisenhammer bivalve operating proctoscope. Examine the fissure to exclude induration suggestive of an underlying intersphincteric abscess.

3 Remove hypertrophied anal papillae or a fibrous anal polyp, sending them for histopathological examination. Remove a sentinel skin tag.

4 Rotate the operating proctoscope to demonstrate the left lateral aspect of the anal canal. Palpate the lower border of the internal sphincter muscle. Replace the Eisenhammer retractor with a Parks' retractor, which permits outward traction, making the internal sphincter more obvious.

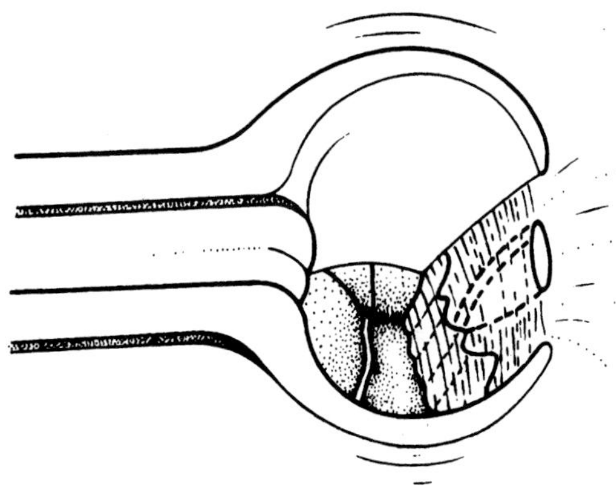

Fig. 18.12 Lateral partial internal sphincterotomy.

5 Make a small incision 1 cm long in line with the lower border of the internal sphincter. Insert scissors into the submucosa, gently separating the epithelial lining of the anal canal from the internal sphincter, and also into the intersphincteric space to separate the internal and external sphincters.

6 If you make a hole in the mucosa open it completely to avoid the risk of sepsis.

7 Clamp the isolated area of internal sphincter with artery forceps for 30 seconds. This markedly reduces haemorrhage.

8 With one blade of the scissors on each side of it, divide the internal sphincter muscle up to the level of the top of the fissure (Fig. 18.12).

KEY POINTS Limit the sphincteric division

- Do not extend the division of the internal sphincter above the upper limit of the fissure.
- Never extend it above the line of the anal valves.

9 Press on the area for 2–3 minutes to stop the bleeding. The wounds do not normally need to be closed.

10 Do not apply a dressing unless there is excessive bleeding that will be controlled by pressure from it. The dressing exacerbates postoperative pain.

11 Apply a perineal pad and pants.

Aftercare

1 Prescribe a bulk laxative such as sterculia (Normacol) 10 ml once or twice a day.

2 Bruising under the perianal skin signifies a haematoma, but it requires no treatment.

ANAL ABSCESS AND FISTULA

Appraise

1 Most abscesses and fistulas in the anal region arise from a primary infection in the anal intersphincteric glands. Furthermore, they represent different phases of the same disease process. An acute-phase abscess develops, when free drainage of pus is prevented by closure of either the internal or external opening of the fistula, or both, which is the chronic phase.

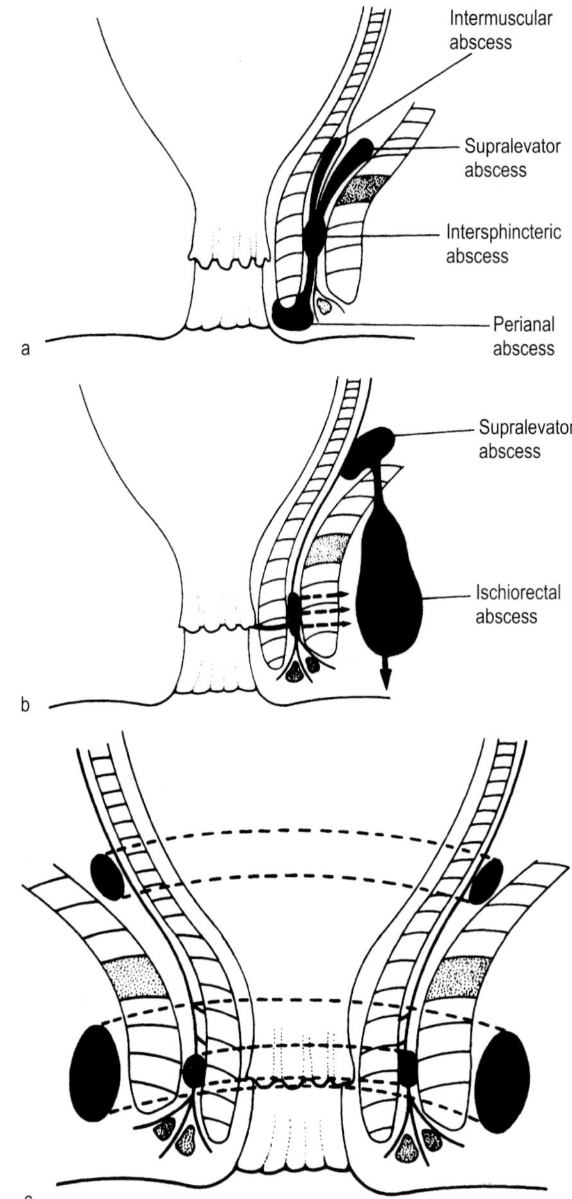

Fig. 18.13 Spread of intersphincteric abscess. (a) Vertical spread upwards and downwards from a primary intersphincteric abscess. (b) Horizontal spread from infection medially across the internal sphincter into the anal canal, upwards into the supralevator space. (c) Circumferential spread.

2 Other causes of sepsis in the perianal region include pilonidal infection, hidradenitis suppurativa, Crohn's disease, tuberculosis and intrapelvic sepsis draining downwards across the levator ani.

3 Once established, an intersphincteric abscess may spread vertically downwards to form a perianal abscess or upwards to form either an intermuscular abscess or supralevator abscess, depending upon which side of the longitudinal muscle spread occurs (Fig. 18.13a). Horizontal spread medially across the internal sphincter may result in drainage into the anal canal, but spread

laterally across the external sphincter may produce an ischiorectal abscess (Fig. 18.13b). Finally, circumferential spread of infection may occur from one intersphincteric space to the other, from one ischiorectal fossa to the other and from one supralevator space to the other (Fig. 18.13c).

4 Once an abscess has formed surgical drainage must be instituted; antibiotics have no part to play in the primary management. As the tissues are inflamed and oedematous, do the minimum to promote resolution of the infection. More tissue can be divided later to resolve the condition. Send a specimen of pus to the laboratory for culture. The presence of intestinal organisms suggests the presence of a fistula.

5 Avoid preoperative preparation of the bowel as it causes unnecessary pain.

6 Place the anaesthetized patient in the lithotomy position and now shave the operation area.

Perianal abscess

1 Recognize the abscess as a swelling at the anal margin.

2 Make a radial incision and excise overhanging edges. Allow pus to drain and send a sample to the laboratory.

3 Gently examine the wound to see if there is a fistula.

4 Insert a gauze dressing soaked in normal saline solution and surrounded by Surgicel. Do not pack the wound tightly.

Intermuscular abscess

1 Recognize the abscess as an indurated swelling, sometimes mobile within the lower rectal wall.

2 As this is an upward extension of an intersphincteric abscess, manage it similarly, but the upper limit of division of the internal sphincter and/or circular muscle of the rectum is higher.

3 Control bleeding from the divided edges of the rectal wall.

4 Insert a gauze dressing soaked in normal saline to the upper limit of the wound. Do not pack the wound tightly.

Supralevator abscess

1 This is recognizable as a fixed indurated swelling palpable above the anorectal junction.

2 Drainage of a supralevator abscess extends upwards to a similar level as an intermuscular abscess, except that the whole rectal wall needs to be divided.

3 Insert a gauze dressing soaked in normal saline, surrounded by Surgicel, into the anal canal to the upper limit of the wound. Do not pack the wound tightly.

Ischiorectal abscess

1 Recognize this as a brawny inflamed swelling in the ischiorectal fossa.

2 An ischiorectal abscess often spreads circumferentially from one side to the other, so carefully examine the patient under anaesthesia to determine if this has occurred. Recognize the abscess by feeling the induration inferior to the levator ani muscle.

3 For the same reason, employ a circumanal incision to establish drainage. Excise the skin edges to create an adequate opening and send a specimen of pus to the laboratory.

KEY POINTS Gentleness

- Be very careful when exploring the cavity with your finger. You may spread infection, damage the levator ani or injure the rectum itself.
- Never use a probe.

4 Gently insert a gauze dressing soaked in normal saline surrounded by Surgicel to the upper limit of the wound. Do not pack the wound tightly.

Postoperative

1 Remove the dressing on the second postoperative day while the patient lies in the bath, having been given an intramuscular injection of pethidine 100 mg or papaveretum 7–15 mg.

2 Initiate a routine of twice-daily baths, irrigation of the wound and the insertion of a tuck-in gauze dressing soaked in physiological saline or 1:40 sodium hypochlorite solution.

3 If the patient has evidence of persistent local or systemic sepsis, administer systemic antibiotics guided by the culture report. Metronidazole is effective against anaerobic organisms.

4 Assess the patient for the possible presence of a fistula detected at the time of abscess drainage, or a history of recurrent abscesses, or palpable induration of the perianal area, anal canal and lower rectum, or the presence of gut organism in the pus. If so, plan to re-examine the patient under anaesthesia and carry out the appropriate treatment.

FISTULA

Appraise

1 A fistula is an abnormal communication between two epithelial-lined surfaces. Therefore, in the context of fistula in ano, there should be an external opening on the perianal skin, an internal opening into the anal canal and a track between the two.

2 There may be no external opening, or it may be healed over. Likewise there may be no internal opening as the sepsis arises in the area of the intersphincteric gland, which is the primary site of infection. It may not drain across the internal sphincter into the anal canal. Finally, the track may follow a very complicated path.

3 The presence of infection is characterized by the physical sign of induration, detected by palpation with a lubricated, covered finger.

SUPERFICIAL FISTULA

Assess

1 Place the anaesthetized patient in the lithotomy position. Always perform sigmoidoscopy, looking especially for inflammatory bowel disease.

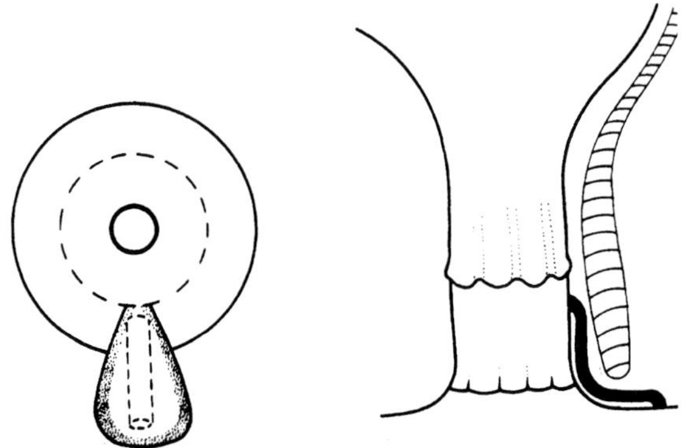

Fig. 18.14 A diagram to show a superficial fistula and the pear-shaped wound required to treat it.

2 Palpate the perianal skin, anal canal and lower rectum to detect induration. This is confined to the distal anal canal and localized to one area, as superficial fistulas are really fissures covered with skin and lower anal canal epithelium (Fig. 18.14).

Action

1 Insert a bivalve operating proctoscope and pass a fine probe along the track.

2 Lay open the fistula using a no. 15 bladed knife or electrocautery.

3 Curette the granulation tissue and send a specimen for histopathology.

4 If there is no induration deep to the internal sphincter, fashion the external skin wound so that it becomes pear-shaped and perform a lateral sphincterotomy (see above).

5 Insert a gauze dressing soaked in normal saline solution and surrounded by Surgicel to the upper limit of the wound.

INTERSPHINCTERIC FISTULA

1 An intersphincteric fistula results when the sepsis is inside the striated muscle of the pelvic floor and the anal canal (Fig. 18.15).

Assess

1 Have the anaesthetized patient in the lithotomy position. Perform sigmoidoscopy in all cases, especially looking for inflammatory bowel disease.

2 Palpate carefully for induration. There is often a long subcutaneous perianal track leading to the external opening. You can feel induration in the wall of the anal canal between a finger in the anal canal and the thumb externally. If there is an upward extension, you feel induration in the rectal wall. Although the internal opening into the rectum may be above the anorectal ring, laying it open is not difficult as the striated muscle will not be divided. Remember that there may not be an internal opening.

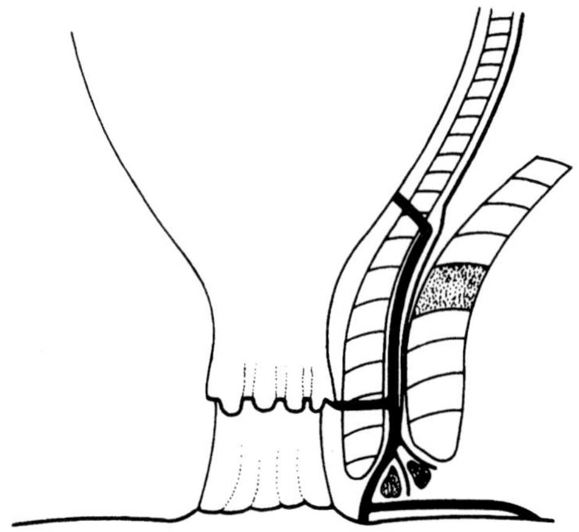

Fig. 18.15 Intersphincteric fistula. Note how the track may extend upwards into the rectum above the level of puborectalis and subcutaneously some distance from the anus.

Action

1 Insert a bivalve operating proctoscope and pass a fistula probe, such as Lockhart–Mummery's, or Anel's lacrimal probe, along the track. This runs parallel to the long axis of the anal canal.

KEY POINT Gentle manipulation

- Never force a probe or you may create false passages.

2 If there is a long subcutaneous track, the probe is directed from the external opening towards the anus. Lay it open and remove the granulation tissue with a curette. The upward extension between the sphincters becomes apparent as granulation tissue exudes from the opening.

3 Divide the internal sphincter as high as the tip of the probe. Again remove granulation tissue by curettage. If no granulation tissue protrudes from a residual part of the track, and palpation reveals no more induration, do nothing more.

4 If necessary, totally divide the internal sphincter and the muscle of the lower rectum completely, to lay open the fistula.

5 Create an adequate external wound to allow drainage.

6 Insert a gauze dressing soaked in normal saline solution surrounded by Surgicel. Do not pack the wound tightly.

7 Apply a perineal pad and pants.

TRANS-SPHINCTERIC FISTULA

1 In a trans-sphincteric fistula, the primary track passes across the external sphincter from the intersphincteric space to the ischiorectal fossa. The infection may also have drained across the internal sphincter into the anal canal, where you find the internal opening of the fistula, which is usually at the level of the anal valves (Fig. 18.16).

Assess

1 Have the anaesthetized patient in the lithotomy position with the buttocks well down over the end of the table. Invariably

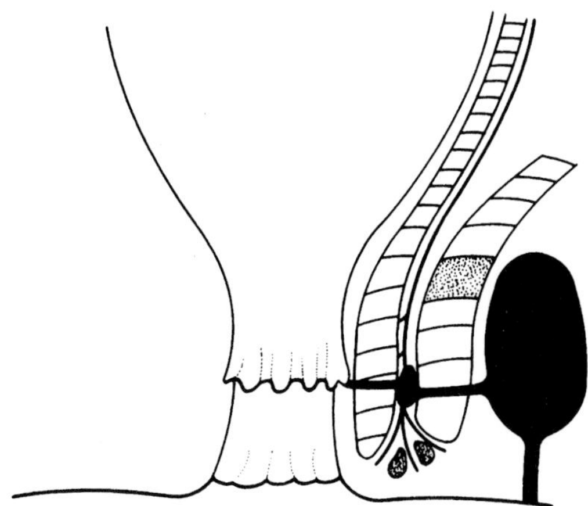

Fig. 18.16 Trans-sphincteric fistula.

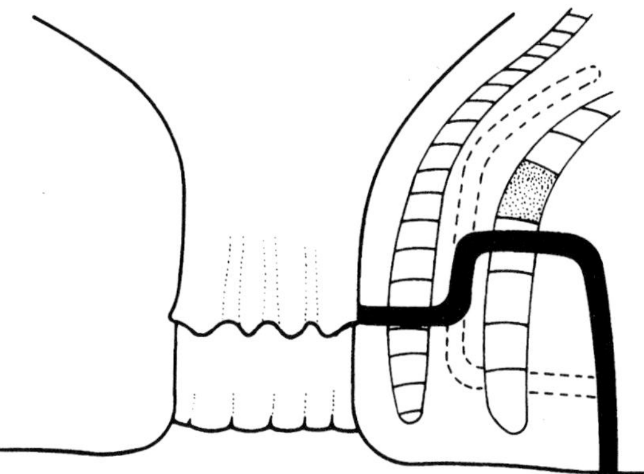

Fig. 18.17 The level at which the primary track crosses the external sphincter is not necessarily at the same level as the internal opening into the anal canal. It may be higher or lower; furthermore, there may be an upward intersphincteric extension.

perform sigmoidoscopy, especially looking for inflammatory bowel disease.

2 Palpate carefully for induration. The external opening(s) are usually laterally placed and indurated, but there is not usually any induration extending towards the anus subcutaneously in a trans-sphincteric fistula. You may palpate induration within the wall of the anal canal, the site of the primary anal gland infection. Induration is also detected under the levator ani muscles and is often circumferential. Palpate between a finger in the lower rectum, and thumb on the perianal skin, for a large area of induration. This is especially obvious if circumferential spread has not occurred and the contralateral side is normal.

KEY POINTS Complex presentations

- Remember that there may be no internal opening—the infection has not crossed the internal sphincter.
- If there is an internal opening at the level of the anal valves, the level at which the primary track crosses the external sphincter may not be the same—it may be lower or higher (Fig. 18.17).
- Infection can spread vertically in the intersphincteric space and open into the rectum, in addition to spreading across the external sphincter.
- Circumferential spread of infection and other secondary tracks may also develop.

Action

1 Pass a bivalve operating proctoscope in order to try and identify the internal opening.

2 Pass a Lockhart–Mummery probe into the external opening. It may extend several centimetres and can be felt very close to a finger in the rectum. Do not force the probe, and do not pass it into the rectum, as this is never the site of the internal opening.

3 If there is spread of infection towards the midline posteriorly, direct the probe previously inserted into the external opening, posteriorly towards the coccyx. With a scalpel (no. 10 blade) in the groove of the probe divide the tissue between the skin and the probe; divide skin and fat only, you should not divide any muscle. Apply tissue-holding forceps to the skin edges and secure any major bleeding points. Alternatively, perform the laying open with electrocautery.

4 Curette away granulation tissue, sending some for histopathological examination, and look for a forward extension from the site of the external opening. Lay it open.

5 Seek any extension of the sepsis to the opposite side by palpation, probing and looking for granulation tissue pouting from an opening in the previously curetted track. Use a no. 10 bladed knife or electrocautery to divide skin and fat to lay open any further tracks.

6 Insert the bivalve proctoscope again and re-identify the internal opening. It may or may not be possible to pass a probe either through the internal opening into the previously opened tracks or from the previously opened tracks into the anal canal.

7 Divide the anal canal epithelium and the internal sphincter to the level of the internal opening, if present, with a no. 15 bladed knife or electrocautery, thus opening up the intersphincteric space. If there is no internal opening, open the intersphincteric space in a similar way, to the level of the anal valves. Curette any granulation tissue.

8 Now identify the primary track across the external sphincter. If it is at or below the line of the anal valves, divide the muscle. If it is higher, as it often is, it may be possible to divide the muscle, but determining this requires considerable experience. It is often safer to drain the track by inserting a length of fine silicone tubing (1 mm diameter) or no. 1 braided suture material (seton). Monofilaments such as nylon are often uncomfortable for the patient because of the sharp ends beyond the knot.

? DIFFICULTY

1. Accurate definition of a complex fistula can be difficult. Do not be tempted to risk causing incontinence by dividing the external sphincter.
2. Insert a loose seton (Latin: *seta*=bristle; a ligature threaded through the track), and order a magnetic resonance imaging (MRI) scan to clarify the situation; you can then plan effective and safe definitive treatment.

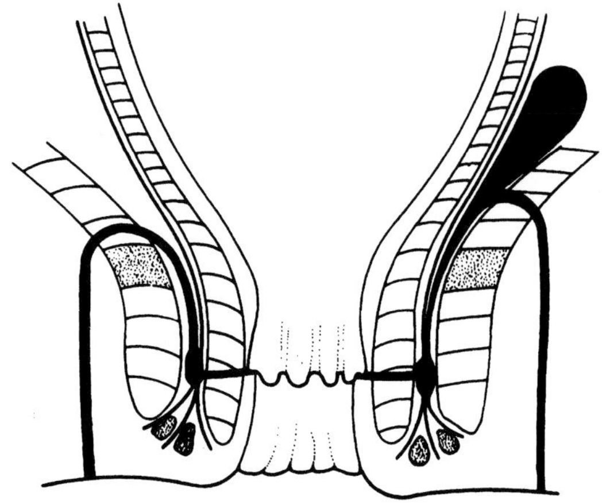

Fig. 18.18 Suprasphincteric fistula. There may be an associated supralevator abscess.

9 Once all the septic areas have been drained, fashion the wound so that drainage can continue and the wound can heal from its depths. You almost certainly need to trim the skin and fat.

KEY POINTS The phases of the procedure

- Drain the secondary tracks
- Drain the intersphincteric abscess of origin
- Drain the primary track, either by dividing the muscle or by inserting a seton.

10 Insert gauze dressings soaked in normal saline surrounded by Surgicel into the wounds and the anal canal. Do not pack the dressings tightly.

11 Apply a perineal pad and pants.

SUPRASPHINCTERIC FISTULA

- In a suprasphincteric fistula, the primary track crosses the striated muscle above all the muscles of continence (Fig. 18.18). As this is a variant of a 'high' trans-sphincteric fistula, manage it on similar principles.
- This is a very rare form of fistula. When possible refer the patient to a surgeon specializing in this field.

EXTRASPHINCTERIC FISTULA

1 An extrasphincteric fistula arising from an upward extension of infection from the ischiorectal fossa is also unusual, possibly due to the injudicious use of a probe during operation.

2 Create a defunctioning loop colostomy as a preliminary to closing the opening in the rectum and treat the fistula along the lines indicated above.

3 Manage a fistula arising from pelvic sepsis from, for example, acute appendicitis, Crohn's disease or diverticular disease, and not, therefore, of anal gland origin, by treating the primary disease (see Chs 14, 16).

POSTOPERATIVE

1 Remove the dressing on the second or third postoperative day after giving an intramuscular injection of pethidine 100 mg or papaveretum 7–15 mg. Carry out the first dressing in the operating theatre under general anaesthesia if the wound is very extensive.

2 Initiate a routine of twice-daily baths, irrigation of the wound and insertion of gauze soaked in physiological saline.

3 Inspect the wound at regular intervals until healing is complete.

4 Encourage the bowel movements to coincide with these dressing times by giving laxatives. If they do not coincide, arrange bath–irrigation–dressing routines as necessary.

5 If there is voluminous discharge of pus, review the wound in the operating theatre under general anaesthesia after 10–14 days. In patients with large wounds, this may need to be repeated. Lay open any residual tracks and curette away the granulation tissue.

6 Administer antimicrobial agents such as erythromycin 250 mg 8-hourly and metronidazole 400 mg 8-hourly for up to 28 days, to assist in the elimination of the sepsis.

7 A seton does not complicate the postoperative routine. Allow the wound to heal around it; this may take 3 months. Then, under general anaesthesia, remove the seton and curette its track free of granulation tissue. Spontaneous healing occurs in approximately 40% of patients. If healing does not occur, lay open the residual track. The advantage of this staged division of the external sphincter is that healing occurs around the 'scaffolding' of the external sphincter. When it is subsequently divided—and this is not always necessary—its ends separate only slightly. This produces a better functional result than if it were divided at the outset.

COMPLICATIONS

1 Failure to heal may be from inadequate or inappropriate drainage of intersphincteric abscess of origin, or of secondary tracks, or of the primary track. Give the nurses clear instructions and advice about the dressings. Inadequate postoperative dressings allow bridging of the wound edges and pocketing of pus. If there is excessive growth of granulation tissue, cauterize it with silver nitrate or curette it away under general anaesthetic.

KEY POINTS Slow healing?

- Is the patient malnourished or suffering from zinc deficiency?
- If hairs are growing into the wound, shave the area.
- Have you missed a specific cause for the fistula, such as Crohn's disease?

2 Secondary haemorrhage may occur from any potentially septic open wound, healing by second intention.

3 Anal incontinence of varying degrees may follow division of the sphincter muscles. If all the sphincter complex has inadvertently

been divided, consider repairing it once the sepsis has been eradicated and healing has occurred.

4 Successful fistula surgery depends upon accurate definition of the pathological anatomy, drainage of the intersphincteric abscess of origin, the primary and secondary tracks, and excellent postoperative wound care.

OTHER PROCEDURES

- A tight seton is designed to cut through the fistula track slowly, in the hope of reducing the separation of muscle ends. Apply it firmly but not tightly. Replace it at monthly intervals.
- Specialist colorectal surgeons may create advancement flaps to avoid sphincter division and employ an intersphincteric approach and core-out fistulectomy. About 50% only succeed. They are employed particularly in high trans-sphincteric fistulae, especially when situated anteriorly in women, who have a short anal canal.

PILONIDAL DISEASE

A simple pilonidal sinus detected as a chance finding during routine examination probably does not require treatment. Operate only if it is painful or infected, producing a pilonidal abscess.

Prepare

Place the anaesthetized patient in the left lateral position with the right buttock strapped to hold it up. Elastic adhesive strapping is adequate and adheres better if the skin has been sprayed with compound tincture of benzoin. Carefully shave the area.

Action

1 Determine the extent of sepsis by palpation for induration and by using probes.

2 Completely excise the skin of the septic area.

3 Curette away the granulation tissue and embedded hairs.

4 Check with a probe in the base of the wound to detect any side tracks, and look for any residual granulation tissue that may be pouting from a side track.

5 Fashion the wound so that there are no overhanging edges.

6 Stop bleeding.

7 Dress the wound with gauze soaked in physiological saline solution and apply pressure to it.

Postoperative

1 Initiate a twice-daily routine of bath, irrigation and dressing.

2 Keep the wound edges shaved.

3 Cauterize any excess granulation tissue with silver nitrate.

4 Complications include haemorrhage, delayed healing and recurrence. If necessary, repeat the operative procedure to get healing.

OTHER PROCEDURES

1 Lay open a simple pilonidal sinus and marsupialize (Latin: *marsupium*=pouch; create a pouch with an open mouth) the wound. This keeps the wound open until the interior has filled up.

2 In Bascom's operation each pit is excised with a no. 11 bladed knife. Drain the cavity through a laterally placed incision.

3 Various rotation flaps can be used, all having the objective of avoiding a midline suture line.

HIDRADENITIS SUPPURATIVA

Appraise

1 Hidradenitis (Greek: *hidros*=sweat+*aden*=gland+*itis*=inflammation) suppurativa (Latin: =pus-forming) is a septic process that involves the apocrine (Greek: *apo*=off+*krinein*=to separate; the secretion is a breakdown product of the cell) sweat glands. It occurs in the perineum as well as the axillae.

2 Recurrent abscess formation often results from inadequate drainage. There is no communication with the anal canal and the infection is superficial. Occasionally, hidradenitis occurs in association with Crohn's disease and lithium therapy.

3 Combine surgical treatment of acute abscesses with continuing dermatological input as topical or systemic antimicrobial agents, retinoids, hormonal therapy and immunosuppressive medications may also help to control the disease.

Action

1 Drain the pus from each abscess. They are often multiple and may intercommunicate.

2 Curette away all the granulation tissue.

3 Remove all overhanging skin.

4 Allow the defect to heal by second intention.

5 In very severe cases it may be necessary to excise and graft an area most affected in order to prevent multiple recurrences.

ANAL MANIFESTATIONS OF CROHN'S DISEASE

Appraise

1 These occur in approximately 50% of patients affected with Crohn's disease.

2 The perianal area has a bluish discoloration and there may be oedematous skin tags. Ulceration, which can be extensive, may involve the perianal skin, anal margin and anal canal. Sepsis may occur in the form of either an abscess or a fistula (Fig. 18.19).

KEY POINT Suspect Crohn's disease

- Always think of the possibility of anal Crohn's disease. This may be the first manifestation of the condition.

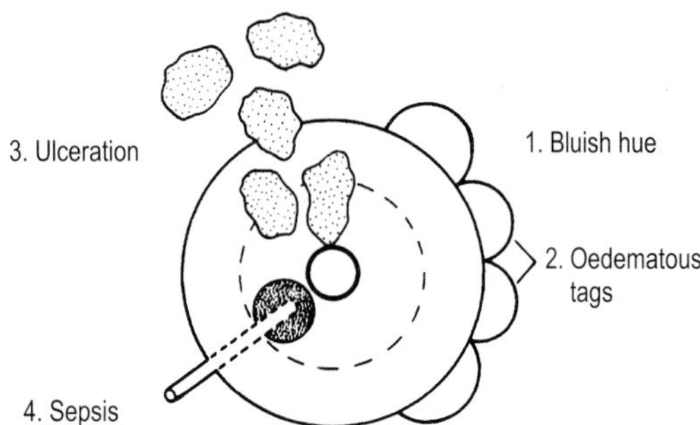

Fig. 18.19 Diagram to show the anal manifestations of Crohn's disease.

Action

1 Remove a small biopsy specimen of a skin tag, or granulation tissue together with a rectal mucosal biopsy for histopathological examination.

2 Drain any abscess in the usual way, taking care not to divide any muscle.

3 For long-term seton drainage of fistulae prefer a soft suture material such as no. 1 Ethibond. By using 2/0 silk a secure knot can be tied without the need for too many 'throws' that would create a bulky knot. Finally turn the knot so that it lies within the track, leaving only a smooth loop of suture on the outside.

4 Fully investigate the patient.

CONDYLOMATA ACUMINATA

Appraise

1 Condylomata acuminata (warts) result from human papillomavirus (HPV) infection of the squamous epithelium. Papilliferous lesions may develop on the perianal skin, within the anal canal and on the genitalia. Exclude other forms of sexually transmitted disease and attempt to trace contacts.

2 Treat scattered lesions by applying 25% podophyllin in compound benzoin tincture. Treat more extensive lesions by operation—a technique of scissors excision.

Action

1 Have the anaesthetized patient placed in the lithotomy or prone jack-knife positions.

2 Infiltrate a solution of 1:300 000 adrenaline (epinephrine) in normal saline under the epithelium bearing the perianal lesions, to reduce bleeding when you excise the warts, and to separate the individual lesions to preserve the maximum amount of normal skin.

3 Hold the warts with fine-toothed forceps and remove them with pointed scissors.

4 Remove intra-anal canal warts in the same way after inserting a bivalve operating proctoscope. There is often a confluent ring of lesions in the upper anal canal. Totally remove these and then join the mucosa of the lower rectum to that of the anal canal at the dentate line with sutures (Fig. 18.20). In addition to achieving mucosal apposition, this mucosal anastomosis is haemostatic.

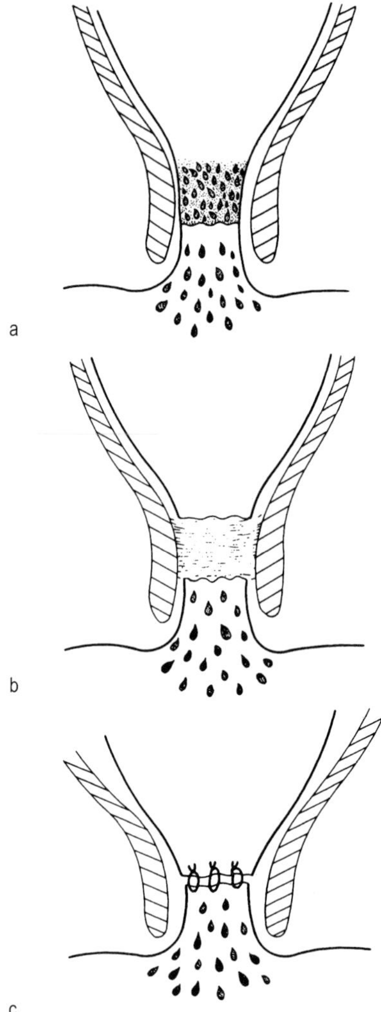

Fig. 18.20 (a) Confluent intra-anal canal warts above the dentate line. (b) The warts, together with all the mucosa, are removed, leaving a section of muscle denuded of mucosa. (c) The lower rectal mucosa is attached to the dentate line by means of a series of catgut sutures.

5 Send the excised lesions, particularly the intra-anal ones, for histopathological examination.

Postoperative

1 No special measures are needed.

2 Carry out regular examinations to detect further wart formation, which usually occurs within the first 3 months. Treat scattered lesions with podophyllin. More extensive recurrences require further inpatient treatment.

ANAL TUMOURS

Tumours in this region may be divided into two groups, although opinions differ as to the anatomical level of division.

For the purposes of this chapter anal canal tumours arise from the dentate line and above. Anal margin tumours arise below the dentate line.

ANAL MARGIN TUMOURS

Appraise

1 These may be benign or malignant. Condylomata acuminata, kerato-acanthoma, apocrine gland tumours, premalignant Bowen's disease and Paget's disease are benign.

2 Excise condylomata acuminata (warts) with scissors as above.

3 Totally excise other tumours. If the defect is not too large allow the wound to heal by second intention. Close large defects with split skin grafts.

4 Histopathological information is essential in deciding whether or not any further treatment is required.

5 Malignant tumours of the anal margin are mainly squamous cell carcinomas, although basal cell carcinoma can occur. Induration suggests malignancy. Small microinvasive carcinomas can be adequately treated by wide local excision, but more advanced cancers require a combination of radiotherapy and chemotherapy (see below).

ANAL CANAL TUMOURS

Appraise

1 These are almost always malignant and include squamous cell carcinoma, basaloid carcinoma, adenocarcinoma and malignant melanoma.

2 Examine the tumour under anaesthesia and remove a biopsy specimen.

3 There is virtually no indication for local excision in infiltrative squamous carcinoma of the anal canal, which may be treated conservatively in the majority of cases, by primary radiotherapy with chemotherapy. Reserve operation for dealing with residual tumour, complications of therapy or subsequent tumour recurrence.

4 If surgery is indicated after failed combined modality therapy, then this usually requires abdominoperineal excision of the rectum (see Ch. 16) and anal canal, widely excising the perianal skin, ischiorectal fossa fat and the levator ani muscles near the lateral pelvic wall. Ensure that you have positive histology after radiochemotherapy of a squamous carcinoma prior to performing an abdominoperineal resection.

RECTAL ADENOMAS

Appraise

1 Adenomas of the rectum may be classified on a histopathological basis into tubular, tubulovillous and villous. From the clinical viewpoint these three types of adenoma are similar in their behaviour as there is no invasion of neoplastic cells across the muscularis mucosae. A more useful classification is according to their clinical appearance; for example, are they pedunculated or sessile?

2 Are there any other neoplastic lesions—benign or malignant—in the large intestine? In patients with lesions more than 2 cm in diameter, there is an incidence of further tumours of 25% (benign 18%, malignant 7%). Order a colonoscopy.

> **KEY POINT Familial disease?**
>
> - Multiple small adenomatous polyps in the rectum suggest the diagnosis of familial adenomatous polyposis.

3 Is the lesion totally benign or does it have malignant areas? There is a 50% chance of malignant areas in patients with lesions larger than 2 cm in diameter.

4 Be sure to remove the whole lesion, a total excision biopsy, which is diagnostic as well as therapeutic if the lesion proves to be totally benign. Do not perform an incision biopsy as it is not representative of the whole lesion and makes subsequent submucosal excision difficult.

Action

1 Totally remove lesions less than 5 mm across, by twisting with a pair of Patterson biopsy forceps.

2 Employ diathermy snare excision for those that are pedunculated.

3 Submucosally excise those that are sessile, non-circumferential and confined to the lower two-thirds of the rectum (see below).

4 Those in the lower third of the rectum that are circumferential may be suitably excised by a modified Soave operation (see below).

5 Employ anterior resection for sessile non-circumferential tumours with the lower border in the upper third of the rectum, and circumferential tumours with the lower border in the upper two-thirds of the rectum.

SUBMUCOSAL EXCISION OF SESSILE ADENOMA

Appraise

1 Undertake this technique only if there are no malignant lesions at a higher level. Resect a carcinoma of the sigmoid colon first.

2 Undertake this technique provided the tumour does not feel indurated on palpation with the finger or the end of the sigmoidoscope, suggesting malignant change.

Prepare

1 Order full bowel preparation.

2 Place the patient in the lithotomy position or the jack-knife position, which is especially suitable for anterior lesions.

Action

1 Insert a bivalve operating proctoscope and ensure that illumination is adequate. You may find it advisable to wear a headlamp.

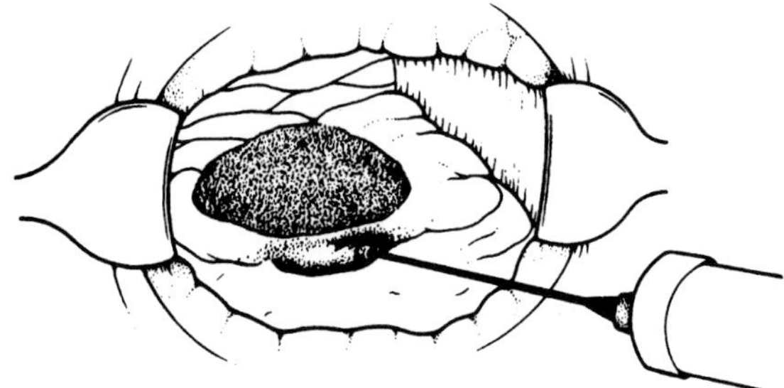

Fig. 18.21 1:300000 adrenaline (epinephrine) in normal saline is injected into the submucosa to elevate the mucosa and the tumour within it. This will prove difficult if there has been a previous incision biopsy, or malignancy is present.

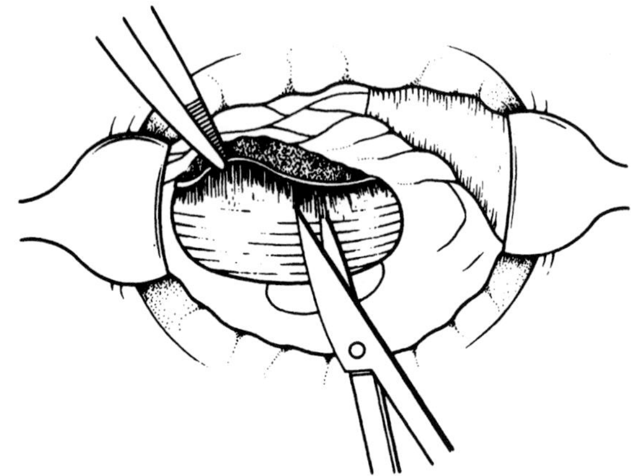

Fig. 18.22 The mucosa is dissected from the underlying circular muscle (white fibres).

2 Inject 1:300000 adrenaline (epinephrine) in physiological saline into the submucosa under the tumour.

KEY POINT Cause for suspicion

- Benign tumours are entirely mucosal; therefore, if you find it difficult to create artificial oedema in the submucosa, suspect malignant invasion (Fig. 18.21).

3 With sharp scissors or electrocautery incise the mucosa approximately 1 cm from the edge of the tumour and then dissect it free of the circular muscle of the rectum, which appears as white fibres in the distended submucosal layer (Fig. 18.22).

4 Seal bleeding points with diathermy.

5 Allow the wound to heal spontaneously without suturing it. Close any defect you inadvertently created in the muscle with sutures.

6 Pin the specimen to a cork board before fixing it, so that the pathologist can determine whether or not there is any malignant invasion, by taking serial sections (Fig. 18.23).

Postoperative

1 No special measures need be adopted other than to ensure that constipation does not occur.

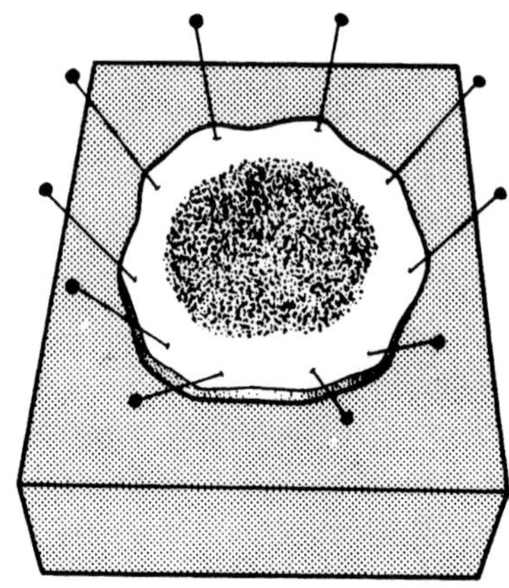

Fig. 18.23 The specimen with a margin of normal mucosa is pinned to a cork board prior to fixing to assist the histopathologist.

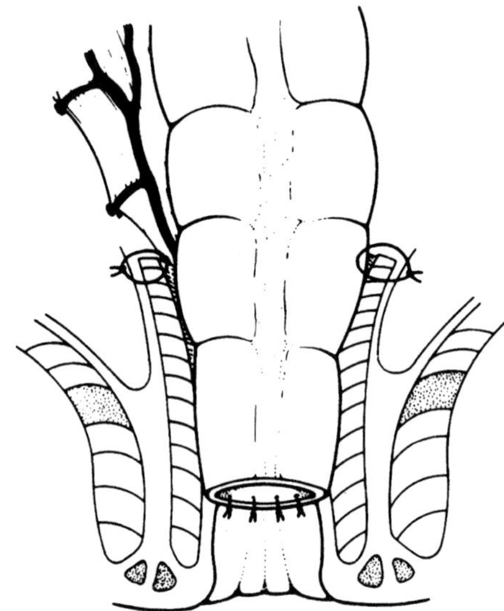

Fig. 18.24 Modified Soave operation. The mucosa has been removed from the distal rectum by both the abdominal and perineal surgeon. The descending colon is now passed into the muscle tube and sutured at the dentate line.

2 Haemorrhage is a rare complication.

3 Study the histopathological report. If there are malignant foci, decide whether or not to proceed to a more radical procedure.

4 Follow up the patient to detect any recurrence and metachronous (sequential but separated by appreciable intervals) lesions.

5 Stenosis of the rectum may develop if excision was performed for too large a lesion.

MODIFIED SOAVE OPERATION

1 Reserve this operation for large circumferential lesions with their lower border in the lower third of the rectum and extending into the upper third.

2 In principle, all the tumour is excised submucosally by a combined abdominal and per-anal approach. The rectal muscular tube is relined with descending colon, anastomosed through the anus to the level of the dentate line (Fig. 18.24).

3 Circumferential lesions extending over only a few centimetres can be treated by submucosal excision, with plication of the muscle tube to allow mucosal anastomosis.

4 This is an unusual operation best reserved for performance in a specialist centre.

RECTAL PROLAPSE

Appraise

1 The symptom of prolapse (i.e. tissue slipping through the anus) may result from causes other than complete rectal prolapse. Distinguish haemorrhoids, anal polyps, mucosal prolapse and rectal adenomas.

2 Treatment consists of control of the prolapse, re-education of the bowel habit and improvement, if necessary, of sphincter function.

3 First control the prolapse. While an internally intussuscepted rectum lies in the lower third of the rectum (the first phase of prolapse), sphincter function is inhibited, as it will be as a complete prolapse passes through the anal sphincter and keeps it open. Many operations have been described to achieve control. In the UK, complete rectal prolapse is usually treated either by abdominal rectopexy or by perineal mucosal sleeve resection (Delorme's procedure, see below).

4 Abdominal rectopexy is associated with unpredictable postoperative constipation, which in some patients can be severe. There are claims that concomitant sigmoid resection (resection rectopexy, also known as the Frykman–Goldberg operation) reduces this risk.

5 After rectopexy only a few patients have sphincter dysfunction severe enough to produce significant incontinence. Pelvic floor physiotherapy, faradism and electrical stimulators give little long-term benefit. The problem is anatomically the result of pelvic floor neurogenic myopathy producing a shortened anal canal with widening of the anorectal angle. Postanal pelvic floor repair reduces the anorectal angle and lengthens the anal canal, restoring satisfactory continence in some patients.

6 All abdominal pelvic dissection in male patients has the potential to cause either erectile or ejaculatory dysfunction. Because of this it is now required that the aspect has been mentioned and recorded when obtaining informed consent.

ABDOMINAL RECTOPEXY

Prepare

1 Order full bowel preparation (see Ch. 16). Warn the nurses that as these patients have defective sphincter function they may be incontinent during preparation.

2 Order metronidazole 500 mg intravenously and gentamicin 80 mg intravenously at induction of anaesthesia.

3 The patient should be catheterized.

4 Place the anaesthetized patient in the Lloyd-Davies (lithotomy Trendelenburg) position.

Action

1 Make a midline or Pfannenstiel incision.

2 Carry out full exploration.

3 Mobilize the sigmoid colon by dividing the congenital adhesions.

4 Starting at the level of the sacral promontory, incise the peritoneum beside (but not damaging) the superior haemorrhoidal artery. The ureters lie laterally on both sides, but always check their position. The presacral nerves lie just behind the superior haemorrhoidal artery; take care to preserve them. Extend the peritoneal incision to the bottom of the prerectal pouch, then across the midline between the rectum and vagina or bladder, so that the rectum may be separated from them.

5 Enter the postrectal space and open it up by dissection, holding the rectum forward with your left hand or a tipped anterior St Mark's retractor. Exert adequate tension on the rectum to display the areolar tissue. Seal any vessels with diathermy.

6 Now that the anterior and posterior dissection of the rectum is complete its only attachments are the two lateral ligaments. It is arguable whether or not these should be divided.

7 Achieve perfect haemostasis.

8 Place two no. 1 nylon stitches between the upper parts of the lateral ligaments on each side and the vertebral disc just distal to the sacral promontory; avoid the median sacral artery. These will suspend the rectum while scarring fixes it in place.

9 Observe whether the sigmoid loop is redundant. If it is, and particularly if there is a background history of constipation, perform sigmoid resection with end-to-end anastomosis. Otherwise it is not worth resecting the sigmoid colon (Fig. 18.25).

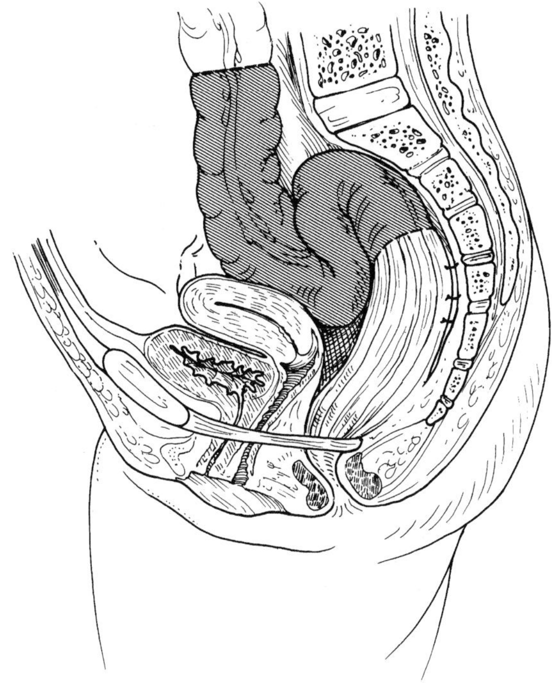

Fig. 18.25 Abdominal rectopexy can be done with or without sigmoid resection and is now usually achieved simply with a series of non-absorbable sutures rather than as previously with sponge or mesh.

10 A drain is not usually necessary, but if there is a persistent collection of blood and fluid in the pelvis, insert a tube drain for 24 hours.

11 Close the abdominal wound.

Postoperative

1 Maintain the patient on intravenous fluids. Allow the patient to drink when there are good bowel sounds and flatus has been passed.

2 Remove the catheter on the fifth postoperative day after sending a sample of urine for culture.

3 Avoid constipation. Give a mild osmotic laxative such as milk of magnesia to initiate bowel movement. Subsequently use suppositories such as glycerine and bisacodyl.

Complications

1 Haemorrhage may lead to a pelvic haematoma.

2 Postoperative constipation is unpredictable and can be troublesome.

MUCOSAL SLEEVE RESECTION (DELORME)

The functional results of this procedure (Fig. 18.26) are good and it is particularly useful if the prolapse is small or incomplete and in high-risk patients who are unsuitable for abdominal surgery.

Prepare

1 Order a full bowel preparation.

2 The patient is given general or regional anaesthesia and lies in the lithotomy position.

Action

1 Reproduce the prolapse and infiltrate the submucosal plane with saline containing 1:300 000 adrenaline (epinephrine) to facilitate the dissection and to limit bleeding.

2 Make a circumferential incision through the mucosa 1 cm proximal to the dentate line.

3 Develop the submucosal plane circumferentially using either scissors dissection or electrocautery until you reach the apex of the prolapse.

4 Continue the dissection back up inside the prolapsed rectum until close to the level of the anus. Unless you do this, only half of the prolapse will have been treated.

5 Re-approximate the mucosal edges using interrupted 2/0 polyglactin 910 (Vicryl) sutures, which are also used to plicate the denuded rectal wall. Ensure that each suture takes several bites of the rectal wall in order to obliterate any potential dead space beneath the mucosa.

6 The plicated rectal wall returns to the pelvis and lies above the sphincter, preventing further prolapse.

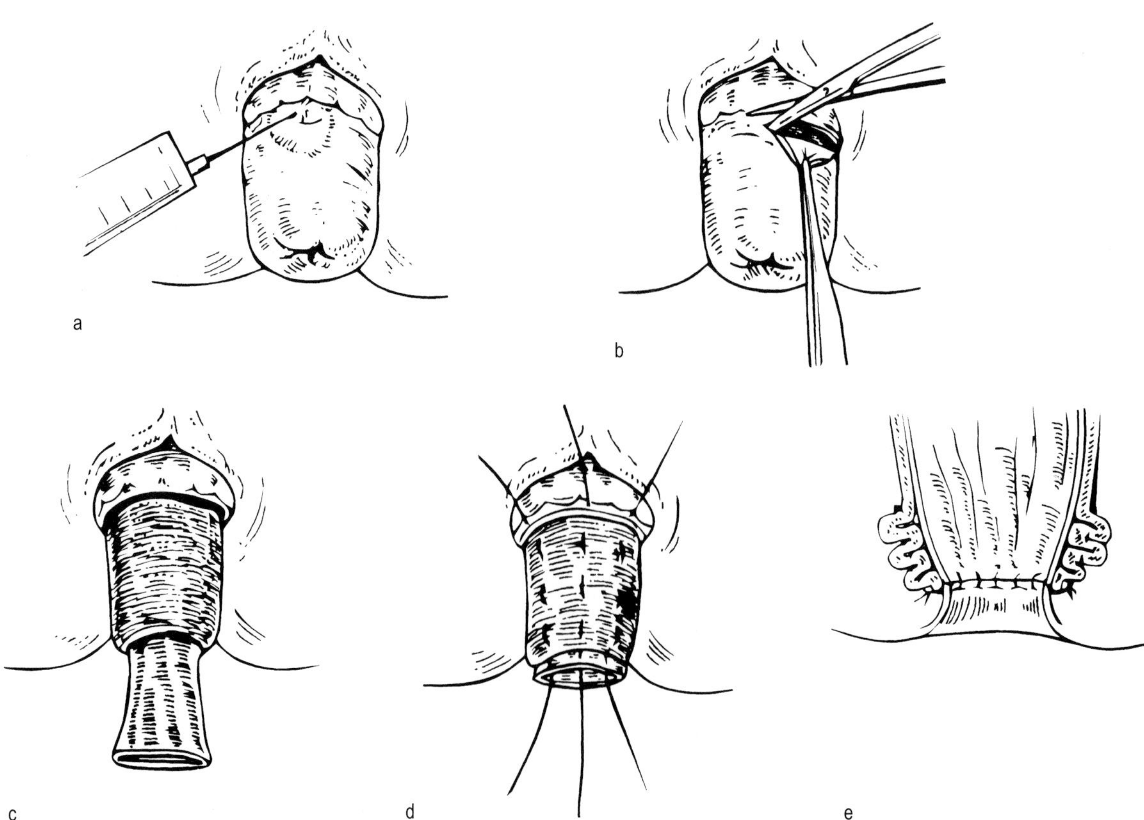

Fig. 18.26 Delorme's procedure. The mucosal prolapse has been excised and interrupted sutures used to re-approximate the mucosal edges and plicate the rectal wall.

Postoperative

1 Avoid constipation by using an osmotic laxative.

2 Complications can include haemorrhage, anastomotic breakdown and stricture formation.

FAECAL INCONTINENCE

Appraise

1 Determine the cause of faecal incontinence. If the anal sphincter is normal consider causes such as faecal impaction or irritable bowel. If the anal sphincter is abnormal consider the possibility of a congenital abnormality, complete rectal prolapse (see above), a lower motor neurone lesion, disruption of the sphincter ring due to trauma (including surgical and obstetric trauma) or muscle atrophy.

2 Operative treatment may be employed for the correction of some congenital abnormalities, complete rectal prolapse and simple disruption of the external sphincter (sphincter repair). Severe incontinence may need to be treated with the implantation of an artificial bowel sphincter. Sacral nerve stimulation is an alternative approach which is gaining in popularity.

3 Disruption of the sphincter ring may be suggested by a history of trauma—accidental, obstetric or surgical—and diagnosed by detecting a defect in the sphincter ring. Such a defect is best demonstrated using endoanal ultrasound.

INJECTION OF BULKING AGENTS

1 The use of polytetrafluoroethylene (Teflon or polytef) was first reported in the context of a weakened or defective internal anal sphincter muscle by Shafik in 1993.

2 Other reports are limited in number and restricted to pilot studies. They include injections with autologous fat, glutaraldehyde cross-linked collagen injection (Contigen), polydimethylsiloxane (PTP) implants and Durasphere.

3 New agents are now under trial in both the urinary and the faecal incontinence setting. Contigen and Durasphere have FDA approval in the USA; only PTP implants are currently licensed for use in the UK.

Prepare

1 The patient should be put onto laxatives 2 days pre-injection to continue for a week after injection.

2 An enema can be given preprocedure.

3 If the procedure is to be performed under local anaesthesia, a local anaesthetic cream can be used prior to injection of the anaesthetic agent.

4 Antibiotics are given intravenously at the time of the first injection and continued orally for a week after.

Action

1 There is little agreement on the optimal injection methodology.

2 The patient may be in the prone jack-knife, lithotomy or left lateral position.

3 Injections are sometimes given circumferentially in all patients and sometimes only into a defect in those with a single internal anal sphincter defect.

4 Trans-sphincteric injection may reduce infection when compared to direct anal canal injection.

5 The site of the injection may be guided by the index finger to avoid any dispersal of product; however, some centres prefer to use a retractor or ultrasound guidance.

OVERLAPPING SPHINCTER REPAIR

A colostomy is necessary only in complex cases, such as patients with Crohn's disease, a rectovaginal fistula, or where the injury is very extensive (e.g. cloacal).

Prepare

1 Order a full bowel preparation.

2 The patient is given a general anaesthetic and lies in the supine position for construction of the loop sigmoid colostomy (see Ch. 17). Then place the patient in the lithotomy position for the sphincter repair.

3 Pass a urinary catheter.

Action

1 Make an incision following the slight pigment change seen around the anus. Centre it on the point of injury; it usually extends 180° (Fig. 18.27).

2 Dissect out into ischiorectal fat. This means that the anal sphincter now lies between the depths of the wound and the anal canal (Fig. 18.28).

3 For an anterior, usually obstetric, injury mobilize the anus from the vagina. It helps to place two fingers in the vagina and two Allis forceps on the anal margin of the wound. The plane lies fractionally posterior to any large veins (because these will be paravaginal veins) (Fig. 18.29).

4 Split the muscle scar down its length and develop the plain between the anal mucosa and the muscle on either side.

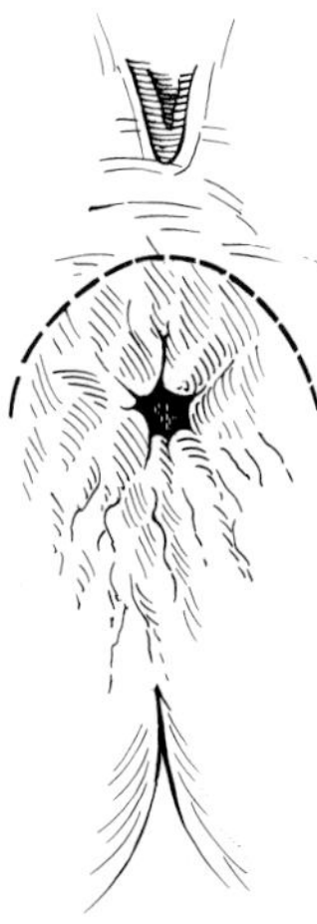

Fig. 18.27 The incision should follow the slight pigment change seen around the anus. It should be centred on the point of injury and will usually extend 180°.

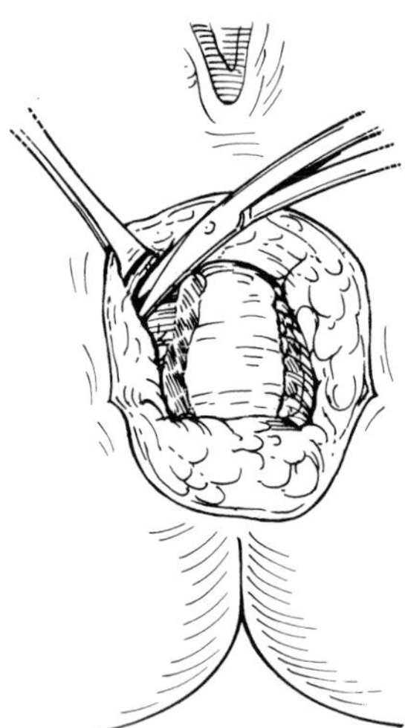

Fig. 18.28 Dissect out laterally into ischiorectal fat. This means that the anal sphincter now lies between the depths of the wound and the anal canal.

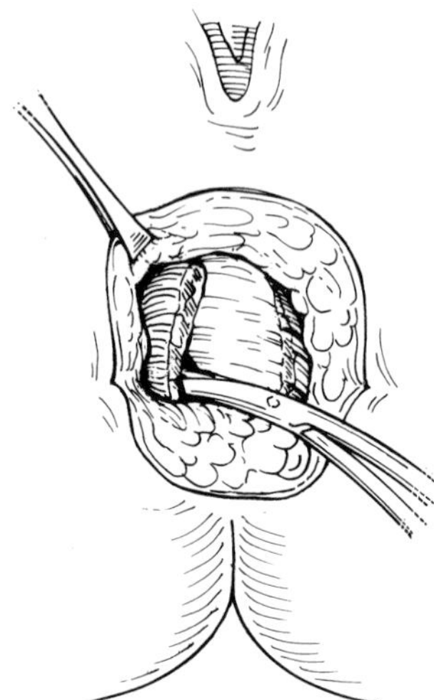

Fig. 18.29 Next, dissect close to the anal mucosa. This leaves a bulk of tissue between the lateral ischiorectal plane and the perianal plane that will contain the divided ends of internal and external sphincter.

5 After sufficient mobilization you can achieve a muscle overlap of about 2 cm, extending the length of the anal canal. Suture with 2/0 polydioxanone (PDS) (Fig. 18.30).

6 When possible, close the wound. Otherwise leave it open to heal by second intention (Fig. 18.31).

Postoperative

1 The patient can eat and drink normally and does not need confinement of the bowels.

SACRAL NERVE STIMULATION

1 This is performed in two stages: a temporary testing phase and a permanent implant for those patients who are found to gain benefit during the testing phase.

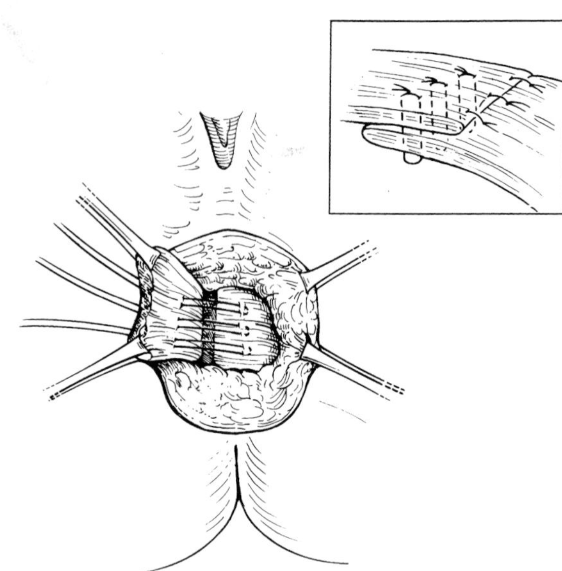

Fig. 18.30 After sufficient mobilization a muscle overlap of about 2 cm can be achieved extending the length of the anal canal. Suture with 2/0 polydioxanone (PDS).

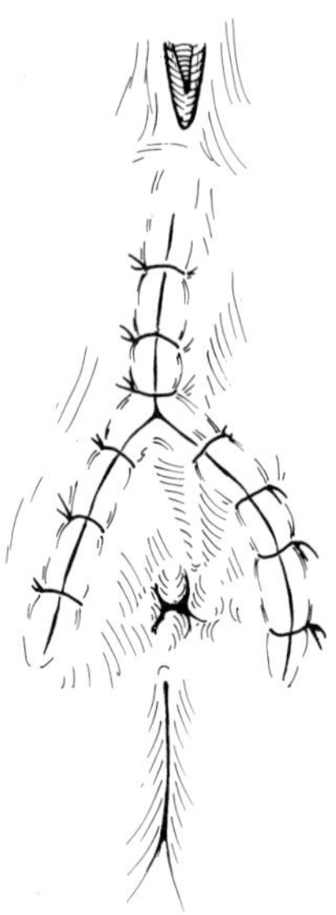

Fig. 18.31 When possible, close the wound. It may help to close it in an inverted 'Y' fashion allowing reconstruction of the perineal body and lengthening the distance between the posterior forchette and the anal canal. Otherwise leave it open to heal by second intention.

2 There is no need for any bowel preparation.

3 The patient is given a general anaesthetic without muscle relaxants and lies in the prone jack-knife position. The anus and the big toes should be visible.

TEMPORARY TEST WIRE INSERTION

Action

1 Mark out the bony landmarks for the position of the S3 foramina. They are typically 1 cm cephalad to the crest of the sacrum and 1 cm lateral to the midline.

2 Insert the 20G, 3.5-inch (9-cm) spinal insulated needles (Medtronic 041828-004) into S3 on either side and find the best response to stimulation using an external, hand-held neurostimulator (Medtronic Model 3625 Screener). The current used for stimulation usually ranges from 0.5 to 2 mA at a rate of 20 Hz and a pulse width of 200 seconds.

3 Response to the stimulus is assessed clinically, looking for deepening and flattening of the buttock groove from lifting and dropping of the pelvic floor—known as a 'bellows' action—and a flexion of the big toe.

4 If the response if suboptimal it may be necessary to insert the needles into S2 or S4. Stimulation at the level of S2 usually causes a clamp-like contraction of the anal sphincter with rotation of the leg, ankle flexion and calf contraction. S4 is associated with a 'bellows' action and a pulling sensation on the perineum but not with any toe movement.

5 Using the foramen of maximal response, thread a temporary percutaneous stimulator test lead (Medtronic 3057) down through the needle and re-test the adequacy of the stimulation with the external stimulator and the wire. If a good response is still obtained slide the needle out over the wire being very careful not to dislodge the wire. Secure the wire.

Postoperative

1 When the patient is awake and co-operative, attach the wire to the external stimulator (Medtronic Model 3625 Screener).

2 The stimulus employed for the 3-week temporary test phase is that which is the maximum comfortably tolerated by the patient, and usually ranges between 0.5 and 3 mA at 15 pulses/second with a pulse width of 210 microseconds.

THE PERMANENT IMPLANT

The decision to proceed to permanent implantation is based on the patient's and the doctor's subjective assessment of a significant improvement and on a 50% quantitative improvement in episodes of faecal incontinence—either frequency or amount lost.

Action

1 The initial steps taken to find the correct foramen during the test are repeated. The permanent electrode (Medtronic 3093) is then inserted instead of the wire and this self-secures itself with barbs. This is then tunnelled subcutaneously out to the permanent stimulator which is implanted in the buttock.

2 The stimulator is left turned off until the patient is awake and responsive.

Postoperative

The stimulator is externally programmed using telemetry. The current required for stimulation is usually between 0.5 and 2 volts at a frequency of 15 pulses/second and a pulse width of 210 microseconds.

ARTIFICIAL BOWEL SPHINCTER (THE ACTICON)

The operation to implant the Acticon is relatively simple; however, infection is a major hazard and preoperative preparation should be meticulous.

Prepare

1 Order a full bowel preparation.

2 Irrigate the rectal and vagina with Betadine wash-outs.

3 Get the patient to shower in antiseptic.

4 Swab the patient for MRSA (methicillin-resistant *Staphylococcus aureus*).

5 Plan to use adequate antibiotic cover in the perioperative period.

Action

1 Make an incision similar to that for an anterior overlapping repair arcing around the front of the anus.

2 A tunnel is then created around the outside of the anal sphincters to accommodate the hydraulic cuff. Sizers can be used to assess the size of the cuff to be implanted. All parts of the sphincter are carefully primed with radio-opaque fluid with the exclusion of all air bubbles prior to implantation.

3 A further 'bikini-line' incision a few centimetres long is then made on the side chosen for implantation of the pump (this depends on whether the patient is right- or left-handed).

4 The connector tube from the cuff is tunnelled up to the abdominal incision; the pump and the preperitoneal reservoir are implanted through the same incision. The pump sits in the labia majorum in women and in the scrotum in men. All three major components are connected by fully implanted silicone tubing.

5 The pump is squeezed to achieve cuff deflation via a temporary transfer of fluid into the balloon. A push-button device on the pump locks the pump closed until healing has occurred at about 6 weeks.

Postoperative

1 Continence is restored by re-activating the pump with a sharp squeeze in the clinic setting at about 6 weeks.

2 Time must be spent with the patient to ensure his full understanding of the pump mechanism or he may not be able to pass stools on discharge.

FURTHER READING

Beck DE, Wexner SD 1998 Fundamentals of anorectal surgery, 2nd edn. Saunders, Philadelphia

Fielding LP, Goldberg SM 1993 Rob and Smith's operative surgery, 5th edn. Butterworth-Heinemann, Oxford

Goldberg SM, Gordon PH, Nivatvongs S 1980 Essentials of anorectal surgery. Lippincott, Philadelphia

Goligher JC 1984 Surgery of the anus, rectum and colon, 5th edn. Baillière Tindall, London

Henry MM, Swash M 1992 Coloproctology and the pelvic floor, 2nd edn. Butterworth-Heinemann, Oxford

Keighley MRB, Williams NS 1999 Surgery of the anus, rectum and colon, 2nd edn. Saunders, London
Martin M-C, Givel J-C 1990 Surgery of anorectal diseases. Springer-Verlag, Berlin
Nicholls RJ, Dozois RR 1997 Surgery of the colon and rectum. Churchill Livingstone, Edinburgh
Phillips RKS 1998 Colorectal surgery: a companion to specialist surgical practice. Saunders, London
Sir Alan Parks Symposium Proceedings 1983 Annals of the Royal College of Surgeons of England (Supplement)
Thomson JPS, Nicholls RJ, Williams CB 1981 Colorectal disease. Heinemann Medical Books, London
Todd IP, Fielding LP 1983 Rob and Smith's operative surgery: alimentary tract and abdominal 3. Colon, rectum and anus, 4th edn. Butterworths, London.

19

Open biliary operations

R.C.N. Williamson, L.R. Jiao

CONTENTS

INTRODUCTION

1 This chapter concentrates on open operations for gallstones, since until lately these have been by far the most common indication for 'open' biliary surgery. Introduced as recently as 1987, laparoscopic cholecystectomy has rapidly been taken up by many centres throughout the world. At present almost all elective cholecystectomies are carried out by the laparoscopic route (Ch. 20), but open operation is still commonly performed in some developing countries and also in difficult or complicated circumstances when it cannot be completed with a laparoscopic approach.

2 Biliary diversion undertaken as part of a palliative procedure for pancreatic cancer is described in Chapter 21; likewise resection of malignant strictures of the lower bile duct.

3 When operating on the biliary tract, always ensure that the patient is positioned on the operating table so that the upper abdomen overlies a radiolucent tunnel. Alert the radiographer and theatre staff in advance that an operative cholangiogram may be required.

4 Routine antibiotic prophylaxis is a wise precaution in biliary surgery. Choose a broad-spectrum agent excreted in bile, such as one of the cephalosporins. A single parenteral dose given shortly before operation may suffice, unless the bile is obviously infected.

5 Carry out thromboprophylaxis routinely unless there is a specific contraindication. We use subcutaneous low-dose heparin and below-knee compression stockings.

OPEN CHOLECYSTECTOMY

Appraise

1 Whether symptomatic or 'silent', gallstones are the overwhelming indication for cholecystectomy. Their prevalence makes cholecystectomy the second most common intra-abdominal operation in Western countries after appendicectomy. Cholecystectomy is occasionally indicated for acalculous cholecystitis, gallbladder carcinoma or cholecystoses (cholesterosis, adenomyosis), or during the course of partial hepatectomy or pancreatoduodenectomy. As a rule, remove a diseased gallbladder encountered incidentally at operation provided there is adequate access and an additional procedure would not be inappropriate (Table 19.1).

2 Although cholecystectomy can safely be performed by the laparoscopic route in many patients (see Ch. 21), certain situations will make it safer to convert to open operation. Difficulties can arise when: the pathology encountered is difficult, such as Mirizzi syndrome; the anatomical anomalies are not clearly understood; or the experience of the surgeon is insufficient to deal with a problem, such as bleeding. To persist with laparoscopic removal in such circumstances is to risk injury to the bile duct (Table 19.2).

3 Dissolution therapy with cheno- or ursodeoxycholic acid is a reasonable alternative to cholecystectomy in very elderly or infirm patients with a functioning gallbladder and a limited number of small, radiolucent calculi. Treatment is often prolonged, and recurrence commonly follows its cessation.[1] Extracorporeal shock-wave lithotripsy[2] and percutaneous cholecystolithotomy (and dissolution) are other methods for dealing with gallstones non-operatively but, unlike laparoscopic cholecystectomy, they have the disadvantage of leaving the diseased gallbladder in situ to form more stones.

4 The earlier lists of absolute contraindications to laparoscopic cholecystectomy have mostly been reduced to relative contraindications as surgical expertise and equipment have improved. Nevertheless, some consideration should be given to open cholecystectomy in cases of previous upper abdominal operations, acute cholecystitis, cirrhosis,[3] pregnancy and cholecystoenteric fistula. Currently, one of the remaining contraindications to laparoscopic cholecystectomy is when a strong suspicion of gallbladder carcinoma exists preoperatively.

5 Acute cholecystitis will generally settle when the patient is treated with rehydration and antibiotics,[4] allowing operation to be delayed for a few days or weeks according to policy (see below). Persistence of fever and local tenderness or evidence of

TABLE 19.1 Indications for open cholecystectomy

Benign conditions

- Symptomatic cholelithiasis
  - Failure of laparoscopic cholecystectomy
  - Contraindication for laparoscopic approach
    - Previous intra-abdominal operation
    - Extensive adhesions
  - Complications of gallstones
    - Choledochoduodenal fistula
  - Patient's choice
- Asymptomatic cholelithiasis
- Failure of laparoscopic cholecystectomy

Malignant conditions

- Gallbladder cancer
- Cholangiocarcinoma
- Pancreatic carcinoma
- Hepatectomy for liver cancer

TABLE 19.2 Indications for conversion of laparoscopic cholecystectomy to open

- Difficulty in establishment of adequate pneumoperitoneum
  - Extensive adhesion
  - Complications of port insertion
- Difficulty in visualization of gallbladder
  - Retracted small gallbladder
  - Adhesion around gallbladder
  - Distended stomach or duodenum
- Difficulty in dissection of gallbladder
  - Technical difficulties
    - Severe inflammation with dense adhesions
    - Friable gallbladder
    - Small retracted gallbladder
    - Incarcerated gallbladder
  - Difficult anatomy
    - Aberrant anatomy related to cystic artery, duct and right hepatic artery
- Complications
  - Haemorrhage
  - Damage to other structure
    - Common bile duct injury
    - Liver injury
    - Intestinal injury
    - Hepatic artery injury
    - Stomach injury
- Unsuspected pathology
- Perforated gallbladder/abscess
- Gallbladder cancer
- Cholangiocarcinoma
- Mirizzi syndrome

spreading peritonism are indications for urgent operation because of the risk of gangrene or perforation (see also the section on cholecystectomy below). About 10% of patients with acute cholecystitis have acalculous disease, and these patients are at particular risk of perforation.

6 The timing of operation after an acute attack of cholecystitis or biliary colic is disputatious. Our preference is to confirm the diagnosis at an early stage by ultrasonography (or contrast radiology) and to put the patient on the next 'cold' operating list. This policy of early cholecystectomy avoids recurrent attacks or complications, such as acute pancreatitis, but occasionally results in a more difficult operation. Often, however, the inflammatory oedema assists dissection of the gallbladder from the liver bed. Recent studies suggest that laparoscopic cholecystectomy is safe in the acute setting, but a higher conversion rate must be expected.[5,6]

7 Transient jaundice is compatible with stones confined to the gallbladder. Continuing jaundice suggests obstruction of the bile duct and requires further investigation, including an 'invasive' cholangiogram (either percutaneous transhepatic or endoscopic retrograde). Perioperative precautions in obstructive jaundice are outlined in Chapter 2.

8 Half the population have some variation from 'normal' in the arterial supply of the gallbladder or the disposition of the bile ducts. Therefore, do not embark upon cholecystectomy without learning the common anatomical variations.[7]

▶ KEY POINT Gallstones may be coincidental

- Gallstones are very common and their symptoms often mimic those of many other diseases. Careful laparotomy after entering the abdominal cavity will identify these conditions.

Prepare

As described above, ensure that the operating table will allow operative cholangiography (if needed) and 'cover' the operation with prophylactic antibiotic therapy.

Access

1 Choose between a right upper paramedian, an oblique subcostal (Kocher's) or a transverse incision, according to your experience and the shape of the patient's abdomen.

2 In a paramedian incision it is simpler to split the fibres of rectus abdominis than to mobilize and retract the muscle belly. In practice, no harm ensues from denervation of the medial portion of the rectus. The incision starts at the costal margin 5 cm from the midline and runs down to just below the umbilicus.

3 Some surgeons prefer Kocher's oblique subcostal incision, which extends parallel to the costal margin for about 15 cm. If the incision is taken further to the right, isolate and preserve the ninth thoracic nerve. Divide the muscles using diathermy in the line of the skin incision. A transverse incision provides a better cosmetic scar at the expense of slightly limited access.

4 'Minicholecystectomy' can be carried out through a short (5 cm) transverse incision with careful retraction, in favourable cases. It gives an excellent cosmetic result but has probably been superseded by laparoscopic cholecystectomy.[8]

Assess

1 Examine the gallbladder to see if it is inflamed, thickened or contains stones. With the patient supine, stones sink to the neck of the gallbladder. If the organ is hard and adherent to the liver, consider the possibility of carcinoma.

2 Gallstone symptoms can mimic those of other diseases. Explore the rest of the abdomen, looking in particular for hiatal hernia, peptic ulcer, diverticular disease of the colon and diseases of the liver, pancreas and appendix.

3 Examine the common bile duct. It should not exceed 6–8 mm in diameter. Insert your left index finger through the epiploic foramen (described in 1732 by the Danish anatomist Jacob Winslow), and feel the duct between finger and thumb. Is it thickened, does it contain stones? Feel the lower duct after splitting the peritoneum in the floor of the foramen with the edge of a finger.

4 Examine the head of pancreas between finger and thumb, again passing your left index finger through the epiploic foramen and down behind the gland. Normal pancreas has a softish nodular feel, but with experience you will learn to detect the induration that denotes chronic inflammation or neoplasia.

Action

1 Place your hand over the liver and gently manipulate the right lobe downwards into the wound.

2 Ask the anaesthetist to empty the stomach by aspirating the nasogastric tube. Divide any omental adhesions to the undersurface of the gallbladder.

3 Place one pack in the subhepatic space to retract the intestines and another just covering the duodenal bulb.

4 Decide whether to commence gallbladder dissection at the fundus or in the region of the cystic duct. We generally prefer to display the structures in Calot's triangle (Fig. 19.1) and to ligate and divide the cystic artery before proceeding to the fundus and working back towards the cystic duct. If chronic inflammation is severe, it is safer to start at the fundus; some surgeons advocate this approach routinely.

5 Cholecystectomy may be performed with you standing on the right- or left-hand side of the operating table. Try both positions on different occasions and see which you find more comfortable.

6 If the gallbladder is very distended, aspirate it before proceeding (Fig. 19.2). The empty gallbladder is easier to grasp for dissection and less likely to contaminate the peritoneal cavity if accidentally entered. Pack off the fundus and insert an Ochsner trocar, which is connected to the sucker tubing. Alternatively, use a syringe and wide-bore needle. Afterwards, seal the defect by grasping it with tissue-holding forceps.

'Duct-first' technique

1 The first assistant's left hand draws the duodenal bulb downwards, while a retractor draws the liver upwards. Grasp the neck of the gallbladder with sponge-holding forceps and draw it to the patient's right. This three-way traction provides good exposure (Fig. 19.1).

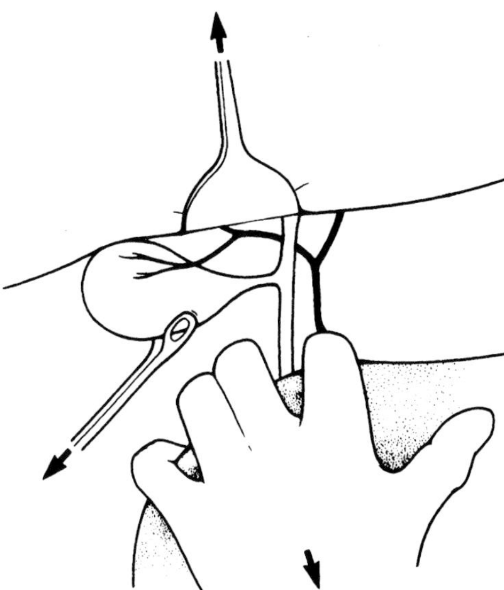

Fig. 19.1 Cholecystectomy. Traction in three directions displays Calot's triangle, which is bounded by the cystic duct, common hepatic duct and inferior border of the liver. The triangle has been extended by mobilization of the neck of the gallbladder. The cystic artery normally arises from the right hepatic artery within Calot's triangle.

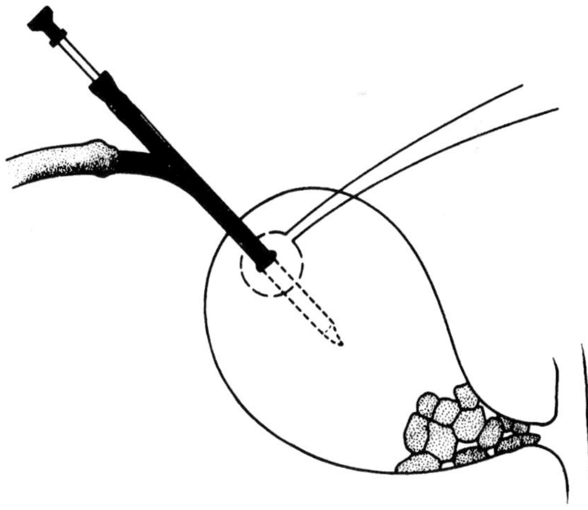

Fig. 19.2 Decompression of an obstructed gallbladder before cholecystectomy (or cholecystostomy). The side-arm of the Ochsner trocar is connected to the sucker tubing.

2 Incise the peritoneum over the neck of the gallbladder and continue for a short distance along its superior border. Using blunt dissection gently open the space between the gallbladder and the liver at this point and expose the cystic artery. Follow the vessel on to the gallbladder wall and confirm that it is the cystic artery and not the right hepatic artery. Ligate the vessel twice in continuity and divide it between the ligatures.

3 Prior division of the cystic artery helps to straighten out the cystic duct. Now expose the duct by a combination of sharp and blunt dissection, and trace it to its junction with the common hepatic duct to form the bile duct. It is vital to display this three-way junction before dividing the cystic duct.

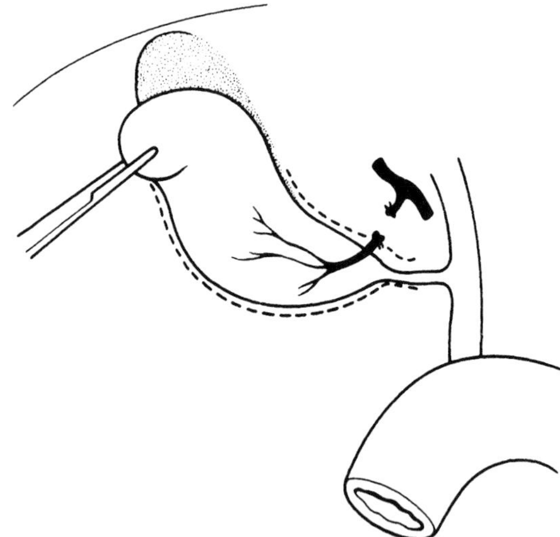

Fig. 19.3 Cholecystectomy: separation of the fundus of the gallbladder from the liver. The lines of peritoneal division are shown. The fundal dissection may be carried out after ligation and division of the cystic artery (as shown) or as the first stage of cholecystectomy.

4 Perform an operative cholangiogram via the cystic duct if required (see next section). Take a swab of the bile for bacteriological culture on opening the duct.

5 While awaiting the X-ray films (this is avoided if you can perform the cholangiogram with real-time fluoroscopic images), proceed to dissect the gallbladder from its liver bed. Leave the cholangiogram catheter in situ but complete the division of the cystic duct, grasping its gallbladder end with Moynihan's cholecystectomy forceps. Incise the peritoneum along the anterior and posterior aspects of the gallbladder, proceeding either towards or away from the fundus. Traction on the fundus assists the dissection (Fig. 19.3).

Numerous small vessels and occasionally accessory bile ducts traverse the areolar tissue between the liver and the gallbladder. Diathermy coagulation is effective to secure these vessels, but it may be simpler to ligate leashes of tissue on the hepatic side and then divide them with scissors. Remove the gallbladder, preserving it for subsequent gross and histological examination.

6 Routinely open the gallbladder, inspect its contents and submit any suspicious nodule or ulcer to urgent frozen-section examination to exclude carcinoma.

7 If the cholangiogram pictures are technically satisfactory, withdraw the catheter and ligate the cystic duct close to the origin of the bile duct. Try and avoid leaving too long a cystic duct stump but do not struggle to place the ligature exactly flush with the bile duct. Avoid tenting or narrowing the bile duct while tying the ligature. We use an absorbable suture material for the ligature, such as 2/0 or 3/0 polyglactin 910 (Vicryl). If the cystic duct is large, use a transfixion suture.

8 Use diathermy to stop any residual oozing from the liver bed. Often the application of a surgical pack to the gallbladder fossa, with or without the aid of a haemostatic agent such as Surgicel for a few minutes, will stop most bleeding. If you observe a leak of bile from a small cholecystohepatic duct, close the duct with a Vicryl stitch. Do not attempt to close the raw area of liver with sutures.

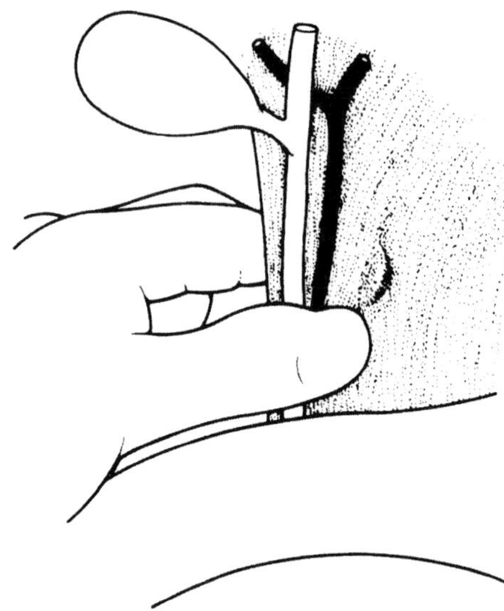

Fig. 19.4 Pringle's manoeuvre. Digital compression of the hepatic artery within the free edge of the lesser omentum controls haemorrhage from branches of the vessel beyond that point.

9 Remove the packs and aspirate any blood.

'Fundus-first' technique

1 Grasp the fundus of the gallbladder with tissue-holding forceps. Incise the peritoneum between the fundus and the liver, using frequent diathermy to secure the many fine vessels. Larger vessels can be ligated on the hepatic side and divided.

2 Extend the peritoneal incision along the anterior and posterior aspects of the gallbladder (Fig. 19.3). Open up the plane between the liver and the gallbladder, and proceed towards the neck of the organ, staying close to the gallbladder. Identify the cystic artery. Ligate and divide the artery close to the gallbladder wall.

3 The advantage of the 'fundus-first' technique is that it brings you directly on to the cystic duct from the safe side and lessens the risk of bile-duct injury. Trace the cystic duct to its junction with the common hepatic duct. Perform a cholangiogram. Ligate and divide the cystic duct and remove the gallbladder.

4 Secure haemostasis in the liver bed. Remove the packs.

KEY POINTS The golden rule: display the ductal anatomy

- Usually straightforward, cholecystectomy can sometimes, unpredictably, be a major technical challenge. Under such circumstances take great care to avert future disaster.
- The golden rule is never to cut any major structure, whether duct or artery, until you have displayed the crucial anatomy—notably the entry of the cystic duct into the bile duct.
- Always call for help from a senior surgeon if you are in trouble.

? DIFFICULTY

1. *Is the gallbladder stuck to the duodenum or transverse colon and obscured by inflammatory adhesions?* The organ can usually be freed by gentle digital dissection, but remember that calculi may have fistulated into the adherent viscus.
2. *Can you not identify the cystic artery or the three-way union of ducts?* Perhaps the tissues are fibrotic or bleed too easily. The liver may be enlarged and stiff; the gallbladder may be inaccessible because the costal margin is low or the patient obese. Do not proceed until you have improved the view. Enlarge the incision if necessary. Have the light adjusted. Use the sucker. Place and employ your assistants usefully, or summon further assistance.
3. *Can you still not safely progress?* Adopt the 'fundus-first' technique. Seek senior help. If the dissection is very difficult, consider an alternative procedure, either cholecystostomy or subtotal cholecystectomy.
4. *Are you proceeding with the dissection, but the anatomy is anomalous or confusing?* In these circumstances do not divide any structure until you have fully displayed the anatomy, and you understand it. Remember the common variations, summon a textbook of surgical anatomy or seek assistance from a senior surgeon. If you can confidently identify the cystic duct, perform cholangiography in order to clarify the remaining ductal anatomy.
5. *Do you suspect damage to the common hepatic duct or the bile duct?* If the possibility exists, you must declare the issue and not just hope for the best. Enlist the help of the most experienced surgeon available and discuss the case with a regional hepatopancreatobiliary centre. Cholangiography may be helpful. Repair partial division of the main duct immediately using fine absorbable sutures, and place a T-tube across the anastomosis through a separate stab incision. It is often better, following complete transection, and particularly resection of a length, of duct, to perform a hepaticojejunostomy repair using a Roux loop of jejunum. Anastomosis can be difficult with a normal bile duct. Do not undertake this procedure unless you are fully trained to do it; otherwise, discuss the problem with a hepatopancreatobiliary specialist. Resolve to make accurate notes, with drawings to display the exact situation.
6. *Severe bleeding?* Do not panic and apply haemostats blindly or use inappropriate diathermy; the situation is almost certainly recoverable. Control the bleeding by local pressure. Arrange for blood to be available and for arterial sutures, tapes and bulldog clamps. Summon further advice and assistance if necessary.
   - If the bleeding is arterial, compress the free edge of the lesser omentum between finger and thumb or apply a non-crushing intestinal clamp just tightly enough to control bleeding (Pringle's manoeuvre; Fig. 19.4). Dissect out and control the hepatic artery, which normally lies on the left-hand side of and below the bile duct. Remember that accessory hepatic arteries arising from the left gastric or superior mesenteric arteries are not controlled by occluding the main hepatic artery. Expose the damaged vessel. If it is large, repair it with arterial sutures; if it is small, ligate each end. You may find that you have pulled the cystic artery off the right hepatic artery. If so, suture the defect in the parent vessel. In the absence of jaundice or hypotension, ligature of the right hepatic or even the common hepatic artery, although best avoided, does not lead to infarction of the liver.
   - If the bleeding is venous, control it by compression for 5 minutes timed by the clock, then explore, evaluate and repair the damage as necessary.
7. *Can the gallbladder not be separated from the liver?* Suspect carcinoma, and consider frozen-section examination if the diagnosis is equivocal. Resect carcinoma of the gallbladder if you are able to achieve a curative resection. This usually necessitates resection of the gallbladder bed and the nodes at the porta hepatis. This decision is often guided by the depth of tumour invasion into the gallbladder wall on histology. Although some surgeons favour partial hepatectomy, any attempted resection is best performed by a fully trained hepatobiliary surgeon. If severe but benign fibrosis makes it extremely difficult to develop a safe plane of dissection, be willing to leave the back wall of the gallbladder attached to the liver and destroy the exposed mucosa with diathermy current.

Checklist

1 Review the clinical and radiological criteria for continuing to exploration of the bile duct (see below).

2 Examine the gallbladder bed, the common duct and the ligatures on the cystic duct and cystic artery.

Closure

1 Place a tube drain or fine-bore suction drain to the subhepatic pouch if you are concerned about possible biliary leak from the gallbladder bed on the liver, or if the area is oozing and there is the possibility of haematoma formation.

2 Close the abdominal wall in layers as for a standard laparotomy incision (see Ch. 4).

Aftercare

1 The nasogastric tube can usually be removed at 12–24 hours and the drain at 48 hours. In straightforward cases introduce a light diet at 24–36 hours and discharge patients at 3–8 days.

2 A small amount of bile may drain at first from the raw surface of the liver but ceases spontaneously within a few days. Regard a larger leak of more than 100 ml bile per day or a persistent fistula as a complication and manage it accordingly.[9]

KEY POINTS Initial management of a postoperative bile leak

- In the setting of postoperative biliary ascites and sepsis, first control the bile leak and treat the sepsis. This can often be achieved by positioning a percutaneous drain.
- Before contemplating re-operation and repair you must carry out imaging of the bile ducts, either from above by percutaneous transhepatic cholangiography or HIDA (hepatobiliary iminodiacetic acid) scan, or from below by endoscopic retrograde cholangiography, and often both.

Complications

1 Copious bile drainage through the wound or drain site suggests unrecognized injury to the bile duct or a slipped ligature on the cystic duct. Under these circumstances a retained calculus in the bile duct may be associated with persistence of the biliary fistula. Damage to the main duct is often accompanied by jaundice. Confirm the diagnosis by cholangiography, obtained either by transhepatic needling or by retrograde cannulation of the ampulla. Endoscopic retrograde cholangiopancreatography (ERCP) is extremely valuable for both diagnosis and treatment of postoperative bile leak. The only action needed may be decompression of the bile duct with the insertion of a temporary stent to control a leak from either the cystic duct or a small tear in the bile duct. Re-operation is needed if the leak continues. A small defect in the bile duct may be amenable to repair over a T-tube, after ensuring that there are no ductal calculi, but a larger defect or complete transection requires Roux-en-Y hepaticojejunostomy (see later).

2 Wound infection is uncommon unless the bile duct is explored or there is severe acute cholecystitis.

3 Subhepatic abscess occasionally results from an undrained collection of blood or bile; management is considered in Chapter 8. True subphrenic abscess is rare, likewise septicaemia.

4 The mortality rate of cholecystectomy is well under 1%. Most deaths occur in the elderly, those with gangrene or perforation of the gallbladder or those with concomitant ductal stones. Most postcholecystectomy symptoms result from unrecognized intercurrent disease.

REFERENCES

1. Lanzini A, Northfield TC 1994 Pharmacological treatments of gallstones. Practical guidelines. Drugs 47:458–470
2. Sackman M 1992 Gallbladder stones: shockwave therapy. Baillière's Clinical Gastroenterology 6:697–714
3. Yerdel MA, Koksoy C, Aras N et al 1997 Laparoscopic versus open cholecystectomy in cirrhotic patients: a prospective trial. Surgical Laparoscopy and Endoscopy 7:483–486
4. Westphal JF, Brogard JM 1999 Biliary tract infections: a guide to drug treatment. Drugs 57:81–91
5. Kiviluto T, Siren J, Luukkonen P et al 1998 Randomised trial of laparoscopic versus open cholecystectomy for acute and gangrenous cholecystitis. Lancet 351:321–325
6. Lo CM, Liu CL, Fan ST et al 1998 Prospective randomized study of early versus delayed laparoscopic cholecystectomy for acute cholecystitis. Annals of Surgery 227:461–467
7. Smadja C, Blumgart LH 1994 The biliary tract and anatomy of biliary exposure. In: Blumgart LH (ed.) Surgery of the liver and biliary tract, 2nd edn. Churchill Livingstone, Edinburgh, pp 11–25
8. McGinn FP, Miles AJ, Uglow M et al 1995 Randomised trail of laparoscopic cholecystectomy and mini-cholecystectomy. British Journal of Surgery 82:1374–1377
9. Brugge WR, Rosenberg DJ, Alavi A 1994 Diagnosis of postoperative bile leaks. American Journal of Gastroenterology 89:2178–2183

OPERATIVE CHOLANGIOGRAPHY

Appraise

1 Cholangiography is an integral part of cholecystectomy and should be carried out at an early stage of the operation, unless preoperative visualization of the ducts by, for example, retrograde cholangiography, has been excellent and they are normal. This policy of routine cholangiography has been challenged in the laparoscopic era (Ch. 20) but, as most cases performed with open operation are likely to represent the more difficult cases, we still believe that this traditional teaching holds true during open cholecystectomy.

2 The justification for this policy of routine cholangiography is that it will detect ductal stones that have been missed by inspection or palpation of the bile duct. However, good technique is required to obtain X-rays of good quality and to avoid artefacts such as air bubbles that can lead to negative exploration of the duct. In experienced hands, a selective policy is acceptable, in which cholangiography is reserved for those patients with a history of jaundice or recent acute pancreatitis and those with laparotomy findings suggestive of ductal stones such as a dilated bile duct or a short, wide cystic duct with multiple gallbladder stones.

3 Whatever your policy, always obtain an operative cholangiogram to display the ductal anatomy if there is any suspicion of an anomalous arrangement. If necessary, obtain a check film by cannulating the gallbladder without the need for formally exposing the cystic duct.

4 Warn the X-ray department preoperatively. Ensure that the patient is correctly placed on the operating table, with the upper abdomen overlying a radiolucent tunnel. An image intensifier can facilitate visualization of the biliary tree, but it is still best to obtain 'hard-copy' X-rays for record purposes, unless video records are available.

5 As a rule obtain cholangiograms via the cystic duct. Alternatively, contrast material can be injected directly into the common hepatic or bile ducts. If ductal stones are obviously present at operation, it may still help to discover their number and size, and the state of the duct, before proceeding to exploration.

6 After choledocholithotomy, always check that all stones have been removed by repeating the cholangiogram.

Action

1 Fill a 20-ml syringe and attached fine plastic cannula with saline, making sure no air bubbles remain in the syringe or tubing. Prepare a second syringe filled with 25% sodium diatrizoate (Hypaque) and clearly marked.

2 Isolate 2 cm of cystic duct and ligate it on the gallbladder side. Pass a second ligature around the duct, but do not tie it. Partly divide the cystic duct between these ligatures about 2 cm from its entry into the main duct (Fig. 19.5)

3 Pass the cannula down the cystic duct for about 2 cm and ligate it in situ. If you encounter difficulty from the valvular effect of spiralling ductal mucosa (described in 1720 by the German anatomist and surgeon, Lorenz Heister), withdraw the cannula, gently pass a probe and try again.

4 Check the patency of the cannula when it is tied in place. Inject a small quantity of saline, or detach the syringe and observe bile pass back up the tubing.

5 Remove instruments and swabs from the field. Cover the wound with a sterile towel and allow the radiographer to position the X-ray machine. Have spectators, assistants and nursing personnel leave the operating theatre or take their place behind a lead screen. The anaesthetist remains for the moment to control the patient's respiration.

6 Inject 3–4 ml of contrast medium and have an X-ray film exposed. Insert a further 5–10 ml and obtain a second film.

7 Other techniques are convenient in particular circumstances. The contrast material can be injected directly into the main duct through a fine 'butterfly' needle. Alternatively, clamp the neck of the gallbladder and inject contrast immediately beyond this point. When duodenotomy has been performed, you can obtain a retrograde cholangiogram by cannulating the papilla.

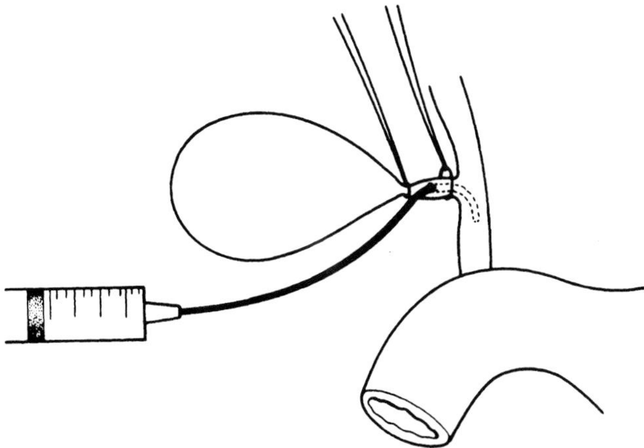

Fig. 19.5 Operative cholangiography. Through a small opening in the cystic duct, a fine polythene cannula is passed into the bile duct and secured in position by tightening a ligature around the cystic duct.

8 Post-exploratory films are obtained via a T-tube inserted into the bile duct. Take care to clear the tube and the ductal tree of air. Repeatedly irrigate the T-tube during closure of the choledochotomy incision. Insert and tie the last stitch under water. Obtain one or two films after injecting 10–20 ml of 25% Hypaque.

9 If the films are technically unsatisfactory, do not hesitate to repeat them. Use further contrast material to try and clear any air bubbles or to obtain better filling of the hepatic ducts.

Interpretation

1 Inspect the films carefully. Make sure that the right and left hepatic ducts are displayed together with their tributaries. The bile duct usually overlies the spine, and occasionally this can obscure certain features. If necessary, obtain further films with the operating table rotated 15° to the right to throw the bile duct clear of the spine; indeed, some surgeons adopt this precaution routinely. In some patients it may be difficult to demonstrate the intrahepatic bile ducts; in this situation, a degree of head-down tilt will facilitate contrast flowing into the proximal ducts. Take care to study the film closely, as many anomalies can occur.[1]

2 On the pre-exploratory films, exclude the following features: filling defects, obstruction of a major hepatic radicle, dilatation of the bile duct (> 10 mm), failure of contrast to enter the duodenum. Remember that the bile duct normally tapers before smoothly entering the duodenum. If you suspect spasm rather than organic obstruction of the papilla, consider obtaining a further X-ray after an intravenous injection of hyoscine hydrobromide (Buscopan) or glucagon.[2]

3 On the post-exploratory films the most important feature is the presence or absence of a filling defect, consistent with a residual calculus. It is quite common for contrast not to enter the duodenum at this stage, especially after instrumentation of the papilla.

REFERENCES

1. Puente SG, Bannura GC 1983 Radiological anatomy of the biliary tract: variations and congenital abnormalities. World Journal of Surgery 7:271–276
2. Al-Jurf A 1990 A simplified technique to relax the sphincter of Oddi during intraoperative cholangiography. Surgery, Gynecology and Obstetrics 170:163–164

EXPLORATION OF THE BILE DUCT

Appraise

1 Absolute indications for exploration of the bile duct at laparotomy are stones unequivocally shown on a preoperative or operative cholangiogram, stones that can be palpated within the bile duct and stones causing obstructive jaundice. Preoperatively detected stones should usually be treated by ERCP and stone

extraction unless the patient is to be subjected to open operation anyway. The detection of duct stones during laparoscopic cholangiography is usually not an indication to convert to an open procedure as in most cases the duct can be cleared by laparoscopic duct exploration or postoperative ERCP. In the latter case, a transcystic duct drain can be left in situ to provide adequate drainage until the ERCP is organized. This strategy may be appropriate in the elderly patient, although the mortality rate of open common bile duct exploration is low at 1%.[1]

2 Relative indications for choledochotomy are any abnormalities shown on operative cholangiography apart from obvious stones. If the radiological criteria are doubtful, the following clinical factors tend to favour exploration of the duct:
- A history of jaundice or acute pancreatitis.
- Dilatation and opacification of the wall of the bile duct.
- Multiple small calculi in the gallbladder.
- A short wide cystic duct.

3 If narrowing of the terminal bile duct is the only abnormality, it is sometimes possible to rule out appreciable stenosis by passing a soft Jacques catheter (no. 8F) through the cystic duct stump and into the duodenum. Ultrathin choledochoscopes are becoming available for passage through the cystic duct.

4 If doubt remains, explore the duct. Negative exploration is safer than ignoring disease—usually stones but conceivably tumour.

5 Remember that a jaundiced patient needs proper perioperative precautions taken (see Ch. 4).

6 Endoscopic papillotomy may avoid the need for laparotomy in selected patients with bile duct stones, especially those without a gallbladder (see below).

Access

1 If continuing on from cholecystectomy, make sure the existing incision is adequate; otherwise, extend it.

2 If you intend exploring the duct from the start, choose a right upper paramedian incision unless there is a convenient scar to re-open from a previous operation.

3 At re-operation there may be dense adhesions. Find the liver at the upper end of the wound and trace its undersurface, where stomach, small bowel or transverse colon may be adherent. Identify the stomach, follow it distally to the duodenum and draw this downwards to display the region of the common duct.

KEY POINTS In difficult circumstances stay in contact with the liver

- Where the anatomy is difficult to follow and in the presence of dense adhesions, find the liver and stay in contact with it.
- If you wander away, you risk damaging nearby structures.

Assess

1 During abdominal exploration pay particular attention to the extrahepatic biliary tree, liver and pancreas. Decide whether or not to remove a liver biopsy (see Ch. 22).

2 Expose the supraduodenal portion of the bile duct by carefully dissecting within the free edge of the lesser omentum. Carefully examine the duct. Split the peritoneum in the floor of the epiploic foramen to feel its lower end.

3 If previous cholecystectomy has been performed, it may or may not be necessary to obtain operative cholangiograms, depending upon the adequacy of preoperative investigation. Otherwise proceed to cholecystectomy and operative cholangiography, as described above.

Action

1 Place two Vicryl stay sutures in the wall of the supraduodenal bile duct. This low approach gives the option of converting to a choledochoduodenostomy should this be required (see below) and also to performing a proximal hepaticojejunostomy at a later date if a ductal stricture were to develop at the choledochotomy site. Incise the duct vertically between the sutures (Fig. 19.6) and take a culture swab of the bile. Extend the choledochotomy for 15–20 mm. Achieve haemostasis from the cut edges of the duct. Although diathermy current can be used it is generally safer with fine absorbable sutures as this does not result in transmitted diathermy injury to the bile duct vasculature.

2 Remove any obvious stones with forceps. Palpate the duct and try to milk stones towards the choledochotomy. Gently explore the biliary tree upwards and downwards, using Desjardins's or Randall's forceps with the appropriate degrees of angulation. Reconcile the calculi extracted with the cholangiographic appearances.

3 Pass a soft polyethylene catheter (Jacques no. 8F) connected to a 50-ml syringe upwards into the hepatic ducts. Irrigate briskly with saline and repeat until the returning fluid is entirely clear. Now pass the catheter downwards and irrigate the bile duct. If there are multiple stones and gravel, it is sensible to occlude the common hepatic duct with a bulldog clip or tape during this procedure.

4 Pass the catheter through the papilla and into the duodenum, where it can be felt by rolling the bowel between finger and

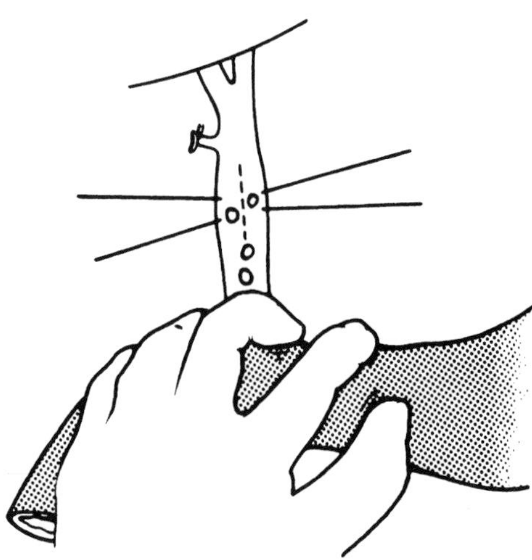

Fig. 19.6 Exploration of the bile duct. Stay sutures are placed and a vertical choledochotomy is performed.

thumb. Failure to pass the catheter suggests either a calculus impacted at the ampulla or some other obstruction, such as papillary fibrosis. Mobilize the duodenum, using Kocher's technique. It may be possible to disimpact the calculus or crush it with forceps (if it is soft) and wash out the fragments. Passage of graded Bakes metal dilators may overcome papillary stenosis, but perform this manoeuvre with great care.

5 After all apparent stones have been removed, insert a choledochoscope if one is available, to check that the ducts are clear. Both rigid and flexible endoscopes require a free flow of irrigant to distend the ductal tree to allow adequate inspection. Temporarily occlude the choledochotomy by crossing the stay sutures.

6 Insert the T-piece of a latex T-tube into the bile duct and close the duct with a running 2/0 Vicryl suture, so that the tube emerges from the lower end of the suture line (Fig. 19.7). The T-tube diameter is normally between sizes 10F and 16F, depending on the size of the duct. Primary closure of the duct without a T-tube has been reported and appears to be safe.[2]

7 Whether or not choledochoscopy has been performed it is sensible to obtain a post-exploratory T-tube cholangiogram, unless no stones are found in the duct and the original grounds for exploration were equivocal.

8 Bring the T-tube directly to the surface of the abdominal wall to exit through a separate stab incision. Suture the tube to the skin and connect it to a drainage bag.

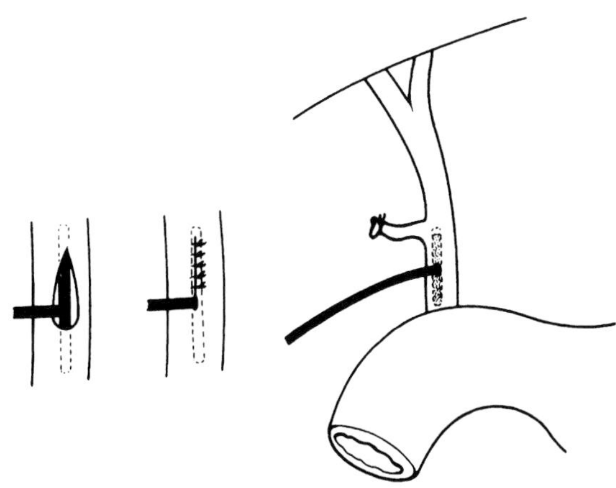

Fig. 19.7 T-tube drainage of the bile duct. The tube is brought out through the lower end of the sutured choledochotomy.

? DIFFICULTY

1. *Do adhesions from previous biliary operations make the bile duct difficult to find?* Explore the area with a syringe and fine needle, aspirating to see if you obtain bile.
2. *Are there multiple stones present with or without biliary mud and gravel?* It is obviously difficult to ensure complete clearance of the dilated ductal tree. Perform a permanent drainage operation, either choledochoduodenostomy or transduodenal sphincteroplasty (see below). Greater readiness to take this step undoubtedly reduces the incidence of retained calculi, which is usually about 10%.
3. *Is there a problem at the lower end of the bile duct?* You cannot remove an impacted calculus or manage to pass an instrument through the papilla. The patient may be jaundiced. Proceed to transduodenal sphincteroplasty (see next section), although this is rarely necessary.[3]

Aftercare

1 Leave the T-tube on free dependent drainage for 3 days, then lift the bag level with the wound for 2–3 days and elevate to the shoulder thereafter. Output of bile will decrease, provided there is no residual obstruction in the duct. If pain develops after elevating the bag, return to dependent drainage.

2 Obtain a T-tube cholangiogram 7–10 days after operation. Check the films to ensure that there is free drainage of contrast into the duodenum and there are no filling defects. Repeat the X-ray if appearances are equivocal.

3 If the X-rays are satisfactory, spigot the T-tube and remove it on the tenth postoperative day. A firm pull is usually required. Observe the patient overnight before discharge from hospital.

Complications

1 Wound infection and intra-abdominal sepsis are more common when the bile duct is explored than after cholecystectomy alone. Be sure to obtain a bile culture at operation, and consider extending the course of prophylactic antibiotics if sepsis is anticipated.

2 A retained calculus may be shown on the postoperative T-tube cholangiogram. If it is clear that you have left a stone behind, do not remove the T-tube. Small stones can sometimes be cleared by flushing the duct with normal saline. Give an antispasmodic to relax the sphincter of Oddi and infuse 1 litre of saline from a bag suspended 1 m above the wound. If this technique fails, leave the T-tube in situ for 6 weeks to obtain a mature fibrous track and repeat the X-ray. It may now be possible to pass a steerable catheter down the T-tube track and remove residual calculi under X-ray control (Burhenne technique). Flexible choledochoscopy along the T-tube tract can also be successful.[4] Other treatment options for retained stone include endoscopic papillotomy and re-operation, but prevention is very much better than cure.

REFERENCES

1. O'Sullivan ST, Hehir DJ, O'Sullivan GC et al 1996 Open common bile duct exploration: end of an epoch? Irish Journal of Medical Science 165:32–34
2. Tu Z, Li J, Xin H et al 1999 Primary choledochorrhaphy after common bile duct exploration. Digestive Surgery 16:137–139
3. Thompson JE, Bennion RS 1989 The surgical management of impacted common bile duct stones without sphincter ablation. Archives of Surgery 124:1216–1219
4. Chueng MT 1997 Postoperative choledochoscopic removal of intrahepatic stones via a T-tube tract. British Journal of Surgery 84:1224–1228

INTERNAL DRAINAGE FOR DUCTAL STONES

Appraise

1 Some form of permanent drainage operation is indicated during exploration of the bile duct when multiple stones and biliary mud are encountered, or when papillary stenosis impedes the onward passage of contrast or instruments. Such patients are likely to have a history of jaundice and dilatation of the extrahepatic biliary tree.

2 In the presence of suppurative cholangitis any form of internal surgical drainage is probably inadvisable. Content yourself with removing obstructing calculi from the duct, irrigation and insertion of a T-tube. In many circumstances this can be achieved endoscopically if appropriate expertise is available. If necessary, further procedures may be attempted when the emergency has passed.

3 A calculus that is impacted in the ampulla and cannot be extracted is a clear indication for *transduodenal sphincteroplasty*. The intention is to create a passage into the duodenum equal in size to the diameter of the bile duct, so that any remaining stones can enter the duodenum. Correctly performed, this is probably the procedure of choice for establishing long-term drainage of the duct. Indeed, a few surgeons use the transduodenal approach for routine exploration of the bile duct. Sphincteroplasty implies suturing the bile duct mucosa to the duodenal mucosa. It is preferable to operative sphincterotomy alone, since the sutures are haemostatic and also help to prevent renewed stenosis of the papilla.

4 *Choledochoduodenostomy* is a satisfactory alternative, especially in the elderly.[1] Create an ample side-to-side anastomosis, bypassing the lower part of the bile duct. Occasionally, stasis in the bypassed duct leads to recurrent cholangitis ('sump' syndrome), which can easily and effectively be dealt with by endoscopic papillotomy.[2] Provided the bile duct is dilated, this operation is technically simpler to perform in most cases than sphincteroplasty and may therefore be appropriate if the operating surgeon has little experience of transduodenal sphincteroplasty. Other types of biliary bypass, such as end-to-side choledochoduodenostomy or choledochojejunostomy, offer little advantage over the side-to-side procedure in calculous disease.

5 *Endoscopic papillotomy* can provide ductal drainage without the need for a major surgical operation and is therefore particularly useful in the elderly or infirm. The diathermy incision usually abolishes the pressure gradient between the duodenum and the bile duct and is therefore a form of sphincterotomy. Calculi can often be extracted by retrograde instrumentation or will pass spontaneously. Endoscopic papillotomy is probably the treatment of choice for bile duct stones unless an open operation was contemplated for the gallbladder, including retained stones discovered in the early aftermath of cholecystectomy, unless a T-tube track is available for percutaneous extraction. In experienced hands it is safer than open operation for ductal stones that are causing deep jaundice or acute cholangitis, especially in the elderly or infirm.[3] In the era of laparoscopic surgery, common bile duct stones detected preoperatively can be successfully removed endoscopically before you undertake cholecystectomy.

? DIFFICULTY

1. Thorough mobilization of the duodenum is important to create a safe anastomosis.
2. If the duodenum and/or the bile duct are grossly adherent to surrounding structures and cannot be approximated without tension, choledochoduodenostomy is inadvisable.
3. Consider leaving a T-tube in situ and proceeding to endoscopic papillotomy at a later date.

CHOLEDOCHODUODENOSTOMY

Action

1 First thoroughly mobilize the duodenal loop using Kocher's manoeuvre.

2 If you consider this before exploring the bile duct, make a vertical incision low down in the supraduodenal portion of the duct to avoid subsequent tension on the anastomosis (Fig. 19.8).

3 Incise the duodenum longitudinally at the junction of its first and second parts. Pass a finger downwards to examine the ampulla and exclude a lesion at this site.

4 Roll the duodenum upwards and create a side-to-side anastomosis with the bile duct, using one layer of fine absorbable sutures, either continuous or interrupted. It is important to create a stoma that is at least 2.5 cm in diameter.

5 Place a drain into the subhepatic pouch.

Complications

1 The most serious complication is anastomotic leakage and formation of a duodenal fistula. Treat a high-output fistula with nasogastric intubation and parenteral nutrition; re-operation may well be needed if it fails to close.

2 Anastomotic dehiscence should not occur in the absence of suppurative cholangitis if you avoided creating tension at operation.

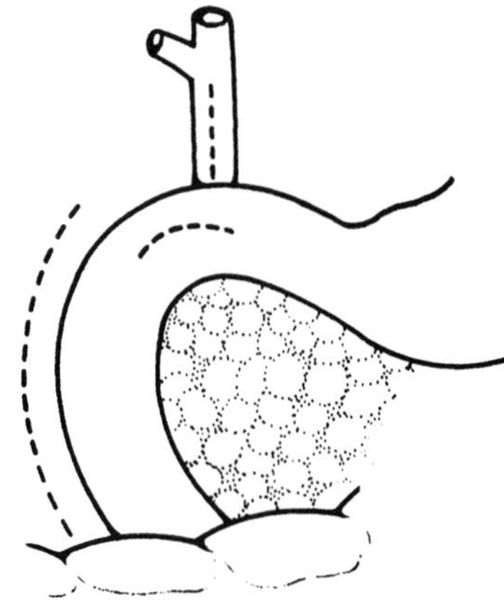

Fig. 19.8 Choledochoduodenostomy. The bile duct and duodenum are opened as shown and then approximated. Kocherization of the duodenum reduces tension on the anastomosis.

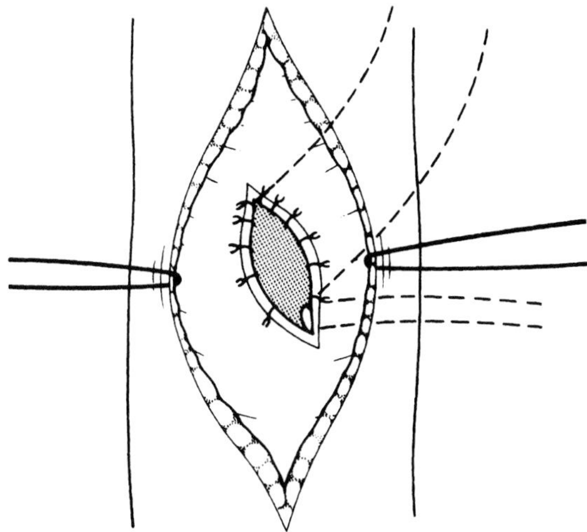

Fig. 19.9 Transduodenal sphincteroplasty. The papilla is approached via a longitudinal duodenotomy and is incised. Interrupted sutures coapt the mucosa of the terminal bile duct and duodenum. The orifice of the major pancreatic duct can be seen at the lower end of the sphincteroplasty.

TRANSDUODENAL SPHINCTEROPLASTY

Action

1 Mobilize the duodenal loop and make a longitudinal duodenotomy incision, about 4 cm long, opposite the papilla (Fig. 19.9). The papilla can usually be palpated in the descending duodenum, especially if it is diseased. Otherwise it can be localized by passing a catheter or bougie down the bile duct via a supraduodenal choledochotomy.

2 Once the duodenum has been opened, grasp the mucosa with Babcock's forceps and search for the papilla on the posteromedial wall. Again, an instrument passed from above may be of assistance.

3 Pass a blunt-nosed polyethylene cannula (no. 8F) through the papilla from above. If necessary, first make a short relieving incision to allow extraction of an impacted calculus or dilate a stenosed papilla gently under direct vision. Cut off the end of the cannula, insert a grooved hernia director into its lumen and withdraw the cannula so that the director enters the lower bile duct with its groove towards the liver.

4 Use the groove to insert two 3/0 absorbable sutures into the papilla at about 10 o'clock and 12 o'clock. Tie these sutures and divide the papilla for a short distance between them, using sharp scissors. Now place and tie two further stay sutures towards the apex of the cut and proceed methodically in this manner until you have created a wide stoma, which usually accepts the tip of the little finger. Each suture unites the lax, pink intestinal mucosa to the paler and tighter mucosa of the terminal bile duct. Insert the final stitch into the apex of the 'V'.

5 Search for the orifice of the major pancreatic duct. The orifice can nearly always be found on the lower lip of the papilla at about 5 o'clock. Clear juice can usually be seen emerging from the duct. Ensure that the opening is in no way obstructed by the sutures. If appropriate, gently pass a fine polythene cannula (no. 4F or 5F) to check the patency of the duct and consider if retrograde pancreatography is indicated.

6 Close the duodenotomy in the line that it was created, using a running suture of 2/0 or 3/0 polyglactin 910 (Vicryl). Place the second, seromuscular, layer of sutures with care to avoid excessive narrowing of the duodenum.

7 Though T-tube drainage of the supraduodenal duct is not essential after carrying out an adequate sphincteroplasty, it does provide a safety-valve if the stoma is narrowed by postoperative oedema and it permits subsequent cholangiography. We always insert a T-tube, therefore.

8 Drain the subhepatic pouch as before.

? DIFFICULTY

1. Do not hesitate to pass an instrument from above if you cannot find the papilla after opening the duodenum.
2. Facilitate display of an inaccessible papilla by placing retractors inside the duodenum.
3. The 'stitch-and-cut' technique described controls haemorrhage and allows you to create and suture a precise incision.

Complications

1 The most serious complication is acute pancreatitis, although duodenal fistula can also arise from the medial or lateral wall. Acute pancreatitis can be avoided by ensuring that the orifice of the major pancreatic duct is not occluded by sutures.

2 Treat established pancreatitis along standard lines (see Ch. 21).

ENDOSCOPIC PAPILLOTOMY

Action

1 Do not attempt endoscopic papillotomy until you are fully proficient at both gastroduodenoscopy and ERCP.

2 As a rule, carry out diagnostic ERCP before performing papillotomy. If a stone is impacted at the papilla it may be impossible to cannulate either ductal orifice until the stone has been extracted, in which case make a 'pre-cut' through the papilla using a needle knife.

3 Treat this procedure like a surgical operation. Admit the patient to hospital, check the coagulation status and platelet count. Group and save serum in case emergency blood transfusion becomes necessary. Starve the patient for 6 hours beforehand. Obtain a preliminary X-ray of the upper abdomen. Sedate the patient with intravenous midazolam, titrated carefully to the desired level of sedation. Give intravenous hyoscine butylbromide (Buscopan, 40 mg) or glucagon (2 mg) to inhibit duodenal peristalsis. Give prophylactic antibiotics when there is bile duct obstruction.

4 Pass a long, insulated, side-viewing duodenoscope through the pylorus and into the descending duodenum. Turn the patient prone. Rotate the instrument to bring the lens 'face-on' to the

papilla, which can be identified as a pink nipple partly covered by a proximal transverse fold of mucosa.

5 Cannulate the bile duct by inserting a diathermy catheter into the papilla along the axis of the duct (i.e. in a retrograde fashion). Insert a small quantity of water-soluble contrast such as Conray 420 under fluoroscopic control to check that the correct duct has been cannulated.

6 Partly withdraw the cannula and exert traction, so that its contained wire arches against the roof of the ampulla at about 1 o'clock. Using alternative bursts of cutting and coagulation current, make a 10–15-mm incision and secure haemostasis.

7 Remove calculi by atraumatic balloon catheters or baskets, but you can leave small stones to pass spontaneously. Sometimes repeated endoscopic examinations or instrumentation can be avoided by leaving a catheter in the bile duct after sphincterotomy and bringing it out through the patient's nose. This allows lavage with saline and the performance of check cholangiograms. Consider contact lithotripsy and endoscopic stenting for unfit patients with large calculi that cannot be extracted from the duct.

KEY POINTS Watch the patient as well as the papilla

- Endoscopic papillotomy and stone retrieval is a difficult procedure suitable only for those with proper experience with this technique.
- The procedure is often performed in a dimly lit room.
- Carefully monitor the patient's vital observations. In elderly patients or those with sepsis, it may be useful to enlist the assistance of an anaesthetist to supervise the patient's sedation.

? DIFFICULTY

1. Remember that attempts at cannulation are doomed to failure unless the papilla is seen 'face-on'.
2. Expertise is needed to achieve successful papillotomy before the patient and the endoscopist become fatigued.
3. Tight stenosis of the ductal orifice and a peri-ampullary diverticulum may make it difficult to cannulate the bile duct and proceed to safe papillotomy.

Complications

1 The complication rate is 5–10% and the mortality rate approximately 1%.

2 Bleeding occasionally requires emergency operative intervention, as does frank perforation, although minor leaks may settle with conservative management.

3 Acute cholangitis is less likely if the duct is cleared of stones.

4 Transient elevation of serum amylase may follow the procedure, but clinical acute pancreatitis is uncommon.

REFERENCES

1. De Almeida AC, dos Santos NM, Aldeia FJ 1996 Choledochoduodenostomy in the management of common duct stones or associated pathology: an obsolete method? HPB Surgery 10:27–33
2. Mavrogiannis C, Liatsos C, Romanos A et al 1999 Sump syndrome: endoscopic treatment and late recurrence. American Journal of Gastroenterology 94:972–975
3. Choudari CP, Fogel E, Kalayci C et al 1999 Therapeutic biliary endoscopy. Endoscopy 31:80–87

ALTERNATIVES TO CHOLECYSTECTOMY

Appraise

- *Cholecystostomy* is a temporary expedient for draining an obstructed or infected gallbladder to the exterior. Consider it when gross disease of the gallbladder or intercurrent illness make cholecystectomy unsafe. In the very elderly or infirm with empyema of the gallbladder or necrotizing cholecystitis, open cholecystostomy under local anaesthetic can be life-saving.[1] If cholecystectomy is planned, but obesity and/or severe inflammation cause serious technical difficulties, cholecystostomy is a reasonable option, especially if you are inexperienced. However, a second operation may well be needed at a later date.
- Cholecystostomy is sometimes performed to relieve obstructive jaundice before proceeding to resection of a periampullary cancer (see Ch. 21) or to drain an obstructed biliary tree, or if gallstones are encountered during laparotomy for severe acute pancreatitis.
- *Subtotal cholecystectomy* may be a better option than cholecystostomy if you encounter difficulty in removing the entire gallbladder for stones. It avoids the need for further surgery.
- *Percutaneous cholecystostomy* may be a better option than open cholecystostomy in a patient with severe acute cholecystitis, especially the acalculous type, who is unfit for operation,[2] and occasionally in a child who develops acute dilatation (hydrops) of the gallbladder.

PERCUTANEOUS CHOLECYSTOSTOMY

Access

1 This technique is carried out by an interventional radiologist in the X-ray department, using local anaesthetic with or without intravenous sedation.

2 Under ultrasound guidance a fine needle is inserted into the gallbladder, using the transhepatic route to reduce the risk of bile leakage.

Action

1 Once access has been gained to the gallbladder, a sample of bile is aspirated for bacteriological culture.

2 A guide-wire is placed through the needle, which is then removed, and dilators are used to dilate the track and allow insertion of a cholecystostomy catheter.

3 A catheter cholecystogram is performed at 24–48 hours to evaluate the cystic duct and confirm the presence of gallstones. Once the patient improves, a choice can be made whether to

proceed to cholecystectomy or attempt percutaneous extraction of the stones.

? DIFFICULTY

In difficult cases, the transperitoneal route can be used to puncture the gallbladder, but loss of access and bile leakage are greater risks by this route.

Complications

- There is a small risk of a vasovagal response and cardiac arrest.
- Bile leakage can occur if the catheter becomes dislodged.

OPEN CHOLECYSTOSTOMY

Access

Carry out planned cholecystostomy through a short transverse incision in the right upper quadrant. Place the incision over the fundus of the gallbladder when this is palpable.

Action

1 Protect the margins of the wound and pack off the area of the gallbladder to prevent contamination by infected bile. Free adhesions sufficiently to expose the fundus of the gallbladder.

2 Aspirate the fluid contents of the gallbladder by suction through an Ochsner trocar and cannula or syringe and wide-bore needle.

3 Grasp the partly collapsed fundus with tissue-holding forceps to control the organ and prevent it from retracting. Make a short incision in the fundus and obtain a culture of the bile. Suck out residual bile.

4 Explore the lumen of the gallbladder with a finger and extract all the stones. Saline irrigation may help or insert a gauze swab to trap small calculi. If the patient's condition allows, try and determine the presence or absence of gangrene, or perforation. If there are obvious calculi in the cystic duct or Hartmann's pouch, they may be gently disimpacted and milked towards the fundal incision.

5 After the gallbladder has been cleared of stones, insert a large Foley or Malecot catheter into the lumen and secure it with Vicryl sutures to effect a watertight closure (Fig. 19.10). The Foley catheter needs to be brought through the abdominal wall via a separate stab incision immediately over the gallbladder before placement. Insert a corrugated drain into the subhepatic space if there has been an extensive dissection.

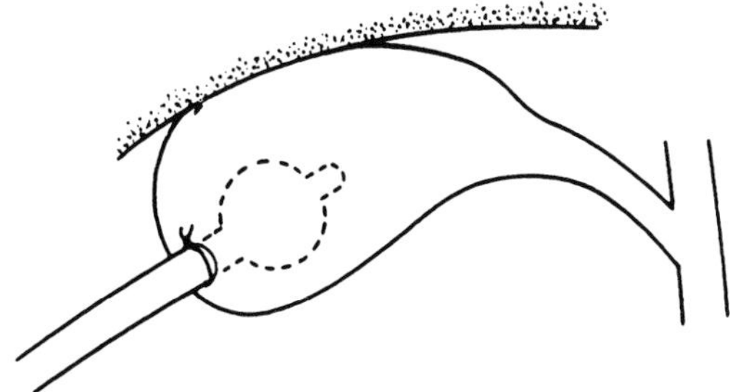

Fig. 19.10 Cholecystostomy. A large Foley catheter is sutured into the gallbladder, taking care not to puncture the balloon when inserting the stitches.

? DIFFICULTY

1. *Is the gallbladder friable or necrotic and does it tear during the dissection?* Excise devitalized segments and close the remnant around the tube. If the cystic duct is cleared of stones and bile flow is re-established, subtotal cholecystectomy without external tube drainage is a reasonable alternative in unfavourable circumstances (see below).
2. *Cannot calculi be disimpacted easily from the depths of the gallbladder?* The options are to remove as much debris as possible and insert a tube as before or proceed to subtotal or complete cholecystectomy despite the patient's poor condition.

Aftercare

1 Record the amount of cholecystostomy drainage and replace electrolytes as needed. Obtain a tube cholecystogram at 7–10 days. If there are no residual stones and contrast enters the bile duct, clamp and then remove the tube. Consider elective cholecystectomy at a later date.

2 Residual stones are a clear indication for re-operation when the patient's condition allows.

SUBTOTAL CHOLECYSTECTOMY

Assess

1 During an attempted cholecystectomy consider this procedure when gross oedema and fibrosis in Calot's triangle make recognition of the surgical landmarks very difficult.[3] To persist with total cholecystectomy in such circumstances risks injury to the hepatic artery and the bile duct.

2 By leaving the posterior wall of the gallbladder in situ, subtotal cholecystectomy may reduce the severity of haemorrhage in a cirrhotic patient with gallstones. It may also be appropriate when you discover a gangrenous gallbladder during planned cholecystostomy.

Action

1 Make no attempt to dissect the cystic artery in Calot's triangle. Aspirate the gallbladder contents and then open the organ. Remove it piecemeal leaving part of the posterior wall attached to the liver. Under-run bleeding vessels with sutures, and cauterize the retained mucosa with diathermy current if it is oozy.

2 It may be possible to obtain a cholangiogram by cannulating the cystic duct via the neck of the opened gallbladder, but in the absence of jaundice you can abandon this step if necessary. Close the orifice of the cystic duct with a purse-string suture inserted within the gallbladder lumen.

Aftercare

1 Leave a drain to the subhepatic space and remove it when appropriate.

2 It should not be necessary to perform any further procedure unless ductal stones have been left behind.

REFERENCES

1. Spain DA, Bibbo C, Ecker T et al 1993 Operative tube versus percutaneous cholecystotomy for acute cholecystitis. American Journal of Surgery 166:28–31
2. Sugiyama M, Tokuhara M, Atomi Y 1998 Is percutaneous cholecystostomy the optimal treatment for acute cholecystitis in the very elderly? World Journal of Surgery 22:459–463
3. Katsohis C, Prousalidis J, Tzardinoglou E et al 1996 Subtotal cholecystectomy. HPB Surgery 9:133–136

HEPATICOJEJUNOSTOMY FOR BENIGN BILE DUCT STRICTURE

Appraise

- This section is chiefly concerned with *traumatic biliary stricture*, which almost always results from inadvertent injury to the bile duct during cholecystectomy. The condition is now also seen following laparoscopic cholecystectomy. Immediate recognition and careful repair of the injured duct at the original operation reduce but do not abolish the risk of subsequent stenosis. Suspect it following cholecystectomy, if there is early development of obstructive jaundice with or without fever. An external biliary fistula strongly suggests an injury to the duct.
- Investigation begins with an ultrasound scan to show any dilatation of the proximal biliary tree and to exclude a collection of bile in the subhepatic space. A good-quality cholangiogram is needed to delineate the stricture, either by percutaneous transhepatic cholangiography (PTC) or endoscopic retrograde cholangiography (ERC) according to the height of the structure and available expertise. For strictures involving the hilus, PTC is superior because it demonstrates the proximal hepatic ducts with greater clarity. Occasionally bilateral PTC is required with separate puncture of the right and left liver. For a complex injury, consider angiography to exclude concomitant vascular damage.
- The best chance of a successful outcome is when the first repair is carried out by an experienced hepatobiliary surgeon. There is little role for the non-operative stenting of benign strictures, except perhaps in high-risk patients. The fundamental principle is to resect the strictured area of duct, leaving a healthy segment of proximal duct for precise anastomosis to a Roux loop of jejunum. When the stricture involves the confluence of hepatic ducts, it is necessary to lower the hilar plate, dividing the connective tissue that covers the biliary confluence and the extrahepatic portion of the left hepatic duct, and to dissect out the right and left hepatic ducts for separate or combined hepaticojejunostomies.[1] There is probably little place nowadays for Smith's mucosal graft procedure, in which a sleeve of jejunal mucosa is sutured to a transhepatic tube and drawn up into the intrahepatic biliary tree; recurrent stricture is common because of the lack of precise mucosal coaptation.
- For a difficult high stricture, and especially when operating for recurrent stricture, it is wise to create a jejunal access loop. This allows the radiologist to approach the anastomosis from below, should subsequent dilatation and calculus extraction be needed.[2]
- *Sclerosing cholangitis* is sometimes amenable to a surgical approach entailing resection of a dominant stricture at or below the hilus with reconstruction by means of hepaticojejunostomy Roux-en-Y. Exclude cholangiocarcinoma as far as possible by operative biopsy.
- Kasai's hepatic portoenterostomy may permit surgical correction of otherwise non-correctable *congenital biliary atresia*. The atretic ducts are followed to the porta hepatis, and a small disc of liver tissue is excised at this point, revealing small bile ducts. The end of a Roux loop is then sewn to the surrounding liver capsule.
- The most common type of *choledochal cyst* can be likened to a fusiform aneurysm of the extrahepatic bile duct. Resect it with hepaticojejunostomy at or just below the hilus. Internal drainage of a choledochal cyst is inadequate because of the subsequent risks of cholangitis and cholangiocarcinoma.

The operation of hepaticojejunostomy for iatrogenic biliary stricture will now be described, but similar principles apply to the surgical management of the other benign conditions of the bile duct.

Prepare

1 Control sepsis with drainage of any subhepatic collection of infected bile and with appropriate antibiotics.

2 Correct any electrolyte imbalance and malnutrition.

3 Unless there is complete occlusion of the extrahepatic biliary tree, jaundice may not be particularly severe. Take perioperative precautions in jaundiced patients.

4 It is usually better to spend time in thorough investigation and preoperative preparation than rush to re-explore.

Access

1 It is usually possible to use the old cholecystectomy incision, but do not hesitate to extend it as required or start afresh with a right subcostal incision if the previous incision is inappropriate.

2 There are likely to be extensive adhesions in the right upper quadrant and possibly also residual collections of extravasated bile. Locate the right lobe of the liver and detach adherent organs, such as stomach, duodenum and transverse colon, from its lower border. Identify and mobilize the duodenal loop, and explore carefully above this point to find the bile duct. Be prepared to aspirate any potential tube with syringe and needle, looking for bile.

Assess

1 Except for an early and very localized stricture well below the hilus, resection of an established stricture with direct end-to-end anastomosis is unlikely to produce a successful long-term result, unlike primary repair at the time of injury.

2 Remember that the objective is to free-up an adequate length of healthy proximal bile duct and to fashion an accurate and watertight anastomosis to the jejunum with the complete avoidance of tension.

Action

1 Dissect out the supraduodenal portion of the bile duct and encircle it with a sling, taking care not to injure the portal vein lying posteriorly.

2 The site of the stricture can usually be identified from without, but, if not, open the duct low down and explore gently with probes. Recurrent stricture following a previous repair is almost always at the site of biliary–enteric anastomosis, so trace the bowel upwards to this point.

3 Divide the bile duct below the stricture or detach it from the bowel anastomosis. Obtain a culture of bile. Should you remove a liver biopsy specimen? Oversew the distal end of the duct. Holding the proximal end with a pair of artery forceps dissect upwards, keeping close to the duct, to expose at least 1 cm of healthy duct above the fibrotic or inflamed area of the stricture. It may be necessary to transect the duct at progressively higher levels until you are satisfied with the mucosal appearances.

4 Resect the strictured segment. If the proximal duct is undilated, consider whether incising it for a few millimetres in the anterior midline would make for an easier and wider anastomosis. It is suggested that anastomotic strictures occur as a result of ischaemia and the recommendation is that the anastomosis be fashioned with proximal rather than distal hepatic duct.[3]

5 Select a length of upper jejunum for conversion into a Roux loop (see Ch. 14). Transilluminate the mesentery, ligate and divide two or three arterial arcades, transect the bowel and close the distal cut end with a double layer of sutures. Create a mesocolic window and bring the Roux loop up behind the transverse colon, so that it reaches the common hepatic duct without tension.

6 Make a small enterotomy some 3 cm from the closed end of the Roux loop. Make the incision slightly shorter than the diameter of the bile duct, bearing in mind that an enterotomy will stretch.

7 Fashion the hepaticojejunostomy using a single layer of interrupted 3/0 or 4/0 polyglactin 910 (Vicryl) sutures.[4] Insert the corner stitches followed by the back row. Clip each stitch and do not tie until the entire back row has been inserted.

8 If the anastomosis has been difficult to create, for example with a small or rather fibrotic duct, it is wise to splint it with a fine tube. Use a transhepatic tube brought out through the liver parenchyma by means of a blunt introducer (Fig. 19.11). Other surgeons prefer a tube brought out through the jejunum well below the anastomosis. In either case, bring the tube to the exterior; it can be used to obtain a postoperative check cholangiogram.

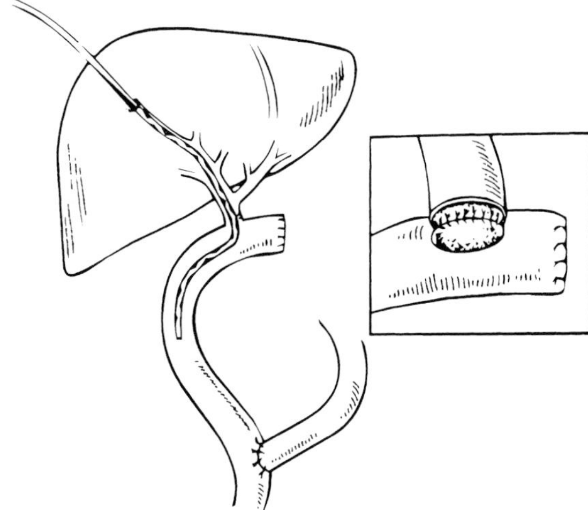

Fig. 19.11 Hepaticojejunostomy Roux-en-Y. A retrocolic jejunal conduit has been brought up for anastomosis to the upper common hepatic duct. A transhepatic splinting tube has been placed across the anastomosis. Side holes are created in those segments of the tube destined to lie within the liver and jejunum. An alternative ploy is to position the upper end of the tube within the intrahepatic biliary tree and bring the lower end out through the jejunum below the anastomosis. The insert shows a close-up of the biliary–enteric anastomosis after tying the posterior row of sutures (and with the tube omitted for the sake of clarity).

9 Now complete the anterior row of interrupted Vicryl sutures to create a watertight anastomosis.

10 Restore intestinal continuity by end-to-side jejunojejunostomy.

11 Close the abdomen with a drain to the subhepatic space.

Approach to the left hepatic duct (Fig. 19.12)

1 Divide the ligamentum teres and free the falciform ligament from the abdominal wall back to the diaphragm. Be willing to divide the narrow bridge of tissue connecting the left lateral segment of liver to the quadrate lobe to further improve exposure.

2 Retract the quadrate lobe, and make an incision through the connective tissue at its base where Glisson's capsule blends with the lesser omentum (Fig. 19.12a).

3 The hilar plate is lowered by deepening this incision to expose the main left hepatic duct, which runs almost horizontally at this point and lies outside the liver substance (Fig. 19.12b).

4 Follow the left duct to the right to expose its confluence with the right hepatic duct, which can then itself be mobilized. If necessary, gain further exposure of the left duct by dissecting it to the left towards the umbilical fissure.

? DIFFICULTY

1. High strictures involving the confluence of the hepatic ducts are particularly demanding. Tackle them only if you have experience with this type of surgery. The usual principles apply; prepare healthy ducts above the stricture for anastomosis to a jejunal loop. Problems arise from difficult access, small undistensible ducts affected by secondary sclerosing cholangitis and, in late cases, secondary biliary cirrhosis and portal hypertension.
2. Most hilar strictures can be dealt with by dissecting out the left hepatic ductal system, as described below. Occasionally further access to the right hepatic duct may be gained by splitting the liver in the principal plane (hepatotomy) or, in particularly difficult cases, the hilar dissection can be abandoned and an approach made to the segment III duct in the umbilical fissure. These techniques are outlined in the next section.
3. If the main confluence of the hepatic ducts has to be resected, repair can often be effected by suturing together the medial walls of the right and left hepatic ducts and then anastomosing the united duct to the Roux loop. If the ducts are widely separated, individual anastomosis will be required. Many surgeons use bilateral transanastomotic stents to cover this type of high repair. If recurrent stricture seems likely, for example in the presence of extensive fibrosis or after a previous failed repair, create an access loop.

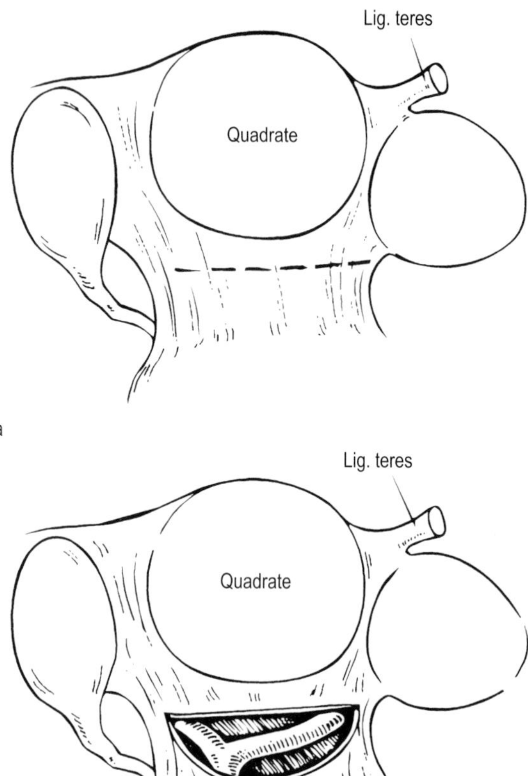

Fig. 19.12 Lowering the hilar plate during an approach to the left hepatic duct. (a) After elevating the quadrate lobe, the peritoneum is incised horizontally at the point at which the lesser omentum fuses with the liver capsule. (b) The left hepatic duct has been traced to the right to expose its confluence with the right hepatic duct.

Creation of an access loop (Fig. 19.13)

1 Hepaticojejunostomy is carried out to the apex of the jejunal loop, leaving approximately 15 cm of bowel beyond the anastomosis, so that the closed upper end can be brought up to the abdominal wall without tension but also without redundancy.

2 If a transanastomotic stent has been employed, bring out the tube close to the apex of the bowel. Using stainless-steel wire, place a purse-string suture through the bowel at this point and tie it to produce a marked ring 3 cm in diameter. Suture the apex of the jejunum to the undersurface of the abdominal wall. Place a row of metal clips along the serosa to mark each border of the access loop.

3 If stenosis subsequently develops at the biliary–enteric anastomosis, the radiologist can percutaneously puncture the access loop through the marker ring and use the metal slips as 'landing lights' to advance a guide-wire up the access loop and through the anastomosis.

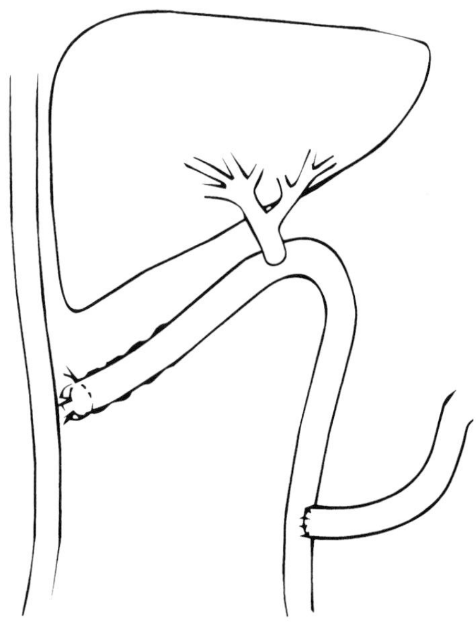

Fig. 19.13 Hepaticojejunostomy with a jejunal access loop. The top of the Roux loop is anchored to the peritoneum of the anterior abdominal wall, and it is marked with a circular stainless-steel suture and metal clips to show the axis of bowel leading to the anastomosis. The radiologist can subsequently use these radio-opaque guides for a percutaneous approach via the jejunal loop to the anastomosis.

Aftercare and complications

1 Potential complications of hepaticojejunostomy are wound infection, cholangitis, subhepatic abscess and a biliary fistula from an anastomotic leak. Most of the serious complications and deaths occur in patients with difficult hilar strictures,

especially after repeated operations and in those with portal hypertension.

2 Postoperative cholangiography is carried out through one or more transanastomotic stents 7–10 days after the operation. If the anastomosis is intact, you can make a decision on whether to remove the stent at this stage or, following a difficult repair, to leave it in situ for several weeks.

3 The incidence of late restricture varies widely according to the length and thoroughness of follow-up and the proportion of difficult cases included in any one series. Serial liver function tests and cholescintigraphy with iminodiacetic acid derivatives can be used to assess the patency of the repair.

REFERENCES

1. Sutherland F, Launois B, Stanescu M et al 1999 A refined approach to the repair of postcholecystectomy bile duct strictures. Archives of Surgery 134:299–302
2. McPherson SJ, Gibson RN, Collier NA et al 1998 Percutaneous transjejunal biliary intervention: 10 year experience with access via Roux-en-Y loops. Radiology 206:665–672
3. Terblanche J, Worthley CS, Spence RA et al 1990 High or low hepaticojejunostomy for bile duct strictures. Surgery 108:828–834
4. DiFronzo LA, Egrari S, O'Connell TX 1998 Safety and durability of single layer, stentless, biliary–enteric anastomosis. American Surgeon 64:917–920

OPERATIONS FOR HILAR CHOLANGIOCARCINOMA

Appraise

- Malignant stricture of the bile duct at the level of the hilus is caused by cholangiocarcinoma, direct invasion of gallbladder carcinoma or nodal metastasis from a primary carcinoma elsewhere such as breast, stomach, pancreas. Of these, primary cholangiocarcinoma is the most amenable to surgical cure, because it is relatively slow-growing and can remain localized for a long time, but less than one-third of patients have disease amenable to curative resection.[1]
- The level, nature and extent of a malignant bile-duct stricture can generally be determined preoperatively by a combination of ultrasound and CT (computed tomography) scan, PTC (sometimes bilateral) and angiography. CT and magnetic resonance cholangiography with three-dimensional reconstruction are proving to be useful non-invasive investigations. Also assess the patient's suitability for major hepatobiliary surgery. In recent years, positron emission tomography (PET) has also proved to be valuable in preoperative diagnosis and staging of cholangiocarcinoma.[2]
- For resectable cholangiocarcinomas a choice has to be made between local excision of the hilus, central hepatic resection (local excision plus quadrate lobectomy) and a major hepatectomy comprising right or left hemihepatectomy, or even extended hepatectomy. The choice depends largely on the extent of ductal disease but partly on the involvement of vascular structures and hepatic parenchyma. You may be able to make the final decision only at operation. Sometimes local excision of the hilus is a reasonable option even if residual disease at the resection margin makes this purely palliative. It is generally agreed that resection of segment I (caudate lobe) is necessary to achieve curative resection.[3] The role of total hepatectomy and liver transplantation in cholangiocarcinoma has been reported from a large series of 207 transplanted patients, but the long-term results are poor due to a high incidence of local and systemic recurrence.[4]
- Irresectability of a cholangiocarcinoma is generally indicated by hepatic or distant metastases, by a large mass, by involvement of the main trunk of the hepatic artery or portal vein and by strictures extending up to involve the second-order ducts on both sides. For irresectable tumours a choice has to be made between non-operative stenting on the one hand, usually by percutaneous insertion of an endoprosthesis such as an expandable metal stent, and surgical bypass on the other hand. Preoperative PTC should indicate whether there is a dilated segment of left hepatic duct or its tributary (the segment III duct) that is available for a left hepaticojejunostomy.[5] The Longmire procedure can occasionally be used for patients with advanced disease at the hilus (see below). Nowadays there is very little place for operative intubation, since stenting can be achieved more simply by the percutaneous or endoscopic route.
- From the above comments you realize that patients with malignant bile-duct stricture should be managed jointly by yourself and the interventional radiologist. The radiologist plays a crucial role in preoperative imaging and, by stenting the stricture, can obviate the need for a major operative procedure in an unfavourable case. He can also provide preoperative biliary decompression if this is considered desirable (see below).
- Tackle operations on the hepatic hilus only if you have adequate experience. Techniques for the resection and bypass of a malignant hilar stricture are outlined in this chapter. Hepatectomy is considered in Chapter 22. For more detailed descriptions of these operations, consult a specialist text.

KEY POINT Palliating hilar cholangiocarcinoma

- Most patients with hilar cholangiocarcinoma are not resectable for cure, and adequate palliation depends on draining functional liver volume. This goal can be reliably achieved by stenting and only occasionally is surgical bypass required in patients who are initially explored for potential resection.

Prepare

Correct anaemia and coagulopathy preoperatively. Acute cholangitis and incipient renal failure are indications for emergency biliary decompression either from above (at PTC) or, if necessary, from below (at ERCP). Many surgeons proceed without such decompression, preferring to operate on a dilated and uninfected proximal biliary tree.

Access

1 The standard approach is via a bilateral subcostal ('high gable') incision, which can be extended upwards in the midline or laterally into the right flank to increase exposure.

2 Full mobilization of the liver is required if you need to undertake major hepatectomy.

Action

1 *Local excision of hilar stricture*. The technique is similar to that described above for a benign stricture involving the confluence of the hepatic ducts. Mobilize the gallbladder and dissect the common hepatic duct upwards. Lower the hilar plate to improve exposure. If resection seems feasible, divide the common hepatic duct low down, oversew the distal end, and exert gentle traction on a clip applied to the proximal end so as to facilitate the posterior dissection. Carefully dissect the ductal confluence off the bifurcations of the hepatic artery and portal vein, which lie behind it. Transect the right and left hepatic duct or their major tributaries at a convenient level above the upper extent of carcinoma. The resection margin of the duct can be sent for frozen-section examination if there is any doubt. Sometimes access to the right hepatic duct can be improved by hepatotomy, that is splitting the liver deeply in the principal plane just to the left of the gallbladder fossa. Alternatively, resect the quadrate lobe which opens up the centre of the liver like a book. Sometimes part or even all of the caudate lobe must be removed to clear a tumour extending posteriorly. The drawback of dividing liver tissue is the increased blood loss entailed. After excising the tumour, prepare a Roux loop for hepaticojejunostomy with or without bilateral transanastomotic stents, which should be placed before commencing the anastomosis (see previous section). It may be possible to approximate the two or more hepatic ducts with sutures and then sew them as a single duct to the Roux loop. If access is limited, it often helps to place the anterior row of sutures through the ductal mucosa before placing and tying the posterior row; then insert the anterior sutures into the bowel to complete the anastomosis.

2 *Excision of the hilus with major liver resection*. This approach may be indicated to achieve complete clearance of a cholangiocarcinoma extending asymmetrically to involve second- or third-order ducts on one side only. Unilateral occlusion of the relevant hepatic artery or portal vein branch is not a contraindication. Right hemihepatectomy may be extended to include segment IV (quadrate) if necessary to obtain tumour clearance, provided the patient is a good surgical risk and has sufficient hepatic reserve. Left hemihepatectomy can likewise be extended to the right. Resect the ductal confluence together with the appropriate liver segments en bloc. Reconstruction involves anastomosis to the retained left or right hepatic duct. The principles of hepatic resection are described in Chapter 22.

3 *Palliative bypass to the left hepatic ducts*. Traced upwards from the confluence, the right hepatic duct plunges almost vertically into the liver but the left hepatic duct runs horizontally within the hilar plate before branching and entering the liver tissue near the umbilical fissure. By lowering the hilar plate, you can often expose a 2–3-cm segment of dilated main left duct that lies away from the hilus and is therefore free of tumour and suitable for anastomosis. Proper decompression of one-half of the liver will usually bring about the resolution of jaundice. The undrained segments atrophy, while those that are drained undergo compensatory hyperplasia. If the main left duct is involved by cancer, it may still be possible to relieve jaundice by carrying out an anastomosis to the segment III duct, which lies within the umbilical fissure. Divide the narrow bridge of liver tissue joining the quadrate lobe to the left lateral segment, and then pull the round ligament (ligamentum teres) downwards. Incise the peritoneum overlying the left side of its base and deepen the incision, taking care to secure bleeding vessels. Expose the segment III duct as it lies just above the portal vein branch to the lateral segment. Open the duct in its long axis and anastomose it to a jejunal loop over a splinting tube.

4 *Longmire procedure*. A small segment at the tip of the right or left liver is resected to expose dilated intrahepatic ducts, which can be used for a palliative peripheral hepaticojejunostomy (Fig. 19.14). The procedure is occasionally indicated for an

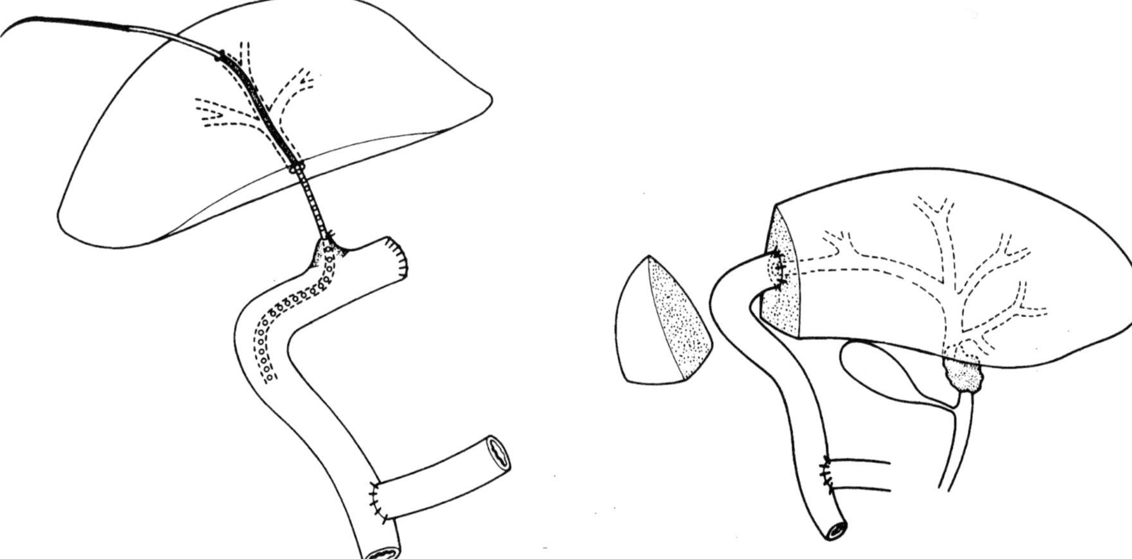

Fig. 19.14 Longmire's operation for irresectable tumour at the hilus of the liver. After resection of the lateral pole of the right (and/or left) hepatic lobe, a Roux loop of jejunum is sutured around the exposed dilated bile ducts.

irresectable hilar tumour if access to the main left duct or its branches is difficult, for example in a patient with an atrophic right liver and gross hypertrophy on the left.

Aftercare and complications

1 Complications are similar to those described after hepaticojejunostomy for bile duct stricture, with the added risks of bleeding and liver failure if a major hepatectomy is included (see Ch. 22).

2 In skilled hands the mortality rate of a hilar resection including hepatectomy is approximately 10%.

REFERENCES

1. Burke EC, Jarnagin WR, Hochwald SN et al 1998 Hilar cholangiocarcinoma; patterns of spread, the importance of hepatic resection for curative operation, and the presurgical clinical staging. Annals of Surgery 228:385–394
2. Kluge R, Schmidt F, Caca K et al 2001 Positron emission tomography with ^{18}fluor-2-deoxy-D-glucose for diagnosis and staging of bile duct cancer. Hepatology 33:1029–1035
3. Nimura Y, Hayakawa N, Kamiya J 1994 Hilar cholangiocarcinoma: the surgical therapy. In: Serio G, Huguet C, Williamson RCN (eds) Hepatobiliary and pancreatic tumours. Graffham Press, Edinburgh, pp 116–122
4. Meyer CG, Penn I, James L 2000 Liver transplantation for cholangiocarcinoma: results in 207 patients. Transplantation 69:1633–1637
5. Jarnagin WR, Burke E, Powers C et al 1998 Intrahepatic biliary enteric bypass provides effective palliation in selected patients with malignant obstruction at the hepatic duct confluence. American Journal of Surgery 175:453–460

FURTHER READING

Adam A, Roddie ME 1991 Acute cholecystitis: radiological management. In: Williamson RCN, Thompson JN (eds) Gastrointestinal emergencies: part II. Baillière Tindall, London, pp 787–816

Baker AR, Neoptolemos JP, Leese T et al 1987 Choledochoduodenostomy, transduodenal sphincteroplasty and sphincterotomy for calculi of the common bile duct. Surgery, Gynecology and Obstetrics 164:245–251

Blumgart LH, Fong Y 2000 Surgery of the liver and biliary tract, 3rd edn. Saunders, London

Boggi U, Candio G, Campatelli A et al 1999 Percutaneous cholecystectomy for acute cholecystitis in critically ill patients. Hepatogastroenterology 46(25):121–125

Bornman PC, Terblanche J 1985 Subtotal cholecystectomy: for the difficult gallbladder in portal hypertension and cholecystitis. Surgery 98:1–6

Csendes A, Burdiles P, Diaz JC 1998 Present role of open choledochostomy in the surgical treatment of patients with common bile duct stones. World Journal of Surgery 22:1167–1170

De Aretxabala X, Bahamondes J C 1998 Choledochoduodenostomy for common bile duct stones. World Journal of Surgery 22:1171–1174

D'Angelica MI, Jarnagin WR, Blumgart LH 2004 Resectable hilar cholangiocarcinoma: surgical treatment and long-term outcome Surgery Today 34:885–890

Ebata T, Nagino M, Kamiya J et al 2003 Hepatectomy with portal vein resection for hilar cholangiocarcinoma: audit of 52 consecutive cases. Annals of Surgery 238:720–727

Frazee RC, Van Heerden JA 1989 Cholecystectomy with concomitant exploration of the common bile duct. Surgery, Gynecology and Obstetrics 168:513–516

Gonzalez-Koch A, Nervi F 1998 Medical management of common bile duct stones. World Journal of Surgery 22:1145–1150

Gouma DJ, Obertop H 1992 Acute calculous cholecystitis. What is new in diagnosis and therapy? HPB Surgery 6:69–78

Kondylis PD, Simmons DR, Agarwal SK et al 1997 Abnormal intraoperative cholangiography. Treatment options and long term follow-up. Archives of Surgery 132:347–350

Krige JEJ, Bornman PC, Harries-Jones EP et al 1987 Modified hepaticojejunostomy for permanent biliary access. British Journal of Surgery 74:612–613

Launois B, Sutherland FR, Harissis H 1999 A new technique of Hepp-Couinaud hepaticojejunostomy using the posterior approach to the hepatic hilum. Journal of the American College of Surgeons 188:59–62

Lillemoe KD, Pitt HA, Cameron JL 1992 Current management of benign bile duct strictures. Advances in Surgery 25:119–174

Marcos-Alvarez A, Jenkins RL 1996 Cholangiocarcinoma. Surgical Oncology Clinics of North America 5:310–316

Matsuoka J, Sakagami K, Gouch A et al 1994 A safe, easy technique for transduodenal sphincteroplasty. Journal of the American College of Surgeons 179:474–476

Maudar KK 1996 Evaluation of surgical options in difficult gallbladder stone disease. Journal of the Indian Medical Association 94:138–140

Metcalfe MS, Wemyss-Holden SA, Maddern GJ 2003 Management dilemmas with choledochal cysts. Archives of Surgery 138:333–339

Munson JL, Sanders LE 1994 Cholecystectomy. Open cholecystectomy revisited. Surgical Clinics of North America 74:741–754

Nagino M, Nimura Y, Kamiya J et al 1998 Segmental liver resections for hilar cholangiocarcinoma. Hepatogastroenterology 45:7–13

Pappas TN, Slimane TB, Rooks DC 1990 100 consecutive common duct explorations without mortality. Annals of Surgery 211:259–262

Pernthaler H, Sandbichler P, Schmid T et al 1990 Operative cholangiography in elective cholecystectomy. British Journal of Surgery 77:399–400

Schmidt SC, Langrehr JM, Hintze RE et al 2004 Management and outcome of patients with combined bile duct and hepatic arterial injuries after laparoscopic cholecystectomy. Surgery 135:613–618

Strasberg SM 1998 Resection of hilar cholangiocarcinoma. HPB Surgery 10:415–418

Toouli J, Wright TA 1998 Gallstones. Medical Journal of Australia 169:166–171

Traynor O, Castaing D, Bismuth H 1987 Left intrahepatic cholangioenteric anastomosis (round ligament approach): an effective palliative treatment for hilar cancers. British Journal of Surgery 74:952–954

Widdison AL, Norton S, Armstrong CP 1995 Open cholecystectomy in the age of the laparoscope. Annals of the Royal College of Surgeons of England 77:256–258

Williamson RCN 1988 Acalculous disease of the gallbladder. Gut 29:860–872

Williamson RCN, Abdulhadi ALY 1994 Recent advances in diagnosis and treatment of carcinoma of the gallbladder. In: Serio G, Huguet C, Williamson RCN (eds) Hepatobiliary and pancreatic tumours. Graffham Press, Edinburgh, pp. 127–138

Winkler E, Kaplan O, Gutman M et al 1989 Role of cholecystostomy in the management of critically ill patients suffering from acute cholecystitis. British Journal of Surgery 76:693–695

20

Laparoscopic biliary surgery

J.N. Thompson, S.G. Appleton

CONTENTS

LAPAROSCOPIC CHOLECYSTECTOMY

Appraise

1 Laparoscopic cholecystectomy is now the treatment of choice for patients with symptomatic gallstones. Additional indications for the operation include selected patients with gallstones who have no symptoms but are at risk of severe complications and those who have no stones but suffer severe 'biliary' symptoms.[1]

2 There are few absolute contraindications to laparoscopic cholecystectomy. Cirrhosis with portal hypertension is dangerous because of the substantial risk of uncontrollable bleeding during the operation, which may also precipitate hepatic failure. Sustained carbon dioxide pneumoperitoneum can cause significant cardiovascular changes in patients with ischaemic heart disease and significant hypercarbia in patients with respiratory disease. If carcinoma of the gallbladder is diagnosed preoperatively, avoid laparoscopic excision.

3 Contraindications to the laparoscopic technique may become apparent during the procedure. These include:
- Discovery of a different pathology from that expected.
- An inability to identify the anatomy safely, usually because dense adhesions make safe dissection impossible.
- Uncontrollable bleeding and damage to adjacent structures or organs.

KEY POINTS Respond to circumstances

- In the face of these findings, convert to an open procedure sooner rather than later.
- Conversion to an open cholecystectomy is not a failure of surgical technique but safe practice.

4 Some centres now perform laparoscopic cholecystectomy as a day-case procedure, although this requires appropriate facilities and good postoperative support.

5 Laparoscopic cholecystectomy has rendered virtually obsolete non-operative treatments of gallstones such as lithotripsy or dissolution therapy.

6 Mini-cholecystectomy performed through a 5-cm right upper quadrant incision is an alternative to laparoscopic cholecystectomy and has comparable results. However, as with the laparoscopic procedure, special instruments and training are required.

Prepare

1 Obtain informed consent for laparoscopic cholecystectomy, including discussion of:
- The possibility of conversion to an open operation during the procedure, which varies from unit to unit but is of the order of 5%.
- The risks of bleeding, infection, bile leak and ductal injury.
- If operative cholangiography is to be performed, the possibility of finding common bile duct stones (10%) and their management.

2 Institute thromboprophylaxis with subcutaneous heparin and compression stockings because the reverse Trendelenburg position, together with a positive-pressure pneumoperitoneum, encourages the development of deep venous thrombosis.

3 General anaesthesia is required, with endotracheal intubation and muscle relaxation.

4 Biliary tract surgery rarely involves anaerobic microorganisms and satisfactory prophylaxis is achieved with a cephalosporin alone. Give a prophylactic antibiotic such as cefuroxime 1.5 mg intravenously as a single dose at the induction of anaesthesia. If there is leakage of bile during the operation, give a further two postoperative doses.

5 Place the patient supine on a radiolucent operating table that allows on-table cholangiography. The patient's upper abdomen and lower chest lie over the radiolucent section. There should be room for the C-arm of the image intensifier both above and below the table.

6 Pass a nasogastric tube to deflate the stomach. This decreases aspiration associated with the pneumoperitoneum, reduces the risk of accidental perforation by a trocar and improves visibility during the procedure. Similarly, if you use a closed technique for inserting the initial trocar, pass a catheter to empty the urinary bladder and avoid accidental perforation.

7 Most surgeons stand on the patient's left with the first assistant opposite (Fig. 20.1). Alternatively, the patient may be placed in the Lloyd-Davies position while you operate from the foot of the table between the patient's legs.

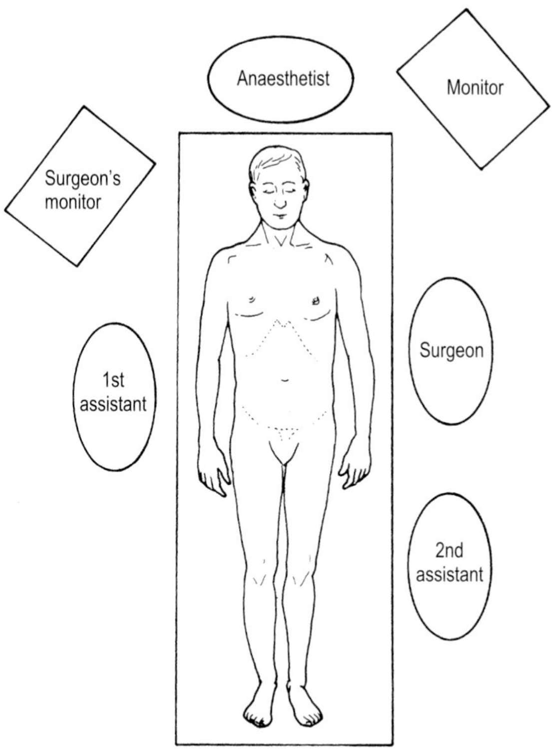

Fig. 20.1 Position of personnel for laparoscopic cholecystectomy.

8 Prepare the skin of the abdomen from the nipples to the suprapubic region using 10% povidone–iodine in alcohol (Betadine) or other cleansing agent. Ensure the skin is prepared up to the posterior axillary line on the patient's right side, for the lateral port. Similarly, ensure that the drape at the top end extends above the level of the xiphisternum and that the right drape is placed as far lateral as possible.

9 Arrange the various leads and tubes that may be required before establishing the pneumoperitoneum; these include the gas tubing, diathermy lead, light source and irrigation–suction tubing. Secure them with clips or tape to the surgical drapes around the operating field, to minimize tangling.

Access

1 We use an 'open' laparoscopic technique to access the peritoneal cavity, insert the primary subumbilical cannula and establish a pneumoperitoneum.[2] A Veress needle is used to establish a pneumoperitoneum in the closed technique, followed by blind insertion of the initial trocar and cannula (see Ch. 5). Insert all subsequent trocars under direct vision. Maintain an intra-abdominal pressure of 10–14 mmHg throughout the procedure.

2 A 30° laparoscope is better than a 0° scope for obtaining 'angled' views and for 'looking down' onto Calot's triangle (described by the French surgeon Jean Francois Calot, 1801–1844)—the triangle bounded above by the liver, below by the cystic duct and medially by the common hepatic artery, although other definitions exist.

3 Four ports are required initially (Fig. 20.2): a 10-mm umbilical port for the camera; a 5-mm lateral port to retract the fundus

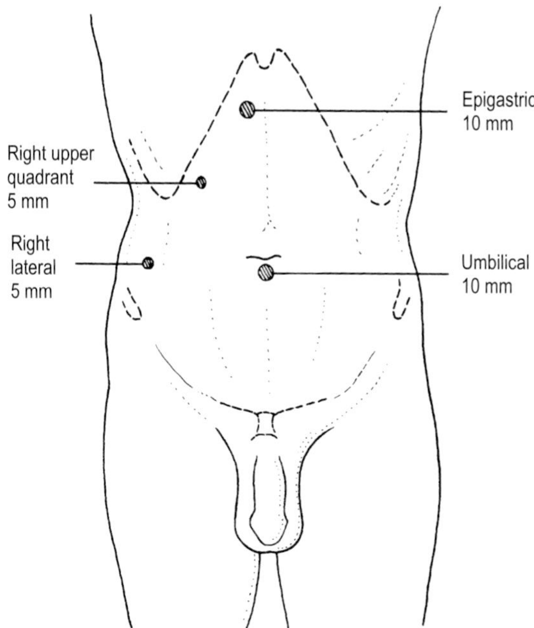

Fig. 20.2 Positions of port sites for laparoscopic cholecystectomy.

of the gallbladder; a 5-mm right upper quadrant port placed in the midclavicular line to manipulate the neck of the gallbladder; a 10-mm cannula with a 5-mm reducer or a 5–12-mm disposable port in the epigastrium, just to the right of the midline and 2–5 cm below the xiphisternum.

4 Introduce the epigastric port into the abdominal cavity through or just to the right of the ligamentum teres. It is the main port for dissecting instruments, diathermy, clip applicators, suction and irrigation.

5 A large or floppy left lobe of the liver occasionally obstructs the view of Calot's triangle. Overcome this with a liver retractor placed through an additional 5-mm port in the left upper quadrant.

Assess

1 As in a laparotomy, the initial task is to examine the abdominal cavity. Carry out a systematic inspection of the contents of the four quadrants and pelvis. This is equivalent to the exploratory laparotomy in open biliary surgery. Note common disorders of a benign nature, for example colonic diverticular disease, pelvic adnexal disease in the female, but these do not preclude the performance of laparoscopic cholecystectomy. More serious findings, particularly if you suspect neoplasia, may necessitate conversion to open laparotomy or postponement of the surgical treatment pending further investigations and preparation of the patient.

2 Facilitate your assessment of the subhepatic region by tilting the operating table 25–35° head up and 10–15° sideways to the left; this encourages the abdominal contents to fall away from the area.

3 *Assess feasibility of laparoscopic cholecystectomy*. This is an assessment of the technical difficulty and safety of gallbladder

excision using the laparoscopic method. To a large extent, the decision is influenced by your experience of laparoscopic surgery. The situations that may be encountered are:

- *Easy cases*. The patient is thin and the intraperitoneal fat is minimal. The gallbladder is floppy and non-adherent. When the gallbladder is lifted and retracted upwards by a grasping forceps, the cystic pedicle—the fold of peritoneum covering the cystic artery, duct and lymph node—is readily identified as a smooth triangular fold between the neck of the gallbladder, the inferior surface of the liver and the common bile duct. These patients are undoubtedly better served by laparoscopic than by open cholecystectomy.
- *Feasible but more difficult cases*. These include obese patients in whom the cystic pedicle is fat-laden. A gallbladder containing a large stone load may be difficult to grasp and this can cause problems with retraction and exposure. The gallbladder may be distended by cholecystitis or because of a stone impacted in the neck. Difficulties may also be encountered due to adhesions from previous surgery. Provided you are experienced and prepared to proceed carefully, laparoscopic cholecystectomy can be accomplished with safety and a good outcome.
- *Cases of uncertain feasibility—trial dissection*. This group includes patients with dense adhesions, those in whom the cystic pedicle cannot be visualized and patients with contracted fibrotic gallbladders where the neck or Hartmann's pouch appears to be adherent to the common bile duct. If you are experienced, it is reasonable to perform a careful trial dissection. The feasibility or otherwise of the operation becomes apparent as the dissection proceeds.

KEY POINTS Be willing to convert

- Trial dissection does not equate with a long or hazardous procedure.
- If you cannot clearly identify and expose the structures of the cystic pedicle in Calot's triangle, convert to an open procedure.

- *Unsuitable cases*. These include patients with the following findings:
  i. Severe acute cholecystitis with gangrenous patches or a gross inflammatory phlegmon obscuring the structures of the porta hepatis
  ii. Chronically inflamed gallbladder with the neck adherent to the common hepatic duct, indicative of the syndrome described in 1948 by the Argentinian surgeon Pablo Mirizzi. This was obstructive jaundice caused by compression of the common hepatic duct by a stone on the cystic duct or neck of the gallbladder; variations have subsequently been described.
  iii. Cirrhosis with established portal hypertension and large high-pressure varices surrounding the gallbladder and cystic pedicle.

In patients with severe acute cholecystitis that precludes safe dissection, a laparoscopic cholecystostomy may be performed, with interval cholecystectomy at a later date (see later). It is foolhardy to attempt laparoscopic cholecystectomy in patients in whom the gallbladder neck/Hartmann's pouch is densely adherent or fistulated into the common hepatic duct, since the risk of damage to the bile duct is considerable. These patients are best served by open operation (see Ch. 19).

4 If the gallbladder is not visible then use blunt-tipped grasping forceps or a probe in the lateral port to gently sweep away omentum, colon or small bowel. Alternatively, insert grasping forceps under the edge of the liver and gently lift it to expose the fundus of the gallbladder.

5 Grasp the fundus of the gallbladder with self-retaining toothed grasping forceps inserted through the lateral port. Gently push the gallbladder up over the liver towards the diaphragm as far as it will comfortably go and have your assistant hold it in this position.

6 It is difficult to grasp a distended and tense gallbladder so decompress it with a Veress needle or a 16G Abbocath passed through the abdominal wall just below the costal margin in the midclavicular line. Aspirate gallbladder contents using a 20-ml syringe or suction tubing put in the barrel of a 10-ml syringe with the plunger removed. Send the bile to microbiology for culture and sensitivity. Withdraw the Veress needle or Abbocath and place the grasping forceps over the puncture site in the gallbladder to limit further bile spillage.

7 If the gallbladder has been previously inflamed, adhesions are commonly found to its serosal surface. Flimsy adhesions may pulled off with fine non-toothed grasping forceps whereas thicker more vascular adhesions require diathermy division close to the gallbladder wall. Take care to avoid the hepatic flexure of the transverse colon laterally, and the duodenum medially, both of which may be closely adherent to the gallbladder.

Action

Dissecting Calot's triangle

1 Hold the neck of the gallbladder with grasping forceps, fairly close to the origin of the cystic duct, if visible. This is probably the most important instrument in the initial dissection, as it allows the structures in the cystic pedicle to be exposed under tension and the gallbladder neck can be moved up and down so you can see both superior and inferior surfaces of Calot's triangle.

KEY POINTS Anatomy

- You must never embark on this dissection unless you know the anatomy intimately.
- Make certain what the structure you intend to cut is before you cut it.

2 A stone impacted in the neck of the gallbladder may be massaged back into the body with forceps. If this fails, the grasping forceps may be positioned just behind the stone and still permit adequate movement of the gallbladder. Alternatively, replace the 5-mm port in the right upper quadrant with a 10-mm port and use heavy grasping forceps to hold the stone within the gallbladder.

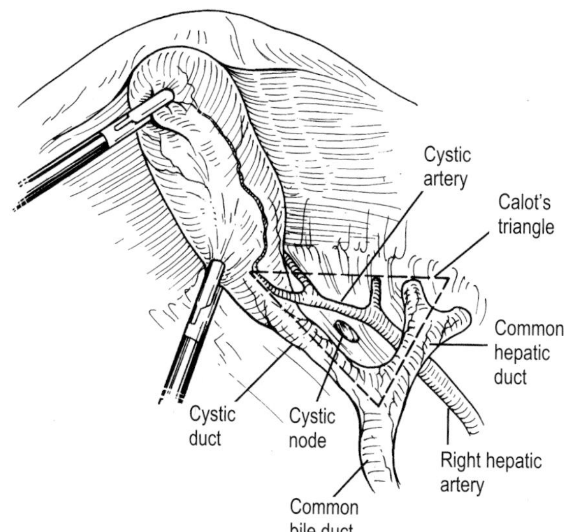

Fig. 20.3 Gallbladder retracted to show anatomy of Calot's triangle.

3 Begin the dissection by using the diathermy hook or scissors to make a small hole in the peritoneum overlying the cystic duct close to the gallbladder neck.

4 Proceed with dissection of Calot's triangle (Fig. 20.3) in one of three ways.

- Grip the free edge of peritoneum just created with fine-tipped, straight or curved grasping forceps and peel the peritoneum medially to expose the structures of the cystic pedicle. Sometimes the peritoneum peels back easily to reveal the cystic duct and cystic artery but if you feel any resistance it is safer to proceed to one of the following methods.
- With the diathermy hook divide the peritoneum on the undersurface of Calot's triangle, aiming posterolaterally towards the junction of gallbladder wall and liver. Remember to keep the peritoneum under tension using the grasping forceps on the neck of the gallbladder and to keep close to the gallbladder wall. When you reach the sulcus between the body of the gallbladder and the liver, continue dividing the peritoneum along the inferior border of gallbladder and liver for about 1–2 cm laterally. Move the neck of the gallbladder down and divide the peritoneum over Calot's triangle in a similar manner laterally towards the junction of gallbladder and liver, again taking care to keep close to the gallbladder wall. Continue the dissection for 1–2 cm laterally along the gallbladder–liver junction to open out Calot's triangle and improve the view.
- Employ a similar approach as above but use dissecting scissors attached to diathermy instead of the hook. This technique demands careful attention to ensure that you know what is between the blades of the scissors before you cut.

5 The aim of the dissection is to identify and clear the cystic duct and cystic artery so they may be clipped and divided safely. Frequently, this requires a disjointed dissection that alternates between the superior and inferior aspects of Calot's triangle, which is why the grasping forceps on the neck of the gallbladder is so important.

6 The cystic duct and artery usually run parallel to each other. The peritoneum overlying them will have been divided at right-angles to these structures but create the window between them by inserting the tips of the scissors or dissecting forceps and opening them parallel to the duct and artery.

7 Diathermize any small bleeding vessels immediately; blood quickly obscures the view of Calot's triangle. It also absorbs the light from the camera, so darkening the view considerably. Remove clots with the suction/irrigation device. In difficult cases 'hydrodissection' of the tissues with the irrigation device may be helpful.

8 Clear and skeletonize the cystic duct close to the neck of the gallbladder for 1–1.5 cm if possible. Ensure that the structure you think is cystic duct is entering the gallbladder and has no 'branches' or other connections. There is no advantage in dissecting out the junction of cystic duct and common hepatic duct; you are more likely to injure the bile duct if you attempt to identify the T-junction.

KEY POINT Anatomy

- **To ensure it is the cystic artery that has been identified, and not the right hepatic artery, follow the vessel to the gallbladder wall.**

9 Sometimes the cystic artery can be seen to divide into its terminal anterior and posterior branches; this may occur more medially than anticipated and require distal clips on each of the branches before dividing the artery. To confirm a structure as an artery, observe it carefully and closely, to detect visible pulsation.

10 When clipping either artery or duct, ensure that both tips of the clip applicator can be seen behind the structure being clipped in order to avoid inadvertently clipping important adjacent structures such as the common hepatic or common bile duct. When there is a short cystic duct avoid placing clips close to the junction with the common duct; instead, divide the neck of the gallbladder and use an Endoloop suture ligature.

Peroperative cholangiogram

1 The necessity and indications for peroperative cholangiography during laparoscopic cholecystectomy are fiercely debated. Peroperative cholangiography may be performed routinely, selectively or rarely.

- *Routinely*. Some surgeons routinely perform cholangiography during laparoscopic cholecystectomy. They argue that it allows for the detection of bile duct stones and, by identifying the anatomy of the biliary tree, guards against damage to the extrahepatic ducts. It may also be useful training.
- *Selectively*. A cholangiogram is performed if there is a preoperative suggestion of bile duct stones such as a history

of jaundice, dilated common bile duct on ultrasound or abnormal liver function tests. Any identified ductal stones may then be dealt with at the time of the operation, either by laparoscopic or open bile duct exploration, or postoperatively by endoscopic retrograde cholangiopancreatography (ERCP).

- *Rarely*. Surgeons who rarely or never perform cholangiography depend on a pre- or postoperative ERCP to deal with bile duct stones and argue that identifying the anatomy does not alter the incidence of bile duct injury. They may use magnetic resonance cholangiopancreatography (MRCP) for preoperative cholangiography in patients with risk factors for ductal stones.

2 Although we use a selective approach, we suggest that you should be familiar with the technique of laparoscopic cholangiography.

KEY POINTS Learn laparoscopic cholangiography

- Learn the technique even if you do not use it on a regular basis.
- You occasionally encounter aberrant or uncertain ductal anatomy.
- Imaging of the biliary ducts during operation may be very helpful.

3 Cholangiography is usually performed via the cystic duct.

4 Once the cystic artery has been divided place a clip on the cystic duct at its junction with the gallbladder.

5 Insert the cholangiogram catheter introducer through the abdominal wall 2 cm below the right costal margin in the anterior axillary line. The introducer we use has a curved bevelled tip that produces a bend in the cholangiogram catheter as it is extruded. Attempt to have the cholangiogram catheter and cystic duct parallel to each other as it is difficult to manipulate the cannula into the duct at an angle.

6 Keep the cystic duct under tension and with the scissors (concavity to the left) make a cut in the duct close to the clip at the gallbladder–cystic duct junction. A small leak of bile indicates when you have reached the lumen. The cut should involve one-third to a half of the duct's circumference.

7 Position the tip of the catheter introducer next to the cut. Flush the cholangiogram catheter with saline to avoid introducing air bubbles into the ductal system, since these can be mistaken for stones. Advance the catheter so it emerges from the introducer in the direction of the cystic duct. Slide the catheter into the cystic duct and advance it by about 3 cm if possible. This may require some manipulation. If the catheter does not slide into the duct easily, try:

- Flushing the catheter with saline as you advance it in an attempt to open up the cystic duct.
- Having your assistant release some of the tension on the cystic duct.
- Turning the introducer through 180° so the catheter comes out to hit the back wall of the cystic duct first, and then manipulate it around to pass down the duct.

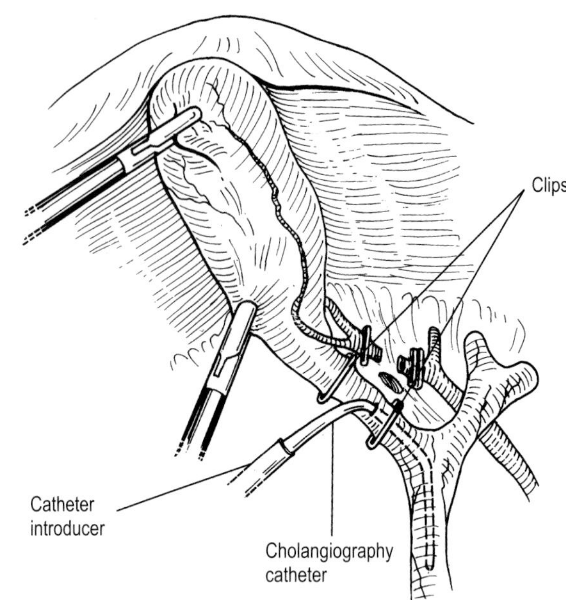

Fig. 20.4 Insertion of catheter for cholangiography.

8 If a cholangiogram catheter is unavailable, use a 4F Cook or Bard ureteric catheter.

9 Once in place, secure the catheter by placing a clip across the cystic duct medial to the incision (Fig. 20.4). You must place this sufficiently firmly to secure the cholangiogram catheter, but not so tight as to obstruct the flow of contrast medium. Inject saline as you apply the clip to warn if this point has been passed. Similarly, look for bile reflux up the catheter on gentle aspiration.

10 Alternatively, use a cholangiography carrier cannula (Storz). This consists of forceps with a central channel and basket-type jaws at the end. Insert the instrument through the right upper quadrant port and pass the cholangiogram catheter through the central channel. Position the catheter in the cystic duct as described above. Once it is in position, advance the cholangiography cannula and close its jaws over the cystic duct and catheter to secure them.

11 Flush the catheter with saline while observing the cystic duct to ensure there is no leakage of contrast. If you see saline reflux back into the abdominal cavity then reapply the clip securing the catheter or reposition the catheter.

12 Remove the catheter introducer if appropriate, taking care not to displace the catheter. Remove, withdraw or displace any other metal instruments or trocars that will obscure the X-ray image. Deflate the pneumoperitoneum for the duration of the X-ray. Allow the radiographer to position the X-ray machine. Apply a 20° lateral tilt of the operating table to the left to eliminate overlap of ductal contrast on the vertebral column. Ensure all personnel either leave the theatre or are protected behind lead screens or aprons while the X-ray images are being obtained.

13 If you are using plain X-ray films, inject 3–4 ml of dilute contrast (50:50 mixture of Omnipaque and normal saline) and

have an X-ray film exposed. Inject a further 5–10 ml of dilute contrast and obtain a second film.

14 If possible, use image-intensification facilities as dilute contrast medium can then be injected continuously while the image is being 'screened'. The common bile duct should be seen to fill down to the ampulla. If the ampulla is patent, contrast flows into the duodenum, which is easily recognized by its mucosal folds. Continue injecting contrast to fill the main intrahepatic ducts as well as the common duct. Obtain some permanent images as a record. If the images are unsatisfactory, repeat them.

15 Following cholangiography, re-establish the pneumoperitoneum and re-introduce the instruments and laparoscope. Remove the clip securing the cholangiogram catheter and withdraw the catheter under direct vision.

Gallbladder resection

1 Close the medial end of the cystic duct in one of three ways:

- *Clips*. Use metal (titanium) clips or absorbable polydioxanone (Ethicon) clips to close the cystic duct stump. Apply these at right-angles to the duct and check that they occlude the whole width of the duct. Failure to do this could result in a postoperative bile leak. Most surgeons use two clips on the medial cystic duct stump for added safety. Do not squeeze the clips too tightly—a particular hazard with reusable instruments—because they may 'cut through' the duct.
- *Endoloop*. Apply a 2/0 polyglactin 910 (Vicryl) endoloop once the cystic duct has been divided. This is particularly useful for a wide, oedematous or inflamed cystic duct where clips are liable to slip or cut through. Pass the endoloop through the epigastric port. Pass the tips of dissecting forceps through the endoloop and pick up the cystic duct stump. Apply enough tension on the cystic duct to slide the endoloop down over it without tenting up the bile duct. Tighten the endoloop securely around the cystic duct stump and then cut the ligature.
- *Ligate in continuity*. Pass a length of 2/0 polyglactin 910 (Vicryl) thread behind the intact cystic duct. The duct can then be ligated in continuity using intra- or extracorporeal knotting techniques.

2 When the medial end of the cystic duct has been secured the duct can be divided using scissors. The gallbladder is now detached from the structures of the porta hepatis.

3 Gallbladder dissection from the liver can be relatively straightforward in a non-inflamed gallbladder, especially one attached to the liver by a mesentery. However, more often than not, the gallbladder is chronically inflamed, contracted, adherent or partially buried in the liver bed.

4 Keep the gallbladder on the stretch using grasping forceps attached to the fundus and neck respectively. Divide the serosa along the upper and lower junctions of gallbladder and liver using scissors or the hook attached to diathermy. Coagulate any obvious vessels before dividing the peritoneum.

5 Retract the gallbladder neck laterally (Fig. 20.5). This raises the neck of the gallbladder from the liver bed and reveals the loose fibrous tissue plane that separates the gallbladder wall from the liver parenchyma. Divide this fibrous tissue using a combination of blunt and sharp dissection with scissors and diathermy using scissors and/or hook (Fig. 20.6).

6 Stay close to the gallbladder wall; if the dissection is allowed to wander too close to the liver parenchyma, considerable

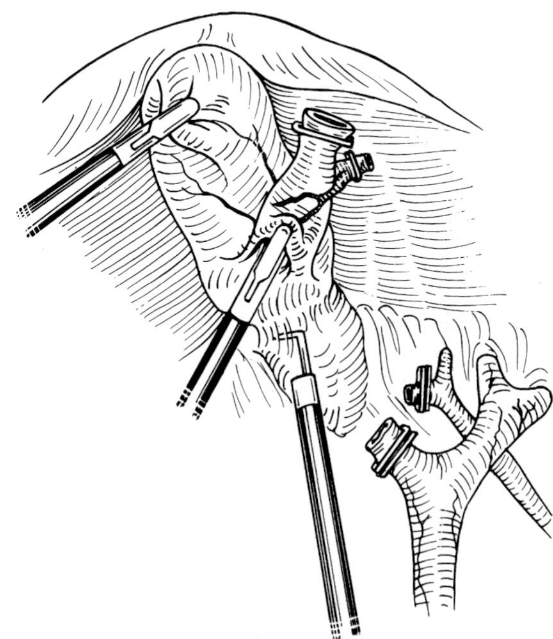

Fig. 20.5 Retraction of gallbladder neck to expose fibrous tissue connecting gallbladder to liver.

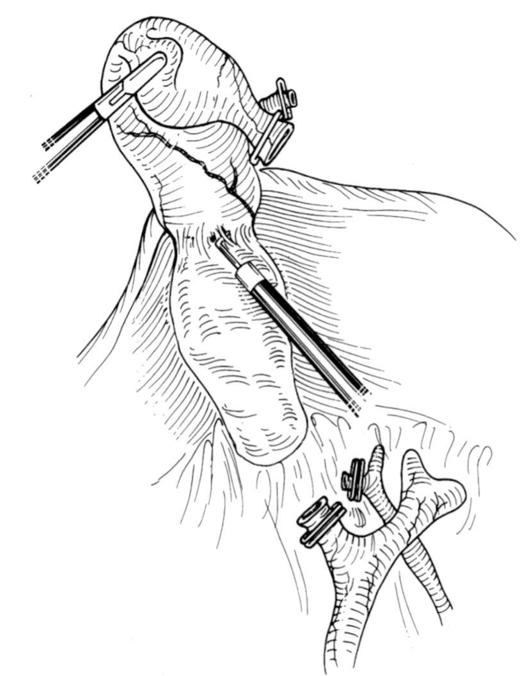

Fig. 20.6 Grasping forceps on the under-surface (liver aspect) of the gallbladder to aid dissection of the fundus from the liver.

bleeding can occur. If bleeding does occur push the gallbladder back into the gallbladder fossa to compress the area for a few minutes until the bleeding has stopped or has slowed enough for bleeding points to be identified and diathermized.

7 Midway through dissection of the gallbladder from the liver bed move the grasping forceps from the neck of the gallbladder to its undersurface—the liver aspect. This allows better control of dissection for the lateral half of the gallbladder.

8 Occasionally you encounter the small cystohepatic bile duct of Luschka (German anatomist, 1820–1875) entering the gallbladder directly from the liver parenchyma. If you recognize it clip it to avoid a troublesome postoperative bile leak.

9 Before the gallbladder is completely detached, push it up over the liver towards the diaphragm. This retracts the liver edge and exposes the gallbladder fossa, allowing you to thoroughly inspect and coagulate residual bleeding points. Pay particular attention to the cut peritoneum at the edge of the gallbladder fossa. Irrigating the gallbladder fossa with saline under pressure helps to identify bleeding points, which may occasionally need clipping. This manoeuvre also allows inspection of the cystic pedicle to check the clips on the cystic duct and artery.

10 Dissecting the fundus of the gallbladder can be difficult, particularly if the gallbladder is large or embedded in the liver. Techniques that may be helpful include:
- Retract the fundus of the gallbladder medially and the under-surface laterally to reverse the usual position of the gallbladder
- Remove the grasping forceps from the fundus and place them on the under-surface of the gallbladder to push it upward over the liver edge. Frequently a combination of manoeuvres is required to detach the fundus completely.

11 Once detached, place the gallbladder out of the way on the superior surface of the liver.

12 Use blunt-tipped grasping forceps or a probe to lift up the liver edge to allow a final inspection of the gallbladder fossa and cystic pedicle for any bleeding or bile leaks. Aspirate any remaining blood or clots from the subhepatic fossa, over the right lobe of the liver and the right paracolic gutter.

Extracting the gallbladder

1 The gallbladder may be removed via the epigastric or umbilical port sites.

2 We routinely place the gallbladder in a retrieval bag before removing it. In any case use a bag if the gallbladder has been perforated during the procedure or is very distended with bile or stones, or you risk perforation and spillage during extraction. A number of bags are available, some attached to introducing instruments. We use a Bert bag. Moisten a fabric bag with saline to ease its manipulation. Insert fine grasping forceps into the base of the bag and then twist it around the shaft of the forceps. Insert the bag and forceps through the epigastric port and place it on top of the liver. Unfurl the bag and have your assistant grab one edge of the open end with grasping forceps in the lateral port while you grab the other edge to open out the bag. Using the forceps in the right upper quadrant port, guide the gallbladder into the bag either fundus or cystic duct first. Grab the edges of the retrieval bag with alligator forceps and extract both the bag and gallbladder in the manner described below.

3 *Gallbladder removal through the epigastric port.* This is suitable for small, non-distended gallbladders. Insert a pair of heavy, self-grasping, toothed (alligator) forceps through the epigastric port. Bring the bag, or gallbladder, into view and grasp the edge, or the clipped cystic duct end. Under direct vision, gently withdraw the bag or gallbladder into the epigastric cannula as far as it will go. Slide the cannula and alligator forceps out of the abdominal cavity. Grasp the exteriorized edge of the bag or neck of the gallbladder, on the abdominal surface with a pair of Kocher's forceps or a heavy arterial forceps to prevent retraction back into the abdominal cavity. Release the alligator forceps and, with a combination of gentle rotation and traction, extract the bag or gallbladder. If you have not used a bag, avoid excessive traction on the gallbladder as this may cause perforation with intraperitoneal spillage of bile and stones.

4 *Gallbladder removal through the umbilical port.* Remove the laparoscope from the umbilical port and replace it in the epigastric port. Insert alligator forceps into the umbilical port and under direct vision follow them up to the liver. Grasp the bag or clipped cystic duct end of the gallbladder, and withdraw it through the umbilical port in the manner described above. We prefer to use the umbilical port, since fascial closure is easier.

5 If the intraperitoneal portion of the gallbladder is distended with bile, grasp the exteriorized neck between two clips. Cut between them to enter the lumen of the gallbladder and insert the suction device to aspirate the bile and allow extraction of the gallbladder.

6 If the gallbladder has a large stone load that prevents extraction, open the exteriorized neck, aspirate the bile and insert a Desjardins or Spencer–Wells forceps into the gallbladder lumen to crush or extract the stones. You risk perforating the fundus of the gallbladder with resultant stone spillage and wound contamination especially if you have not used a bag.

7 You may insert large forceps such as Spencer–Wells down the outside of the partially extracted bag or gallbladder. When you see the tips laparoscopically in the abdominal cavity, open the forceps. This may stretch the port site sufficiently to allow you to remove the gallbladder.

8 To remove larger stones that are heavily calcified or impacted you may need to enlarge the trocar site by cutting it. Take care to suture-repair the defect in the linea alba to prevent subsequent herniation.

Checklist

1 Re-establish the pneumoperitoneum after extracting the gallbladder, and insert the laparoscope to make a final check for bleeding or bile leak.

2 Check that there is no previously unnoticed damage to other organs, including the liver such as lacerations or tears, transverse colon and duodenum including diathermy burns, or small bowel, by trocar injuries.

? DIFFICULTY

1. Convert to an open operation if laparoscopic cholecystectomy proves to be too difficult, if bleeding cannot be controlled or if you damage any viscera.
2. If a thin-walled gallbladder is perforated during the procedure, bile and often also small stones spill into the peritoneal cavity. Insert the suction device into the perforation to aspirate the gallbladder to dryness before sucking out as much of the escaped bile as possible. Multiple small stones may be more easily aspirated using a 10-mm suction device. Prevent further escape of stones by closing the perforation with grasping forceps or metal clips. Try to locate and remove all stones from the peritoneal cavity. Larger stones may be placed in a retrieval bag with the gallbladder, for extraction.
3. *Retrograde (fundus-first) cholecystectomy*. This is a useful technique in experienced hands when the gallbladder is acutely inflamed or when dense adhesions distort Calot's triangle. When necessary, use it with caution and not as an alternative to conversion to open operation. Insert a retractor through the lateral port. Position it under the liver to the left of the gallbladder and lift up the liver edge. It is then possible to start the dissection at the fundus of the gallbladder and work down towards its neck. Mobilize the gallbladder fully. Retract the mobilized gallbladder laterally and in a caudal direction to open out Calot's triangle, which assists in identifying the anatomy. Since the cystic artery is patent, you may encounter heavier than usual bleeding during dissection of the gallbladder.
4. *Partial cholecystectomy*. In chronic fibrotic cholecystitis, when the gallbladder is very adherent to the liver, dissection of the gallbladder can produce significant bleeding and result in damage to the hepatic parenchyma. In these circumstances it is acceptable to perform an incomplete cholecystectomy. After dividing the cystic duct, open the gallbladder with scissors close to its junction with the liver. Aspirate the gallbladder to dryness and remove any stones with grasping forceps or suction. Cut along the gallbladder wall close to its junction with the liver and follow this all the way round, so leaving the back wall of the gallbladder in situ. Coagulate the mucosal surface of the residual gallbladder with diathermy to prevent mucus production.
5. *Subtotal cholecystectomy*. If Calot's triangle is obliterated or considered hazardous to dissect, divide the gallbladder with scissors at the level of Hartmann's pouch. Extract stones and place them in a retrieval bag, and aspirate bile. It is usually possible at this stage to dissect out a short length of Hartmann's pouch/cystic duct, in order to ligate it with an endoloop or oversew it. Dissect the body and fundus of the gallbladder from the liver in the usual way and place it in a bag for extraction.

Closure

1 *Drains*. Many surgeons do not use a subhepatic drain after routine laparoscopic cholecystectomy unless there is concern about bleeding or bile leakage. Routine drainage overnight has the advantage of detecting the occasional postoperative bile leak at an early stage, thus avoiding inappropriate early discharge from hospital. A suction or non-suction drain can be inserted through the lateral or right upper quadrant port and placed in the subhepatic space with grasping forceps inserted through the epigastric port. Secure the drain to the skin with a suture.

2 Remove the cannulas under vision and ensure there is no bleeding from the abdominal wall puncture sites.

3 Deflate the pneumoperitoneum as much as possible to reduce referred pain to the shoulder after operation.

4 Close wounds greater than 1 cm in the linea alba under direct vision with 0 polyglactin 910 (Vicryl) or PDS to avoid subsequent hernia formation.

5 Infiltrate the skin wounds with long-acting local anaesthetic such as bupivacaine, and approximate the edges using sutures, skin tapes or staples.

Postoperative

1 Remove the nasogastric tube at the end of the operation.

2 Following reversal of muscle relaxation and extubation, insert an oropharyngeal airway. Administer oxygen by mask for the first 3 hours.

3 Remove the drain, if inserted, on the day following operation if there is no bile in it and blood loss of less than 50 ml per 24 hours.

4 The majority of patients are ready for discharge from hospital on the day following operation.

Complications

- *Bile leak*. If a drain has been placed then this complication is usually recognized by the presence of bile in the drain bottle on the day following operation. In the absence of a drain the patient may be discharged from hospital only to return unwell 3–5 days following operation with pain and tenderness in the right upper quadrant of the abdomen and jaundice. Biliary leaks may arise from the cystic duct stump, divided cystohepatic duct of Luschka in the gallbladder bed, or injury to a major bile duct (see below). An ultrasound or CT scan helps determine the size and position of any intra-abdominal collections and they can also be drained under imaging control. If a significant bile leak continues after drainage, undertake early ERCP to demonstrate the site of the leak and determine if any significant bile duct injury has occurred. The majority of minor biliary leaks seal in time with external drainage alone; however, a temporary biliary stent inserted endoscopically decompresses the biliary system, hastening closure of the leak and shortening hospital stay.

- *Major bile duct injury*. The incidence of bile duct injury was initially higher following laparoscopic cholecystectomy than following open operation, but the incidence is now comparable at 1 in 300–500 operations. Major bile duct injuries include complete transections and clipping the common duct.

KEY POINT Accept your limitations

- The management of major bile duct injuries is complex and best dealt with in a unit specializing in their treatment.

REFERENCES

1. Schwesinger WH, Diehl AK 1996 Changing indications for laparoscopic cholecystectomy. Surgical Clinics of North America 76:493–504
2. McMahon AJ, Baxter JN, O'Dwyer PJ 1993 Preventing complications of laparoscopy. British Journal of Surgery 80:1593–1594

LAPAROSCOPIC EXPLORATION OF THE COMMON BILE DUCT

Appraise

1 The finding of stones in the common bile duct on peroperative cholangiography occurs in up to 10% of patients undergoing laparoscopic cholecystectomy. Clearance of the ducts requires either laparoscopic or open exploration of the ducts at the time of surgery, or postoperative ERCP. The decision rests primarily on the expertise available locally. Several units have reported series of laparoscopic duct exploration with duct clearance rates of over 90%, a figure that compares well with the results of an expert endoscopist. Laparoscopic exploration of the common bile duct may be performed by either the transcystic duct approach or by choledochotomy.

2 The *transcystic duct approach* is the most commonly used and is suitable for small ductal stones of less than 8 mm in diameter. Stones lying above the cystic duct/common hepatic duct junction are difficult to remove by the transcystic route and usually require choledochotomy. Stone clearance via the cystic duct can be performed under X-ray image intensification and/or direct visual guidance using a narrow flexible choledochoscope. Both techniques are performed after cholangiography but before cystic duct continuity is lost or before commencing dissection of the gallbladder from the liver bed.

3 *Laparoscopic choledochotomy* is technically more difficult than the transcystic approach because of the need to suture the bile duct incision. However, it does allow full inspection of the extrahepatic ducts and removal of larger stones. As with open operation, do not perform laparoscopic choledochotomy unless the common bile duct measures at least 10 mm in diameter.

Action

Transcystic approach: radiological

1 Remove the cholangiogram catheter and any retaining clip from the cystic duct. Use dissecting forceps to gently squeeze the cystic duct in a medial to lateral direction to clear it of any debris. Irrigate the cystic duct opening to obtain a clear view. Disposable catheter kits are available to facilitate removal of ductal stones. They allow passage of a guide-wire through the cystic duct into the common duct to maintain access. An access sheath may be inserted into the cystic duct to give easy repeated instrumentation of the common duct. Insert a Dormier basket in its closed position through the cystic duct and into the contrast-filled common bile duct under fluoroscopic control with the C-arm image intensifier. Ensure that the tip of the basket is at the level of the ampulla and open the basket. Slowly withdraw it to trawl the duct stones into the basket. At the level of the cystic duct close the basket over the stones to retain them and then withdraw the basket and stone through the cystic duct. Once extracted the stones may be removed individually by grasping forceps through the 10-mm epigastric port or placed in a retrieval bag.

2 If the stones are too large to pass through the cystic duct then either close the basket tightly to crush them or apply non-traumatizing forceps on to the cystic duct to achieve a similar effect. Alternatively, dilate the cystic duct with a balloon catheter to allow removal of medium-sized stones (5–8 mm). Several passes of the basket may be required to clear the stones.

3 A Fogarty-type balloon catheter can be used to trawl the common bile duct of stones (see below) via the transcystic route. However, if you use this technique you risk displacing stones from the common bile duct into the common hepatic duct. Confirm duct clearance by repeat cholangiography.

Transcystic approach: direct vision

1 Use a 6-mm or 3-mm flexible choledochoscope to visualize the common bile duct. This is facilitated by using a second camera system attached to the head of the telescope, and a video mixer that displays both the laparoscopic and choledochoscopic images on the same monitor simultaneously.

2 Insert the flexible choledochoscope through a metal reducer in the epigastric cannula. Keep the tip of the epigastric cannula close to the cystic duct to prevent intra-abdominal looping of the shaft of the choledochoscope. Pass the scope into the cystic duct while irrigating continuously with saline. If the cystic duct is too narrow to allow passage of the scope then it can be dilated with a balloon catheter as described previously. Within the common bile duct, combine rotation and withdrawal of the scope to yield a view of the lumen. Advance the scope down to the ampulla. Stones may be pushed or flushed through the ampulla or withdrawn along the common bile duct and cystic

duct using a stone extraction basket. Thread the extraction basket through the choledochoscope and under direct vision advance it beyond the stone or stones. Open the basket then draw back against the scope to grasp and secure the stones. Withdraw the choledochoscope, stone basket and stones together out of the abdominal cavity through the epigastric port. Re-introduce the scope into the common bile duct to confirm that there are no further stones. The smaller 3-mm scope can be passed through the ampulla into the duodenum to ensure that the duct is completely clear.

3 View the common bile duct as you withdraw the choledochoscope. Within a dilated common bile duct it is possible for a stone to lie adjacent to the scope and be missed while a more distant stone is being retrieved.

4 Clip or ligate and then divide the cystic duct in the manner described previously prior to completion of the cholecystectomy.

Laparoscopic choledochotomy

1 Identify the common bile duct. Minimal dissection is required because only the anterior wall needs to be identified. Stay sutures are unnecessary. Make a 1-cm choledochotomy incision in the anterior wall of the common bile duct. Carefully coagulate any bleeding points along the cut edge.

2 The majority of stones can be expressed through the choledochotomy incision by:

- *Suction extraction*. Insert the tip of the suction device just into the choledochotomy incision, aiming towards the ampulla, and apply low-pressure suction. This enables small stones to be sucked to the tip of the device for removal with grasping forceps.
- *Duct massage*. Insert blunt-tipped grasping forceps through the epigastric and right upper quadrant ports on each side of the common bile duct, to massage larger stones to the choledochotomy incision for extraction.
- *Balloon catheter*. Cannulate the common bile duct with a biliary Fogarty-type balloon catheter and advance it through the ampulla into the duodenum. Inflate the balloon and withdraw until you feel resistance at the ampulla. Deflate the balloon enough to allow it to re-enter the common bile duct and then re-inflate it. As you withdraw the balloon catheter, stones trapped behind the balloon are delivered to the choledochotomy incision for individual removal with grasping forceps.

3 Failure of the above techniques to remove the stones requires the insertion of the choledochoscope as previously described for stone removal under direct vision. The advantage of the choledochotomy is that the common hepatic, left and right intrahepatic and common bile ducts can all be visualized.

4 Because of the ampullary oedema associated with supraduodenal choledochotomy and bile duct exploration, the duct may become obstructed in the first few days postoperatively unless you insert a T-tube or biliary stent. Introduce a precut T-tube into the abdominal cavity through a stab incision in the right upper quadrant. Keep each limb of the T-tube fairly short (about 1 cm) and, with the help of dissecting forceps introduced through the epigastric and right upper quadrant ports, feed the limbs into the common bile duct through the choledochotomy incision. Close this incision above or below the long limb of the T-tube with two to three interrupted 3/0 or 4/0 absorbable sutures such as polyglactin 910 (Vicryl). Confirm the patency of the T-tube by flushing it with saline. Secure the T-tube to the abdominal wall after desufflation of the pneumoperitoneum. Alternatively place a biliary stent into the bile duct and through the ampulla via the choledochotomy. Fully close the choledochotomy. Remove the stent endoscopically 2–3 weeks postoperatively.

Postoperative care

Order a T-tube cholangiogram between days 7 and 10 to confirm ductal clearance. In the absence of stones, remove the T-tube by simple traction after removing the securing stitch in the abdominal wall. Deal with residual stones discovered postoperatively by percutaneous stone extraction through the T-tube track or at ERCP.

LAPAROSCOPIC CHOLECYSTOSTOMY

Appraise

- Early laparoscopic removal of an acutely inflamed gallbladder is practised by some surgeons.[1] This is often a technically demanding operation, however, with a higher morbidity than an elective procedure. Inflammatory oedema and adhesions frequently distort and obscure the anatomy to an extent that makes dissection difficult, bloody and, at times, hazardous.
- Percutaneous cholecystostomy under ultrasound control is often used to decompress the gallbladder and relieve symptoms in poor-risk and elderly patients with acute cholecystitis. Although not generally used as an alternative in these patients because of the risk of general anaesthesia, laparoscopic cholecystostomy does have a role when acute inflammatory changes are found at operation.

KEY POINT Respond to the findings

- If you are a relatively inexperienced laparoscopist and discover at initial laparoscopy a distended and severely inflamed gallbladder with areas of patchy necrosis of its wall and vascular adhesions, proceed to laparoscopic cholecystostomy.

Action

1 Insert a 5-mm epigastric port and a 5-mm port in the right midclavicular line just above the level of the umbilicus. Pass a 12F or 14F latex Foley catheter into the peritoneal cavity through a stab incision in the abdominal wall directly over the fundus of the gallbladder as identified by finger pressure.

2 As previously described, aspirate the gallbladder using a Veress needle or a 16G Abbocath inserted at the fundus of the gallbladder. Send the bile for microbiological studies.

3 Direct the tip of the Foley catheter to the puncture site on the gallbladder using dissecting forceps in the right upper quadrant port. Grasp the fundus of the gallbladder gently and enlarge the puncture site with scissors.

4 Introduce the catheter into the lumen of the gallbladder and inflate the balloon with 5–10 ml of saline. Apply gentle traction to produce an adequate seal.

5 Deflate the pneumoperitoneum and secure the external part of the Foley catheter to the abdominal wall.

Postoperative

1 Leave the catheter for 2–3 weeks or until you carry out elective cholecystectomy.

2 At the elective procedure, you will find that the gallbladder fundus is adherent to the anterior abdominal wall at the site of insertion of the catheter but this can be dissected off with scissors or hook diathermy.

REFERENCE

1. Kiviluoto T, Siren J, Luukkonen P et al 1998 Randomised trial of laparoscopic versus open cholecystectomy for acute and gangrenous cholecystitis. Lancet 351:321–325

LAPAROSCOPIC CHOLECYSTOJEJUNOSTOMY

Appraise

1 Laparoscopic techniques can be used to diagnose and stage pancreatic malignancies but view them as complementary to other imaging modalities including ultrasound, CT scanning, MRI and endoscopic ultrasound.[1]

2 Staging a patient with pancreatic malignancy requires a careful laparoscopic examination of the abdominal cavity. At laparoscopy you may identify small liver and peritoneal metastases, missed on other imaging techniques, that make the cancer inoperable. This spares the patient an unnecessary laparotomy.

3 Laparoscopic palliative biliary bypass may be performed at the time of the staging laparoscopy. The alternative, and more commonly used, method of relieving jaundice in patients with pancreatic cancer is the placement of an endoscopic or percutaneous biliary stent. These methods do not rely on the presence of a patent cystic duct.

4 If you are considering laparoscopic cholecystojejunostomy, arrange imaging such as preoperative MRCP or peroperative cholecystography to evaluate the anatomy of the cystic duct and its patency into the common duct. If tumour encroaches on or near the entry point of the cystic duct into the common duct, it is more appropriate to perform a bypass to a more proximal part of the extrahepatic biliary tree, or rely on biliary stenting.

Action

1 This procedure is greatly facilitated by the use of a 30-mm endoscopic linear stapling device. Introduce a 30° laparoscope through the umbilical port and a retractor through the right lateral port to elevate the liver edge medial to the gallbladder. A 10-mm epigastric port accommodates instruments and the endoscopic linear stapling device. A 5-mm right upper quadrant port accommodates grasping forceps and needle-holders.

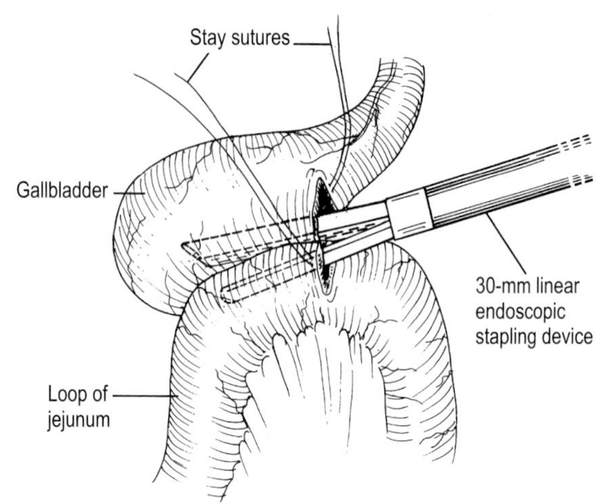

Fig. 20.7 Formation of cholecystojejunostomy.

2 Identify the start of the jejunum using dissecting grasping forceps. Unite a loop of jejunum, approximately 50 cm from the duodenojejunal flexure, to the anterior aspect of the neck or body of the gallbladder with two 2/0 polyglactin 910 (Vicryl) sutures placed 2 cm apart. Decompress the gallbladder using a Veress needle or a 16G Abbocath.

3 With scissors or hook diathermy, make adjacent holes in the gallbladder and jejunum large enough to pass the arms of the stapling device. Insert the 30-mm linear endoscopic stapling device through the epigastric port and create a stapled side-to-side anastomosis between gallbladder and jejunum (Fig. 20.7). Remove the stapling device and close the enterotomy with full-thickness 2/0 polyglactin 910 (Vicryl) laparoscopic sutures.

4 If the patient also has gastric outlet or duodenal obstruction, you may also perform a gastrojejunostomy in a similar fashion.

REFERENCE

1. Bogen GL, Mancino AT, Scott-Conner CEH 1996 Laparoscopy for staging and palliation of gastrointestinal malignancy. Surgical Clinics of North America 76:557–569

FURTHER READING

Chitre VV, Studley JGN 1999 Audit of methods of laparoscopic cholecystectomy. British Journal of Surgery 86:185–188

Cueto JG, Jacobs M, Gagner M 2002 Laparoscopic surgery. Higher Education, New York

Gallegos N 1998 Biliary tract and gallbladder: laparoscopic cholecystectomy. In: Hobsley M, Treasure T, Northover J (eds) Laparoscopic surgery. The implications of changing practice. Edward Arnold, London

Geoghegan JG, Keane FBV 1999 Laparoscopic management of complicated gallstone disease. British Journal of Surgery 86:145–146

MacFayden BV, Arrequi ME, Eubanks S et al (eds) 2003 Laparoscopic surgery of the abdomen. Springer-Verlag, Berlin
Nathanson L 2001 Gallstones. In: Garden OJ (ed.) Hepatobiliary and pancreatic surgery: a companion to specialist surgical practice, 2nd edn. Baillière Tindall, London
Scott-Conner CEH, Cuschieri A, Carter F (eds) 2000 Minimal access surgical anatomy. Lippincott Williams & Wilkins, Philadelphia

INTERNET WEB SITES

www.limit.ac.uk
www.websurg.com
www.laparoscopy.com
http://consensus.nih.gov/cons/090/090_intro.htm

21

Pancreas

R.C.N. Williamson, A. Shankar

CONTENTS

INTRODUCTION

1 Operations on the pancreas are some of the most challenging in abdominal surgery for the following reasons:

- The pancreas is relatively inaccessible in its retroperitoneal position. The neck, body and tail lie behind the lesser sac while the head is obscured by the greater omentum and transverse colon. Thus the approach to the pancreas requires a good deal of mobilization.
- The pancreas is intimately related to major blood vessels, notably the splenic and superior mesenteric veins, which unite to form the portal vein behind its neck. Adherence to the superior mesenteric vessels can make for a difficult dissection in inflammatory or neoplastic diseases of the pancreas. The pancreas has a rich arterial supply: the right pancreas (the head) receives blood from the pancreaticoduodenal arcades and the left pancreas (body and tail) from the splenic artery. Its venous drainage to the portal system is by a number of quite large but thin-walled veins.
- Shared blood supply and a close anatomical relationship mean that adjacent organs are routinely removed as part of a pancreatic resection. Thus the spleen is generally included in a distal pancreatectomy. More importantly, the duodenum and lower bile duct are excised during proximal pancreatectomy, necessitating a complex reconstruction thereafter.
- Resection of the head of the pancreas is followed by anastomosis between the pancreatic stump (a solid organ) and a hollow tube (generally the jejunum). If this anastomosis leaks, powerful digestive enzymes are liberated in active form and can cause severe tissue destruction.
- Acute and chronic pancreatitis are some of the most difficult inflammatory conditions to manage anywhere in the body. Likewise, pancreatic cancer is often advanced by the time of diagnosis and its surgical eradication requires an extensive operation.
- Diseases of the head of pancreas commonly present with obstructive jaundice. The function of many of the body's systems is impaired in deeply jaundiced patients, notably the kidneys, reticuloendothelial system and coagulation pathways, as well as the liver itself. Thus special precautions are required when undertaking major procedures on such patients.

KEY POINT Expertise

- It follows that you should undertake pancreatic operations only after adequate training in the field and decidedly not if you are inexperienced.

2 Pancreatic imaging has been dramatically improved over the last two decades with the introduction of ultrasonography, spiral computed tomography (CT), endoscopic retrograde cholangiopancreatography (ERCP), endoscopic ultrasound, percutaneous transhepatic cholangiography (PTC) and magnetic resonance imaging/cholangiopancreatography (MRI/MRCP).[1] Three-dimensional reconstructions of images obtained during CT or MRI[2] may provide a totally non-invasive way of imaging not only the biliary and pancreatic ducts but also the vascular anatomy in this area.

Some form of vascular imaging is required prior to pancreatic surgery in order to determine operability and delineate vascular anomalies. Visceral angiography has to a large extent been superseded by three-dimensional reconstruction during CT and MR angiography.

3 Pancreatic endocrine tissue is scattered through the gland in islets described in 1869 by the Berlin physician and anatomist, Paul Langerhans (1847–1888), with a relative preponderance in the body and tail. A major pancreatic resection can impair both endocrine and exocrine function sufficiency to cause diabetes and/or steatorrhoea. Particularly in chronic pancreatitis, where there may be pre-existing insufficiency, it is good practice to measure pancreatic function before and after operation.

4 We routinely employ a transverse ('gable') incision for pancreatic surgery, that is a curved bilateral subcostal incision. Pancreatic operations should be covered by appropriate broad-spectrum antibiotics, such as a cephalosporin. If there is any likelihood of operative cholangiography or pancreatography

being required, place the patient on an operating table with X-ray tunnel.

EXPLORATION OF THE PANCREAS

Access

1 Examination of the pancreas is usually performed as part of a general abdominal exploration.

2 If examination of the whole pancreas is the major purpose of the operation, select either a bilateral subcostal, 'gable' incision or a curved transverse incision midway between umbilicus and xiphoid and convex upwards.

3 Adequate inspection and palpation of the whole pancreas requires both mobilization of the duodenum and entry into the lesser sac.

Assess

1 Before approaching the pancreas, pay particular attention to the duodenum, liver, spleen and bile duct.

2 Mobilize the duodenal loop and pancreatic head by Kocher's manoeuvre (Fig. 21.1). Gently clear the omentum from the anterior aspect of the head of pancreas, which can now be directly inspected and palpated between finger and thumb.

3 Expose the body and tail of the pancreas through the lesser sac, which can be entered through the greater or lesser omentum. Separate the congenital adhesions between the stomach and the pancreas. If necessary, divide the peritoneum along the superior border of the pancreas, so that you can insinuate a finger beneath the gland.

4 The inferior border of the pancreas can also be mobilized by dividing the overlying peritoneum; take care not to wound the superior or inferior mesenteric veins. Trace the middle colic vein downwards to find the superior mesenteric vein.

5 Lying at the splenic hilum, the tail of pancreas is the least accessible part of the gland. It can usually be approached by dividing the greater omentum and retracting the stomach upwards.

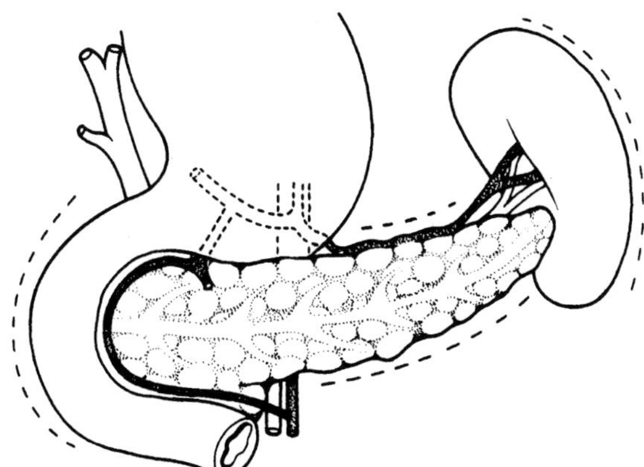

Fig. 21.1 Exposure of the pancreas. The lines of peritoneal incision are shown. The head of the pancreas and uncinate lobe are supplied by the superior and inferior pancreaticoduodenal arteries and the body and tail by the splenic artery.

You may need to divide several short gastric arteries and the attachments of the splenic flexure of the colon from the spleen. If necessary be willing to divide the peritoneum lateral to the spleen and lift the spleen and tail of pancreas forwards into the wound.

6 Learn to recognize the firm, nodular consistency of normal pancreas by palpating the gland during all upper abdominal operations. You should then be able to differentiate the hard sclerotic gland of chronic pancreatitis or a localized tumour, which may be hard as in carcinoma or soft, cystic. The pancreatic duct is not palpable unless it is dilated.

7 If you feel a mass in the region of the ampulla, it may assist diagnosis to open the duodenum and directly visualize the pancreatic papilla. Confirm suspected carcinoma at this site by removing a suitable biopsy for immediate frozen-section histology, if endoscopic biopsy has not already provided the diagnosis.

KEY POINTS Access to the pancreas

- You cannot adequately examine the pancreas without full (Kocher's) mobilization of the duodenum along with exploration of the lesser sac.
- Mobilize the lateral attachments of the spleen if necessary, to facilitate examination of the pancreatic tail.
- You may also need to divide the peritoneum along the upper and lower borders of the pancreas.

REFERENCES

1. Fayad LM, Kowalski T, Mitchell DG 2003 MR cholangiography: evaluation of common pancreatic diseases. Radiological Clinics of North America 41:97–114
2. Takeshita K, Furui S, Takada K 2002 Multidetector row helical CT of the pancreas: value of three dimensional images, two dimensional reformations and contrast enhanced multiphasic imaging. Hepatobiliary Pancreatic Surgery 9:576–582

PANCREATIC BIOPSY

Appraise

- No method of biopsying the pancreas is devoid of risk, yet a positive tissue diagnosis is particularly important for the proper management of suspected malignant disease.
- Cancer in the head of the pancreas usually obstructs the pancreatic duct, leading to a type of chronic pancreatitis in the upstream gland. At operation it can be difficult or even impossible to distinguish the induration of obstructive pancreatopathy from that of malignant infiltration, and this difficulty introduces a sampling error. Likewise, on pancreatic imaging there is often no sharp distinction between tumour and adjacent pancreatitis.
- Percutaneous biopsy of the pancreas can be carried out under ultrasound or CT scan guidance by directly inserting a fine needle for cytology, or wider-bore needle for histology, into the mass that has been demonstrated. In expert hands this is quite a sensitive technique, though you may need more than one pass of the needle to obtain a positive answer. Although

percutaneous biopsy of the pancreas is a relatively safe and sensitive technique, as a rule limit it to patients with unresectable tumours or those patients in whom operative treatment is not indicated.[1]

- At ERCP pure pancreatic juice may be obtained or brushings can be taken from strictures of the bile duct or pancreatic duct. Cytological examination of this material may reveal malignant cells. The majority of pancreatic cancers exhibit a mutation in the gene K-*ras*; this may yet prove to be a valuable diagnostic test, although its lack of specificity has limited its usefulness.[2] When pancreatic cancer invades the duodenum, it can be directly biopsied through the endoscope.
- At laparotomy the safest method of confirming the diagnosis of cancer is to sample a site of possible metastasis, usually a liver nodule, peritoneal deposit or lymph node adjacent to the pancreas (see Chapter 22 for the technique of liver biopsy). If there are no obvious metastases, do not hesitate to biopsy the primary pancreatic tumour itself.
- The usual indication for pancreatic biopsy is to confirm carcinoma in a patient whose tumour is deemed irresectable, since in a resectable case the specimen itself provides ample histological material. Because of the sampling error you must obtain pathological confirmation of carcinoma before closing the abdomen, and this need may govern the choice between fine-needle aspiration biopsy and the use of a Tru-cut needle. In many hospitals it is easier to obtain urgent frozen-section histology, as from a Tru-cut specimen, than an urgent cytological opinion.

Action

1. Using a fine (18–20G) needle and a 20-ml syringe, aspirate the site of the lesion. Apply strong suction while advancing and withdrawing the needle within the lesion, then release the suction and remove the needle and syringe. Eject the material in the needle track on to a glass slide and make a smear for cytological examination.
2. If the surface of the pancreas is diseased, perform a 'shave' biopsy with a scalpel. Remember the possibility that an inflammatory 'halo' may surround the actual neoplastic tissue.
3. You can obtain a core of tissue for histological examination using a Tru-cut needle. If the lesion is in the head of the pancreas you can approach it transduodenally, avoiding the risk of pancreatic fistulae, or insert the needle directly into the pancreas.
4. If the above techniques are inadequate and a biopsy is essential, incise the gland directly over the lesion and obtain a small piece of tissue. However, it may be better to carry out a formal partial pancreatectomy under these circumstances.
5. The complications of biopsy include acute pancreatitis and pancreatic fistula. If pancreatic juice escapes from the site of incision or the needle puncture, consider pancreatectomy or Roux-en-Y drainage of this area.

REFERENCES

1. Ihse I, Axelson J, Dawiskiba S et al L 1999 Pancreatic biopsy: why? when? how? World Journal of Surgery 23:896–900
2. Moore PS, Beghelli S, Zamboni G et al 2003 Genetic abnormalities in pancreatic cancer. Molecular Cancer 2:7

OPERATIVE PANCREATOGRAPHY

Appraise

- Preoperative endoscopic pancreatograms with or without MRCP now usually provide adequate information on the pancreatic duct in patients with chronic pancreatitis to make on-table ductography largely obsolete. However, in some instances it is still necessary, so have patients placed on an X-ray table. Ductography may also be useful during operations for carcinoma and pancreatic trauma.
- The choice of route depends upon the operation being performed.[1] During operations on the biliary tract, obtain a retrograde pancreatogram by transduodenal cannulation of the papilla. If you suspect ductal disease in the head of pancreas after resection of the distal gland, the duct can be cannulated at the site of amputation. In chronic pancreatitis or carcinoma, a dilated duct may be palpable as a soft cord in a sclerotic gland. Obtain pancreatograms either by needle puncture of the duct or occasionally by incision and intubation in the body of the pancreas.
- Operative cystography may be useful to delineate pancreatic pseudocysts and their ductal communication.
- Use a dense water-soluble contrast medium, such as Conray 420 or Omnipaque. Be careful not to overdistend the ductal tree, especially during retrograde pancreatography, since there is a risk of inducing acute pancreatitis.
- Image intensifier facilitates on-table pancreatography but is by no means essential.

Action

Retrograde pancreatography (Fig. 21.2a)

1. Sphincterotomy is helpful but may not be essential.
2. The major pancreatic duct enters the duodenum horizontally and its orifice is located at about 5 o'clock on the lower lip of the papilla. You can usually pass a 5F umbilical catheter for 2–3 cm, but you need to occlude the orifice around the catheter to prevent spillage of contrast; we use Babcock's forceps. Obtain the first picture after introducing 1–2 ml of contrast.
3. Retrograde ductography may also be obtained by cannulating the accessory papilla, usually in patients with pancreas divisum, or cannulation of the main duct in the neck of pancreas after proximal pancreatectomy, usually in patients with chronic pancreatitis.

Prograde pancreatography (Fig. 21.2b)

1. The pancreas has been divided across the body or neck.
2. Search carefully for the transected duct. Pass a fine catheter down it for 1–2 cm and suture the duct around the catheter to effect a watertight seal.
3. Then instil contrast as before.

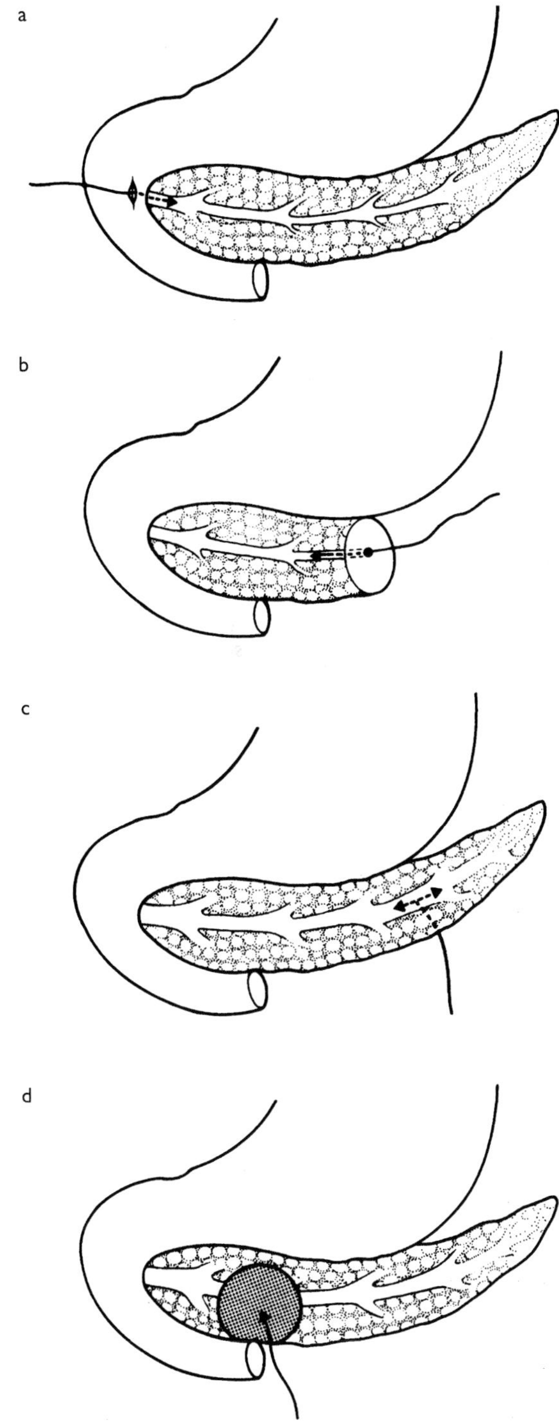

Fig. 21.2 Various methods of operative pancreatography: (a) transduodenal (retrograde) cannulation; (b) prograde cannulation following distal pancreatectomy; (c) ambigrade pancreatogram obtained by cannulation of a distended duct in the body of the gland; (d) pancreatic cystogram.

Ambigrade pancreatography (Fig. 21.2c)

1 Mobilize the body of the pancreas and feel carefully for the softer sensation of a dilated duct. This can be aided by the use of intraoperative ultrasound.

2 Insert a butterfly needle into the duct and observe the colourless pancreatic fluid flow back into the tubing. Several millilitres of contrast medium may be needed to fill a dilated ductal system, but do not continue injecting if pressure builds up.

3 If needle puncture is unsuccessful and pancreatography is necessary, make a short vertical incision in the body of pancreas and deepen it until you enter the duct. Insert a fine T-tube into the duct and close the gland about the tube. Afterwards, you must either resect the gland distal to the point of incision or drain the duct into a Roux loop of jejunum.

Pancreatic cystography (Fig. 21.2d)

1 Intrapancreatic pseudocysts are found in chronic pancreatitis and have a softer texture than the surrounding gland. Extrapancreatic pseudocysts generally follow an attack of acute pancreatitis and are situated in the lesser sac.

2 To obtain a cystogram, partly aspirate the cyst contents and introduce a similar quantity of contrast material.

Interpretation

The normal pancreatic duct tapers from a diameter of 3–4 mm in the head to less than 2 mm in the tail. Ductal anomalies in the main channel described by the Bavarian anatomist Wirsung in 1642, and the accessory channel described by the Venetian anatomist Santorini in 1724, and their communication and drainage are common. Look for sites of stricture and dilatation in both the main duct and its side-branches.[2] Contrast injected by the prograde route should enter the duodenum.

Determine the size of a cyst and the number of loculi, its relation to the gland and the presence or absence of any communication with the main duct.

REFERENCES

1. Cooper MJ, Williamson RCN 1983 The value of operative pancreatography. British Journal of Surgery 70:577–580
2. Axon ATR, Clasen M, Cotton PB et al 1984 Pancreatography in chronic pancreatitis: international definitions. Gut 25:1107–1112

LAPAROTOMY FOR ACUTE PANCREATITIS

Appraise

1 *Diagnostic laparotomy* should now be rare in patients with acute pancreatitis. With widespread availability of abdominal CT, diagnostic laparotomy is rarely necessary. Despite this, you may be confronted occasionally by acute pancreatitis during a laparotomy for other presumed pathologies, such as small-bowel infarction and leaking abdominal aneurysm.

2 Avoid laparotomy in the first week of acute pancreatitis, as it is too early for a safe, effective debridement, and formal resection carries a formidable mortality rate. Patients with proven severe gallstone pancreatitis may, however, benefit from early ERCP and stone extraction if ductal calculi are suspected, as this may lower both morbidity and mortality.[1]

3 Laparotomy, often with debridement, for patients with established necrotizing pancreatitis, is now being reserved primarily for those with infected necrosis.[2] Determine the presence of

infection preoperatively by percutaneous radiological fine-needle aspiration. In some specialist units open 'necrosectomy' for infected necrosis is being superseded by percutaneous drainage. Here percutaneous radiological drains are inserted under local anaesthetic, with the tracts subsequently dilated up to a size to permit passage of a nephroresectoscope. The necrotic tissue can then be resected using the telescopic instrument after which irrigation catheters can be inserted. Initial publications suggest an associated reduction in mortality and morbidity with this minimally invasive approach.[3] Other complications of acute pancreatitis such as pseudocysts, bleeding and abscesses are now often managed radiologically, with surgery reserved for complications not amenable to radiological intervention, or in those patients with infective necrosis not amenable to percutaneous techniques. This multidisciplinary care of patients with severe acute pancreatitis, especially with increased use of interventional radiology, suggests that such patients should be cared for in specialist units.

4 If you detect gallstones it is wise to carry out this *prophylactic* operation after the patient has recovered from pancreatitis but before going home, so as to prevent another acute attack (see Ch. 19). Prior to operation, have the bile duct imaged using either MRCP, or ERCP if the patient has a high chance of ductal calculi, to avoid leaving occult ductal calculi.

Prepare

1 Hypovolaemia is a consistent feature of acute pancreatitis and may be profound. Make sure that the fluid depletion has been fully corrected by intravenous administration of colloid and crystalloid solutions before embarking on the operation. Monitor the central venous pressure and urine output during resuscitation in the elderly or those with severe fluid loss.

2 Look for and treat early complications such as hypoxaemia, hypocalcaemia and incipient renal failure.

3 Give prophylactic broad-spectrum antibiotics.

Access

1 If the cause of peritonitis was uncertain, the patient is likely to have had a midline or right paramedian incision performed for abdominal exploration. If necessary, extend the incision upwards to permit examination of the biliary apparatus and pancreas.

2 When operating for established pancreatitis, use a transverse ('gable') incision.

Assess

1 Bloodstained free fluid is usually present in the abdominal cavity in acute pancreatitis. Whitish plaques of fat necrosis are visible on serosal surfaces, especially in the region of the pancreas.

2 Lift up the greater omentum and transverse colon. There is oedema and blackish discoloration of the retroperitoneal tissues. The pancreas itself is swollen and may be haemorrhagic or even necrotic.

3 Examine the gallbladder and, if possible, the bile duct to determine if these organs are diseased. A more thorough examination is required if the patient has obstructive jaundice.

4 In a case of infected pancreatic necrosis, extensively explore the retroperitoneal tissues to carry out a full assessment.

Action

For diagnostic laparotomy

1 Once you have made the diagnosis, do nothing unless there is a definite indication. Attempts at debridement of the pancreas at this stage can be disastrous. Formal exploration of the pancreas is usually unnecessary to obtain a diagnosis and may be meddlesome.

2 The management of coincidental gallstones is controversial, so be prepared to seek senior advice. In oedematous (mild) pancreatitis it is correct to carry out cholecystectomy with operative cholangiography and proceed to exploration of the duct and even transduodenal sphincteroplasty, if necessary (see Ch. 19). In haemorrhagic, severe pancreatitis, extensive ductal exploration and duodenotomy are best avoided. If ductal stones are present, remove them gently if possible and leave a T-tube to drain the duct.

3 It is unusual to encounter loculated fluid or pus during the first week of an attack of acute pancreatitis, but drain any such collection to the exterior.

4 Consider placing a peritoneal dialysis catheter through a stab incision into the pelvis for postoperative peritoneal lavage. This treatment has not been shown to be of definite value but may be useful if the pancreatitis is complicated by renal failure.

5 Wound dehiscence is common following laparotomy for acute pancreatitis. Take extra care in closing the linea alba or rectus sheath, and consider inserting tension sutures.

For infected pancreatic necrosis

1 Enter the lesser sac by dividing the greater omentum. The lesser sac is often obliterated by the inflammatory process and you quickly enter a large cavity containing pus and necrotic debris. Although the pancreas itself can undergo haemorrhagic infarction in a severe case of pancreatitis, more often the gland is viable and there is peripancreatic necrosis affecting the retroperitoneal fat.

2 Digitally explore the necrotic cavity and remove all dead tissue. The cavity may ramify extensively. Be prepared to explore upwards to the diaphragm, downwards behind the left or right colon to the pelvis, backwards to the perirenal areas and forwards into the transverse mesocolon and the root of the small bowel mesentery. Where possible, avoid sharp dissection and use your fingers to separate the solid necrotic material. A gently used 'blunt-tipped' sucker often provides a good method of atraumatic dissection. Send samples of fluid and necrotic material for bacteriological examination. The main risk is of bleeding, so be gentle but thorough.

3 Check the viability of the small and large intestine. The right colon in particular can become ischaemic following thrombosis of its blood supply. In these circumstances proceed to right

hemicolectomy but do not restore intestinal continuity. Bring out the terminal ileum as an end ileostomy (Ch. 14) and the transverse or descending colon as a mucous fistula, using separate small incisions for each stoma. Placement of a gastrostomy avoids long-term nasogastric intubation and the placement of a jejunostomy tube aids early enteric feeding.[4]

4 Irrigate the large retroperitoneal cavity thoroughly with warm saline and secure haemostasis. You must now choose between closing the abdomen with generous drainage and leaving it open as a 'laparostomy'. Each technique has its advocates. The closed technique is easier to manage with regard to nursing care, but up to one-third of patients require one or more repeat laparotomies for further debridement. The open technique allows inspection of the abdominal contents on a daily basis with ready drainage of further collections, but at the expense of a higher incidence of postoperative bleeding and intestinal fistula. Some surgeons reserve laparostomy for the most severe cases and use the closed drainage technique when necrosis is less extensive.

5 In the *closed* technique it is vital to ensure adequate drainage of the retroperitoneal cavity and lesser sac. We place four wide-bore drains, bringing two out as far posteriorly as possible, one on each side. If the necrotizing process is limited to the lesser sac, it is helpful to 'compartmentalize' the abdomen by suturing the greater omentum to the peritoneum along the lower border of the transverse incision. Postoperatively the lesser sac can then be irrigated in isolation from the remaining abdominal viscera. Take care closing the abdomen because of the risk of subsequent wound dehiscence. Insert deep tension sutures in a severe case.

6 In the *open* technique make no attempt to suture the abdominal wall. One or two drains may be placed in the depths of the cavity and brought out through stab incisions. Cover the exposed viscera with several packs wrung out in saline. Consider placing a large piece of adherent plastic sheeting over the entire wound to prevent leakage of fluid. Surprisingly, evisceration is seldom a problem.

Aftercare

1 Continue standard supportive measures for acute pancreatitis, with intravenous fluids and nasogastric suction as required. Patients with a severe attack will require total parenteral nutrition. Antibiotic therapy is needed to manage septic complications, the choice of agent being tailored to the organism cultured. Recent evidence suggests that, in cases of severe pancreatitis, early prophylactic antibiotics decrease the incidence of septic complications and there may be a corresponding decrease in mortality rate.[5]

2 On admission or following a diagnostic laparotomy, it is helpful to assess the severity of acute pancreatitis, using multiple laboratory criteria, such as the Ranson or Imrie scoring systems, and/or serial measurements of C-reactive protein and white cell count. All patients with severe acute pancreatitis should be managed in an intensive therapy unit. Ultrasound and CT scans may be used to detect the development of complications, notably pseudocyst, bleeding and infected pancreatic necrosis.

3 Following a closed drainage procedure for necrotizing pancreatitis, institute saline lavage down two of the four drains, using the other two for egress of the fluid. Commence lavage with warm isotonic fluid either at the end of the operation or after overnight recovery, allowing the peritoneum to 'seal'. Infuse between 50 and 200 ml/hour, depending upon the size of the cavity and the degree of contamination. Continue lavage at least until the effluent becomes clean. Monitor the serum albumin level, because prolonged lavage will exacerbate protein depletion. Use clinical judgement and weekly CT scans to assess progress and the necessity or otherwise for repeat laparotomy and debridement.

4 Following laparostomy, inspect the abdominal cavity. Nearly all these patients will require mechanical ventilation in an intensive therapy unit, and the packs can usually be changed in this setting without the need to take the patient back to the operating theatre. Intravenous sedation will generally suffice. Remove the packs and examine the abdominal viscera. Gently insinuate your hand into the cavity, drain any pus and tease out any further necrotic tissue. Wash out the cavity and place fresh packs. If the patient's condition improves, consider secondary suture of the abdominal wall at a later date.

KEY POINTS Surgical intervention in acute pancreatitis

- Patients with severe pancreatitis require combined specialist care by surgeons and intensivists.
- In most cases of sterile necrosis, operation is not required but you must be mindful of other complications occurring such as infarction of bowel or gastrointestinal haemorrhage that need urgent surgical attention.

Complications

1 Infected pancreatic necrosis is a difficult and dangerous condition. The mortality rate is at least 20–30% in most published series. A successful outcome requires good surgical and nursing care, which often needs to be continued for several weeks. Supportive measures include intravenous fluids, parenteral nutrition and antibiotics as required.

2 There are many potential complications, and their management can be summarized as follows.

- *Respiratory failure/adult respiratory distress syndrome (ARDS)*. Continue assisted respiration under the supervision of an experienced anaesthetist, and consider tracheostomy after 10–14 days of endotracheal intubation (see Ch. 2).
- *Renal failure*. Haemofiltration or haemodialysis are generally be required unless the infracolic compartment of the abdomen can be used for peritoneal dialysis. Dopamine and dobutamine may be used to improve renal blood flow.
- *Myocardial failure*. Pressor support may be required to maintain an adequate blood pressure and peripheral circulation.
- *Continuing sepsis*. This is the single most important factor underlying multiple organ failure. Hectic fever and leucocytosis indicate active infection. Remember the possibility of septicaemia from a contaminated central venous line.

Obtain blood cultures and consider the need to change the line. Repeat the chest X-ray to look for a focus of infection. Perform ultrasound, CT or isotope scans to image the abdominal cavity, and consider whether percutaneous drainage or repeat laparotomy are needed to deal with further collections.

- *Intestinal.* Prolonged ileus is common in patients with abdominal sepsis, especially those on a ventilator. Remember the possibility of colonic, or small-bowel, ischaemia, which may require repeat laparotomy. Very occasionally a prolonged duodenal ileus necessitates a gastroenterostomy. These patients are prone to peptic stress ulceration, institute prophylaxis with topical agents such as sucralfate or intravenously with H_2-receptor antagonists or proton-pump inhibitors.
- *Haemorrhage.* Bleeding follows arterial or venous erosion in the wall of the infected cavity and blood may escape into the gut, into the abdominal cavity or down the drain. Resuscitate the patient and, if there is gastrointestinal haemorrhage, consider endoscopy to look for erosive gastritis (see Ch. 13). If there is evidence of intra-abdominal bleeding the patient should have a CT scan with vascular reconstruction. In most instances this reveals the site of bleeding and identifies the feeding vessel. This can then be followed by visceral angiography and transcatheter embolization. If radiology is unsuccessful then a laparotomy may be required, with suture of the bleeding vessel and occasionally formal resection. Such operative procedures carry a high morbidity and mortality.
- *Pancreatic fistula.* Survivors may develop a pancreatic fistula from the abscess cavity along a drain track to the skin. Most of these fistulas heal spontaneously with the passage of time and can simply be managed in the interim by collection into a stoma bag. Manage an intestinal fistula or mixed fistula along standard lines (see Ch. 14).

REFERENCES

1. Fogel EL, Sherman S 2003 Acute biliary pancreatitis: when should the endoscopist intervene. Gastroenterology 125:229–235
2. Werner J, Uhl W, Hartwig W et al 2003 Modern phase-specific management of acute pancreatitis. Digestive Diseases 21:38–45
3. Carter CR, McKay CJ, Imrie CW 2000 Percutaneous necrosectomy and sinus tract endoscopy in the management of infected pancreatic necrosis: an initial experience. Annals of Surgery 232:175–180
4. Al-Omran M, Groof A, Wilke D 2003 Enteral versus parenteral nutrition for acute pancreatitis. Cochrane Database Systematic Review CD002837
5. Bassi C, Larvin M, Villatoro E 2003 Antibiotic therapy for prophylaxis against infection of pancreatic necrosis in acute pancreatitis. Cochrane Database Systematic Review CD002941

DRAINAGE OF PANCREATIC CYSTS

Appraise

- True cysts are congenital or neoplastic and are rare. Cysts complicating acute or chronic pancreatitis and pancreatic trauma are 'false' pseudocysts, in that they have no epithelial lining. Both types are best diagnosed by ultrasound and CT scanning of the upper abdomen.
- A collection of fluid around the pancreas is quite a common sequel of acute pancreatitis, but most of these resolve spontaneously. Drainage is required for an expanding mass, which often causes pain, or for vomiting and jaundice, or for a mass that fails to resolve or becomes infected. Within 4–5 weeks of the acute attack, the cyst wall is unlikely to be sufficiently mature to take sutures, and external drainage is required. Thereafter, internal drainage becomes feasible, either cystgastrostomy or cystjejunostomy Roux-en-Y. Reserve cystgastrostomy for moderate-sized cysts that are closely applied to the back of the stomach on imaging. Both endoscopic and laparoscopic methods are now available to avoid open operation for internal cyst drainage (see below).
- Percutaneous aspiration of pancreatic pseudocysts is becoming increasingly popular. The procedure is carried out under ultrasound or CT control. A pigtail catheter can be inserted for external drainage, or a percutaneous transgastric approach can be used to position a stent in the cystgastrostomy position.[1] Percutaneous needling and drainage may be suitable for small cysts discovered in the early weeks after an attack of acute pancreatitis. Surgical drainage seems a more appropriate technique for large, mature or recurrent cysts and for those that communicate with the pancreatic duct.
- Sometimes an encysted collection of blood and/or pancreatic fluid may follow blunt abdominal trauma. Traumatic cysts are prone to complications and require early drainage, usually to the exterior.
- Pseudocysts developing in association with chronic pancreatitis are generally contained within the pancreas and frequently communicate with the main ductal system. They may develop insidiously with gradual expansion of the pancreas, sometimes at multiple sites, or rapidly after an attack of acute-on-chronic pancreatitis, in which case they contain some necrotic material. Endoscopic retrograde pancreatography therefore runs the risk of introducing infection into the cyst cavity so give prophylactic antibiotic cover. It is a useful investigation because a dilated pancreatic duct also requires drainage. Smaller cysts can be resected together with diseased pancreas or drained into the duct and thence to a Roux loop of jejunum. Treat larger cysts by cystenterostomy, unless a preoperative angiogram shows an arterial pseudo-aneurysm in the wall, in which case resection may be safer.
- Never assume that a cystic mass in or adjacent to the pancreas is an inflammatory pseudocyst unless there is clear evidence of acute pancreatitis, for example recent pain and hyperamylasaemia, or chronic pancreatitis, from a consistent history and imaging. There are several varieties of cystic neoplasm, including serous and mucinous cystadenoma, mucinous cystadenocarcinoma and cystic endocrine tumour. Always obtain a biopsy of the cyst wall at operation, and arrange frozen-section examination if there is any suspicion of neoplasia.[2] Resect neoplastic cysts if possible.
- Endoscopic techniques have recently become available for internal drainage of a pseudocyst, using endoscopic ultrasound guidance. With a diathermy wire passed down the operating channel of an endoscope, the endoscopist creates an opening from the cyst into the stomach or duodenum.[3] It is even possible to

drain a communicating pseudocyst into the duct via a nasopancreatic tube or short pancreatic stent passed per endoscope. These methods are gaining popularity, but no randomized trials have been performed to compare them to traditional methods.

Prepare

1 In patients with a chronic pseudocyst, do not embark on an operation for the cyst without fully investigating the pancreas.

2 Bleeding can be a problem during operations for pseudocyst, so ensure that cross-matched blood is available beforehand.

3 Remember that intraoperative cystography or ductography may be required, and make the necessary arrangements.

KEY POINTS Drainage of pseudocysts

- The techniques of percutaneous or endoscopic cystgastrostomy require the posterior wall of the stomach to be adherent to the pseudocyst. This is often not the case in pseudocysts associated with chronic pancreatitis where the lesser sac is patent.
- Furthermore, patients with chronic pancreatitis often have varices around the stomach, adding further hazard to this technique.

Assess

1 After an acute attack of pancreatitis or pancreatic trauma an encysted collection of fluid may be entered on approaching the pancreas. This type of collection is usually best drained to the exterior. The resultant pancreatic fistula does not cause skin excoriation, since the pancreatic enzymes are not activated, and it will nearly always close spontaneously. If a large cyst is palpable within the lesser sac, try and determine whether the posterior wall of the stomach is adherent to the front of the cyst, in which case cystgastrostomy may be appropriate. If not, internal drainage into a Roux loop of jejunum is a satisfactory method of dealing with a mature cyst.

2 During laparotomy for chronic pancreatitis, plan your attack according to the operative findings in the underlying pancreas, supplemented by a knowledge of pancreatic ductal anatomy obtained from either ERCP, MRCP or ductography (see above). A cyst in the head of the pancreas can sometimes be marsupialized into the duodenum. Elsewhere in the gland, cystjejunostomy Roux-en-Y is the best option, unless complete resection can be safely achieved.

3 Try and create a good-sized stoma between the cyst and the viscus chosen for internal drainage, so that tube drains are not needed.

Action

Cystgastrostomy (Fig. 21.3)

1 This is only indicated for effusions into the lesser sac that have been present long enough to have developed a fibrous wall. The stoma will probably close once the cavity has filled in after drainage.

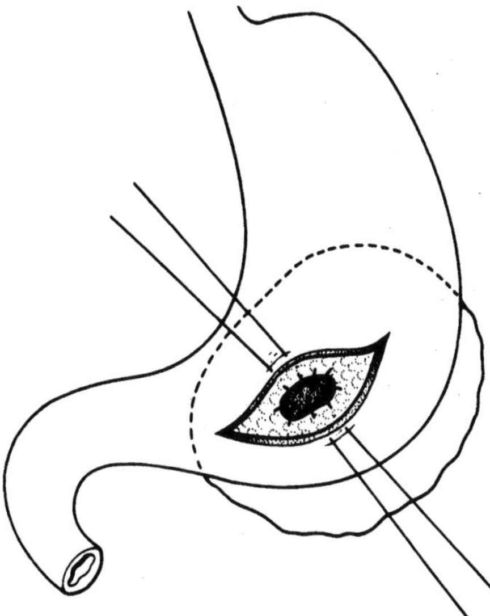

Fig. 21.3 Pancreatic cystgastrostomy. The anterior wall of the stomach is held open by stay sutures. A collection of pancreatic fluid in the lesser sac ('pseudocyst') is drained into the stomach through a posterior gastrostomy.

2 After packing off the stomach, make a longitudinal incision through the anterior gastric wall fairly close to the greater curvature and opposite the incisura angularis. Suck out the gastric contents.

3 Now incise the posterior gastric wall for a short distance opposite the anterior gastrotomy. Deepen the incision and enter the cyst, obtaining samples of the fluid for culture and chemical analysis. Evacuate the contents of the cyst and gently break down any loculi with your finger.

4 Insert a running polyglactin 910 (Vicryl) suture round the margins of the posterior gastrotomy, ensuring a stoma at least 4 cm in diameter. Close the anterior gastrotomy in two layers and close the abdomen with drainage.

Cystduodenostomy

1 Reserve this procedure for a small cyst in the head of pancreas close to the duodenal loop.

2 Make a longitudinal duodenotomy opposite the cyst. Inset a needle into the cyst. Aspiration of bile warns you that the bile duct is nearby and you should not proceed.

3 If the aspirate is clear, leave the needle in place and incise the duodenal wall to enter the cyst. Suture the margins of the opening as above. Close the duodenum in two layers, taking care not to narrow its lumen. Close the abdomen with drainage.

Cystjejunostomy (Fig. 21.4)

1 This technique is applicable to all types of cyst with walls thick enough for suturing. It is the most likely method to obtain dependent drainage and avoid the potential problem of food debris contaminating the pseudocyst cavity.

2 Mobilize the pancreas and if preoperative ductal imaging is unclear obtain an operative cystogram. Now incise the anterior wall of the cyst, sample and drain its contents and explore its recesses for any obvious ductal communication.

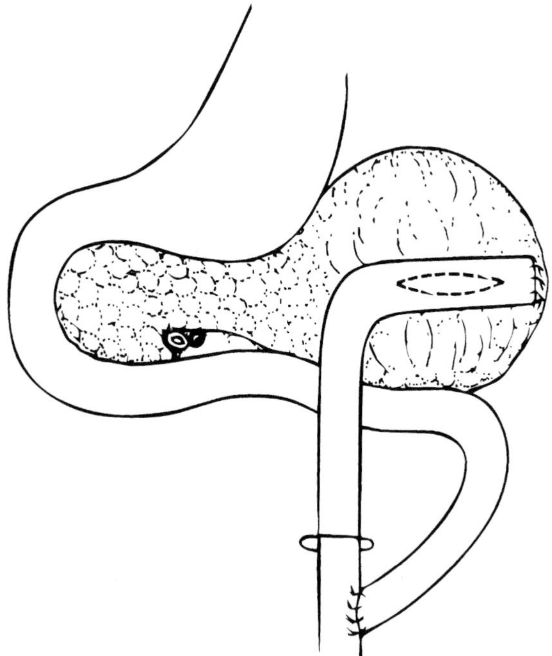

Fig. 21.4 Pancreatic cystjejunostomy. A retrocolic Roux loop of jejunum has been anastomosed to a large cyst within the tail of pancreas.

3 Create a Roux loop of jejunum (Ch. 14) and close its end. Approximate the upper end of the Roux loop to the front of the cyst without tension. Create a generous side-to-side anastomosis between the opening into the cyst and a longitudinal jejunotomy. Use one or two layers of suture according to the thickness of the cyst wall, but use polyglactin 910 (Vicryl) for the inner layer.

4 Restore intestinal continuity by jejunojejunostomy at the base of the Roux loop. Drain the abdomen through a stab incision as above.

Laparoscopic techniques

Both cystgastrostomy and cystjejunostomy have been performed using laparoscopic surgery.[4] Although these techniques may provide adequate internal drainage, they do not allow for full assessment of the pseudocyst to exclude neoplasia, and resection of a pseudocyst would be extremely difficult using laparoscopic methods.

Nevertheless, in properly selected cases laparoscopy may provide a way of achieving good internal drainage in a minimally invasive way and warrants further investigation.

KEY POINT Drainage versus resection of pseudocysts

- The decision to drain or resect a chronic pseudocyst will depend on several factors: its position in the gland, the general condition of the patient, the patient's endocrine and exocrine function, the presence or absence of varices, the extent of disease in the underlying pancreatic tissue and the degree of suspicion of neoplasia.

Complications

1 Decompression of a pseudocyst into the gut may be followed by haemorrhage if there was a pre-existing pseudo-aneurysm, although angiography, whether derived from CT, MRI or visceral angiography, should always be undertaken before drainage of a chronic cyst. Once bleeding occurs the patient requires a CT scan, with an emphasis on the arterial phase, to determine the site of origin, proceeding to a angiogram and transcatheter embolization. If this fails, re-operation is required, sometimes with formal resection.

2 Pancreatic fistula is seldom troublesome, because the enzyme content of pancreatic juice is low in patients with chronic pancreatitis. Treat a gastric or intestinal fistula along standard lines.

REFERENCES

1. Vidyarthi G, Steinberg SE 2001 Endoscopic management of pancreatic pseudocysts. Surgical Clinics of North America 81:405–410
2. Spinelli KS, Fromwiller TE, Daniel RA et al 2004 Cystic pancreatic neoplasms: observe or operate. Annals of Surgery 239:651–659
3. Beckingham IJ, Krige JE, Bornman PC et al 1999 Long term outcome of endoscopic drainage of pancreatic pseudocysts. American Journal of Gastroenterology 94:71–74
4. Siperstein A 2001 Laparoendoscopic approach to pancreatic pseudocysts. Seminars in Laparoscopic Surgery 8:218–222

DRAINAGE OF THE PANCREATIC DUCT

Appraise

1 Ductal drainage is preferable to resection for the relief of pain in chronic pancreatitis, since it preserves the remaining functioning tissue. However, only an anastomosis between the pancreatic duct and adjacent viscus that is several millimetres in diameter is likely to remain patent. Therefore do not ordinarily undertake a drainage operation unless the duct is two to three times its normal diameter.

2 The operation of choice is longitudinal pancreaticojejunostomy, which creates a long side-to-side anastomosis between the incised duct and a Roux loop of jejunum. Often this may be combined with a 'coring' out of the head of the pancreas, a so-called 'Frey modification'. A lateral anastomosis between the amputated body of pancreas and a Roux loop is less likely to stay open unless the duct is grossly dilated at the site of transection, in which case it should probably be opened up in the proximal gland. Sometimes it is reasonable to combine conservative distal resection with a limited longitudinal pancreaticojejunostomy.

3 Formerly popular for the treatment of chronic pancreatitis, sphincteroplasty has in fact little to offer. It is reasonable to consider biliary sphincteroplasty (Ch. 19), followed by a similar procedure to widen the orifice of the pancreatic duct, when there is moderate dilatation of the whole duct tapering to a stricture at its orifice, but this is an uncommon situation in chronic pancreatitis. Pancreatic sphincteroplasty may be indicated for patients with recurrent acute pancreatitis or chronic abdominal pain and stenosis in the terminal pancreatic duct. In pancreas

divisum, accessory pancreatic sphincteroplasty is sometimes helpful.

4 Drainage of an obstructed distended duct into the back of the stomach (pancreaticogastrostomy) is quite a simple technique that may bring worthwhile relief of pain from irresectable carcinoma of the head of pancreas.

5 Techniques for draining normal-calibre and dilated pancreatic ducts after proximal pancreatectomy (Whipple resection) are considered at the end of this chapter.

Prepare

1 Do not operate on patients with chronic pancreatitis unless you have some experience of this disease and are capable of carrying out pancreatectomy.

2 Ensure that preoperative imaging and pancreatic function tests have been adequately undertaken.

3 Arrange for cross-matched blood to be available, together with the facilities for operative pancreatography, and give prophylactic antibiotics perioperatively.

Access

Operations for chronic pancreatitis require generous access to the upper abdomen. Excellent exposure is afforded by a transverse subcostal incision that divides both recti and is gently curved with an upward convexity ('gable' incision).

Assess

1 Expose the pancreas carefully but completely and examine it thoroughly. Is the gland indurated throughout, or is the disease partly localized? Can you feel the pancreatic duct as a soft dilated tube in the body of the gland? Are there any associated cysts? If there is serious suspicion of carcinoma, obtain a biopsy.

2 Look for evidence of gallstones, which are quite commonly associated with chronic pancreatitis. The bile duct may be slightly dilated, with a thickened, opaque wall. Examine the stomach and duodenum for peptic ulcer disease. Exclude cirrhosis of the liver, portal hypertension and splenomegaly. Perform liver biopsy if the patient is an alcoholic.

3 Do not hesitate to obtain an operative pancreatogram if you are in any doubt about the best procedure for chronic pancreatitis if the preoperative ductal imaging is uncertain. If the disease is not very severe, amputate the tail of the pancreas for histological examination; also, prograde pancreatography may provide useful information for subsequent clinical management.

KEY POINTS Indications for drainage procedures in chronic pancreatitis

- Although drainage procedures are the optimal operations in chronic pancreatitis because they can relieve pain without exacerbating functional insufficiency, they require a 'target' to drain, either a pseudocyst or a dilated duct.
- Otherwise some form of resection is required, tailored to the site of maximal disease.

Action

Pancreatic sphincteroplasty

1 Expose the papilla by a transduodenal approach and carry out biliary sphincteroplasty.

2 Look for the orifice of the major pancreatic duct on the lower lip of the papilla. Magnifying spectacles may be helpful. Pass a soft umbilical catheter (4–6F) and obtain a retrograde pancreatogram if ERCP or MRCP were inadequate. If you cannot locate the orifice, ask the anaesthetist to give an intravenous injection of secretin (1 unit/kg) and look for the flow of pancreatic juice within 30–60 seconds.

3 Divide the common septum between the terminal portions of the bile duct and pancreatic duct for a distance of about 10 mm. Obtain a tiny biopsy if the septum appears scarred. Facilitate the septotomy by placing fine (5/0) sutures on either side of the proposed line of incision, tying them and dividing the septum between them, using straight iris scissors.

4 Suture the mucosa of the pancreatic duct to that of the bile duct using 5/0 polyglactin 910 (Vicryl) sutures.

5 A similar technique should be used for accessory sphincteroplasty, but here it is often necessary to give secretin to identify the tiny ductal orifice.

6 Close the duodenum and leave a drain to the subhepatic pouch, as for biliary sphincteroplasty.

Longitudinal pancreaticojejunostomy (Fig. 21.5)

1 Expose the body, neck and part of the head of pancreas through the lesser sac. It is usually not necessary to mobilize the gland completely. If needle pancreatography has been performed, leave the needle in position as a guide to the duct.

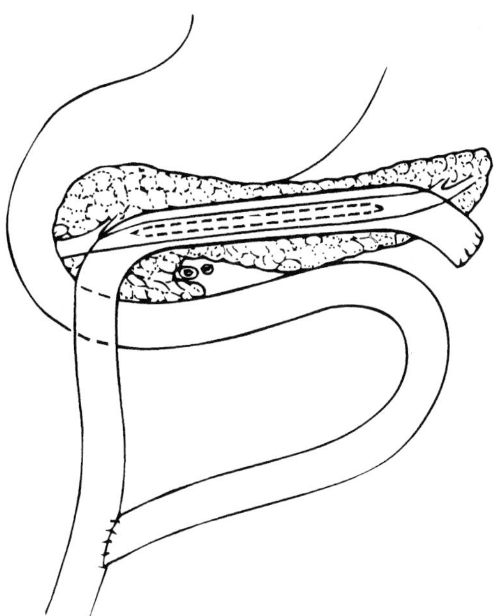

Fig. 21.5 Longitudinal pancreaticojejunostomy Roux-en-Y. The dilated duct is opened widely and a long side-to-side anastomosis is created.

2 Incise the front of the pancreas between stay sutures at a convenient place in the body of the gland. If the duct is clearly dilated, make the incision in the long axis of the gland. If not, make a small exploratory incision across the axis. Intraoperative ultrasound can be helpful in identifying an impalpable duct.

3 On entering a dilated ductal system, aspirate the pale, greyish pancreatic juice. Extend the incision in each direction, using scalpel or pointed scissors, and under-run any major bleeding vessel. Ensure that the gastroduodenal artery is properly controlled where it is divided in the neck of the gland. Open the duct widely from head to tail. Remove all calculi and try to open any cysts into the main duct.

4 Select a Roux loop of jejunum and close its end. Bring the loop through a mesocolic window so that it lies comfortably along the entire pancreas. Insert interrupted silk sutures to approximate the fibrotic 'capsule' of the pancreas and the seromuscular layers of the jejunum. Now make a long jejunotomy to match the incision in the pancreatic duct and place a running all-coats suture between the two, using 3/0 polyglactin 910 (Vicryl). The ductal lining is tough and takes sutures quite well. Finish with an anterior seromuscular layer of silk.

5 Restore intestinal continuity by end-to-side jejunojejunostomy. Close the abdomen with a drain to the region of the pancreas.

Lateral pancreaticojejunostomy (Fig. 21.6)

1 Reserve this procedure for draining a dilated duct in the neck or proximal body of pancreas after distal resection. It may be sensible to open up the duct at the site of transection by incising for a few centimetres through its anterior wall and the overlying pancreas.

2 Fashion a retrocolic Roux loop of jejunum as above and close its end. Make a small subterminal jejunotomy to match the diameter of the duct and insert an all-coats suture, using fine non-absorbable stitches. Tack the peripheral pancreatic substance to the seromuscular layer of jejunum with a second layer of similar sutures.

3 Restore intestinal continuity as usual.

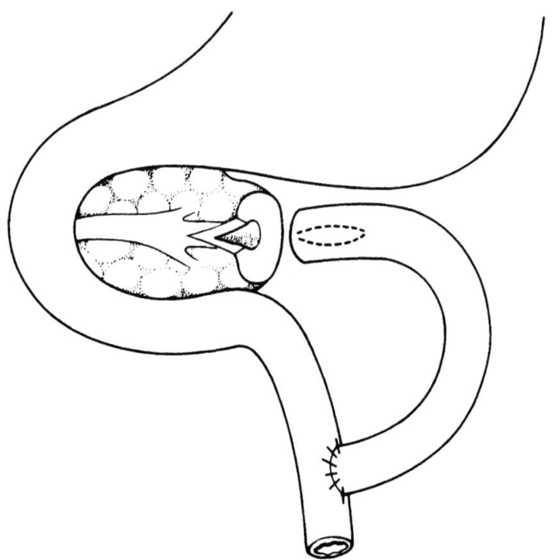

Fig. 21.6 Lateral pancreaticojejunostomy Roux-en-Y. Following distal pancreatectomy a dilated pancreatic duct is opened for a short distance and sutured to the Roux loop.

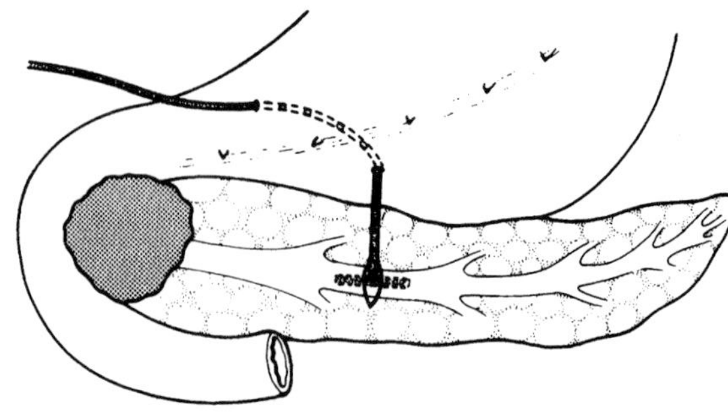

Fig. 21.7 Intubated pancreaticogastrostomy. In an attempt to relieve back pain from an irresectable carcinoma of the head of pancreas, the obstructed pancreatic duct is decompressed into the stomach. The small incisions in the back of the stomach and the front of the pancreas are approximated and the T-tube is brought to the exterior.

Intubated pancreaticogastrostomy (Fig. 21.7)

1 Examine the body of pancreas for the tell-tale sensation of a dilated duct. Needling the duct, with or without pancreatography, will help to confirm your finding.

2 Make a short vertical incision across the body of pancreas and deepen this until you enter the duct. Insert a T-tube into the duct; suture the gland around the entry of the tube. Make tiny posterior and anterior gastrotomies several centimetres apart. Bring the tube through each wall of the stomach and thence by a stab incision to the exterior. Make sure there are two or three holes in the tube within its intragastric course, and tighten a purse-string suture around the anterior gastrotomy. By traction on the tube, draw the stomach down on to the front of the pancreas, and approximate the two organs with a few tacking sutures.

3 Postoperatively the T-tube may drain the stomach in preference to the nasogastric tube, but it can usually be clamped with safety after flatus has been passed per rectum.

Complications

1 These are uncommon, but reactive haemorrhage and pancreatic fistula are theoretical risks, as after a cyst drainage procedure (see above).

2 Acute pancreatitis should not follow a sphincteroplasty unless the ductal orifice has been inadvertently occluded.

3 A transient rise in serum amylase following manipulation of the pancreas and/or pancreatography is of little importance.

LAPAROTOMY AND BYPASS FOR PANCREATIC CANCER

Appraise

- Ductal adenocarcinoma of the pancreas is both common and difficult to treat. Its cause is largely unknown. Most tumours are irresectable by the time they are diagnosed, and this is particularly so for cancers of the body and tail of pancreas, where early symptoms are scarce and non-specific. When the tumour is within the head of pancreas, the patient may present with obstructive jaundice while the tumour is still relatively small and localized.

- Some patients with cancer of the head of pancreas require laparotomy to confirm the diagnosis, determine the potential resectability of the tumour and allow a choice to be made between resection and bypass. Despite the scale of the operation required, carry out resection for potentially curable tumours in those of reasonable general health, since this policy offers the only chance of cure. Less aggressive cancers such as neuroendocrine tumour or cholangiocarcinoma may be difficult or impossible to differentiate from pancreatic cancer on either preoperative or operative assessment, and the same can hold true for the benign condition of chronic pancreatitis.
- Staging laparoscopy, possibly in combination with laparoscopic ultrasound, may allow detection of peritoneal deposits, small liver metastases and even portal venous invasion, but the number of patients in which this will add extra information above that obtained from conventional imaging is controversial. Some authors claim that laparoscopic examination excludes an extra 30% of patients from curative resection. Most series suggest that 14% of patients can be spared an unnecessary laparotomy,[1] and if one considers that laparoscopy may in fact provide the opportunity to institute palliative bypass then this technique of 'preoperative' staging becomes attractive.
- Most patients with cancer of the body or tail of pancreas do not require laparotomy because the tumour either metastasizes or encases the superior mesenteric vessels at an early stage and is therefore seldom resectable. Moreover, jaundice and duodenal obstruction occur late if at all. Thus optimal management comprises obtaining a tissue diagnosis by means of guided percutaneous needle biopsy, confirming the irresectability of the tumour by CT scan and considering non-operative measures such as radiotherapy and chemotherapy, especially for younger patients and those with troublesome back pain. However, if imaging leaves you in any doubt about the nature or resectability of the tumour, perform laparotomy.
- Preoperative investigation of a patient with obstructive jaundice starts with liver function tests and ultrasound scan to exclude hepatocellular disease and show a dilated biliary tree consistent with a 'surgical' cause of obstruction. Ultrasound and CT scan may show gallstone disease, a pancreatic or periampullary mass, nodal or hepatic metastases and major vascular involvement. PTC and ERCP are invaluable for showing the level and the nature of bile duct stricture, but one or other test will generally suffice. PTC gives better visualization of the proximal biliary tree, which is useful for a high stricture, whereas ERCP can provide an additional pancreatogram, which is useful to confirm pancreatic cancer or chronic pancreatitis. If combined with endoscopic ultrasound, this can visualize the adjacent vascular structures and aid in the assessment of operability.[2] Endoscopic-ultrasound-guided fine-needle aspiration can provide a cytological diagnosis without risking tumour seeding outside the pancreas. If preoperative jaundice is not deep and stenting not required, then non-invasive imaging with MR or spiral CT may be sufficient. Delineation of the adjacent venous and arterial anatomy is important both in determining operability and in identification of anatomical anomalies. This can usually be achieved non-invasively using three-dimensional reconstructions of CT,[2] but may require formal visceral angiography. Preoperative percutaneous biopsy is unnecessary in patients who are proceeding to laparotomy.
- It is debatable whether non-operative stenting or surgical bypass is the better option for irresectable cancer of the pancreatic head. Stenting can be achieved by either the percutaneous transhepatic route or the endoscopic transpapillary route depending on available local expertise. In expert hands the two procedures have similar morbidity and mortality rates, which are equivalent to those of surgical bypass. The recent introduction of expandable metal stents seems likely to reduce the problem of stent clogging, which leads to cholangitis and recurrent jaundice. Metal stents should only be placed if the patient is deemed to be inoperable. The longevity of metal stents is an important consideration because repeated admissions for clearing or replacement of blocked stents can outweigh any advantage gained by avoiding the initial recovery period in hospital that follows a surgical bypass. It is not acceptable simply to stent a patient who might otherwise be suitable for resection without thorough assessment of the case. In general, very elderly or infirm patients and those with advanced carcinoma should be managed by non-operative stenting. For younger patients, those with a potentially resectable tumour and those without extensive distal spread or incipient duodenal obstruction, operative bypass is preferable. The ability to perform biliary and gastric bypass by laparoscopic techniques,[3] along with increasing expertise with expandable metal stents in the biliary tract and more recently in the duodenum, means that the surgeon has a wider choice of palliative options and patient selection becomes even more important.

KEY POINT Surgery versus stenting

- If any doubt exists about the diagnosis or the resectability of the tumour then patients should undergo a laparotomy and trial dissection. If unresectability is confirmed, then the option of a double surgical bypass should be considered.

Prepare

1 Patients with prolonged obstruction of the extrahepatic biliary tree tolerate major resectional procedures very poorly. The following specific problems should be anticipated and countered:

- *Coagulopathy*. If hypoprothrombinaemia is present, give sufficient parenteral vitamin K to restore the prothrombin time of the blood to normal. Routine preoperative administration of vitamin K is a sensible precaution in any jaundiced patient.
- *Hepatorenal syndrome*. Preoperative rehydration is the simplest and most important precaution. In deeply jaundiced

patients, renal failure may be precipitated by intraoperative hypotension, and this should be avoided as far as possible. Catheterize the patient after induction of anaesthesia, ensure adequate hydration and administer intravenous mannitol (40 g) to achieve an osmotic diuresis during the operation.

- *Sepsis*. Though infected bile is more likely with gallstones than a malignant stricture, 'invasive' cholangiography or operation may provoke infection in any obstructed biliary tree. Both procedures should therefore be covered by prophylactic antibiotics.
- *Malnutrition*. Decreased hepatic synthesis of albumin inevitably follows obstructive jaundice and may not improve until the obstruction has been relieved. Consider parenteral nutrition postoperatively if convalescence is prolonged.
- *Wound failure*. The healing of wounds is impaired in jaundiced patients. Take particular care with abdominal closure.

2 Preoperative decompression of the obstructed biliary tree is controversial. External transhepatic drainage may improve general health at the risk of various complications (e.g. infection, bile leakage, electrolyte loss). In general, we reserve preoperative biliary stents for patients with deep and prolonged jaundice or those with complications such as renal insufficiency and cholangitis. Internal decompression by transhepatic or endoscopic retrograde intubation of the stricture is safer but requires appropriate expertise.

3 If radiological or endoscopic skills are not available, staged resection is a reasonable alternative for patients with unrelenting obstructive jaundice for more than 2–3 weeks. At the first operation, determine that the tumour in the region of the pancreatic head is mobile and potentially resectable. Do not prolong the dissection but carry out cholecystojejunostomy. Reoperate at 3–4 weeks when serum bilirubin levels have fallen and serum albumin has risen.

Access

1 A right subcostal incision will suffice for cholecystojejunostomy alone.

2 If, as is usual, further bypass procedures or pancreatectomy are indicated, extend the incision across the midline, dividing both recti to complete a gable incision.

Assess

1 *The gallbladder is distended and there is such diffuse metastatic spread that the patient is unlikely to live very long*. Relieve obstructive jaundice by the simple expedient of cholecystojejunostomy (see Ch. 19). If you are in doubt about the patency of the cystic duct, consider obtaining an operative cholecystogram via a Foley catheter inserted into the fundus. Cholecystojejunostomy is generally best avoided. Patients with carcinomatosis are better served by non-operative stenting, whereas for those with a better prognosis but irresectable tumours prefer to use the common hepatic duct for anastomosis since it prevents recurrence of jaundice from encroachment of tumour on the cystic duct.

2 The tumour is clearly irresectable but not as advanced as the above; alternatively, the gallbladder is collapsed or contains calculi. Do not use the gallbladder for anastomosis. More lasting biliary diversion is achieved by choledochojejunostomy Roux-en-Y (see Ch. 19), dividing the bile duct above the 'leading edge' of tumour to limit upward spread. Cholecystectomy generally facilitates the operation and is certainly advisable if the gallbladder is obstructed.

3 The tumour could be resectable and there is no overt metastasis. Embark upon a trial dissection. If the superior mesenteric and portal veins can be separated from the neck of pancreas, proceed to pancreatoduodenectomy (see next section).

4 *You have decided against resection*. Be sure that you obtain a positive tissue diagnosis by appropriate biopsy with frozen-section confirmation. Consider palliative procedures to relieve jaundice, vomiting and pain. Carry out biliary diversion as described in paragraphs 1 and 2 above. Unless the prognosis is extremely limited, create an antecolic gastroenterostomy (see Ch. 13) to bypass present or future duodenal obstruction (Fig. 21.8). Alternatively, use the same Roux loop for biliary and gastric bypass (Fig. 21.9).

5 Options for pain relief include intubated pancreaticogastrostomy, if the pancreatic duct is clearly dilated, or coeliac plexus block; postoperative radiotherapy may also help. An intraoperative nerve block involves injection of 15–20 ml of 50% alcohol on each side at the level of the diaphragmatic crura. Aspirate the syringe each time to ensure that the needle has not entered the aorta or vena cava. Another option is division of the splanchnic nerves within the chest using thoracoscopy (thoracoscopic splanchnicectomy). This minimally invasive procedure has been shown to provide pain relief in some patients with pancreatic cancer.

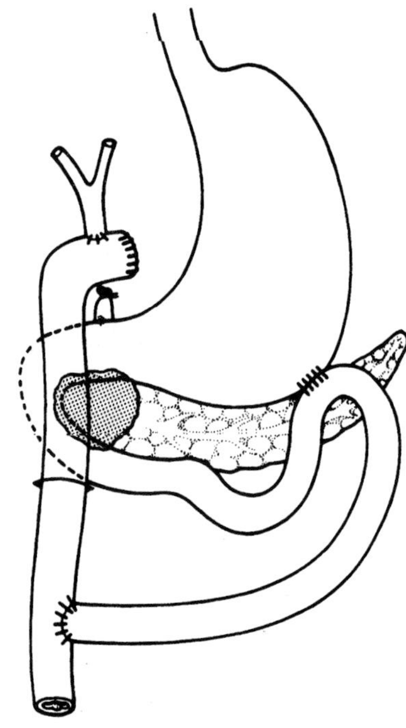

Fig. 21.8 Bypass procedures for an irresectable carcinoma of the head of pancreas. The bile duct is transected well above the tumour, cholecystectomy is performed and biliary drainage is achieved by hepaticojejunostomy Roux-en-Y. An antecolic gastroenterostomy is included.

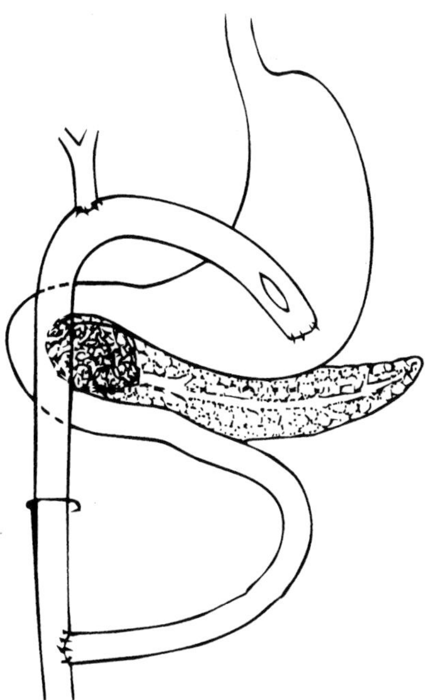

Fig. 21.9 Single-loop biliary and gastric bypass for an irresectable carcinoma of the head of pancreas. This procedure is an alternative to that shown in Figure 21.8.

6 Palliative resection can no longer be justified for adenocarcinomas of the pancreas, as positive margins are one of the strongest predictors of poor outcome and survival in this patient group is no better than those undergoing bypass alone.

Aftercare and complications

1 Once the patient recovers from operation and there is an unequivocal tissue diagnosis, consider the advisability of radiotherapy and/or chemotherapy.

2 There is a low risk of leakage from the biliary anastomosis following palliative bypass. Should the leak persist it should be investigated by fistulography and if necessary PTC, with the option for percutaneous stenting of the anastomosis.

3 Occasionally, patients with advanced carcinoma of the pancreas continue to vomit postoperatively despite one or two patent gastric outlets, that is pylorus and stoma. One possible mechanism for delayed gastric emptying is autovagotomy caused by extensive lymph-node spread. Exclude a mechanical obstruction by means of barium meal and/or endoscopy and administer prokinetic agents such as metoclopramide, domperidone, cisapride and erythromycin.

REFERENCES

1. Hennig R, Tempia-Caliera AA, Hartel M et al 2002 Staging laparoscopy and its indications in pancreatic cancer patients. Digestive Surgery 19:484–488
2. Kalra MK, Maher MM, Mueller PR et al 2003 State of the art imaging of pancreatic neoplasms. British Journal of Radiology 76:857–865
3. Urbach DR, Swanstrom LL, Hansen PD 2002 The effect of laparoscopy on survival in pancreatic cancer. Archives of Surgery 137:191–199

DISTAL PANCREATECTOMY

Appraise

1 Distal pancreatectomy is undertaken for chronic inflammation, trauma or tumour in the body and tail of the gland or as part of a radical gastrectomy for carcinoma of the stomach. In chronic pancreatitis indications include scarring and calcification that predominate to the left of the midline, ductal stricture in the neck or body of pancreas and a pseudocyst in the body or tail. Visualization of the surrounding vasculature should be performed preoperatively, using CT or angiography, to look for splenic artery pseudo-aneurysm or splenic vein thrombosis. CT scan, ERCP, MRCP and tests of endocrine and exocrine pancreatic function help in assessing the patient and choosing the best surgical option in chronic pancreatitis.

2 Complete distal hemipancreatectomy by dividing the gland in front of the portal vein, but you may extend the resection to include the neck and part of the head of pancreas. Occasionally performed for diffuse pancreatitis, a subtotal pancreatectomy removes upwards of 80% of the gland. Take care to preserve the bile duct and at least one of the pancreaticoduodenal arteries. Anticipate varying degrees of pancreatic insufficiency such as diabetes, steatorrhoea, depending on the functional status of the residual pancreas. In such extensive disease proximal pancreatoduodenectomy or even total pancreatectomy may be better options (see below).

3 *Conventional* distal pancreatectomy includes splenectomy. This procedure is indicated for the limited number of ductal carcinomas that are resectable and for most cases of chronic pancreatitis, especially when associated with severe inflammation, pseudocyst and/or splenic vein thrombosis.

4 *Conservative* distal pancreatectomy involves separating the distal pancreas from the splenic vessels and preserving the spleen. It may be indicated for less severe cases of chronic pancreatitis and for endocrine tumours in the body and tail. It is useful to preserve the immunological function of the spleen and avoid the large dead space that follows splenectomy.

Prepare

1 Distal pancreatectomy can be a difficult and bloody operation. Ensure that cross-matched blood is available.

2 Immunize the patient with the polyvalent anti-pneumococcal vaccine Pneumovax, since these organisms are the most common cause of overwhelming postsplenectomy infection. Current guidelines also include immunization with meningococcal and *Haemophilus influenzae* type b vaccines.[1] Try to give the vaccines 2–4 weeks before operation for maximum effect.

Access

1 Good exposure of the upper abdominal cavity is essential for any type of pancreatectomy.

2 Probably the best access is provided by the transverse or curved gable incision.

Assess

1 In operations for chronic pancreatitis the likelihood and extent of resection are indicated by preoperative investigations, including endoscopic pancreatography, MRCP, CT and pancreatic function tests. At laparotomy, however, examine the entire gland. Perform operative pancreatography if there is any chance of a dilated ductal system, not identified on preoperative imaging, since drainage might be more appropriate than resection in such a case.

2 When operating for upper abdominal trauma, first inspect the liver, spleen and mesentery and deal with any site of bleeding. Pancreatic or duodenal injury should be suspected if there is a retroperitoneal haematoma. Mobilize the duodenum and inspect both surfaces. Enter the lesser sac and examine the pancreas thoroughly. Major contusion or fracture of the pancreatic neck should be treated by distal pancreatectomy.

3 Resection of carcinoma of the body of pancreas is nearly always precluded by direct involvement of the superior mesenteric vessels and/or metastatic spread. Follow the middle colic vein back to find the superior mesenteric vein and establish the relation of this vessel to the tumour. If the main vessels are uninvolved, distal pancreatectomy may will be appropriate.

4 Many surgeons remove the left pancreas in a *prograde* fashion, starting with the tail and proceeding towards the midline; this technique is described below. Increasingly the authors carry out much of the dissection in a *retrograde* fashion, mobilizing and dividing the neck of the pancreas at an early stage and, if possible, securing the splenic vessels before elevating the pancreatic tail and body.

Action

Conventional distal pancreatectomy (Fig. 21.10)

1 Start by freeing the neck of pancreas from the underlying portal vein. Trace the middle colic vein downwards to the root of the transverse mesocolon. To display its junction with the superior mesenteric vein, it is necessary to incise the peritoneum along the inferior border of the neck and proximal body of pancreas. In chronic pancreatitis this can be a slow and difficult dissection, and a number of small vessels on the pancreas need to be secured. Once the superior mesenteric vein has been exposed, gently develop the plane between the vein and the pancreas. Pass a finger upwards through this tunnel and expose the tip of your finger by dividing the peritoneum along the superior border of the neck of pancreas. Now that the superior mesenteric and portal veins have been freed, it is safe to proceed to mobilize the tail and body of pancreas towards the midline. Alternatively, continue the dissection to the left to identify, ligate and divide the splenic artery and vein before mobilizing the tail of pancreas (see 'assess' section, paragraph 4).

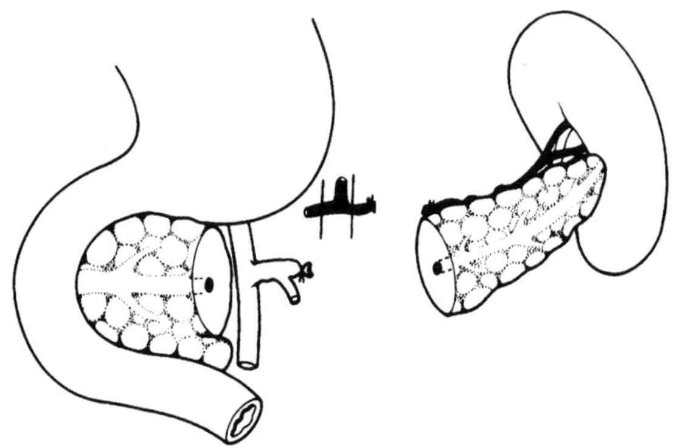

Fig. 21.10 Conventional distal pancreatectomy including splenectomy. Transection just to the right of the portal vein removes about 60% of the gland.

2 In chronic pancreatitis, especially if there is a pseudocyst, the posterior surface of the stomach and the transverse mesocolon and splenic flexure can become adherent to the distal pancreas and need to be dissected free.

3 Mobilize the spleen upwards by dividing its posterior peritoneal attachment—the posterior layer of the lienorenal ligament. The greater omentum will have been partly divided already in entering the lesser sac; now complete the division. Ligate and divide the short gastric vessels. If the spleen is torn during the dissection, ligate its vascular pedicle and complete the splenectomy at this stage.

4 The pancreatic tail lies at the splenic hilum and has already been partly mobilized. Divide the peritoneum along the upper and lower borders of the distal pancreas. Several small vessels need to be ligated or coagulated by diathermy. Continue the dissection towards the midline, lifting the body and tail of pancreas forwards and to the right. Severe chronic inflammation binds the pancreas firmly to its bed, and sharp dissection is needed to free it posteriorly.

5 As the prograde pancreatic dissection approaches the midline, search for the splenic artery as it reaches the posterior surface of the gland near its upper border. Encircle the vessel with a right-angled Lahey forceps and tie it with stout ligatures (2/0 polyglactin 910 or silk), doubly ligating on the proximal side. Ideally, the artery should be tied before the vein to prevent congestion of the spleen, but sometimes it is necessary to ligate and divide the splenic vein first if the artery is encased and inaccessible.

6 The splenic vein can be seen running along the posterior surface of the body of pancreas. As it approaches its right-angled junction with the superior mesenteric vein, it is usually joined by the inferior mesenteric vein. Carefully insert a pair of Lahey forceps between the pancreas and the splenic vein. Ligate and divide the splenic vein, if possible preserving the entry of the inferior mesenteric vein. The pancreas can now be lifted gently off the portal vein. Great care must be taken in the presence of chronic inflammation, since it is easy to tear the great veins.

7 Decide where to transect the pancreas. Division in front of the portal vein is usually considered to represent hemipancreatectomy. Insert 2/0 silk stay sutures at the upper and lower border of the pancreas at this point and place a soft intestinal clamp across the neck (the clamp is optional). Divide the pancreas to the left of the clamp and stay sutures and remove the specimen. Be careful not to injure the underlying vein during transection of the gland.

8 Remove the clamp and secure haemostasis. Look for the amputated main pancreatic duct, which normally measures 2–3 mm in diameter at this point. Consider operative pancreatography,

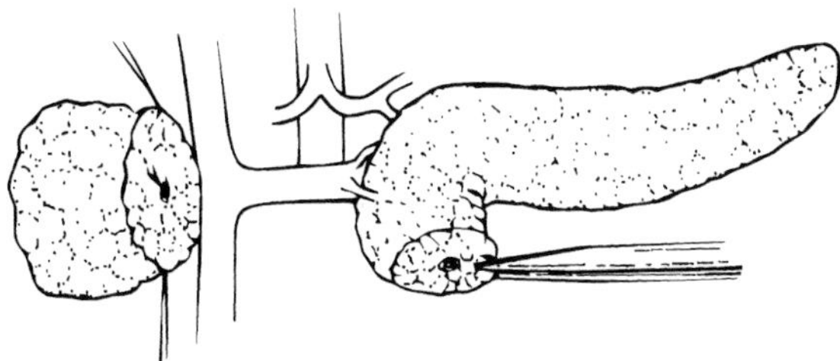

Fig. 21.11 Conservative distal pancreatectomy preserving the spleen. The pancreas is transected at its neck and peeled off the splenic artery and vein from right to left, dividing the numerous vascular branches.

and a drainage procedure, if the duct is dilated. Otherwise, under-run the duct and close over the pancreatic stump, using 3/0 silk sutures.

9 Check that the splenic bed and pancreas are dry. Insert one or two tube drains and close the abdomen.

Conservative distal pancreatectomy (Fig. 21.11)

1 The principles of the operation are similar to those for conventional resection, except that an attempt is made to preserve the splenic vessels and spleen. The dissection can be either prograde or retrograde—that is towards, or away from, the midline, or a combination of both. The operation is carried out entirely within the lesser sac without any mobilization of the spleen. This procedure is ideally suited for benign disease and is associated with a significantly lower morbidity rate.[2]

2 Start by freeing the neck and proximal body of pancreas from the underlying great veins, as described above. Select the site of pancreatic transection and insert stay sutures on either side, approximately 1 cm apart, one pair on the upper border and one pair on the lower border. Place a Kocher's director beneath the pancreas to protect the great veins, then incise through the gland with a scalpel on to the director.

3 Secure haemostasis from each cut surface of the pancreas. Identify the proximal pancreatic duct and under-run it with a 3/0 silk suture. Oversew the pancreatic stump at this point with interrupted 3/0 silk sutures.

4 Gently elevate the distal pancreas from the underlying splenic vein. Identify the splenic artery as it passes from the coeliac axis to reach the pancreas to the left of the midline. Proceed slowly to free the pancreas from the splenic vessels, ligating and dividing the several arterial and venous branches that connect them.

5 If the pancreas is very adherent to the splenic vessels, it may help to elevate the tail of the gland and dissect progradely towards the site of adherence, thereby approaching it from both sides. It is not uncommon to pull a small branch off the splenic artery or vein and then encounter bleeding. Using a sucker to obtain exposure, close the defect(s) in the vessel with fine sutures (e.g. 4/0 or 5/0 silk or polypropylene). Sometimes the parent vessel has been sufficiently exposed for a soft vascular clamp to be used for temporary control.

6 Complete the dissection, remove the specimen, check for haemostasis and close the abdomen, leaving a tube drain to the pancreatic bed.

Other techniques

1 If there is concern about the extent of distal resection and the potential for endocrine or exocrine failure, then a middle segment pancreatectomy may be performed.[3] Transect the pancreas to the right of the portal vein as described and then, once the gland is mobilized off the splenic vessels, transect it again. Close the proximal stump as for a distal pancreatectomy and anastomose a Roux-en-Y loop of jejunum to the tail (see below).

2 Distal pancreatectomy has been performed using laparoscopic techniques with both conventional and spleen-preserving approaches described.[4] This procedure is clearly for advanced laparoscopists only and is currently not recommended for malignant disease.

KEY POINT Splenectomy versus splenic preservation in distal pancreatectomy

- Although splenic preservation is usually associated with a lower morbidity rate, the risk of major intraoperative blood loss probably outweighs this benefit and, if bleeding becomes a problem, then sacrifice the spleen and draw the operation to an end.

? DIFFICULTY

1. Even with a normal pancreas, the conservative technique is seldom easy. Do not attempt it until you have some experience of conventional distal pancreatectomy. If you encounter serious bleeding, it is better to abandon the attempt to preserve the spleen. In fact, it is usually possible to ligate the splenic artery, with or without the vein, yet retain the spleen, provided that the site of ligation is away from the splenic hilum.
2. Bleeding is the main problem with conventional distal pancreatectomy also, especially in severe pancreatitis. If you encounter serious haemorrhage, control it with pressure while taking the usual steps: ensure that access and lighting are optimal and that you have adequate assistance and a functioning sucker. Then remove the pack, identify the source of haemorrhage and control it with sutures. It is usually a tear in the splenic vein that is to blame, and there is a risk that this can extend into the portal vein. It is for this reason that we prefer to expose the portal vein as the first step in the operation, so that any bleeding can be controlled under direct vision.
3. If you are uncertain about the security of stump closure, start the patient on octreotide, 100 micrograms three times a day by subcutaneous injection, and continue the drug for up to 7 days to decrease pancreatic exocrine secretion and reduce the occurrence of pancreatic fistula and other complications, although this practice is not supported by all studies.[5]

Aftercare

1 Leave the drain(s) for a minimum of 5 days, especially after splenectomy, then shorten them and remove them over a period of 2–3 days.

2 If preoperative pancreatic function was normal, a 50–60% distal resection will seldom precipitate serious endocrine or exocrine insufficiency. In a patient with prediabetes or a more extensive pancreatectomy, the blood glucose should be monitored particularly closely and insulin may be required. In any case, repeat exocrine and endocrine function tests before allowing a patient with chronic pancreatitis to return home.

Complications

1 Even with a drain there is a chance of haematoma in the splenic bed and a subsequent left subphrenic abscess. Suspect the diagnosis if the patient develops fever, leucocytosis and a pleural effusion at the left base. Ultrasound or CT scan confirms the diagnosis and allow percutaneous drainage of the collection.

2 A few patients develop a pancreatic fistula from the cut end of the pancreas, sometimes after percutaneous drainage of a collection. Provided that there is no ductal obstruction in the head of pancreas—and pancreatic ductal imaging with ERCP, MRCP or ductography, should have declared this issue—the fistula will close spontaneously and usually within a month of operation. The somatostatin analogue octreotide may possibly hasten the closure of the fistula. If the fistula persists, place a pancreatic stent endoscopically or institute nasopancreatic drainage to speed closure.

REFERENCES

1. Funk EM, Schlimok G, Ehret W et al 1997 The current status of vaccination and antibiotic prophylaxis in splenectomy. I: Adults. Chirurg 68:586–590
2. Benoist S, Dugue L, Sauvanet A et al 1999 Is there a role of preservation of the spleen in distal pancreatectomy? Journal of the American College of Surgeons 188:255–260
3. Warshaw AL, Rattner DW, Fernandez-del Castillo C et al 1998 Middle segment pancreatectomy: a novel technique for conserving pancreatic tissue. Archives of Surgery 133:327–331
4. Vezakis A, Davides D, Larvin M et al 1999 Laparoscopic surgery combined with preservation of the spleen for distal pancreatic tumors. Surgical Endoscopy 13:26–29
5. Stojadinovic A, Brooks A, Hoos A et al 2003 An evidence based approach to the surgical management of resectable pancreatic adenocarcinoma. Journal of the American College of Surgeons 196:954–964

PROXIMAL PANCREATECTOMY

Appraise

- Proximal pancreatectomy is undertaken for:
  i. Carcinoma of the head of pancreas.
  ii. Other less-aggressive tumours in this region, loosely called periampullary cancers and including distal cholangiocarcinoma, carcinoma of the ampulla, carcinoma of the duodenum and large neuroendocrine tumours of the pancreatic head.
  iii. Severe chronic pancreatitis preferentially involving the head of pancreas and sometimes complicated by bile duct stricture or pseudocyst.
- All these conditions can present with obstructive jaundice, and the investigation of jaundice has been described previously. Particularly for pancreatic cancer, attempt to assess resectability before operation, using ultrasound, CT scan and/or angiography to determine the size and extent of the tumour, the presence or absence of lymph node and liver metastases and the all-important relationship of the tumour to major vascular structures, notably the portal vein. Vascular imaging is also useful to show anomalies in arterial supply, notably the right hepatic or common hepatic artery arising from the superior mesenteric artery and running up behind the portal vein, which is present in about 25% of subjects.
- Ordinarily offer proximal pancreatectomy for resectable tumours of the pancreatic head, provided that on-table assessment (see below) confirms the absence of distal metastases. There is no absolute upper age limit, but pay particular consideration to patients over the age of 70–75 years because of the extent of the operation required. Palliative procedures for pancreatic cancer have already been described.
- Typically, neoplastic and inflammatory conditions of the pancreatic head present in very different ways. In pancreatic cancer there is a short history of progressive obstructive jaundice with minor or moderate pain, a discrete non-calcified mass on CT scan and an irregular stricture on cholangiography. In chronic pancreatitis there is a long history of abdominal pain associated with weight loss and alcoholism, the jaundice is less severe, remitting or absent, and imaging reveals calcification and/or pseudocyst and a smooth tapering stricture in the bile duct. However, the clinical features of the two conditions can overlap sufficiently to be indistinguishable. Resection is the best treatment in either case, and it obviates the need for biopsy.
- There is lively debate regarding the best operation for the various conditions described above, but controlled data are scarce. The extent of the operation can be considered under three headings:
  i. *The extent of pancreatic resection*. For cancer most surgeons perform hemipancreatectomy rather than total pancreatectomy, but for chronic pancreatitis tailor the resection to the distribution of the disease. This question is considered further under 'Total pancreatectomy'.
  ii. *The extent of gastroduodenal resection*. The occasional benign tumour of the ampulla and small localized ampullary carcinomas in elderly patients may be suitable for a *transduodenal ampullectomy*, in which the ampulla is circumcised and the terminal portions of bile duct and pancreatic duct are resutured to the duodenal mucosa. The operation of *duodenum-preserving resection*[1] of the head of pancreas has recently been advocated for chronic pancreatitis. The central portion of the head of pancreas is removed, leaving a rim within the duodenal loop, and a Roux loop of jejunum is brought up for anastomosis to the pancreatic duct on either side and sometimes also to the bile duct, if this is strictured or has been entered. With these exceptions, which will not be discussed further because of their limited application,

resection of the pancreatic head involves excision of the duodenal loop and terminal bile duct. This *pancreatoduodenectomy* may be accomplished by conventional or conservative techniques, as described below.

iii. *The extent of resection of other organs*. The gallbladder is frequently removed in the hope of improving the radical cure of cancer by dividing the bile duct at a higher level. Some surgeons advocate resection of the portal vein en bloc for locally invasive tumour, with end-to-end venous reconstruction. Others are prepared to resect and reconstruct the superior mesenteric artery or even the coeliac axis, while others will carry out a radical lymphadenectomy, removing most of the para-aortic nodes. With the exception of cholecystectomy, all these procedures increase the length of the operation and the risk of complications and death. We are not convinced that these disadvantages are outweighed by improved chances of cure.

- The *conventional* type of pancreatoduodenectomy (Fig. 21.12), described in 1935 by the New York surgeon Allen O. Whipple (1881–1963), includes a distal hemigastrectomy for the following reasons:
  i. It removes lymph nodes along the greater and lesser curves of the stomach, yet these nodes are very seldom involved until the tumour has widely disseminated.
  ii. Antrectomy reduces the risk of erosive gastritis and postoperative bleeding, yet retention of the pylorus will prevent alkaline reflux and modern acid-reducing drugs give added protection.

  Whipple's operation is indicated for carcinoma of the upper portion of the pancreatic head or neck and for chronic pancreatitis complicated by duodenal ulcer disease or duodenal stenosis.

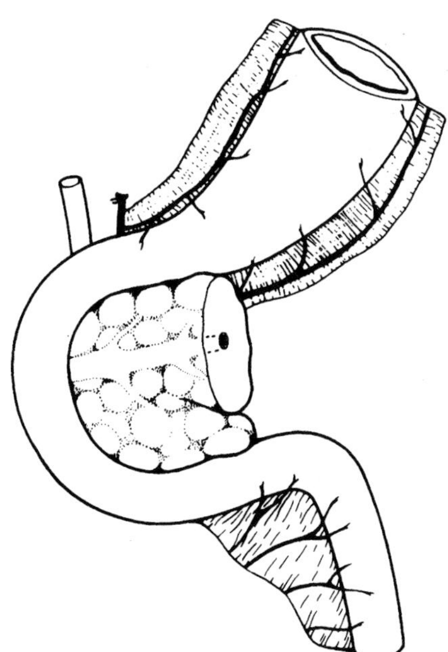

Fig. 21.12 Conventional pancreatoduodenectomy (Whipple's operation). The resection specimen is shown and includes the distal half of the stomach, the duodenal loop and duodenojejunal flexure, the terminal bile duct and the head and uncinate process of the pancreas.

- The *conservative type* of pancreatoduodenectomy retains the entire stomach and duodenal cap and is termed pylorus-preserving proximal pancreatoduodenectomy (PPPP). It has the theoretical advantage of allowing better postoperative nutrition and weight gain and the duodenal anastomosis is easier to construct, but delayed gastric emptying is sometimes a problem in the early postoperative period, although the delay in return to normal diet would seem to be no different.[2] PPPP is indicated for most patients with chronic pancreatitis and periampullary cancer and for those with pancreatic cancer arising from the lower part of the head and uncinate process, providing similar local control and long-term survival.[3]
- As mentioned earlier, many types of pancreatic operation have been carried out laparoscopically and pancreatoduodenectomy is no exception.[4] Considerable concern still exists about the oncological soundness of laparoscopic surgery, and clearly this technique currently has limited application only to benign disease in a few specialist centres. As for all types of laparoscopic pancreatic surgery, the advantage over the open procedure is yet to be established.

Prepare

1. Pancreatoduodenectomy is a major undertaking. Detailed pancreatic imaging should be accompanied by thorough assessment of the patient's general health. Ensure that at least 4 units of cross-matched blood are available. Cover the procedure with broad-spectrum antibiotics.
2. The perioperative precautions to be taken in deeply jaundiced patients and the role of preliminary biliary decompression have been discussed earlier.
3. On-table pancreatography may be needed in patients with chronic pancreatitis although increase use of less-invasive imaging such as MRCP makes this less common.

Assess

As for all major pancreatic operations, the bilateral subcostal approach gives the best access, but a vertical midline or transverse incision can also be employed.

Access

1. In a case of suspected or proven *neoplasia*, start by making a detailed search for metastatic disease. Look and feel for hepatic metastases, peritoneal seedlings and lymph nodes. Pancreatic cancer spreads first to lymph nodes in the anterior and posterior duodenopancreatic grooves and along the hepatic artery, and then to nodes around the origin of the coeliac axis and superior mesenteric artery. Select one or more suitable metastases for biopsy to confirm the diagnosis. Nodes adjacent to the pancreas can be resected en bloc, but more distant disease means that resection should be abandoned except in highly selected patients, for example those with neuroendocrine cancer.

> **KEY POINTS Intraoperative staging of pancreatic cancer**
>
> - Undertake a thorough search for extrapancreatic tumour deposits before attempting resection, including the liver, all peritoneal surfaces, the coeliac nodes and the inferior surface of the transverse mesocolon near the ligament of Treitz.
> - Sample any suspicious deposits and subject them to frozen-section examination.

2 Ensure that the primary tumour can be mobilized. The usual problem is posterior fixity to the preaortic fascia, which is often heralded by back pain. If the tumour is irresectable by virtue of local invasion or distant metastasis, proceed to bypass surgery. Do not forget to obtain a positive tissue diagnosis before closing the abdomen.

3 In a favourable case, now proceed to establish whether the portal vein is free of the cancer. Preoperative vascular imaging should have indicated this point, but there is no substitute for a trial dissection to make sure. Enter the lesser sac by dividing the greater omentum outside the gastroepiploic arcade or elevate the omentum off the transverse colon in the avascular plane. Use the middle colic vein(s) to guide you to the superior mesenteric vein below the neck of pancreas. Carefully divide the peritoneum and fascia over the vein until the vessel wall is clearly exposed, then use gentle blunt dissection to develop the tunnel upwards behind the neck of pancreas.

4 If the tumour lies close by, or obstructive pancreatitis hampers this dissection, it may be safer to expose the portal vein above the neck of pancreas before proceeding from below. Divide the peritoneum overlying the free edge of the lesser omentum, securing the superficial blood vessels. Identify and expose the common bile duct, encircle it with a right-angled forceps and pass a soft tube around the duct as a sling. Dissect out the gastroduodenal artery, which arises almost invariably from the apex of a right-angled bend (or 'genu') of the main hepatic artery. Sling these vessels also. Now, pulling gently on the slings, separate the structures and dissect deeply between them to expose the front of the portal vein. The gastroduodenal artery can be ligated and divided at this point to provide better exposure to the portal vein.

5 Gently establish the tunnel between the neck of pancreas in front and the portal vein behind, using your two index fingers passed one from above and one from below (Fig. 21.13). As long as you stay directly in front of the vein you will not encounter any pancreatic venous branches. If there is clear-cut invasion of the portal vein, abandon the resection and proceed to a bypass. If not, proceed to pancreatoduodenectomy (see 'Action' below).

6 In a case of *chronic pancreatitis* carry out a general laparotomy; in particular examine the liver (and consider biopsy), gallbladder, bile duct, spleen, stomach and duodenum. Peptic ulcer, cirrhosis, gallstones and splenomegaly can all be associated with pancreatitis. Mobilize and examine the pancreas from head to tail. Some form of operative pancreatography may be needed, depending upon the presence or absence of pseudocyst or a palpable pancreatic duct and the quality of the preoperative imaging. It is almost always possible to resect the head of pancreas in chronic pancreatitis, even if a small portion of tissue has to be left to protect the great veins, so a trial dissection as such is unnecessary. It is often easier to create the tunnel from above and divide the neck of the pancreas onto a right-angled clamp passing inferiorly, without first dissecting from below. The inferior tunnel is often impossible to create safely from below.

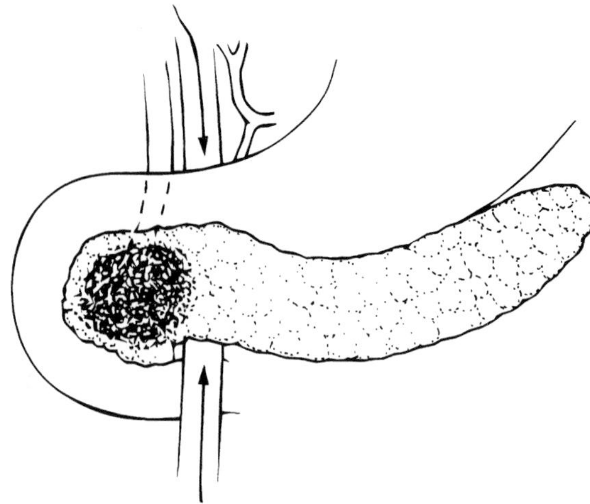

Fig. 21.13 Trial dissection to establish the resectability of a carcinoma of the head of pancreas. One finger is passed along the portal vein from above and another finger along the superior mesenteric vein from below to establish a safe plane behind the neck of pancreas.

7 Sometimes there is a mass in the head of pancreas, but it is impossible to be certain whether it is inflammatory or neoplastic. Remember that induration of the body of pancreas could represent either ductal obstruction by tumour or primary chronic pancreatitis. Resection is the best treatment in either case, so do not waste time with a biopsy. If you have the necessary expertise, proceed to pancreatoduodenectomy. If not, carry out a cholecystojejunostomy in the presence of jaundice and then refer the patient elsewhere.

8 Make a choice between conservative or conventional pancreatoduodenectomy. For myself, the standard procedure is now PPPP, and we perform distal gastrectomy only if there is concomitant duodenal disease, if the cancer lies close to the pylorus or if the pancreatitis is so severe that the duodenum cannot easily be separated. There are several different techniques for reconstruction after pancreatoduodenectomy, but our standard procedure will be described.

Action

Conservative pancreatoduodenectomy

1 Once the trial dissection has been completed, you are well under way. In chronic pancreatitis, however, it may require a long and rather hazardous dissection to clear the portal vein. Attempt this procedure only if you have had adequate experience. If you have not already done so, dissect out the structures

in the free edge of the lesser omentum. Doubly ligate the gastroduodenal artery, with two ligatures on the proximal side, making sure that you have identified and preserved the main hepatic artery.

2 Begin to separate the first part of the duodenum from the underlying pancreas, securing the numerous vessels that run between the two. Keep close to the duodenal wall, proceeding either towards or away from the pylorus as you prefer. Ligate and divide the right gastroepiploic artery and vein close to their origin on the pancreas. Aim to mobilize the pylorus and the proximal 6 cm or so of duodenum. Apply a light crushing clamp to the duodenum at least 5 cm beyond the pylorus and cut the bowel flush with the clamp, using a non-crushing clamp temporarily to occlude the pylorus. Now suck out the stomach, cover the duodenal stump with a swab wrung out in antiseptic solution and held in place with Babcock's forceps and displace the stomach to the left side of the abdomen. Frozen-section examination of the duodenal resection margin may be necessary and can be carried out at this time. Quickly oversew the distal duodenum so you can remove the crushing clamp.

3 You have now exposed the pancreatic neck and can divide it under direct vision. Complete the mobilization of its upper and lower borders. Insert and tie four stay sutures of 2/0 silk, one on each side of the proposed line of transection (Fig. 21.14). Place a Kocher's director in front of the portal vein and divide the pancreatic neck on to the director. Apply a soft intestinal clamp to the pancreas on one side or the other if there is marked bleeding from the gland. Using diathermy and sutures if necessary, stop the bleeding from each cut surface. Identify the pancreatic duct, which will often be dilated. In a potential case of cancer take a generous biopsy from the transected neck of pancreas for frozen-section pathology.

4 Proceed to separate the head and uncinate process of the pancreas from the portal and superior mesenteric veins. Tease out, ligate and divide the pancreatic veins, usually one from the superior aspect of the gland and two or three lower down. These are fragile vessels and bleed profusely if damaged. Have fine sutures available such as 4/0 silk or 5/0 polypropylene (Prolene) to close any holes in the portal vein. Throughout this dissection use your left hand to grasp, steady and retract the head of pancreas. Compress the portal vein using your left hand to control venous bleeding that may occur. This is why it is so important to Kocherize the duodenum prior to creating the portal vein 'tunnel'.

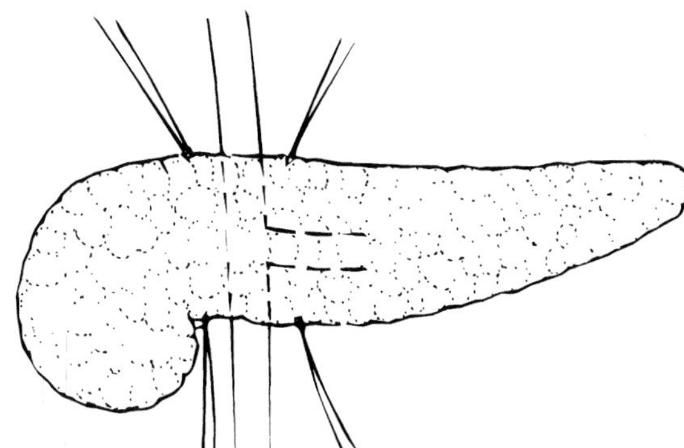

Fig. 21.14 Preparing to transect the neck of pancreas. Stay sutures are placed on the upper and lower borders of the pancreas on either side of the proposed line of transection.

5 Mobilize the bile duct prior to dividing it either low down in chronic pancreatitis or generally at a higher level in carcinoma of the pancreas; in this case perform cholecystectomy. Apply a small vascular clamp or bulldog clip to the bile duct and cut across the duct below this point, taking a culture swab of bile. If a stent is in situ it will have to be removed at this point and can also be sent off for microbiological examination. Frozen-section of the bile duct can be arranged at this point if required.

6 Now free the pancreas from its attachment to the preaortic fascia, ligating and dividing the connective tissue in leashes just beyond the gland. During this manoeuvre control the specimen with your left hand as before, taking care not to injure the superior mesenteric artery, which can be pulled underneath the vein by traction on the specimen. One (or more) leash of tissue will contain the inferior pancreaticoduodenal branch(es) of the artery.

KEY POINT Mobilization of the pancreatic head

- During division of the deep attachments of the pancreatic head, it is helpful if the operator's left hand is placed behind the head of pancreas and duodenum in order to elevate the specimen out of the wound, thereby facilitating the dissection and maintaining vascular control in case of venous bleeding. During this procedure care must be taken not to damage the superior mesenteric artery, which can easily be rotated from its normal position and pulled into the field of dissection.

7 Mobilize the ligament of Treitz below the transverse mesocolon, Gently draw the upper jejunum through the congenital retrocolic 'defect' and into the supracolic compartment. Complete the mobilization of the uncinate process. Ligate and divide the mesentery to the duodenojejunal flexure. Complete the resection by dividing the upper jejunum and its mesentery at a convenient point. The end of the jejunal loop is then brought into the supracolic compartment through a window created in the transverse mesocolon, although the congenital retrocolic defect can be used. If the transverse colon mesentery is short you may need to bring the jejunal loop antecolically.

8 You must now embark on the reconstruction, joining the pancreatic neck, bile duct and duodenal stump to the upper jejunum in that order (Fig. 21.15a). First, elevate the body of pancreas posteriorly for about 4 cm, carefully dividing one or two tributaries of the splenic vein. This manoeuvre allows you to create an invaginating anastomosis.

9 *Pancreatic anastomosis.* The technique varies according to the disease process and the calibre of the pancreatic duct. We grade the difficulty of this anastomosis into three groups and deal with each in a slightly different way. In a patient with cancer

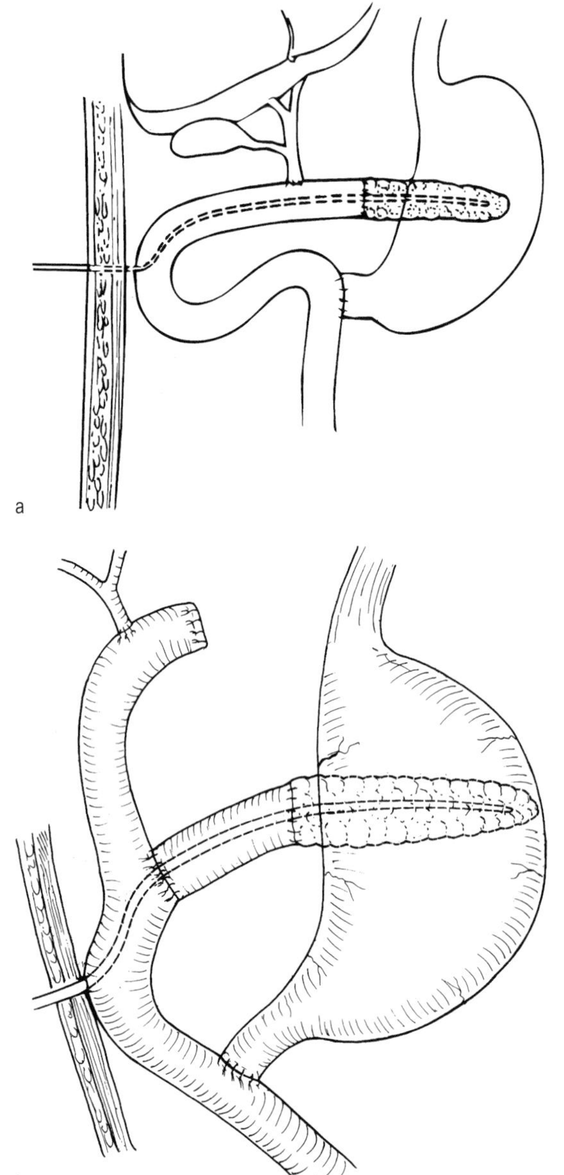

Fig. 21.15 Reconstruction following pylorus-preserving pancreatoduodenectomy (PPPP): (a) the pancreatic anastomosis is protected by a fine-bore tube brought to the exterior and sutured into the duct; (b) if the pancreas is soft and its duct is tiny, it may be safer to perform the pancreaticojejunostomy using a separate Roux loop.

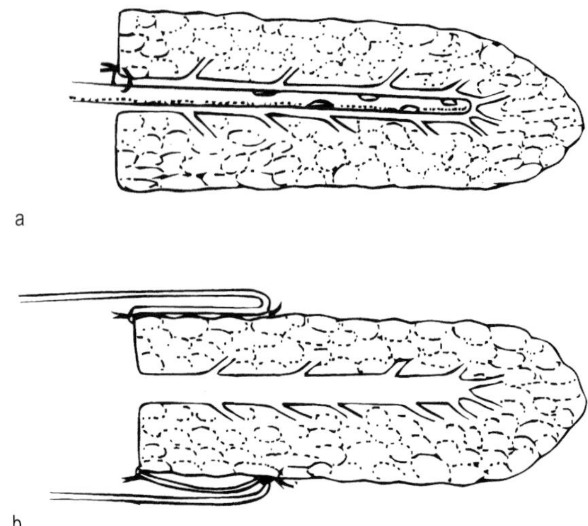

Fig. 21.16 Pancreaticojejunostomy following resection of the pancreatic head: (a) insertion of a transanastomotic stent; (b) two-layer invaginating anastomosis.

(soft gland) and a small pancreatic duct, we use a transanastomotic stent and a separate Roux loop to reduce the risk of leakage of activated pancreatic juice from the anastomosis (Fig. 21.15b). Check that a 4F or 6F infant-feeding tube will pass well down the pancreatic duct (Fig. 21.16a). Now introduce the tube, first into the abdomen through a stab incision below the right-hand end of the main wound and then into the upper jejunum through a tiny incision about 30 cm distal to the cut end of bowel; use a long pair of forceps thrust down the bowel to grasp the tube and draw it out. Insert the tube right down the pancreatic duct and suture it firmly in place with two 3/0 polyglactin 910 sutures that pick up the ductal mucosa. Alternatively, the tube can be secured by transfixing it with a double-ended suture, then passing each needle through the duct and out through the anterior surface of the gland; tie the suture over a small 'buttress' of muscle taken from the abdominal wall. In a patient with cancer and a degree of obstructive pancreatopathy, where both the duct is somewhat enlarged and the gland firmer than normal, a separate Roux loop is unnecessary and a transanastomotic stent usually suffices because many of the sutures can incorporate the duct and hold it open. In chronic pancreatitis the fibrotic nature of the gland along with the ductal dilatation and the low enzymatic content of the pancreatic juice make serious leakage unlikely, so in this case the anastomosis can be accomplished without the need for a stent. With or without a stent, use interrupted 3/0 silk sutures to create a two-layer invaginating end-to-end pancreaticojejunostomy (Fig. 21.16b). Starting posteriorly with the inner layer, place a row of interrupted stitches between the pancreas—parenchyma above and below, duct centrally—and the full thickness of the jejunum. Take generous bites of pancreas to avoid the sutures cutting out. Now tie this row of sutures and complete an anterior row. Starting posteriorly, place a second row of interrupted sutures circumferentially between the outer aspects of the pancreas and jejunum at least 1 cm from the cut edge. When this outer layer of stitches is tied it will draw the jejunum over the pancreas like a sheath. Alternative anastomoses are end-to-side pancreaticojejunostomy (see Fig. 21.17) and end-to-side pancreaticogastrostomy, in which the pancreatic stump is joined to the back of the stomach[5] (Fig. 21.18).

10 *Biliary anastomosis*. Carry out an end-to-side choledochojejunostomy with one layer of interrupted 3/0 polyglactin 910 sutures. Insert stay sutures in the bile duct, remove the clamp, suck out the bile and secure any bleeding vessels. Now place the posterior row of sutures, tie them and complete the anastomosis anteriorly. In most patients with cancer the anastomosis is easy because the duct is dilated, but in chronic pancreatitis the

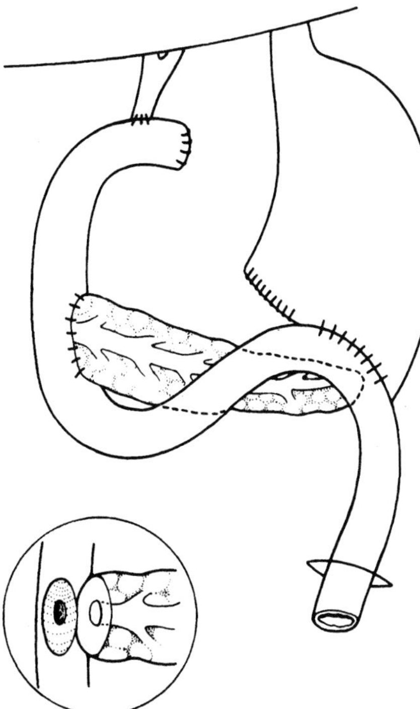

Fig. 21.17 Reconstruction after conventional pancreatoduodenectomy with an end-to-side pancreaticojejunostomy. To create the pancreatic anastomosis (inset), the pancreatic duct is sutured directly to the jejunal mucosa; the anastomosis can be splinted by a fine polythene tube.

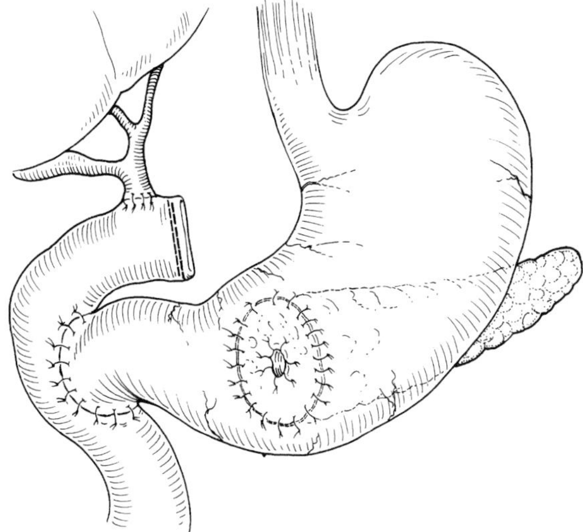

Fig. 21.18 Reconstruction following pylorus-preserving proximal pancreatoduodenectomy (PPPP). Pancreaticogastrostomy has been described as a safe alternative.

wall may be thick and the lumen narrow; consider using a fine-bore T-tube inserted through a stab incision in the duct with the lower limb of the 'T' placed across the anastomosis. Bring the long limb of the tube out through a stab incision in the abdominal wall. Another option is to pass a stent as per the pancreatic anastomosis, bringing it our through the same enterotomy. If a pancreatic stent has been used, suture the jejunum to the abdominal wall at the exit point well below the biliary anastomosis.

11 *Duodenal anastomosis*. Check the viability of the duodenal stump and be prepared to sacrifice the terminal 1–2 cm. Try to preserve a minimum of 2–3 cm of healthy bowel between pylorus and anastomosis. Now carry out a two-layer end-to-side duodenojejunostomy, using polyglactin 910 sutures. The duodenal anastomosis should be 25–30 cm distal to the biliary anastomosis.

Conventional pancreatoduodenectomy

1 The only difference from PPPP is that the distal 30–50% of stomach is resected, together with the pylorus and entire duodenum.

? DIFFICULTY 21.2

1. Pancreatoduodenectomy is generally easier in cancer than it is in chronic pancreatitis, when severe inflammatory adherence can make for a particularly difficult dissection. Be prepared to leave a small amount of inflamed pancreatic tissue to protect the portal and superior mesenteric veins if necessary.
2. If bleeding occurs from the portal vein, do not panic. Control the bleeding with packs, then try to identify the source and suture it. It is seldom necessary (or easy) to clamp the main portal vein above and below the source of haemorrhage.
3. If, after dividing the neck of pancreas and mobilizing the head, you find invasion of the superior mesenteric vein in the region of the uncinate process, it is occasionally appropriate to resect a short segment of vein en bloc and restore continuity by end-to-end anastomosis. More often it will become apparent that the origin of the superior mesenteric artery is also encased and that the resection is therefore palliative. Mark the residual tumour with metal clips and consider postoperative radiotherapy.
4. If the pathologist reports that there is carcinoma at the transection line in the pancreas, proceed to total pancreatectomy (see below).
5. *The pancreas is soft and the sutures keep cutting out.* Take deeper bites with mattress sutures. Stent the anastomosis and invaginate the bowel thoroughly. If all else fails, perform total pancreatectomy.
6. *There is a low entry to the cystic duct.* Either remove the gallbladder or divide the septum between cystic duct and common hepatic duct to create a common biliary channel for anastomosis.
7. *After PPPP the duodenal stump looks blue.* Resect back towards the pylorus until bleeding is encountered from the end. If the duodenum is clearly non-viable, convert to conventional (Whipple) resection.

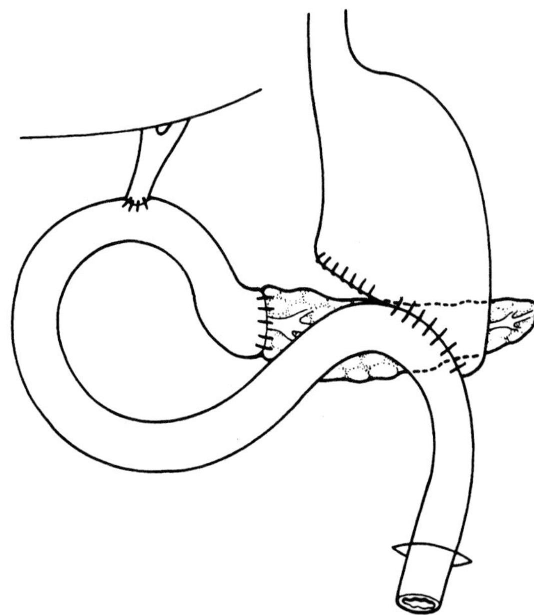

Fig. 21.19 Reconstruction after conventional pancreatoduodenectomy with an end-to-end pancreaticojejunostomy.

2 After freeing the portal vein, divide the greater and lesser omentum along the antrum (see Ch. 13). Cut across the stomach between clamps or TA90 staple lines. Now displace the gastric stump to the left to expose the neck of pancreas, and proceed as before.

3 At the end of the operation carry out gastrojejunostomy rather than duodenojejunostomy, as described for Polya gastrectomy in Chapter 13. Use a two-layer anastomosis to create a generous stoma (Fig. 21.19).

Closure

1 Check carefully for haemostasis and consider washing out the upper abdomen. Place two soft tube drains to the region of the pancreatic anastomosis.

2 Consider the need for a feeding jejunostomy, particularly in elderly patients or those with a low preoperative serum albumin level. We use a 14F latex T-tube placed in the infracolic jejunum and then sutured to the abdominal wall.

3 Close the abdominal wall in layers, taking particular care to achieve a sound closure in a jaundiced patient, in whom impaired healing can be anticipated.

Aftercare

1 Watch the patient closely for the first 48 hours after this major procedure. Check the postoperative haemoglobin levels and correct any anaemia promptly. Monitor the serum amylase level also, together with urea and electrolytes.

2 Keep a close eye on the drain output. Brownish fluid may indicate a developing pancreatic fistula (see below) and a high amylase level in the effluent will confirm this fact.

3 Pancreatic stents should drain a variable quantity of clear juice but if they slip out into the jejunum the fluid becomes bile-stained. Consider performing an X-ray down the tube after 5–7 days. Thereafter it may well be possible to clamp the tube before removing it at 10–12 days.

4 Some surgeons give octreotide routinely for 5–7 days postoperatively (200 micrograms t.d.s. subcutaneously, or by intravenous infusion) starting immediately before operation. Others reserve the drug for 'high-risk anastomoses', that is those with a soft pancreas and a tiny duct, which are especially prone to leak.

Complications

1 The most serious complication is leakage from the pancreatic anastomosis, which can result in sepsis and serious haemorrhage. The fistula usually declares itself about 5 days postoperatively. If the output is low and the patient's general condition is satisfactory, it is reasonable to consider conservative treatment with antibiotics, octreotide and parenteral nutrition. In the presence of bleeding or sepsis the patient should have a CT scan. If a collection is present it should be drained percutaneously. If bleeding has occurred an arterial reconstruction should be done from the CT and if possible transcatheter embolization performed. If this fails then perform laparotomy. If anastomotic dehiscence is confirmed, the safest measure is to remove the remaining pancreas and to under-run the bleeding vessel. The commonest vessel is the gastroduodenal artery stump which lies adjacent to the pancreatic anastomosis.

2 The other anastomoses may also leak, causing biliary or duodenal fistulas, but the consequences are seldom as serious unless internal sepsis leads to secondary breakdown of the pancreaticojejunostomy. Thus conservative measures may suffice to allow spontaneous closure.

3 Reactive haemorrhage, chest infection and wound infection are possible complications of any upper abdominal procedure of this extent.

4 Approximately 10% of patients develop delayed gastric emptying after PPPP and require continued nasogastric intubation. Institute parenteral nutrition and give prokinetic drugs such as metoclopramide, domperidone, cisapride and erythromycin. A feeding jejunostomy is particularly helpful in this situation. Carry out a barium study to see if any contrast leaves the stomach and rule out a mechanical obstruction. Gastric tone will eventually recover.

REFERENCES

1. Beger HG, Schlosser W, Siech M et al 1999 The surgical management of chronic pancreatitis: duodenum-preserving pancreatectomy. Advances in Surgery 32:87–104
2. Halloran CM, Ghaneh P, Bosonet L et al 2002 Complications of pancreatic cancer resection. Digestive Surgery 19:138–146
3. Yamaguchi K, Kishinnaka M, Nagai E et al 2001 Pancreatoduodenectomy for pancreatic head carcinoma without pylorus preservation. Hepatogastroenterology 48:1479–1485
4. Masson B, Sa-Cunha A, Laurent C et al 2003 Laparoscopic pancreatectomy: report of 22 cases. Annales de Chirugie 128:452–456
5. Aranha GV 1998 A technique for pancreaticogastrostomy. American Journal of Surgery 175:328–329

TOTAL PANCREATECTOMY

Appraise

- Total pancreatectomy has sometimes been recommended for the routine management of resectable cancers on the grounds that it avoids the problems of multifocal origin of ductal carcinoma and potential leakage from the pancreaticojejunostomy. The counter-arguments are that it increases the risks of the procedure, conveys no actual survival advantage and renders the patient an obligate diabetic. Reserve the procedure for bulky tumours encroaching on the neck, for cancer in diabetics and for the occasional patient in whom frozen-section examination is positive during partial pancreatectomy. There is no evidence to suggest that total pancreatectomy for cancer provides any survival advantage, and in fact it may be associated with a worse outcome.[1]
- Total pancreatectomy is occasionally indicated in patients with end-stage chronic pancreatitis and may be combined with pancreatic transplantation, especially if lesser procedures have failed or there is generalized disease with pre-existing endocrine and exocrine failure.[2,3]
- Completion pancreatectomy may be the wisest move if a fistula develops from a leaking pancreaticojejunostomy anastomosis in a patient requiring re-laparotomy (see previous section).
- Duodenal resection is virtually always a part of total pancreatectomy. In our experience[3] most of these procedures have been carried out for chronic pancreatitis, and here it is usually possible to preserve the pylorus and sometimes possible to preserve the spleen.

Assess

1 Patients who are candidates for total pancreatectomy should have thorough preoperative investigation to determine the structure and residual function of the gland.

2 At laparotomy the surgeon should assess whether the appearances of the pancreas are consistent with the previous imaging, whether any lesser procedure than total pancreatectomy might be appropriate and whether the stomach or spleen can be retained.

Action

1 The operation is essentially an amalgam of proximal and distal pancreatectomy, as described above. It is generally best to start by freeing the pancreatic neck from the subjacent portal vein, then to proceed with mobilization of the head and conclude by resecting the body and tail. Sometimes you may embark on an extended distal resection but later appreciate that the head of pancreas is so diseased that it should also be removed.

2 Following pylorus-preserving total pancreatectomy, the neatest reconstruction is an end-to-end duodenojejunostomy followed by biliary anastomosis a few centimetres downstream (Fig. 21.20).

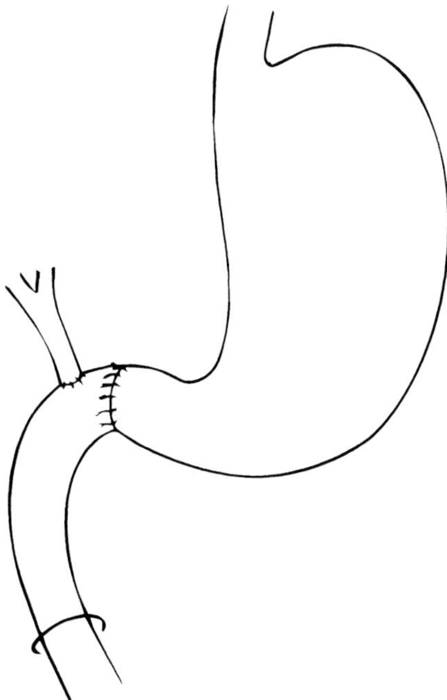

Fig. 21.20 Reconstruction following pylorus-preserving total pancreatectomy. The gallbladder has been included in the resection specimen.

Aftercare and complications

1 There is no pancreatic anastomosis to leak, but biliary and intestinal fistulas can arise from the other two anastomoses and there is clearly some risk of reactive haemorrhage and subphrenic abscess.

2 The early management of diabetes is not usually difficult provided that glucose and insulin therapy are modulated to avoid the chance of hypoglycaemia. Aim to keep the blood sugar on the high side of normal and do not worry about precise control until the patient is eating normally. Involve a diabetologist in the subsequent management and do not allow the patient home until he has been taught how to measure blood and urine sugar levels and how to self-administer insulin.

3 Exocrine pancreatic supplements will also be required for the rest of the patient's life, the exact dose varying widely from one individual to another. In addition, a low-fat diet and acid-reducing drugs will often be needed to control steatorrhoea and allow proper weight gain.

REFERENCES

1. Ihse I, Anderson H, Andren-Sandberg 1996 Total pancreatectomy for cancer of the pancreas: is it appropriate? World Journal of Surgery 20:288–293
2. Clayton HA, Davies JE, Pollard CA et al 2003 Pancreatectomy with islet autotransplantation for the treatment of severe chronic pancreatitis: the first 40 patients at the Leicester general hospital. Transplantation 76:92–98
3. Fleming WR, Williamson RCN 1995 Role of total pancreatectomy in the treatment of patients with end stage chronic pancreatitis. British Journal of Surgery 82:1409–1412

LAPAROTOMY FOR ISLET CELL TUMOUR

Appraise

- *Insulinoma* is the commonest islet cell tumour. It is usually solitary and benign. It presents with episodic hypoglycaemia and the diagnosis is confirmed by finding a low blood sugar and an inappropriately high serum insulin either spontaneously or after provocation by fasting. Most insulinomas are sufficiently vascular to be localized as a 'blush' on selective pancreatic arteriography.[1] Local excision is sufficient.
- *Gastrinoma* can arise in the pancreas, the duodenal wall or sometimes further afield. It presents with theZollinger–Ellison syndrome of intractable peptic ulceration and diarrhoea. The diagnosis is confirmed by finding high basal gastric acid with hypergastrinaemia on radioimmunoassay. The ulcer diathesis should be controlled preoperatively by ranitidine or omeprazole while an attempt is made to localize the tumour by arteriography, endoscopic ultrasonography andcontrast-enhanced CT scan. Many gastrinomas are malignant, with lymph node or even liver metastases.[2] The best surgical treatment is to identify and resect all tumour tissue, but subtotal or even total gastrectomy is sometimes required.
- Glucagonoma, somatostatinoma and other hormone-secreting tumours are rare entities, but a more common condition is the *non-functioning neuroendocrine tumour* of the pancreas. This presents as a relatively slow-growing mass with pain or jaundice or bleeding, and imaging usually shows a sizeable tumour, which is hypervascular and may be calcified or partly cystic. It is often worth resecting these tumours even in the presence of metastases[3] as sometimes residual disease will respond to chemotherapy.
- Some patients with islet cell tumour, especially gastrinoma, have coincident tumours of the parathyroid or pituitary gland as a part of *multiple endocrine neoplasia* (MEN I—multiple endocrine neoplasia type I). There is usually a positive family history, and the pancreatic tumours are often multiple.[4]

Assess

1. To find a small islet cell tumour, you must be prepared to mobilize and examine the entire pancreas. Inspect and palpate the anterior and posterior surfaces from head to tail. Even if one tumour has been identified preoperatively and you find it quickly, remember that these lesions can be multiple (especially in MEN I) and continue to examine the rest of the gland. Preoperatively all attempts should be made at localization employing, CT, MRI, endoscopic ultrasound, isotope scans and provocative arteriography. This latter technique involves injecting calcium into the pancreatic feeding vessels whilst measuring the plasma hormone levels, to determine the part of the pancreas in which the tumour is located.
2. Intraoperative ultrasound scanning can be extremely useful, allowing identification of previously unseen lesions, exclusion of multifocal disease and relationship of tumours to the pancreatic duct, which is important when deciding between resection and enucleation.
3. If you do not find the tumour, repeat the digital examination and the ultrasonography if you have it available. If you are searching for a gastrinoma remember that there may be a tiny tumour in the duodenal wall; mobilize and examine the duodenum thoroughly. There is little role for 'blind' pancreatic resection in the management of insulinoma, unless there has been confident preoperative localization but you are unable to feel the tumour. It may be better to close the abdomen and

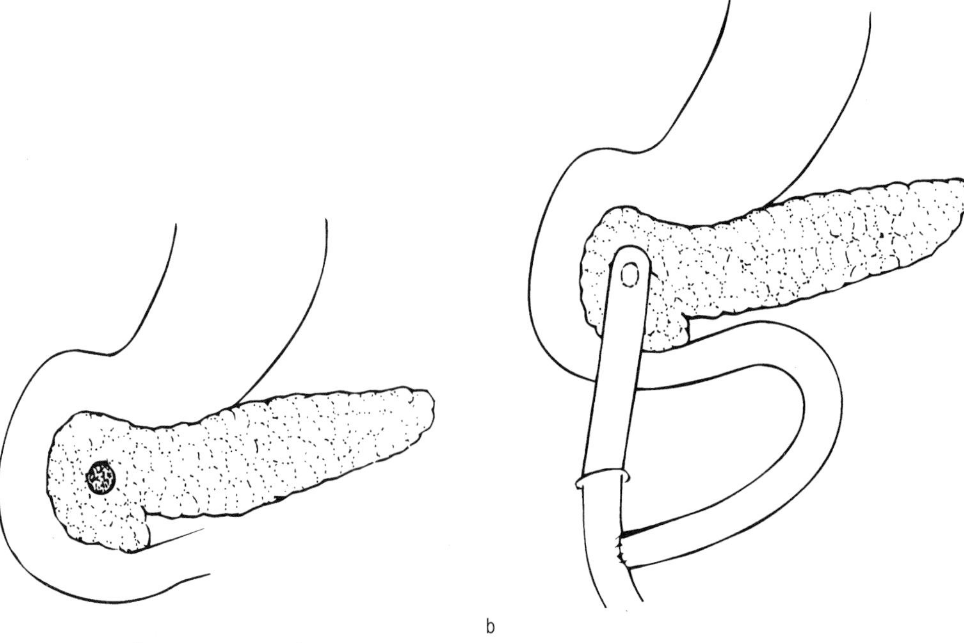

Fig. 21.21 Surgical management of an insulinoma in the pancreatic head: (a) enucleation of the adenoma; (b) a retrocolic Roux loop is brought up and sewn to the margins of the defect.

reinvestigate the patient, including transhepatic portal venous sampling.

4 For large non-functioning tumours, assess the patient at operation as you would for ordinary pancreatic cancer except that the presence of distant metastases should not necessarily preclude resection. You may enucleate liver secondaries or even carry out partial hepatectomy in suitable cases.

Action

1 For insulinoma or gastrinoma in the head or neck of pancreas, *enucleation* is the best option. Incise the pancreas over the tumour and shell the lesion out with a small cuff of normal tissue. Send the lesion for immediate frozen-section pathological examination. Secure haemostasis. If removal of the tumour has left quite a cavity within the gland and, in any case, if you open the pancreatic duct, it is safer to create a Roux loop of jejunum and suture it to the margins of the defect (Fig. 21.21); otherwise a pancreatic fistula may result. Successful removal of an insulinoma may be followed by rebound hyperglycaemia within 30–45 minutes. A small gastrinoma in the duodenal wall is also suitable for local excision unless metastases limited to pancreaticoduodenal lymph nodes make pancreatoduodenectomy advisable.

2 For an islet cell tumour in the distal body or tail of pancreas, conservative distal pancreatectomy is often the best option.

3 For non-functioning tumours some form of major pancreatic resection is usually indicated.

4 A laparoscopic approach for resection of islet cell tumours has been used and both enucleation and partial resection have been reported.[5] With the addition of laparoscopic ultrasound it may be possible to find moderate-sized tumour but there is no substitute for palpation during open exploration.

REFERENCES

1. Geoghegan JG, Jackson JE, Lewis MP et al 1994 Localization and surgical management of insulinoma. British Journal of Surgery 81:1025–1028
2. Kisker O, Bastian D, Bartsch D et al 1998 Localization, malignant potential, and surgical management of gastrinomas. World Journal of Surgery 22:651–658
3. Cheslyn-Curtis S, Sitaram V, Williamson RCN 1993 Management of non-functioning neuroendocrine tumours of the pancreas. British Journal of Surgery 80:625–627
4. Mignon M, Ruszniewski P, Podevin P et al 1993 Current approach to the management of gastrinoma and insulinoma in adults with multiple endocrine neoplasia type I. World Journal of Surgery 17:489–497
5. Jaroszewski DE, Schlinkert RT, Thompson GB et al DK 2004 Laparoscopic localisation and resection of insulinomas. Archives of Surgery 139:270–274

FURTHER READING

Aldridge MC, Williamson RCN 1991 Distal pancreatectomy with and without splenectomy. British Journal of Surgery 78:976–979

Beger HG, Buchler M, Bittner R et al 1998 Necrosectomy and post operative lavage in necrotising pancreatitis. British Journal of Surgery 75:207–212

Boyle TJ, Williamson RCN 1994 Bypass procedures. Current Practice in Surgery 6:154–160

Bradley EL III 1987 Long-term results of pancreaticojejunostomy in patients with chronic pancreatitis. American Journal of Surgery 153:207–213

British Society of Gastroenterology 1998 United Kingdom guidelines for the management of acute pancreatitis. United Kingdom guidelines for the management of acute pancreatitis. Gut 42 (Suppl 2):S1–S13

Buchler MW, Friess H, Müller MW et al 1995 Randomized trial of duodenum-preserving pancreatic head resection versus pylorus-preserving Whipple in chronic pancreatitis. American Journal of Surgery 169:65–69

Buchler MW, Gloor B, Muller CA et al 2000 Acute necrotising pancreatitis: treatment strategy according to status of infection. Annals of Surgery 232:619–626

Buter A, Imrie CW, Carter CR et al 2002 Dynamic nature of early organ dysfunction determines the outcome in acute pancreatitis. British Journal of Surgery 89:298–302

Cooper MJ, Williamson RCN, Benjamin IS et al 1987 Total pancreatectomy for chronic pancreatitis. British Journal of Surgery 74:912–915

Cuschieri A, Jakimowicz JJ, van Spreeuwel J 1996 Laparoscopic distal 70% pancreatectomy and splenectomy for chronic pancreatitis. Annals of Surgery 223:280–285

Dimagno EP 1998 A perspective on the use of tubeless pancreatic function tests in diagnosis. Gut 43:2–3

Fernandez-del Castillo C, Warshaw AL 1995 Cystic tumours of the pancreas. Surgical Clinics of North America 75:1001–1016

Frey CF, Mayer KL 2003 Comparison of local resection of the head of the pancreas combined with longitudinal pancreaticojejunostomy (Frey procedure) and duodenum preserving resection of the pancreatic head (Beger procedure). World Journal of Surgery 27:1217–1230

Grace PA, Williamson RCN 1993 Modern management of pancreatic pseudocysts. British Journal of Surgery 80:573–581

Grant CS 1998 Insulinoma. Surgical Clinics of North America 7:819–844

Huang JJ, Yeo CJ, Sohnn T et al 2000 Quality of life and outcomes after pancreaticoduodenectomy. Annals of Surgery 6:890–898

Isenman R, Rau B, Beger HG 1999 Bacterial infection and extent of necrosis are determinants of organ failure in patients with acute necrotising pancreatitis. British Journal of Surgery 86:1020–1024

Kaplan EL, Horvath K, Undekwu A et al 1990 Gastrinomas: a 42-year experience. World Journal of Surgery 14:365–376

Keith RG 1995 Surgery for pancreas divisum. Gastrointestinal Endoscopy Clinics of North America 5:171–180

Kimura W, Inoue T, Futakawa N et al 1996 Spleen-preserving distal pancreatectomy with conservation of the splenic artery and vein. Surgery 120:885–890

Kozarek RA, Taverso LW 1996 Pancreatic fistulas: etiology, consequences and treatment. Gastroenterologist 4:238–244

Lillemoe KD, Barnes SA 1995 Surgical palliation of unresectable pancreatic carcinoma. Surgical Clinics of North America 75:953–968

Lillemoe KD, Pitt HA 1996 Palliation. Surgical and otherwise. Cancer 78 (3 Suppl):605–614

Mason GR 1999 Pancreaticogastrostomy as reconstruction for pancreatoduodenectomy: review. World Journal of Surgery 23:221–226

McCarthy MJ, Evans J, Sagar G et al 1998 Prediction of resectability of pancreatic malignancy by computed tomography. 85:320–325

Merchant NB, Conlon KC 1998 Laparoscopic evaluation in pancreatic cancer. Seminars in Surgical Oncology 15:155–165

Mertz HR, Sechopoulos P, Delbeke D et al 2000 EUS, PET, and CT scanning for evaluation of pancreatic adenocarcinoma. Gastrointestinal Endoscopy 52:367–371

Neoptolemos JP, Russell RC, Bramhall S et al 1997 Low mortality following resection for pancreatic and periampullary tumours in

1026 patients: UK survey of specialist pancreatic units. UK Pancreatic Cancer Group. British Journal of Surgery 84:1370–1376

Newell KA, Liu T, Aranha GV et al 1990 Are cystgastrostomy and cystjejunostomy equivalent operations for pancreatic pseudocysts? Surgery 108:635–640

Norton JA 1998 Gastrinoma: advances in localization and treatment. Surgical Clinics of North America 7:845–861

Park A, Schwartz R, Tandan V et al 1999 Laparoscopic pancreatic surgery. American Journal of Surgery 177:158–163

Park BJ, Alexander HR, Libutti SK et al 1998 Operative management of islet-cell tumours arising in the head of the pancreas. Surgery 124:1056–1061

Povoski SP, Karpeh MS, Conlon KC et al 1999 Preoperative biliary drainage: impact on intraoperative bile cultures and infectious morbidity and mortality after pancreaticoduodenectomy. Journal of Gastrointestinal Surgery 3:496–505

Smedby O, Riesenfeld V, Karlson B et al 1997 Magnetic resonance angiography in resectability assessment of suspected pancreatic tumours. European Radiology 7:649–653

Sohn TA, Yeo CJ, Cameron JL et al 2000 Resected adenocarcinoma of the pancreas in 616 patients: results outcomes and prognostic indicators. Journal of Gastrointestinal Surgery 4:567–616

Spivak H, Galloway JR, Amerson JR et al 1998 Management of pancreatic pseudocysts. Journal of the American College of Surgeons 186:507–511

Tagaya N, Kasama K, Suzuki N et al 2003 Laparoscopic resection of the pancreas and review of the literature. Surgical Endoscopy 17:201–206

Takada T, Yasuda H, Amano H et al 2004 A duodenum preserving and bile duct preserving total pancreatic head resection with associated pancreatic duct–duct anastomosis. Journal of Gastrointestinal Surgery 8:220–224

Tillou A, Schwartz MR, Jordan PH 1996 Percutaneous needle biopsy of the pancreas: when should it be performed? World Journal of Surgery 20:283–286

Trede M, Schwall G 1988 The complications of pancreatectomy. Annals of Surgery 207:39–47

Trede M, Saeger HD, Schwall G et al 1998 Resection of pancreatic cancer: surgical achievements. Langenbecks Archiv für Chirurgie 383:121–128

Usatoff V, Brancatisano R, Williamson RC 2000 Operative treatment of pseudocysts in patients with chronic pancreatitis. British Journal of Surgery 87:1494–1499

Watanapa P, Williamson RCN 1992 Pancreatic sphincterotomy and sphincteroplasty. Gut 33:865–867

Watanapa P, Williamson RCN 1992 Surgical palliation for pancreatic cancer: developments during the past two decades. British Journal of Surgery 79:8–20

Watanapa P, Williamson RCN 1993 Single-loop biliary and gastric bypass for irresectable pancreatic carcinoma. British Journal of Surgery 80:237–239

Williams DB, Sahai AV, Aabakken L et al 1999 Endoscopic ultrasound guided fine needle aspiration biopsy: a large single centre experience. Gut 44:720–726

Williamson RCN 1984 Early assessment of severity in acute pancreatitis. Gut 25:1331–1339

Williamson RCN, Bliouras N, Cooper MJ et al 1993 Gastric emptying and enterogastric reflux after conservative and conventional pancreaticoduodenectomy. Surgery 114:82–86

22

Liver and portal venous system

S. Bhattacharya

CONTENTS

INTRODUCTION

The liver is considered by many surgeons to be a hallowed organ, and one that presents them with insurmountable problems. They fear massive haemorrhage after any violation of the capsule and dread the thought of attempting any elective procedure. These are unfounded myths: the liver is as amenable to surgery as any other organ, providing you respect certain principles.

TRAUMA

The most frequent and frightening procedure you are called upon to perform on the liver is to arrest haemorrhage following trauma or spontaneous rupture of a tumour.

Liver injuries can result from penetrating trauma such as stab or gunshot injuries, usually producing liver laceration, although high-velocity bullets may also cause significant contusion.

Blunt trauma, often sustained in road traffic accidents, is usually associated with contusions and haematomas. Contusion carries a very high mortality rate, directly related to the severity and number of other affected organs. Some recent reviews of the management of liver trauma are referenced below.[1-4]

Appraise

1 The patient may present with a typical history, in a shocked state. Maintain the patient's airway, breathing and circulation (ABC), following the principles of advanced trauma life support (ATLS). After ensuring normal cardiorespiratory function, carry out a secondary survey, examining the head, spine, chest and limbs as well as the abdomen. If the external injuries do not conform to the degree of shock, assume there is internal bleeding. Stop external haemorrhage by direct pressure, splint any broken limbs, protect a fractured spine, treat a crushed chest by mechanical ventilation and assess any head injury. Now direct your attention to the internal bleeding.

2 In case of doubt about intra-abdominal bleeding in a severely shocked patient, obtain an urgent contrast-enhanced computed tomography (CT) scan, to demonstrate liver parenchymal injury. Emergency portable abdominal ultrasound may also demonstrate a ruptured liver. Failing that, insert a wide-bore (14G) needle attached to a 20-ml syringe into each of the four quadrants of the abdomen—four-quadrant tap. The diagnosis is confirmed if you aspirate blood or heavily blood-stained fluid. Alternatively, perform a diagnostic peritoneal lavage, although this test is often oversensitive.

3 If you remain in doubt and the patient fails to respond to normal resuscitation, consider performing an emergency laparotomy.

4 Treat penetrating injuries in general, and gunshot wounds in particular, by laparotomy. Treat conservatively only selected patients with stab injury who are haemodynamically stable and in whom there is no evidence of hollow viscus perforation.

5 Treat conservatively those patients with blunt trauma who are haemodynamically stable, even if there is demonstrable liver injury on CT or ultrasound scan. Monitor the patient with repeated clinical assessment and scans. If the patient becomes haemodynamically unstable or develops signs of impending peritonitis, proceed to a laparotomy. Carry out urgent laparotomy on a shocked patient who fails to respond adequately despite aggressive initial fluid replacement.

KEY POINTS Emergencies

- Spontaneous rupture of an occult liver tumour may present with shock and a distending abdomen, or an 'acute abdomen' of unknown cause.
- Carry out urgent laparotomy.

EXPLORATION OF A DAMAGED LIVER

Prepare

1 Have you booked an intensive care unit bed if needed postoperatively?

2 You are about to embark on a major surgical procedure, carrying a high mortality rate. As far as possible, ensure you have an experienced anaesthetist, competent assistant and experienced scrub nurse.

3 Pass a bladder catheter. To avoid the complication of renal failure it is important to monitor urine flow during major liver surgery and ensure adequate fluid volume replacement.

4 Place a central venous line, wide-bore peripheral venous lines, and ideally an arterial catheter to allow constant measurement of arterial pressure.

5 Ensure there are at least 12 units of blood available, together with fresh-frozen plasma (FFP) and platelets to replace lost clotting products.

Access

1 If you suspect the diagnosis preoperatively, use a right subcostal incision 3 cm below the costal margin. If necessary extend the incision across the midline 3 cm below the left costal margin as an inverted 'V,' or vertically upwards as a low sternal split. If you need to gain access above the liver, create a second incision in the tenth rib bed from the anterior axillary line to join the original subcostal incision at right angles. This allows you to open the chest, divide the costal margin and so gain control of the inferior vena cava (IVC) above the diaphragm.

2 If you discover the rupture at diagnostic laparotomy through a midline incision, create a transverse lateral extension to the costal margin to gain access and assess the need for further extensions.

3 If you discover the rupture through a totally inappropriate lower abdominal incision, close it and re-explore the abdomen through an appropriate incision.

4 Prefer a self-retaining retractor that can be fixed to the operating table and provides forcible upward retraction of the costal margins, such as Thompson's retractor (Rocialle Medical). It crucially reduces the need for manual assistance, greatly improves access and usually eliminates the need for thoracic extensions.

Assess

1 There is usually much blood clot in the peritoneal cavity and probably some fresh bleeding. Remove clot with your hands and a sucker.

2 Look systematically for damage to the liver, the gut from oesophagus to rectum, spleen, pancreas, anterior and posterior abdominal wall and the diaphragm. If necessary pack the abdominal cavity with sterile packs, removing them serially, inspecting each of the four quadrants in succession.

Action

1 If there is obvious damage to, and haemorrhage from, another intra-abdominal viscus such as the spleen, and that is the primary source of bleeding, surround the damaged area of the liver with large sterile packs and have an assistant apply gentle pressure to control the bleeding. Attend to the lesion in the other organ first, and then turn your attention to the liver.

2 Remove blood and blood clot to gain adequate exposure of the bleeding area of the liver. Control the haemorrhage. Most patients do not require major surgical procedures. Attempt only the minimum surgery necessary to control haemorrhage.

3 Avoid exploring and rough handling of sites of injury that are not bleeding at the time of exploration provided the blood pressure is normal. If the patient is hypotensive there is risk of reactionary haemorrhage when the patient becomes normotensive.

KEY POINT Remember to stick to essentials

- Your primary aims are, in order: to stop the bleeding, to remove obviously devitalized liver tissue and to stop bile leaks.

4 Explore the tear of the liver locally and remove any avascular tissue. If the laceration still bleeds and extends deeply into the liver parenchyma, gently explore the depth of the wound but avoid creating further damage. This procedure is very important in contusion injuries, for major branches of the liver vessels may be ruptured, producing large areas of devascularized tissue. Do not be tempted to explore tears that are not bleeding, since you only encourage further bleeding.

5 Identify bleeding points and apply fine haemostatic forceps. Ligate them with fine synthetic absorbable material such as polyglactin 910 (Vicryl) or polydioxane sulphate (PDS) or use titanium Ligaclips. Suture-ligate larger vessels with PDS or Vicryl.

6 If there is vascular oozing from a large raw area of liver, cover it with one layer of absorbable haemostatic gauze (Surgicel) and apply a pack. Fibrin sealants such as Floseal (Baxter) may help in stopping the ooze from a raw surface. Avoid using deep mattress sutures to control such bleeding, since they may produce areas of devascularization which predisposes to subsequent infection.

? DIFFICULTY

1. *Is there uncontrolled haemorrhage from torn liver?* If haemorrhage is massive, attempt control by inserting a finger through the opening into the lesser sac behind the hepatic hilar structures and apply a Satinsky or other vascular clamp across them. If you do not have vascular clamps available, carefully apply a non-crushing intestinal clamp. This is the Pringle manoeuvre and stops bleeding from branches of the hepatic artery and portal vein.
2. Try to identify any large vessels crossing the tear in the liver and ligate them or suture any tears in their walls. If bleeding persists despite the Pringle manoeuvre, either the patient has an aberrant arterial supply such as an accessory left hepatic artery to the left lobe, or an aberrant right hepatic artery arising from the superior mesenteric, or, more commonly, the bleeding is from the hepatic veins or the inferior vena cava.
3. Injuries involving the major hepatic veins or the inferior vena cava are very difficult to treat and even in experienced hands they are associated with high mortality. Bleeding from such injuries are not controlled by clamping the liver hilum. Attempt to

mobilize the inferior vena cava above and below the liver, identify the caval tear in order to suture it. Unless you are very experienced, do not attempt total vascular isolation of the liver by using intracaval shunts. They are rarely necessary and, even when inserted by experienced surgeons, still have a 60–70% mortality rate.

4. Although a normal liver can tolerate normothermic ischaemia for up to 1 hour, after clamping the liver hilar vessels, it is advisable to release them every 15 minutes timed by the clock.
5. Before releasing any vascular clamps after prolonged clamping, warn the anaesthetist, who may wish to take precautionary measures against the effects of massive acidosis and potassium release, which can cause cardiac arrest.
6. *Packing*. If you cannot achieve control using the described techniques, do not attempt a major resection as an emergency procedure without the assistance of an experienced hepatic surgeon. This is rarely necessary in an emergency and has a high mortality rate. It has been shown in several studies that control is better achieved by packing around the liver with gauze rolls. Do not insert gauze into the depths of a liver laceration. Gently place the packs above, behind and below the liver to compress the bleeding areas (Fig. 22.1).
7. Having gained control, close the abdomen. This allows time to assess the next move and possibly to carry out a contrast-enhanced CT scan and a hepatic angiogram. You may then choose to re-explore in 48–72 hours to remove the packs and re-assess, or transfer the patient to a specialist liver surgery unit.
8. *Is there damage to the extrahepatic biliary tree?* Attempt reconstruction by anastomosing cut ends of the bile duct end-to-end over a T-tube splint inserted through healthy bile duct. Use interrupted absorbable sutures such as Vicryl or PDS. If the damage to the duct is excessive, identify the most distal section of duct which is undamaged below the liver and divide it there. Suture-ligate the distal stump of the bile duct. Anastomose the proximal end of the bile duct to the side of a loop of jejunum, preferably a Roux-en-Y loop, using interrupted sutures of Vicryl or PDS for a single-layer anastomosis.
9. If the patient is very ill and unstable, there is no urgency in carrying out a biliary anastomosis. Leave a tube drain through the abdominal wall down to the site of biliary leak; the repair can be carried out by an expert at a later date.

Check

1 When you have gained control of the bleeding from the liver, carry out a full, careful and gentle exploration for other intraperitoneal injuries if you have not done so already (Chs 3, 4). Explore the entire gut from the oesophagus to rectum and pay special attention to the retroperitoneal duodenum, the pancreas and the spleen.

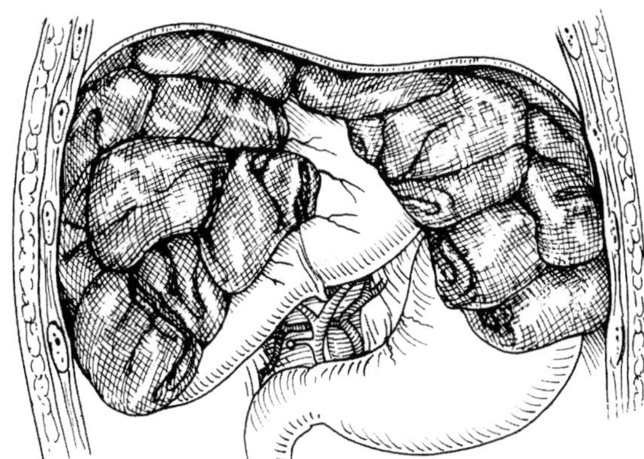

Fig. 22.1 Placement of packs around a ruptured liver. (Adapted from Blumgart LM (ed.) 1994 Surgery of the liver and biliary tract. Churchill Livingstone, Edinburgh, p 1230.)

2 When you are certain that haemorrhage is controlled and that other lesions have been appropriately dealt with, inspect it once more, unless you needed to pack the liver to control haemorrhage. If there are devascularized areas, remove them to prevent infection.

KEY POINTS Decision

- If you have had no experience of liver resection operations it is safer to close the abdomen.
- Either transfer the patient to an experienced colleague or seek advice before re-exploring the liver yourself after a few days when the patient's condition is stable.
- If you find bile leaking from damaged intrahepatic bile ducts, ligate or suture them.

Closure

1 Before you close, mop the peritoneal cavity dry with surgical swabs, or carry out a gentle lavage with warm normal saline and then suck out all the fluid.

2 Close the abdomen 'en masse' in standard fashion.

3 If you have operated on any part of the biliary tract insert a drain, preferably with a closed system. If there is liver parenchymal damage only, then a drain is probably unnecessary in the absence of an obvious biliary leak.

Aftercare

1 Admit the patient to an intensive care unit or high-dependency nursing area.

2 If further operation is required, for example because packs were inserted to control haemorrhage, arrange transfer to a specialist unit if possible.

3 Mechanically ventilate the patient electively and maintain the blood gases within normal range until the patient is haemodynamically stable, other injuries have been treated and the

core temperature has returned to normal. Correct any remaining electrolyte imbalance. Measure blood sugar hourly and treat any abnormality immediately.

4 Evaluate biochemical liver function daily.

5 Maintain intravascular volume and normal clotting. Transfuse with blood and FFP as required.

6 Maintain urine flow. If it falls below 30 ml/hour, first check that the circulating blood volume is adequate, with normal blood pressure and central venous pressure. If you are in any doubt about this, give a 'fluid challenge' of 250 ml of colloid-containing fluid intravenously. If this fails to stimulate urine flow despite an adequate blood pressure and normal central venous pressure, consider giving a low-dose dopamine infusion. If this fails to improve urine flow give 40 mg of furosemide (frusemide) intravenously and seek the advice of a renal physician.

7 Give a versatile antibiotic mixture such as a combination of cefuroxime and metronidazole.

8 If gastrointestinal activity does not return within 2–3 days, institute intravenous nutrition.

9 Sudden collapse suggests that the patient has developed further internal bleeding or septicaemia. If this is associated with abdominal swelling, resuscitate with intravenous blood or colloid, and FFP if the clotting screen is abnormal. Order a contrast-enhanced CT scan if possible to confirm haemorrhage and return the patient to the operating room in order to carry out a further gentle careful, exploration and attempt to control bleeding.

10 If you suspect septicaemia then start full investigations to determine the source. Culture blood, urine and any leaking body fluid. Order a chest X-ray and carry out an ultrasound or CT scan of the abdomen to look for an abscess. Give appropriate versatile antibiotics. Drain an intraperitoneal abscess either by a further operation or by ultrasound-guided needle aspiration. If the patient is very shocked and the diagnosis uncertain, it is safer to re-explore the abdomen than to wait. Intra-abdominal sepsis is very common following liver trauma and devascularized areas of the liver may become necrotic and infected.

KEY POINT Better to look and see than wait and see

- If you are in any doubt about further bleeding or sepsis, re-exploration is safer than waiting. If you fail to recognize and treat it, the patient may die.

RE-EXPLORATION

Prepare

1 If possible, obtain a hepatic arteriogram before re-exploration to fully assess any vascular damage and so allow you to prepare for appropriate surgical management and, if necessary, obtain expert help.

2 Ensure that the patient is stable and correct biochemical and haematological abnormalities. Discuss any clotting impairment with the haematologists and give cryoprecipitate or FFP before surgery.

3 Order 12 units of blood and some platelets and FFP.

Access

1 Gently and carefully open the previous incision.

2 Soak the packs with saline before you attempt to remove them. Remove them slowly and gently. Send a piece immediately for microbiological culture.

Assess

As a rule everything is dry. Avoid any major exploration of the liver.

Action

1 If bleeding recurs, suture-ligate the bleeding point with a fine suture or apply haemostats to any obvious bleeding vessels and ligate them.

2 Aspirate any bile collections and attempt to ligate or suture any leaking bile ducts.

3 If major bleeding starts again, attempt to identify the main vessel and suture it. On rare occasions you may carry out lobectomy (see below) if the injury is confined to one lobe.

4 Occasionally, following a severe blunt crushing injury, the damage is so great that no surgical procedure can save the patient's life, even in the most expert of hands.

Closure

1 If you are sure there are no more local problems, perform a warm saline peritoneal lavage, close the abdomen without drainage and continue antibiotic therapy, adjusted in due course when the results of the culture of the removed packs are available.

Aftercare

As before.

REFERENCES

1. Trunkey DD 2004 Hepatic trauma: contemporary management. Surgical Clinics of North America 84:437–450
2. David Richardson J, Franklin GA, Lukan JK et al 2000 Evolution in the management of hepatic trauma: a 25-year perspective. Annals of Surgery 232:324–330
3. Marr JD, Krige JE, Terblanche J 2000 Analysis of 153 gunshot wounds of the liver. British Journal of Surgery 87:1030–1034
4. Parks RW, Chrysos E, Diamond T 1999 Management of liver trauma. British Journal of Surgery 86:1121–1135

PRINCIPLES OF ELECTIVE SURGERY

Appraise

KEY POINT Caution

- Complex hepatic surgery should, as far as possible, be carried out in specialist units.

- Do not undertake an elective operation on the liver without complete preoperative investigation and a fairly certain working diagnosis. Occasionally, an isolated hepatic lesion may be identified during a scan carried out for another reason. If you discover a lesion in the liver during a laparotomy, carefully consider the risks before trying to excise or biopsy it or you may expose the patient to serious risks. Operation on a patient with impaired liver function can be very hazardous and carries a high morbidity and mortality.
- The history is crucial. The cause of a space-occupying lesion may be suggested if the patient lived in an area where hydatid disease, amoebiasis, schistosomiasis or other liver parasitic infections are endemic. Suspect an hepatic cell adenoma in a woman who has taken high-oestrogen-containing contraceptive pills. Carefully assess each patient to make the diagnosis but also to assess fitness for surgery. Typical findings are jaundice, systemic signs of chronic liver disease, a mass or tenderness in the right upper quadrant of the abdomen.
- Carry out biochemical liver function tests. Measure the alphafetoprotein (AFP) and carcinoembryonic antigen (CEA) if you suspect a malignant primary or secondary liver tumour. Order a hepatic virus screen for evidence of present or past infection with hepatitis B virus (HBV) or hepatitis C virus (HBC).
- Arrange for ultrasound and CT scans of the upper abdomen. These demonstrate the size of the liver and the biliary ducts within and outside it, and may show gallstones or tumour. Patency of major vessels and the presence of any space-occupying lesions in the liver can be assessed. A picture characteristic of cirrhosis may be seen. Some centres use magnetic resonance imaging (MRI) rather than CT.
- Selective coeliac and superior mesenteric angiography demonstrates the arterial anatomy outside and within the liver, and the vascularization of any intrahepatic lesion. Reserve this for selected cases, but it may be of great value in determining operability, and provides useful anatomical knowledge for the operation. Furthermore, the venous phase of the angiograms demonstrates patency or distortion of the portal vein. It also demonstrates the position and nature of any abnormal portasystemic shunts in the presence of portal venous hypertension.
- Always obtain histological confirmation of the nature of any underlying parenchymal liver disease. First, correct any clotting or platelet abnormalities. The biopsy can be carried out percutaneously, by blind insertion, with CT or ultrasound direction, at peritoneoscopy, or at laparotomy. Use either a Tru-cut or a Menghini needle. The needle track can be embolized by injecting Gelfoam suspension into the needle sheath as it is removed. If clotting cannot be corrected, an expert can obtain a transjugular biopsy using a special catheter introduced into an hepatic vein branch through a jugular vein puncture.
- Be cautious about performing percutaneous biopsy of a liver tumour. Malignant cells have been seeded along the track made by both conventional and even fine needles. This jeopardizes the patient's outlook. Consider the need for absolute histological confirmation in the light of the results of the other investigations. In major centres, the morbidity and mortality of a liver resection is very low—less than 5%. The risk of seeding an otherwise curable cancer must be weighed against this. If the liver is cirrhotic, the resection carries a much higher complication rate, and biopsy of a suspicious lesion is probably indicated.
- Consider portal pressure measurement. This can be gauged from wedged hepatic venous pressure (WHVP) measurements. The presence of a raised WHVP is said to indicate a poorer prognosis in patients undergoing hepatic resection. Intraoperative measurement of portal pressure may be valuable during shunt procedures designed to produce portal decompression when a fall in pressure indicates a successful operation.
- Before undertaking any operative procedure on a patient with a liver disease, check the blood film, platelet count and clotting profile and correct any abnormality, if possible by giving blood products. Rarely are platelet infusions necessary, but all patients undergoing liver surgery, especially if jaundiced or with severe biochemical dysfunction, benefit from injections of vitamin K_1. If the clotting profile is badly deranged, the patient may need an infusion of FFP and occasionally cryoprecipitate.

OPERATIVE LIVER BIOPSY

Prepare

This is rarely carried out as an isolated procedure. Check the patient's blood group. If you anticipate a more major procedure than a simple biopsy, cross-match an adequate quantity of blood and platelets and have available some FFP for replacement therapy during surgery.

Access

This depends on which procedure you intend to perform apart from the liver biopsy. Prefer to use a midline or right subcostal incision.

Action

1. Take the liver biopsy early during laparotomy. Prolonged liver trauma during laparotomy can produce changes that make histological interpretation of the specimen difficult.
2. Select an area of diseased liver or an edge that presents easily through the incision.
3. Place two mattress stitches of 3/0 Vicryl or PDS on an atraumatic round-bodied needle to form a 'V', the apex of this pointing towards the hilum of the liver (Fig. 22.2a).
4. Gently but firmly tie these stitches (Fig. 22.2b) and remove the wedge of tissue between them with a sharp knife (Fig. 22.2c). The cut edges of the liver should be dry. Insert another suture of similar material if haemostasis is not complete or use diathermy coagulation to establish haemostasis.
5. You may also use a Tru-cut needle to take a liver biopsy. If you are not familiar with the needle, rehearse your movements before inserting it into the liver. After removing the needle, check that you have an adequate core of tissue. Gently shake or tease the core of tissue into a pot of formalin, taking care not to crush it. The puncture site occasionally requires a

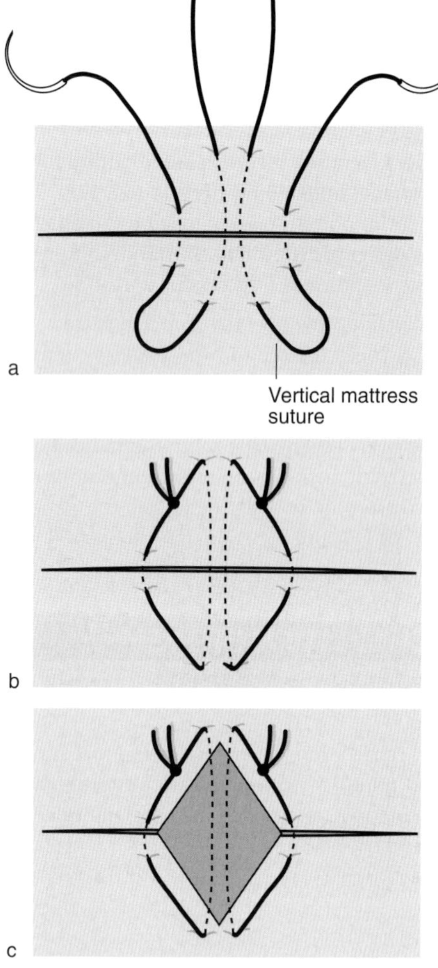

Fig. 22.2 Technique for wedge liver biopsy: (a) initial placement of two mattress stitches; (b) tie each firmly; (c) remove the wedge of tissue between them.

figure-of-eight or Z-stitch with 4/0 Vicryl or PDS to obtain haemostasis.

6 Complete your examination of all abdominal structures.

7 Close the incision in the standard fashion.

INFECTIVE LESIONS

BACTERIAL LIVER ABSCESS

Appraise

- Open surgical drainage of liver abscesses is rarely necessary. The standard treatment is aspiration of the pus under imaging guidance, and antibiotic therapy after localizing it with ultrasound or CT scanning, using a large-bore percutaneous needle.
- Until the exact nature and antibiotic sensitivities of the causative organism are known, administer an intravenous third-generation cephalosporin with metronidazole, possibly with gentamicin. Keep in mind the nephrotoxicity of gentamicin and measure its blood levels regularly.
- You may have to aspirate the abscess several times, but if it fails to respond to repeated aspiration and antibiotics or the percutaneous insertion of a drain, then very rarely you may be forced to operate. Localize the abscess first with ultrasound or CT scans. Administer intravenous antibiotics. Cross-match 4 units of blood and have available FFP. Avoid surgical exploration if possible, because it may be complicated by difficulty in finding the abscess, hepatic haemorrhage or local and systemic sepsis. Use intraoperative ultrasound, if available, to identify the site of an intrahepatic lesion.

Access

1 Use a right subcostal incision 3 cm below the costal margin for an anterior abscess.

2 Approach a posterior abscess through the bed of the right posterior 12th rib.

Action

1 Isolate the peritoneal contents from the area of the abscess by packs.

2 Insert a needle into the abscess, aspirate some of the contents to send for immediate examination and culture, including anaerobic culture, to confirm the diagnosis.

3 Incise the abscess and suck out the contents. Gently insert a finger to identify and breakdown all loculi.

4 Wash out the cavity with physiological saline.

5 Insert a tube drain, preferably as a closed system such as a Robinson drain. Pass the distal end of the drain through the abdominal wall at a suitable site, not through the incision.

6 Achieve haemostasis at the edge of the liver incision by using 3/0 Vicryl or PDS mattress sutures on an atraumatic needle or diathermy coagulation.

7 If possible, draw some omentum into the abscess cavity.

8 Close the abdomen.

9 Leave the drain until drainage ceases and the cavity is demonstrably collapsed on ultrasound, CT or a sinogram. Until then continue appropriate antibiotics.

AMOEBIC ABSCESS

Appraise

- This rarely requires surgical treatment.
- Positively confirm the diagnosis by identifying trophozoites (Greek: *trophe* = nourishment + *zoon* = animal; adult of the asexual cycle) in the aspirate, or a positive serological test. The presence of amoebae in stools or a rectal biopsy is very indicative, but absence of organisms does not exclude the diagnosis.
- Treatment is with metronidazole, 400–800 mg orally 8-hourly in an adult for at least 7 days. Resolution of the abscess can be monitored using regular ultrasound screening. If it becomes secondarily infected or is discovered at laparotomy then treat it like any other liver abscess.

HYDATID CYST

Appraise

- Suspect a hydatid cyst in patients who present with a liver mass and who live or have lived in an endemic area. Confirm it by the presence of eosinophilia, positive hydatid serology and classic ultrasound and CT appearances.
- Past treatment was mainly surgical. There is growing evidence that percutaneous treatment, combined with antihelminthic drug therapy is safe and effective in selected patients with uncomplicated cysts.[1] Consider it only if the cyst does not communicate with the biliary system on ERCP (endoscopic retrograde cholangiopancreatography). Remember that this procedure carries a low but definite risk of anaphylaxis. Administer an initial course of albendazole, followed by puncture of the cyst under imaging guidance, aspiration of the cyst contents, instillation of hypertonic saline into the cyst cavity, and then re-aspiration—the acronym is PAIR. In some centres, sclerosing agent is finally injected into the cyst cavity, followed by a further course of albendazole. Albendazole alone, without percutaneous intervention, is not considered ideal therapy; use it only if PAIR or surgery is not possible. Surgery, in the form of cystectomy and omentoplasty, is still preferred by many clinicians who feel there is insufficient evidence for the routine use of PAIR. It is certainly the standard treatment for complicated cysts, cysts that communicate with the biliary tree and where percutaneous therapy has failed.

Prepare

1. Give at least a 4-week cycle of albendazole tablets (10 mg/kg/day in divided doses for an adult) before and after surgery to prevent growth of any spilt protoscolices (Greek: *protos* = first + *scolex* = a worm). You may administer up to three cycles of 4 weeks each, with a 2-week gap between cycles. Some surgeons additionally cover the perioperative period with another drug, praziquantel.
2. Visualize the biliary tract preoperatively with ERCP, especially if there is any history of attacks of jaundice or cholangitis, suggesting a communication between the cyst and the biliary tree.
3. Have available fluid with which to wash out the cyst to kill any remaining scolices. This can be absolute alcohol, 1% cetrimide, 10% formalin solution, 0.5% silver nitrate solution, or sterile 20% saline, which is the safest.
4. Have available sterile black towels (see below) with which to pack off the surrounding tissues. Some surgeons soak these in formalin solution.
5. If possible have available a refrigerated funnel—a 'cryofunnel'—or suction funnel.
6. Warn the anaesthetist to be prepared for sudden anaphylactic shock if there is inadvertent spillage of cyst contents into the peritoneal cavity, although this is a rare.

Access

1. If possible arrange for the incision to overlie the cyst.
2. Use an extended right subcostal incision 3 cm below the costal margin or, if the abscess lies posteriorly, a tenth-rib thoracoabdominal incision.

Action

1. When you reach the cyst, take care in handling it to avoid rupture. It is usually attached to surrounding tissues by fibrinous adhesions which you must gently separate.
2. Isolate the cyst from the rest of the peritoneal or chest contents with packs. Traditionally, these are covered with black towels, which are claimed to make any spilt daughter cysts or scolices visible.
3. A metal 'cryofunnel' has a 5-cm diameter narrow end fused to a circular metal tube through which liquid nitrogen can be passed. Place the narrow cooled end of the funnel on the exposed cyst and pass through liquid nitrogen. Freezing unites the cyst wall to the lower end of the funnel, preventing any spilt contents from contaminating surrounding structures. You can carry out all the operative procedures through the funnel. A modification of this funnel—the Aarons cone—employs suction to attach the funnel to the cyst. Unfortunately, many cysts are so sited that the bony chest wall prevents the use of these funnels.
4. Insert a wide-bore needle into the cyst and carefully aspirate as much as possible of the contained fluid.
5. Incise the wall of the cyst and gently remove the yellow-grey cyst membrane, together with any free daughter cysts.

KEY POINTS Avoid spillage

- Do not spill any of the cyst fluid, daughter cysts or membranes.
- They can infect any other part of the abdomen.

6. When the cyst is empty fill it with a fluid—ideally 20% saline—that will destroy any remaining protoscolices. Leave the fluid in the cyst for at least 10 minutes, then aspirate it and repeat the procedure. Take great care when using any of the other irritant solutions, especially formalin, to prevent them leaking into the biliary tree, where they can cause sclerosing cholangitis. The preoperative ERCP should have demonstrated any communications between the cyst and the biliary tree and warned you of the possibility. Seal them using an absorbable suture such as Vicryl or PDS before irrigating the cavity.
7. Finally aspirate the fluid. If you used a 'cryofunnel', turn off the liquid nitrogen and allow the contact between funnel and liver to thaw. Remove the packs carefully to prevent any contamination.
8. Unroof the cyst as much as possible—a technique known as saucerization—to allow omentum and other peritoneal contents to fill the cavity easily and so avoid the problems associated with delayed healing and infection of intrahepatic fibrous-walled cavities with a narrow neck. The omentum may be tacked into place with a few absorbable sutures (omentoplasty).

9 The value of inserting a drain into the cyst cavity is controversial. If it is possible to saucerize it then do not drain. If you leave the cavity with a narrow neck you can insert a closed drainage system.

10 If you have demonstrated any evidence of communication between the cyst and biliary tree, consider performing an operative cholangiogram to ensure that you have closed it and that the biliary tree is free from any obstructing daughter cysts, which will need to be removed.

11 Ensure that haemostasis is complete. Wash out the peritoneal cavity with large volumes of physiological saline.

Technical points

1 Some surgeons advocate excision of the cyst intact, including the 'pericyst'. In some circumstances this is possible, but it can cause severe bleeding. Attempt it only if you are experienced.

2 If there has been spillage of cyst contents into the peritoneal cavity, washing with sterile water may reduce the likelihood of further infestation because of the toxic osmotic effect of water on the protoscolices.

Postoperative

Watch for hypernatraemia if you have used large volumes of 20% saline.

OTHER CYSTS

Appraise

- The majority of liver cysts are totally asymptomatic and are discovered only at autopsy or during a routine laparotomy. When symptoms develop, they include right upper quadrant abdominal swelling, discomfort or acute pain associated with haemorrhage into the cyst or rupture of the cyst.
- Massive polycystic disease of the liver is rare but can cause severe pain. In 50% of patients with polycystic disease, there is associated polycystic renal disease. The renal lesions are more serious and life-threatening than are the liver lesions. Some patients also have associated pancreatic cysts. These patients should be treated only in major centres since they may ultimately require liver transplantation.
- Occasionally, cysts become infected or the patient may have recurrent cholangitis due to biliary tract narrowing from pressure.
- A very rare liver cyst is caused by a biliary cystadenoma—a premalignant lesion—and this needs excising.
- Symptomatic cysts are diagnosed before surgery is undertaken as a result of investigation of the symptoms, especially by ultrasound and CT scans.
- Before attempting diagnostic percutaneous aspiration of a cyst, consider if it is hydatid (see section on hydatid cyst).

Access

Use an extended right subcostal incision 3 cm below the costal margin.

Action

1 Carry out a thorough abdominal exploration, particularly palpating the kidneys and pancreas even though preoperative scans should have warned you of any pancreatic or renal lesions.

> **KEY POINT Hydatid disease?**
>
> - If you cannot exclude hydatid disease, manage the cyst as if it were a hydatid cyst.

2 If you are certain the cyst is not hydatid, aspirate fluid with a needle and send the fluid for cytological, microbiological and chemical analysis.

3 If you discover an asymptomatic cyst less than 8 cm in diameter incidentally during a laparotomy for something else, leave it alone.

4 If the cyst is symptomatic or large, carefully unroof it, allowing it to drain freely into the peritoneal cavity. You may gently pack omentum into it. Such a cyst may recur but can then be treated by percutaneous aspiration or formal resection. If you are experienced in laparoscopic surgery you may elect to de-roof a symptomatic superficial liver cyst by a minimal access approach.

5 If the cyst is superficial, carry out simple wedge excision if you are experienced in this technique.

6 If the lesion is large, multilocular, or appears to be vascular, then it is probably wise not to attempt further action at this stage. Close the abdomen and await the results of the tests on the cyst fluid. Later, you can treat the lesion electively following investigations.

REFERENCE

1. Khuroo MS, Wani NA, Javid G et al 1997 Percutaneous drainage compared with surgery for hepatic hydatid cysts. New England Journal of Medicine 337:881–887

NEOPLASMS

Appraise

1 Liver neoplasms can be solid or cystic, benign or malignant, primary or secondary, single or multiple.

2 Preoperative assessment (see section on principles of elective surgery above) is essential to determine the need for surgical treatment. Particularly valuable are AFP and CEA levels, which may indicate if the lesion is a primary or secondary tumour. Ultrasound, CT and MR scans, angiograms and biopsy are valuable, but remember the risk of needle-track tumour dissemination.

3 Not every neoplasm requires excision once it can be proved to be benign, unless it is causing symptoms. However, consider for laparotomy patients with malignant, suspected malignant or symptomatic benign disease.

4 Administer intravenous prophylactic antibiotics with the premedication, such as a cephalosporin and metronidazole and plan to maintain this postoperatively for 3 days.

Prepare

1 If a major liver resection is possible, advise your anaesthetist and order 6 units of blood. Warn the blood bank that you may need platelets and FFP.

2 Correct any clotting abnormality before surgery. Give jaundiced patients vitamin K_1 injections.

3 Assess the state and function of the unaffected liver with biochemical liver function tests and, if necessary, by studies of functional reserve capacity (usually available only in major centres) and by histological examination to exclude cirrhosis. Partial resection of a cirrhotic or poorly functioning liver carries a high morbidity and mortality and needs to be balanced against the prognosis following attempted resection.

4 Have available a Thompson-type self-retaining retractor, which can be fixed to the operating table. It provides forcible upward retraction of the costal margin, facilitating the operation by improving access and reducing the need for manual assistance. Have available vascular clamps and sutures, if possible also an ultrasonic dissector with which to cut liver parenchyma, and an intraoperative ultrasound probe.

5 Have the anaesthetist insert a central venous catheter and an arterial cannula for pressure measurements.

6 Pass a bladder catheter to allow urine flow to be monitored.

7 Plan for postoperative analgesia with your anaesthetist. We routinely use epidural analgesia, the catheter for which is placed after the patient is anaesthetized. The anaesthetist may prefer you not to administer subcutaneous heparin as antithrombotic prophylaxis until the epidural catheter is inserted.

WEDGE EXCISION OF SOLITARY LIVER LESION

Access

1 First create a right subcostal incision 3 cm below the costal margin to explore the lesion. This can be extended across the midline below the left costal margin as an inverted 'V' to gain greater exposure.

2 Add a vertical extension from the midpoint to the xiphisternum—Mercedes Benz incision—to gain even greater exposure. You will rarely need to split the sternum or open the chest through a tenth rib extension.

Assess

1 Carry out a general exploration to exclude other intra-abdominal pathology.

2 Identify the site of the liver tumour and decide if your incision is adequate to allow safe resection. If it is too small, extend it.

3 Explore the liver hilum. Identify the hepatic artery, portal vein and common bile duct and pass a tape around them. This allows a vascular clamp to be applied to control haemorrhage during liver resection—the Pringle manoeuvre.

4 If it is available, use an ultrasound imaging probe to examine the entire liver and identify the number, site and vascular relations of the tumours.

Action

1 Incise the liver capsule at least 1 cm away from the tumour. Gently apply a vascular clamp across the hilar vessels (see above). Although the normal liver can tolerate up to 60 minutes of warm ischaemia, to reduce hepatocellular damage to a minimum release the clamp for 5 minutes every 15 minutes.

2 Divide the liver substance using a finger-and-thumb pinch technique or a small haemostat, identifying major ductal or vascular structures crossing the line of incision. Clip these with fine haemostats, divide them and coagulate or ligate them.

3 If it is available, use an ultrasound dissector. With experience you can divide the liver parenchyma and easily identify the ducts and vessels crossing the line of transection. Blood loss is reduced using this instrument but the operating time is increased.

4 Remove the tumour, and ligate any remaining ducts and vessels held in the haemostats with fine Vicryl or PDS. Coagulate with diathermy any remaining small bleeding points. Remove the clamp from the hilum.

5 If the cut surface of the liver is not dry, cover it with absorbable haemostatic gauze (Surgicel) and apply a pack. After 10 minutes, gently remove the pack. The area should be dry. Coagulate any remaining bleeding points.

Check

1 Carefully inspect the liver hilum to ensure that no major structures have been damaged.

2 Perform cholangiography if there is any question of biliary tract damage.

Closure

1 Once the cut surface of the liver is dry, wash the perihepatic peritoneal cavity with warm saline.

2 Apply the omentum to the transected surface of the liver and close the wound using a mass closure suture and a subcuticular skin suture.

3 Do not use a drain since there is no evidence that this traditional practice offers any advantage and it may predispose to postoperative problems such as fluid collection and sepsis.

RIGHT OR LEFT HEPATECTOMY

For an extensive discussion of liver resectional techniques refer to Blumgart[1] and Launois.[2]

Anatomy

1 The liver is divided into two anatomical lobes, each being supplied by its own branch of the hepatic artery, portal vein and hepatic duct. The junction of the two lobes is about 4 cm lateral to the right of the attachment of the falciform ligament and in the line of the gallbladder bed (Fig. 22.3a). By ligating hepatic artery and portal vein branches supplying either lobe, it is possible to see the junction between them as a fairly sharp colour change.

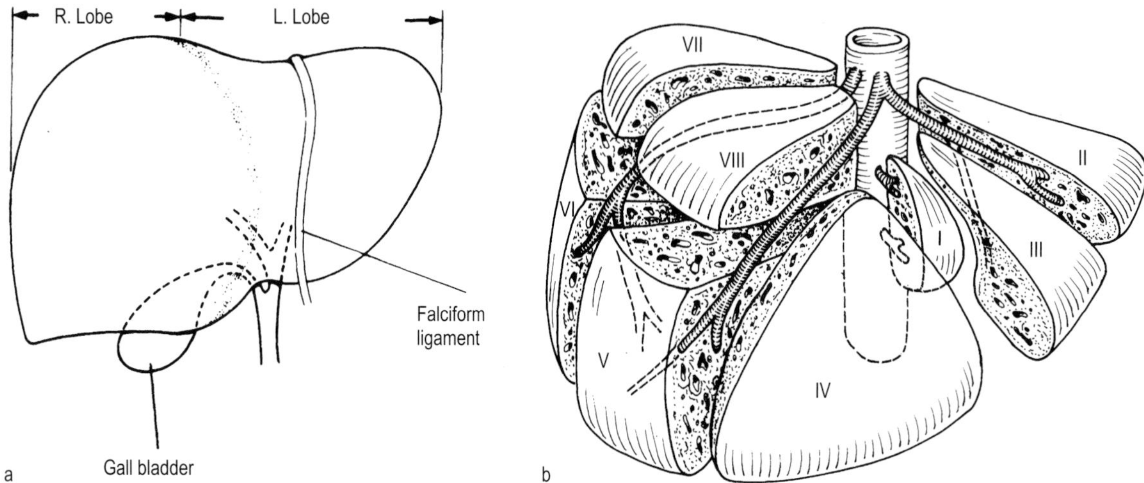

Fig. 22.3 Anatomy of the liver: (a) the main lobes of the liver; (b) diagrammatic representation of the segments of the liver. (Adapted from Launois B, Jamieson GG 1993 Modern operative techniques in liver surgery. Churchill Livingstone, Edinburgh, p 7.)

2 The liver is further divided into eight segments, described initially by Couinaud[3] in 1957 (Fig. 22.3b). Segment I, adjacent to the IVC, is also known as the caudate lobe, and segment IV, between the falciform ligament and the main lobular division, is known as the quadrate lobe.

3 As a result of the hepatic architecture it is possible to divide the liver through the main plane separating the right and left lobes. It is also possible to remove segments of the liver. Removal of all the liver tissue to the right of the falciform ligament (right lobe plus segment IV) is called an extended right hepatectomy or trisegmentectomy. This resection is, however, difficult to perform. Do not undertake it if you are inexperienced.

4 Removal of segments II and III of the left lobe, that part of the liver to the left of the falciform ligament, is comparatively straightforward.

Appraise

Left, right or extended right hepatectomy can be carried out depending on the location of the tumour and the desired clearance margin, which is ideally at least 1 cm.

Access

This is as for a wedge excision but it is necessary to extend the incision for this more radical operation.

Action

1 After full exploration of all abdominal viscera, divide the falciform ligament on the anterior surface of the liver as far as the suprahepatic IVC. This will allow you to mobilize the liver.

2 Dissect the hepatic hilum and identify the branches of the hepatic artery, portal vein and bile duct supplying and draining the affected lobe. If the right lobe is to be removed, also identify and dissect the cystic duct and artery.

3 Doubly ligate with Vicryl or PDS, and divide the structures supplying the lobe to be removed (Fig. 22.4a).

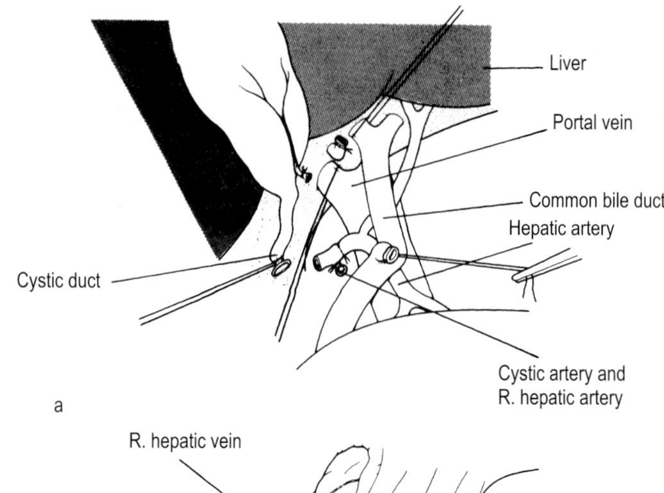

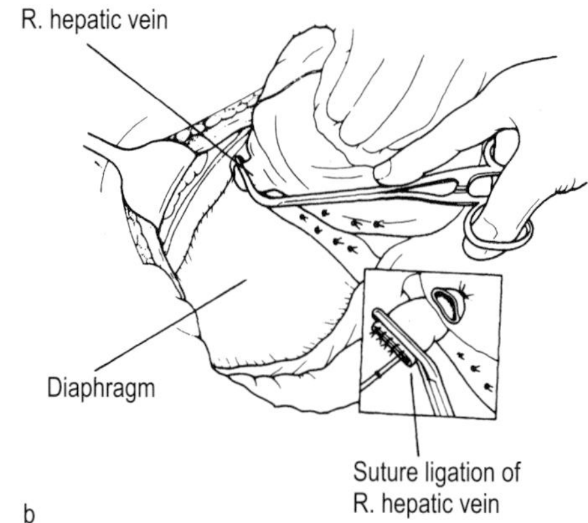

Fig. 22.4 Right hepatectomy: (a) the vessels supplying the lobe to be removed are ligated; (b) the hepatic veins from the lobe to be removed are ligated.

4 Divide the peritoneal reflections between the back of the liver lobe and the diaphragm and retract the lobe from the diaphragm and posterior abdominal wall until you see the IVC.

5 Identify the small veins from segment I (the caudate lobe), entering the IVC. Dissect, ligate and divide them (Fig. 22.4b).

Carefully dissect the main right, middle or left hepatic veins, closing them with vascular clamps before dividing them. Use vascular suture to close the ends (Fig. 22.4b). You may use an endovascular stapler, if one is available, to divide and staple the hepatic veins.

6 Return to the anterior surface of the liver. You should be able to identify a demarcation line between the devascularized lobe to be removed and the normal vascularized liver which is to remain.

7 Cut through the capsule just on the vascularized side of this demarcation line.

8 Use a finger-and-thumb pinching technique, dissect with a small haemostat, or use the ultrasonic dissector if it is available, to divide the liver substance between this incision and the IVC.

9 Doubly clip with fine haemostats any vascular or biliary tract structures crossing the line of transection as you encounter them.

10 Remove the diseased lobe and ligate with fine Vicryl or PDS the vessels or ducts held in haemostats on the remaining liver.

11 Control any smaller bleeding points by diathermy coagulation.

12 Cover the raw area of the liver with absorbable haemostatic gauze (Surgicel) and apply a pack for 10 minutes.

Check

1 When haemostasis is complete, explore the hilar structures to ensure that no major damage has occurred.

2 Consider on-table cholangiography if there is any doubt about damage to the biliary system.

Closure

1 Gently flush the peritoneal cavity with warm saline.

2 Cover the transected area of liver with omentum and close the abdomen. Place a soft, wide-bore tube drain only if you expect a significant collection of blood or bile.

Technical point

T-tube drainage of the biliary tract is unnecessary unless you suspect some distal obstruction, or if there has been damage to the common bile duct.

Aftercare

1 The initial postoperative management of these patients is critical, and is best carried out in an intensive care or high-dependency unit for the first 24 hours, or at least until the patient is warm, extubated, self-ventilating and haemodynamically stable.

2 The broad principles of management are as outlined in the aftercare of major liver trauma.

REFERENCES

1. Blumgart LH, Fong Y (eds) 2000 Surgery of the liver and biliary tract, 3rd edn. Harcourt, London, pp 1639–1798
2. Launois B, Jamieson GG 1993 Modern operative techniques in liver surgery. Churchill Livingstone, Edinburgh
3. Couinaud C, Le Foie 1957 Etudes anatomiques et chirurgicales. Masson, Paris

SURGICAL MANAGEMENT OF HAEMORRHAGE FROM OESOPHAGEAL VARICES

The most life-threatening complication of portal hypertension that requires surgical treatment is bleeding from oesophageal varices. While the majority of patients do stop bleeding spontaneously, the in-hospital mortality from the first bleed is in the region of 50%.

Management is complex and is ideally undertaken by a specialist team including a medical hepatologist, specialist radiologist and a surgeon.[1,2]

Appraise

1 Aim to resuscitate the patient, find the cause of the bleeding and stop it. These three processes must be carried out in parallel. The prognosis is directly related to the severity of any underlying liver disease. Minimal hepatocellular damage carries a good prognosis; if it is severe, the prognosis is poor. As there is no way of predicting which patients will fare badly or well, initially treat them all actively.

2 Resuscitate by infusing compatible blood, platelets and clotting products given as FFP. If intravenous fluid is needed while the blood is being cross-matched, maintain the circulating volume with colloid.

3 Endoscope a patient admitted to hospital with massive upper gastrointestinal haemorrhage. This is the most certain way of discovering if bleeding is from ruptured oesophageal varices.

KEY POINTS Accurate diagnosis

- Although a previous history and clinical examination may suggest variceal bleed, you must directly visualize the bleeding area before starting treatment.
- Especially alcoholics with known varices bleed from other gastrointestinal lesions.

4 If you confirm variceal bleeding at endoscopy, perform sclerotherapy by injecting sclerosing agents into or around the varices, or obliterate the varices by variceal banding by placing a constricting rubber-band at the base of the varix. You need to be experienced in the appropriate techniques. Although you may control bleeding in most patients, there is a significant risk of re-bleeding, and of complications such as oesophageal ulceration and perforation. Occasionally you need to repeat sclerotherapy or ligation in the acute phase to control bleeding.

5 If bleeding persists despite endoscopic attempts at control or if endoscopy is not available, then give a vasoactive drug such as vasopressin to reduce splanchnic blood flow, thereby reducing portal flow and pressure. Administer vasopressin as a continuous intravenous infusion at 0.4 units/minute, increasing if necessary to 0.6 units/minute and continuing until bleeding has stopped for 24 hours. Vasopressin can cause myocardial ischaemia, arrhythmias, heart failure, mesenteric ischaemia, limb ischaemia, pulmonary oedema and cerebrovascular

accidents, so use it with caution. Be willing to administer simultaneous nitroglycerine sublingually, intravenously or transdermally. Alternatively give terlipressin, somatostatin, or its synthetic analogue octreotide. Although it is expensive, somatostatin is the safest and probably the best option; give it as a 250-μg bolus and a 250–500-μg/hour infusion, continued for 2–5 days if it is beneficial.

6 If the vasoactive drugs fails, control bleeding for up to 24 hours maximum by oesophagogastric tamponade using an orogastric triple lumen balloon tube (Sengstaken–Blakemore tube). This has a gastric balloon, an oesophageal balloon and a channel for draining the stomach. In the four-lumen Minnesota version there is also a channel for oesophageal drainage. After passing the tube, inflate the gastric balloon with 250–300 ml of air and apply gentle traction to the tube. The patient may wear a motorcycle helmet. After pulling on the tube, tape it to the bar across the face. This tamponades (French: *tapon* = a plug) the oesophagogastric junction and the fundus. If bleeding continues, as signalled by fresh blood emerging up the gastric channel, then connect the oesophageal balloon to a manometer with a 'Y'-connection and fill it with air to a pressure not exceeding 40 mmHg. Deflate the oesophageal balloon for 30 minutes every 4–6 hours and remove the tube after 12 hours. Balloon tamponade is unlikely to be curative; expect half the patients to re-bleed when the tube is removed. It 'buys time' while deciding on more definitive measures. Dangers include oesophageal perforation and aspiration pneumonia.

7 As soon as you have controlled the bleeding investigate liver pathology and function, and the anatomical patency of the liver blood supply using ultrasound and Doppler angiography.

8 If variceal bleeding persists despite all the conservative measures, consider performing a transjugular intrahepatic portasystemic shunt (TIPSS). This is performed in the radiology suite by a specialist interventional radiologist. A transjugular catheter is passed from a major hepatic vein through liver parenchyma into a major branch of the portal vein. The track is then dilated by a forced balloon angioplasty and an expandable metallic stent 8–12 mm in diameter is placed along the track. This creates a portasystemic shunt and provides immediate decompression of the portal system. Problems associated with TIPSS resemble those following surgical shunts, including hepatic encephalopathy (20–40%) and progressive shunt occlusion. Where it is available, assess cirrhotic patients who receive a TIPSS as potential liver transplant recipients. Orthotopic (Greek: *orthos* = straight, right + *topos* = place; placed in the usual site) liver transplantation itself provides excellent portal decompression. However, it is rarely available following an emergency variceal bleed because of the need for an extensive preparation and also because there is a severe shortage of organs.

9 If TIPSS is not available, after resuscitation and full assessment, decide if a surgical procedure is required. This can be either a 'veno-occlusive' procedure designed to stop the venous haemorrhage, such as oesophageal disconnection or oesophagogastric devascularization, or a 'portal decompression' procedure, namely a portasystemic shunt.

KEY POINTS Select a procedure within your expertise and available facilities

- Initially prefer a veno-occlusive technique which carries less risk than other procedures. The exact choice of technique depends on your expertise and facilities. It is better to attempt to stop the bleeding initially by a veno-occlusive technique.
- Emergency portal decompression is associated with a 50% mortality rate and a 40% chance of portasystemic encephalopathy in survivors.
- Bleeding from gastric fundal varices is difficult to control by sclerotherapy or banding and, if TIPSS is not possible, operation remains the only effective treatment.

OESOPHAGOGASTRIC DISCONNECTION

Appraise

- The portal vessels feeding the varices or the varices themselves can be ligated by a variety of thoracic or abdominal surgical approaches. When emergency control of variceal bleeding is required after failed endoscopic sclerotherapy/ligation, a simple and effective way of doing this is oesophagogastric disconnection and re-anastomosis using a circular stapling device (EEA Autosuture, or Proximate ILS Ethicon). If a stapler is not available it is possible to achieve the same effect by transection and sutured re-anastomosis but this is a difficult procedure. The transaction is best performed leaving a cuff of 1 cm of stomach attached to the oesophagus, since the gastric wall holds sutures more securely than the oesophageal wall. If you encounter concomitant bleeding from gastric fundal varices that stapled disconnection alone will not control, a more extensive devascularization procedure is indicated.
- Oesophagogastric devascularization may be performed electively to prevent recurrent variceal re-bleeding:
    i. When extrahepatic portal hypertension involves thrombosis of splenic and mesenteric veins so there are no suitable veins into which the portal system can be shunted.
    ii. In schistosomiasis, in which there is mild liver dysfunction with splenomegaly and hypersplenism.
    iii. Where there exists a high probability of encephalopathy with a shunt.
- Oesophagogastric devascularization may be achieved by the Hassab procedure. The distal oesophagus is mobilized, all of its feeding vessels are ligated and disconnected. Splenectomy is carried out, the left gastric (coronary) vein is ligated, and the greater and lesser curves of the entire proximal stomach are devascularized. Sugiura described a more extensive operation which was originally performed as a two-stage procedure. Through a thoracotomy, the lower oesophagus is devascularized and oesophageal transaction carried out. After 6 weeks, through an abdominal approach, the stomach is devascularized, splenectomy carried out, followed by vagotomy and pyloroplasty. The procedure has now been modified to a one-stage transabdominal operation. The distal oesophagus is mobilized transhiatally and devascularized, followed by a stapled

transection, then gastric devascularization and splenectomy are performed.

- The technique to be described involves performing a stapled oesophagogastric disconnection in an emergency, together with the outline of a more extensive devascularization should it be necessary. It has been shown to be as safe as endoscopic sclerotherapy and may be slightly more effective in preventing rebleeding in the long term.[3]

KEY POINTS Future liver transplant recipient?

- Before undertaking any surgical procedure involving a laparotomy, and especially any dissection in the region of the liver hilum, consider carefully the possibility that the patient may in due course need a liver transplant.
- Try not to jeopardize this by generating vascular adhesions.

Prepare

1 This procedure, designed to occlude all veins filling the oesophageal plexus from below, is best carried out using a mechanical circular stapling instrument such as EEA Autosuture or Proximate ILS Ethicon. Have available disposable circular stapling instruments (sizes 25, 28 and 31 or similar) and the accompanying measuring bougies.

2 Have the anaesthetist give a single prophylactic intravenous injection of a cephalosporin and metronidazole at the start of the operation.

Access

1 Rotate the patient slightly to the right with wedges placed under the left shoulder and left side of pelvis.

2 Use a left subcostal incision 3 cm below the costal margin.

Assess

1 Aspirate ascitic fluid from the peritoneal cavity and measure the volume carefully. This helps you to calculate subsequent fluid replacement. Replace it with an adequate volume of colloid, preferably albumin, not with crystalloid solution.

2 Carry out a general exploration and perform a liver biopsy if histological diagnosis of the liver disease is in doubt.

Action

1 Identify the oesophagogastric junction by palpation after the anaesthetist has passed a nasogastric tube.

2 Gently retract the left lobe of the liver from this region using a Deaver retractor.

3 Incise the peritoneum in front of the lower end of the oesophagus, coagulate any bleeding vessels and gently pass a finger behind the oesophagus and immediate peri-oesophageal tissues. Encircle these structures with a tape.

4 Extend the oesophageal mobilization proximally and distally until you can easily pass two fingers around the whole of the lower oesophagus. You do not need to separately identify the vagi unless they prevent adequate mobilization, in which case exclude them from the mobilized tissues.

5 Make a vertical gastrotomy in the anterior stomach wall 10–15 cm from the oesophagogastric junction and insert through this one of the measuring bougies. Start with the 31-mm bougie and introduce it into the lower oesophagus to ensure that the lumen is large enough to accommodate it and thus the 31-mm staple instrument. It usually passes easily but, if not, do not force; instead try one of the smaller ones.

6 Unpack and remove the staple gun of the same size.

7 Remove the tape from the lower oesophagus and replace it with a stout thread ligature.

8 Pass a finger through the gastrotomy and into the lumen of the lower oesophagus. Have the anaesthetist slowly withdraw the nasogastric tube until the tip just disappears proximally up the oesophagus.

9 Pass the well-lubricated head of the selected staple gun into the lower oesophagus and separate the anvil from the staple cartridge by adjusting the screw on the handle. Have an assistant steady the instrument and palpate the groove between the separated head and anvil through the wall of the oesophagus.

10 Tie the thread ligature firmly in this groove and cut the ends (Fig. 22.5a). It takes time to ensure that the ligature is firmly tied.

11 While protecting the lower end of the oesophagus with a hand placed around it, tighten the screw to bring the staple cartridge and anvil together. Check the mobility of the lower oesophagus and actuate the staple instrument. Carry out this manoeuvre very gently and carefully to avoid damaging the lower oesophagus which is usually very delicate, especially following recent endoscopic sclerotherapy.

12 Unscrew the nut in the handle of the instrument by two turns to slightly separate anvil from staple cartridge. Firmly hold the lower oesophagus and, with a gentle twisting motion, remove the instrument via the gastrotomy.

13 Place a large pack into the upper peritoneal cavity in the region of the transection while you inspect the instrument. Separate the anvil and staple cartridge, remove the anvil and the plastic ring. Within the circular knife blade you will find the resected portion of oesophagus. Remove this and ensure that a complete 'doughnut' of oesophageal wall has been obtained (Fig. 22.5b).

? DIFFICULTY 22.2

1. If the doughnut is incomplete, it means that there is a portion of the oesophageal wall that has not been adequately stapled, and patent varices may still be present.
2. When you remove the pack from the upper abdomen, bleeding may not be fully controlled. If so, carefully inspect the anastomosis to identify where the transection is incomplete, or determine the site of bleeding.
3. In both cases insert some additional mattress sutures of Vicryl through the entire thickness of the oesophageal wall to control bleeding from any remaining vessels and seal the anastomosis. If the transection is complete the area will be dry.

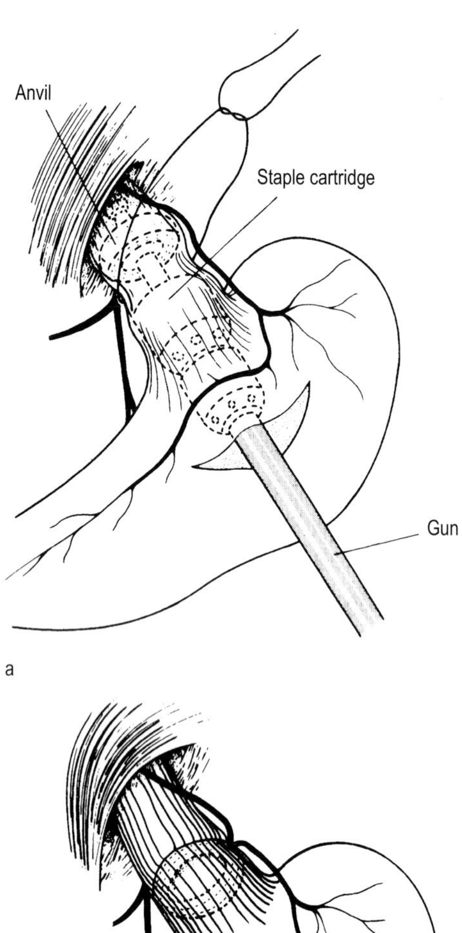

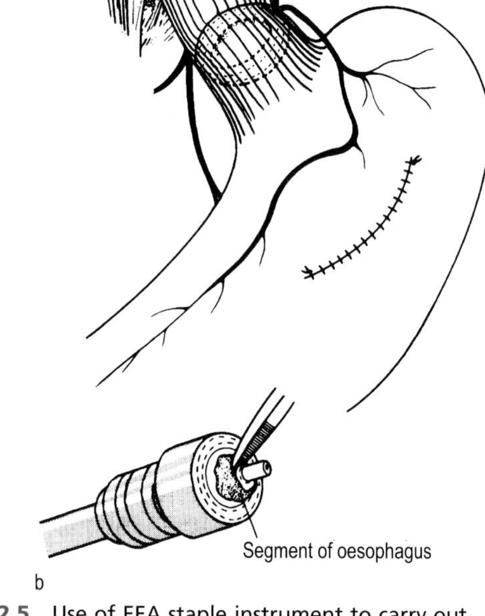

Fig. 22.5 Use of EEA staple instrument to carry out oesophagogastric transection: (a) the instrument is passed into the lower oesophagus, the staple cartridge and anvil are separated and a ligature is tied around the entire oesophagus in the groove between the two; (b) after firing the gun the instrument is removed.

14 Pass a finger through the gastrotomy into the lower oesophagus across the line of transection, have the anaesthetist slowly re-pass the nasogastric tube and, with your finger, guide it back into the lumen of the stomach.

15 Close the gastrotomy in one or two layers with absorbable sutures.

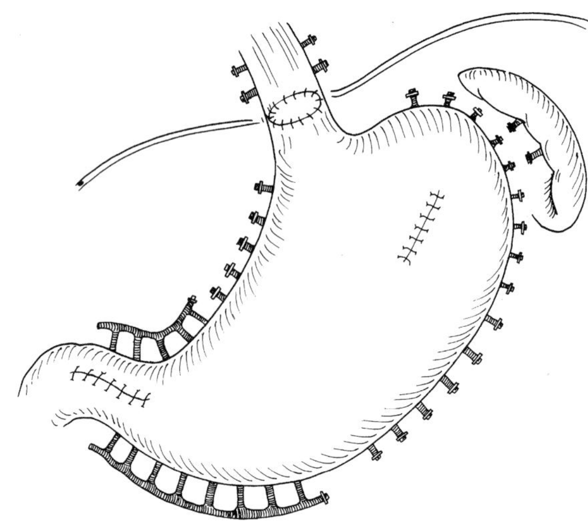

Fig. 22.6 Oesophagogastric devascularization.

16 If there is bleeding from fundal varices, undersew them or carry out gastric devascularization coupled with splenectomy (Fig. 22.6). Mobilize the spleen as for splenectomy (see Ch. 23). Ligate and divide the vessels in the splenic pedicle. Identify, dissect, ligate and divide all the short gastric vessels between the greater curvature of the stomach and the spleen. Remove the spleen. Check the rest of the greater curvature of the stomach and dissect, ligate and divide any remaining vessels between it and the diaphragm. On the lesser curve of the stomach identify, ligate and divide any vessels passing to it from the lesser omentum. Continue this dissection down to the region of the antrum. The entire proximal stomach should now be separated from any feeding vessels along its greater and lesser curves. Fortunately, the internal vascularization of the stomach is almost always adequate to prevent any avascular necrosis.

Closure

1 Flush the area gently with 2–3 litres of warm saline.

2 Close the abdominal incision en masse in the usual way without drainage.

Postoperative

1 Since the stomach has been opened and the contents have flooded the peritoneal cavity despite the saline toilet, continue the prophylactic antibiotic regimen started with the operation for 3 days afterwards.

2 Arrange initial management in an intensive care unit with the help of medical hepatologists (see section on aftercare following liver trauma and liver resection).

REFERENCES

1. Stanley AJ, Hayes PC 1997 Portal hypertension and variceal haemorrhage. Lancet 350:1235–1239
2. Sherlock S, Dooley J 2001 Diseases of the liver and biliary system, 11th edn. Blackwell Science, Oxford
3. Burroughs AK, Hamilton G, Phillips A et al 1989 A comparison of sclerotherapy with staple transection of the oesophagus for the emergency control of bleeding from esophageal varices. New England Journal of Medicine 321:857–862

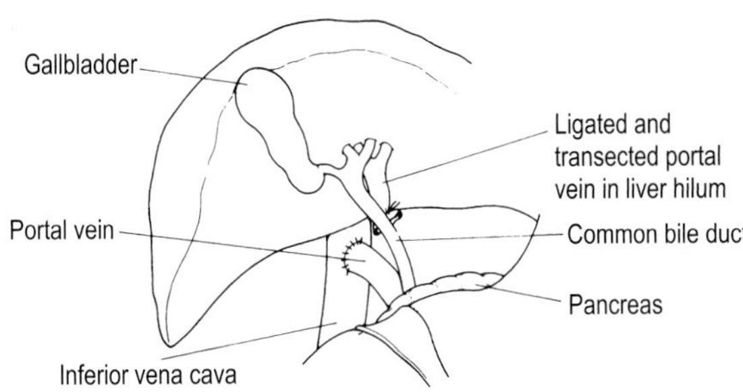

Fig. 22.7 End-to-side portacaval shunt.

PORTAL DECOMPRESSION

Appraise

- Portal decompression can be portacaval, which may be end-to-side or side-to-side (Fig. 22.7), mesocaval, which may be side-to-side or with a synthetic PTFE 'H' graft (Fig. 22.8a), proximal splenorenal (Fig. 22.8b) or distal splenorenal (Fig. 22.8c). The last one, also known as the Warren shunt, is called a 'selective' shunt, as it decompresses only the varix-bearing area of the portal bed. There is no evidence to suggest that any one operation is in the long term any better than any of the others, so choose the one with which you have had most experience. In poor-risk patients perioperative mortality is 50%; in good-risk patients, around 5%.
- The incidence of the major complication, portasystemic encephalopathy, is similar (20–40% over 1 year) after any of these operations, although it may be less in the early days following the Warren shunt and perhaps following the small-diameter mesocaval shunt.
- A problem with all shunts is that they are liable to occlude.
- Do not attempt portal decompression without full preoperative investigations, including consultation with an experienced hepatologist. Investigate liver function, identify the nature of the liver pathology and the vascular anatomy. This means that it is rarely a procedure that can be entertained in an emergency. Patients who tolerate this operation well with minimal encephalopathy are those with good liver function, such as patients with portal vein occlusion, primary biliary cirrhosis or hepatic fibrosis. Do not undertake a shunt operation lightly; there is a risk of encephalopathy and consequent intellectual impairment.

5 Shunt procedures are carried out infrequently now since patients with poor liver function and bleeding oesophageal varices are often candidates for TIPSS in the first instance and liver transplantation in the long term. Therefore the description will be limited to the traditional end-to-side portacaval shunt.

PORTACAVAL SHUNT

Appraise

- This is the time-honoured operation for achieving portal decompression, although it is now rarely performed. It shunts all the portal blood into the infrahepatic vena cava, totally reduces the portal hypertension and stops bleeding from oesophageal varices.

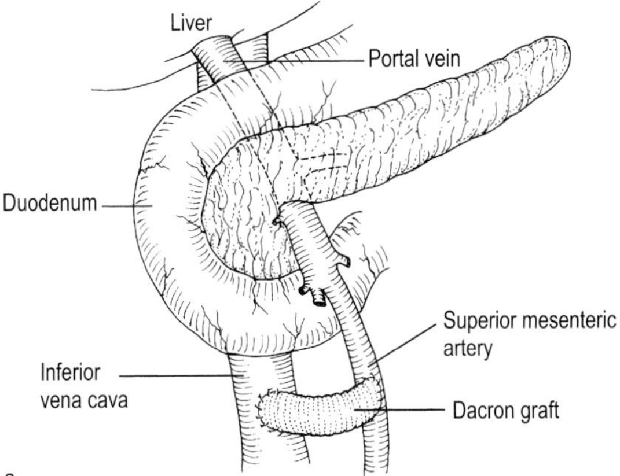

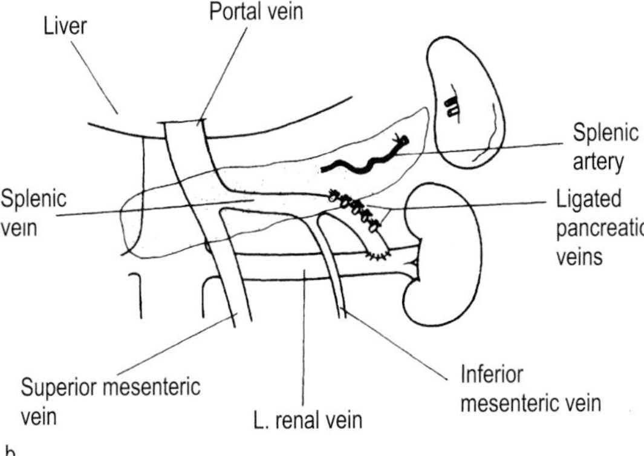

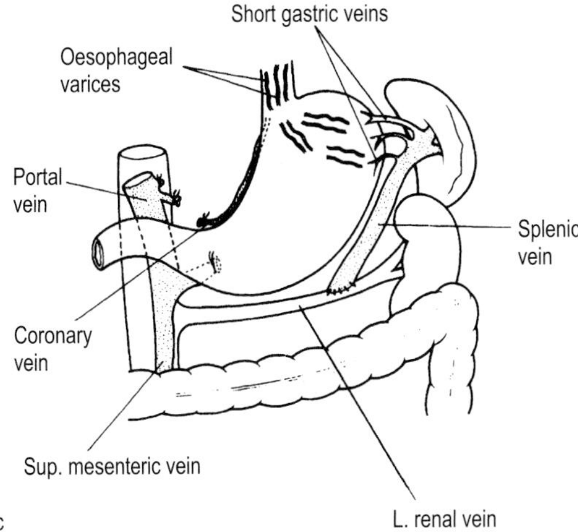

Fig. 22.8 Mesocaval and splenorenal shunts: (a) Drapanas 'H' mesocaval shunt; (b) proximal splenorenal shunt; (c) Warren distal splenorenal shunt.

- The problems are:
  - i. There is a high incidence (30–40%) of portasystemic encephalopathy.
  - ii. The operation involves extensive dissection of the liver hilum, which may make subsequent liver transplantation difficult.
- It is still a very useful operation for treating portal hypertension in patients with good liver cell function.

Prepare

1 Preoperative hepatic angiography is mandatory. Especially, you must have good images of the splenic, superior mesenteric and portal veins.

2 Correct any electrolyte or blood clotting imbalance preoperatively. Order 6 units of blood, some FFP and platelets, and warn the blood bank that you may need more.

3 Have available vascular instruments and sutures.

Access

1 Place the patient supine on the operating table with sandbags under the right shoulder and pelvis to rotate the patient slightly towards the left.

2 Use a right subcostal incision 4 cm below the costal margin and extending from the left costal margin to the right mid-axillary line.

Assess

1 Aspirate and measure the volume of any ascitic fluid. This helps in calculating the postoperative fluid requirements.

2 Thoroughly explore the abdomen to exclude any incidental serious intra-abdominal pathology that may make you review the decision to perform a portacaval shunt.

3 If histological assessment of the liver pathology has not been made, take a liver biopsy.

Action

1 Mobilize and retract distally the hepatic flexure of the colon. Mobilize the duodenum using Kocher's manoeuvre by dividing the peritoneal reflection between it and the posterior abdominal wall. Identify and expose the IVC below the liver. There are usually dilated portasystemic venous anastomotic vessels in this tissue, which may require individual ligation. Diathermy coagulation alone is frequently inadequate to secure haemostasis.

2 Incise the edge of the hepatoduodenal ligament between liver and duodenum and identify the portal vein behind the common bile duct.

3 Dissect the portal vein free of attachments from its origin up to its bifurcation. There are frequently one or two branches entering it from the pancreas. Doubly ligate and divide them. You can gain extra length by gently dissecting the vessel from the pancreas. During this dissection retract the common bile duct anteriorly and to the left, taking care not to damage the blood supply to its wall.

4 Pass a tape around the portal vein.

5 Dissect the anterior surface of the IVC from the suprarenal vein to the lower edge of the liver.

6 Clamp the portal vein just above the pancreas with a Satinsky or DeBakey clamp.

7 Encircle the hepatic end of the portal vein with a stout ligature or preferably a suture-ligature, and tie it firmly. Transect the portal vein cleanly, immediately below this ligature. Flush the now collapsed segment of portal vein distal to the clamp with a solution of heparin 1:500 000 in physiological saline.

8 Draw the vein to the IVC. Apply a Satinsky clamp to the anterior surface of the IVC without totally occluding the lumen.

9 Trim the end of the portal vein obliquely so that it will join the anterior wall of the IVC in a gentle curve without kinking.

10 Remove an oval segment of the anterior wall of the IVC the same size as the oblique cut end of the portal vein.

11 Using standard vascular anastomotic techniques, suture the end of the portal vein to the side of the IVC with 4/0 polypropylene or similar vascular suture material. Just before completing the anastomosis flush the lumen of the portal vein and the occluded segment of the IVC with heparinized saline.

12 Complete the anastomosis. Remove the clamp on the IVC followed by the clamp on the portal vein.

Check

1 Confirm a good flow through the shunt by feeling for a venous thrill or preferably by observing a measured fall in portal pressure when the clamps are removed. It should be only slightly higher than the IVC pressure.

2 Check that haemostasis is complete.

Closure

1 Close the abdominal wall in a standard manner, without drainage.

2 For a description of other portasystemic shunts, refer to Blumgart.[1]

Postoperative

Because the liver loses part of its vascular inflow, a degree of hepatic decompensation may develop. To anticipate and manage this:

- Manage the patient initially in the intensive care unit with help from an expert medical hepatologist.
- Maintain accurate water, electrolyte and colloid balance and correct abnormal clotting.
- Take steps to prevent or control hepatic encephalopathy. In consultation with the hepatologist prescribe twice-daily phosphate enemas to keep the colon empty, and oral lactulose or lactitol when gastrointestinal activity returns, at a dose producing one or two soft motions a day. Restrict protein intake, starting at 20 g/day and increasing by 10 g every second day. Patients with chronic encephalopathy will probably tolerate no more than 40–60 g/day. In some severe cases of portasystemic encephalopathy the patient needs additional oral non-absorbed antibiotics such as neomycin 1 g four times a day for a week.

REFERENCE

1. Blumgart LH, Fong Y (eds) 2000 Surgery of the liver and biliary tract, 3rd edn. Harcourt, London, pp 1799–2030

MANAGEMENT OF ASCITES

- The management of ascites is mainly medical, and consists of a low-sodium diet, fluid restriction, diuretics and concomitant potassium replacement if necessary. Paracentesis with colloid replacement is the next step if medical management does not succeed. Monitor progress by weighing the patient daily, measuring urine volume and checking for electrolyte imbalances, azotaemia and encephalopathy. If repeated paracentesis proves difficult, consider ordering a TIPSS procedure.
- Another option is a surgical peritoneovenous shunt (LeVeen shunt). This involves placement of a tube extending from the peritoneal cavity to the jugular vein through a subcutaneous track in the anterior chest wall; interposed in the tube is a one-way valve that opens only to pressure exceeding 2–4 cmH_2O and allows drainage of ascitic fluid into the circulation. The Denver version of the shunt has a pumping mechanism within the valve. A peritoneovenous shunt is indicated only in cirrhotic patients with intractable ascites unresponsive to medical therapy. Contraindications include very poor liver function with encephalopathy, infected ascites, coagulopathy and cardiac failure. Complications are common with peritoneovenous shunts, and include shunt blockage, infection, thrombocytopenia and occasionally disseminated intravascular coagulation. The operation is rarely performed these days.

23

Spleen

R.C.N. Williamson, A.K. Kakkar

CONTENTS

ELECTIVE SPLENECTOMY

Appraise

- The spleen is an important organ. Do not lightly remove it. It has haematological functions in the maturation of red blood cells and the destruction of effete forms. Of greater importance in surgical practice, it has certain immunological functions, notably production of opsonins (tuftsin, properdin) for the phagocytosis of encapsulated bacteria. When possible, conserve at least part of the spleen, as opposed to total splenectomy. This may protect against serious post-splenectomy sepsis (see below). *Streptococcus pneumoniae* is the most common infecting organism, less commonly *Neisseria meningitidis* and *Haemophilus influenzae*.
- Elective splenectomy may be indicated for certain lymphomas and leukaemias, for haemolytic anaemias such as acquired autoimmune, hereditary spherocytosis, for idiopathic thrombocytopenic purpura, for other types of splenomegaly with hypersplenism and occasionally for conditions such as cyst, abscess, haemangioma or splenic artery aneurysm.
- Splenectomy is sometimes carried out as a part of other operations, such as total gastrectomy, radical proximal gastrectomy, distal pancreatectomy and 'conventional' splenorenal shunt.
- Before the advent of computed tomography (CT), staging laparotomy played an important role in determining the extent of intra-abdominal disease in patients with Hodgkin's lymphoma. The increasing use of combination chemotherapy has reduced the need for precise staging, although it is occasionally needed for those who might be treated with radiotherapy alone. Staging laparotomy entails splenectomy, multiple liver biopsies and sampling of any palpable lymph nodes.
- An alternative to elective open splenectomy is laparoscopic splenectomy. The indications are identical for each approach; the operative method is described in Chapter 24.

Prepare

1. Patients with hypersplenism, anaemia, thrombocytopenia and coagulopathies require preoperative correction. Arrange for immunocompromised patients to receive prophylactic antibiotic cover.
2. Risk of post-splenectomy sepsis necessitates prophylactic immunization against *Streptococcus pneumoniae, Haemophilus influenzae* type b and meningococcal strains A and C. Organize vaccination 3–4 weeks before operation, except in children under the age of 2 years or those who are immunocompromised, such as patients with Hodgkin's disease who have received extensive chemotherapy.
3. Make sure that, in obtaining informed consent from the patient, you have included advice on the risks of post-splenectomy sepsis.

Access

1. As a rule make an upper midline, left upper paramedian or left subcostal incision.
2. When removing a very large spleen a left thoracoabdominal approach often facilitates the procedure.
3. Use a long midline incision when carrying out a staging laparotomy.

Assess

1. Explore the whole abdomen, particularly noting the liver and any enlarged lymph nodes. Take appropriate biopsies.
2. Make a careful search for accessory spleens (splenunculi). These are usually to be found near the splenic hilum, in the gastrosplenic ligament or greater omentum. Remove all splenunculi if you are performing splenectomy for a blood dyscrasia.

Action

1. If the spleen is enormous, first tie the splenic artery in continuity (Fig. 23.1). Enter the lesser sac by dividing 8–10 cm of greater omentum between ligatures, keeping to the colic side of the gastroepiploic vessels. Divide the adhesions between the back of the stomach and the front of the pancreas. Palpate along the superior border of the body of pancreas for arterial pulsation. Incise the peritoneum at this point, mobilize the vessel with right-angled forceps and ligate it with 0 or 1 silk.

KEY POINT Reduce the size of a very large spleen

- Consider injecting 1 ml of 1:10 000 adrenaline (epinephrine) into the splenic artery immediately before ligating it. This can shrink the size of a massive spleen and facilitate the subsequent dissection.

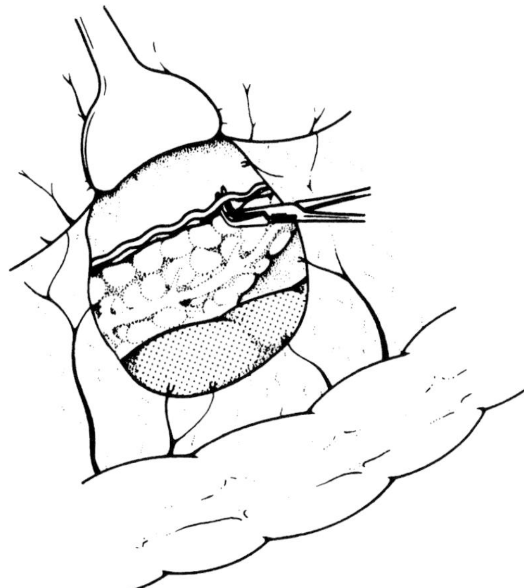

Fig. 23.1 Ligation of the splenic artery at the superior border of the body of pancreas. Part of the greater omentum has been divided, allowing access to the lesser sac.

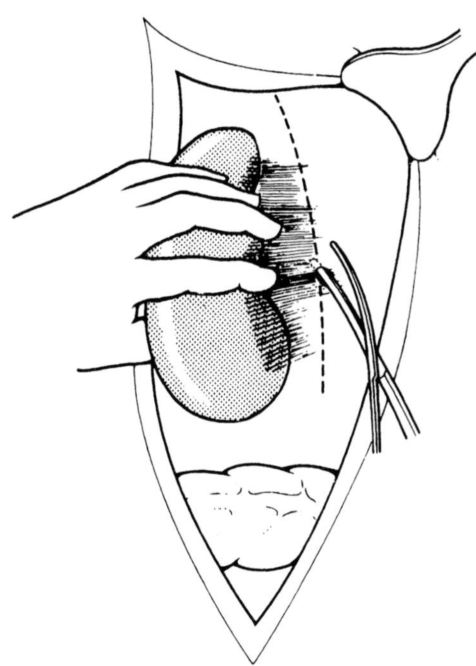

Fig. 23.2 Division of the left peritoneal leaf of the lienorenal ligament as a preliminary to mobilization of the spleen.

2 Pass your left hand over the top of the spleen to draw it medially, and have the left side of the abdominal wall retracted. Coagulate and divide any adhesions between the convex surface of the spleen and the parietal peritoneum.

3 Swab any blood from the groove behind the spleen, then cut through the peritoneum just lateral to the spleen; this is the left leaf of the lienorenal ligament, slitting it upwards and downwards (Fig. 23.2).

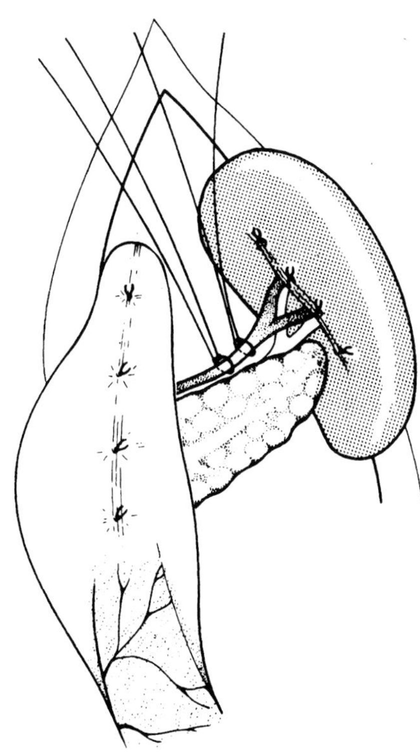

Fig. 23.3 Exposure of the splenic artery and vein after prior division of the gastrosplenic ligament. Two ligatures have been passed around the splenic artery.

4 Gently mobilize the spleen forwards and medially, using the fingers of your left hand. Identify the left colic flexure and free it from the spleen. Identify the tail of pancreas as it turns forwards into the splenic hilum, and gently dissect it free. Place a pack in the splenic bed while you complete the splenectomy.

5 Proceed to free the spleen from its attachments to the diaphragm (avascular) and greater curvature of the stomach, containing the vasa brevia. Carefully incise the anterior peritoneal leaf of the gastrosplenic ligament. Identify, ligate and divide the short gastric vessels, taking care not to include any of the stomach wall in the ligatures. Sometimes it is easier to delay this manoeuvre until you have dealt with the splenic artery and vein.

6 Control the vascular pedicle of the spleen between fingers and thumb and dissect away the fatty tissue to expose the splenic artery and vein (Fig. 23.3). Doubly clamp, ligate and divide each vessel. Be careful not to injure the tail of pancreas at this point. After dividing the remaining peritoneal attachments—the right leaf of the lienorenal ligament—you can remove the spleen. Platelet transfusions may now be given in thrombocytopenic patients.

7 Place a pack in the splenic bed, then remove the pack and obtain haemostasis.

KEY POINT Gastric injury?

- In dividing and ligating the short gastric vessels during splenic mobilization, take care not to include any of the stomach wall within the sutures. Otherwise you may risk causing a gastric fistula.

? DIFFICULTY

1. Especially with a massive spleen (larger than 1.5 kg), you may encounter troublesome bleeding from vascular adhesions to the diaphragm or parenchymal tears.
2. Enlarge the incision or ligate the splenic artery above the pancreas to improve control. Alternatively, mobilize the spleen and bring it up to the surface as soon as possible.
3. Improve the exposure by having an assistant strongly retract the left costal margin.

Closure

1 Remove the pack, inspect the splenic bed and coagulate any oozing vessels.

2 Examine the ligatures on the main vascular pedicles.

3 Make sure that the adjacent viscera are undamaged.

4 Place a suction drain in the splenic bed. If there is an enormous cavity or if the stomach or pancreas have been wounded, prefer a wide-bore tube drain.

5 Consider nasogastric intubation for 24–28 hours.

Aftercare

1 Remove the nasogastric tube when gastric aspirates diminish and the patient passes flatus.

2 Remove the drain when the discharge has almost ceased

3 Check the blood haemoglobin, white cell and platelet counts postoperatively. Leucocytosis and thrombocythaemia nearly always ensue, with peaks at 7–14 days. Persistent leucocytosis and pyrexia suggest the possibility of a subphrenic abscess.

4 Consider some form of prophylactic anticoagulation if the platelet count exceeds 1000×10^9 per litre.

5 If you have previously overlooked it, start immunization with anti-pneumococcal vaccine. Children should receive prophylactic penicillin for 2 years to prevent post-splenectomy sepsis. Advise adults to take an antibiotic such as amoxicillin at the first sign of any infective illness. Immunocompromised patients should receive either penicillin V (250 mg b.d.) or amoxicillin (250 mg o.d.) as routine prophylaxis against post-splenectomy sepsis.

Complications

1 *Respiratory.* Chest infection may result from splinting of the left diaphragm causing atelectasis. You may avoid the need to give antibiotics if the patient receives vigorous physiotherapy. Occasionally a left pleural effusion requires aspiration.

2 Suspect subphrenic abscess if there is fever and leucocytosis. Ultrasonography will confirm the diagnosis and permit percutaneous drainage.

3 Reactive haemorrhage may be caused by a slipped ligature, necessitating re-operation.

4 Gastric or pancreatic fistula is rare. It may close with conservative management including parenteral nutrition, but otherwise re-operate to deal with it.

Developments

Radiofrequency ablative techniques to perform partial splenic resection have recently been described, but their use requires specialist equipment that is not routinely available.

EMERGENCY SPLENECTOMY

Appraise

- Emergency splenectomy may be indicated for traumatic rupture. Enlarged spleens are at increased risk of rupture, which may even occur spontaneously. Most cases of ruptured spleen follow road traffic accidents.
- Classically, patients are shocked, with pain in the left hypochondrium and shoulder-tip and with evidence of left lower rib fractures. Diagnostic paracentesis may confirm a haemoperitoneum, and urgent laparotomy is normally required after initial resuscitation.
- Some minor splenic injuries can be managed conservatively with vigilant clinical observation and blood transfusion. Appropriate patients are less than 60 years of age, haemodynamically stable, with a blood transfusion requirement not exceeding 3–4 units and computed tomography (CT) scan evidence that the spleen has not been fragmented. Failure of conservative treatment is indicated by renewed evidence of bleeding or spreading peritonism. In this case carry out laparotomy.
- Accidental splenic injury sustained during operations such as vagotomy or left hemicolectomy was formerly an indication for splenectomy, but the bleeding can usually be controlled by lesser means (see below).

Access

1 Use a midline upper abdominal incision.

2 Do not hesitate to make a T-shaped extension towards the left costal margin if access is difficult and the patient is exsanguinating.

Assess

1 First check that a ruptured spleen is the source of bleeding. It is often easier to feel than to see whether the spleen is intact.

2 Remove or repair a ruptured spleen without further ado, postponing exploration of the rest of the abdomen until later.

3 Particularly in young children try to avoid total splenectomy if at all possible, because they are at particular risk of post-splenectomy sepsis. If the spleen is shattered or bleeding profusely, however, you have no alternative but to remove it promptly to save life.

Action

1 Quickly but carefully mobilize the spleen and bring it forwards into the abdominal wound. In ruptured spleen it is often pos-

sible to break down the left peritoneal leaf of the lienorenal ligament using your fingers. If splenic repair is at all likely, however, try to avoid further injury to the spleen during this manoeuvre.

2 Once the spleen has been brought up into the wound, compress its vascular pedicle between finger and thumb to control the bleeding. Inspect the organ thoroughly and assess the extent of damage.

3 If total splenectomy is inevitable, proceed as for an elective operation, securing the splenic artery and vein at an early stage. Consider placing thin slices of splenic tissue in omental pockets at the end of the operation to encourage splenic regeneration (splenosis). Conservative splenic operations are described later in this chapter.

KEY POINTS Obtain good exposure

- In emergency splenectomy a good view is essential.
- Have the left costal margin lifted by a retractor.
- Scoop and suck blood and clot from the left hypochondrium.
- Control the splenic hilar vessels with your hand if necessary to stop bleeding.

? DIFFICULTY

1. *The patient is bleeding to death from the spleen, but you cannot identify the precise source of haemorrhage.* There may not be time to summon senior help. Consider extending the incision as described. Place your hand over the top of the spleen, break down its posterior attachments and deliver it into the wound as quickly as possible. Now compress or clamp the pedicle, and you will bring the situation under control.
2. *You have inadvertently injured the stomach or pancreas during splenectomy*, usually because of inadequate mobilization of the spleen. Remove the spleen and place a pack in the splenic bed. Inspect the damage carefully. Repair a gastric defect in two layers. Repair or resect the tail of pancreas, using non-absorbable sutures. Ask the anaesthetist to insert a nasogastric tube. Drain the splenic bed.

Closure, aftercare and complications

These are essentially the same as for elective splenectomy. Give triple vaccine immunization during the recovery period plus prophylactic penicillin as an additional precaution in children or the immunocompromised.

CONSERVATIVE SPLENIC SURGERY

Appraise

- Following splenectomy there is a 1.0–2.5% risk of developing overwhelming septicaemia from encapsulated bacteria, especially the pneumococcus, usually within 2 years of operation.

TABLE 23.1 A grading system for splenic trauma

Grade	Injury	Action
I	Capsular injury not actively bleeding	No intervention
II	Capsular or minor parenchymal injury	Topical haemostatic agents
III	Moderate parenchymal injury	Suturing and haemostatic agents
IV	Severe parenchymal injury	Partial splenic resection
V	Extensive injury	Splenectomy

The mortality rate of post-splenectomy sepsis is high. The risk is higher in young children and after splenectomy for haematological disease, but fatal cases have occasionally been reported in adults after removal of a ruptured spleen.

- Non-operative management may be appropriate for lesser degrees of splenic injury, especially in children. Embolization therapy has been attempted in hypersplenism. With these exceptions, alternatives to total splenectomy can be assessed only at laparotomy, but they may be feasible in at least 40% of patients with blunt splenic trauma.
- Anatomically, there are between three and seven well-defined splenic segments, each with an independent blood supply. Thus partial splenectomy is a practical proposition.
- A grading system for splenic trauma is summarized in Table 23.1.

Assess

1 At operation for abdominal trauma, remove forthwith a spleen that is either fragmented or avulsed from its vascular pedicle. Under these circumstances consider autotransplantation of some splenic pulp into the peritoneal cavity (see above). If the extent of damage and bleeding is less severe, gently mobilize the spleen into the wound after dividing its peritoneal attachments. Remove attached clot and examine the organ thoroughly. Decide whether topical haemostatic agents, partial splenectomy or some form of splenic repair (splenorrhaphy; Greek: *rhaphe*= a seam) might be feasible, with or without ligation of the splenic artery or its branches.

2 Capsular tears and other minor injuries to the spleen inadvertently sustained at operation seldom necessitate splenectomy. Retract or extend the incision adequately to inspect the spleen without mobilizing it. Application of a haemostatic agent usually suffices, with or without suturing.

3 Remove the spleen along with adjacent viscera, either to widen the extent of lymph-node clearance, as in gastrectomy for cancer, or for technical reasons, as in distal pancreatectomy or 'conventional' splenorenal shunt. Make sure that these indications are relevant in each individual case.

4 Removal of the entire organ can sometimes be avoided in certain elective operations on the spleen. Thus marsupialization

(Greek: *marsyppion*=a pouch) may be adequate for congenital splenic cysts and segmental splenectomy for tropical splenomegaly.

Action

1 To avoid the need for splenectomy try applying haemostatic applications to superficial lacerations of the capsule or splenic pulp. Full mobilization of the spleen is unnecessary if the damaged area is accessible, but use suction to obtain a clear view. Fibrin glue may be sprayed over the injured site or injected into a splenic laceration. Apply an appropriate disc of gelatin sponge to the laceration and maintain light pressure until the sponge soaks up the blood and becomes adherent. Alternatively, sprinkle some microfibrillar collagen powder over the site of injury. Gently pack off the area and leave if for 5–10 minutes before checking that you have achieved haemostasis.

2 Deeper or more extensive lacerations may still be suitable for repair. Mobilize the spleen, at least in part. As in operations on the liver, use synthetic absorbable sutures swaged on to a long blunt needle. Take deep bites of splenic tissue on either side of the tear, and tie the sutures snugly. Use omentum or Teflon buttresses to prevent the stitches cutting through (Fig. 23.4a), together with a topical haemostatic agent to control surface bleeding. Alternatively, wrap the organ in an absorbable polyglycolic acid mesh. Consider ligating the splenic artery along the superior border of the pancreas.

3 For partial splenectomy, fully mobilize the organ and carefully dissect in the splenic hilum to identify and ligate the segmental arteries and veins. Then incise the capsule at the point chosen for transection of the organ and use a finger-fracture technique to resect the upper or lower pole (Fig. 23.4b). Secure haemostasis by means of synthetic absorbable sutures.

? DIFFICULTY

1. If bleeding continues despite these endeavours, you should probably proceed to total splenectomy.
2. Be sure to leave a drain to the area of the spleen following conservative operations.

Aftercare

1 Monitor the haemoglobin level and remove the drain when it ceases to function. Splenic size and function can be checked by serial scintiscans and haematological investigations.

2 Immunological function after splenorrhaphy or partial splenectomy is uncertain, so prophylactic measures should probably be taken against post-splenectomy sepsis (see above).

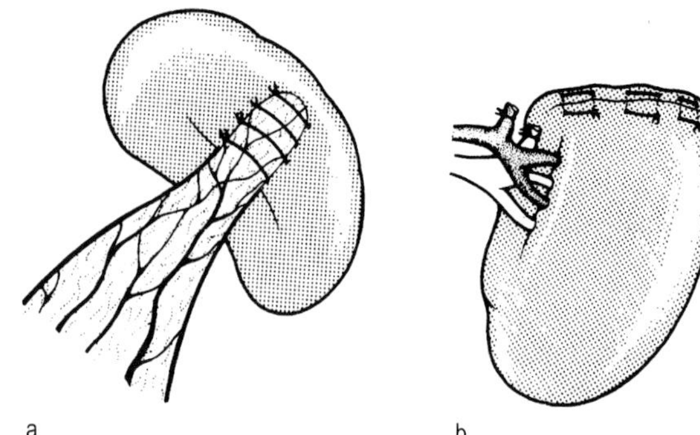

Fig. 23.4 Alternatives to total splenectomy: (a) a laceration of the splenic pulp has been sutured over a tongue of greater omentum; (b) resection of the upper pole of the spleen with ligation of its feeding vessels.

FURTHER READING

Büjükünal C, Danismend N, Yeker D 1987 Spleen-saving procedures in paediatric splenic trauma. British Journal of Surgery 74:350–352

Clarke PJ, Morris PJ 1994 Surgery of the spleen. In: Morris PJ, Malt RA (eds) Oxford textbook of surgery. Oxford University Press, Oxford, pp 2121–2130

Cooper MJ, Williamson RCN 1983 Splenectomy: indications, hazards and alternatives. British Journal of Surgery 71:173–180

Dawson AA, Jones PF, King DJ 1987 Splenectomy in the management of haematological disease. British Journal of Surgery 74:353–357

Feliciano DV, Spjut-Patrinely V, Burch JM et al 1990 Splenorrhaphy. The alternative. Annals of Surgery 211:569–582

Gilchrist BF, Trunkey DD 1990 Injuries to the spleen and pancreas. In: Williamson RCN, Cooper MJ (eds) Emergency abdominal surgery. Churchill Livingstone, Edinburgh, pp 36–51

Habib NA, Spaulding D, Navarra G et al 2003 How we do a bloodless splenectomy. American Journal of Surgery 186:164–166

Holdsworth RJ, Irving AD, Cuschieri A 1991 Postsplenectomy sepsis and its mortality rate: actual versus perceived risks. British Journal of Surgery 78:1031–1038

Longo WE, Baker CC, McMillen MA et al 1989 Nonoperative management of adult blunt splenic trauma. Criteria for successful outcome. Annals of Surgery 210:626–629

Pachter HL, Spencer FC, Hofstetter SR 1990 Experience with selective operative and nonoperative treatment of splenic injuries in 193 patients. Annals of Surgery 211:583–591

Redmond HP, Redmond JM, Rooney BP et al 1989 Surgical anatomy of the human spleen. British Journal of Surgery 76:198–201

Shackford SR, Sise MJ, Virgilio R et al 1981 Evaluation of splenorrhaphy: a grading system for splenic trauma. Journal of Trauma 21:538–542

Shaw JHF, Clark M 1989 Splenectomy for massive splenomegaly. British Journal of Surgery 76:395–397

Velanovich V, Weaver M 2003 Partial splenectomy using a coupled saline–radiofrequency hemostatic device. American Journal of Surgery 185:66–68

Wilhelm MC, Jones RE, McGehee R et al 1988 Splenectomy in hematologic disorders. The everchanging indications. Annals of Surgery 207:581–589

24

Laparoscopic splenectomy

S.J. Nixon, A. Rajasekar

DESCRIPTION OF OPERATION

Appraise

- A laparoscopic approach is now accepted as the standard procedure for elective splenectomy. Technical developments and surgical experience have overcome most of the practical difficulties. Long-term follow-up of patients with idiopathic thrombocytopenic purpura (ITP) and autoimmune haemolytic anaemia, the two most common indications, have shown identical results to open operation. The short-term benefits of laparoscopic over open surgery are those seen in other areas.
- Several factors can add to the technical difficulty of the procedure. The spleen is located in the deep recess of the left subphrenic space. Adhesions may impede access and reduce splenic mobility, particularly at the posterior pole of the spleen. Proximity of the stomach, colon and pancreas can lead to accidental injury. Splenic capsular or vascular damage can result in rapid haemorrhage and loss of vision.
- The indications for laparoscopic splenectomy include ITP, which may be HIV-related, autoimmune haemolytic anaemia, hereditary spherocytosis, thalassaemia, malignancy and splenic cysts. Several studies have shown identical response rates in ITP.[1–4]
- There are no absolute contraindications to laparoscopic splenectomy and few relative contraindications. Gross obesity, peritoneal adhesions and the presence of inflammation add to the technical challenges. Many laparoscopic procedures have been successfully performed in pregnant women but there is no report of laparoscopic splenectomy. Splenectomy for splenic trauma has been reported. Rupture of splenic artery aneurysm during the dissection can be catastrophic. Spleen size is a major factor. Massive splenomegaly presents you with difficulties of access to the vessels lying beneath it, difficulty in manoeuvring the spleen due to its physical size and weight and problems with retrieval. In our view, a spleen that extends beyond a point half way between the costal margin and umbilicus is best removed by open operation. Preoperative intra-arterial embolization has been described in an attempt to reduce the splenic size and operative bleeding. Laparoscopic splenectomy has not been reported in cases of portal hypertension.
- Advantages include reduced pulmonary complications, less postoperative pain, early recovery of bowel function, reduced hospital stay and early return to normal activities. In patients with AIDS there may be less risk of exposure of theatre staff. Significant mortality has been reported following open splenectomy in patients with AIDS. Both patient and theatre staff may benefit from a minimal-access approach.
- Elective splenectomy is a relatively uncommon procedure. In our own area, with a population of 1 million, only 10 cases are referred annually. This limits learning and teaching of the procedure, and laparoscopic splenectomy should be performed by surgeons expert in the technique. With experience, total procedure time including anaesthesia has fallen to 90 minutes. Identification of accessory spleens may be less thorough than in open surgery but long-term results are the same.
- The rate of conversion to open splenectomy varies from 0% to 19%. Haemorrhage is the most common reason for conversion, followed by difficulty in mobilizing the spleen due to adhesions or spleen size, and injury to adjacent organs. The mortality and morbidity rate range from 0% to 6% and 5% to 20%, respectively.

Prepare

1 Give Pneumovax (Pasteur Mérieux, UK) 0.5 ml subcutaneously or intramuscularly 2 weeks prior to the operation. In an emergency, vaccinate the patient once fully recovered. Administer prophylactic antibiotics such as cephalosporin, at induction of anaesthesia.

2 Reserve packed red blood cells for all patients and platelets for thrombocytopenic patients. Preoperative medical therapy (e.g. IgG therapy or increasing steroids) may elevate platelet count transiently in ITP cases. Give parenteral steroid coverage in patients with ITP or other haematological disease on long-term corticosteroids. Involve the haematologist in the pre- and postoperative care of the patient. If the platelet count is low, transfuse platelets intraoperatively after division of hilar vessels to prevent rapid sequestration.

3 Obtain informed consent both for laparoscopic splenectomy and for open splenectomy. Inform the patient about overwhelming post-splenectomy infection (OPSI) and the importance of lifelong prophylactic antibiotics.

KEY POINTS Risks of overwhelming post-splenectomy infection

- In adults, the lifetime risk of OPSI is said to be less than being involved in a fatal traffic accident.
- In children the risk may be higher.

4 The operation of laparoscopic splenectomy is performed under general anaesthesia with endotracheal intubation. A nasogastric tube may be needed to decompress the stomach but is not routinely necessary.

5 When operating on HIV patients, take universal precautions by using double gloves, face shields, masks and disposable gowns.

6 There are two operative techniques described in the literature: the anterolateral approach, which we prefer, and the posterior approach. The anterolateral approach is associated with decreased operative time, postoperative stay, transfusion and the required number of trocars.[5]

KEY POINT Progressive learning

- Initially select patients with normal-sized spleens. Once adequate experience is gained, larger spleens can be removed safely.

Access

Anterolateral approach[6]

1 Place the patient supine with right lateral rotation, slightly head up, with a 10° break in the table and left arm elevated to provide exposure. Ensure that the patient is securely strapped to the table.

2 Avoid excessive forward rotation which causes the spleen to fall forwards towards you and impairs access, especially if the spleen is large.

3 Place the monitor at the head end, to the patient's left. Place the instrument tray at the left foot end. You and the camera operator/assistant all stand on the patient's right side.

4 Establish pneumoperitoneum and introduce a 10-mm cannula in the left mid-axillary line at the level of the umbilicus. Introduce a 0° or 30° telescope.

KEY POINTS Technical considerations

- Before inserting the accessory ports, assess the possibility of completing the procedure laparoscopically.
- Inserting a Veress needle in the mid-axillary line is surprisingly easy since the anterior and posterior rectus sheaths are clearly felt as the needle passes through.
- We initially described placing the telescope port at the umbilicus but a more lateral insertion improves vision, particularly of the lienorenal ligament.

5 Place two 5-mm cannulas 3 cm below the costal margin to form a triangle with the telescope port. When you are learning you may find it easier to use three ports, the exact mirror image of those for laparoscopic cholecystectomy (Fig. 24.1) which gives an additional port for retraction. In difficult cases introduce a 10-mm cannula in the epigastrium rather than the 5-mm cannula through which to introduce a large fan retractor. There may be a peritoneal reflection holding the splenic flexure of colon, so limiting access behind the spleen. Divide this before placing the lateral port.

6 Place a diathermy hook (or scissors) in the lateral port and an atraumatic grasper in the medial port (or two graspers if three ports have been used).

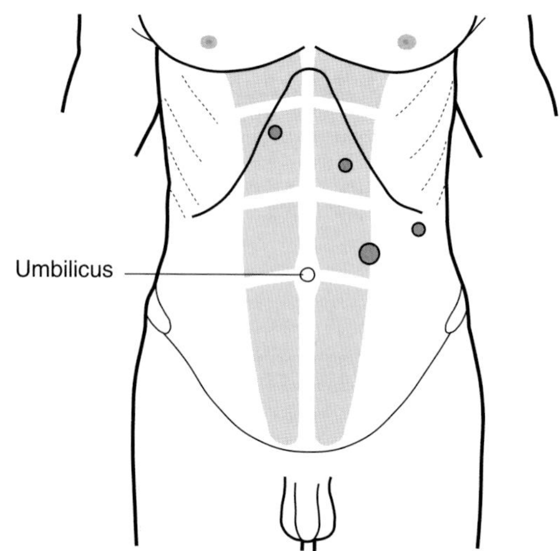

Fig. 24.1 Operating port positions for anterolateral approach laparoscopic splenectomy.

Assess

Assess the size of the spleen and the anterior and posterior adhesions to the spleen. Inspect the other abdominal contents.

KEY POINTS Accessory spleens?

- Accessory spleens normally lie deep to the spleen but may lie in the mesentery. Look for these and remove any if found
- At the end of the procedure, search again in the hilar area, gastrosplenic ligament, splenocolic ligament, splenorenal ligament and greater omentum.

Action

1 The intention is to roll the spleen towards the patient's right side, divide the lienorenal ligaments under direct vision, thereby thinning the hilar structures. Then divide the hilar vessels using a vascular stapling gun.

2 Elevate the left posterior margin of the spleen with the right-hand instrument and place the left-hand grasper along the spleen's left edge to maintain rightward retraction. Have the lienorenal ligament held under tension. Begin division of the lienorenal ligament with hook or scissor diathermy, keeping close to the spleen. Alternatively use a harmonic scalpel if available. The spleen becomes increasingly mobile. Continue this dissection as high as possible since posterior adhesions prevent downwards retraction of the spleen and impede positioning of the staple gun at a later stage.

KEY POINT Improve access?

- Division of the left triangular ligament of the liver may improve access but is not routinely necessary.

3 Protect the hilar vessels and the pancreas which will come into view.

4 Replace the spleen into its original position.

5 Elevate the right anterior border and divide any adhesions between the spleen and stomach or omentum—they are not usually present.

6 Introduce atraumatic graspers in the lateral and medial ports and place them on either side of the hilum. Use both the graspers to elevate the spleen (Fig. 24.2). It is now possible to estimate if sufficient thinning of the hilar structures has been achieved to allow placement of the EndoGIA-2 stapling gun (Auto Suture, UK). The modern staple gun opens more widely than previous models and is designed to apply clips more securely.

7 Replace the lateral 5-mm cannula with a 15-mm Versaport (US Surgical Corporation), able to take instruments from 5 to 15 mm in diameter. Introduce the EndoGIA with a 60-mm vascular cartridge, open the stapler and carefully place it across the hilum close to the spleen using the left-hand retractor(s) to aid positioning (Fig. 24.3).

8 Once you are satisfied with the position, close the stapler and fire it. The initial firing should have divided all the branches of the splenic artery and vein but may not have reached the short gastric vessels. Carefully open the stapler and withdraw it. Reassess the remaining attachments of the spleen to the stomach and decide on an appropriate cartridge reload, such as 30, 45 or 60 mm. In most cases, two firings will completely separate the spleen from its blood supply and attachments.

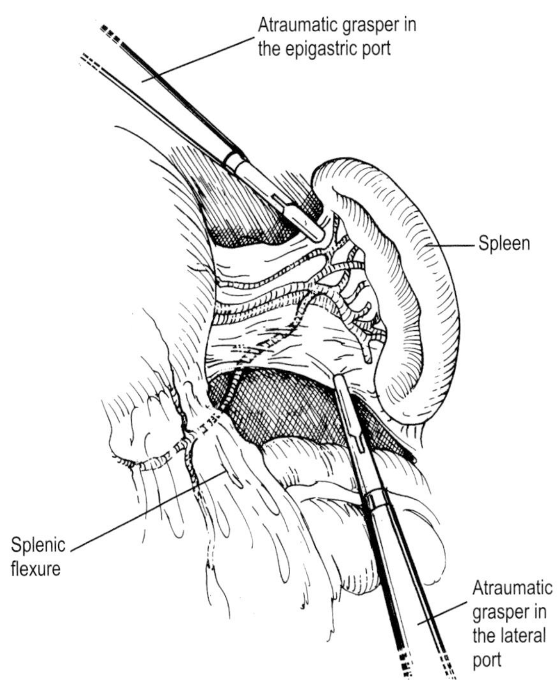

Fig. 24.2 Elevation of the spleen using two atraumatic graspers.

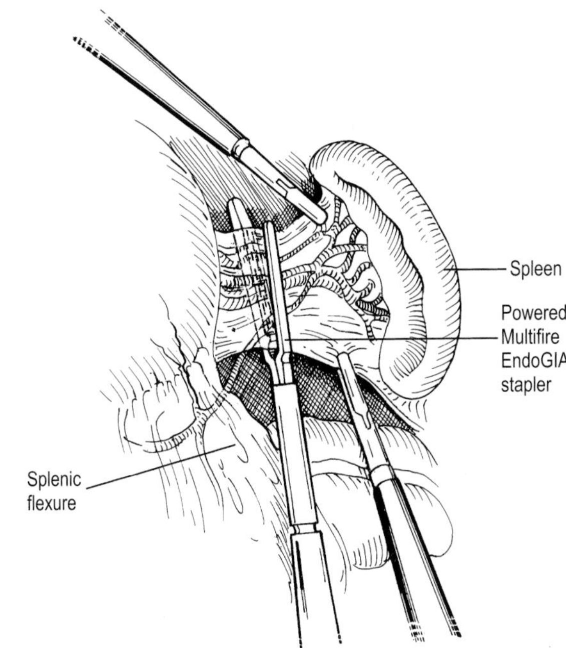

Fig. 24.3 Ligation of hilar vessels.

KEY POINTS Precautions

- Try to avoid damaging the splenic capsule.
- While stapling the hilum, take extra care not to injure the fundus of the stomach or the tail of the pancreas. Position the stapler correctly before closing it, because reopening the stapler for repositioning is dangerous and may damage the hilar vessels.
- Occasionally the stomach is so close to the spleen that a cuff of stomach will be incorporated into the staple line. This should present no problems.

9 The spleen is now free. Introduce a large retrieval bag (Endo-Catch II, Auto Suture, UK) via the Versaport, open it and place the spleen within it. This manoeuvre is facilitated if you hold the spleen by grasping the hilar staple line. Withdraw the bag and remove the spleen piecemeal after morselating it with sponge-holding forceps (Fig. 24.4). Use an electromechanical morselator if one is available.

10 If the spleen is required intact for histological examination or is too large to be placed in a retrieval bag, remove it through a small Pfannenstiel incision.

Posterior approach[7]

1 With the patient supine, stand on the patient's left, or between the legs with the patient in a modified lithotomy position. The assistant and the camera operator stand on the right with the scrub nurse at the foot. Exposure of the spleen may be improved by a slight reverse Trendelenburg tilt and rotation with elevation of the patient's left side.

2 Place monitors at the head of the operating table and the instrument tray at the foot.

3 After insufflating the peritoneum, introduce a 10-mm port at the umbilicus. Insert the laparoscope and video camera through the umbilical port. Place two ports in the upper midline for

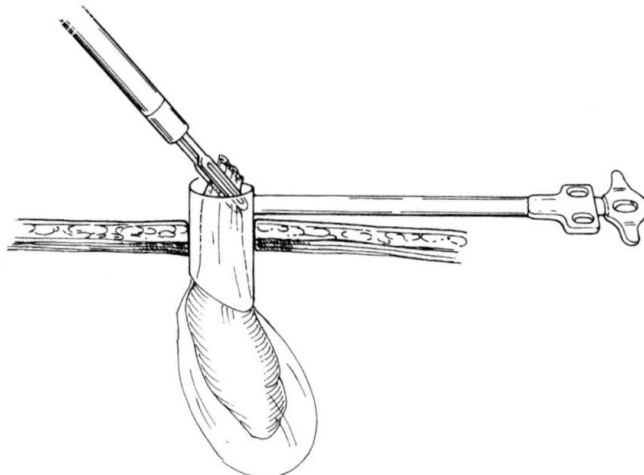

Fig. 24.4 Morselation of the spleen using sponge-holding forceps.

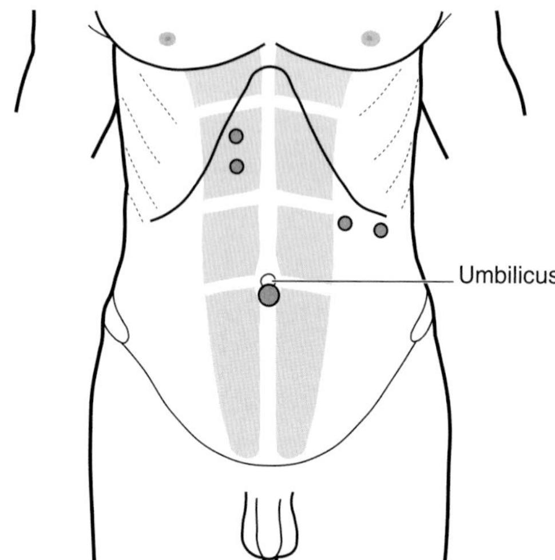

Fig. 24.5 Operating port positions for posterior approach laparoscopic splenectomy.

retraction and exposure of the operative field. Position two further ports for dissection in the left subcostal region, near the costal margin and 12 cm apart. The size of these ports depends on the instruments used but one of the lateral ports needs to be at least 12 mm for introduction of the EndoGIA stapler (Fig. 24.5).

4 Search for accessory splenunculi and remove any that you find. Use atraumatic graspers to retract the stomach and colon. Divide the lienocolic ligament and control bleeding using surgical clips or electrocautery. Dissect the medial aspect of the inferior pole and proceed in a cephalad direction. Ligate the inferior polar vessels using surgical clips.

5 Use dissectors to open the peritoneum overlying the splenic vessels. Use the suction/irrigation catheter to blunt-dissect the anterior and posterior extent of the hilar structures. Now ligate the splenic artery and vein using the EndoGIA stapler. Before closing the stapler ensure that the tail of the pancreas and the greater curvature of the stomach are not included in it. If you prefer, individually dissect and ligate the splenic vessels using surgical clips.

6 Continue the dissection cephalad along the medial border of the spleen. Retract the greater curvature of the stomach, expose the short gastric vessels and ligate them using the linear stapler.

7 Now the spleen is completely detached from the diaphragm and the stomach. Dissect the lateral splenic attachments and free the spleen. Through one of the subcostal ports introduce a large extraction bag. Place the spleen into the bag. Before drawing the bag out, irrigate and inspect the splenic bed for haemostasis. Grasp the drawstring of the extraction bag through the umbilical port and elevate the bag with the specimen towards the abdominal wall. Open the bag and fragment the spleen using scissors or fingers and remove them piecemeal until the bag can be extracted.

? DIFFICULTY

Do not hesitate to convert the procedure into an open operation if you encounter uncontrollable bleeding, visceral injury, difficulty in handling the spleen, or when dense posterior adhesions are present between the spleen and the diaphragm.

Checklist

1 Ensure that haemostasis is satisfactory by performing saline lavage after retrieval of the spleen.

2 Check for injury to the pancreas, the stomach and the splenic flexure of the colon.

3 Make sure that accessory splenunculi are removed.

4 Place a small drain in the splenic bed for detection of bleeding or pancreatic injury, which is very rare.

Closure

1 Withdraw the accessory ports under vision. Withdraw the telescope and the large Versaport.

2 Infiltrate bupivacaine 0.5% into the wounds up to a total volume of 20 ml.

3 Close the larger port sites using 2/0 polyglactin 910 (Vicryl) on a J-shaped needle. Close the skin with adhesive strips (Steri-Strip).

Postoperative

1 Give parenteral pain medication until the patient takes liquids by mouth. Most people require oral analgesics for 2 or 3 days.

2 Allow the patient to eat and drink on recovery from the anaesthetic, usually the same evening as the operation.

3 Check the drain for active bleeding. Remove it in 12 hours if the drainage is less than 50 ml.

4 Check all the appropriate blood tests before discharge.

5 Liaise with the haematologist regarding continuation of any medical therapy such as steroids and completion of vaccination programme.

6 If the patient is mobile, managing to eat and drink and with adequate pain control, arrange discharge on the first postoperative day. The majority of patients go home within 2 days.

7 Follow the patient in the outpatient clinic in about 6 weeks time.

8 The haematologists usually arrange for long-term follow-up, depending upon the disease.

Complications

- *Postoperative bleeding*. If the patient becomes unstable, or if the drain produces a large amount of fresh blood, anticipate postoperative bleeding. If the patient is stable, repeat the laparoscopy to look for the site of bleeding. The usual sites are the hilar or short gastric vessels or from the lateral port site. If you identify the bleeding vessel, clip it or suture it. If the patient is unstable perform a laparotomy and control the bleeding site.
- *Injury to the adjacent organs*. The splenic flexure of the colon, the greater curvature of the stomach or the tail of the pancreas could be damaged during the operation. Laparotomy may be required to inspect the damage. The colonic and stomach injury can be successfully closed using serosubmucosal absorbable sutures. Injury to the tail of pancreas may require either primary repair or resection. Undetected pancreatic injury may later present as pancreatic ascites, a subphrenic collection or pancreatic fistula. All such injuries should be very rare.
- *Subphrenic collection*. This may develop due to minor bleeding or serous oozing from the raw area in the diaphragm and retroperitoneum. If this happens, carefully monitor the platelet count and clotting parameters. Confirm your clinical suspicion by ultrasonography or CT (computed tomography) scan. If the collection is significant, perform percutaneous drainage under X-ray control with antibiotic cover.
- *Subphrenic abscess*. A subphrenic collection may become an abscess which can usually be drained percutaneously but may require a laparotomy.
- *Thrombocytosis* can occur following splenectomy, leading to deep venous thrombosis and pulmonary embolus. We recommend routine subcutaneous heparin prophylaxis and compression stockings.
- *Portal vein thrombosis* has been reported. It is a difficult diagnosis to make as symptoms are of vague abdominal pains. In cases of slow recovery, consider this possibility with a radiologist and arrange ultrasound or CT scan, which can establish the diagnosis.
- *Overwhelming post-splenectomy infection* (OPSI) has been reported in 1% of adults and in 10% of children under 5 years of age. This is mostly during the first 2 years postoperatively, although cases have been reported after even 20 years. Give advice regarding immunization, foreign travel and lifelong prophylactic antibiotics. Advise patients to carry an information card at all times. If signs of infection develop, they should take a course of appropriate antibiotics immediately. If the infection does not settle, then admit and treat the patient with parenteral antibiotics.

REFERENCES

1. Friedman RL, Fallas MJ, Carroll BJ et al 1996 Laparoscopic splenectomy for ITP: the gold standard. Surgical Endoscopy 10:991–995
2. Delaitre B, Pitre J 1997 Laparoscopic splenectomy versus open splenectomy: a comparative study. Hepatogastroenterology 44:45–49
3. Watson DI., Coventry BJ, Chin T et al 1997 Laparoscopic versus open splenectomy for immune thrombocytopenic purpura. Surgery 121:19–22
4. Kathouda N, Hurwitz MB, Rivera RT et al 1998 Laparoscopic splenectomy: outcome and efficacy in 103 consecutive patients. Annals of Surgery 228:568–578
5. Trias M, Targarona, EM, Espert JJ et al 1998 Laparoscopic surgery for splenic disorders. Lessons learned from a series of 64 cases. Surgical Endoscopy 12:66–72
6. Miles WFA, Greig JD, Wilson RG et al 1996 Technique of laparoscopic splenectomy with a powered vascular linear stapler. British Journal of Surgery 83:1212–1214
7. Flowers JL, Lefor AT, Steers J 1996 Laparoscopic splenectomy in patients with haematologic diseases. Annals of Surgery 224: 19–28

FURTHER READING

Choy C, Cacchione R, Moon V et al 2004 Experience with seven cases of massive splenomegaly. Journal of Laparoendoscopic & Advanced Surgical Techniques. Part A 14:197–200

Friedman RL, Phillips EH 1997 Laparoscopic splenectomy. In: Ponsky JL (ed.) Complications of endoscopic and laparoscopic surgery: prevention and management. Lippincott Raven, Philadelphia, pp 159–170

Rege RV, Merriam LT, Joehl RJ 1996 Laparoscopic splenectomy. Surgical Clinics of North America 76:459–468

Wu JM, Lai IR, Yuan RH 2004 Laparoscopic splenectomy for idiopathic thrombocytopenic purpura. American Journal of Surgery 187:720–723

Internet web sites

http://www.edu.rcsed.ac.uk/video_album_menu.htm
An example of the lateral approach with a stapling gun.

http://www.edu.rcsed.ac.uk/gem%20videos.htm
An example of a more anterior approach using the harmonic scalpel.

25

Breast

R. Sainsbury

CONTENTS

MANAGEMENT OF BREAST SYMPTOMS

Assessment

1 You need a scheme of management for patients presenting with a breast complaint (Fig. 25.1).

2 Common symptoms include breast pain, lumps, lumpiness and nipple changes including inversion, bleeding and discharge. Be suspicious of carcinoma if an older woman presents with recent nipple inversion. Exclude carcinoma or other causes of breast pain and lumpiness before deciding on conservative management.

3 Is a lump truly discrete? If there is diffuse nodularity, arrange ultrasound examination. If this is normal in a younger woman, re-examine her at a different point in the menstrual cycle and if this is also normal, reassure her.

4 Refer women over the age of 35 years for mammography and/or ultrasound to complement clinical examination of the 'difficult' breast. Select ultrasound for women below 35 years.

5 For discrete lumps ultrasound differentiates cystic from solid lesions. Prepare a cytological smear from solid lesions. Completely aspirate a cyst then re-examine the breast to exclude a residual lump.

6 Breast cysts often sudden appear suddenly and are of concern to the patient. They are most common before and around the menopause but occur at any age. Cyst drainage usually establishes the diagnosis and 'cures' the condition so the patient can be immediately reassured.

KEY POINTS Caution

- If the fluid from the cyst is bloody, or if there is a residual lump, perform formal biopsy.
- Cytology of cyst fluid is worthwhile only if it is bloodstained or there is a residual mass after aspiration.

7 If the lump is solid, declared benign on cytology, excise it if the woman is age 35 years or older, if the lump increases in size or is associated with pain, if the cytology is equivocal or if the patient requests it. For a confirmed fibroadenoma in a younger patient, offer the alternatives of observation or ablation by means of laser thermocoagulation.

8 Perform triple assessment—examination, imaging and histology or cytology—on patients with discrete areas of breast abnormality. Histology of a core biopsy, usually taken using a spring-loaded device, may be helpful.

9 If the diagnosis remains doubtful, determine to remove a biopsy as soon as possible.

10 At open biopsy do not, as a rule, rely on frozen-section histology; prefer to await paraffin-section histology. Lesions that have defied diagnosis by standard triple assessment are also difficult to interpret by the pathologist and require an optimum specimen. Frozen-section is occasionally valuable when imaging or cytology are equivocal in suspicious lesions.

11 Assess the risk for patients with a family history, and devise a stratagem for regular follow-up, or reassure and discharge them

12 Patients present with cosmetic problems including hypertrophy or unevenness of the breast. If you are not appropriately trained refer them to a plastic surgeon.

BIOPSY

ASPIRATION CYTOLOGY

1 In the outpatient clinic this has the advantage of being applicable for all breast lumps and requiring the minimum of special equipment.

2 It has the disadvantage of requiring the special skills of an experienced cytologist and the quality of the aspirate is operator-dependent, demanding experience and skill.

3 The cytological aspirate is usually reported as containing no cells (C_0), blood and debris (C_1), benign epithelial cells (C_2), atypical cells (C_3), cells suspicious of carcinoma (C_4) or carcinoma (C_5). Methods of reporting vary from centre to centre.

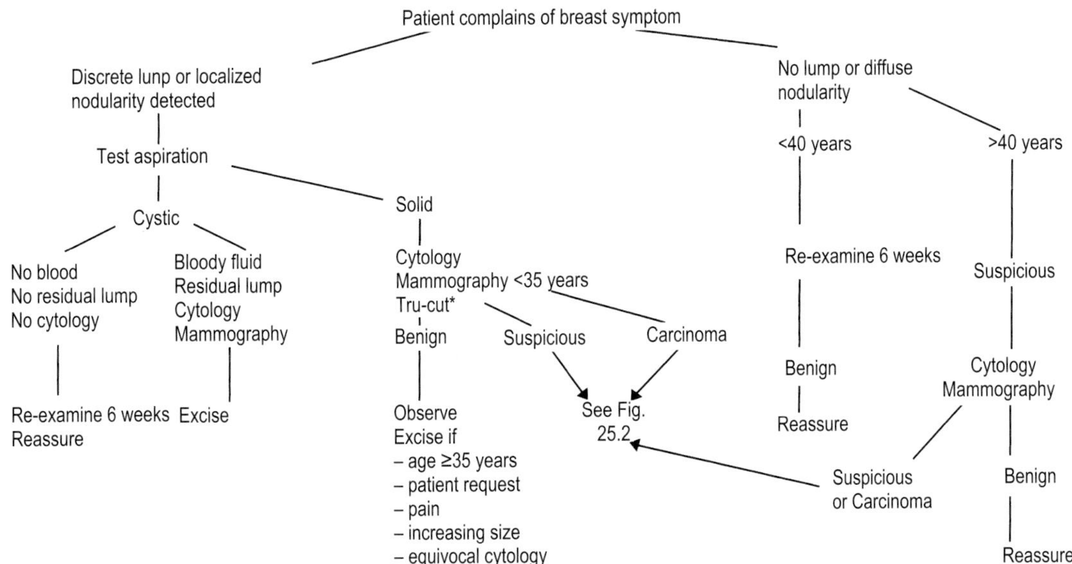

Fig. 25.1 Scheme of management for patients presenting with a breast symptom.*Tru-cut is difficult unless lump is greater than 2 cm.

4 A preoperative diagnosis of carcinoma can usually be made by combining clinical assessment, cytodiagnosis and imaging, enabling appropriate patient counselling and planning of the operation list.

Action

1 Attach a 21G (green) or 23G (blue) needle to a 10-ml syringe. You may wish to insert the syringe into an extractor 'gun'.

2 Clean the overlying skin then fix the lump between thumb and index finger of the non-dominant hand.

3 Insert the needle into the middle of the lump and apply suction to the syringe plunger. Move the needle in several different directions through the lump while maintaining negative pressure. Do not allow the needle point to leave the skin or air enters the needle and the aspirated material is drawn into the syringe, becoming difficult to remove.

KEY POINT Pleural damage

- Avoid penetrating the intercostal space.

4 Release the pressure and then withdraw the needle. Ask the patient or your assistant to apply pressure to the breast for 2 minutes to avoid haematoma formation.

5 Eject a drop of aspirate onto the end of a dry microscope slide. Gently spread this out with another slide to create a thin smear without repeated smearing, to avoid creating artefactual changes, which confuse interpretation.

6 Immediately and accurately label the slide, ensuring that no material falls onto the table, which could then be picked up onto the back of the next set of slides. The slide may be sprayed with, or immersed in, a fixative. Send the slide for reporting.

7 If you obtain no aspirate repeat the procedure.

? DIFFICULTY

1. Obtaining good samples for cytology demands practice. A consistent report of C_I 'inadequate' may indicate that the sampled area contains no breast epithelial cells (e.g. a lipoma).
2. If you remain doubtful, proceed to a core-cut biopsy or excision biopsy.

CORE-CUT OR 'TRU-CUT' NEEDLE BIOPSY (Fig. 25.2)

Action

1 Infiltrate the skin over the lump with 1% lidocaine. Introduce the needle into the breast, to inject local anaesthetic deep into the breast tissue to enter the tumour.

2 Wait 2 minutes for the anaesthetic to work.

3 Make a small nick in the skin with the tip of a sharp-pointed scalpel (no. 11 blade).

4 Fix the tumour yourself or have an assistant fix the tumour within the breast between finger and thumb, to provide a static target.

5 The best approach to the lump is often from the side to avoid firing the needle backwards.

6 Push the needle, in its closed position, through the skin incision until you reach the edge of the tumour.

7 A spring-driven biopsy needle can obtain a sample more rapidly than one obtained by hand and causes less discomfort for the patient.

8 If microcalcification is a dominant feature, X-ray the specimen to ensure you have obtained the correct specimen.

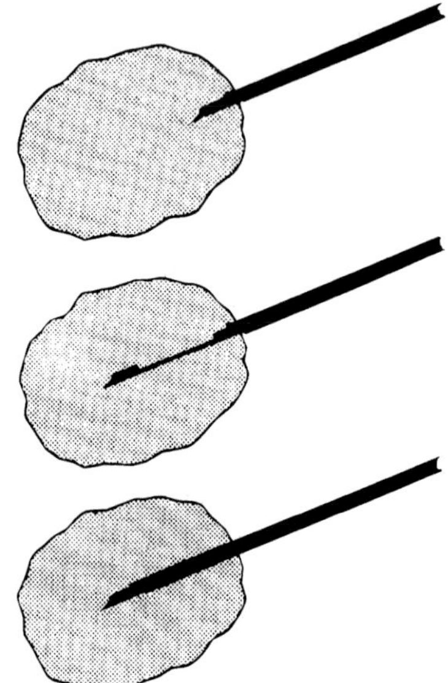

Fig. 25.2 Tru-cut needle.

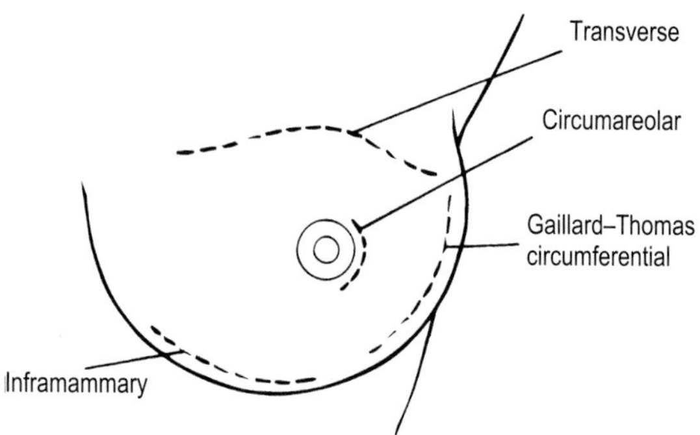

Fig. 25.3 Incisions for removal of a lump from the left breast.

OPEN BIOPSY

Rarely an open biopsy will be required to make a diagnosis. If a lesion is very large then a thin slice may be taken through the lesion, or part of the lesion may be taken if an operation is planned.

The term 'lumpectomy' is best reserved for a definitive operation to remove a benign lump, and the term 'wide local excision' to remove a carcinoma with some surrounding normal tissue.

NEEDLE-LOCALIZATION BIOPSY

Collaborate with your radiologist to consistently remove impalpable but suspicious mammographically detected lesions.

An initial specimen radiograph ensures that you have removed the suspicious area, and subsequent radiographs of the sliced specimen ensure that the pathologist examines the radiologically abnormal sections.

Prepare

1. Inspect the original mammograms with the radiologist who is to insert the localization needle and wire.
2. Discuss the needle-insertion site, direction and depth with the radiologist, and the type of wire used, such as simple hook, Reidy or Nottingham needle. It is helpful if the distance between the needle entry site and the lesion is as short as possible.
3. Ensure that the original mammograms, and films taken in two planes following wire insertion, are taken to the operating theatre.
4. Do not arrange frozen-section histology. You need carefully examined paraffin sections to decide regarding further surgery.

Access

Plan a cosmetically satisfactory incision (Fig. 25.3) and estimate the likely surface marking of the lesion from the preoperative mammograms. The incision need not be placed at the point of wire entry.

Action

1. Raise a skin flap between the chosen incision and the needle entry site until you reach the subcutaneous wire. Grasp the wire with an artery forceps and cut off the excess wire flush with the skin.
2. Follow the wire down towards the site of the lesion by sharp dissection, gently moving the wire to facilitate the dissection. Prefer a scalpel to heavy scissors, which could bend or cut the wire inadvertently.
3. Once you reach the point of the wire, grasp it and adjacent tissue in order to excise the area thought to contain the lesion. Mark the specimen with metal clips to facilitate orientation and send it to be X-rayed.
4. Achieve perfect haemostasis, and search the cavity for any residual suspicious tissue.
5. Examine the radiograph of the specimen to confirm that it contains the mammographic lesion. If the lesion is not present, excise a further specimen of breast tissue, searching particularly for areas that look or feel suspicious. Repeat the specimen radiography until you find the lesion.
6. Close the wound as for excision biopsy.
7. Newer techniques are being developed for obtaining cores of tissue from impalpable lesions, or completely excising small impalpable lesions. The radiologist may insert a small metallic marker if he has removed all the microcalcifications to allow subsequent localization of an abnormal area.

KEY POINTS Correct specimen?

- If you are removing a lesion that mammographically contains calcification, ensure that this is present on the specimen radiograph and in the final histology report.
- If you are removing a mammographically suspicious lesion that is not calcified, ensure that the radiographers performing the specimen X-ray are aware of this and are able to compare the specimen X-ray with the earlier mammogram.

BREAST ABSCESS

Appraise

- Breast abscess develops most commonly during lactation. Empty the affected breast by manual pressure, but encourage the mother to continue feeding.
- Early infection can be treated with antibiotics alone but do not wait for fluctuation, as widespread destruction of the underlying breast tissue may have developed by then. Prefer co-amoxiclav and start it early. If an abscess is present clinically or on ultrasound, aspirate it using a wide-bore needle, repeated as necessary; the abscess cavity can be washed out with a combination of antibiotic dissolved in local anaesthetic.
- If the skin over the abscess has become thinned, it is usually simple to drain it under general anaesthesia using a no. 11 blade knife to make a very small incision.

Access

If the abscess cavity is longstanding, incision and drainage may be required, although this can often be avoided.

Action

1. Site the incision over the point of skin thinning, but if it is near the nipple use a periareolar incision.
2. Send pus for culture and antibiotic sensitivities. If necessary, change to the appropriate antibiotic.
3. Introduce a gloved finger into the abscess cavity and rotate it to break down all loculi in a potentially multiloculated cavity.
4. If the cavity allows, introduce a retractor and examine the walls. Stop any bleeding with diathermy.
5. If this is a lactational abscess cavity it is not necessary to remove biopsy specimens. Otherwise remove a specimen to exclude a carcinoma.
6. Ensure that the incision is sufficiently long to allow the wound to heal from the deepest parts upwards, to prevent the development of a chronic abscess.
7. Insert a drain only if not all pus is drained. Alternatively, loosely pack the cavity.
8. Apply a non-adhesive dressing.
9. Advise the patient to wear a supportive brassiere to diminish the risk of haematoma developing.
10. Allow bilateral breastfeeding to recommence as soon as it is comfortable.

▶ KEY POINTS Prefer aspiration to incision

- Incision and drainage should be a last resort.
- If possible rely on repeated aspirations of the abscess of the cavity.

DUCT ECTASIA AND MAMILLARY DUCT FISTULA

Appraise

- Duct ectasia (Greek: *ex*=out+*tenein*=to stretch; dilatation) is the collection of thick, toothpaste-like material in the terminal ducts. It may become infected, causing areas of redness or abscesses.
- Occasionally, a fistula develops between a duct and the skin at the areolar margin. This discharges pus, often heals spontaneously before breaking down again. It is now acknowledged to be smoking-related, so dissuade the patient from smoking.
- If a mamillary duct fistula does not heal, it may require laying open (see below).

Action

1. If this is a fistula, insert a probe through the external opening and hook it up though the nipple. Cut around the areola, extending to no more than a quarter of the nipple and excise the fistulous track to the back of the nipple.
2. Obtain perfect haemostasis.
3. Close the wound with interrupted absorbable sutures.
4. If you are operating to excise the major ducts (Hadfield's operation), you need a longer incision (but no more than three-fifths of the circumference of the areola).
5. Cut the subcutaneous tissue down to the duct system.
6. Use blunt dissection to reach the plane circumferentially around the terminal lactiferous ducts, just deep to the areola and nipple.
7. Divide the ducts close to the nipple and remove them with a conical wedge of tissue including the distal 1–2 cm of the subareolar tissue, including the major lactiferous ducts and sinuses.
8. If there is a fistulous tract ensure this is excised in its entirety with all granulation tissue.
9. Send all tissue for histological examination.
10. Insert a small vacuum drain and close the wound with 3/0 subcuticular absorbable sutures or interrupted 4/0 polypropylene.

NIPPLE DISCHARGE AND BLEEDING

Appraise

1. If the nipple discharge is serous, serosanguineous or frank blood arising from a solitary duct, then manage as below for nipple bleeding.
2. Test for blood. This is usually done using Dip-Stix.
3. If one duct is involved and imaging is negative, then a microdochectomy may be required.
4. If bilateral longstanding nipple discharge occurs which is an embarrassment, then a Hadfield's operation may be the preferred choice.
5. Multiduct multicolour nipple discharge is often physiological and does not need intervention.

NIPPLE BLEEDING

Appraise

1 Determine which duct the blood is coming from.

2 Arrange an ultrasound scan and a mammogram to exclude underlying malignancy.

3 Send the material for cytology; it may yield papillary cells or, very occasionally, carcinoma cells.

4 Surgically explore the breast unless the bleeding occurs during pregnancy, frequently with bilateral bleeding, which stops spontaneously after parturition, or in someone who is taking anticoagulants.

Prepare

1 Mark the site of the affected duct on a diagram.

2 Discuss the operation and the possible implications with the patient. Warn specifically about alterations in nipple sensation.

3 Mark the site and side of the lesion with a skin pencil on the patient herself.

Access

1 The procedure may be done under a local or general anaesthetic.

KEY POINTS Cannulate the duct

- Cannulate the affected duct with a fine lacrimal probe to assist in dissecting it out.
- Insert the cannula when the patient is on the operating table, beforehand.

2 Infiltrate the area with bupivacaine 0.25% and adrenaline (epinephrine) 1:200 000 to minimize bleeding and postoperative pain.

3 When you pick up the nipple between finger and thumb, you may feel thickening along one duct, or feel the probe within the duct.

Action

1 Make a circumareola incision and dissect down to expose the duct.

2 Excise the duct with a small amount of surrounding breast tissue and send it for histology.

3 Obtain haemostasis.

CARCINOMA

Establish the diagnosis preoperatively in nearly all cases, by means of triple assessment. Counsel the patient about treatment options and arrange for a meeting with the Breast Nurse. Discuss the alternatives to primary surgery with wide local excision or mastectomy, by, for example, primary medical treatment. Document your discussions

When carcinoma has been detected as a result of screening, a preoperative diagnosis should have been made by percutaneous biopsy. Occasionally you need to perform a localization biopsy for diagnosis as opposed to therapy.

Appraise

- The local management of breast carcinoma demands excision of the tumour with clear margins. If the tumour is small in comparison with the total breast volume and sited peripherally, this can be achieved by wide local excision. Up to 10% of breast volume can be removed without significant cosmetic differences being observed by the patient. The long-term survival after wide local excision and radiotherapy equals that of a mastectomy. Some form of axillary dissection is still required to stage the patient and to treat the axilla. The importance of axillary node staging is reinforced by the evidence that adjuvant cytotoxic chemotherapy can reduce the relative risk of death by 20–25% in the node-positive population. A similar benefit is seen in a patients who have hormone-responsive tumours if given tamoxifen or the newer aromatase inhibitors. Sentinel node is increasingly replacing traditional axillary dissection as a method of staging the axilla (see below).
- Modified radical (or Patey) mastectomy (see later) provides good locoregional control, with acceptable morbidity, for patients unsuitable for breast conservation and may be indicated for patients with a large operable primary tumour, multifocal disease or central tumours.
- Simple mastectomy is rarely indicated in patients with breast cancer. It has very few advantages over a well-performed modified radical mastectomy and the major disadvantage of not staging or treating the axilla. The only indications for its performance in patients with breast cancer are for isolated breast recurrence after breast-conserving surgery, when the axilla has been previously treated, large phyllodes (Greek: *phyllon* = leaf + *eidos* = like; showing a lobulated, leaf-like appearance) tumours, multifocal duct carcinoma in situ, and for those rare elderly frail women who are medically unfit for a modified radical mastectomy.
- Mastectomy with immediate reconstruction, using either an implant or a myocutaneous flap, is being increasingly used by trained breast surgeons (oncoplastic surgery) and sometimes in conjunction with plastic surgery colleagues. This procedure is also valuable in the management of extensive intraduct carcinoma and as a prophylactic procedure in patients with a very strong family history. This will be discussed in further detail below.
- Primary medical therapy with tamoxifen may be used in frail elderly patients, and primary cytotoxic chemotherapy may be appropriate for locally advanced cases such as 'inflammatory' carcinoma. In patients with large tumours that are operable by mastectomy, primary (or neoadjuvant) chemotherapy may be used to shrink the tumour and allow breast conservation in up to 50% of cases.

PAGET'S DISEASE

1 When this disease is suspected, take a biopsy of the nipple area under local anaesthetic to prove the diagnosis histologically. It

may also be possible to do so with imprint cytology of the nipple.

2 When Paget's cells are demonstrated there is always an underlying intraduct carcinoma, which is invasive in 50% of cases.

3 Mastectomy is usually recommended, but primary radiotherapy or wide excision of the nipple and underlying breast tissue are possible alternatives.

EXCISION BIOPSY AND WIDE LOCAL EXCISION FOR CARCINOMA

EXCISION BIOPSY

Appraise

1 Normally reserve this for patients with a solid breast lump that is clinically benign. The aim is to extract the lesion with the narrowest margin and least cosmetic defect, consistent with establishing a histological diagnosis and removing the palpable abnormality.

KEY POINT Inadequate surgery

- Excision biopsy is insufficient for removal of carcinoma.

2 Preliminary excision biopsy is occasionally necessary for that minority of patients with a breast carcinoma in whom the diagnosis cannot be established by preoperative cytology, core-cut needle biopsy and/or mammography. Definitive operation is then required as a second procedure after paraffin-section examination. It has the advantage of allowing another opportunity for counselling prior to the definitive operation.

Prepare

1 Check that the lesion is still present on admission. Occasionally, lesions disappear. Check also that no new lesion has appeared in either breast.

2 Mark the exact site of the lesion on the breast with the patient lying in the position she will occupy on the operating table, otherwise you may be unable to find the mass once the patient is anaesthetized.

3 Obtain consent for the operation and carefully explain the potential risks.

4 Check that you have the right patient in the anaesthetic room and are operating on the correct side.

Access (Fig. 25.3)

1 Incise over the region of the lump. Place the incision to minimize scarring.

2 Periareolar incisions heal with least visible scars, but may not always be suitable.

3 Incisions in the medial half of the breast have a tendency to develop keloid scars.

4 Avoid radial incisions except medially.

5 Place the incision within the area of skin that would be included within a mastectomy if it is required subsequently. This avoids an unnecessary scar complicating the mastectomy scar.

Action

1 If possible excise the lump completely without cutting into it. While aiming to excise it, if necessary make a thin slice through the lesion. Use sharp dissection with scissors or knife, while holding the specimen with Lane or Allis tissue forceps or by inserting a suture through the lesion.

2 Try not to cut into the specimen. The pathologist needs to report on the margins of excision and so needs to incise the lesion. Palpate the resected specimen to make sure you have removed the palpable abnormality.

3 If mammary duct ectasia is present, a toothpaste-like substance may issue from transected ducts at the edge of the cavity adjacent to the nipple.

4 When you are operating on a benign lesion, resecting cavity margins is unnecessary.

5 Sometimes it is impossible to remove all the abnormal tissue, particularly with fibrocystic disease, which tends not to have a well-defined edge. Under these circumstances, remove the most severely affected tissue and obtain a representative biopsy.

6 Determine to obtain perfect haemostasis. Try using the spray setting, if there is one, on the diathermy machine. Spray diathermy, also called fulguration mode, employs a high voltage. The electrode is held 2–4 mm from the tissue so that the current jumps across the air gap and spreads to create widespread coagulation. It is useful to cauterize small vessels without the need to pick them up in forceps.

Closure

1 If you have achieved perfect haemostasis you do not need to introduce a drain. Otherwise insert a small suction or corrugated drain to reduce the risk of a haematoma.

2 Close the skin using a subcuticular suture of 3/0 synthetic material. Support the closed wound with Steri-Strips for 10 days.

WIDE LOCAL EXCISION FOR CARCINOMA

Appraise

This is a therapeutic operation for the excision of a carcinoma with clear surrounding margins. As an extra precaution the cavity walls can be re-resected, thus increasing the chance of achieving clear margins and so reducing the need to return the patient to theatre for a further resection. It does have the potential disadvantage of prejudicing the cosmetic appearance.

The breast-conserving operation against which other procedures are measured in the treatment of early cancer is the 'quadrantectomy'. It is upon this operation that most of the published data comparing breast-conserving therapy with mastectomy in randomized trials have been based. Quadrantectomy is the most certain means of obtaining microscopically clear margins, and with postoperative breast irradiation gives local recurrence rates equivalent to those obtained by primary mastectomy. In contrast, wide local excision results in a higher incidence of local recurrence, even following adjunctive radiotherapy to the primary site that has been employed in the treatment protocol. The local recurrence rate is higher in younger women.

QUADRANTECTOMY

Prepare

1 Check that the diagnosis of breast carcinoma has been confirmed by cytology, Tru-cut biopsy or previous excision biopsy.

2 Check that the patient is suitable for breast-conserving surgery by clinical examination. Ensure that the mammogram does not reveal multifocal disease.

3 Confirm that the Nurse Counsellor has discussed the diagnosis and treatment with the patient.

4 Mark the side and site of the carcinoma.

Access

1 Position the patient supine on the table, with the arm on the operative side extended on an arm board.

2 Prepare the skin and place the towels to allow access to the breast and axilla. Wrap the arm separately to facilitate axillary dissection (see below).

3 With a skin-marking pen, mark the position of the lump. Draw on the skin the edges of a quadrant of breast tissue that encompasses the lump at its centre. You thus draw two radial lines extending out from the nipple at right-angles to each other towards the periphery of the breast.

4 Draw the chosen incision line on the skin. A circumferential incision is best, approximately midway between the nipple and the periphery of the breast, extending from one radial line to the other of your previously outlined quadrant. The incision ideally lies directly over the lump, allowing an ellipse or crescent of skin overlying the carcinoma to be removed in continuity, but its position should allow good access to both the central and peripheral parts of the breast. Do not normally remove skin unless the carcinoma directly involves it, because this distorts the position of the nipple, spoiling the cosmetic result.

Action

1 Elevate two skin flaps centrally towards the nipple, so you can remove the subareolar major duct system of the quadrant. Elevate them peripherally to the edge of the breast disc, exposing it along a quarter of its outside circumference.

2 Dissect along the edge of the breast disc down to the underlying pectoral fascia and muscle. You can now create a submammary plane of cleavage between the breast and pectoral fascia. Gradually lift the breast tissue free from the chest wall. Employ blunt dissection, but ligating or diathermizing perforating vessels before dividing them with scissors.

3 Use the two radial lines marked on the skin to define the edges of the quadrant. Cut vertically through the breast tissue along these radii as far as the pectoral fascia so that the quadrant is freed from the chest wall. Continue the dissection along the two radii until they meet behind the nipple, and you excise the major duct system in continuity with the rest of the quadrant.

4 Mark the specimen with sutures to denote its three planes: superior–inferior, medial–lateral and superficial–deep.

5 Send the specimen for histology. Do not incise it in the theatre to inspect it. You may contaminate the operative field with viable malignant cells and it prevents adequate assessment of margins of clearance by the pathologist, since the intact specimen is dipped in ink to outline the margins in histological sections.

6 Achieve complete haemostasis.

7 Pack the cavity with a dry swab and proceed to perform the axillary dissection that usually accompanies a quadrantectomy.

Closure

1 Remove the swab, and ensure that haemostasis remains perfect.

2 A drain is rarely needed.

3 Close the skin edges using subcuticular sutures.

4 Wound closure without drainage produces a good early cosmetic appearance. The large quadrantic cavity is full of air, subsequently filling with serous fluid, which gradually becomes organized into fibrous tissue, filling in the cavity.

5 If the quadrantectomy cavity is in continuity with the axillary dissection cavity, suture the edges of the axillary skin to pectoralis major muscle. A suction drain placed in the axilla is prevented from sucking out the air and seroma fluid from the breast cavity.

KEY POINTS Breast volume

- As a rule do not approximate the residual breast tissue at the edges of the cavity.
- However, this may leave an unacceptably large defect.
- If you mobilize the residual breast and approximate the edges with absorbable sutures this restores shape but produces a greater loss of breast volume.

AXILLARY SURGERY

- Axillary nodal status remains the most important prognostic factor for determining survival and is combined with size and grade to form the Nottingham Prognostic Index.
- If the patient presents with palpable nodes, then perform axillary clearance. Consider fine needle cytology of palpable nodes and make a diagram.
- Ultrasound scanning and to some extent magnetic resonance imaging (MRI) demonstrate nodal status but, like clinical examination, do not rely upon them.
- In the absence of a palpable axillary node, apart from full clearance you may perform nodal sampling or a sentinel node biopsy.

AXILLARY CLEARANCE

Appraise

- While a limited 'axillary sampling' operation to biopsy a few lymph nodes in level I (lateral to pectoralis minor) may give valuable staging information, the advantage of a formal level II (up to the medial border of pectoralis minor) or level III (beyond the medial border of pectoralis minor) axillary clearance is that the operation is also therapeutic, providing local disease control without the need for axillary irradiation.
- Because 70–80% of breast cancer patients have a negative axillary dissection, novel methods are being studied with the intention of avoiding full axillary surgery in these patients. The technique most commonly practised is sentinel lymph node biopsy, in which the first node in the axilla draining the breast tissue around a tumour is identified perioperatively using a combination of radioisotope and blue dye. This node can then be removed; if it is not involved it is unlikely that further axillary nodes are involved.
- The combination of axillary surgery and irradiation is associated with the highest risk of long-term lymphoedema.

Prepare

1 Shave the axilla.

2 Warn the patient about the possibility of postoperative numbness if the intercostobrachial nerve is damaged, and of lymphoedema.

3 Encourage the patient to move the shoulder fully before operation and arrange for her to be taught shoulder exercises to perform after operation.

Access

1 Axillary clearance performed through an oblique incision just behind, and parallel to, the lateral edge of the pectoralis major muscle provides good access but has the disadvantage of producing an ugly scar and limitation of shoulder abduction. Prefer a transverse incision with its anterior corner at the pectoral edge and the posterior angle just crossing the anterior border of latissimus dorsi, running 3 cm below and parallel to the axillary vein with the arm abducted at 90°. Cosmetically this produces an excellent result.

2 Use a combination of sharp and blunt dissection at either end of the axillary incision, to identify the lateral border of pectoralis major and the anterior border of latissimus dorsi muscles. These landmarks form the anterior and posterior limits of your axillary dissection.

3 Dissect up and down along the lateral border of pectoralis major muscle and identify the underlying pectoralis minor muscle. Insinuate a finger under the insertion of pectoralis minor to separate it from the underlying structures and have your assistant retract the muscle forwards and medially in order to expose the axillary contents of level II.

4 If you intend to carry out a level III clearance, define both borders of pectoralis minor muscle. It may be necessary to divide the insertion into the coracoid process but with good assistance it is usually possible to dissect behind the muscle.

5 Flex and abduct the shoulder and flex the elbow so that the forearm lies across the patient's towelled-off face to facilitate exposure of the subpectoral area. Have the arm supported by an assistant or sling it from the crossbar of the anaesthetist's drape support.

KEY POINTS Preserve structures

- Carefully follow and preserve the thoracodorsal trunk down into latissimus dorsi muscle; it may be required if you later use a latissimus flap.
- Also avoid damaging the lateral division of the medial pectoral nerve and the long thoracic nerve.
- Identify and carefully ligate the angular vein which runs anteriorly into the thoracodorsal trunk.

6 Gently 'stroke' the axillary contents away from the chest wall and off the subscapularis muscle using a gauze swab or 'peanut' swab, to identify the nerve to serratus anterior in the posterior axillary line, and the nerve to latissimus dorsi travelling with the subscapular vessels.

7 Identify the intercostobrachial nerve and dissect it free from the axillary contents, preserving as many branches as feasible.

8 Now you have defined the limits of the dissection and the nerves, you can complete the removal of the axillary contents.

9 Achieve complete haemostasis.

? DIFFICULTY

1. If you are unable to remove the axillary contents without severing the intercostobrachial nerve, do not hesitate to divide it; afterwards inform the patient that she is likely to experience a little numbness on the medial aspect of her upper arm.
2. Axillary vein damage should not happen, but occasionally an over-enthusiastic assistant can tear a vein. This should be mended promptly and help from an experienced vascular surgeon may be needed. A short course of postoperative anticoagulation may be required if significant venous injury has occurred.
3. If there is heavy nodal involvement in the axilla excise all the palpable lymph nodes together with any soft tissue disease.
4. Only rarely is tumour found encasing the axillary vein and it is usually fairly easy to dissect off. If you have to leave any tumour behind, mark it with surgical clips to allow planning of any future radiotherapy.

Closure

1 Insert a vacuum drain into the axilla and suture the skin with subcuticular sutures.

2 Personally supervise the dressing of the wound. In particular, squeeze out all blood and air from under the flaps into the

vacuum containers in order to avoid the subsequent development of an axillary seroma.

3 Before sending the specimen to the pathology laboratory mark the apex of the specimen with a stitch and mark the junction of level I with level II with a second stitch. This helps the pathologist to orientate around the specimen and subsequently report on it.

SENTINEL NODE BIOPSY

The sentinel (Italian: *sentinella*=on guard) node is the first node to which the lymph drainage of the breast goes. With a patient who has a clinically uninvolved axilla, sentinel node biopsy is replacing conventional axillary dissection. The node is identified by injecting a radioisotope (usually technetium combined with colloidal albumin particles) some hours before operation, combined with a blue dye (Patent Bleu V) injected when the patient is on the operating table.

Prepare

1 Discuss with the patient if you should proceed to a full axillary clearance if you discover positive nodes, so you have informed consent.

2 Warn the patient about the need for a second operation if the sentinel node is found to be positive.

3 Mention that the injection of blue dye will cause the urine to become green.

Access

1 Allow enough time for the blue dye to travel from the injection site to the axilla. This is of the order of 5–10 minutes.

2 Make a short incision over the site of maximum radioactivity as detected by the gamma probe.

3 If no clear signal is obtained, make the incision just below and medial to the edge of the hair-bearing skin.

Action

1 When you open the axilla you usually see lymphatic vessels with blue dye in them. Follow these to the relevant node. The node can also be localized using the gamma probe.

2 Gently remove the node without damaging it.

3 When you have excised the node, carefully check that there are not other sentinel nodes present.

4 Achieve perfect haemostasis.

5 Close the wound using subarticular soluble stitches.

Postoperative

1 Following wide local excision and sentinel node biopsy you can usually discharge the patient on the same day.

2 If facilities are available, an interoperative diagnosis may be attempted by means of imprint cytology from the nodes.

MODIFIED RADICAL (OR PATEY) MASTECTOMY

Appraise

1 Check that the diagnosis of breast carcinoma has been confirmed by cytology or core-cut biopsy or previous excision biopsy.

2 If the diagnosis rests on positive cytology, are you satisfied clinically and radiologically that this is invasive carcinoma prior to undertaking an axillary dissection?

3 In case of doubt perform a preliminary biopsy for paraffin sections to be examined.

KEY POINT Diagnosis certain?

- Routine of 'Frozen section? Proceed' operation is no longer acceptable.

Prepare

1 Confirm that the patient has seen the Nurse Counsellor and has had an opportunity to discuss her diagnosis and treatment fully.

2 Breast reconstruction should be available for every patient undergoing mastectomy. Ensure that the patient is aware of this, offered either immediately or after an interval.

3 Mark the side and site of the carcinoma.

4 Cross-matched blood is seldom necessary but establish the patient's blood group.

Access

1 Place the patient on the table in the supine position, with the arm on the operative side extended on an arm board.

2 Prepare the skin and place the towels to allow access to the breast and axilla. Wrap the arm separately to facilitate axillary dissection (see below).

3 With a skin-marking pen, mark the position of the lump. Draw on the skin your chosen ellipse for the incision, lying transversely and encompassing approximately 5 cm of skin around the lesion and also the nipple (Fig. 25.4).

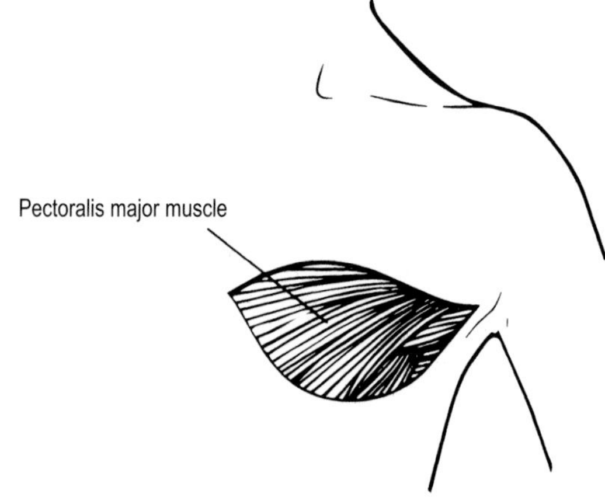

Fig. 25.4 Elliptical incision for Patey mastectomy.

4 If a transverse incision is impracticable, then make an oblique incision, but do not take it up as far as the clavicle or across to the upper arm; this type of scar is still seen on elderly patients who had a mastectomy many years ago but it is unnecessarily ugly and may be responsible for stiffness of the shoulder.

5 Ensure that you will be able to approximate the wound edges at the end of the operation before you make the incisions along your marked lines.

Action

1 Elevate the skin flaps in the plane between subcutaneous fat and mammary fat. This can be facilitated by subcutaneous infiltration with 1:400 000 adrenaline (epinephrine) in saline or 0.25% bupivacaine (Marcaine) and adrenaline (epinephrine).

2 Have your assistant hold up the skin flaps and check after every few cuts with the scalpel or scissors that you are not in danger of making the flap too thin, resulting in 'button-holing'. However, ensure that you do not leave any breast tissue in the flaps.

KEY POINTS Skin care

- Do not allow traumatizing tissue forceps to be placed on the skin flaps.
- Insist on the use of skin hooks into the cut edge, or apply Allis forceps to the rolled-back edges of the skin.

3 Raise the upper flap to the upper limit of the breast. This is usually 2–3 cm below the clavicle but varies from patient to patient. A good guide is the second intercostal space.

4 Catch any bleeding points with fine forceps and apply diathermy current to them. Take care not to burn the skin itself by contact with the diathermy needle. If skin is inadvertently burned, cut away the damaged area, bevelling it off so that it will not be demonstrable later (Fig. 25.5). Burnt skin takes many weeks to heal and is painful.

5 Raise the lower flap in a similar manner, to the lower limits of the breast.

6 Place a large tissue forceps, such as Lane's, on the breast which is to be removed, handing it to an assistant to hold, thus facilitating the subsequent dissection.

7 Return to the uppermost part of the breast and dissect down until you see the fascia of pectoralis major. Introduce a finger covered by a swab and find a submammary plane of cleavage between the fascia and the breast, as discussed under quadrantectomy.

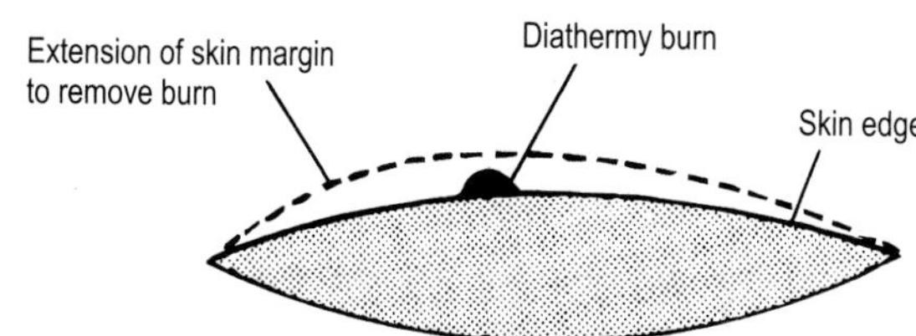

Fig. 25.5 Removal of accidental diathermy burn.

8 Proceed in this plane in a downwards direction, catching and ligating the perforating vessels as they appear, before cutting them; this reduces the amount of operative bleeding considerably.

9 If the tumour appears to infiltrate into the pectoralis muscle, then excise a portion of this muscle with the specimen.

10 Continue downwards, elevating the breast alternatively laterally and medially but leaving the axillary tail of the breast in continuity with the axillary contents.

11 The medial end of the dissection proceeds to the lower limit of the breast. Elevate the breast laterally to complete its removal from the chest wall. The breast is now only attached at the axilla. Take care to identify and ligate one or two major perforating vessels passing through the second and third intercostal spaces.

12 Place dry packs under each skin flap.

13 Identify the lateral border of pectoralis major and clear the axillary tail of the breast and the axillary contents from along this border.

14 Identify latissimus dorsi and clear the axillary contents from its anterior border.

15 Proceed as for an axillary clearance; a satisfactory result can be achieved by preserving the pectoralis minor muscle and dissecting up to level II (Fig. 25.6).

Closure

1 Insert two vacuum drains, one for the flaps and a second for the axilla.

2 Suture the skin edges with subcuticular sutures. If there is a discrepancy between the lengths of the two flaps, close the wound using interrupted sutures placed halfway along the incision then halfway between these lengths and so on, thus avoiding a 'dog-ear' at one end.

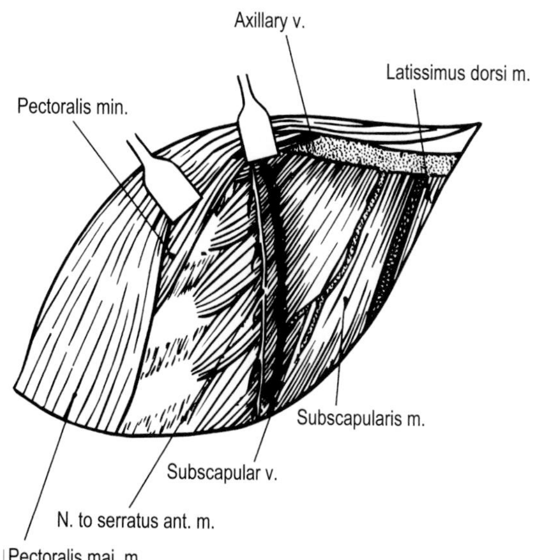

Fig. 25.6 Left Patey's operation with preservation of pectoralis minor.

3 After completing the closure, activate the vacuum drains and squeeze out all the fluid and air from beneath the skin flaps so that they adhere to the chest wall.

? DIFFICULTY

1. Rarely, you may have to apply a split skin graft to part of the wound if the skin edges cannot be opposed without tension. If so, the surgery has probably been too radical or the case selection inappropriate.
2. A myocutaneous flap gives a better cosmetic result in these circumstances.

Aftercare

1 Supplying and arranging the fitting of a breast prosthesis for the patient is really within the operation considerations.

2 Artificial breasts are now available that are of a weight and consistency comparable with the removed breast. They change shape with the patient's change of posture and they take on body temperature. It is almost impossible to tell which is the side of the mastectomy when feeling through a patient's clothes, and this is of very great importance to her as a woman. She can buy clothes as anyone else does, and also wear swimsuits and evening dresses without calling attention to her deficiency.

3 Make yourself aware of the range and variety of prostheses available. In the UK, under Health Service regulations, any woman is entitled to the type and size of prosthesis of her choice. In addition, these may be replaced as frequently as necessary. If you are unaware of the variety available, delegate the responsibility to the Appliance Officer.

4 Many centres now employ mastectomy counsellors who, as well as providing psychosocial rehabilitation of the patient, are responsible for the physical rehabilitation. This includes the prescription of a soft temporary prosthesis immediately postoperatively, which can be worn for about 6 weeks until the wound is no longer sore and then replaced by the permanent prosthesis worn within the brassiere.

5 No woman should leave hospital with a stiff shoulder following mastectomy. Commence active physiotherapy within 24 hours of operation and provide the patient with a list of exercises for abduction of the arm. Encourage her to brush her hair and fasten the back of her dress.

BREAST RECONSTRUCTION

- In order to undertake breast reconstruction you need skill in assessing the patient's suitability for the various procedures as well as in the technical performance of a procedure.
- While most patients with operable breast cancer can now be treated by breast-conserving surgery, careful attention must be paid to patient selection and technique to achieve optimal cosmetic results. All patients undergoing mastectomy should be offered the option of a reconstruction, as either an immediate or a delayed procedure. Fears about hiding local recurrence or affecting survival are unfounded and have been disproved.
- The aims of a breast reconstruction are to achieve symmetry, provide a lasting result and satisfy the patient's requirement for a pleasing aesthetic result in terms of shape, form, consistency and size. These demand a skilled, experienced surgeon specializing in breast reconstruction. There are many available techniques, including the insertion of a submuscular silicone implant, placement of a tissue expansion device with subsequent implant insertion, implantation of a 'permanent' expander, and autogenous tissue transfer using either the latissimus dorsi myocutaneous flap with a silicone implant or the transverse rectus abdominis muscle (TRAM) flap, which has the advantage of not requiring an implant.
- The patient may want construction of a new nipple/areola complex and may need adjustment of the contralateral breast.
- Loss of more than 10% of the breast volume is associated with a cosmetic defect. Some patients may be suitable for 'fill' procedures such as latissimus dorsi mini-flap without transposition of skin.

BREAST RECONSTRUCTION WITH A 'PERMANENT' TISSUE EXPANDER

Appraise

- Prior chest wall irradiation is a relative contraindication to this procedure.
- Following mastectomy a breast mound can be recreated using a subpectoral silicone prosthesis. This can be done either at the time of mastectomy or as a delayed procedure at any time later.
- Note that only a very moderate degree of ptosis can be achieved by an implant and there is a limit to the size of breast mound that can be made. In patients with large and/or ptotic breasts either a myocutaneous flap such as the TRAM flap may be indicated. Alternatively, the contralateral breast can be reduced or lifted.

KEY POINTS Suitability?

- Involve the Breast Counsellor Nurse.
- Have the patient assessed as to her suitability for breast reconstruction and the choice of method.
- Show her photographs of your results, let her read any literature on the subject and if possible meet a patient who has had the procedure.
- This ensures that she has realistic expectations and is likely to be satisfied with the result.

Prepare

1 Discuss the operation and complications with the patient, including any concerns she may have about silicone. You can reassure the patient that silicone leakage does not cause problems.

2 Order the implants if a bank of implants if not available. To gain enough expertise in reconstruction operations, it is likely you will be working a unit that has access to these facilities.

3 Preoperatively, mark the breast borders, including the position of the inframammary fold.

4 Administer antibiotics with induction of anaesthesia.

Action

1 If the procedure is being performed at the same time as mastectomy, following removal of the breast and axillary dissection make an incision in the line of the fibres of pectoralis major at about the level of the sixth intercostal space.

2 If the procedure is delayed, open the old mastectomy scar and free skin flaps from underlying fascia and muscle using sharp dissection.

3 Form a pocket between pectoralis major and the underlying ribs and intercostal muscles. Use a combination of blunt and sharp dissection, including cutting diathermy.

KEY POINTS Technical aids

- Make sure you have good lighting. A head-light may be a valuable aid.
- Carefully arrange suitable retraction.
- Maintain good haemostasis.

4 You may need to employ sharp dissection under the fibres of rectus abdominis muscle.

5 Open the implant and soaked it in an iodine solution. Remove all air from the implant and insert it into the submuscular pocket (see Fig. 25.7).

6 One-stage implants such as the Becker or McGhan implants have a silicone shell and saline-filled cavity, which is inflated over time to expand the tissues. Inflation is performed through the subcutaneously implanted port. The port and its tubing are brought out of the submuscular pocket at the lateral side of the chest wall, through pectoralis major muscle. You need to form a subcutaneous pocket using dissecting scissors, well away from the implant.

7 Suture the port in place.

8 Close the pectoralis muscle over the implant. Inflate the implant with up to 100 ml of saline provided the muscle tension allows this.

? DIFFICULTY

1. If the pectoralis muscle is somewhat atrophied in the lower part, it can be completely detached from its lower border and either the muscle can be closed over the prosthesis or it can even be left so that the lower part of the implant is subcutaneous.
2. If you make small holes in the muscle when forming the subpectoral pocket, repair them using absorbable sutures.
3. You may improve the cosmetic result by reconstructing a submammary fold using absorbable sutures from the muscle to the subcutaneous tissue.

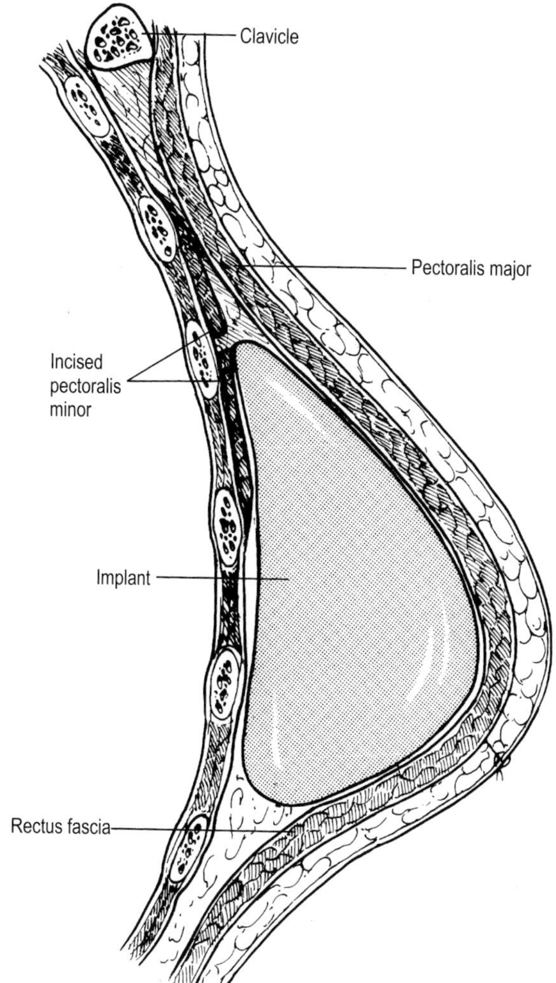

Fig. 25.7 Subpectoral silicone implant.

Closure

1 Insert two vacuum drains, one submuscularly over the implant and the other subcutaneously.

2 Close the wound in two layers uniting subcutaneous tissues deeply and closing the skin with subcuticular sutures.

Aftercare

1 Arrange for the patient to wear a firm brassiere or compression garment for at least 2 weeks.

2 Once the wound has healed and the sutures are removed, commence expansion of the prosthesis as an outpatient procedure under sterile conditions. Insert a butterfly needle into the port at the side of the chest wall and inject 50–100 ml of saline. Repeat this at weekly or longer intervals until you achieve the correct volume to match the opposite breast. Some devices, such as the Becker, require over-expansion for a time.

3 Warn the patient that full ptosis takes up to 1 year.

LATISSIMUS DORSI RECONSTRUCTION

1 The latissimus dorsi is generally a safe flap and within the expertise of an experienced breast surgeon (see Ch. 39).

You should have observed a number of operations before attempting it.

2 Develop the ability to think in three dimensions so you can assess which skin, if necessary, needs to be rotated to fill the defect.

3 The flap area can be used without skin to fill large defects.

DEVELOPMENTAL ABNORMALITIES

Appraise

- Mastitis neonatorum occurs in the first few days of life, is associated with maternal hormones and subsides spontaneously. Rarely, infection supervenes, requiring surgical drainage.
- Extra or supernumerary breasts and/or nipples are encountered along the milk line from midclavicular region to groin. Do not intervene unless they become involved with a disease process such as may affect normal breast tissue or unless the size is cosmetically unacceptable. Lactation may occur with pregnancy, and carcinoma occasionally arises in a supernumerary breast. Treatment is as for any breast disease.
- With the onset of puberty, one breast disc may enlarge in a young girl from the age of 8 years onwards. If the disc is excised, no breast will develop on this side of the body; if it is biopsied, the developed breast may be deformed.

KEY POINTS Preserve children's breasts

- Do not excise unilateral breast enlargements thinking they are neoplasms.
- Neoplasms are almost unknown before the age of 12 years.
- See the child again in 2 months; usually the other breast disc has begun to enlarge.
- Reassure the mother and child.

- In some racial groups (Afro-Caribbean and some Indian/Pakistani groupings), axillary accessory breast tissue can be a problem. This accessory tissue is occasionally removed for cosmesis or if it enlarges extensively during pregnancy. The scars are often unattractive and may become infected so counsel the patient beforehand.
- Poland's syndrome is an uncommon congenital chest-wall deformity characterized by unilateral absence of the sternal head of the pectoralis major muscle, deficiency of the breast and nipple, chest-wall deformity and abnormalities of the upper extremity including finger-shortening and syndactyly. Correction is difficult and requires specialist expertise.
- Breast size is rarely uniform and you may be consulted by patients asking for a procedure to make them even. Should you enlarge the smaller breast or reduce the larger breast? Generally, prefer the latter unless the smaller breast is very undeveloped. Timing is important. The under-developed breast may catch up towards the end of puberty; balance this against the embarrassment that unevenness may cause during this period of a girl's life.

OTHER BREAST PROCEDURES

BREAST AUGMENTATION

This requires insertion of prostheses either in the submammary or subpectoral plane in order to enhance the breast size. This operation is not generally available on the UK Health Service. Take care in counselling these patients. Determine what exactly the patient's expectations are. Unless you are expert, refer these patients to a specialist.

BREAST REDUCTION

This operation is allowed on the National Health Service and is generally of great benefit to the patient. Increasingly a minimum of about 500 g must be removed on each side before the Health Service is willing to allow the procedure to be undertaken.

From the various techniques that are available you need to make a suitable selection for each patient after discussion of the scars, alteration of nipple sensation, potential loss of the nipple, and prospects of breast feeding. Show pictures of previous patients following this procedure. Warn patients that the breast tissue may grow back.

GYNAECOMASTIA

Appraise

- This is frequently unilateral and may occur in boys and young men, either following minor trauma or spontaneously. It usually settles without treatment.
- If it does not settle, it may be necessary to excise the breast disc on one or both sides. Carry this out through a periareolar incision without leaving a noticeable scar but there is a high incidence of postoperative haematomas. It is best to leave a nubbin of breast tissue attached to the areola for best cosmetic results.
- Gynaecomastia also occurs in old age, associated with drugs given for hypertension or congestive cardiac failure. Less frequently nowadays it is seen in men treated with high doses of oestrogens for prostatic cancer and in men suffering from alcoholic cirrhosis. Occasionally, subcutaneous mastectomy is indicated if the condition is an embarrassment or is causing pain and tenderness. The commonest cause now is cannabis usage.
- Operations for gynaecomastia are often performed badly and patient dissatisfaction is high. You must warn the patient about the likely outcome and, if you feel that the patient has inappropriate expectations, refer him to a specialist. Newer techniques of endoscopic surgery and liposuction are available.

FURTHER READING

Bostwick J III 1997 Plastic and reconstructive breast surgery. Quality Medical Publishing, St Louis

Curran D, van Dongen JP, Aaronson N et al 1998 Quality of life of early stage breast cancer patients treated with radical mastectomy or breast conserving procedures. European Journal of Cancer 34:307–314

Dixon M 1995 ABC of breast disease. BMJ Publishing Group, London

Early Breast Cancer Trialists' Collaborative Group 1995 Effects of radiotherapy and surgery in early breast cancer. New England Journal of Medicine 333:1444–1455

Early Breast Cancer Trialists' Collaborative Group 1996 Ovarian ablation in early breast cancer: an overview of the randomised trials. Lancet 348:1189–1196

Early Breast Cancer Trialists' Collaborative Group 1998 Polychemotherapy for early breast cancer: an overview of the randomised trials. Lancet 352:930–942

Early Breast Cancer Trialists' Collaborative Group 1998 Tamoxifen for early breast cancer: an overview of the randomised trials. Lancet 351:1451–1467

Fisher B, Redmond C, Poisson R et al 1989 Eight year results of a randomized trial comparing total mastectomy and lumpectomy with or without radiation in the treatment of breast cancer. New England Journal of Medicine 320:822–828

Harris JR, Hellman S, Henderson IC et al 1987 Breast diseases. Lippincott, Philadelphia

Hermon C, Beral V 1996 Breast cancer mortality rates are levelling off or beginning to decline in many western countries: an analysis of time trends, age-cohort and age-period models of breast cancer mortality in 20 countries. British Journal of Cancer 73:955–960

Hughes LE, Mansel RE, Webster DJT 1989 Benign disorders and diseases of the breast: concepts and clinical management. Baillière Tindall, London

Keshtgar MRS, Ell PJ 1999 Sentinel lymph node detection and imaging. European Journal of Nuclear Medicine 26:57–67

Mariani L, Salvadori B, Marubini E et al 1998 Ten year results of a randomised trial comparing two conservative treatment strategies for small size breast cancer. European Journal of Cancer 34:1156–1162

Silverstein MJ 1998 Ductal carcinoma in situ of the breast. British Medical Journal 317:734–739

26

Thyroid

R.E.C. Collins

CONTENTS

INTRODUCTION

- Thyroid disorders fall broadly into two categories:
  Swellings which can be solitary or multinodular.
  Graves' disease, described by the Irish physician in 1835, is usually, but not always, associated with diffuse enlargement of the gland.
- Thyroid surgery is increasingly performed in major centres by specialist surgeons. Successful thyroid surgery requires judgement as to whether surgery is required and, if so, which is the appropriate operation. For example, there has been a significant movement away from partial thyroidectomy for multinodular goitre, towards total thyroidectomy. The presence of a colloid goitre is not an automatic indication for thyroidectomy. When possible, adhere to evidence-based and consensus management. The British Association of Endocrine Surgeons (BAES) has produced guidelines for the investigation, management, operative selection, perioperative care and subsequent follow-up.
- Exclude, confirm and evaluate thyrotoxicosis with thyroid function tests [thyroid-stimulating hormone (TSH), thyroxine/tri-iodothyronine (T4)/T3)], calcium/albumin and thyroid antibodies. Different laboratories have different ranges for normality so familiarize yourself with local interpretation of results.
- Inappropriate or poorly performed thyroid surgery is reprehensible and invites litigation. Operative complications, particularly damage to the recurrent laryngeal nerve and to parathyroid glands, are potentially so disabling that occasional thyroidectomy is increasingly deprecated. If you carry out thyroid surgery in the UK, you should submit your results to the national audit organized by BAES. If you do not, you expose yourself to adverse legal comment in the event of poor outcomes.

Investigate

1 *Fine-needle aspiration cytology*. Ask the patient to lay supine. Gently extend the neck. Local anaesthesia is unnecessary as the procedure is not painful or distressing. Perform the aspiration free hand, aiming at the dominant nodule. Smear the aspirate, from two or three passes to the nodule, onto a slide and allow it to dry in the air. Use either a 5-ml syringe and green no. 1 needle or a special 'aspiration gun'. Skin preparation is traditionally an alcohol swab but its value is uncertain. Closely co-operate with the cytologist. Cytology may not distinguish between benign and malignant disease in follicular lesions or between a colloid nodule and a follicular neoplasm. Interpretation of the tests is facilitated if the reports are standardized according to the classification of the Association of British Pathologists.

2 *Ultrasound-guided cytological biopsy* is valuable if the nodule is small and difficult to palpate, and is usually conducted by a radiologist in the X-ray department.

3 *Ultrasound scanning*, performed by the radiologist, helps distinguish solitary from multiple nodules, solid from cystic lesions and is a useful adjunct to cytology.

4 *Computed tomography* (CT) scanning clearly defines the relationship of the gland to the trachea and its retrosternal progression, in cases where you suspect malignant disease with lymphatic involvement, or in the presence of large, multinodular goitres.

5 *Routine radio-isotope imaging* of euthyroid multinodular goitres is unnecessary, but it is valuable in toxic disease to identify the site of the toxic focus, which is not always in the dominant nodule.

6 *Laryngoscopy*. Many surgeons routinely employ this preoperatively but others confine themselves to doing it only when there is a history of voice change, previous thyroid surgery or when thyroid malignancy has been already established.

7 *Pulmonary function tests* are valuable in the presence of multinodular goitre and indicate the degree of tracheal compression.

Prepare

1 Offer thorough counselling and consent prior to operation and record the discussion so it can be seen to have been done. Discuss the implications of recurrent laryngeal nerve damage and be prepared to give your own figures. BAES reports an incidence of approximately 5%; a higher rate is unacceptable. Damage from neuropraxia is transient. Subtle changes of timbre of the voice can occur in the absence of obvious damage to the recurrent laryngeal nerve, sometimes from external laryngeal nerve damage. Discuss the small but definite risk of postoperative haemorrhage. There is an inevitable visible scar, sometimes with temporary surrounding numbness. Following in particular total thyroidectomy, temporary or permanent hypoparathyroidism may develop, requiring vitamin D or calcium supple-

ments. Lifelong T4 supplements are needed following total thyroidectomy and in about 20% of patients following hemi-thyroidectomy. If the operation is for malignant disease, warn that adjunctive treatment may be indicated. BAES supplies useful, simple, explanatory leaflets for your patients outlining the operation and its risks.

2 Low-dose heparin prophylaxis against deep vein thrombosis is of unproven value and it may increase perioperative bleeding. However, external pneumatic compression boots may be valuable.

KEY POINTS Record consent discussion

- Record that you have fully explained the risks of thyroidectomy.
- List the precise complications you have discussed.

THYROID NODULE DISEASE

There are three slightly different conditions encompassed by the heading thyroid nodule disease:

- The multinodular goitre.
- The management of a dominant nodule within a multinodular goitre.
- The management of a solitary nodule.

Assess

1 The predominant symptom is of swelling and, only in extreme examples, disorders of swallowing or breathing. Occasionally relatively moderate-sized multinodular goitres may cause surprisingly undue symptoms, particularly if a nodule is situated behind the trachea. This can cause unpleasant symptoms of wanting to cough and tracheal irritation. In more advanced cases, particularly in possible malignancy, seek possible changes in voice from damage to the recurrent laryngeal nerve, and compression, or rarely invasion, of the trachea.

2 Dysphagia is rare. If present exclude globus hystericus and primary oesophageal disease.

3 Sudden pain and swelling is produced by haemorrhage into a cystic component of the goitre.

4 Note the approximate size of the goitre. Is the trachea deviated to one side or compressed? Is there retrosternal progression?

5 Look for venous engorgement.

Appraise

1 The presence of a multinodular goitre is not of itself an indication for surgery.

2 The following are indications for surgery:

- Cytological features of a follicular lesion (adenoma or carcinoma), medullary cancer or papillary cancer.
- Clinical suspicion of malignancy persisting in spite of negative cytology. Remember, fine-needle aspiration cytology (FNAC) is not an exact science and the distinction between a benign colloid nodule and a follicular tumour can be very subtle.
- Mismatch between clinical and investigatory evidence such that malignancy cannot be eliminated.
- Pressure signs or symptoms on trachea or venous return.
- Toxicity, although other treatment modalities need to be discussed.
- Progressive enlargement of a retrosternal goitre.
- Continuing discomfort associated with a goitre.
- Patient preference after thorough and proper counselling. Some patients are intolerant of a persistent neck lump.

GRAVES' DISEASE

Appraise

- Management of Graves' disease demands a multidisciplinary team, including an endocrinologist, a specialist in nuclear medicine, surgeon and anaesthetist. Operation is one of several treatment options, which include antithyroid drugs, beta-blocking drugs and radioactive iodine ablation. A non-surgical team member should participate in recommending operation after the other options have been discussed with the patient, whose views must be taken into account.
- Consider operative treatment only after other treatments have failed, been dismissed by the patient, or in a pregnant woman or one hoping for pregnancy in the near future. Preoperatively, point out to these patients the operative risks, including hypoparathyroidism resulting from radical surgery. Eye signs, such as exophthalmos associated with Graves' disease, may not regress postoperatively—indeed, rarely, in the short term, it may worsen.
- Inform the patient from the unit's records of the likelihood of becoming euthyroid or hypothyroid. Because of the tendency to offer more radical operations in younger patients, recurrent thyrotoxicosis is unlikely.
- The classic operation is subtotal thyroidectomy, designed to render the patient euthyroid. Plan to leave a total thyroid mass of about 4 grams, retaining 2–3-gram remnants of each lobe posteriorly.
- A few patients subsequently develop recurrent thyrotoxicosis; consequently, there is a tendency for more radical surgery. Total thyroidectomy is sometimes recommended especially for young people.
- A compromise is hemi-thyroidectomy on one side, leaving a small remnant on the other side to minimize the danger of post-operative hypoparathyroidism and bilateral recurrent laryngeal nerve damage.

Prepare

1 Render patients euthyroid preoperatively, with antithyroid drugs such as carbimazole, the dose being adjusted for each patient. Alternatively you may institute a 'block and replace' regimen, giving large doses of antithyroid drugs and replacement using T4, while giving beta-blocking drugs, such as propranolol, to reduce the risks of thyrotoxic crisis. Otherwise, give beta-blockers to overcome parasympathetic overactivity.

2 Oral iodine, such as Lugol's iodine, 1 ml daily for 10 days preoperatively, reduces the vascularity of the gland at operation and in theory should reduce blood loss.

OPERATIONS ON THE THYROID

Access

1 Lay the patient supine on the table with a sandbag between the shoulders and a ring or some such securing device under the head so that the neck is extended. Take care in elderly patients not to over extend the neck, since this is associated with postoperative neck stiffness. Raise the head to about 15° to minimize neck vein engorgement. Apply external pneumatic compression boots to the legs.

2 Infiltrate the fascia and platysma under the skin of the neck along the intended incision with 20–30 ml of 1:400 000 adrenaline in physiological saline, prepared by mixing 1 ml of 1% adrenaline (epinephrine) in 400 ml of saline.

KEY POINTS Check the solution

- The adrenaline (epinephrine) solution reduces bleeding from the skin flaps you will create, including platysma, by producing vascular constriction.
- Check the solution yourself, to ensure that it is correct.

3 Standard advice is to make a transverse incision about two finger-breadths above the clavicle. However, this does not allow for variations in the shape of the neck or the nature of the goitre. Carefully inspect the neck and the goitre to estimate where the superior thyroid pedicle lies. Place the incision (Fig. 26.1) such that this can be ligated comfortably and securely with Vicryl at an early stage in the procedure, thus controlling the vessels that may otherwise bleed throughout the operation.

4 Deepen the incision through platysma and to the lateral border of the sternomastoid muscles. Achieve haemostasis using diathermy coagulation or by tying off the larger vessels with Vicryl.

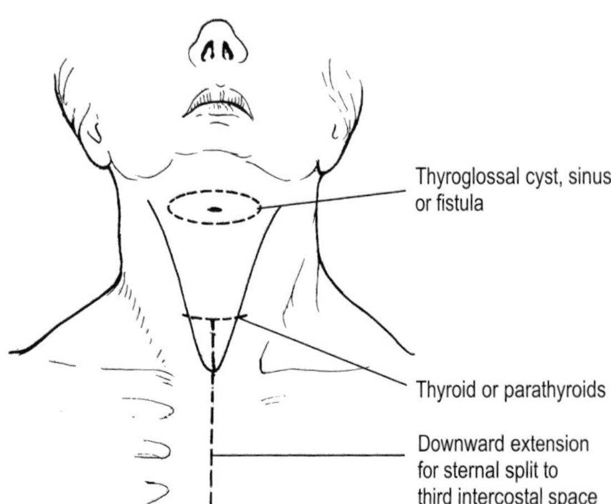

Fig. 26.1 Incisions for operations on the thyroid, parathyroids and thyroglossal lesions.

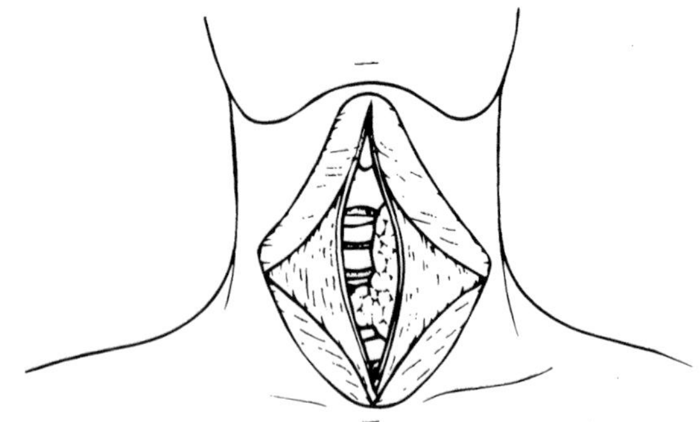

Fig. 26.2 Separation of strap muscles to expose isthmus and larynx.

5 Lift the platysma muscle of the superior flap upwards with Allis forceps, dissecting using coagulating diathermy in the subplatysmal plane. Identify and avoid damaging the anterior jugular veins and cutaneous nerves which lie superficial to the strap muscles. Raise the upper flap as far as the thyroid cartilage.

6 Similarly, raise the lower flap as far down as the sternal notch. When this is completed insert a Joll's or similar self-retaining retractor to the platysma and subdermal tissues at the midpoint of each flap and open it fully to expose the strap muscles.

7 Identify the pale midline raphe between the strap muscles and incise along it using diathermy. Now separate the strap muscles by incising along this line using diathermy, until you see the thyroid gland beneath (Fig. 26.2). At this stage apply an Allis forceps on each side to the medial edge of the strap muscles on the side of the goitre or the dominant or bigger side. Have an assistant lift the strap muscles vertically while you apply pressure on the thyroid gland, pulling it towards you.

8 Create a tissue plane between the strap muscles and the thyroid gland.

9 There are several flimsy layers of fascia to negotiate and this is aided by having the strap muscles lifted off the gland. As the last flimsy layer is divided the vessels on the surface of the thyroid bulge as the restraining pressure is released from them. Once you have established a good tissue plane, remove the Allis forceps from the strap muscles, replacing them with Langenbeck retractors.

10 Dissection should be completely bloodless. Achieve this by applying the diathermy forceps to grasp and seal individual small vessels. Tie larger vessels using fine polyglycolic acid ligatures.

OPERATION FOR BENIGN NODULAR DISEASE

Appraise

- Subtotal lobectomy for nodular goitre results in a 15% recurrence rate, ultimately requiring re-operation. Recurrent nerve palsy rates are higher at re-operation. Subtotal lobectomy is not suitable for the majority of cases of benign nodular disease and its use is confined to Graves' disease.
- There is no place for enucleation of solitary thyroid nodules. Carry out total lobectomy with isthmusectomy. Frozen-section is not recommended.

Action

1 Stand on the opposite side of the patient from the lesion

2 Expose the gland on the affected side, initially retracting the gland medially and vertically upwards.

3 Identify the middle thyroid veins. They are very variable and may be multiple, lying along the anterolateral border of the thyroid or condensed into one or two bigger vessels.

4 Before ligating them, search for the inferior parathyroid gland. It usually lies anteriorly and inferiorly on the capsule of the thyroid gland, but is variable and may lie distinct and separate from the gland, in the fat between the thyroid and thymus. It is tongue-like and 'pinky'-brown. Cautiously and gently free it off the thyroid capsule using diathermy, carefully preserving its own blood supply.

5 Divide the inferior thyroid veins between double ligatures, close to the capsule of the gland.

6 Now that this space is clear, concentrate on securing the superior thyroid artery (Fig. 26.3). Place a small Langenbeck retractor superiorly and a large Langenbeck retractor laterally. Gently push the upper pole of the thyroid laterally and create a tissue plane between the cricothyroid muscle and the superior thyroid vessels, using dissecting scissors. Look out for a small vessel running obliquely across this space and be prepared to control it with a fine ligature. By pulling the vessels laterally away from the cricothyroid you minimize the risk of damaging the external laryngeal nerve, since this usually lies either on, or deep to, the covering of the cricothyroideus muscle. Gently dissect free the vascular pedicle both medially and laterally, using a combination of sharp scissor and gauze pledget dissection. Gently insinuate a Lahey or similar angled forceps, under direct vision, underneath the superior thyroid vessels and draw three 3/0 absorbable ligatures around the vessels. Tie them so you can divide the vessels between the middle and lower ligatures, thus leaving a double tie on the proximal stump.

7 Promptly apply an artery forceps onto the distal, thyroid end of the vessel, otherwise the ligature tends to pull off. The forceps can now be used to apply gentle traction, pulling the upper pole of the thyroid laterally and downwards. Now mobilize the upper part of the thyroid. Look for the tongue-like, pinky-brown, upper parathyroid gland; it is usually adherent to the upper, posterolateral surface of the thyroid. It rarely looks like a nodule or lymph node. Carefully ease the parathyroid gland off the capsule of the thyroid while retaining its own blood supply to preserve its function.

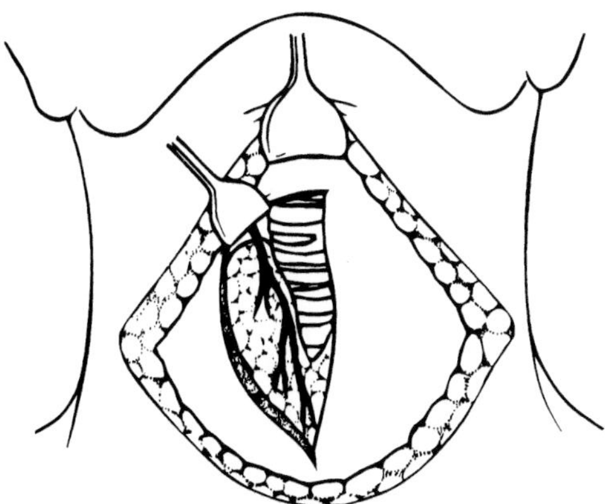

Fig. 26.3 Retraction of strap muscles to expose superior pole and blood supply.

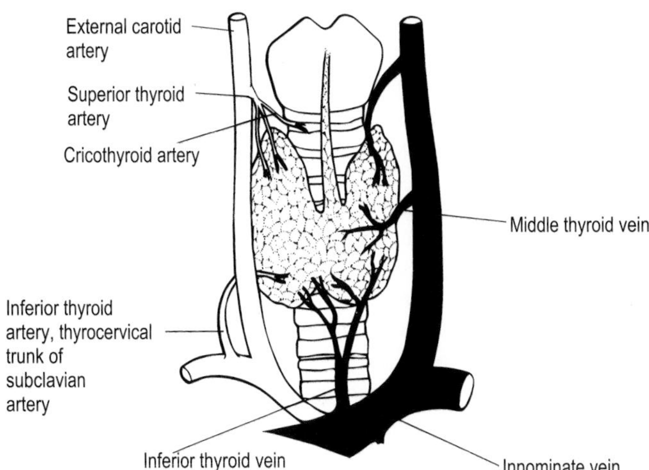

Fig. 26.4 Arterial supply and venous drainage of thyroid.

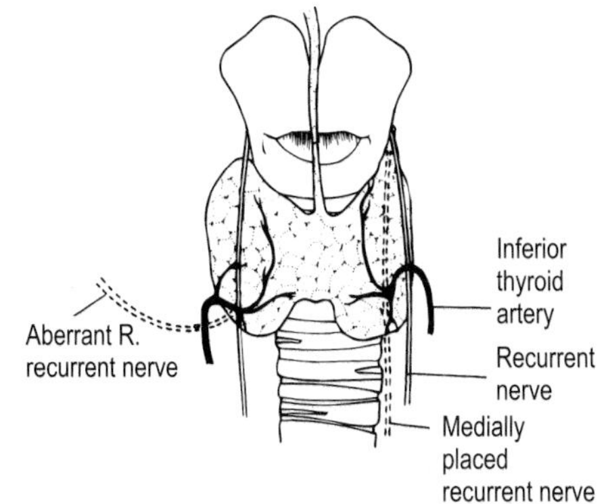

Fig. 26.5 Position of recurrent nerves in relation to inferior thyroid artery and some variations.

8 Now secure the branches of the inferior thyroid artery (Fig. 26.4) on the capsule of the thyroid and identify the recurrent laryngeal nerve. The nerve lies posteriorly and medially in the tracheo-oesophageal groove. Its position is very variable anatomically; although it usually lies deep to the branches of the inferior thyroid artery, occasionally it lies in front of, or between, its branches (Fig. 26.5). In 17% of cases the recurrent laryngeal nerve is bifid for 1–2 cm before entering the cricothyroideus muscle. The nerve appears white, usually with a small red vessel running on its surface. On the right side only, the nerve may be non-recurrent, coming directly either downwards or laterally across from the main vagal trunk.

KEY POINTS Preserve the recurrent laryngeal nerves

- The anatomy of the nerves varies. Learn the normal and variant sites.
- Do not assume where the nerves lie, look widely for them. Do not cut anything until you are certain.

9 Individually ligate with fine Vicryl the branches of the inferior thyroid artery. Tiny branches lying at a distance from the nerve may be cautiously sealed with diathermy current. The ultrasonic harmonic scalpel may be used to seal small vessels but there is still a risk of damaging contiguous tissues, putting the recurrent laryngeal nerve at risk. Avoid undue stretching of the nerve by tenting it up as you retract the thyroid towards you. Follow the nerve up to its point of entry into the larynx close to the lateral thyroid ligament (of Berry). Use a small curved haemostatic clip to create a tunnel parallel to the nerve between the oesophagus and the gland, thus keeping it free of damage. Do not apply a sling or retract the nerve.

10 Dissect across the front of the trachea, separating the gland, using diathermy when necessary; continue, to include the isthmus. There is frequently a pyramidal lobe going between the two main lobes superiorly, upwards high into the neck. Follow it as high as practical and as close to the hyoid bone as possible; then divide it between ligatures. It tends to run to one side or other. If it runs on the affected side, take it with the specimen.

11 The lobe to be removed, and the isthmus, are now free. Place an artery forceps across the contralateral side of the isthmus, divide the gland and remove the specimen. Oversew the remnant capsule with a running Vicryl suture.

Check

1 With the gland divided, check the anatomy, confirm the viability of the parathyroids. If one parathyroid gland is doubtful, remove it, mince it into small pieces and re-implant these either in the sternomastoid or a strap muscle, marking its position with a black silk suture.

2 Assiduously seek and seal any bleeding points.

Drain?

1 Drainage is rarely necessary.

2 If you are in doubt, insert a fine tube drain, taking care not to have the drain end impinge on the recurrent laryngeal nerve.

Closure

1 Approximate the strap muscles using a Vicryl suture.

2 Carefully close the platysma muscle with a continuous Vicryl suture.

3 Use staples or subcuticular absorbable sutures for the skin closure.

RETROSTERNAL MULTINODULAR GOITRE

Appraise

- Most extensions are into the anterior and superior mediastinum. Deliver them into the neck with gentle traction.
- Occasionally they extend behind the trachea, enter into the posterior mediastinum and become intimately related to major vascular structures within the chest. In about 3%, blood supply is from the aortic arch—so-called thyroidea ima (Latin: =lowest). Anticipate, identify, doubly ligate and divide it. If you are not highly skilled and experienced, do not attempt this.
- You may rarely need to divide the sternum to gain access to the superior mediastinum in order to mobilize a largely intrathoracic goitre shaped like a tear-drop, with a narrow neck and wider, inferior bulk.

KEY POINTS Risks of bleeding

- Even though the patient is euthyroid, the blood supply to the gland is often abnormally increased.
- Be obsessive about haemostasis throughout.

SUBTOTAL THYROIDECTOMY FOR GRAVES' DISEASE

Action

1 Expose the whole thyroid gland as for total thyroidectomy.

2 Ligate both superior thyroid poles.

3 Do not divide the inferior thyroid artery. Tie it in continuity, lateral to the recurrent laryngeal nerve avoiding damage to the nerve. There is a theoretical possibility of damage to the blood supply of the parathyroid gland but this is not borne out by comparative studies looking for subsequent hypoparathyroidism.

4 Divide the isthmus and mobilize each lobe laterally.

5 The procedure entails slicing across each lobe from the lateral edge towards the trachea, leaving intact the posterior capsule with the attached remnant of thyroid gland. Leave the thickest part of the remnant laterally, so that it can be folded over medially, allowing the lateral capsular edge to be sutured to the medial capsule.

6 A variety of techniques is available for the actual resection of the gland. A popular method is to place the tips of a series of artery forceps to the capsule from the lateral aspect, around the periphery of the segment to be resected, demarcating the outer edge.

7 While steadying the posterior capsule and attached gland with these forceps, cut within the ring of forceps tips with a scalpel, from lateral to medial, leaving intact the posterior capsule still held with the forceps, covered with the chosen volume of gland remnants, from lateral to medial.

8 As a guide, the remnant strip is often recommended to be 3 cm × 1 cm on each side, bearing in mind that it is easier to treat myxoedema than thyrotoxicosis.

9 Achieve haemostasis using diathermy or suture ligation.

10 Rather than cut the area flat, it helps subsequent closure of the capsule if a deeper area is incised in the middle of the section to be removed. There is thus a thicker remnant of the gland adherent to the lateral remnant of posterior capsule than to the medial part.

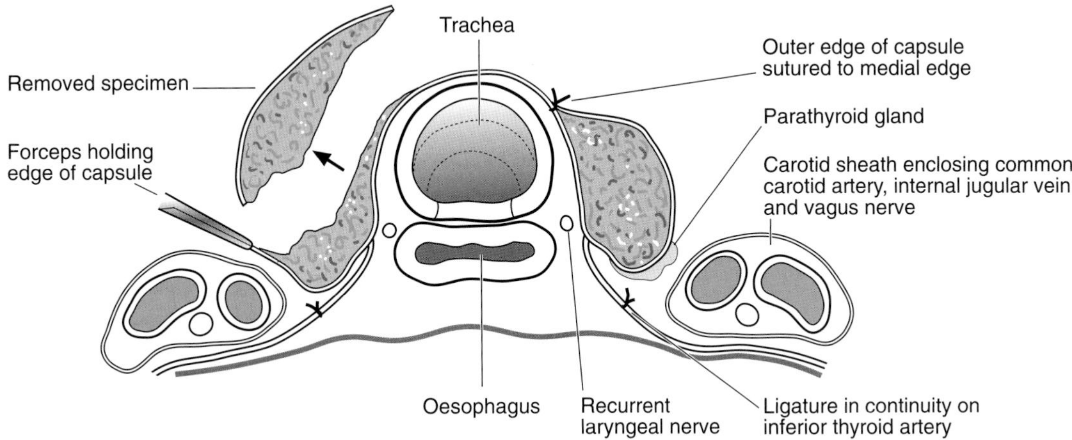

Fig. 26.6 Subtotal thyroidectomy. The diagram shows a transverse section. On the left is the posterior capsule and glandular remnant, thicker laterally. On the right, the posterior capsule and thyroid remnant have been folded medially and sutured to the medial capsular remnant and tracheal adventitia.

11 Close the remnant capsule with a continuous Vicryl suture by folding the lateral edge medially, after reassuring yourself again that you have achieved perfect haemostasis (Fig. 26.6).

12 Even though you took care to control all bleeding throughout, do not close the skin until you have thoroughly re-checked every part of the operative site for bleeding points.

TOTAL THYROIDECTOMY

Action

1 Repeat the process employed for a unilateral lesion on the other side. Follow exactly the same precautions as on the first side.

KEY POINTS Conserve parathyroid function

- Preserve at least one viable gland.
- In case of doubt, remove a doubtful gland, mince it and implant pieces into the sternomastoid or a forearm muscle.
- Following implantation, function takes 3 months to recover.

2 In the presence of malignant disease there are theoretical objections to implanting cells from a potentially malignant field into a new area. I do not recommend it when malignant disease is a possibility.

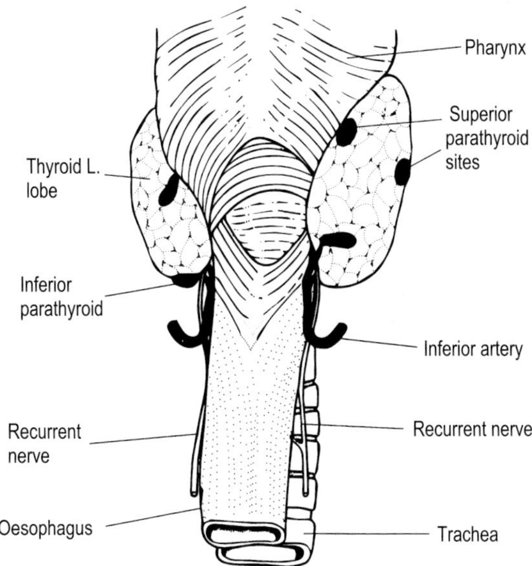

Fig. 26.7 Thyroid and parathyroids seen from behind. Variable positions of parathyroid glands.

MALIGNANT DISEASE

Appraise

- Well-differentiated tumours greater than 2 cm diameter and all medullary carcinomas demand total thyroidectomy as described.
- Treatment of papillary carcinoma, and to a lesser extent follicular carcinoma, is still controversial. One option is lymph node dissection of the central inferior cervical compartment. This entails removing all perithyroid tissues, skeletonizing the trachea and oesophagus while removing lymphatics and the upper thymus, and clearing everything between the recurrent laryngeal nerves and the trachea. There is a risk of damaging aberrant low parathyroid glands with subsequent hypoparathyroidism (Fig. 26.7).
- If there is macroscopic evidence of lymphatic spread in the deep cervical chain in papillary tumours, carry out a limited dissection of the obviously involved glands in this chain. Initial radical neck dissection is rarely indicated.
- In medullary thyroid cancer it is essential that a central lymph node dissection is carried out, as the incidence of local recurrence in this area is high. This condition should only be treated by those with a special experience of it. Remember to screen preoperatively for a phaeochromocytoma as part of a MEN (multiple endocrine neoplasia) syndrome, and if positive deal with the adrenal gland first.

- Anaplastic carcinoma is rarely resectable and attempts to do well-meaning but inappropriate surgery should be resisted.
- There is no place for resectional surgery in thyroid lymphoma. The diagnosis should be made by needle-core biopsy.

MINIMALLY INVASIVE TECHNIQUES

1 A variety of techniques have been developed to remove part or all of the thyroid gland.

2 Laparoscopic instruments can be introduced through the axilla, the anterior chest wall or via periareola incisions in the nipples.

3 Reports of Australian experience suggest a high incidence of recurrent laryngeal nerve damage. Studies of outcome are underway.

4 At present the technique must be restricted to specialist units.

THYROIDECTOMY UNDER LOCAL ANAESTHESIA

The operation was initially performed under local anaesthesia before methods were available to control hyperthyroidism. This continues in a few centres.

A disadvantage is the risk of bilateral paralysis of the recurrent laryngeal nerve resulting from blockade with the local anaesthetic, with consequent difficulty in breathing postoperatively.

RE-OPERATIVE THYROID SURGERY

Appraise

- This is dangerous because you may have no idea of the procedure and of the technical competence of the previous surgeon. The records of the previous operation may not be available. You cannot know how many parathyroid glands are still in present and whether the tissue planes are obliterated. Mid-20th century surgeons sometimes uttered the adage, 'Never re-operate on the thyroid'.
- The exception to this advice is completion thyroidectomy after an original thyroid lobectomy demonstrates the presence of malignant disease demanding a more radical procedure. This is usually carried out shortly after the original procedure, and usually by the same surgeon who knows the circumstances of the original operation.
- Re-operation on benign multinodular goitres is also necessary when the trachea is seriously compromised.
- Alert the patient to the increased risk of damage to recurrent laryngeal nerves and parathyroid glands.
- Always perform preoperative laryngoscopy.

POSTOPERATIVE

1 Impress on nurses and resident doctors the importance of close monitoring to detect difficulty with breathing resulting from blockage of the airway during the next 12 hours following thyroid surgery. This can be due to haematoma formation and subsequent laryngeal oedema. It is life-threatening and frightening for the patient and also the attendants alike. It requires immediate recognition and corrective action.

2 Keep clip-removing forceps by the bedside when clips have been used for closure. Remove clips immediately in order to evacuate the clot.

COMPLICATIONS TO THYROID SURGERY

- *Haemorrhage*. The presence of a vacuum drain does not insure against catastrophic haemorrhage. Bleeding within a closed neck can rapidly lead to laryngeal oedema and tracheal obstruction from clot and blood. Serious respiratory distress or sudden swelling of the neck demand immediate removal of the clips or stitches at the bedside and removal of the sutures apposing both platysma and strap muscles. Ideally intubate patients before returning them to the operating theatre.

KEY POINTS Decompression

- Removing skin clips or stitches alone, is insufficient.
- Remove stitches closing platysma and strap muscles so you can evacuate accumulated clots and blood.

- *Tracheomalacia* (Greek: *malakia*=softness). This rare complication of thyroid surgery results from long-standing pressure on the trachea, usually from large multinodular goitres in countries where treatment is not available. The trachea becomes floppy and collapses after operation, demanding intubation or tracheostomy. Some surgeons doubt its existence.
- *Thyroid crisis*. Imperfectly controlled thyrotoxic patients who undergo operation may develop an acute form of thyrotoxicosis, with hyperpyrexia, tachycardia, respiratory distress and agitation. Treatment is by intravenous beta-blockers, oxygen therapy, sedation and the intravenous administration of sodium iodide solution. Monitor the patient in an intensive care unit.
- *Hypocalcaemia*. Check the blood calcium after all operations for Graves' disease, since there is an incidence of 30% transient hypocalcaemia, following total thyroidectomy. The peak time for hypocalcaemia is probably on the fourth or fifth day postoperatively, by which time many patients may have been discharged if they are otherwise well. Check serum calcium on the first postoperative visit, since latent and undiagnosed hypoparathyroidism can lead to clinical problems such as cataract formation.
- *Postoperative pain*. Thyroid surgery is usually well tolerated and not particularly painful. Nurse patients propped up in bed, the position described by the New York surgeon George Fowler in 1900 for the management of pelvic peritonitis.
- *Hoarseness*. Assume that hoarseness lasting more than 2–3 days is due to recurrent nerve palsy. Request the opinion of an ear, nose and throat surgeon. Most cases result from neuropraxia which is a physiological derangement of normal function; recovery is likely but may take up to 2 months. In addition to huskiness of voice there will be difficulty in the power of cough and this can sometimes lead to respiratory difficulty in the immediate postoperative period.
- *Wound infection*. This should be a rarity.
- A small percentage of thyroidectomy scars develop *keloid*.

- *Hypothyroidism*. All patients having total thyroidectomy need lifetime T4 replacement. Following total thyroidectomy for malignant conditions it is preferable to give T3 rather than T4 because of its much shorter half-life. This allows easier and earlier treatment with radio-iodine ablation for any residual thyroid tissue in the postoperative period.

THYROGLOSSAL CYSTS

Appraise

- These are situated above the thyroid and below the hyoid bone. Although considered midline swellings, they are usually just off the midline to one side and they usually present as painless lumps that move on swallowing or protruding the tongue.
- They are usually excised both for cosmesis (*Greek*: *cosmeein*=to adorn; beautify) and because they occasionally become uncomfortable or infected.
- Occasionally they can discharge in the neck, forming a thyroglossal sinus.
- Cyst excision is advisable (described by the American surgeon Walter Sistrunk in 1920).

Access

1. Position the patient as for a thyroidectomy.
2. Make a skin crease incision over the cyst.

Action

1. Dissect out the cyst to define the tract in its upper position.
2. Separate the strap muscles and trace the tract up to the hyoid bone.
3. Excise the middle portion of the hyoid bone, since thyroglossal tracts have a complex relationship to the back of the body of the hyoid bone. Transect the hyoid bone using small bone-cutting forceps just lateral to the cyst on each side (Fig. 26.8).
4. Follow the tract up into the neck to the base of the tongue.

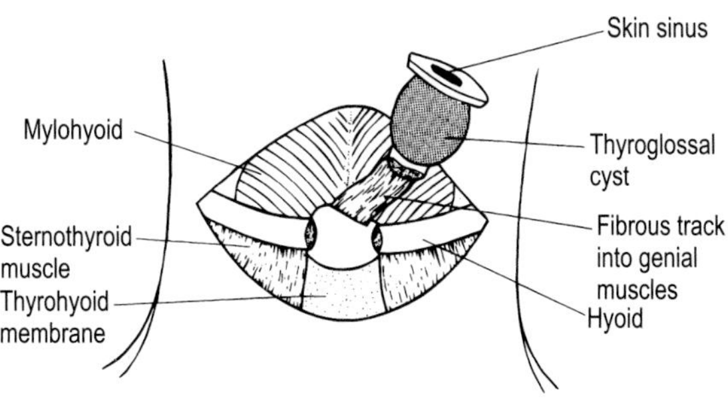

Fig. 26.8 Excision of thyroglossal cyst with sinus, showing excision of hyoid bone.

KEY POINT Haemostasis

- Anticipate, avoid or control bleeding, especially if there has been infection in the cyst or tract.

Closure

1. Re-approximate the strap muscles and the platysma.
2. Insert clips or a subcuticular suture in the skin.

FURTHER READING

Col NF, Surks MI, Daniels GH 2004 Subclinical thyroid disease: clinical applications. JAMA 291:239–243

Denham DW, Angelos P 2003 The pathologist's role in the management of thyroid and parathyroid lesions: the surgeon's perspective. Pathology Case Reviews 8:16–21

Surks MI, Ortiz E, Daniels GH et al 2004 Subclinical thyroid disease: scientific review and guidelines for diagnosis and management. JAMA 291:228–238

Internet web sites

www.BAES.info

Guidelines for the surgical treatment of endocrine disease and training requirements for endocrine surgery. British Association of Endocrine Surgeons, 2004.

27

Parathyroid

R.E.C. Collins

CONTENTS

HYPERPARATHYROIDISM AND PARATHYROIDECTOMY

Hyperparathyroidism is usually classified into primary, secondary or tertiary disease. In practice, secondary hyperparathyroidism is nearly always associated with chronic renal failure and its treatment.

The distinction between secondary and tertiary hyperparathyroidism is often blurred and it may be simpler to refer to primary hyperparathyroidism or hyperparathyroidism associated with renal disease.

In primary hyperparathyroidism a benign adenoma of a single gland is the usual cause, but in 10–15% of cases hyperplasia of more than one gland is the cause and, very rarely, probably less than 1%, the cause is a parathyroid carcinoma. The presence of more than one adenoma has been reported, especially in patients aged over 80 years, but is still rare.

Appraise

- Classic symptoms of hypercalcaemia may be marked or very vague. They are classically described as:
  Moans (neuropsychiatric disorders).
  Bones (osteitis fibrosis cystica and bony pains).
  Stones (renal).
  Abdominal groans (abdominal pain, constipation, pancreatitis and a variety of vague, non-specific abdominal symptoms).
- Many patients are diagnosed co-incidentally with hyperparathyroidism from serum chemistry performed for other medical conditions.
- The surgeon has a responsibility to ensure that, whatever the referral pathway, alternative courses of hypercalcaemia have been excluded. It is also worth noticing that a small percentage of people will have hyperparathyroidism as a feature of one of the multiple endocrine neoplasia (MEN) syndromes. Also occasionally familial hypercalcaemic hypocalciuria can be a catch as it presents a similar biochemical profile, and it is therefore important that urinary calcium estimations are done to exclude this condition.

Investigations

The biochemical diagnosis of hyperparathyroidism requires demonstrating persistently raised levels of serum calcium with an associated high serum parathormone (PTH) level or a level that is inappropriately normal in the presence of high serum calcium levels. Normocalcaemia does not exclude hyperparathyroidism and some patients with renal stones have been shown to have high PTH levels in the presence of a normal serum calcium. Hypocalciuria (less than 2 mmol/day) should prompt the diagnosis of familial hypercalcaemic hypocalciuria.

Preoperative localization. Technetium-99^{m}-labelled sestamibi radionuclear scanning and high-resolution ultrasonography have now been developed with acceptable levels of accurate forecasting of the site of a parathyroid adenoma. These techniques, which were not used regularly by many surgeons, are being developed because of appreciation that this now allows minimally invasive surgery to take place which seems to be beneficial to patients without detriment to the incidence of cure. In secondary hyperparathyroidism, four-gland enlargement is the norm and the surgery will be the same as for hyperplasia due to primary hyperparathyroidism. The indications for a surgical attack very much rely on the indications from the renal physicians where a chronic imbalance of hypercalcaemia and or hyperphosphataemia causes a secondary increase in parathyroid secretion. This can make control of dialysis programmes difficult and can produce significant pathological bone change. It is often accompanied by severe pruritus, muscle weakness and sometimes with soft-tissue calcification.

Indications for surgery

Over the last few years a more liberal approach to surgery for patients with asymptomatic hyperparathyroidism has been developing. There are no clear means to predict which patients will deteriorate if left unoperated upon and there is now some evidence to suggest that patients aged 70 years or less have a higher mortality with untreated disease and that this can be reversed by successful parathyroid surgery.

Cardiac changes have been shown to be reversed after treatment of asymptomatic disease, and symptoms of depression and anxiety may be reversed. Loss of bone mineral content is partially reversible and this is becoming an increasingly important factor in postmenopausal women.

There is no adequate medical therapy that will permanently correct hypercalcaemia preoperatively. Many patients today have relatively mild disease, but a serum calcium level in excess of 3.0 mmol/litre is considered to be an absolute indication for surgery. The patient will require to be hydrated well and if the patient has been admitted in a hypercalcaemic crisis then a period of re-hydration will be mandatory before attempting surgery. If there is evidence of bone disease then preoperative treatment with 1α-hydroxycholecalciferol for a few days may help 'hungry-bone syndrome' in the postoperative period. In other words, by giving preoperative One-Alpha vitamin D, the risk of catastrophic falls in calcium postoperatively because of the bones re-absorbing calcium from the blood can be minimized.

The standard operation to correct hyperparathyroidism is through a cervical collar incision made in a similar way for exploring the thyroid (see Ch. 26). Operations should seek to cure the disease in over 97% of first-time neck explorations. Preoperative counselling should be thorough and should explain the same potential risks as can occur after thyroid surgery. There is also the additional risk of failing to find the gland at the first operation because it may be in an ectopic site such as the mediastinum.

KEY POINTS Experienced?

- Do not attempt parathyroidectomy on an occasional basis.
- Before embarking on this operation seek special training and experience.

STANDARD OPERATION

Access

1. Incision and exposure are as for thyroidectomy (see Ch. 26).
2. To define the parathyroid glands (Fig. 27.1) dislocate the thyroid lobe medially and anteriorly whilst the strap muscles of the neck are retracted laterally in the opposite direction. It is often necessary to divide the middle thyroid veins and the operation should proceed with absolutely meticulous haemostasis.

Intraoperative localization of parathyroids

- In 1971, Dudley introduced the methylthioninium chloride (methylene blue) total-body infusion technique. The standard dose that he described was 5 mg/kg body weight, but Rowntree modified this later to 7.5 mg/kg body weight, particularly in females. Methylthioninium chloride is set up in an infusion of 5% dextrose and usually 500 ml is infused in the hour or so prior to surgery. In patients with chronic renal disease where rapid changes of fluid balance are not sensible, a much smaller volume, normally about 200–250 ml, can be accommodated satisfactorily. In greater than 90% of cases this technique rapidly stains abnormal parathyroid glands a dark blue. It is very exceptional for parathyroid tissues not to be stained and to be very distinctive from the general background blue tones otherwise noted in the tissues. Anaesthetists will need to be warned that this can have an effect on oxygen saturation but it is not a significant problem. Occasionally a few patients having this infusion can experience adverse reactions and therefore they need to be monitored carefully by the nursing staff in the period prior to surgery. If any adverse reaction is noted then the infusion is immediately stopped. Anaphylaxis is extremely rare and would be treated as in any other circumstance.
- Other techniques have been described using radionuclear sestamibi scans and a special probe. There is no evidence that they produce anywhere near as consistently good results as methylthioninium chloride staining and they are much more expensive and time-consuming. A significant number of surgeons, however, use no form of intraoperative localization either through design or ignorance.
- At operation, the parathyroid glands, if methylthioninium chloride has been used, will be readily identified. The *lower gland* is usually situated at the anterior-inferior aspect of the thyroid capsule although in about 15% of cases it can be distinctly separate from the gland and in the upper pole of the thymus. Occasionally the lower gland is situated a little higher, closer to the inferior thyroid artery. The *upper parathyroid gland* is usually situated very high and very posterior on the capsule of the thyroid gland close to the cricothyroidius muscle and usually just above the point of entry of the branch of the inferior thyroid artery into the capsule of the gland. It can be very closely adherent to the recurrent laryngeal nerve but there is normally a distinct tissue plane separating it from that structure. When the upper gland is ectopic it tends to progress inferiorly and posteriorly. Lower glands if they become ectopic go further down to the thymus and are virtually always situated in the anterior mediastinum whereas upper glands are situated in the posterior mediastinum. A common source of intrathoracic glands is in the aortopulmonary window. On occasions ectopic glands can appear just about anywhere else in the neck from inside the carotid sheath to almost up to the base of the skull although these truly difficult ectopic glands are extremely rare.
- In young people with a positive sestamibi and/or ultrasound scan showing a single abnormal gland it is now considered acceptable by many to explore just the one side of the neck and to remove the offending adenoma and to confirm another normal gland. Other surgeons would still explore the contralateral side, particularly in older patients because of the small chance of detecting a second adenoma.
- An increasingly difficult problem in older people with milder disease forms who are now being operated on earlier in their

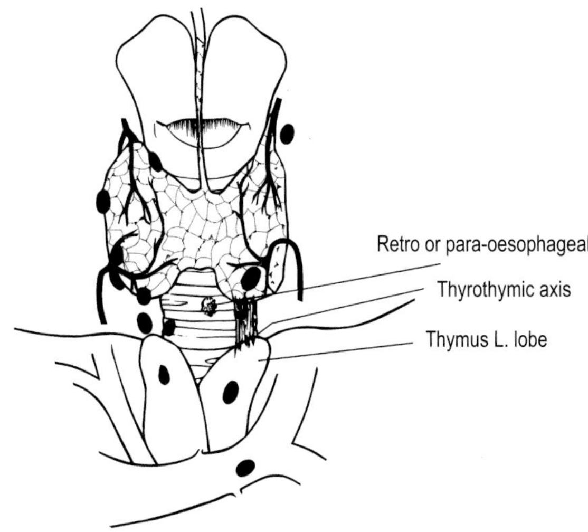

Fig. 27.1 Various positions for parathyroid glands.

disease process than they were hitherto is that the distinction between a solitary adenoma and three 'normal glands' can be difficult to detect from hyperplasia affecting mainly one gland with mild hyperplasia of the other three. This requires great judgement and in cases of doubt it is recommended that three and a half glands would be removed. If more than one gland is clearly involved, or in fact we are dealing with hyperplasia due to either primary or secondary hyperparathyroidism, then it is usual to remove three and a half glands. Some authorities would remove all four and run the patient postoperatively on calcium and vitamin D supplements.

KEY POINTS Four-gland hyperplasia

- In four-gland hyperplasia it is sensible to not leave the half gland left behind to be the last gland to be operated upon.
- Just occasionally this fourth gland can in fact be damaged by the technique and will need complete removal. It is better, therefore, to do this earlier on with either the first or second gland to be removed so that, if there is a mishap, a portion of one of the other glands can still be left behind.

- The glands are enclosed in a little envelope of fat that moves separately from the thyroid. If methylthioninium chloride is not used they can be identified because they are a pale brown or tan colour. It is sometimes difficult to decide whether a large nodule is a thyroid nodule (part of a colloid nodule or even an adenoma) or whether it is pathological parathyroid gland. In these situations the thyroid nodule when cut virtually always demonstrates an irregular surface almost as it if follicles can be identified with the naked eye. In parathyroid disease, however, it is rather like cutting across a blancmange as the consistency is homogeneous. Parathyroid glands have a very rich blood supply and tiny vessels can be seen coursing across the surface. There is usually a small feeding vessel which can be gently touched with the diathermy of course making sure that the gland is not in close proximity to the recurrent laryngeal nerve. If there is any doubt a tiny silver clip can be placed over the feeding vessel.
- Some surgeons send the glands for frozen-section histological evaluation, but many surgeons do not. The histological interpretation of tiny pieces of tissue with all the artefacts of frozen section is not always reliable and a competent experienced parathyroid surgeon can virtually always satisfactorily identify parathyroid glands.

KEY POINTS Description of parathyroid glands

- Parathyroid glands are like little tongues. They are not usually round and globular unless they are significantly enlarged and their consistency is quite different from that of lymph nodes.
- Lymph nodes very rarely pick up methylthioninium chloride.

- Sometimes, in spite of a positive sestamibi scan and/or an ultrasound localization, the gland cannot be identified at operation. Rarely this is because the parathyroid adenoma is intrathyroid. True intrathyroid parathyroids are very rare and they are usually situated in little clefts in the surface of the gland, but on some occasions they can be truly within the gland substance itself. In this situation it would be acceptable to perform a hemithyroidectomy if there was a clear-cut preoperative localization study indicating the site of the lesion. In incidences where the lower gland cannot be found, it may well be acceptable to pull the thymus gently up into the neck and remove as much of it on that side as is possible.

LATERAL APPROACH TO THE PARATHYROIDS

- Some surgeons, through a collar incision, instead of separating the strap muscles and going to look for the parathyroids between the thyroid and the strap muscles, actually develop a tissue plane between the strap muscles and the sternomastoid and then come in behind the strap muscles to look for parathyroids on each side.
- This approach is the basis of the increasingly popular localized lateral approach for parathyroid surgery. This is gaining popularity following the rapidly gaining experience and increasing confidence in preoperative localization techniques such as sestamibi scanning and high-definition ultrasonography. The lower glands are much more accessible and easily found with this technique than the upper ones although many surgeons are now using it for both upper and lower glands. Essentially an incision about 2.0 cm long is made transversely across the neck just in front of the sternomastoid muscle on the side of the suspected adenoma. With good imaging the size and structure of the thyroid can be seen from the scan and this can be readily transposed to the operative situation so that the incision can be placed over the lower or upper pole of the thyroid whichever seems appropriate. A tissue plane is then created lateral to the strap muscles and between them and the sternomastoid. The thyroid capsule is found and then the lower or upper parathyroid is searched for. This approach is greatly enhanced by the use of intraoperative methylthioninium chloride staining and the use of a headlight for the operating surgeon also makes life much easier.
- Having removed the gland there is only need just to close the platysma and oppose the skin either with sutures, staples or just sticky-paper dressings. The operation can be done in straightforward cases by an experienced surgeon in under 10 minutes and the patient can be allowed home later the same day.

OTHER MINIMALLY INVASIVE TECHNIQUES

These are being developed particularly in Italy and France and use laparoscopic-type equipment to create a small defect in the neck to again enter the same tissue planes as for the lateral approach and the glands can be removed in the same way.

There have been other approaches for those patients who feel strongly about not having a scar in their neck to approach the thyroid through incisions made either in the axilla or, in some case reports, via the periareola incision made around one of the nipples.

In general terms, however, the small localized lateral cervical incision heals so beautifully that it is virtually invisible within a few weeks of surgery.

THE USE OF INTRAOPERATIVE PTH SERUM ASSAY

There has recently been a vogue which has risen and fallen again to do rapid serum assay estimations of PTH levels to confirm that the offending gland has been removed and that no other glands are left hypersecreting.

Although different units report different experiences, there now seems to be sufficient experience to suggest that false positives and false negatives can occur with this technique and it does add a significant cost to the procedure without clearly demonstrating benefit to the patient.

Once an adenoma has been removed, it is not usually now considered necessary to biopsy the normal glands. This produces an increased incidence of postoperative hypocalcaemia.

PARATHYROID CARCINOMAS

Parathyroid carcinomas are usually associated with extremely high calcium levels and sometimes with a palpable gland in the neck preoperatively.

The tumours can be identified at operation because they tend to invade neighbouring structures, particularly the thyroid gland and on occasions the recurrent laryngeal nerve. Indeed, someone presenting with hypercalcaemia and voice changes should always be considered to have a parathyroid carcinoma and counselling should be given preoperatively that there may be risks of permanent changes to the voice.

The usual recommended procedure if parathyroid carcinoma is suspected is to perform a hemithyroidectomy on the same side and also to remove any tissues nearby that are clearly macroscopically affected. This would include any obviously enlarged lymph nodes but it is not usual at the first operation to recommend radical removal of lymphatic tissue in the neck.

RE-OPERATION

Re-operation for persistent or recurrent hypercalcaemia should only be performed by experts, and it is considered mandatory to attempt localization studies beforehand. In addition to ultrasonography and sestamibi scanning, the use of CT (computed tomography), PET (positron emission tomography) scanning, arteriography and venous sampling in the neck all have their advocates. In general, the more investigations that can be done in these cases the better.

The most usual place for a missed parathyroid gland at the original surgery is in one of the standard anatomical positions; parathyroid glands in extremely ectopic positions are extremely uncommon.

CLOSURE AND POSTOPERATIVE CARE

1 The wound of the standard cervical incision is closed in the usual way for a thyroid operation.

2 It is not necessary usually to put drains in, but certain patients with renal disease who have been on steroids are hypertensive and those who have had a difficult neck dissection may benefit from a small suction drain for a day or so.

3 The vast majority of patients undergoing parathyroid surgery do not run into problems with hypocalcaemia postoperatively. A small number do and these can sometimes be predicted. They are those who have significant bone disease, those who have significant metabolic biochemical disorders and those who start with calcium levels in excess of 3.25 mmol/litre.

4 It is traditional to believe that serum calcium levels fall within the first 24 hours and occasionally they can be low, but in practice the time of maximum fall of calcium levels is usually on postoperative day 5, by which time most patients have been discharged. It is therefore important that patients are warned of symptoms of tingling in the hands or tetany, and that if there are any adverse occasions if they have been discharged early they should be encouraged to report back to hospital.

5 Asymptomatic hypocalcaemia to a level of about 2.0 mmol/litre does not usually need any specific treatment and usually spontaneously corrects within 24–48 hours. Calcium levels below 2 mmol/litre, or where there are symptoms of hypocalcaemia such as tetany and tingling, are usually treated with a combination of intravenous infusion of calcium gluconate plus the oral administration of various calcium supplements and One-Alpha vitamin D (One-Alpha calciferol). Patients can safely be discharged on this; then, at follow-up within a week or two in outpatients, their calcium levels can be monitored and attempts made to withdraw the supplements.

6 In the case of solitary adenomas it is usual to see patients once more at about 3 months when they can safely be discharged. Patients who have hyperplasia, however, should be kept under permanent review because as the years go by there is a tendency for the remnant half gland to enlarge and become reactive. This only happens in a small percentage of people but prudence dictates that it is sensible to follow up such patients for life.

FURTHER READING

Armstrong J, Leteurtre E, Proye C 2003 Intraparathyroid cyst: a tumour of branchial origin and a possible pitfall for targeted parathyroid surgery. Australian and New Zealand Journal of Surgery 73:1048–1051

Borley NE, Collins RE, O'Doherty M et al 1996 Technetium-99m sestamibi parathyroid localisation is accurate enough for unilateral neck exploration. British Journal of Surgery 83:989–991

Dudley NE 1971 Methylene blue for rapid identification of the parathyroids. British Medical Journal 3:680–681

Irvin GL, Molinari AS, Figueroa C et al 1999 Improved success rate in reoperative parathyroidectomy with intraoperative PTH assay. Annals of Surgery 229:874

Palazzo FF, Sadler GP 2004 Minimally invasive parathyroidectomy. British Medical Journal 328:849–850

Internet web site

www.BAES.info

Guidelines for the surgical treatment of endocrine disease and training requirements for endocrine surgery. British Association of Endocrine Surgeons, 2004.

28

Adrenalectomy

R.E.C. Collins

CONTENTS

INTRODUCTION

Adrenalectomy is most commonly undertaken for a benign unilateral adrenal adenoma that is usually functional, patients presenting with the consequence of excessive secretion of hormone rather than the mechanical effect of the adrenal tumour. Bilateral adrenal surgery is sometimes undertaken for simultaneously occurring bilateral adrenal tumours or for hypersecreting states associated with certain types of Cushing's syndrome associated with an excess of ACTH (adrenocorticotrophin) production.

Rare tumours such as carcinoma occasionally present, offering the chance of surgical removal. Laparoscopic approaches are increasingly used. Do not embark on this demanding area without adequate training in open or laparoscopic techniques. Patients with functional secreting endocrine tumours require adequate preparation. Closely co-operate with endocrinology and anaesthesiology colleagues.

Appraise

- *Phaeochromocytomas* (Greek: *phaios*=dusky) arise in the adrenal medulla and secrete adrenaline, noradrenaline or dopamine. They present with episodic headaches, palpitations, hypertension and various syndromes involving apprehension and fear. Confirm the diagnosis by detecting increased levels of urinary catecholamines and by finding a tumour on computed tomography (CT), magnetic resonance imaging (MRI) or meta-iodobenzylguanidine (MIBG) imaging. 10% of phaeochromocytomas do not arise in the adrenal gland, 10% are bilateral, 10% are malignant and 10% occur in childhood. Noradrenaline-secreting tumours are most frequent and require adequate, preoperative alpha-adrenergic blockade using appropriate agents. Occasionally propranolol can be used to produce beta-blockade. Try to achieve normotension with preoperative medication over a period of 2–4 weeks. It is usual to give preoperative fluid loading with intravenous normal saline or dextrose for 24 hours preoperatively.

KEY POINTS Diagnosis

- Many diagnostic tests must be performed while the patient is off any antihypertensive therapy.
- Consult with an endocrinologist to confirm the appropriate diagnosis.

- *Conn's syndrome*, described by the Ann Arbor physician in 1955, usually results from an adenoma arising from the zona glomerulosa—the outer layer of the adrenal cortex and which secretes mineralocorticoids. Hyperaldosteronism produces hypertension with associated hypokalaemia (serum potassium less than 3.5 mmol/litre) which is often resistant to normotensives. Confirm the diagnosis by detecting raised levels of plasma aldosterone with decreased plasma renin. Estimate the size of the adenoma with CT and MRI. The demonstration of a cortical adenoma on scanning is not proof that it is Conn's syndrome. There are other causes of hypertension with a non-functioning, benign cortical adenoma.
- Prepare the patient for 2–3 weeks before operation with spironolactone as an antagonist of aldosterone.
- *Cushing's syndrome* was described in 1932 by the American neurosurgeon. Adenomas arise in the zona fasciculata and secrete excess glucocorticoids. Make the diagnosis by detecting raised plasma cortisol with loss of a normal diurnal variation and an increased 24 hour urinary cortisol. A dexamethazone suppression test helps confirm the diagnosis. In Cushing's disease, a pituitary adenoma produces ACTH with bilateral adrenal cortical hyperplasia. Plasma concentrations of ACTH are raised and can be suppressed by high-dosage dexamethazone. Preoperatively, you may give metyrapone, a competitive inhibitor of 11β-hydroxylation in the adrenal cortex, thus inhibiting the production of cortisol, to control the symptoms. Patients with adrenal hyperplasia from ACTH hypersecretion require bilateral adrenalectomy with hydrocortisone during and after the operation. In the presence of unilateral adenoma, steroid production from the other gland may be suppressed for up to 12 months before normal function resumes. Appropriately administered hydrocortisone is also needed for those having single-side adrenalectomy. These patients, like those with a phaeochromocytoma, need regular perioperative blood sugar determinations. Most require postoperative monitoring in an intensive care or high dependency unit.
- *Virilizing* (Latin: *virilis*=man) *and feminizing syndromes* are rare and can be produced by excessive sex steroid secretion from an

adenoma in the inner zona reticularis. There is a high incidence of malignancy.

- *'Incidentalomas'* are adrenal cortical tumours discovered by chance, often as a result of CT or MRI scans performed for the diagnosis of other conditions. Investigations demonstrate that some are functional, so they all must be screened for hormonal activity. Some are associated with metastatic malignant disease. However, it is rare for a solitary adrenal metastasis to be detected on MRI scanning without finding an associated primary lesion if it had not been detected previously. Non-functioning tumours less than 5 cm diameter can usually be left but monitored regularly. Because of the increased risk of malignancy in tumours larger than 5 cm, remove them.
- *Adrenocortical carcinoma and other rare tumours*. Adrenocortical carcinoma is often highly malignant. Adrenalectomy is the one hope of cure but the 5-year survival rate is in the region of only 20–35%.

ADRENALECTOMY

DECIDE

1 As a rule treat solitary tumours by total removal of the affected adrenal gland. Where there is adrenal hyperplasia in Cushing's disease, remove all adrenal tissue. Subtotal excision of an adrenal tumour is inappropriate.

2 Laparoscopic removal is increasingly employed for small tumours. Prefer open operation for removal of malignant, large tumours and when there are difficulties such as adhesions following previous operations.

PREPARE

1 Bring the patient to the best possible condition before operation.

2 Order thromboprophylaxis during the perioperative period.

3 Prescribe prophylactic antibiotics for patients with Cushing's disease or syndrome.

LAPAROSCOPIC APPROACH

There are two routes: the transperitoneal and the retroperitoneal.

TRANSPERITONEAL APPROACH

Right side

1 Elevate the side to be operated upon with a combination of sandbags and table-tilting to position the patient half-way between true lateral and fully supine. It is useful to 'break' the operating table. Create a pneumoperitoneum, usually using a Veress needle. Create four or five ports situated in the subcostal space between the midline and the axillary fold. Occasionally a lower port may be preferable for a camera.

2 Now retract the liver with a rigid steel rod or a Nathanson retractor. Carefully dissect off the peritoneum overlying the tumour and vena cava, using diathermy and an ultrasonic scalpel, which is particularly useful for sealing small vessels.

KEY POINTS Dissect carefully

- Avoid damaging the vena cava.
- Confirm the anatomy, particularly the relation of the tumour to the renal vessels.

3 Continue the dissection between the vena cava and the gland or tumour to identify the main adrenal vein. Apply three occluding clips and divide the vein leaving two clips on the caval side. Continue the dissection close to the tumour and divide all other vessels with diathermy, scissors or an ultrasonic dissector. Large aberrant vessels may develop in the presence of phaeochromocytomas; they also need to be clipped.

4 Gently mobilize the tumour, leaving the diaphragm intact and free from diathermy injury. Now remove the tumour within a bag through a widened port site.

Left side

1 Reverse the position of the patient on the operating table, otherwise the approach is identical to that for the right gland.

2 Expose the gland in one of two ways. You may bring the spleen forward with the tail of the pancreas, then approach the adrenal gland between the spleen and the diaphragm. Sometimes, after carefully retracting the spleen laterally, you can approach the adrenal gland above the pancreas. In either approach you must free the splenic flexure of the colon to gain access. Clip the vessels similarly to those on the right side.

RETROPERITONEAL APPROACH

1 Place the patient semiprone, so you can insert ports posteriorly into the retroperitoneal fat just below the costal margin. This is a valuable approach for particularly large patients with Cushing's disease, or in the presence of previous upper abdominal surgery.

2 Create an artificial space, either with an inflatable balloon or by using higher-pressure insufflation than that used in an intraperitoneal approach, rising up to 19–20 mmHg.

4 Identify the gland in the same manner as in the open approach.

5 Control the vessels with clips, diathermy or harmonic scalpel.

OPEN APPROACHES

POSTEROLATERAL APPROACH

1 This is the most popular open route for patients with large, potentially malignant tumours.

2 Position the patient lying on one side with the affected side uppermost. Support the patient with sandbags or supports in front and behind. A strap usually secures the patient's pelvis. Place the upper arm in a suitable arm rest at the same height as that shoulder. You may 'break' the table to tense the skin and fascia on the operative side.

3 Make an incision over the eleventh rib from the lateral edge of the paravertebral muscles to the lateral rectus sheath margin. Divide latissimus dorsi and serratus posterior muscles with cutting diathermy and incise the periosteum of the eleventh rib

using a diathermy point. Strip the periosteum from the rib throughout its length, freeing the deep attachments to the rib with a gauze swab. Dissect the rib free anteriorly first, elevating it as the dissection proceeds.

KEY POINTS Anatomy

- Do not damage the intercostal neurovascular bundle, lying immediately inferior to the rib margin.
- Do not injure the underlying pleura, which is vulnerable posteriorly.

4 Cut through the rib costal cartilage with scissors and remove it. Sweep the pleura superiorly and posteriorly and similarly sweep the peritoneum anteriorly, using gauze swabs.

5 Identify the kidney, lying inferiorly. Incise the deep fascia, allowing the retroperitoneal fat to bulge out. Have the kidney retracted inferiorly, while you proceed carefully by blunt dissection of the fat above and medial to the kidney, using light scissors (Fig. 28.1).

6 The right adrenal tends to cap the upper pole of the kidney whereas on the left side it is more related to the upper medial border. Feel and see large tumours with small veins coursing away from the gland, particularly in phaeochromocytomas; they demonstrate that the dissection is adjacent to the adrenal gland.

KEY POINTS Look for a golden edge

- The adrenal gland has a characteristic golden colour quite distinctive from surrounding fat.
- Once you find this edge the operation becomes easier as you dissect along the edge.

7 You may be unable to identify any normal adrenal gland in the presence of a large phaeochromocytoma. Handle the gland carefully. Do not grasp it with forceps. Prefer retracting it by inserting 5–6 continuous bites of Vicryl or monofilament nylon suture held up and clipped. Since the force is distributed through several points the gland remains intact. Be patient. Skilful dissection of an adrenal gland is a slow process, particularly in very fat patients with Cushing's syndrome. Avoid haste.

Right-sided gland

1 Concentrate on safely ligating the adrenal vein that empties directly into the inferior vena cava. It was formerly advised that this was achieved early, to minimize release of active hormones into the venous system. With the availability of modern blockades this is less essential, but ligate it early if this can be achieved easily (Fig. 28.2).

2 Handling of certain phaeochromocytomas produces significant swings of blood pressure. The other vessels may not be easily identifiable. There are usually three arteries and veins. Divide smaller branches using diathermy and scissors or harmonic scalpel. The adrenal vein is often worryingly short and wide. If you are anxious, place a Satinsky clamp on the side of the inferior vena cava, remove the tumour, then repair the vein with 5-0 Prolene suture.

3 If you damage the adrenal vein haemorrhage is profuse. Avoid grabbing the vena cava wildly with artery forceps. Pack the wound carefully and arrange for blood transfusion. Ensure that the suckers work effectively and that you have adequate exposure. Then carefully remove the packs, apply a Satinsky clamp to the damaged area of the vena cava and repair it with 5-0 Prolene.

Left-sided gland

Although laparoscopic left-sided gland removal tends to be difficult, open removal is usually easy. The vessels are usually smaller and there is no risk of damage to the vena cava. Deal cautiously with a low vein entering into the left renal vein but this is usually long and amenable to ligation.

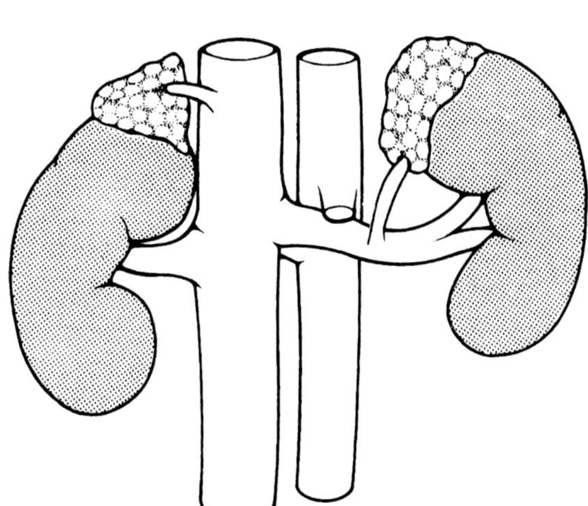

Fig. 28.1 Position and venous drainage of the adrenal glands.

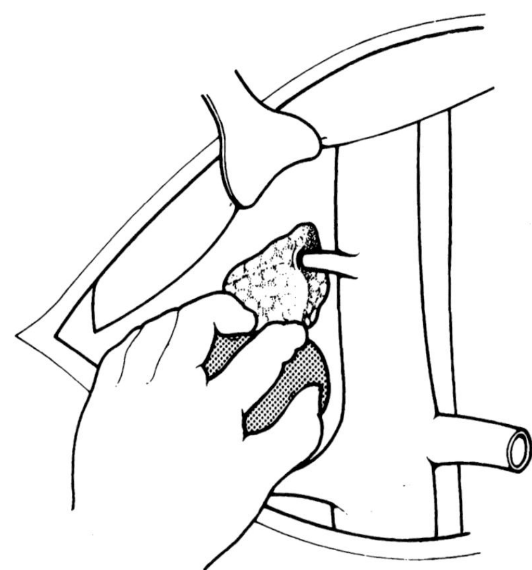

Fig. 28.2 Exposure of the right adrenal vein, which enters the vena cava directly after a short extraglandular course.

POSTERIOR APPROACH

1 Use this for small tumours up to 5–6 cm in diameter, when there is little risk of malignancy. Place the patient prone, with good support under the shoulders and hips, with no abdominal contact. Break the table to tense the lumbar fascia. Place the patient's arms alongside the head, carefully supported.

2 Make a horizontal incision over the eleventh rib, extended medially and superiorly over the paravertebral muscles. Excise the rib, carefully avoiding damage to the neurovascular bundle at the inferior margin of the rib. Try not to damage the pleura, but, if you do, reconstitute it at the end of the procedure. Do not insert a chest drain, provided you have expressed all the air from the pleural cavity by expanding the lungs at the end of the procedure.

3 Dissect the glands as in the lateral approach.

ANTERIOR TRANSPERITONEAL APPROACH

1 This was formerly employed for bilateral disease and is still occasionally used for bilateral large phaeochromocytoma.

2 Use either a rooftop (chevron) incision or a long midline incision. Approach the right adrenal gland by performing Kocher's manoeuvre to mobilize the duodenum and by retracting the liver upwards with a long deep retractor.

3 The right adrenal vein can be difficult to control, particularly in some large tumours which extend behind the vena cava. On the left, improve access by incising the lienorenal ligament to release the splenic flexure, then incise the lateral colonic reflection, thus sweeping the viscera forward.

4 Avoid injury to the spleen, splenic vessels and the tail of the pancreas. Identify the adrenal gland by finding the golden edge. The pancreas is a creamy or pinkish white.

CLOSURE

1 Close in layers.

2 Take care to close the pleura if it was opened, after asking the anaesthetist to expand the lungs.

3 Drains are not usually necessary.

4 As a rule, order a chest X-ray in the recovery ward to exclude a significant pneumothorax. A small amount of air in the pleural cavity can be tolerated.

POSTOPERATIVE

1 This must be in an intensive care unit.

2 Epidural anaesthesia is valuable, particularly following the removal of a phaeochromocytoma.

3 Anticipate a liability to profound swings of blood pressure in either direction and have available appropriate pharmacological drugs and fluid infusions.

4 Glucocorticoids are required following bilateral adrenalectomy for Cushing's disease.

5 Following bilateral adrenalectomy, give fludrocortisone 0.1 mg, orally.

KEY POINTS Special considerations

- Collaborate with endocrinologists and anaesthetists for functioning endocrine tumour management.
- Manipulation of hormonal activity is a skilful job requiring care and expertise.
- Do not perform adrenal procedures on an occasional basis.

FURTHER READING

Janetschek G 1999 Surgical options in adrenalectomy: laparoscopic versus open surgery. Current Opinion in Urology 9:213–218

Sidhu S, Gicquel C, Bambach CP et al 2003 Clinical and molecular aspects of adrenocortical tumorigenesis. Australia and New Zealand Journal of Surgery 73:727–738

INTERNET WEB SITE

www.BAES.info

British Association of Endocrine Surgeons Guidelines for the Surgical Treatment of Endocrine Disease and Training Requirements for Endocrine Surgery, 2004.

29

Arteries

P.L. Harris

CONTENTS

INTRODUCTION

As a consequence of the high prevalence of arterial disease in Western countries, and the lack of effective medical treatment, arterial operations have come to represent a considerable proportion of the total surgical workload. Accordingly, this aspect of general surgery has evolved into a speciality with a degree of complexity that is recognized in the training programmes of those who wish to make the management of vascular disease a major part of their practice. However, given the ubiquitous nature of arteries, all competent surgeons should be familiar with the basic principles of arterial repair and reconstruction.

KEY POINTS Indications for operation

There are three main reasons for operating on an artery:

- Injury.
- Aneurysmal dilatation.
- Occlusion.

INDICATIONS FOR OPERATION

- *Injury*. This may result from sharp or blunt trauma. It can occur in association with fracture of long bones, especially the femur and humerus. Increasingly common are iatrogenic injuries resulting from the use of arterial access routes for various forms of investigation or treatment, and self-induced injury in mainline drug abusers.
- *Aneurysm*. During the last few decades there has been a dramatic increase in the number of operations for atherosclerotic aneurysms of the abdominal and thoracic aorta. The incidence of aneurysms of the popliteal artery is also rising. Dissecting aneurysms of the aorta are a distinct pathological entity for which vascular surgical intervention is sometimes required. Mycotic aneurysms are seen occasionally. *Staphylococcus aureus*, *Streptococcus* spp and *Salmonella* spp together account for approximately 50% of these aneurysms. In another 25% of apparently infected aneurysms no organisms are isolated.
- *Occlusion and stenosis*. Most arterial occlusions result from thrombosis of a stenosed vessel, the underlying disease being atherosclerosis. In many people this is a slowly progressive condition that is part of a natural ageing process and it does not always require surgical intervention. Critical limb ischaemia is a very strong indication for operation, but patients with intermittent claudication require careful assessment in order to balance the potential benefits and risks before any surgical intervention is advised for them. Occasionally an artery becomes acutely occluded by an embolus. Sudden occlusion of an otherwise normal major artery is a catastrophe that threatens both the viability of the limb and the life of the patient. Urgent treatment is required, directed towards removal or dissolution of the occluding embolus. The management of acute and chronic ischaemia is therefore quite different. Less commonly, acute limb-threatening ischaemia develops following sudden occlusion by thrombosis of a previously diseased artery or a bypass graft. The acute-on-chronic ischaemia that results poses a specially difficult problem of management since it cannot usually be treated effectively by thrombectomy alone. Because of its inherently dangerous nature, the urgency, which precludes detailed preoperative preparation, and the elderly frail condition of most of the patients, the mortality risk associated with acute arterial occlusion is high. Furthermore, the urgency of the situation may make it necessary for these patients to be treated in non-specialist units.

GENERAL PRINCIPLES

SPECIAL EQUIPMENT

1 To achieve the best results, modern arterial surgery requires a technically sophisticated operating environment. The increasing application of endovascular techniques, either as the sole method of intervention or in combination with open surgical procedures, requires that fluoroscopic imaging of high quality should be available. A cell-saver to limit the demand for homologous blood, as well as monitoring equipment for quality control, such as intraoperative and transcranial Doppler, are also highly desirable.

2 Not all surgeons who undertake operations on arteries have access to a complete range of these facilities but, provided you are endowed with a 'good pair of hands' and adhere closely to the basic principles described here, you should be able to achieve acceptable results with many of the arterial operations described. Patients who require complex procedures, for example endovascular or thoracoabdominal repair of aneurysms, should be referred to specialized vascular units. But, it is essential for all surgeons to understand the potential and drawbacks of these operations and for this reason I have included brief descriptions of them.

Instruments

- *Clamps*. A good selection of lightweight vascular clamps is essential. The DeBakey Atraugrip range is suitable for large intra-abdominal and thoracic vessels. For smaller vessels (e.g. femoral, popliteal, subclavian, brachial and carotid arteries), miniature clamps of the Castaneda type designed for paediatric cardiac surgery are ideal. A selection of small 'bulldog' clamps is useful for controlling back-bleeding from the side-branches of opened arteries and for delicate vessels; I recommend the Schofield–Lewis type.

  Never clamp peripheral arteries such as those distal to the popliteal or brachial, since they are very sensitive to clamp damage. Control these vessels with fine plastic loops, which may be colour-coded for early identification, and by smooth, round-ended atraumatic intraluminal catheters.

- *Dissecting instruments*. Handle arteries gently, and only with non-toothed forceps. The DeBakey Atraugrip range is suitable. In addition to standard dissecting scissors, use Potts scissors angled in two planes for extending arterial incisions. For dissection within the vessel, in order to remove adherent thrombus or endarterectomy, Watson–Cheyne and Macdonald's dissectors are ideal. Long tunnelling instruments are necessary for conveying grafts between unconnected incisions. To assist exposure of the abdominal aorta and its branches, I recommend a fixed self-retaining retractor system of the Omnitract type.

- *Catheters and shunts*. Atraumatic (umbilical) catheters ranging from 3F to 6F in size are needed for intraluminal irrigation and control of small arteries. A similar size range of Fogarty embolectomy catheters is also essential. These should have a central lumen to enable them to be introduced over a guide-wire under fluoroscopic control, which is essential for selective access to calf vessels from the groin. The central lumen can also be used to facilitate intraoperative radiological contrast studies and for the instillation of heparinized saline into the distal vessels. A useful addition is a range of occlusion and irrigation catheters of the Pruitt type, which have control stops incorporated into the irrigation and balloon ports.

  It is sometimes necessary to employ an intraluminal shunt as a temporary bypass during reconstruction of a vessel, most commonly in carotid endarterectomy. Shunts made for this purpose are of two basic types. The simplest is that designed by Javid. This is a slightly tapered plastic tube with an expansion close to each end. It is retained in place by large and small ring clamps, which are applied around the outside of the vessel in proximity to the expanded segments (see Fig. 29.35). The second type is a modification of the Pruitt catheter described above, with a balloon at each end to retain it in place and to control bleeding, and a side-arm for withdrawal of blood or air from the lumen.

  Ensure that you are familiar with endovascular techniques for arterial reconstruction. For the most part, percutaneous procedures are undertaken in the radiology department while combined endovascular and open operations normally take place in an operating theatre. In both cases, close co-operation between vascular surgeon and interventional radiologist is essential. Carefully follow proper procedures for radiation protection and control. You must be in possession of a certificate of training in radiation control. For intraoperative balloon angioplasty you require access to a range of guide-wires from 0.035 mm to 0.025 mm in diameter, including straight and J-wires and those with a low-friction, hydrophilic coating, together with a choice of angioplasty balloon catheters ranging from 4 mm to 10 mm in inflated diameter. In general, balloons 4 cm in length are most suitable, but balloons of 10 cm length should also be available. Always use a valved introducer sheath to minimize trauma to the artery and reduce blood loss. A range of sizes from 5F to 9F is appropriate. You will also require a selection of angiography and guiding catheters of different sizes and shapes. Use a syringe driver that allows a precisely determined pressure to be maintained within the balloon during inflation. These are mostly disposable but re-sterilizable syringe drivers can be obtained.

- *Magnifying loupes*. Most vascular operations can be performed with the naked eye but, since technical perfection is the key to the success of vascular reconstruction, I recommend that 2.5× magnifying spectacles are used to facilitate most anastomoses.

- *Sutures, needle-holders and suture clamps*. Arteries are always sewn with non-absorbable stitches. There are three types. Fine monofilament material such as polypropylene (Prolene) has the advantage of being very smooth and slipping easily through the tissues so that a loose suture can be drawn up tight. The fact that it has a slight 'memory' can easily be compensated for with familiarity of use. Its main disadvantage is that it has a tendency to brittleness and it must never be picked up directly with metal instruments. The second type of suture is braided material coated with an outer layer of polyester to render it smooth. Examples of such sutures are Ethiflex and Ethibond. Sutures of this type do not slip so easily through the arterial wall but are pleasantly floppy to handle and knot easily. Tough atraumatic needles are swaged on to each end of the suture.

Finally, PTFE (polytetrafluoroethylene; Gore-Tex) sutures are designed specifically for use with PTFE grafts. PTFE is non-compliant so that the holes in the graft made by the passage of a needle do not close around the suture, resulting in more bleeding than occurs with other types of graft. In order to overcome this problem the diameter of the needles is made smaller than that of the suture itself. This is at the expense of some loss of strength, and the fragility of these needles precludes their use in tough or calcified arteries. The suture material itself is extremely strong and has excellent handling properties. In general, use the finest suture that is strong enough for the job; as a rough guide, 3/0 for the aorta, 4/0 for the iliacs, 5/0 for the femoral, 6/0 for the popliteal and 7/0 for the tibial arteries are appropriate. For very fine work a monofilament stitch is always necessary.

In the case of double-ended sutures the end that is not being worked with should be kept out of the way by attaching to it a 'rubber-shod' clamp. This is simply a mosquito or other small clamp, the jaws of which have been cushioned with fine rubber or plastic tubing. Never apply unprotected clamps to monofilament sutures. Because arterial suturing varies from relatively crude to extremely fine, have a wide selection of needle-holders. The range must reflect the fact that some anastomoses are virtually on the surface while others may be at considerable depth, so that holders varying in length from 10 cm up to 30 cm are required. They should be fine-pointed to facilitate accurate placement of sutures and have tungsten or other high-quality jaws to ensure a firm grasp of the needle.

Solutions

For local irrigation of opened vessels and instillation into vessels distal to a clamp, use heparinized saline. This is made up from 5000 units of heparin in 500 ml of physiological saline.

Blood transfusion and autotransfusion

1 Arterial operations, particularly emergency procedures, may be associated with significant blood loss.

2 An autotransfusion system or cell-saver reduces the requirement for banked blood and protects the patient from the risk of blood-borne infections.

Grafts and stents

The best arterial substitute is the patient's own blood vessel, usually vein. However, quite often there is no suitable vein available, because it is either absent, too small for the job required or has itself been damaged by varicosities or thrombophlebitis. Under these circumstances a prosthesis has to be chosen and three types are currently available.

- *Dacron*. This is an inert polymer that is spun into a thread and then either woven or knitted into the familiar cloth graft. It is available in tubes from 5 mm to 40 mm in diameter, straight or bifurcated. In general, prefer the knitted variety with a velour lining as its porosity allows tissue ingrowth and better anchoring of the internal 'neointimal' surface. The original knitted grafts needed to be carefully preclotted with blood taken from the patient prior to the administration of heparin and in an emergency such as a ruptured aneurysm it was necessary to use a woven graft, which leaks less. However, most vascular surgeons now use knitted grafts that have been presealed with bovine collagen, gelatin or albumen. These grafts have very low porosity at the time of insertion and so do not require preclotting. Within 3 months the sealant has been absorbed and replaced by natural fibrous tissue ingrowth, thereby providing the advantages of both woven and knitted prostheses. In the future it is likely that additional substances, for example antibiotics, anticoagulants or agents to prevent anastomotic myointimal hyperplasia, may be incorporated within the sealant. Dacron grafts perform extremely well when used to bypass large arteries with a high flow-rate (e.g. the aorta and iliac arteries) and they are the arterial substitute of choice in these situations.
- *Expanded polytetrafluoroethylene (PTFE)*. Grafts made of this material are slightly more expensive than Dacron but their performance is superior for reconstruction of small arteries. In general, Dacron grafts are used above the groin and PTFE below the groin, although some surgeons use Dacron in preference to PTFE for above-the-knee femoropopliteal bypass. PTFE grafts are available with an external polypropylene support to prevent compression or kinking of the graft. It is essential to use this type of graft whenever the knee or any other joint is crossed.
- *Biological*. The first arterial substitutes tried were arterial or venous allografts or xenografts. These rapidly degraded and were abandoned. However, recently developed techniques for cryopreservation of these grafts with dimethylsulfoxide (DMSO) and liquid nitrogen may reduce the host immunological response and they have been advocated by some specifically for arterial bypass in the presence of infection (e.g. in-situ replacement of infected prosthetic grafts). Biological grafts have also been constructed from human umbilical veins. They are treated to make them non-antigenic and then coated with an outer Dacron support to prevent aneurysmal dilatation. These grafts are associated with comparatively good patency rates even in distal sites, but are subject to a risk of aneurysmal degeneration. For this reason few vascular surgeons use them.
- *Preshaped (cuffed) grafts*. This is a recent development in graft technology. There is evidence to show that, when PTFE grafts are anastomosed to small arteries below the level of the knee joint, better rates of patency may be achieved if a cuff, collar or patch of vein is interposed between the graft and the artery at the distal anastomosis (see Femoropopliteal–infrapopliteal bypass, below). Although the mechanism involved remains uncertain, one possibility is that the configuration of a cuffed anastomosis promotes a pattern of blood flow that inhibits or redistributes the anastomotic myointimal hyperplasia that is the principal cause of graft failure. The configuration or shape of an anastomosis is not dependent upon the use of vein. Preshaped grafts have been manufactured from PTFE to reproduce an anastomosis of 'ideal' configuration without the necessity of constructing a cuff from vein. An additional benefit is that the wall of the shaped end is thinner than that of the body of the graft and this facilitates suturing.
- *Compliant grafts*. One reason that prosthetic grafts are said to perform less well than natural vessels is that they are stiff or non-compliant. This makes them inefficient as conduits of pulsatile flow. Grafts with some degree of compliance are now available but their value in clinical practice is unproven.

- *Stents and stent/grafts*. Metallic stents made from either stainless steel or nitinol may be used as an adjunct to balloon angioplasty in order to maintain patency of the vessel or as a framework to support an endovascular graft for exclusion of an aneurysm. They are of two types: balloon-expandable (e.g. Palmaz stent) and self-expanding (e.g. Wallstent). Stents for endovascular aneurysm repair are covered with Dacron, PTFE or other fabric. They are manufactured as straight tubes or with a bifurcated construction for repair of abdominal aortic aneurysms (see Endovascular repair of abdominal aortic aneurysm, below). Small stents 'covered' with PTFE are also available, but these are associated with a higher incidence of myointimal hyperplasia and should not be used in preference to non-covered stents except for specific indications. Drug-eluting stents that release chemicals to inhibit myointimal hyperplasia (e.g. paclitaxel, rapamycin) have proved disappointing in clinical trials.

BASIC TECHNIQUES OF ARTERIAL REPAIR, ANASTOMOSIS AND TRANSLUMINAL ANGIOPLASTY

Arteriotomy

KEY POINTS Longitudinal arteriotomy

Arteries are best opened longitudinally. This is for three reasons:

- A longitudinal arteriotomy is easier to close; any thrombus that accumulates on the suture line has less tendency to narrow the lumen.
- A longitudinal arteriotomy can be rapidly extended if required.
- A transverse arteriotomy is difficult to close because the intima retracts away from the outer layers. This increases the risk of blood tracking in a subintimal plane, resulting in occlusion of the vessel.

Simple suture

1 Longitudinal arteriotomies in large or medium-sized arteries can usually be closed by simple suture (Fig. 29.1).

2 Use the finest suture material compatible with the thickness and quality of the arterial wall. The aim is to produce an everted suture line that is leak-proof. This is quite different from bowel suture, where the mucosa is deliberately inverted into the lumen and the tension on the sutures is kept low to avoid necrosis of the edges. There is no need to use everting mattress sutures, which would narrow the lumen. A simple over-and-over stitch is adequate, provided that care is taken to ensure that the intima turns outwards. The needle must pass through all layers of the arterial wall with every stitch. The inner layers must be included to ensure good intimal apposition and to prevent flap dissection, and the outer layers must be included since the main strength of the arterial wall resides in its adventitia. Keep a firm, even tension on the suture at all times. Experience is required in order to judge the spacing and size of each bite, and this varies with the size and nature of the artery. Occasionally, as, for example, in aortic aneurysm repair, large irregular stitches may be required but, in general, evenly spaced regular stitching is best.

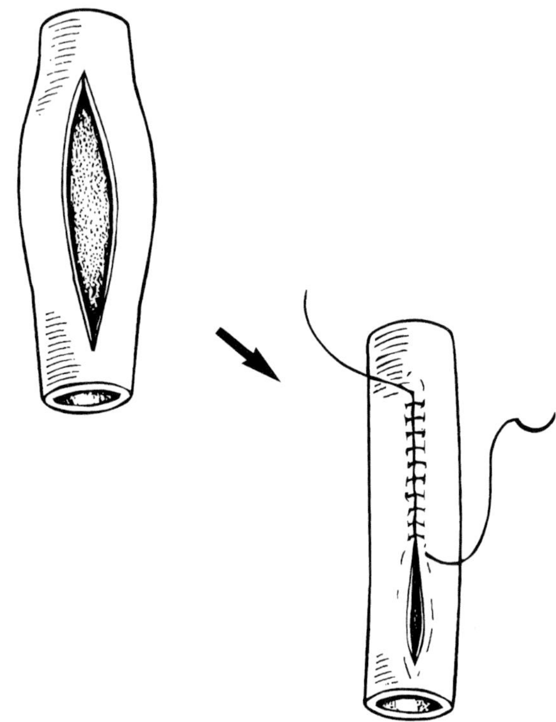

Fig. 29.1 Longitudinal arteriotomy closed by continuous everting arterial suture.

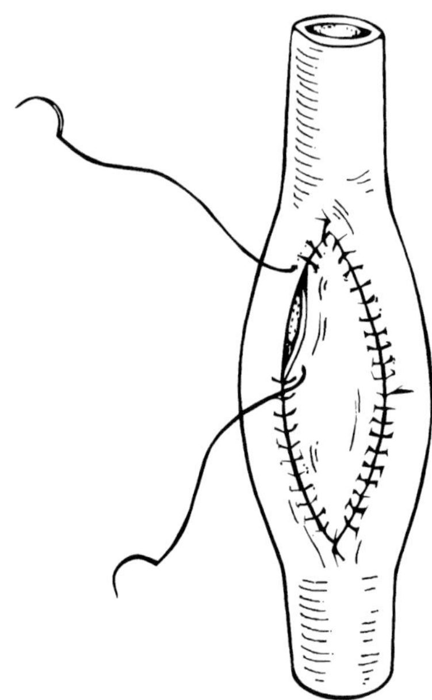

Fig. 29.2 Closure of longitudinal arteriotomy with a patch.

Closure with a patch

1 Close vessels of less than 4 mm in diameter with a patch in order to avoid narrowing of the lumen (Fig. 29.2).

2 This technique may also be used to widen the lumen of a vessel that has become stenosed by disease (e.g. the profunda femoris artery). For small vessels use a patch of autologous vein. Never sacrifice the proximal end of the long saphenous vein for this purpose. Use either a segment taken from the ankle, a tributary or a piece of vein from another site (e.g. an arm vein). For larger vessels prosthetic material (either Dacron or PTFE) may be used. When cutting the patch to shape, always ensure that the ends are rounded rather than being tapered to a sharp point. This is to prevent narrowing of the lumen caused by 'clustering' of sutures at the point. After shaping the patch use just one double-ended stitch commencing close to one end and working around each side. Do not finish the stitching at the apex; carry one of the sutures around to the other margin to complete the closure and tie the knot a short distance to one side. Knots at the apex may be a cause of significant narrowing. This technique permits direct vision of the internal suture line and allows final trimming of the patch to be delayed until closure is nearly complete in order to ensure a perfect match for size.

End-to-end anastomosis

1 For small delicate arteries this is accomplished most safely by applying the principles of the triangulation technique originally described by Carrel.[1] Join the vessels with a suture placed in the centre of the back or deepest aspect of the anastomosis (Fig. 29.3). Be sure to tie the knot on the outside. Place two more sutures so as to divide the circumference of the vessels equally into three. Any disparity in calibre can be compensated for at this stage. Always use interrupted sutures for small vessels, in which case keep the three original stay sutures long and apply gentle traction on them to rotate the vessel and facilitate exposure of each segment of the anastomosis in turn. Complete the back or deep segments first, leaving the easiest segment at the front to be finished last.

2 For larger vessels it is permissible to use continuous sutures. Cut the ends of the vessels to be joined obliquely, then make a short incision longitudinally to create a spatulate shape. Overlapping the two spatulate ends avoids any risk of narrowing at the anastomosis.

3 A different technique of end-to-end anastomosis can be employed with great effect in operation on aneurysms. This is the inlay technique (see Repair of abdominal aorta aneurysm, below).

End-to-side anastomosis

1 This is the standard form of anastomosis for bypass operations. It should be oblique and its length should be approximately twice the diameter of the lumen of the graft. The end of the graft is fashioned into a spatulate shape, which will, on completion of the anastomosis, adopt a 'cobra-head' appearance. The end of the anastomosis in the angle is referred to as the 'heel' and the other end as the 'toe'. The simplest way of completing it is to place a double-ended stitch at the heel and another at the toe and to run sutures along each margin, ending with a knot at the halfway point on each side. However, there is an advantage in keeping the inside of the suture line in view as much as possible. Achieve this by starting with a double-ended suture at the heel. Leave the toe free. Run the suture up each side to beyond the midpoint and then retain in a 'rubber-shod' clamp. Insert a further stitch through the toe and complete and trim the last two quadrants by tying to the previously retained threads. This is sometimes known as the 'four-quadrant technique' (Fig. 29.4).

The 'toe' and 'heel' are the most crucial points of an end-to-side anastomosis. To ensure that the toe is completed as smoothly as possible, offset the starting point of the 'toe', suturing a few millimetres to one side or the other of the apex. In order to further reduce the risk of causing a stricture at this point, some surgeons prefer to place a few interrupted sutures around the toe.

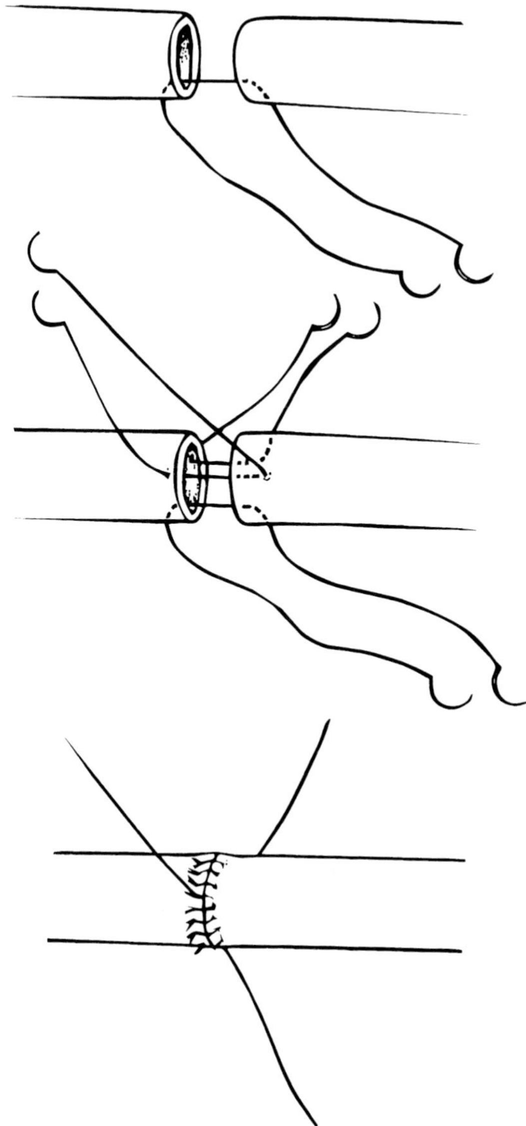

Fig. 29.3 End-to-end anastomosis by the triangulation technique.

2 A stricture of the heel may be avoided by stenting the vessel with an intraluminal catheter of appropriate size until this portion of the anastomosis is complete. An alternative method is the 'parachute' technique (Fig. 29.5). This is particularly useful

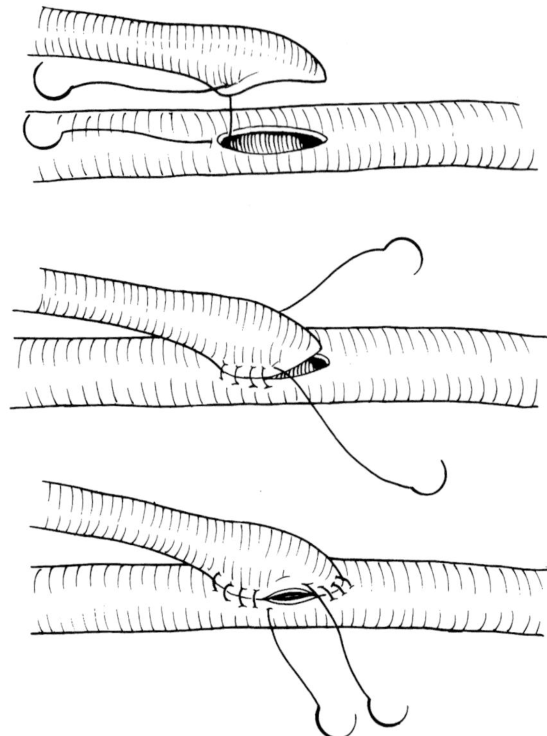

Fig. 29.4 End-to-end anastomosis by the four-quadrant technique.

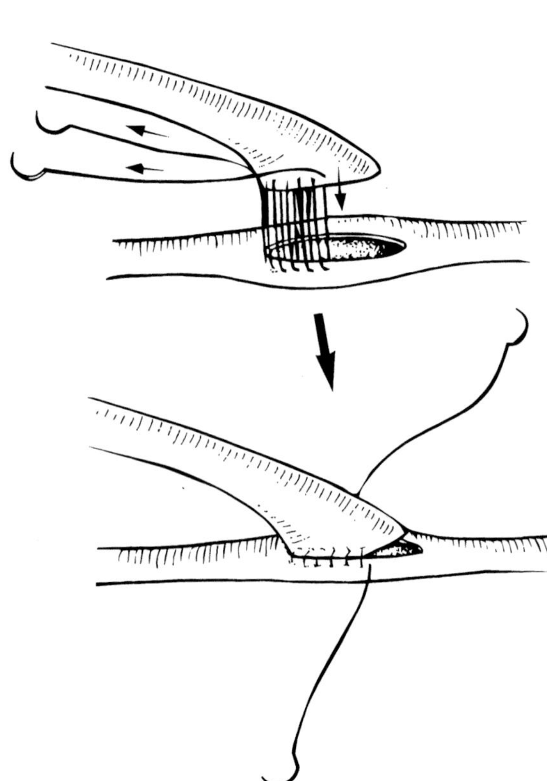

Fig. 29.5 End-to-side anastomosis by the parachute technique.

where access is difficult and good visualization of the anastomosis is impaired, but it is applicable to most situations. With the graft and the recipient artery separated, place a series of running sutures between them at what will become the heel of the anastomosis. These sutures are then pulled tight as the vessels are approximated.

KEY POINT 'Parachute' technique

- It is essential to use a monofilament suture with this method.

Transluminal angioplasty (Fig. 29.6)

1 Approximately half of all patients with symptoms of peripheral arterial occlusion are now treated by this means and the proportion is increasing. Because it is minimally invasive and associated with a low risk of serious complications, patients with disabilities associated with intermittent claudication that would not warrant open bypass surgery may be offered treatment by angioplasty. However, this is controversial—many surgeons do not accept that the long-term results of angioplasty are good enough to warrant this approach. At the other end of the scale, patients with critical ischaemia and co-morbidities that seriously increase the risks of open operation may benefit considerably from an endovascular approach.

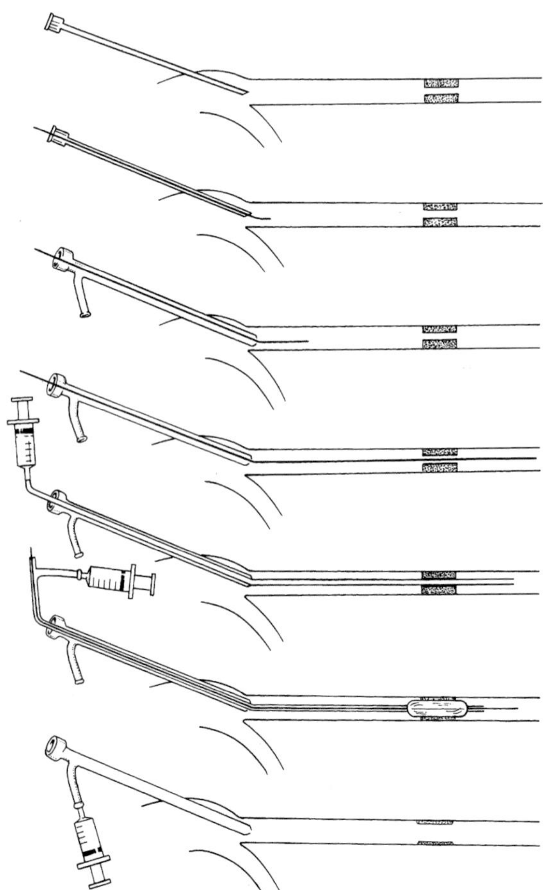

Fig. 29.6 Percutaneous angioplasty.

2 Essential requirements are fluoroscopy with 'subtraction' and 'road-mapping' functions and skilled radiographic assistance. Use a radiolucent operating table.

3 Ensure all operating theatre staff are properly protected against radiation.

4 In the case of elective procedures commence oral antiplatelet therapy at least 48 hours prior to the procedure.

5 Administer mild sedation and oxygen. Monitor heart rate and oxygen saturation using a pulse oximeter. Well-chosen music in the operating room may help patients to relax.

6 Transluminal angioplasty can be undertaken percutaneously or following exposure of an artery. It may be the sole method of treatment or combined with open reconstruction of arteries at other sites (e.g. iliac angioplasty and femorodistal bypass).

7 Always use an introducer sheath. This permits repeated endovascular access with minimal trauma to the vessel. The size of sheath required is indicated by the manufacturers on the packaging of the balloon catheter; 5 to 7F are most common.

8 The common femoral artery is the access vessel for most endovascular procedures and it is important to be familiar with its position with reference to surface landmarks (see Exposure of the common femoral artery, below).

9 For percutaneous access, clean the skin and apply drapes as for an open procedure. Inject a small amount of local anaesthetic at the chosen puncture site and make a nick in the skin with a no. 11 scalpel blade. While palpating the common femoral artery with the fingers of one hand introduce a Potts–Cournand or similar needle. These needles have a central trocar that allows blood to 'flashback' into a chamber on the hub when the lumen of the vessel is entered. Angle the needle to facilitate access of the guide-wire in the direction required. For infra-inguinal procedures, puncture the artery just distal to the inguinal ligament in order to give yourself room to manoeuvre the tip of the needle within the lumen of the common femoral artery when negotiating the guide-wire into the superficial femoral artery. Note that the inguinal ligament lies approximately 2 cm proximal to the groin crease. For access to the upstream iliac arteries the puncture site may be a little lower, but take care to avoid unintended puncture of the superficial or profunda femoral arteries. When no pulse is palpable or percutaneous access is difficult for other reasons use an ultrasound-guided arterial puncture technique whenever this equipment is available. Alternatively 'cut-down' onto the common femoral artery under local infiltration anaesthesia.

10 When 'flashback' occurs, withdraw the trocar and observe strong pulsatile flow from the needle. Unless there is severe inflow obstruction, the absence of pulsatile flow from the needle indicates that the tip is not properly positioned within the lumen. Do not attempt to advance a guide-wire. Re-introduce the trocar and re-position the needle.

11 When satisfied with the position of the needle, withdraw the trocar and insert a short J guide-wire—normally a suitable wire is packaged as a part of the 'introducer set'. A guide-wire that is within the lumen passes without resistance. Therefore, if resistance is encountered do not apply force; this is likely to result in dissection of a subintimal plane. Stop. Withdraw the guide-wire and readjust the position of the needle. For downstream procedures the guide-wire must be manipulated into the superficial femoral artery by adjusting the angle of the needle. This requires that stiff metallic rather than soft plastic or Silastic needles are used. Simple fluoroscopy without contrast is usually sufficient to guide this manoeuvre, but if persistent difficulty is encountered obtain a road-map by injection of contrast through the needle. Never pass a hydrophilic guide-wire through a metallic needle: the hydrophilic coating will be stripped off by the needle when the wire is withdrawn, with potentially dire consequences.

12 If angioplasty is to be performed through the exposed common femoral artery (see Exposure of the common femoral artery, below), do not clamp and open the artery. Place a purse-string suture of 5/0 polypropylene (Prolene) in the front of the artery before puncturing the vessel directly with a Potts–Cournand needle. Then proceed in the same way as for a percutaneous procedure. The purse-string can be snugged to prevent blood loss around the introducer sheath by passing the ends of the suture through a short length of narrow rubber tubing to which a small clamp may be applied.

13 When you are satisfied that the guide-wire is in place, withdraw the needle and insert the introducer sheath with its dilator. Remove the dilator. Flush the sheath with heparinized saline through the side channel, which is fitted with a tap. This channel can be used also for injection of contrast medium in order to obtain an angiographic image of the lesion.

14 Withdraw the short guide-wire and replace it with the wire chosen to attempt navigation of the lesion to be treated. The size of guide-wire required is indicated on the packaging of the balloon catheter—most often 0.35 inches in diameter for peripheral vascular procedures. Introduce it through the sheath floppy end first, using the small plastic introducer cone that comes with the wire to penetrate the valve. If difficulty is encountered in crossing the lesion use a hydrophilic guide-wire. Always wipe the guide-wire with a swab soaked in heparinized saline after removing a catheter over it; dried blood on the surface obstructs the smooth passage of another catheter.

15 Following difficult navigation of the guide-wire pass a 4F angiography catheter across the lesion and obtain an angiogram to ensure that the natural lumen has been entered beyond the lesion before passing a balloon catheter. If a subintimal space has been entered abandon the procedure.

16 For most applications select a balloon catheter of 4 cm in length. For accurate sizing of the balloon obtain an angiogram using a catheter with 1 cm markings. Match the size of the balloon to the diameter of the unstenosed artery. However, this degree of precision is not normally necessary. For lesions in the superficial femoral artery, balloons with a diameter of 6 mm, and for iliac lesions 8 mm, are usually appropriate. Be cautious when selecting catheters for female patients with small arteries.

17 Use a hand-operated syringe driver to inflate the balloon to a pressure of 5–10 atmospheres with a 50/50 mixture of contrast medium and saline. Observe the shape of the balloon as it inflates; 'popping' of the 'waist' caused by the stenosis indicates that the plaque has given way and, usually, a satisfactory

outcome. It is not necessary to maintain inflation of the balloon for more than a few seconds but a second inflation helps smooth the irregularities of the flow surface that result from splitting and fissuring of the plaque.

18 Obtain a completion angiogram to assess the final result. Remember that some irregularity of the flow surface at the site of angioplasty is usual. This tends to remodel naturally within a few weeks. Also, dilatation may continue to occur at the angioplasty site for a short time. If a significant stenosis remains or if a large intimal flap has developed following iliac artery angioplasty, consider the use of an intraluminal stent. Stents do not perform well in the arteries below the groin and should not normally be used in this situation.

19 Following withdrawal of the introducer sheath, in the case of percutaneous procedures apply digital pressure to the puncture site for a minimum of 10 minutes, and longer if needed, before applying a dressing and moving the patient. If the artery has been exposed, tie the purse-string suture to secure haemostasis or apply clamps and proceed with the open procedure.

20 Unless contraindicated, prescribe subcutaneous heparin or low-molecular-weight heparin for 12 hours postoperatively. Monitor peripheral perfusion and the groin for signs of haematoma or formation of a false aneurysm. Commence antiplatelet therapy at least 48 hours before angioplasty and continue it afterwards indefinitely.

REFERENCE

1. Carrel A 1902 La technique opératoire des anastomoses vasculaires et de la transplantation des viscères. Lyon Medicale 99:114–152

EXPOSURE OF THE MAJOR PERIPHERAL ARTERIES

Common femoral artery

1 The common femoral artery needs to be exposed more frequently than any other vessel in the body and it is important to know how to do this swiftly and correctly (Fig. 29.7).

KEY POINT Anatomy

- The surface marking of the artery is at the mid-inguinal point (i.e. halfway between the anterior superior iliac spine and the pubic symphysis). Remember this, since the artery is not always palpable.

2 The groin crease does not correspond in position to that of the inguinal ligament, but lies distal to it by 2–3 cm.

3 Provided that the saphenous vein will not be required during the operation, make a vertical incision directly over the artery. The midpoint of this incision should roughly correspond to the groin crease. Inexperienced surgeons tend to make the incision too low. When limited exposure of the common femoral artery is required (e.g. access for an endovascular intervention), it is permissible to use a transverse incision, which heals better and less painfully than a vertical incision crossing the groin crease.

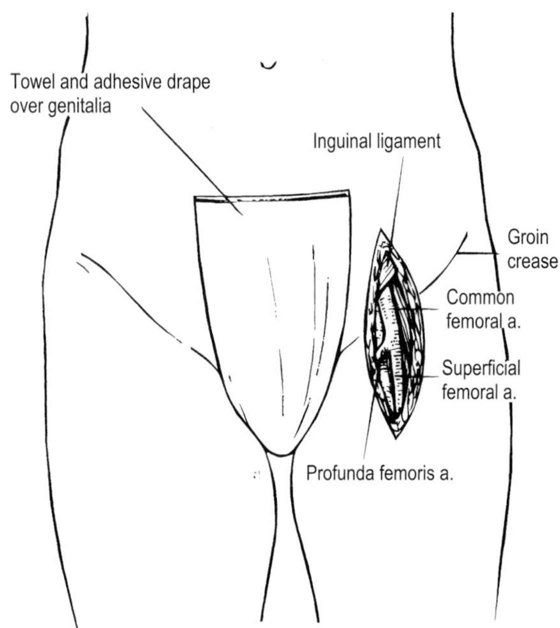

Fig. 29.7 Exposure of the common femoral artery.

Position a transverse incision one finger's breadth above the groin crease.

4 Deepen the incision through the subcutaneous fat, taking care not to cut across any lymph nodes. Expose the femoral sheath and incise it longitudinally to uncover the artery. The femoral vein lies medially and must be protected, but the femoral nerve on the lateral side lies at a deeper plane and is not usually at risk.

5 Pass a Lahey clamp around the back of the artery in order to draw through a plastic sling. Gently lift the artery with the sling, which helps to identify its branches and its bifurcation into the superficial and profunda femoral arteries. Isolate these similarly with slings. Take care to avoid damage to the profunda vein, a tributary of which always passes anterior to the main stem of the profunda artery. For proper exposure of the profunda artery divide this vein between ties.

6 If exposure of the long saphenous vein is required at the same operation make a 'lazy-S' incision, commencing vertically over the artery at the inguinal ligament and then deviating medially over the saphenous vein in the upper thigh.

7 Transection of the many lymphatics in the femoral triangle may cause a troublesome lymphocele or lymphatic fistula after the operation. There is no sure way of avoiding this, but approach the artery from its lateral rather than its medial side and gently reflect any lymph nodes and visible lymph vessels off the femoral sheath with minimal damage.

Popliteal artery

1 The popliteal artery can be exposed above and below the knee by medial approaches. The most inaccessible part lies directly behind the joint line and if its exposure at this level is required a posterior approach is essential (see paragraph 4 below).

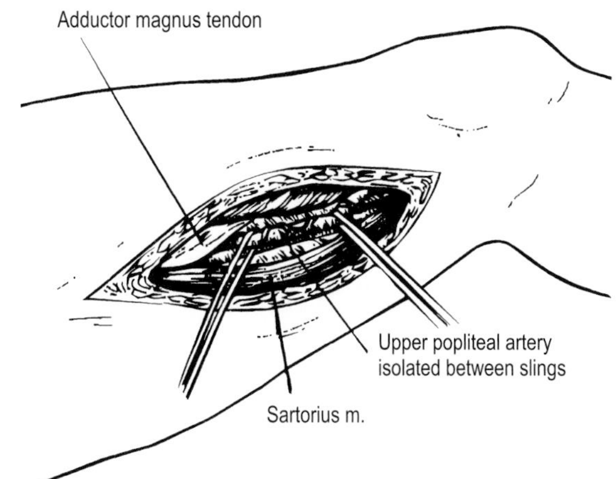

Fig. 29.8 Exposure of the suprageniculate popliteal artery.

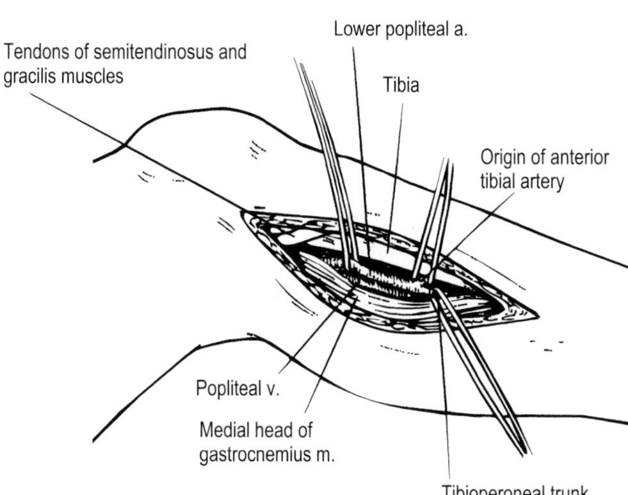

Fig. 29.9 Exposure of the infrageniculate popliteal artery.

2 To expose the suprageniculate artery, make a longitudinal incision over the medial aspect of the lower thigh (Fig. 29.8). If you intend to perform a bypass with a saphenous vein graft, make this incision directly over the previously marked vein. Otherwise the incision should correspond with the anterior border of the sartorius muscle. Inexperienced surgeons tend to place this incision too far anteriorly. Deepen the incision to expose the sartorius muscle, which is retracted posteriorly to reveal the neurovascular bundle enveloped by the popliteal fat pad. The artery lies on the bone. The nerve lies some distance away with the vein in between. The popliteal artery is always surrounded by a plexus of veins, which must be carefully separated and divided in order to avoid troublesome bleeding.

3 In order to expose the infrageniculate popliteal artery, make an incision on the medial aspect of the calf along the border of the gastrocnemius muscle (Fig. 29.9). Continue the dissection between the medial head of this muscle and the tibia to reveal the neurovascular bundle. The vein is exposed first and this has to be lifted carefully away to give access to the artery. By dividing the soleus muscle along its attachment to the medial border of the tibia it is possible to expose the origin of the anterior tibial artery and the whole extent of the tibioperoneal trunk through this incision. Improve the exposure of the popliteal artery proximally by dividing the tendons of sartorius, semitendinosus and gracilis muscles. If necessary, completely divide the medial head of gastrocnemius; this leaves surprisingly little functional disability.

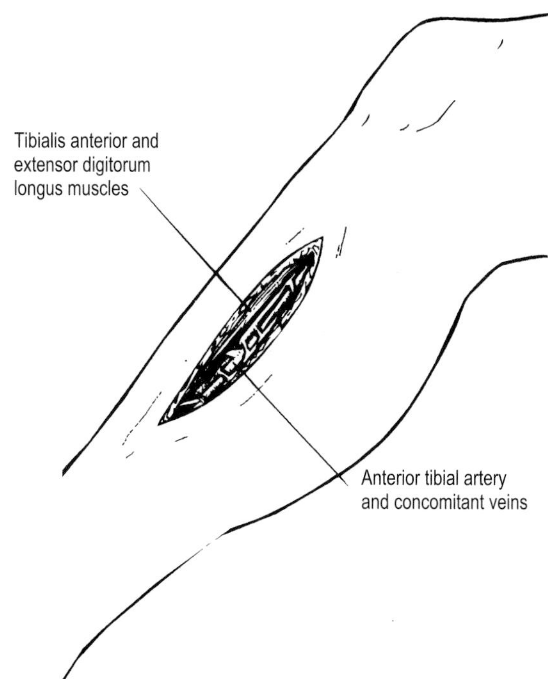

Fig. 29.10 Exposure of the anterior tibial artery.

4 If exposure of the whole length of the popliteal artery is required it is better to use a posterior approach. With the patient lying prone, make a 'lazy-S' incision through the popliteal fossa. Deepen the incision through the popliteal fascia and the fat pad and define the diamond between the hamstring muscles above and the two heads of gastrocnemius below; then follow the short saphenous vein into the neurovascular bundle.

Tibial arteries

1 The proximal end of the anterior tibial artery is relatively inaccessible but the remainder of this vessel and its terminal dorsalis pedis branch can be readily exposed through lateral or anterior incisions made directly over them. Retract the tibialis anterior and extensor digitorum longus muscles anteriorly to reveal the artery lying on the interosseous membrane (Fig. 29.10). If exposure of the proximal anterior tibial artery is required this can be achieved very effectively by excision of the upper part of the fibula with disarticulation of the proximal tibiofibular joint. The common peroneal nerve, which winds around the neck of the fibula, must be protected carefully. This approach destroys the lateral ligament of the knee and, while this is well tolerated in elderly, relatively immobile patients, it is preferably avoided in younger and fitter individuals.

2 The peroneal artery can also be exposed through a lateral incision following resection of a segment of fibula. In most cases,

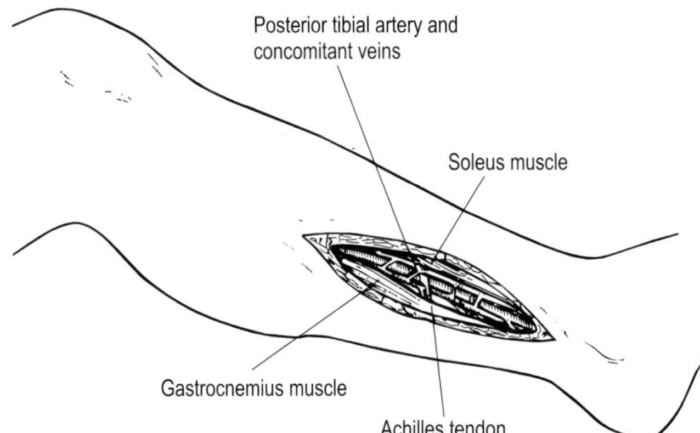

Fig. 29.11 Exposure of the posterior tibial artery.

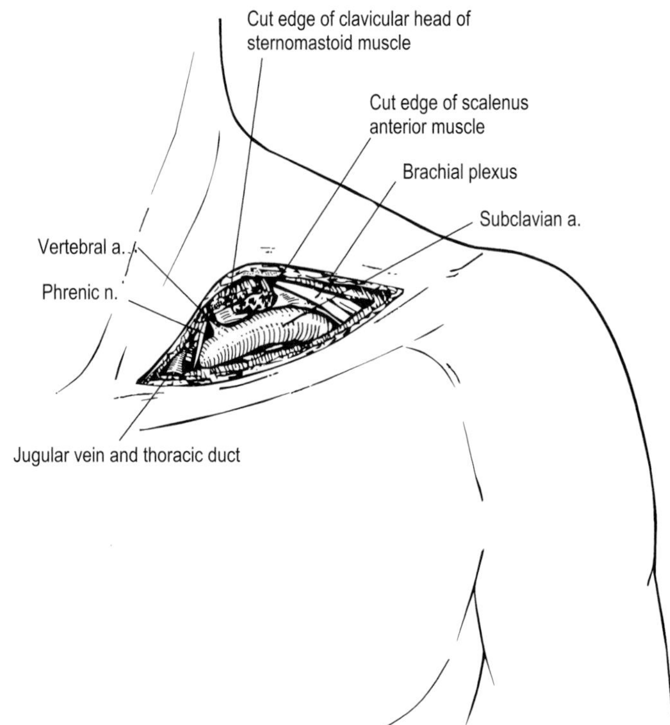

Fig. 29.12 Exposure of the subclavian artery.

however, it is preferable to expose this vessel by a medial approach (see below).

3 To expose the posterior tibial artery, make a longitudinal incision on the medial aspect of the calf centred over the junction between gastrocnemius muscle and its Achilles tendon. Incise the deep fascia and develop the plane between the gastrocnemius and soleus muscles to reveal the posterior tibial vessels and nerve lying on the surface of soleus beneath a layer of fascia (Fig. 29.11). Alternatively, the posterior tibial artery and its terminal lateral plantar branch may be exposed by an incision made directly over it as it lies behind the medial malleolus where it is covered only by deep fascia, and then following it into the foot.

4 To expose the peroneal artery by a medial approach, split the lateral fibres of soleus and flexor hallucis longus muscles. This reveals the artery surrounded by its concomitant veins in the depths of the wound.

Subclavian artery

1 Make a transverse incision 1 cm above the medial third of the clavicle; divide the platysma muscle in the same plane (Fig. 29.12). This exposes the clavicular head of sternomastoid muscle, which is divided, and also a fat pad containing the scalene lymph nodes. Dissect and retract this fat pad superiorly off the surface of the scalenus anterior muscle. Identify the phrenic nerve, which passes obliquely across the front of this muscle to lie along the medial border of its tendon and usually separated from it by a few millimetres. Pass the blade of a MacDonald's dissector behind the tendon of scalenus anterior muscle, in such a way as to protect the phrenic nerve, and divide the tendon by cutting down on to the dissector with a pointed scalpel blade. Retraction of the muscle superiorly exposes the subclavian artery with its vertebral, internal mammary and thyrocervical branches. The first thoracic nerve root and the lower trunk of the brachial plexus cross the first rib above and posterior to the artery. The subclavian vein is deep to the clavicle and is not normally seen through this approach. On the left side the thoracic duct enters the confluence of the internal jugular and subclavian veins. If it is damaged, ligate it to prevent the development of a troublesome postoperative chylous fistula.

2 Extensive exposure of the subclavian artery can be obtained by excision of the inner two-thirds of the clavicle, although this is rarely necessary. The two most common operations on the subclavian artery are carotid–subclavian anastomosis or bypass for a proximal occlusion (subclavian steal syndrome) and repair of a subclavian aneurysm. (This is usually a misnomer since most so-called subclavian aneurysms involve the first part of the axillary artery.) The former is usually completed without difficulty through the approach described above, and the latter is most conveniently accomplished with separate incisions above and below the clavicle to expose the subclavian and axillary arteries (see below).

3 Operations that involve direct exposure of the origin of the subclavian artery have been largely superseded by extrathoracic bypass procedures (carotid–subclavian and subclavian–subclavian bypass). On the rare occasions when direct exposure is considered essential this is best achieved by splitting the manubrium and upper sternum.

Make a right-angled incision with a horizontal component above the medial third of the clavicle and a vertical component in the midline over the manubrium and upper sternum. Complete the supraclavicular exposure of the artery as described above. Deepen the vertical incision through the subcutaneous tissue and periosteum. The periosteum is extremely vascular and diathermy is required to seal the small arteries. Commencing at the suprasternal notch, open a retrosternal plane by finger dissection, and then, with a sternal chisel and hammer or a properly protected reciprocating saw, divide the manubrium and sternum in the midline and spread the edges with a self-retaining retractor. Dissection of the thymus and anterior

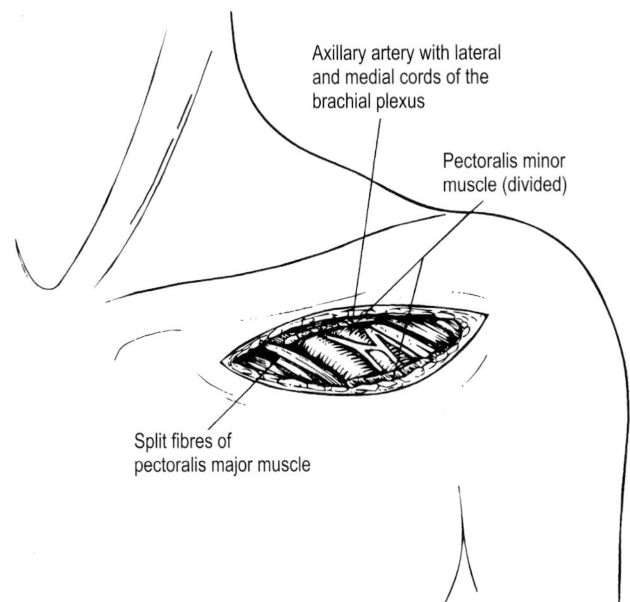

Fig. 29.13 Exposure of the axillary artery.

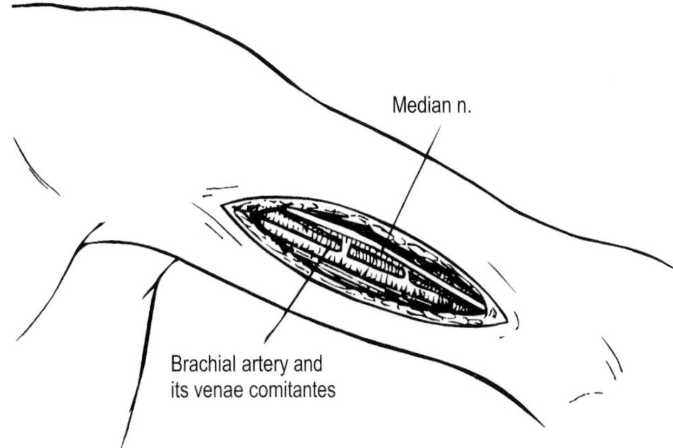

Fig. 29.14 Exposure of the proximal brachial artery.

mediastinal fat is necessary to expose the arch of the aorta and the origins of the supra-aortic vessels. The innominate vein is stretched across the upper part of the incision and must be protected. It is not usually necessary to divide the sternal tendon of the sternomastoid muscle. Close with peristernal wire or strong nylon sutures, taking care to avoid damage to the internal mammary and intercostal arteries when inserting them.

The origin of the left subclavian artery, which arises far back on the aorta arch, can also be exposed through a posterolateral thoracotomy through the bed of the second or third ribs.

Axillary and brachial arteries

1 Access to the axillary artery is most often required for axillofemoral bypass and occasionally for subclavian aneurysm repair (see above). Make a horizontal incision 1 cm below the lateral third of the clavicle, and split the fibres of pectoralis major muscle (Fig. 29.13). This exposes the infraclavicular fat pad, beneath which lies the pectoralis minor muscle. Divide the tendon of this muscle close to its origin at the tip of the acromion process. Some branches of the acromiothoracic vessels may need to be divided. Find the axillary artery surrounded by the cords of the brachial plexus, which must be carefully protected.

2 The proximal brachial artery is found in the groove between biceps and brachialis muscles on the inner aspect of the upper arm (Fig. 29.14). At this point it is still enclosed by cords of the brachial plexus joining to form the median nerve, which crosses it obliquely from the lateral to the medial side. These structures must be carefully separated from it.

3 It is more frequently necessary to expose the bifurcation of the brachial artery in order, for example, to remove surgically a brachial embolus. To do so, make a 'lazy-S' incision in the antecubital fossa followed by division of the biceps aponeurosis (Fig. 29.15). Distal extension of this incision permits the radial, ulnar and anterior interosseous arteries to be followed into the forearm.

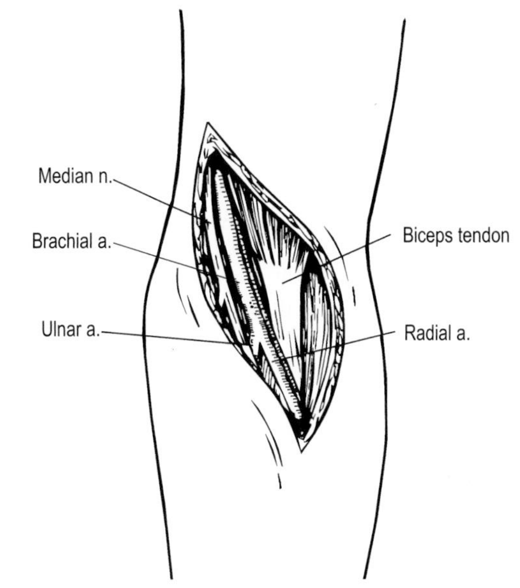

Fig. 29.15 Exposure of the distal brachial artery.

TYPES OF OPERATION

Details of the techniques used to repair or bypass damaged or diseased arteries will be included within the relevant descriptions of specific arterial operations (see below). However, it is useful at this point to summarize the range of procedures available.

- Direct repair, interposition grafting and patch grafting for arterial trauma.
- Surgical embolectomy or thrombectomy.
- Thrombolytic therapy, percutaneous suction and mechanical embolectomy.
- Endarterectomy, which, with the exception of carotid endarterectomy, has now been largely supplanted by bypass surgery as the treatment of choice for occlusive disease.
- Bypass grafting.

- Percutaneous and intraoperative (adjunctive) dilatation angioplasty and endovascular stenting for occlusive arterial disease. The basic technique involves the use of a guide-wire and a balloon dilatation catheter.[1] Devices exist to assist recanalization of resistant occlusions, including lasers, rotational guide-wires, high-frequency electrocoagulation ablators and various types of atherectomy catheters. None of these has yet found a major role in the routine management of vascular disease, and lasers in particular, despite increasing technological sophistication, have so far proved disappointing. The basic technique with balloon catheters has, however, made a major impact in recent years and in some centres more than half of all patients with occlusive disease are treated by these methods.
- Inlay grafting for aneurysms.
- Endovascular stent/graft repair of aortic and peripheral aneurysms.

QUALITY CONTROL

Success in arterial surgery demands technical perfection and this must always be assured as far as is practically possible by appropriate assessment before the patient leaves the operating room. Omission of this step results in a high incidence of early post-operative occlusion and is therefore unacceptable. It is important to appreciate that the presence of a palpable pulse in a graft gives no indication whatsoever that it is technically satisfactory. There may be no mean forward flow through the graft and yet it will be pulsatile. Acceptable methods available for assessing vascular reconstructions at operation include the following:

- *Completion angiography*. This continues to be the 'gold-standard' method. State of the art fluoroscopy is ideal but for infra-inguinal reconstructions 'on-table' angiography is performed very easily using the simple X-ray equipment available in all standard operating theatres.

  Place an X-ray plate wrapped within a sterile Mayo tray cover directly beneath the limb, and take an exposure while injecting 15–20 ml of contrast medium into the proximal end of the graft. Apply a clamp proximal to the injection site during exposure to obviate the necessity for accurate timing of the exposure. Observe proper radiation protection measures during this procedure and further reduce the radiation dose to yourself by interposing a long length of connecting catheter between the syringe and the injection site.

  For more proximal reconstructions, special X-ray equipment is required but other methods of quality control may be effective.
- *Electromagnetic flowmetry*. Based on Faraday's laws of electromagnetic induction, these instruments—although simple in theory—are complicated in practice since they are subject to wide inaccuracies. For meaningful measurement of blood flow they need to be calibrated repeatedly in situ. However, subjective evaluation of the analogue velocity waveforms is useful in that abnormal patterns can easily be recognized with experience.
- *Intraoperative Doppler flowmetry*. Intraoperative Doppler probes are subject to less inaccuracy than electromagnetic flow probes and provide basically the same information. For objective determination of blood velocity the angle of the probe to the direction of flow must be fixed at about 60°; this is achieved by mounting the probe in a plastic holder, which fits snugly around the artery or graft. It is also possible to use a simple hand-held Doppler probe enclosed within the finger of a sterile surgical glove. However, it must be emphasized that the presence of a pulsatile signal is not of itself sufficient evidence of satisfactory function. It is essential to demonstrate also that there is 'adequate' mean forward flow. Unfortunately, this term is difficult to define, since blood flow velocity is only one of a number of factors that affect graft patency.

  Neither electromagnetic nor Doppler flowmetry is as satisfactory as angiography for quality control because certain imperfections within a graft or at the anastomosis may fail to be manifest immediately by obvious malfunction. However, the use of these devices will at least eliminate gross technical error.
- *Angioscopy*. Fibreoptic endoscopes of little more than 1 mm in diameter are now available. Inserted at one end, such instruments will allow direct inspection of the interior of a graft and one anastomosis. Such instruments do traumatize the flow surface and are expensive. For these reasons they have largely been abandoned.
- A satisfactory arterial reconstruction for occlusive disease restores either normal or improved blood flow to the distal circulation, and confirmation that this has occurred is a minimal requirement. The return of palpable pulses to vessels downstream of the reconstruction, for example in the pedal arteries, is a valuable sign and there are a number of simple and inexpensive devices available to supplement clinical assessment, including strain gauge and photoplethysmographs (digital pulse monitors), toe temperature probes, flat and hand-held Dopplers and pulse oximeters. I strongly recommend that one of these be used routinely, since palpation of pulses alone is not always reliable, especially if the vessels distal to the site of reconstruction are diseased.

REFERENCE

1. Gruntzig A, Kumpe DA 1979 Technique of percutaneous transluminal angioplasty with the Gruntzig balloon catheter. American Journal of Radiology 132:547–552

ARTERIAL OPERATIONS

KEY POINTS Factors for success

There are three basic prerequisites for success in arterial surgery. Although the relevance of each varies according to specific circumstance it is a valuable discipline to include an appraisal of all three factors when planning any arterial reconstruction:

- An unimpeded inflow tract—the run-in.
- An adequate outflow tract—the run-off.
- An efficient recanalization or bypass—the conduit.

REPAIR OF ARTERIAL INJURY

Appraise

- Arterial trauma may occur as an isolated event but more often it occurs in association with other injuries, for example fracture of long bones. Under these circumstances there is a danger that the symptoms of ischaemia may be masked and therefore go unrecognized until irreversible tissue damage has occurred. Always assess the distal circulation in cases of fractured long bones or disarticulation injuries, especially those that involve the elbow or knee.

- Arterial injury is manifest by:
  Bleeding, either externally or with the formation of a large haematoma.
  Acute ischaemia with pallor, coldness, loss of sensation, muscle tenderness and weakness, absent pulses and absent or damped Doppler signals with reduced systolic arterial pressure in distal vessels.
- Suspicion of arterial injury is an indication for urgent angiography, except for haemorrhage, in which case proceed directly to surgical exploration.
- Angiographic discontinuity of a major limb vessel always requires urgent surgical exploration. Occlusion of a single tibial or forearm vessel is usually tolerated without ischaemic damage and does not as a rule require reconstruction.
- Beware the concept of 'arterial spasm'. It is true that the smooth muscle of arteries contracts protectively in response to injury so that an important vessel may appear quite small both angiographically and on direct inspection. However, luminal discontinuity is always due to a mechanical fault and demands surgical repair. Never attempt to treat such lesions with vasodilator drugs.
- In the case of multiple injuries, co-operate closely with colleagues of other specialities in planning surgical treatment. Repair of damaged major arteries always takes precedence over orthopaedic fixation of fractures. However, there is a danger that vascular anastomoses may become disrupted during the manipulation of fractures. In these circumstances it may be advisable to restore vascular continuity initially by inserting a temporary intraluminal plastic shunt, and completing the repair once the fractures have been stabilized, when the length of the arterial defect can be accurately measured.
- *Run-in*. This is not usually relevant in arterial trauma.
- *Run-off*. There is a risk that blood clot may form and occlude vessels distal to the site of injury. The procedure must include measures to deal with this problem (see below), otherwise the run-off vessels are usually normal.
- *Conduit*. In the case of limb injuries this is either the original artery repaired directly or an interposition graft of autogenous vein. Since only short segments are required, problems are rarely encountered in finding a vein of suitable quality and calibre.
- For closed injuries to major arteries (e.g. iliac, subclavian) with tearing or rupture of the vessel consider endovascular repair with a covered stent in hospitals with facilities for this type of procedure (see Endovascular repair of aortic and peripheral aneurysms, below).

Prepare

1 Once the presence of major arterial injury has been established, undertake surgical exploration without delay.

2 Have cross-matched blood available and correct serious hypovolaemia.

Access

1 In the case of limb injury, prepare and drape the limb so as to permit direct inspection of skin perfusion and palpation of pulses distal to the site of injury.

2 Consider also the possibility that a segment of healthy undamaged vein of suitable size may need to be harvested for construction of a graft.

3 First, gain proximal control of the artery and then gain distal control. This requires a skin incision that extends well beyond the confines of the injury. Make this incision along the axis of the injured vessel and directly over it.

4 Do not enter the haematoma until the vessel has been dissected and controlled by passing rubber slings around it proximally and distally.

Assess

1 On entering the haematoma there may be brisk fresh bleeding, in which case apply clamps at the proximal and distal control points already prepared.

2 If there is complete disruption of the artery find the ends and apply soft clamps. It is unlikely that they will be actively bleeding at the time of exploration.

3 It is always the case that the vessel is traumatized for some distance proximally and distally from the principal site of injury. Therefore trim each end back a few millimetres at a time until undamaged intima is reached.

4 Assess the length of the defect. Attempt direct end-to-end anastomosis only if there will be no tension. In most cases it is more prudent to insert an interposition graft of autologous vein, even if this is only a centimetre in length.

5 If the artery is in continuity there may be bruising of the adventitia at the site of injury and absence of downstream pulsation. These are sure signs of internal disruption. The intima and inner layers of the media split transversely and the edges roll back to form a flap, which obstructs flow, causing secondary thrombosis. It is never sufficient, therefore, to simply inspect the outer surface of such a vessel and it is totally unacceptable to treat such lesions by topical application of vasodilator substances. Excise the damaged segment completely, cutting back each end of the artery as before to find healthy intima.

6 Active arterial bleeding usually signifies incomplete disruption or a lateral wall defect that inhibits protective retraction and constriction of the vessel.

Action

1 Before commencing repair of the artery pass a Fogarty catheter distally and proximally to withdraw any propagated clot and then instil heparinized saline.

2 If there are associated orthopaedic injuries consider inserting a temporary intraluminal shunt (see above).

3 The adventitia tends to prolapse over the end of a normal artery that has been cut across. Trim this back to prevent it intruding inside the anastomosis.

4 If direct end-to-end anastomosis is possible, accomplish it by the triangulation technique (see Basic techniques) and in most cases employ interrupted sutures in preference to continuous.

5 If the defect is too great to permit direct repair, harvest a segment of vein of appropriate size. Complete the proximal anastomosis first, in end-to-end fashion, using the triangulation technique with interrupted sutures for small or inaccessible vessels or the oblique overlap technique for larger vessels. Remember to reverse the vein to avoid obstruction to blood flow by competent valves. Apply a clamp to the distal end of the graft and allow arterial pressure to distend it in order to determine the optimum length to avoid both excessive tension and kinking. Finally, complete the distal anastomosis.

6 A small puncture or lateral wall defect, as may result from iatrogenic injury following arterial access for investigation or treatment, may be repaired by direct suture or by closing the arteriotomy with a patch.

? DIFFICULTY

1. Technical difficulty may be encountered in effecting satisfactory end-to-end anastomoses, usually because of awkward access. Under these circumstances the ends of the artery may be ligated and the area of trauma bypassed with end-to-side anastomoses at remote, more accessible, sites.
2. Magnification is advisable for small vessel anastomoses.
3. If there is any doubt about the effectiveness of the repair, obtain an on-table angiogram.
4. Recurrent thrombosis despite a technically satisfactory repair warrants immediate systemic heparinization.
5. It may be difficult to decide whether or not to repair associated damage to veins. As a rule, repair major axial veins such as the femoral vein and, in the case of near-amputation of a limb, restore continuity to two veins for each artery repaired. Construct venous anastomoses obliquely and with interrupted sutures.

Closure

1 Where possible, effect primary closure of the incision with suction drainage.

2 In the case of blast injuries and other causes of extensive skin and soft-tissue damage, observe the general principles of wound management. Where primary closure is either not possible or inadvisable, always cover the arterial repair with healthy viable tissue, which in practice usually means a muscle flap.

Aftercare

1 Except in cases where continued bleeding is a serious problem, maintain anticoagulation with heparin for several days.

2 Arrange regular half-hourly observation of the distal circulation during the immediate postoperative period and be prepared to re-explore immediately in the event of recurrent occlusion.

Complications

1 Early thrombosis or bleeding at the site of the repair demands immediate re-exploration and re-assessment.

2 A false aneurysm may result from a contained anastomotic leak and this also requires early re-exploration and repair.

3 The risk of associated deep venous thrombosis is high, so take appropriate preventative measures.

4 Repair of arterial injuries in young, healthy people is usually very successful and long-term disability associated with ischaemia is rare.

SURGICAL EMBOLECTOMY

Appraise

- Embolic occlusion of a major artery results in acute ischaemia, which, if not relieved quickly, may progress to irreversible tissue damage and limb loss.
- The differential diagnosis is from acute thrombosis occurring within an already diseased artery. Differentiation between these two conditions may be impossible on clinical grounds alone, especially since embolization is nowadays more commonly associated with ischaemic heart disease than valvular stenosis, and most patients therefore have generalized arteriosclerosis.
- If there is an immediate threat to the viability of the limb, evidenced by muscle tenderness and paralysis and loss of sensation, then immediate surgical exploration is required irrespective of the cause.
- Revascularization of a limb that is already totally non-viable invariably has fatal consequences and is absolutely contraindicated. Urgent amputation may be life-saving.
- Under other circumstances urgent angiography is indicated to establish the diagnosis and to permit proper appraisal of the various options for treatment.
- Surgical embolectomy is indicated for embolic occlusion of:
  The common femoral artery and vessels proximal to the groin (e.g. saddle embolus).
  The brachial and axillary arteries.
- For patients in whom there is no immediate threat to the viability of the limb, more distal emboli, such as those in the popliteal artery, are more appropriately treated by thrombolytic therapy.

- Preoperative appraisal includes an assessment of the underlying cardiac disease. Surgical embolectomy can be performed under local anaesthesia but general anaesthesia is preferable in the absence of serious anaesthetic risk.
- Run-in, run-off and conduit usually are not relevant to surgical embolectomy in the absence of associated arterial disease.

Prepare

1 The urgency of the situation dictates that preoperative preparation must be limited. Treatment may be required for heart failure or dysrhythmia.

2 Commence systemic anticoagulation with heparin.

Access

1 For lower limb emboli, expose the common femoral artery (see Exposure of the major peripheral arteries, above).

2 For upper limb emboli, expose the brachial artery in the antecubital fossa (see above).

Action

1 Make a short longitudinal arteriotomy. In the case of the femoral artery make this directly over the origin of the profunda artery.

2 Select an embolectomy catheter of a size that is appropriate to vessel: 3F for axillary and brachial arteries, 4F for the superficial and profunda femoral arteries and 5F for the aortic bifurcation.

3 A number of different makes of embolectomy catheter are available. Choose one with a central irrigating lumen that permits injection of heparinized saline or X-ray contrast medium into the vessels beyond the balloon.

4 Pass the uninflated catheter proximally through the vessel beyond the clot. Inflate the balloon and withdraw the catheter slowly while adjusting the pressure within the balloon to accommodate changes in the diameter of the vessel. Avoid severe friction between the balloon and the arterial wall since this can cause serious damage to the vessel.

5 Instruct an assistant to control bleeding from the vessel during this process by applying gentle traction to the rubber sling previously placed around it.

6 Repeat the procedure until no more thrombus is retrieved and forceful bleeding is obtained from the vessel. Avoid all unnecessary passages of the catheter.

7 Instil heparinized saline into the artery and gently apply a clamp.

8 Repeat the same procedure distally.

9 Fill the vessels with heparinized saline and close the arteriotomy. Directly suture the common femoral artery but use a small vein patch for the brachial artery always.

? DIFFICULTY

1. *The catheter will not pass proximally or forceful forward bleeding is not obtained.* This can be due to pre-existing arterial disease or to the catheter having been introduced in a subintimal plane. Avoid direct aortoiliac reconstruction under these circumstances if at all possible and perform either a femorofemoral crossover or an axillofemoral bypass.
2. *The catheter will not pass distally.* Obtain an on-table angiogram. This may show embolus impacted at the popliteal bifurcation and in the tibial arteries, or evidence of atherosclerotic occlusion. Instil a small amount of a thrombolytic agent (streptokinase, urokinase or tPA) locally through a small catheter advanced to the site of occlusion.[1] Then pass a small Fogarty catheter 15 minutes later; more embolus may be retrieved. Alternatively, expose the infrageniculate popliteal artery to enable Fogarty catheters to be introduced directly into the tibial vessels. This requires the administration of a general anaesthetic. If there is a longstanding atherosclerotic occlusion of the superficial femoral artery, restoration of blood flow to the profunda system alone is likely to be sufficient to save the limb. However, if distal perfusion remains poor, then proceed to femoropopliteal bypass. Where facilities for intraoperative fluoroscopy exist, as an alternative to exposure of the popliteal artery for retrieval of emboli from the tibial arteries, pass the embolectomy catheter over a guide-wire negotiated into each vessel in turn. Assess the result by angiography.

Closure

1 Close the wound in layers with interrupted skin sutures or clips after instituting suction drainage.

Aftercare

1 Arrange long-term anticoagulation therapy to prevent recurrent embolization for younger patients. But, in the case of the very elderly, weigh the risks of this strategy against the benefits.

2 Evaluate and treat the underlying cardiac disease.

PERCUTANEOUS THROMBOLYTIC EMBOLECTOMY/THROMBECTOMY

Appraise

See Surgical embolectomy.

Prepare

1 Thrombolytic therapy is contraindicated in patients who have suffered a stroke and in those with intracardiac thrombus. Obtain an echocardiogram to eliminate the latter.

2 Streptokinase is antigenic and may induce severe anaphylactic shock if administered more than once. Therefore ascertain that the patient has never received streptokinase previously. Note

that urokinase and tissue plasminogen activator (tPA) may be given repeatedly without risk of this specific complication, but they are considerably more expensive.

3 Administer systemic anticoagulation with heparin.

Action

1 Puncture the common femoral artery with a Potts–Cournand needle and pass a short guide-wire into the superficial femoral artery.

2 Remove the needle and insert a 6F introducer sheath over the wire.

3 Under X-ray control advance a long guide-wire through the vessel beyond the embolus.

4 Pass a small-bore (4F) catheter over the guide-wire so that the tip enters the clot.

5 Withdraw the guide-wire and infuse the thrombolytic agent according to the manufacturer's instructions. Appreciate that, by infusing the agent locally into the thrombus, relatively small amounts are required. The high incidence of serious bleeding complications associated with systemic administration is thereby reduced.

6 After 30–60 minutes ascertain by X-ray the progress of clot lysis and advance the catheter again over a guide-wire into the embolus. Repeat this process until all blood clot has been dissolved.

7 More rapid and efficient lysis of thrombus can be achieved by the 'pulse-spray' technique. This involves pulsed high-pressure injection of the thrombolytic agent through a catheter with multiple side holes. Special equipment is required that is not available in all hospitals.

8 Finally, withdraw the catheter and apply pressure to the puncture site in the groin for a minimum period of 10 minutes to ensure haemostasis.

9 Thrombosed infra-inguinal bypass grafts are best treated by mechanical thrombectomy in preference to thrombolysis. This avoids haemorrhagic complications and is associated with a reduced risk of embolization of fragmented thrombus into the peripheral vascular bed. The most effective device employs the Bernouilli effect to break up and aspirate the thrombus. A larger sheath is required and excessively prolonged application may induce haemolysis. In most cases adjuvant percutaneous angioplasty will be necessary to deal with causative stenotic lesions due anastomotic intimal hyperplasia or progressive atheroma. Mechanical thrombectomy is not available in all hospitals.

? DIFFICULTY

1. The embolus may fragment and impact in more distal vessels. Further administration of the thrombolytic agent may be effective but it must be infused directly into the clot.
2. Alternatively, small fragments may be removed by suction applied to a larger catheter (suction embolectomy). Provided that the viability of the limb has been secured, small residual fragments of this type may be of no consequence and they may lyse spontaneously in time if left.

Complications

1 In order to minimize haemorrhagic complications, monitor coagulation tests repeatedly and adjust the dose of thrombolytic agent accordingly.

2 There is a risk of blood clot forming around the catheter itself. Therefore maintain heparin anticoagulation throughout the procedure.

3 Groin haematomas will usually resolve spontaneously but expanding haematomas and false aneurysms require surgical repair.

REFERENCE

1. Parent FN, Bernhard VM, Portos TS et al 1989 Fibrinolytic treatment of residual thrombus after catheter embolectomy for severe lower limb ischaemia. Journal of Vascular Surgery 9:153–160

AORTOBIFEMORAL BYPASS

All aortic operations have features in common. These will be described in detail here and will not be repeated in subsequent sections.

Appraise

- The indications for aortobifemoral bypass have diminished considerably since the advent of effective percutaneous angioplasty.
- It is an appropriate procedure for total aortic occlusion, severe aortic bifurcation disease or diffuse widespread aortoiliac disease in patients with critical limb ischaemia or disabling claudication.
- Localized iliac disease, stenoses or short occlusions can be treated very successfully by balloon angioplasty dilatation.
- Manage extensive unilateral iliac disease by either a unilateral extraperitoneal bypass or a femorofemoral crossover graft (see below).
- *Inflow*. This is not a problem in the case of aortic grafts.
- *Outflow*. Very commonly patients with severe symptoms have multilevel disease with involvement also of the femoropopliteal arteries. The profounda femoris artery is nearly always patent but may be stenosed at its origin. There is evidence that the long-term patency of aortofemoral grafts is affected adversely when only one of the run-off vessels is patent.[1,2] Consider concomitant femorodistal bypass, particularly in patients with critical ischaemia. In all other patients it is probably better to confine the operation to the proximal bypass initially and then appraise the merits of a second distal bypass at a later date. However, always correct any profunda origin stenosis at the time of aortofemoral bypass.
- *Conduit*. Use a bifurcated polyester Dacron graft—either 14 mm × 7 mm, 16 mm × 8 mm or 18 mm × 9 mm, depending on the diameter of the native vessels. Knitted grafts are preferred to woven grafts in this situation but otherwise the type of graft used is not important.

Prepare

1 The major risk associated with aortic surgery is that of cardiac complications. It is therefore appropriate for patients to undergo cardiac risk assessment before surgery. This might include: stressed ECG, measurement of left ventricular ejection fraction by echocardiography or radioisotope studies, evaluation of myocardial perfusion by thallium scanning and coronary angiography, depending on the facilities available. An unfavourable result might indicate that:
- Surgery should be abandoned altogether.
- A lesser procedure should be undertaken (e.g. an extra-anatomic bypass).
- Intensive care facilities will be needed postoperatively.
- Coronary artery disease should be treated first.

2 For patients with known myocardial impairment it is essential to optimize left ventricular preload and afterload during the procedure. Monitor these patients throughout the procedure and postoperatively with a Swan–Ganz catheter. Precise information to guide the anaesthetist during and after the operation can be obtained by measuring cardiac output under various degrees of fluid loading preoperatively to determine the optimum conditions for that patient. But this is rarely done in practice.

3 Graft infection is a disastrous complication, although fortunately rare. Administer a large single dose of broad-spectrum antibiotic with induction of anaesthesia.

4 The patient is fully anaesthetized with total muscular relaxation and lies supine on the operating table.

5 Insert arterial, central venous and peripheral venous lines in all patients and a Swan–Ganz catheter in selected patients.

6 Insert a 12F self-retaining Silastic urinary catheter.

7 Prepare the entire area from the level of the nipples to mid-thigh. Cover the genitalia with a small towel and apply an adhesive drape allowing access to the whole of the abdomen and both inguinal regions.

Access

1 Expose the common femoral arteries first.

2 The abdominal aorta may be exposed through a vertical midline incision, a transverse supra-umbilical incision or an oblique muscle-cutting incision in the flank with an extraperitoneal approach. There are advantages and disadvantages associated with each of these. When only one intra-abdominal arterial anastomosis is anticipated, as for example in an aortobifemoral bypass, a transverse incision made directly over the site of the anastomosis gives adequate exposure and heals well with possibly less postoperative pain than a vertical incision (Fig. 29.16).

Make the incision 2 cm above the umbilicus and extending 2–3 cm beyond the rectus sheath on each side. Divide the rectus muscles with diathermy in the same line as the skin incision. Locate and divide the superior epigastric arteries on both sides. Open the posterior rectus sheath and the peritoneum together; vessels in the edge of the falciform ligament should be ligated.

3 Check the abdominal contents to exclude the presence of other pathology (e.g. malignancy), which may influence the decision to proceed.

4 Note the presence of gallstones or peptic ulcer but do not attempt surgical treatment of these at the time of aortic reconstruction.

5 Displace the omentum and transverse colon superiorly, and the small bowel with its mesentery to the right. An efficient fixed self-retaining retractor system such as Omnitract makes it unnecessary to displace these structures outside the abdominal cavity. Keep them in place beneath the retractor blades with large moistened abdominal packs.

6 The aorta lies beneath the posterior parietal peritoneum with the fourth part of the duodenum anterior to it. Incise the peritoneum around the left margin of the duodenum and displace this structure superiorly and to the right to expose the aorta. It is crossed in the upper part of the dissection by the left renal vein.

7 Continue dividing the peritoneum inferiorly to the right of the inferior mesenteric artery to expose the aortic bifurcation and both common iliac arteries (Fig. 29.16).

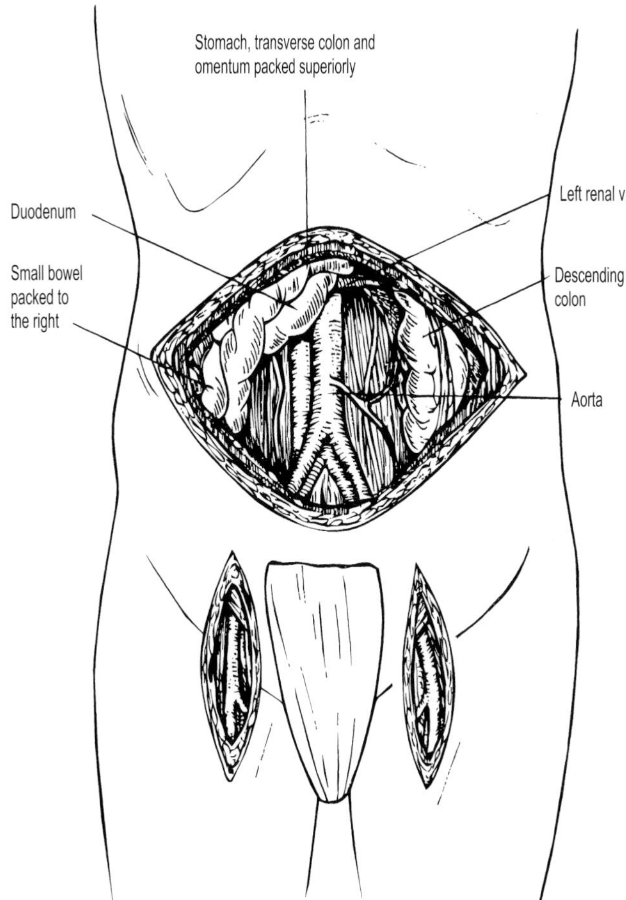

Fig. 29.16 Exposure of the abdominal aorta for aortofemoral bypass.

Assess

1 Palpate the aorta and the iliac arteries to determine the extent of the disease. If there is a very localized block, consider endarterectomy or a local aortoiliac bypass. However, these procedures have largely been superseded by aortobifemoral bypass and, except in very unusual circumstances, it is better to proceed with this standard operation. The crucial point at this stage is to select a site for the proximal anastomosis, avoiding as far as possible large calcified plaques. The segment between the renal vein and the inferior mesenteric artery is usually the most favourable.

2 If there is a total occlusion of the aorta, it is most appropriate to transect it and construct an end-to-end anastomosis with the graft. If the aorta is not totally occluded then many surgeons prefer to construct an end-to-side (onlay) anastomosis in order to preserve perfusion through the natural vessels into the internal iliac arteries. If the external iliac arteries are occluded then an end-to-side anastomosis is certainly to be preferred since there can be no retrograde flow from the distal anastomoses into the iliac system, and ischaemia of the pelvic organs and buttocks may otherwise ensue.

3 Assess the inferior mesenteric artery. If it is a large vessel with a widely patent aortic ostium then preserve it carefully.

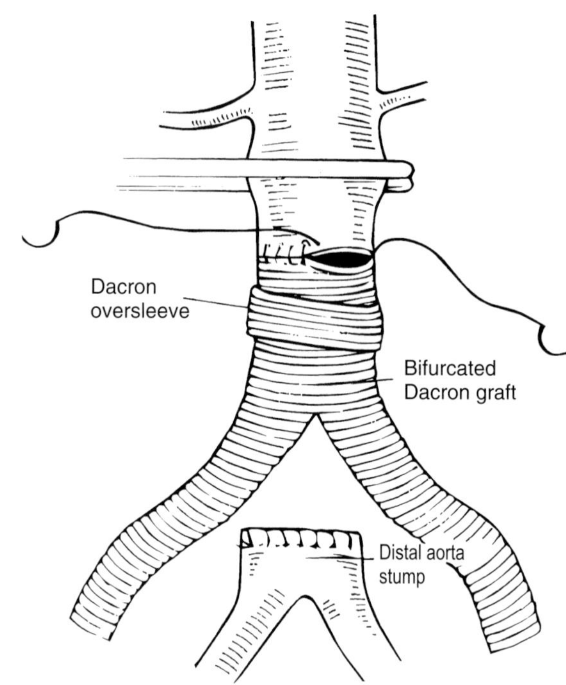

Fig. 29.17 Aortic anastomosis: end-to-end technique.

Action

1 Pass an O'Shaunessy clamp behind the aorta just distal to the left renal vein in order to position a narrow tape, taking care to avoid damage to lumbar veins.

2 Select a bifurcated Dacron graft of appropriate size to match the diameter of the aorta and preclot it if required (see General principles).

3 Give heparin 5000 IU intravenously and allow 3 minutes for it to circulate before applying clamps.

4 If the aorta is occluded apply a suprarenal clamp, transect the aorta 2 cm below the renal arteries, remove the thrombus from the proximal stump, apply an infrarenal clamp and then replace the supra-aortic clamp with one applied to the thrombectomized aorta below the renal arteries. The operation can then proceed in standard fashion. For placement of the suprarenal clamp expose the aorta below the diaphragm. This is achieved by incising the lesser omentum and the posterior parietal peritoneum above the pancreas. Split the fibres of the crus of the diaphragm longitudinally to expose the aorta. Apply a straight aortic clamp vertically, ensuring that it is fully occlusive. It is not necessary to encircle the aorta with a tape. When performing thrombectomy of the infrarenal aortic stump take care to dissect a plane between the thrombus and aortic wall using a MacDonald's or similar dissector. Dissection in the subintimal plane carries a risk of obstruction of the renal arteries by an intimal flap and must be avoided at all costs.

5 Oversew the distal aortic stump with a 3/0 polypropylene (Prolene) stitch. Take the previously prepared Dacron graft. Note that the body of bifurcated grafts is always much longer than is required. Trim away the excess leaving only 1–2 cm otherwise the 'legs' of the graft will come off at a sharp angle and may kink.

Construct an end-to-end anastomosis with 3/0 polypropylene sutures (Fig. 29.17). An oversleeve of graft material may be placed across the anastomosis using a piece trimmed previously. This reinforces the anastomosis, applies tamponade to the suture line and may reduce the risk aortoenteric fistula.

6 If an end-to-side anastomosis is considered appropriate (Fig. 29.18) and the aortic wall is soft it may be possible to apply a partially occluding clamp of Satinsky type. If the aorta is calcified it may be easier to apply two clamps, one above and the other below the anastomosis, but back-bleeding will occur from lumbar arteries in this case on opening the aorta; control these vessels first with sutures. A bifurcated graft of 16 mm × 18 mm size is usually most appropriate. Trim the excess of the body away, cutting it obliquely. Construct an end-to-side anastomosis with 3/0 polypropylene sutures.

7 On completion of the aortic anastomosis apply clamps to each limb of the graft and release the aortic clamp to test its integrity. Additional interrupted sutures may be required at this stage. Once the integrity of the suture line has been secured instil heparinized saline into the graft.

8 Make retroperitoneal tunnels through which to pass the limbs of the graft to the groin incisions. Do this by inserting a finger from the groin to the lateral side of the femoral artery in order to avoid damage to the vein. Insert a finger of your other hand beneath the peritoneum at the aortic bifurcation, ensuring that it passes beneath the ureter, and tunnel both fingers gently until they meet. Then pass a tunnelling instrument from the groin through this channel, attach the limb of the graft and draw it through.

9 Apply clamps to the common, superficial and profunda femoral arteries and make a longitudinal arteriotomy. If there is a pro-

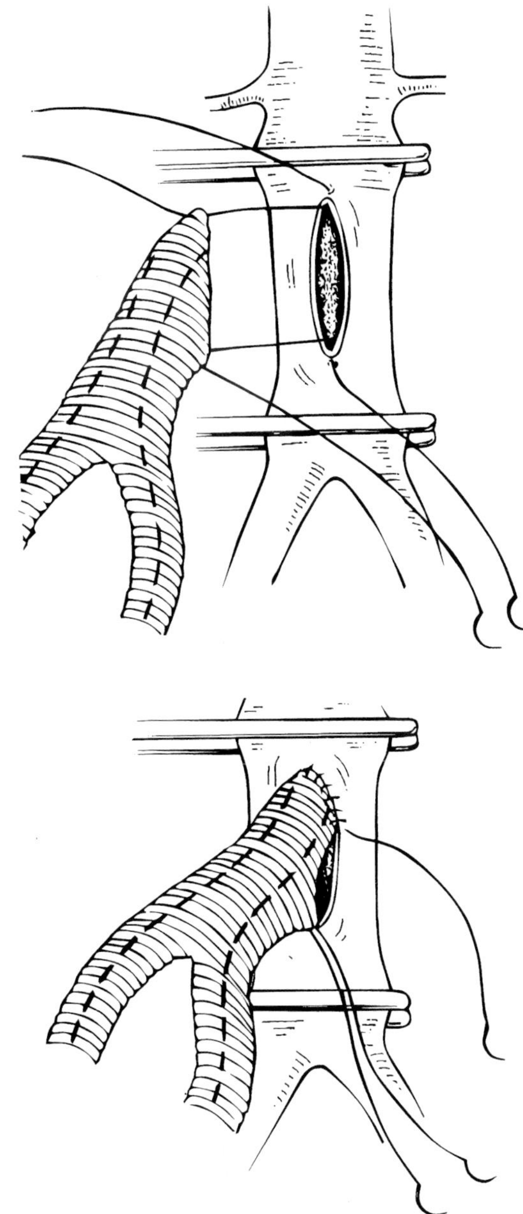

Fig. 29.18 End-to-side 'onlay' anastomosis.

funda origin stenosis extend the arteriotomy across it into the mainstem profunda artery.

10 Apply gentle traction to the limb of the graft, sufficient to just draw out the crimping, then trim it obliquely to the required length and construct an end-to-side anastomosis with 5/0 polypropylene sutures. The distal anastomoses may be constructed simultaneously by two surgeons, but the graft should be vented through one of the anastomoses prior to completion in order to eliminate any clot that may have formed during clamping.

11 Warn the anaesthetist 2–3 minutes before you are ready to release the clamps, so that he may make preparations, and release one limb at a time in order to minimize the risk of declamping shock.

12 Close the posterior parietal peritoneum over the graft. If there is difficulty, cover the graft with omentum to avoid adhesion and erosion of the bowel with the attendant risk of late graft infection.

? DIFFICULTY

1. Calcification in the wall of the aorta may prevent effective application of a clamp, or it may fracture and penetrate the wall, causing a tear, or it may not allow passage of a needle. It is important to avoid large calcified plaques and occasionally it may be necessary to apply a clamp at the level of the diaphragm above the visceral arteries. It is often possible to place sutures around calcified plaques. Exercise caution in removing such plaques because this may result in an extremely thin and friable aortic wall. Carefully repair rupture of the wall by a fractured plaque with adventitial sutures, if necessary buttressed by Dacron pledgets.
2. Beware of trying to close suture-line tears of the aorta with more stitches since this often makes matters worse. Reapply the clamps and carefully place an adventitial mattress suture buttressed with a Dacron pledget across the tear (Fig. 29.19).

Closure

1 Close the abdominal wound in layers, using a non-absorbable nylon stitch for the anterior rectus sheath.

2 Cover the groin anastomosis with two layers of 2/0 synthetic absorbable sutures and subcuticular absorbable sutures for the skin.

3 Drains are not normally required.

Aftercare

1 Carefully monitor cardiac, respiratory and renal function and observe the peripheral circulation. Some patients should certainly be managed initially in an intensive care unit. Most can be looked after satisfactorily in a high-dependency area on a general ward.

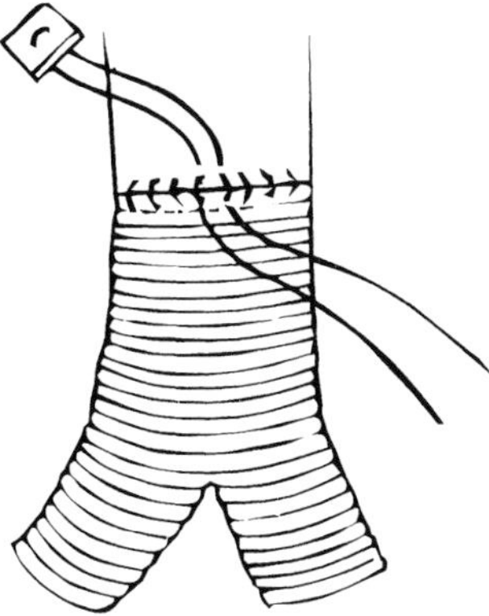

Fig. 29.19 Dacron buttress to control suture line or needle-hole bleeding.

2 All patients develop a postoperative ileus and require parenteral fluid support for 4–5 days.

3 The incidence of postoperative chest infection is particularly high in this group of patients; therefore ensure that they receive regular physiotherapy.

4 Maintain deep venous thrombosis prophylaxis.

5 After discharge from hospital, patients require follow-up visits in the outpatient clinic at about 6 weeks, 6 months and 1 year. The late occlusion rate for these grafts is low and follow-up beyond 1 year is unnecessary.

Complications

Remember five potential complications in particular:

- *Haemorrhage*. A suspicion of intra-abdominal bleeding postoperatively demands immediate re-operation and correction of the fault. 'Haematological' bleeding due to the effect of the heparin or other coagulopathy can be diagnosed by appropriate tests and corrected by administration of fresh-frozen plasma and/or platelets.
- *Graft occlusion*. This results either from embolization of material trapped above the aortic clamp that was not flushed out or from a technical fault at one of the suture lines. This also requires immediate re-exploration. Try passing a Fogarty catheter from the groin first. Recurrent occlusion almost certainly means there is an outflow problem and requires either re-fashioning of the distal anastomosis or even a secondary distal bypass of an occluded femoropopliteal segment.
- *Renal failure*. Application of a juxtarenal clamp nearly always results in some temporary impairment of renal function, probably due to microembolization of the glomeruli. There is no evidence that the routine administration of renal dopamine, mannitol or other diuretic is of any benefit. Renal tubular necrosis may occur postoperatively if there has been excessive blood loss with associated hypotension. It often recovers but a period of supportive haemodialysis or haemofiltration may be required. Total anuria immediately after operation suggests the possibility of occlusion of both renal arteries. Request immediate aortography and if this confirms absence of renal perfusion re-explore urgently with a view to renal artery reconstruction.
- *Myocardial infarction*. This is the most common cause of postoperative mortality; the critical time is the third postoperative day. Maintain cardiac monitoring for 5 days and react promptly to changes in rhythm or other evidence of ischaemia.
- *Infection*. This occurs in 2–3% of aortic grafts and can often be disastrous, resulting in either loss of life or limb. It may become manifest any time from days to years after operation. The symptoms are fever, backache and perhaps a purulent discharge from the wound. If nothing is done, a fatal haemorrhage occurs sooner or later. Computed tomography (CT) and culture of perigraft fluid are useful diagnostic tests. Occasionally infection is confined to one groin, in which case conservative surgery is often successful. Cover the anastomosis with healthy sartorius muscle (sartorius muscle slide operation) and administer local (gentamicin) and systemic antibiotics. But if the whole graft is infected it must be removed and replaced with an extra-anatomical axillofemoral bypass. Occasionally graft infection is associated with erosion of the gastrointestinal tract, usually the duodenum, by the graft and this may result in formation of an aortoenteric fistula. Assume that gastrointestinal bleeding in a patient who has previously had an aortic graft is due to an aortoenteric fistula until proved otherwise. There is no reliable diagnostic test and the diagnosis is therefore made by a process of elimination. Urgent surgical treatment is essential but what form this should take is a matter of some controversy. If the graft is grossly infected it should certainly be removed completely. However, there are many reports of aortoenteric fistulae with local contamination alone being treated successfully by simple closure of the fistula reinforced by an omental patch.

REFERENCES

1. Harris PL, Cave-Bigley DJ, MacSweeney L 1985 Aorto-femoral bypass and the role of concomitant femoro-distal reconstruction. British Journal of Surgery 22:317–320
2. Harris PL, Jones D, How T 1987 A prospective randomised clinical trial to compare in-situ and reversed vein grafts for femoro-popliteal by-pass. British Journal of Surgery 74:252–255

UNILATERAL AORTOFEMORAL/ ILIOFEMORAL BYPASS

Appraise

The indication for this operation is unilateral iliac artery occlusive disease (see Aortobifemoral bypass).

Prepare

See Aortobifemoral bypass.

Access

1 Expose the common femoral artery.

2 Make a gently curved incision in the flank extending from the costal margin superiorly to the lateral edge of the rectus sheath 2–3 cm above the inguinal ligament inferiorly (Fig. 29.20).

3 Divide the external oblique muscle and aponeurosis in the line of its fibres.

4 Cut the internal oblique and transversus muscles in the line of the incision using diathermy. Take care not to open the peritoneum. Repair any inadvertent holes immediately.

5 With finger dissection open up the retroperitoneal space and displace the peritoneal sac and its contents medially. The ureter usually displaces with the peritoneum. Identify it and protect it.

6 Identify the aortic bifurcation and the common and external iliac arteries. Use a fixed self-retaining retractor system to aid exposure.

Assess

Technically, it is easier to make the proximal anastomosis to the common iliac artery than to the aorta. Assess whether or not this is feasible by palpation of the vessels.

Action

1 Select a straight Dacron graft of appropriate size. One of 8 mm in diameter is usually most appropriate, but occasionally grafts

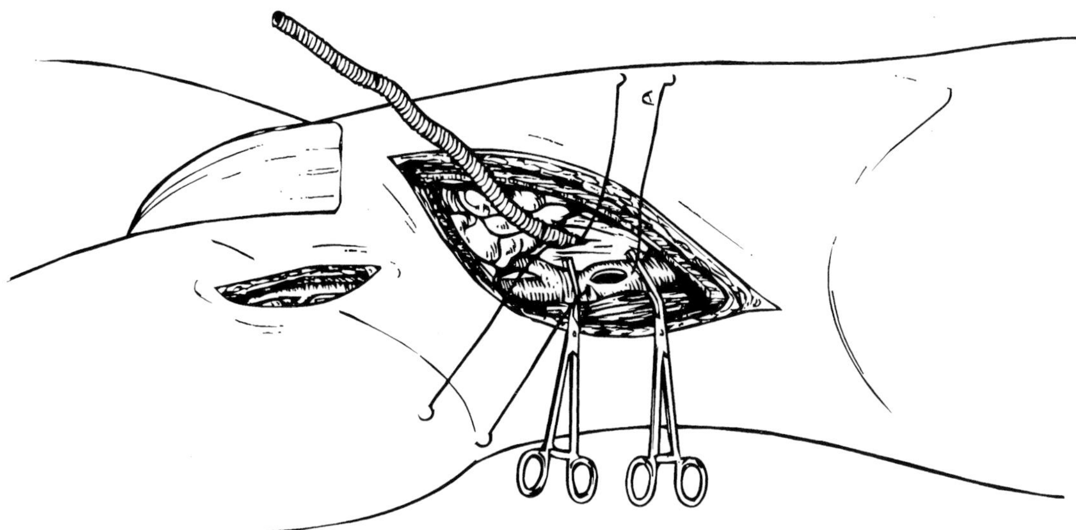

Fig. 29.20 Extraperitoneal iliofemoral bypass.

that are slightly larger or smaller may be required. Preclot it if necessary (see General principles).

2 Administer heparin and allow 3 minutes for it to circulate.

3 For an anastomosis to the common iliac artery apply a clamp to the origin of this vessel and another one at a suitable point distally.

4 For an aortic anastomosis it may be possible to apply a partially occluding clamp of the Satinsky type. If the aorta is calcified, this is unsafe so apply occluding clamps to the aorta and both common iliac arteries.

5 Make a longitudinal arteriotomy approximately 1.5 cm in length.

6 Take the previously prepared Dacron graft and trim the end obliquely to match the length of the arteriotomy.

7 Construct an end-to-side anastomosis with a continuous 4/0 polypropylene suture.

8 Apply a clamp to the graft just beyond the anastomosis and release the arterial clamp to test the suture line. Reinforce it if required (see Aortobifemoral bypass).

9 By finger dissection make a channel through to the groin incision, keeping to the lateral side of the artery to avoid damage to the vein. Draw the graft through this channel using either a tunnelling instrument or a straight aortic clamp.

10 Trim the graft to length and construct an end-to-side anastomosis to the common femoral artery with 5/0 polypropylene sutures (see Aortobifemoral bypass).

? DIFFICULTY

1. In obese patients access may be difficult, especially for an aortic anastomosis. Tilt the table to the side away from you to shift the abdominal contents out of the way, make a generous incision and use a fixed self-retaining retractor system.
2. Aortic or arterial calcification can be a cause of major difficulty (see under aortobifemoral bypass).

Closure

1 Close each muscle layer separately, with interrupted sutures for the transverses and internal oblique and a continuous suture for the external oblique aponeurosis.

2 Close the groin incision in layers (see Aortobifemoral bypass).

3 Drain the retroperitoneal space with a large suction drain.

Aftercare

See aortobifemoral bypass, but recovery is more rapid.

Complications

1 In addition to those described for aortobifemoral bypass, beware of acute arterial occlusion in the opposite limb.

2 Application of clamps at or close to the aortic bifurcation is associated with a high risk of embolic occlusion or thrombosis in the other common iliac artery. This must be checked for and corrected before anaesthesia is reversed.

3 Try passing a Fogarty catheter from the groin first. It this is not successful the best option is a femorofemoral crossover graft.

MINIMALLY INVASIVE AND TOTALLY LAPAROSCOPIC AORTIC RECONSTRUCTION

Appraise

- Minimally invasive techniques for reconstruction of the abdominal aorta and iliac arteries are being developed with the aim of minimizing surgical trauma, recovery time and postoperative complication rates.
- Totally laparoscopic procedures are undertaken by a retroperitoneal approach, with or without gas insufflation. Special instrumentation including aortic clamps has been designed for the purpose. The technical aspects of the operation are

based upon the principles of other established laparoscopic procedures.

- Minimally invasive operations performed through short (8 cm) incisions using retractors designed specially for the purpose represent a compromise between the conventional open and laparoscopic approaches. 'Hand-assisted' laparoscopic reconstruction is a further variation on this theme.
- Obese patients and those with calcified aortas are not suitable for these procedures. Otherwise the factors to be considered preoperatively are the same as those for aortofemoral bypass (see above).
- Facilities for immediate 'conversion' to conventional open surgery, in case of haemorrhagic or other critical intraoperative complications, are essential.
- Because these procedures are still under development and clinical evaluation at the time of writing and their efficacy in comparison to conventional vascular surgery is not established, they will not be described in any further detail here.

FEMOROFEMORAL BYPASS AND ILIOFEMORAL CROSSOVER BYPASS

Appraise

- These are alternative procedures to iliofemoral bypass for unilateral iliac artery disease and the results are comparable in terms of graft patency. Femorofemoral bypass is virtually a subcutaneous procedure and if necessary it can be carried out under local anaesthetic in very unfit patients (Fig. 29.21).

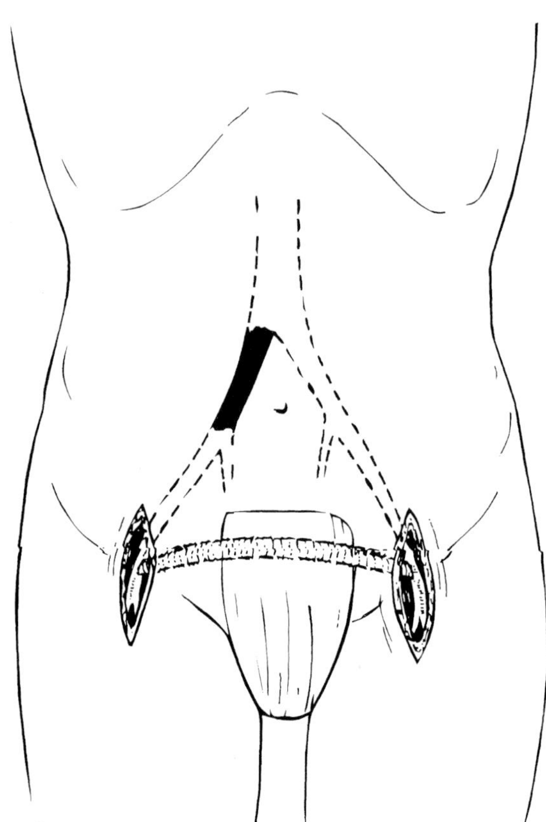

Fig. 29.21 Left-to-right femorofemoral crossover graft.

Iliofemoral crossover bypass has the important advantage of leaving the groin and femoral artery on the donor side undisturbed for possible future procedures. The angle between the graft and the donor artery is also in line with the direction of blood flow and this may have haemodynamic advantages. It is a slightly more invasive operation than femorofemoral bypass and usually requires general anaesthesia.

- *Run-in*. Adequacy of run-in is a crucial factor for the success or failure of these operations as well as their effect on the perfusion of the donor limb. Reliance on subjective assessment of angiograms is unsafe and some objective test of run-in is therefore mandatory. There are a number of methods for doing this but the simplest and most reliable is comparison of radial and femoral arterial pressures. Intra-arterial cannulas are connected to pressure transducers in order to record simultaneously the pressure waves at both sites. There may be a gradient under resting low-flow conditions, in which case inflow to that groin must certainly be judged inadequate. A bolus of papaverine 20 mg is then injected into the femoral artery by means of a three-way tap connected to the pressure line. This causes regional vasodilation and accelerates the blood flow into the limb. A radial to femoral pressure gradient in excess of 20 mmHg developing under high flow conditions is evidence of significant inflow stenosis.

  There are three options possible following a positive pressure test:
  - Abandon the operation completely.
  - Treat the inflow stenosis by balloon angioplasty dilatation either before or during the operation (see below) and then proceed with the femorofemoral bypass.
  - Convert to an axillofemoral bypass.
- *Run-off*. See Aortobifemoral bypass.
- *Conduit*. It is necessary to use a prosthetic graft for this purpose, and 8-mm diameter externally supported Dacron or expanded PTFE grafts are most suitable.

Action

1. For femorofemoral bypass expose both common femoral arteries.
2. For crossover iliofemoral bypass expose the common femoral artery in the recipient limb. On the donor side expose the external iliac artery by making a transverse incision above the inguinal ligament and entering the inguinal canal. Retraction of the spermatic cord and incision of the posterior wall of the inguinal canal reveals the artery in the retroperitoneal space.
3. Select an 8-mm graft.
4. By finger dissection create a tunnel between the two incisions. For femorofemoral bypass make a subcutaneous tunnel just above the superior pubic rami. In the case of crossover iliofemoral bypass make an extraperitoneal tunnel passing deep to the rectus muscles. Draw the graft into the tunnel using either a tunnelling instrument or a large aortic clamp.
5. Give heparin and allow 3 minutes for it to circulate.
6. Apply clamps to the femoral or iliac arteries and make longitudinal arteriotomies of approximately 1 cm length.
7. Trim the ends of the graft obliquely to match the length of the arteriotomies.

8 Fashion end-to-side anastomoses on both sides with 5/0 Prolene, Ethibond or Gore-Tex sutures as appropriate (see General principles). Flush the graft and arteries before completing the anastomosis.

Closure

Close both wounds carefully in layers, without drains.

Complications

1 In addition to the risks of haemorrhage, occlusion and infection (see Aortobifemoral bypass) the main concern is the possibility of ischaemia in the donor limb.

2 Provided that the procedure described here has been followed correctly, inflow obstruction should have been eliminated, but there remains the risk of thrombosis or embolization in the distal vessels.

3 Acute ischaemia requires immediate re-exploration. Less severe ischaemia warrants angiography with a view to further elective surgery.

AXILLOFEMORAL BYPASS

Appraise

- The indications for axillofemoral bypass are:
  Critical lower limb ischaemia in a patient with severe bilateral aortoiliac occlusive disease who will not tolerate safely aortobifemoral bypass (see Aortobifemoral bypass).
  Infection of a previously inserted aortobifemoral bypass.

  Long-term patency rates for axillofemoral grafts are roughly half as good as those for aortobifemoral grafts. Axillobifemoral grafts have better patency rates than axillounifemoral grafts.
- *Run-in.* Although occlusive disease is unusual in the upper limb arteries it is slightly more common on the left than the right side. Therefore, other considerations being equal, use the right axillary artery as the donor vessel. If critical ischaemia is confined to one leg and brachial artery pressures are equal, then use the axillary artery on the same side for the donor vessel.
- *Run-off.* See Aortobifemoral bypass.
- *Conduit.* Preformed axillobifemoral grafts with either right or left side-arms are available. However, construction of the bypass from axillofemoral and femorofemoral components allows more flexible 'tailoring' of the grafts and is therefore to be preferred. Although there is a theoretical risk of compression of the graft against the costal margin when the patient lies on his side, this rarely occurs and the use of externally supported grafts it is not essential.
- When using a preformed graft, trim it in such a way as to ensure that its length from the junction of the side-arm to the distal anastomosis is as short as possible. The reason for this is that the velocity of flow in the graft is potentially halved beyond this point, with a greater risk of thrombosis in this segment. When constructing the bypass from separate axillofemoral and femorofemoral components use a 10-mm diameter graft for the former and an 8-mm graft for the crossover. Construct the crossover bypass first (see above, Femorofemoral bypass) and anastomose the distal end of the axillofemoral component to it in end-to-side fashion. When infection of a pre-existing aortobifemoral graft is the indication for operation use a Dacron graft impregnated with antibiotic. This is prepared by soaking the graft in a solution of rifampicin before implantation. An effectively treated graft turns uniformly brown in colour. A Dacron graft impregnated with 'silver', which is intended to resist infection, is also available commercially.

Prepare

1 Full general anaesthesia is required, with the patient supine on the operating table.

2 It is necessary to prepare the skin and arrange the drapes in such a way as to make available the whole of the trunk and both legs to mid-thigh level. But, keep the donor arm free so that it can be abducted to ensure that there is no tension upon the anastomosis to the axillary artery in this position. Use adhesive drapes to hold the towels in place.

3 Ensure that the anaesthetist places radial or brachial arterial lines on the side that is not going to be clamped.

4 Give prophylactic antibiotics as for aortobifemoral bypass.

Action

1 Expose the axillary artery and both common femoral arteries (Fig. 29.22; see Exposure of the major peripheral arteries).

2 Select 10-mm and 8-mm Dacron grafts of appropriate length or a preformed axillofemoral graft.

3 If possible, it is better to avoid making additional incisions over the course of the graft. Use a long tunnelling instrument inserted from the upper (axillary) incision. Pass it deep to the pectoralis major muscle and then subcutaneously in the anterior axillary line, finally curving forwards above the anterior superior iliac spine to the ipsilateral groin incision. Attach the end of the main stem of the graft to the tunneller and then draw it through to the upper incision. When using a preformed graft continue to pull it through until the junction with side-arm lies at the upper end to the groin incision.

4 Pass the side-arm or femorofemoral component through a subcutaneous suprapubic tunnel (see Femorofemoral bypass).

5 Administer heparin and allow 3 minutes for it to circulate.

6 Apply clamps to the axillary and femoral arteries and make longitudinal arteriotomies approximately 1.5 cm in length.

7 When gauging the length at which trim the proximal end of the graft abduct the arm to ensure that there will be no tension upon the anastomosis in this position.

8 Considerable time is saved if the anastomoses are constructed simultaneously. Trim the ends of the graft obliquely to match the length of the arteriotomies and complete the anastomoses in end-to-side fashion with 5/0 Prolene or Ethibond sutures.

9 Test each anastomosis, flush the graft and fill it with heparinized saline before finally releasing the clamps. Open the circulation into one leg at a time in order to reduce the risk of declamping shock.

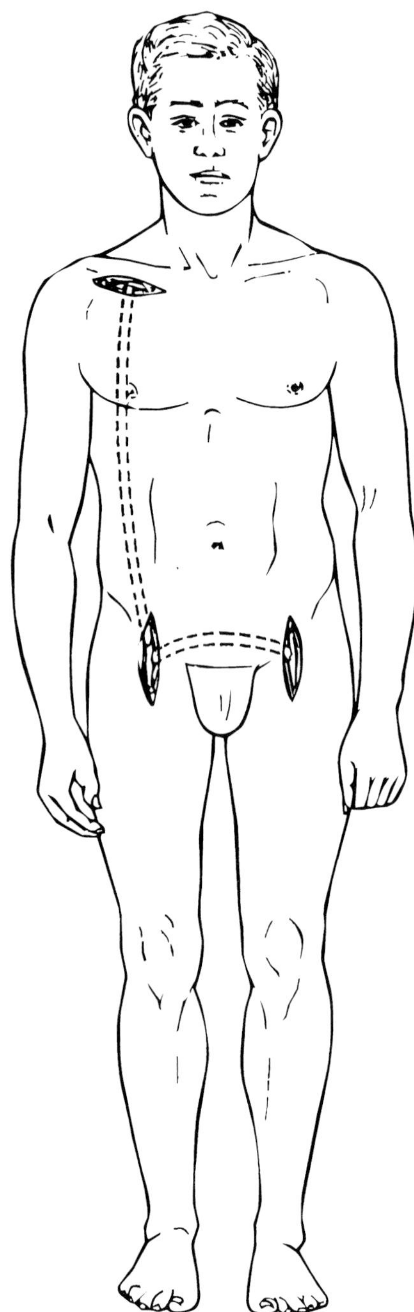

Fig. 29.22 Right axillobifemoral bypass.

Closure

1 Carefully close all three wounds in layers.

2 Drains are not usually necessary.

Complications

1 Occasionally a seroma develops around these grafts. The fluid is initially sterile but there is a risk of secondary infection if it is allowed to discharge spontaneously through any of the wounds. Under strict antiseptic conditions aspirate the fluid with a needle and syringe. This may need to be repeated until no more fluid accumulates or until all wounds are soundly healed.

2 The risk of occlusion by thrombosis is greater than for other proximal bypass procedures. If this occurs, re-establish patency by thrombectomy, ensure there are no technical errors and commence long-term anticoagulation. An important cause of occlusion is angulation due to tension on the axillary artery. This will be apparent on angiography and must be corrected during secondary intervention.

ILIAC ARTERY ANGIOPLASTY AND STENTING

Appraise

- Localized stenoses and short occlusions in the common iliac artery respond well to angioplasty. The addition of an intraluminal stent is indicated when:
  The stenosis is resistant to angioplasty or recurs immediately due to elastic recoil.
  Treatment is being undertaken for a recurrent lesion.

  There is no evidence to support the routine use of stents.
- This procedure may be undertaken as a sole therapeutic intervention and it has largely replaced open surgery for the management of localized iliac artery disease. Alternatively it may be applied to secure an adequate run-in in preparation for infrainguinal arterial reconstruction, in which case it may be undertaken percutaneously prior to operation or through the exposed common femoral artery intraoperatively.

Prepare

1 When undertaken percutaneously prepare the skin and drape the patient as for open iliofemoral bypass (see above).

2 When undertaken intraoperatively prepare the patient as for a femorodistal bypass (see below).

Access

Either

1 Puncture the common femoral artery percutaneously. If there is no pulse palpable in the common femoral artery employ ultrasound guidance (see Basic Techniques, Transluminal angioplasty).

Or

2 Expose the common femoral artery (see Exposure of the major peripheral arteries). Insert a 5/0 polypropylene purse-string suture into the front of the artery.

Assess

1 Puncture the common femoral artery through the purse string and insert a 7F sheath in a proximal direction (see Basic techniques, Transluminal angioplasty).

2 Use a 0.035-mm J-wire to cross the lesion under fluoroscopic control.

3 Pass a 'pigtail' angiography catheter over the wire and, using a pump injector, obtain a digitally subtracted angiogram to visualize the lesion.

4 For further assessment of the lesion record 'pull-through' pressure measurements. Having crossed the lesion with a straight 4F angiography catheter over the guide-wire, connect it to a

pressure transducer to record intraluminal pressure. Withdraw the catheter slowly through the stenosis and record the pressure gradient across it. Any pressure gradient under low-flow conditions is significant. For more accurate assessment repeat the process following injection of a vasodilator (e.g. papaverine 30 mg) intra-arterially into the limb (see above, Femorofemoral bypass, Assess).

Action

1. Select a balloon catheter of appropriate size using the preoperative angiogram as a guide (see Basic techniques). A balloon with an inflated diameter of 8 mm and length of 4 cm is often appropriate but it is essential not to overdilate the artery.
2. Obtain another angiogram to create a 'road map'. This allows a 'live' image of the balloon catheter to be superimposed over a stored image of the lesion to assist accurate positioning of the balloon.
3. Position the balloon over the guide-wire across the lesion and inflate it to the pressure recommended by the manufacturer using a manually operated syringe driver.
4. Use dilute contrast medium to dilate the balloon.
5. Observe the balloon by fluoroscopy as it expands. 'Popping of the waist' signals a good outcome.
6. Replace the balloon catheter with an angiography catheter and obtain a check angiogram to assess the result. If 'pull-through' pressure measurements were made prior to angioplasty repeat these now to ensure that the pressure gradient has been abolished.
7. Remove the introducer sheath and proceed with the femoro-distal bypass procedure.

? DIFFICULTY

1. *Are you unable to cross the lesion with the guide-wire?* Try again with a low friction, hydrophilic wire. Alternatively through an access sheath in the contralateral common femoral artery direct a low-friction hydrophilic guide-wire over the aortic bifurcation with suitably shaped guiding catheters and attempt to cross the lesion in an antegrade direction. If these methods fail or the wires pass subintimally abandon the procedure. Opt for open iliofemoral or femorofemoral bypass to overcome the inflow obstruction.
2. *The lesion is resistant to dilatation or there is a persistent stenosis due to intimal flap formation.* Use an intraluminal stent. For short, hard lesions use a balloon-expandable Palmaz stent. For longer lesions use a self-expanding Wallstent.
3. Lesions at the origin of the common iliac artery do not dilate adequately because displacement of the balloon is accommodated by compression of the opposite iliac artery. There is also a risk that the patency of the contralateral common iliac artery may be compromised. Insert balloon catheters into both common iliac arteries and inflate them simultaneously. This is known as the 'kissing balloons' technique.

Complications

Rupture of the iliac artery is likely to require urgent surgical repair. But, where facilities exist, consider endoluminal repair using a covered stent. (See also Basic techniques and Balloon angioplasty dilatation for femoropopliteal occlusive arterial disease.)

FEMOROPOPLITEAL AND INFRAPOPLITEAL SAPHENOUS VEIN BYPASS

Appraise

- Chronic occlusion of the superficial femoral artery alone seldom if ever results in critical limb ischaemia.
- Most stenoses or short occlusions in the superficial femoral artery can, if deemed appropriate, be treated successfully by percutaneous balloon angioplasty dilatation.
- The patency rates of long femorodistal bypass grafts are not sufficiently good to warrant their application for non-critical disease.
- Therefore the indications for elective femorodistal bypass surgery are critical limb ischaemia associated with extensive superficial femoral, popliteal and tibial artery occlusive disease, or extremely disabling intermittent claudication. Vascular trauma constitutes a frequent indication for emergency femorodistal bypass.
- *Run-in.* An unimpeded inflow is an essential prerequisite for a successful outcome. Objective assessment is essential (see Femorofemoral bypass) and an additional procedure to enhance inflow (e.g. iliac artery angioplasty) is indicated in the event of an adverse result.
- *Run-off.* Poor run-off is a major cause of femorodistal graft failure. It is essential to carefully select the site of the distal anastomosis in order to optimize outflow capacity. When the popliteal artery is visualized angiographically this vessel should normally be used. However, even with digital enhancement, preoperative angiographic assessment of tibial vessels may be unreliable, especially in the presence of critical ischaemia; the absence of images of these vessels on such films must not be accepted as evidence that they are definitely occluded. Objective tests such as pulse-generated run-off assessment[1] have been largely abandoned. Surgical exploration of the distal vessels and on-table angiography is the only reliable method for confirming non-operability. The presence of a Doppler signal will help identify the vessel to be explored first; otherwise start with the posterior tibial artery. (See also Femoropopliteal and infrapopliteal prosthetic bypass.)
- *Conduit.* There are two established methods for using the saphenous vein for femorodistal bypass grafting. These are the reversed and the in-situ techniques. A third method, the non-reversed transposed-vein technique, combines features of both of the original methods. Clinical evidence for the superiority of one of these methods over the others is lacking. Indeed, randomized studies to date indicate that reversed and in-situ grafts perform equally well in both femoropopliteal and infrapopliteal situations.[2] The choice of method, therefore, is a matter of personal preference and, since they appear to have equal merit, both the principal techniques will be described in

detail. The quality of the vein itself, and particularly its diameter, does have an important effect on outcome. This can be assessed preoperatively by duplex scanning. If the saphenous vein is inadequate, alternative sources of autologous vein may be sought or a decision may be made to use a prosthetic graft. If neither of these tests is available this decision must be delayed until the vein has been exposed surgically. An ideal vein has few divisions, is free from postphlebitic thickening of the wall and has a fairly uniform diameter of not less than 4 mm. Unfortunately, not many conform to the ideal and clinical judgement has to be exercised in determining acceptability.

- Note that longer grafts fare less well than shorter grafts and it is permissible in the absence of significant disease in the superficial femoral or popliteal arteries to use a distal donor site as a means of shortening a graft. Most grafts, however, should originate from the common femoral artery.

Prepare

1 Mark the course of the long saphenous vein with indelible ink before operation. If it is not visible on simple clinical examination use a Doppler ultrasound flow probe to follow its course or alternatively arrange for the vein to be 'mapped' by vascular laboratory technologists.

2 The leg is shaved, together with the pubic area and lower abdomen.

3 Under general anaesthesia, the patient lies supine on the operating table. The knee of the affected leg is flexed to about 45° with the hip flexed and slightly externally rotated. Swab the whole area from the umbilicus to the ankle. Enclose the foot in a sterile transparent plastic bag. Place towels under the leg and over the abdomen. Retain the position of the towels over the genitalia and upper thigh with an adhesive drape.

Access/Assess

1 Expose the common femoral artery and the proposed site for the distal anastomosis. If the popliteal artery is occluded and patency of the infrapopliteal vessels has not been determined before operation, expose the posterior tibial, the peroneal and anterior tibial arteries in order. When a patent vessel is found, insert a cannula and obtain an on-table angiogram, from which determine the optimum vessel for the anastomosis (see Quality control, Completion angiography). Ideally, this should communicate directly with the primary pedal arch. Remember when exposing the arteries to make the incisions overlie the saphenous vein wherever possible.

2 Expose a sufficient length of the saphenous vein from the groin distally by making an incision directly over it. Assess its suitability for use as a graft (see above, Appraise).

Action

Reversed saphenous vein graft

1 This is the standard procedure first performed successfully by Jean Kunlin in Paris in 1942.[3]

2 Completely mobilize and remove the long saphenous vein. Ligate the tributaries with fine material a millimetre or so away from its junction with the main trunk to avoid any possibility of narrowing the graft. Transfix the saphenofemoral junction with a stitch.

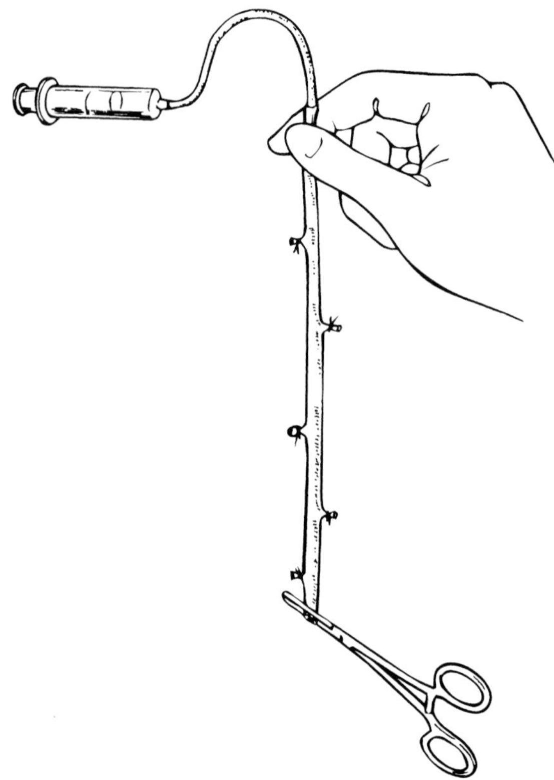

Fig. 29.23 Distending the reversed vein graft with heparinized blood.

3 Insert an umbilical catheter into the distal end of the vein, which will become the proximal end of the graft, and with a clamp at the other end gently distend it with heparinized blood (5000 IU of heparin in 50 ml of blood; Fig. 29.23). Secure any untied tributaries with fine ligatures and any small tears with 6/0 polypropylene mattress or figure-of-eight sutures inserted transversely.

4 Take great care to handle the vein gently at all times. Do not pick it up with metal instruments, do not apply clamps to it (except at the very end during distension—this will be trimmed away prior to construction of the anastomosis), do not overdistend it, do not impact over-large catheters into it, do not allow it to dry out. A traumatized segment of vein may become the site of fibrous stricture formation following implantation and threaten the long-term patency of the graft (see below).

5 Using a long tunneller, place the reversed vein in a route alongside the natural artery through the subsartorial canal and popliteal fossa but outside the abductor magnus tendon. Make sure it passes between the medial and lateral heads of gastrocnemius muscle to enter the popliteal fossa. In the calf, place it in the plane between the gastrocnemius and soleus muscles. Note that it is technically easier to enter this plane with the tunneller inserted from the distal incision and advanced proximally than it is the opposite way round. If the distal anastomosis is to be made to the anterior tibial artery, cross the interosseous membrane just below the popliteal fossa, taking care to avoid damage to the plexus of veins in this area.

6 Take great pains to ensure that the vein does not become twisted when laying it in its tunnel. Check that this has not occurred by gently distending it with heparinized blood after insertion.

7 Give heparin and allow 3 minutes for it to circulate.

8 The anastomoses may be completed simultaneously if two surgeons are available. Otherwise complete the distal anastomosis first. Make an arteriotomy in the recipient vessel about 1 cm in length. Trim the vein graft obliquely to match the length of the arteriotomy and complete the anastomosis in end-to-side fashion with either 6/0 polypropylene for the popliteal artery or 7/0 polypropylene for the infrapopliteal arteries.

9 Remember, do not apply clamps to the small distal arteries (see General principles).

10 On completion of the distal anastomosis the venous valves prevent back-bleeding from the graft; a clamp is not required. Gently flush the graft and the anastomosis with heparinized blood.

11 Apply clamps to the femoral arteries, make an arteriotomy 1 cm in length, trim the graft and construct an end-to-side anastomosis with 6/0 polypropylene sutures.

12 Remove all clamps. Observe the appearance of the graft, the recipient artery and the perfusion of the foot within the transparent plastic bag.

13 If all seems satisfactory, take an on-table completion angiogram before closure of the wounds.

? DIFFICULTY

1. *The vein is inadequate*. Short narrow segments can be resected and replaced with interposition grafts of autologous vein from other sites. If the whole vein is inadequate or missing (having been removed previously), consider using arm veins. This is often possible for femoropopliteal bypass but impractical for grafts that are longer than this. Exercise caution in using the long saphenous vein from the other leg, but this may on occasion be justified. Use a prosthetic graft only if there are no adequate autologous veins available. For distal bypasses where a staging anastomosis is possible, composite prosthetic and autologous vein grafts are preferable to a prosthetic graft alone (Fig. 29.24).
2. *The graft is twisted.* If this occurs despite all precautions, divide the graft at a convenient and readily accessible point, undo the twist and re-anastomose the ends by the triangulation technique with interrupted 6/0 polypropylene sutures.
3. *Completion angiogram shows a technical error at the distal anastomosis.* Take down and reconstruct the anastomosis.
4. *Completion angiogram shows embolic occlusion of the run-off vessels.* Pass a small Fogarty catheter through a short incision in the graft, made directly over the distal anastomosis.

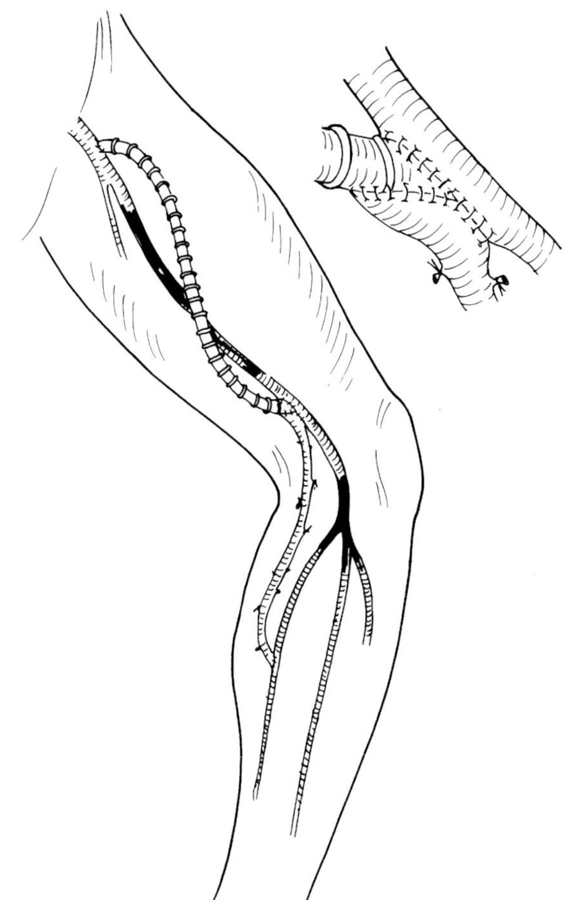

Fig. 29.24 Composite PTFE/autologous vein graft.

In-situ saphenous vein graft

1 In this operation most of the vein is left undisturbed in its natural bed and the valves are destroyed by the passage of a valvulotome (Fig. 29.25).[3,4]

The potential advantages over the reversed operation are:

- It retains its viability and those properties of the vein that depend upon its viability—most importantly an antithrombotic flow surface and a compliant muscular wall.
- The natural taper of the vein matches more closely that of the recipient artery, thereby facilitating the anastomoses and possibly conferring some haemodynamic benefits.
- It is claimed but not yet proven that smaller veins can be made to function more successfully by this technique than by the reversed method.[3]
- Because the graft lies subcutaneously it is easily assessed by simple clinical examination.

On current evidence these advantages would seem to be more theoretical than practical but many surgeons prefer the in-situ operation, particularly for infrapopliteal bypass.

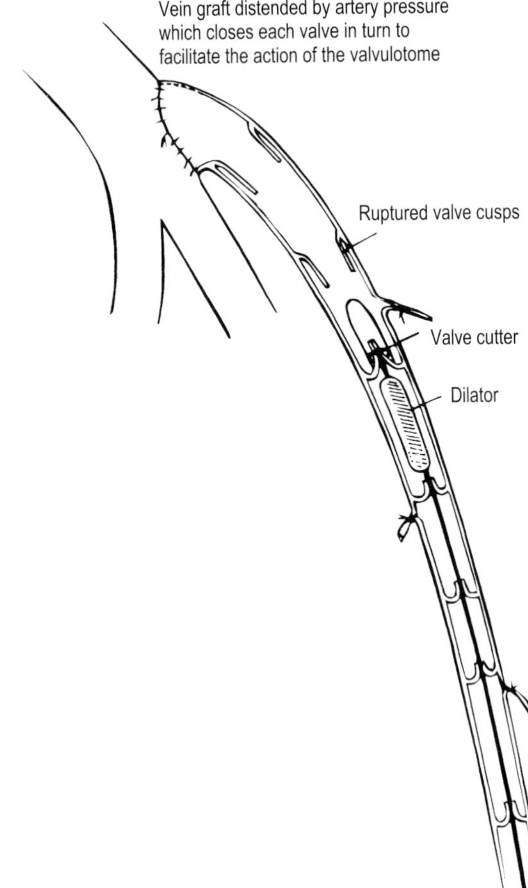

Fig. 29.25 In-situ vein graft. Mode of action of Hall's valvulotome.

2 Expose the vein throughout the required length and tie in continuity all visible tributaries, ensuring that the vein itself is not narrowed by placing the ligatures a millimetre or so away from the main trunk. Preserve the most proximal large tributary in the thigh to allow access of a cannula for on-table angiography later.

3 Carefully dissect the saphenofemoral junction and ligate and divide all tributaries at this level. Apply a paediatric Satinsky-pattern partially occluding clamp to the femoral vein and divide the saphenous vein flush with the junction. Repair the resulting defect in the femoral vein with a continuous 5/0 polypropylene suture and remove the clamp. Mobilize the proximal 5–6 cm of the saphenous vein.

4 Give heparin and allow 3 minutes for it to circulate before application of arterial clamps.

5 With the leg straight, find the point on the femoral artery to which the proximal end of the saphenous vein can be anastomosed without tension. Apply clamps and make a short arteriotomy at this site.

6 Open the proximal end of the saphenous vein, find the first valve and excise its cusps under direct vision with fine scissors.

7 Construct the proximal anastomosis end-to-side with 6/0 polypropylene (Prolene) sutures and release the clamps, allowing the arterial pressure to distend the graft to the level of the first competent valve.

8 Mobilize the distal end of vein and divide it, allowing sufficient length for trimming prior to construction of the anastomosis.

9 Select a valvulotome of the Hall's type of appropriate size. The valvulotome must not impact within the vein and it must not under any circumstances be used as a dilator. Most commonly, the smallest (2.5 mm diameter) instrument will suffice. Pass the valvulotome proximally through the graft to the upstream anastomosis and then withdraw it slowly (Fig. 29.25). Gently tug it as it catches on each valve to break the valve cusps and repeat this process after rotating the valvulotome through 90° to ensure that each of the cusps is ruptured. As the valve is made incompetent, arterial pressure closes the next in line, which once again facilitates the action of the valvulotome. Vigorous pulsatile bleeding on final withdrawal of the instrument indicates that all of the valves have been rendered incompetent. If this does not occur pass the valvulotome again but try to avoid repeated unnecessary passages of the instrument. The absence of pulsatile bleeding despite destruction of the valves is due to persistence of a large perforating vein. Sometimes the presence of a localized palpable thrill will locate it, but if not it will be pin-pointed on the angiogram later.

10 Apply a soft clamp to the graft. Trim the distal end and complete the distal anastomosis in end-to-side manner using 6/0 polypropylene for the popliteal artery or 7/0 polypropylene for the infrapopliteal arteries.

11 If the distal anastomosis is to be made to the anterior tibial artery, it is necessary to mobilize a sufficient length of the vein to allow it to be routed through the interosseous membrane to the lateral side of the calf.

12 For anastomosis to the infrageniculate popliteal artery the end of the vein should simply be turned into the popliteal fossa and a short anastomosis constructed to make a T-junction. An attempt to make this anastomosis oblique is likely to result in kinking and obstruction of the graft.

13 Completion angiography is essential. Introduce a small umbilical catheter into the previously preserved proximal tributary. Insert needles into the wound edges at regular intervals approximately 3 cm apart as radio-opaque markers. Obtain the angiogram as described previously (see Completion angiogram).

14 With the aid of the angiogram locate and ligate all residual tributaries. It may be necessary to repeat the angiogram several times. Finally remove the cannula and ligate the last tributary.

? DIFFICULTY

1. The anatomical relationship between the saphenofemoral junction and the common femoral bifurcation may be such that even after mobilization the saphenous vein will not reach the common femoral artery without tension (short vein). Construct the proximal anastomosis to the superficial femoral or profunda arteries. A limited endarterectomy may be required to ensure a satisfactory inflow.
2. On-table angiography shows an intact valve cusp. Use a tributary to re-introduce the valvulotome, or partially take down the distal anastomosis and re-pass the valvulotome. If both of these are technically difficult, a small incision may be made in the graft itself but great care must be taken not to cause any narrowing upon closure.
3. A tributary protected by a valve at its junction with the main vein will not be visualized on intraoperative angiography. If this valve should later become incompetent under arterial pressure a fistula will develop. Involvement of a superficial tributary causes the development of a painful patch of inflammation in the affected skin, which may progress to skin necrosis. The appearance of these changes postoperatively with an associated overlying bruit is an indication to return the patient to theatre for ligation of the offending tributary under local anaesthesia.
4. See also difficulties associated with reversed saphenous vein bypasses.

Non-reversed transposed saphenous vein graft

1 This method combines features of both the reversed and in-situ techniques.

2 The vein is excised completely and re-sited as appropriate in order to bypass an arterial occlusion. However, it is not inverted.

3 The valves are destroyed by passage of a valvulotome as previously described.

Closure

Close the incisions with absorbable sutures in the subcutaneous tissues and subcuticular monocryl, interrupted monofilament non-absorbable sutures, or clips in the skin. Use two layers of subcutaneous sutures to cover the femoral anastomosis and place a suction drain in the groin wound.

Aftercare

1 Note the state of perfusion of the foot and mark the position of palpable or Doppler-audible pulses for the nursing staff.

2 Evidence of deteriorating perfusion and loss of pulses warrants immediate re-exploration and re-assessment of the graft.

3 Keep the knee slightly flexed for 24 hours. Allow the patient out of bed after 48 hours and allow him to take a few steps on the third postoperative day. Some swelling of the leg is almost invariable after a successful reconstruction. Reassure the patient that this will resolve but may take several weeks to do so. In the meantime he will require periods of rest during the day with the leg in elevation. The patient is usually ready for discharge from hospital within 7 days.

4 Enrol all patients on a postoperative vein graft surveillance programme. 20–30% of grafts develop intimal hyperplastic strictures within the first 6–9 months after implantation and these strictures are associated with a three-fold risk of occlusion during the first 12 months. Prophylactic treatment of such strictures, either by open surgery or balloon angioplasty dilatation, improves secondary patency rates by 10–15% at 12 months.[4] The most effective methods for detecting graft-related strictures are duplex ultrasonic scanning and intravenous digital subtraction angiography. However, there is controversy as to whether it is cost-effective to employ this type of imaging systematically. Where vascular laboratory facilities are not readily available undertake careful examination with resting and post-exercise Doppler pressure measurements in order to identify patients for further assessment by duplex ultrasound scanning or conventional angiography. The most dangerous strictures are those that develop early and those that are most severe. Arrange screening tests at 6 weeks, 3 months, 6 months and 9 months after the operation. Strictures that require treatment are:

- Those that occur at the first screening interval.
- Those causing a stenosis equivalent to a two-thirds reduction on the cross-sectional area of the graft.
- Those that show evidence of progression.

Treat short strictures in the body of the graft or at the distal anastomosis by balloon angioplasty dilatation. For maximum effect, higher than normal inflation pressures may be required (up to 20 atmospheres). Treat strictures over 1 cm in length and those at the proximal anastomosis by patch angioplasty, interposition grafting or jump grafting.

5 Except where specifically contraindicated, all patients should receive regular daily low-dose aspirin or clopidogrel as an antithrombotic agent and all patients should be prescribed a statin in a dose of 40 mg daily.

REFERENCES

1. Beard JD, Scott DJ, Evans JM et al 1988 Pulse generated run-off, a new method of determining calf vessel patency. British Journal of Surgery 75:361–363
2. Harris PL, Jones D, How T 1987 A prospective randomised clinical trial to compare in-situ and reversed vein grafts for femoro-popliteal by-pass. British Journal of Surgery 74:252–255
3. Hall KV 1962 The great saphenous vein used in-situ as an arterial shunt after extirpation of the vein valves. Surgery 51:492–495
4. Leather RP, Powers SR, Karmody AM 1979 A re-appraisal of the in-situ saphenous vein arterial bypass. Its use in limb salvage. Surgery 86:453–461

FEMOROPOPLITEAL AND INFRAPOPLITEAL BYPASS WITH PROSTHETIC GRAFT

Appraise

- The best prosthetic grafts perform almost as well as saphenous vein grafts when anastomosed to the popliteal artery above the knee. However, below the knee they are not nearly as effective as vein grafts and, if the distal anastomosis is to a single tibial or peroneal artery, patency rates at 2 years of approximately half that of veins are to be expected.

- Prosthetic grafts may be considered as a reasonable alternative to autologous vein grafts for above-knee femoropopliteal bypass but their use below the knee is justifiable only if there is no autologous vein available and must be strictly limited to those patients in whom the alternative to reconstruction is a major limb amputation.
- *Inflow.* See Saphenous vein bypass.
- *Outflow.* One reason why prosthetic grafts perform less well than autologous vein grafts is that they require a higher velocity of blood flow through them to prevent blood clot forming on the flow surface. (They have a higher thrombotic threshold velocity.) A restricted outflow tract is therefore less well tolerated. It is possible at operation to calculate the resistance of the peripheral circulation from measurements of the pressure and volume flow of heparinized blood infused at a constant rate into a catheter inserted into the recipient artery. When the peripheral resistance is very high, early graft occlusion is inevitable. In these circumstances primary amputation is clearly the better option. Attempts have been made to overcome the problem by creating an adjuvant arteriovenous fistula at or close to the distal anastomosis, thereby augmenting the run-off, but clinical trials indicate that this manoeuvre does not have sufficient value to justify its routine use.[1]

  A second problem with prosthetic grafts is that platelets react with the alien flow surface. This causes them to adhere, particularly at the distal anastomosis, restricting the outflow further either by initiating thrombosis formation or by the later development of subintimal hyperplasia. The unnatural end-to-side configuration of the anastomosis itself probably also contributes by causing excessive flow disturbance. In order to try to overcome this problem the distal anastomosis has been modified by means of vein patches or cuffs.[2,3] These adjuvant techniques are of proven benefit in terms of short- and long-term graft patency. A recent innovation is the development of PTFE grafts that incorporate a cuff-shaped end for anastomosis to the distal vessel (see Special equipment, grafts).[4]
- *Conduit.* Use an externally supported PTFE graft.

Prepare

1. Commence antiplatelet therapy at least 48 hours before operation. Aspirin in a dose of 75 or 150 mg daily is effective. Clopidogrel is also a very effective antiplatelet agent but some surgeons believe it increases perioperative bleeding significantly. There is no consensus on the issue of whether clopidogrel should be discontinued before operation in patients who are taking it already. However, most agree about the role of low-dose aspirin.
2. Give prophylactic antibiotic cover by administration of a broad-spectrum agent at the time of induction of anaesthesia.
3. For positioning of the patient and preparation of the limb see Femoropopliteal saphenous vein bypass.

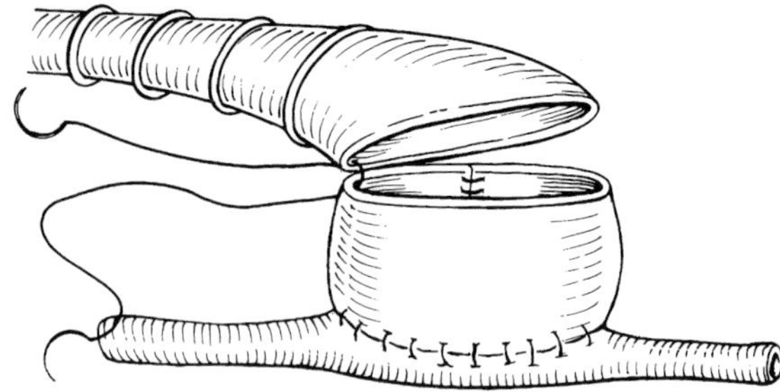

Fig. 29.26 The Miller cuff.

Action

1. Expose the common femoral artery and distal recipient vessel as previously described.
2. Select a graft of either 6 mm or 5 mm internal diameter and, using a long tunnelling instrument, pass it between the two incisions (see Reversed saphenous vein graft).
3. Give heparin and allow 3 minutes for it to circulate before the application of arterial clamps.
4. Construct end-to-side anastomoses to the common femoral and popliteal or tibial arteries using 5/0 and 6/0 sutures respectively. If a PTFE graft has been chosen, use PTFE sutures.
5. If it has been decided to incorporate an interposition vein cuff at the distal anastomosis use the following technique:

   Miller cuff (Fig. 29.26).[2] Obtain a 3-cm length of autologous vein; the distal end of the saphenous vein from the ankle is suitable. Open the vein longitudinally to make a flat strip. Make an arteriotomy 1 cm in length, and suture the strip of vein to the edges of the arteriotomy using 7/0 polypropylene (Prolene) sutures for a tibial artery or 6/0 polypropylene for the popliteal artery. Commence the stitch in the middle of one side and suture the vein to the whole circumference of the arteriotomy. Then trim the excess of the vein strip away and complete the cuff by suturing the free edges together. Finally trim the graft to match the size of the vein cuff and construct an oblique end-to-end anastomosis with a continuous 6/0 PTFE suture.
6. If a precuffed PTFE graft is used it is essential not to trim or adjust the shaped end of the graft in any way. Match the length of the arteriotomy to that of the 'cuff' and not vice versa. Therefore, make an arteriotomy that is slightly shorter than the cuff. Begin suturing at the heel and continue along each side of the anastomosis. Then extend the arteriotomy so that it matches, exactly, the length of the cuff. Finally, complete the anastomosis by suturing around the toe with one needle. Be sure to tie the suture to one side or the other of the toe. Note that when using a precuffed graft it is essential to perform the distal anastomosis before the proximal anastomosis and to draw the graft from the distal to the proximal wound during the tunnelling procedure.

? DIFFICULTY

Note that all anastomoses to tibial arteries must be technically immaculate. Use umbilical catheters of suitable size as stents and fine suture material. Magnification is essential (see General principles).

Closure

Close the wounds in layers with drainage as for saphenous vein bypass.

Aftercare

1 Detailed observation of peripheral perfusion and distal pulses, as for saphenous vein grafts.

2 Continue heparin anticoagulation for 5 days. Maintain aspirin antiplatelet therapy throughout and continue indefinitely. Following this type of bypass, long-term anticoagulation with warfarin, in addition to antiplatelet therapy, is advisable for most patients.

Complications

1 *Early thrombotic occlusion.* In the event of early thrombosis of the graft, return the patient to theatre immediately for thrombectomy and careful reappraisal. If there are no technical faults, consider the addition of an arteriovenous shunt at the distal anastomosis in order to enhance run-off (Fig. 29.27). (This is appropriate only for tibial and peroneal grafts.)

KEY POINT Decision-making

- Avoid repeated over-zealous re-exploration of grafts that are doomed to failure; early amputation is better for the patient.

2 Late occlusion of a prosthetic graft warrants a new angiogram and careful reappraisal. It is often due to subintimal hyperplasia at or close to the distal anastomosis.

The options are:

- Thrombolysis of the graft and dilatation of the outflow tract by balloon angioplasty
- Operative thrombectomy with patch angioplasty or a jump graft at the distal anastomosis
- A combination of thrombolysis and surgical treatment.

Although PTFE grafts can usually be re-opened it is sometimes preferable to replace the whole graft, particularly when it has been occluded for more than 3 weeks.

3 In common with other prosthetic grafts there is a risk of infection (see Aortobifemoral bypass).

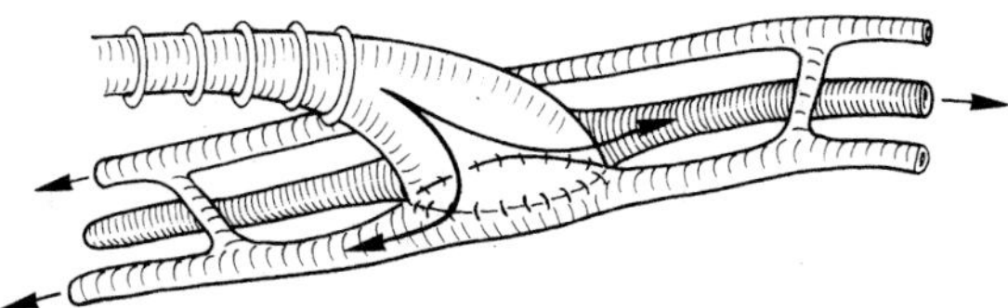

Fig. 29.27 An adjuvant arteriovenous fistula at the distal anastomosis.

PERCUTANEOUS BALLOON ANGIOPLASTY DILATATION FOR FEMOROPOPLITEAL OCCLUSIVE ARTERIAL DISEASE

Appraise

- There is a high failure and recurrence rate associated with the treatment of femoropopliteal occlusions over 10 cm in length. Therefore treat only lesions shorter than this.
- Good results have been claimed following treatment of long femoral lesions using a deliberate subintimal technique.[5] But application of this approach should be left to those with special skills and training.
- Lesions of the common femoral artery, the distal external iliac artery or proximal superficial femoral artery are usually best treated surgically but can be approached by a balloon catheter advanced from the opposite groin over the aortic bifurcation.

Prepare, action and aftercare

See Basic techniques.

Complications

1 Arterial rupture and acute thrombosis require urgent surgical repair under general anaesthesia.

2 Expanding groin haematoma also requires surgical repair but can usually be managed under local anaesthesia.

3 Be aware of the possibility of retroperitoneal haemorrhage if the patient shows signs of hypovolaemia without obvious blood loss. This is most likely to occur if arterial puncture was made proximal to the inguinal ligament. Urgent resuscitation followed by surgical repair under general anaesthesia is required.

4 Occasionally, a false aneurysm develops at the puncture site. In the first place, attempt treatment by manual compression using duplex ultrasound scanning to localize the communication with the arterial lumen. It may be necessary to apply pressure for 30 minutes or more but this technique is usually successful even when applied some weeks after the procedure. Alternatively, undertake open repair under local or general anaesthesia.

5 Stents in the superficial femoral artery tend to cause excessive myointimal hyperplasia and are rarely successful in the long term. Therefore they should not normally be used in this situation.

REFERENCES

1. Hamsho A, Nott D, Harris PL 1999. Prospective randomised trial of distal arteriovenous fistula as an adjunct to femoro-infrapopliteal PTFE bypass. European Journal of Vascular and Endovascular Surgery 17:197–201
2. Miller JH, Foreman RK, Ferguson L et al 1984 Interposition vein cuff for anastomosis of prosthesis to small artery. Australian and New Zealand Journal of Surgery 54:283–286
3. Taylor RS, MacFarland RJ, Cox MI 1987 An investigation into the causes of failure of PTFE grafts. European Journal of Vascular Surgery 1:335–345
4. Brennan JA, Enzler MA, da Silva A et al 1996 New graft design to inhibit myointimal hyperplasia in small vessel anastomoses. British Journal of Surgery 83:1383–1384

5. Bolia A, Fishwick G 1997 Recanalisation of iliac artery occlusion by subintimal dissection using the ipsilateral and the contralateral approach. Clinical Radiology 5:684–687

REPAIR OF ABDOMINAL AORTIC ANEURYSM

Appraise

- The abdominal aorta is the commonest site for aneurysms. These are dangerous lesions, death being the likely outcome in the event of rupture. The rate of growth and the risk of rupture increase exponentially with the diameter of the aneurysm, with a watershed level for serious risk at about 5.5 cm. Therefore, unless the patient is gravely ill from other causes, any aneurysm wider than 5.5 cm should be operated upon electively. The UK Small Aneurysm Trial showed that for smaller aneurysms conservative management with regular surveillance by ultrasound is preferable to operation.[1]
- With improvements in anaesthetic management and progressive modification of surgical technique the mortality rate associated with elective aneurysm surgery is less than 5% in the best centres. In the UK Small Aneurysm Trial the in-hospital mortality rate was 5.8%.

  The important surgical principles are:
  - Minimal dissection.
  - Inlay technique of anastomosis.
  - Use of straight rather than bifurcated grafts whenever possible.
- Emergency operation is indicated for a patient with an aneurysm who develops severe abdominal or back pain with or without circulatory collapse, unless he is already moribund. The mortality risk associated with emergency aneurysm surgery is between 30% and 60%. The overall risk of death from a ruptured aneurysm is, however, more than 90%, since 75% of patients die without reaching hospital.

Prepare

1. Confirm the diagnosis by ultrasound scanning. Computed tomography (CT) and nuclear magnetic resonance imaging give more detailed information if there is a suspicion of visceral artery involvement or perianeurysmal fibrosis (inflammatory aneurysm). CT scanning is essential in order to make precise anatomical measurements if endovascular repair is being considered (see below, Endovascular repair of abdominal aortic aneurysm) and calibrated angiography may provide additional important information. These tests are not necessary if open repair is the only option under consideration.
2. Detailed assessment of cardiac risk is essential before elective operation (see Aortobifemoral bypass).
3. Preoperative assessment of respiratory and renal function is also required.
4. For elective cases the patient is fully anaesthetized with total muscular relaxation. Arterial, central venous or pulmonary artery (Swan–Ganz) catheters are sited and a urinary catheter is positioned in the bladder. The patient lies supine on the operating table with both arms abducted on arm boards. The entire area from the nipples to mid-thigh is prepared. A small towel is placed over the genitalia and an adhesive drape is applied so as to allow access to the whole of the abdomen and both inguinal regions.
5. For emergency cases, all essential vascular access lines and the urinary catheter are inserted, and the abdomen is prepared and draped prior to the induction of anaesthesia. The administration of a muscle relaxant may release tamponade of a retroperitoneal haematoma, with re-bleeding and catastrophic circulatory collapse. Therefore the anaesthetist must not commence anaesthesia until you indicate that you are ready to proceed. While preoperative preparations are being made, maintain the blood pressure at a low level; a systolic pressure of 60 to 80 mmHg is ideal. 'Permissive' hypotension reduces the risk of sudden catastrophic haemorrhage. Good venous access lines are essential at an early stage. But, except in dire emergency, do not infuse fluid to augment the blood pressure until an aortic clamp has been applied.
6. Give, by injection, a broad-spectrum antibiotic with induction of anaesthesia as prophylaxis against graft infection.

Access

1. Make a midline incision extending from the xiphisternum to the pubis, skirting the umbilicus.
2. Check the abdominal contents to exclude the presence of some other condition, such as malignant disease, which might alter the decision to operate on the aneurysm. Note the presence of gallstones or peptic ulcer for future reference only.
3. Displace the omentum and large bowel superiorly and the small bowel with its mesentery to the right. Cover with large moist abdominal packs and retain in place with the blades of a fixed self-retaining retractor system (Omnitract; Fig. 29.28).
4. The duodenum lies across the upper part of the aneurysm and must be displaced. To do this, make an incision in the parietal peritoneum to the left of the duodenum, which is then mobilized upwards and to the right. This completed, place deep narrow retractor blades on each side of the aorta, to expose the neck of the aneurysm and the renal vein crossing it.
5. Continue the incision of the peritoneum longitudinally over the surface of the aneurysm, passing to the right of the inferior mesenteric artery and across the bifurcation.
6. Position additional packs and retractor blades to expose the whole aneurysm and both common iliac arteries (Fig. 29.28). Identify and protect the ureters on each side as they cross the iliac vessels.
7. In the case of an emergency operation for rupture, try to avoid 'crash-clamping' of the aorta without first mobilizing the duodenum and identifying the renal vein. If there is no free bleeding, proceed calmly with the first steps as described above. The presence of a haematoma distorts the anatomy and it is essential to dissect a plane close to the wall of the aorta. Once the neck of the aneurysm has been identified, carefully make a space on each side to accommodate the jaws of a straight clamp and apply this immediately from the front (Fig. 29.29). Then proceed with the remainder of the dissection. If there is free bleeding obtain control initially by manual pressure against the vertebral column while an assistant packs away and retracts the abdominal con-

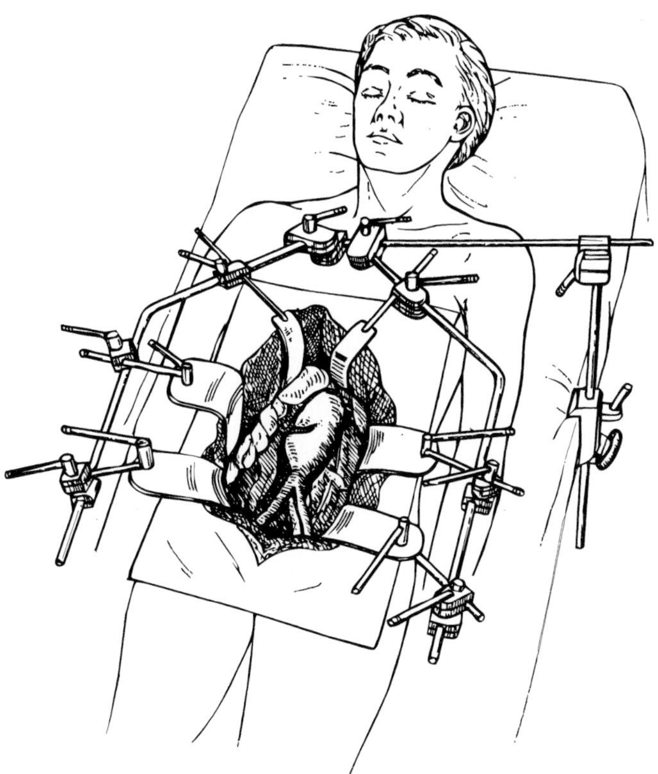

Fig. 29.28 Exposure of the abdominal aorta for resection of an aneurysm.

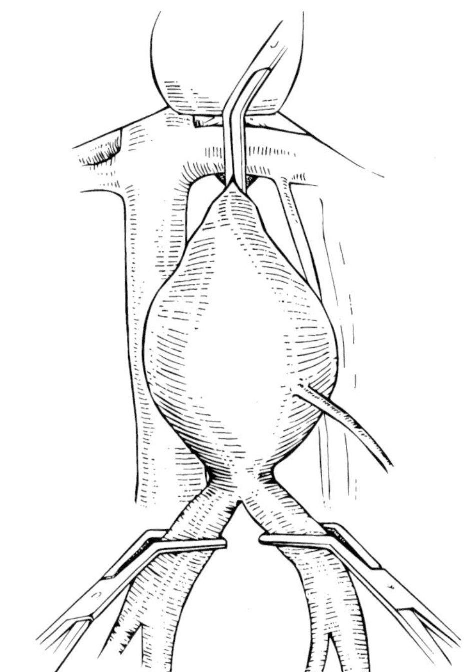

Fig. 29.29 Application of clamps.

tents. In extreme difficulties either apply a clamp at the level of the diaphragm after opening the lesser omentum and splitting the muscular fibres of the crus or use a balloon-occlusion catheter inserted through an incision in the aneurysm itself.

Assess

1 Confirm the position of the neck of the aneurysm relative to the renal arteries; 95% of aneurysms are infrarenal. The minority of aneurysms that involve the visceral arteries, and particularly those extending into the chest, require much more complex and dangerous surgery. Most of these can be diagnosed preoperatively and should be referred to a specialized unit for further assessment and treatment.

2 The left renal vein, which crosses above the neck of most aneurysms can, if necessary, be divided in order to improve access. This should be done well over to the right in order to preserve outflow from the kidney via the adrenal and gonadal veins. Even so, it has been demonstrated that renal function is affected adversely and the vein should therefore be preserved whenever possible.

3 Assess the aortic bifurcation and the iliac arteries. A minor degree of ectasia of the iliac arteries can be accepted and it should be possible to use a straight graft in 60–70% of patients. A bifurcated graft is required if the common iliac ostia have been separated by the aneurysm or if one or both of the iliac arteries are grossly aneurysmal. Occasionally, very severe calcification at the aortic bifurcation makes suturing at this site impossible.

4 Assess the inferior mesenteric artery. Usually it is totally occluded. However, if it is widely patent it is advisable to observe the effect of temporary clamping of this vessel on the bowel circulation before it is finally sacrificed. Ligate it close to the aorta or suture the ostium from within the sac in order to preserve its connections with the superior mesenteric artery via its ascending colic branch.

5 Decide whether to use a straight or bifurcated graft and of what size. Use a low-porosity graft to minimize blood loss and obviate the need for preclotting. Presealed grafts are ideal for this purpose; otherwise use a woven graft.

Action

1 No attempt should be made to encircle either the aorta or the iliac arteries. To do so risks trauma to veins with serious venous bleeding.

2 Carefully dissect a narrow space on each side of the aorta and of both common iliac arteries to permit access for the jaws of straight or slightly angled clamps applied from the front.

3 In elective cases only give heparin intravenously and allow 3 minutes for it to circulate before closing the clamps. Apply only sufficient pressure to occlude blood flow and no more (Fig. 29.29).

4 Open the aneurysm longitudinally and scoop out the laminated thrombus, degenerate atheromatous material and liquid blood it contains. These contents sometimes bear an alarming resemblance to pus. Most aneurysms are in fact sterile but about 10% yield a growth of organisms on culture.

KEY POINT

- Infection? Always send a specimen to the laboratory for microbiological analysis.

5 Control back-bleeding from patent lumbar and median sacral arteries with figure-of-eight sutures of 3/0 polypropylene (Prolene) applied from inside the sac. Insertion of a Travers retractor to hold open the sac is often useful in order to display the ostia of the lumbar arteries and subsequently to facilitate the anastomoses (Fig. 29.30).

6 Infuse 60 ml of heparinized saline into each leg via a catheter inserted temporarily into the common iliac arteries to reduce the risk of intravascular thrombosis during clamping.

7 If a bifurcated graft is to be used, remember to trim it to leave only 3–4 cm of the main trunk above the bifurcation (see Aortobifemoral bypass.).

8 Using 3/0 polypropylene (Prolene) sutures, construct an end-to-end anastomosis to the proximal aorta. This is done from within the sac by the inlay technique (Fig. 29.31). Start suturing, with the parachute technique, to one side of the midline at the back of the graft (see Basic techniques) Stitch from graft to aorta and take large bites to include all layers of the aortic wall each time. Finish in the midline anteriorly.

9 Apply a soft clamp to the graft and gently release the aortic clamp to test the anastomosis. Place additional sutures as required.

10 If a straight tube is to be used, construct a similar anastomosis at the aortic bifurcation.

11 If a bifurcated graft is necessary it may be possible to construct an end-to-end anastomosis by the inlay technique to the iliac bifurcation on both sides. Alternatively, transect the iliac arteries and construct a standard end-to-end anastomosis or pass the limbs of the graft through tunnels to the groin for end-to-end anastomosis to the common femoral arteries (see Aortobifemoral bypass). Try to ensure that one of the internal iliac arteries is perfused orthogradely if at all possible.

12 Before completion of the distal anastomosis flush the graft to eliminate any blood clots and also to ensure that the recipient vessels bleed back satisfactorily. If this is not the case pass embolectomy catheters to retrieve any distal blood clots.

13 Give the anaesthetist several minutes warning before releasing the clamps and re-perfuse one leg at a time in order to minimize the risk of declamping shock. In the case of a bifurcation graft the anastomosis on one side may be completed and this limb perfused before the second anastomosis is constructed. A slight fall in blood pressure on release of a clamp is reassuring evidence that the limb is in fact being adequately perfused.

14 Having made quite certain that all anastomoses are blood-tight and that there is no bleeding from any other source, fold the redundant aneurysm sac over the graft and fix it with a number of synthetic absorbable sutures. Make sure that the graft is covered completely.

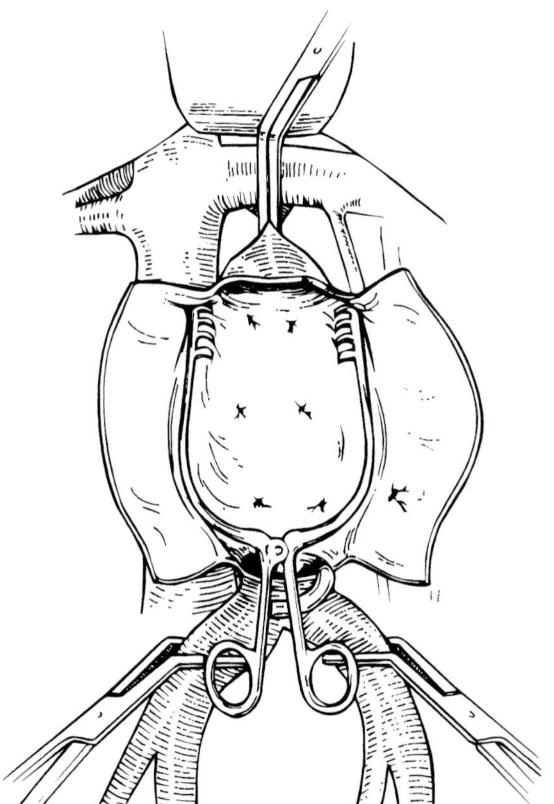

Fig. 29.30 Use of a Travers retractor to display the interior of the aneurysm sac.

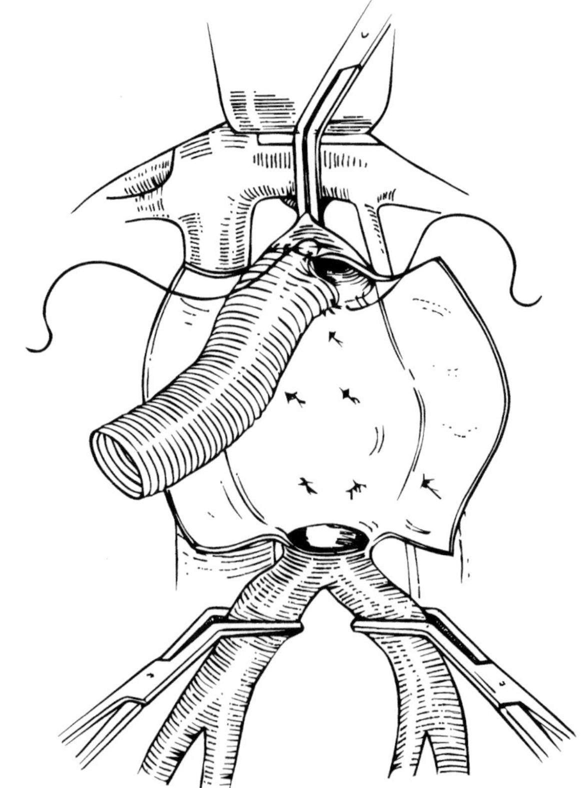

Fig. 29.31 The inlay technique of anastomosis.

? DIFFICULTY

1. If there is difficulty in obtaining control of bleeding from a ruptured aneurysm, see Access.
2. *The left renal vein is torn during application of the clamp.* If possible, repair the vein with 4/0 or 5/0 non-absorbable sutures. The vein may, if necessary, be ligated and divided (see Access). Bleeding from the region of the gonadal or adrenal vein is best controlled by packing in the first place, and sometimes this will be sufficient. If not, apply stitches later.
3. A tear of the iliac veins can produce torrential venous bleeding, the source of which is difficult to identify. If this defect cannot quickly be repaired with sutures, apply local packing and pressure and attend to something else for a while. It may stop spontaneously or be more easily controlled later. Use sutures buttressed with Dacron pledgets.
4. *The neck of the aorta is ectatic and its wall papery thin.* It is usually possible to crimp a large aorta into a smaller graft by the inlay technique of anastomosis and often this is preferable to extending the operation into the suprarenal aorta. If the aorta will not hold stitches, which therefore cut out or tear, it is necessary to transect the aorta and construct an end-to-end anastomosis with a circumferential Dacron buttress and Dacron oversleeve (see Aortobifemoral bypass).
5. If suturing is impeded by calcification in the wall of the vessels, see Aortobifemoral bypass.
6. *The bowel appears ischaemic on completion of the operation.* Re-implant the inferior mesenteric artery.
7. *Venous bleeding occurs from inside the aneurysm on opening the sac.* This signifies an aortocaval fistula. Close the defect from inside the sac with large sutures. If torrential venous bleeding is encountered, secure control first with intraluminal balloon catheters inserted proximally and distally into the cava through the defect.
8. *There is gross perianeurysmal fibrosis (inflammatory aneurysm).* This places at risk structures that are adherent to it—especially the duodenum, the left renal vein and the ureters. Continue the dissection with care. It is often possible to find a safe plane within the wall of the aneurysm, which may be up to 1 cm thick (onion-skin technique). However, if it seems dangerous to proceed it may be more prudent to withdraw, close the abdomen and refer the patient to a specialist unit for further assessment. Administration of steroids for several weeks reduces the fibrosis and thereby facilitates surgery but there are recorded instances of rupture of aneurysms occurring in such patients while on steroids.

Closure

1 Close the posterior parietal peritoneum over the sac, making sure that the duodenum and small bowel cannot gain access to the graft or suture lines with a risk of late graft infection or aortoenteric fistula.

2 Close the abdominal incision in layers after an elective operation, but mass closure is often more expedient following emergency surgery for rupture. Drains are not normally required.

Aftercare

1 Following an emergency operation it is a good policy to maintain positive-pressure ventilation for 12–24 hours after operation. This ensures adequate oxygenation of the blood during a period of potential cardiovascular instability and is also considerably more convenient and kinder to the patient if he has to be returned to theatre for any reason.

2 Maintain cardiac monitoring and regular blood gas analysis for a minimum of 5 days.

3 All patients have postoperative ileus and require nasogastric suction and parenteral fluid and electrolyte infusion.

4 Deep venous thrombosis prophylaxis is necessary until full mobility is re-established.

5 After an uncomplicated recovery the patient is ready for discharge from hospital 8–10 days after operation.

Complications

There are six important potential complications to remember.

- *Haemorrhage.* Early re-exploration is mandatory upon the suspicion of continuing internal bleeding. It may be arising from the anastomosis or from other sources such as a torn mesenteric vessel. 'Haematological' bleeding due to heparin or other coagulopathy can be recognized by appropriate blood tests and can usually be promptly corrected with 1 or 2 units of fresh blood, fresh-frozen plasma or platelets.
- *Occlusion.* This results either from embolization of material trapped above the aortic clamp that was not flushed out, from thrombosis in the distal vessels during clamping or from a technical fault at one of the suture lines. Try passing a Fogarty catheter proximally and distally from the groin first, but be prepared to re-explore the graft if this is unsuccessful.
- *Renal tubular necrosis.* This is common following rupture of an aneurysm and is due to prolonged hypotension. It may be part of a multiple organ failure syndrome, in which case the prognosis is very poor. Isolated renal tubular necrosis often recovers, although a period of support by haemodialysis or haemofiltration may be required. Total anuria immediately after operation suggests the possibility of occlusion of both renal arteries. Request immediate aortography to confirm the problem and re-explore the patient with a view to renal artery reconstruction.

- *Adult respiratory distress syndrome (ARDS).* This is unfortunately not uncommon following emergency operations for ruptured aneurysms, particularly if there has been massive blood loss. It usually becomes apparent within 24 hours but can develop more insidiously over a few days. Mechanical ventilatory support with a high concentration of inspired oxygen and positive end-expiratory pressure is often required to maintain adequate blood gases. The prognosis is generally poor, especially if secondary infection follows.
- *Myocardial infarction.* See Aortobifemoral bypass.
- *Graft infection.* See Aortobifemoral bypass.

REFERENCE

1. The UK Small Aneurysm Trial participants 1998 Mortality results of randomised controlled trial for early elective surgery or ultrasound surveillance for small abdominal aortic aneurysms. Lancet 352:1649–1655

REPAIR OF THORACIC AND THORACOABDOMINAL ANEURYSMS

Appraise

- While repair of a localized aneurysm of the descending thoracic aorta is a relatively straightforward operation, extensive thoracoabdominal aneurysms (type 2) represent a formidable challenge to the vascular surgeon. Both of these procedures require vascular and cardiothoracic surgical facilities and expertise and therefore should be confined to a few highly specialized units. It is inappropriate to describe them in detail here but knowledge of the principles involved is important.
- The application of a clamp to the thoracic aorta increases dramatically the afterload on the heart and is likely to precipitate acute left ventricular failure. At the same time the abdominal viscera and the spinal cord are deprived of a blood supply, with a high risk of multiple organ failure and paraplegia.
- Left heart bypass using an external pump obviates both of these problems.
- Perfusion of the spinal cord during clamping of the thoracic aorta is a function of intra-arterial pressure that is reduced and cerebrospinal fluid pressure that increases. Tapping CSF (cerebrospinal fluid) to keep the pressure at a low level (13 cmH_2O) helps to maintain perfusion of the spinal cord and reduces the incidence of paraplegia.
- Surgical repair of extensive thoracoabdominal aneurysms without left heart bypass and CSF tapping carries a risk of death and paraplegia both in the order of 20%. With the application of these measures the risks may be reduced by half.

Prepare

1. Computed angiography and conventional angiography are required to build up a precise picture of the extent of the lesion preoperatively.
2. Obtain also detailed information about preoperative cardiac, pulmonary and renal function.
3. Following the administration of general anaesthesia a double lumen endotracheal tube is inserted by the anaesthetist and arterial, venous and Swan–Ganz lines are established. Catheterize the bladder.
4. Insert a cannula into the spinal canal at lower thoracic level and connect it to a reservoir the height of which can be adjusted to maintain CSF pressure at the desired level.
5. The patient must be positioned on the table to permit both left thoracotomy and exposure of the abdominal aorta. Support the chest in a left lateral position but rotate the pelvis forward so that the trunk is twisted slightly.
6. Prepare and drape the whole of the chest, abdomen and both groins.

Access

1. For thoracic aneurysms make an incision over the fifth intercostal space. For thoracoabdominal aneurysms make an incision over the sixth or seventh space and extend it across the costal margin to the midline of the abdomen and then inferiorly to the pubis. Divide the diaphragm around its margin to permit the wound to be opened widely with a rib retractor. Do not split the diaphragm into the aortic hiatus. Reflect the spleen, pancreas and left colon to the right to expose the abdominal aorta. The kidney and suprarenal gland may also be reflected or left in situ.
2. Expose the left common femoral artery for access of the arterial line from the extracorporeal pump.

Assess

1. Confirm the extent of the aneurysm and decide upon the site of the anastomoses and clamps.
2. Expose the left pulmonary vein at the hilum of the lung in preparation for insertion of a venous cannula for the extracorporeal circulation.

Action

1. When all dissection has been completed administer heparin to achieve full anticoagulation.
2. Establish left heart bypass (left atrium to left common femoral artery).
3. Apply clamps. In the case of extensive aneurysms isolate the proximal site of anastomosis with clamps in the first place in order to maintain uninterrupted perfusion of the viscera for as long as possible.
4. Open the aneurysm, extract the thrombus and assess the intercostal arteries.

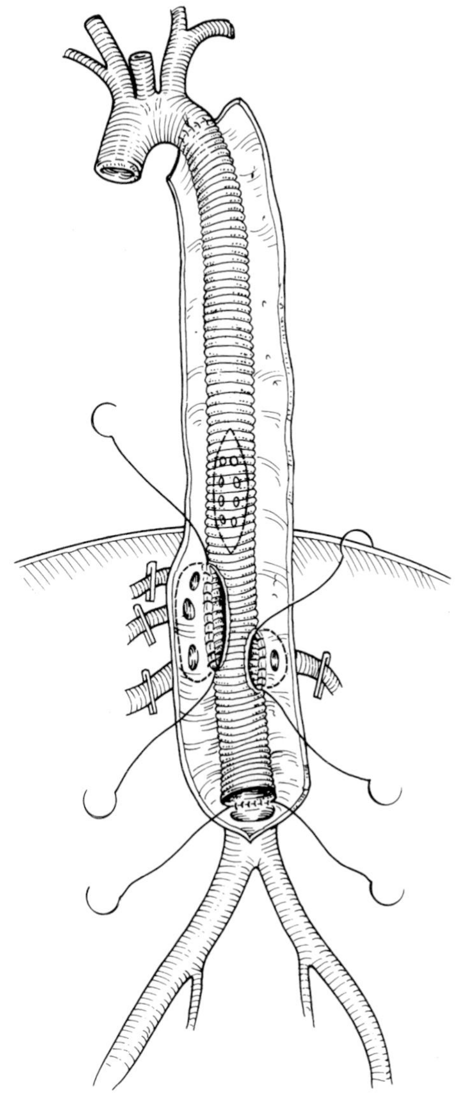

Fig. 29.32 Inlay technique for repair of thoracoabdominal aortic aneurysm.

5 The artery of Adamkewicz that supplies the spinal cord usually arises from one of the intercostal arteries between D8 and D12 level. Widely patent intercostal arteries at this level should be preserved and reimplanted into the graft within a patch of aorta. Smaller intercostal arteries at other levels may be oversewn.

6 Select a graft (usually 28 or 30 mm but may be even larger) and complete the proximal anastomosis with 3/0 polypropylene by an end-to-end inlay technique (Fig. 29.32).

7 Apply a clamp to the graft and check the anastomosis for leaks.

8 Pass the distal end of the graft through the aortic hiatus in the diaphragm.

9 After applying distal clamps, open the remainder of the aneurysm and verify the position of the visceral arteries. Implant these and the intercostals, if patent, using aortic patches. Usually it is possible to include the coeliac axis, superior mesenteric and right renal arteries in one patch, leaving the left renal to be implanted separately. Note that it is not necessary to apply clamps to the visceral arteries which back-bleed very little when the thoracic aorta is clamped. Neither is it necessary to perfuse these arteries with cold saline or other solutions because with left heart bypass the ischaemia time should not exceed 40 minutes.

As an alternative to constructing an aortic patch bearing the abdominal visceral arteries, use a graft incorporating branches of each of the visceral arteries (Coselli). This obviates the risk of subsequent aneurysmal dilatation of the patch.

10 Finally complete the distal aortic or iliac anastomoses and release the clamps.

11 When satisfactory haemostasis has been achieved discontinue left heart bypass, remove the cannulas, repair the access vessels and reverse the heparin.

12 Close the aneurysm sac over the graft.

13 Close the wound in layers taking care to repair the diaphragm. Drain both the chest, via an under-water seal, and the abdomen.

Aftercare

1 Maintain ventilation for 12 hours or until indices indicate that independent ventilation will be possible.

2 Maintain spinal fluid tapping for 3 days.

3 Remove chest and abdominal drains when drainage has ceased.

Complications

1 Haemorrhage, anuria, adult respiratory distress syndrome, myocardial infarction. See Repair of abdominal aortic aneurysm.

2 Paraplegia. Ensure that CSF pressure is optimized. Infarction of the spinal cord is irreversible. Therefore rehabilitation with morale and physical support is the essential and only appropriate response to established paraplegia.

ENDOVASCULAR REPAIR OF ABDOMINAL AORTIC ANEURYSM

Appraise

- The first reported operation to repair an abdominal aortic aneurysm by endovascular deployment of a stent/graft combination within the aneurysm sac was undertaken by Parodi in 1990.[1] Since then the technology of endovascular stent/grafts has evolved rapidly and there are now a large number to choose from.

- Endovascular aneurysm repair has the attributes of a minimally invasive operation. The procedure itself carries a very low risk and the recovery time is much shorter than that associated with conventional open operation. The main drawback of this approach at the present time is that the durability of non-sutured anastomoses and of the stent/grafts themselves is, as yet, unproven.
- For 'fixation' the endograft relies upon a stent with or without hooks or barbs attached, and for 'seal' to exclude the aneurysm sac from the circulation it relies upon firm contact between the fabric of the graft and the vessel wall at each end. These functions demand the existence a 'neck' of at least 15 mm in length between the lowest renal artery and the start of the aneurysm and adequate distal 'landing zones'.
- It is essential to match the size of the endograft to that of the vessels within which it is to be implanted. Over-sizing of the diameter of the stent/graft relative to that of the arteries, in the order of 10–20%, is necessary to ensure adequate fixation and seal. Devices with a diameter at the proximal end up to 36 mm are available.
- The length of the device is critical also. It is permissible to cross the renal arteries with an uncovered stent but in order to achieve an effective seal it is necessary to position the top of the covered part of the stent immediately below the renal arteries without overlapping their ostia. Distally it is permissible to cross one but not both internal iliac arteries.
- Access for the device is via the common femoral artery and it is essential that the iliac arteries can permit the passage of the introducer systems, which vary from 16F to 26F in size. Stenosed, tortuous and especially heavily calcified iliacs may contraindicate this approach although technical resolution of these problems is often possible.
- Bifurcated endografts are to be preferred to tubes. They include one-piece or modular designs, which are assembled in situ during the operative procedure.
- Aneurysms of the descending thoracic aorta can also be repaired successfully by straight endografts introduced from the groin or via the abdominal aorta or an infrarenal aortic graft. The risk of operative complications, including paraplegia and death, appears to be much lower than that associated with open repair.
- Evolving technologies include fenestrated and branched endografts to permit endovascular repair of aneurysms with a very short or no infrarenal neck. These grafts are designed to be deployed across the visceral arteries, perfusion of the organs being maintained via the fenestrations or branches. In the future they may be used also to treat complex thoracic and thoracoabdominal aneurysms. Because they are not yet available for clinical use except in a few investigational centres they will not be described here in any further detail.

Prepare

1. The clinical indications for endovascular repair are similar to those for open repair (see above). However, some patients who are unfit for the open operation may be able to tolerate the less-invasive endovascular procedure.
2. For accurate measurements of the aneurysm and adjacent arteries and assessment of the access route obtain CT scans in a dynamic format which can be viewed on a work station. Angiograms with an intraluminal measuring catheter in situ (calibrated angiogram) may provide useful additional information, but modern dynamic CT angiography obviates the need for this invasive test in all but a few patients. Be sure that the minimal anatomical criteria, as defined by the device manufacturer, are satisfied.
3. Preoperative assessments of cardiac, respiratory and renal function are required as for open aneurysm repair (see above).
4. General anaesthesia is to be preferred. If regional anaesthesia is used, facilities for general anaesthesia must be immediately available in case conversion to open repair becomes necessary.
5. Place the patient supine upon a radiolucent operating table and prepare as for open aneurysm repair, including the administration of a broad-spectrum antibiotic on induction of anaesthesia (see above). Pulmonary artery catheterization is not necessary as a routine for endovascular procedures.
6. Position the X-ray tube, fluoroscopy screens and angiography injector pump. It is especially important to ensure that those performing the operation have unobstructed sight of the screens, which must be directly in front of them to avoid any errors due to parallax. Place a long instrument table with sterile cover at the foot of the operating table to accommodate the guide-wires, catheters and introducer system.

Access

1. For endovascular repair with a bifurcated endograft, access to both common femoral arteries is required. Although percutaneous access is possible with some types of device the benefit is marginal and it is recommended that the common femoral arteries are exposed on both sides. Because the exposure required is limited, use short transverse incisions placed one finger's breadth above the groin crease and directly over the femoral pulse, rather than a classical vertical incision. It is not essential to dissect the profunda femoris artery Apply Silastic loops to the common femoral artery.
2. The choice of side of access for the body and ipsilateral limb of the device is dependent upon the anatomical configuration and distribution of disease in the iliac arteries and the direction of any angulation of the neck of the aneurysm.
3. Having exposed the common femoral arteries give heparin 5000 IU intravenously.
4. Through the contralateral common femoral artery position a pigtail angiography catheter within the aorta just above the

expected level of the renal arteries (see above, Basic techniques, for steps required). Obtain an angiogram to determine precisely the position of the renal arteries relative to bone structures or a radio-opaque measuring scale placed under the patient.

5 Via the ipsilateral side pass first an angiography catheter over a standard 0.35-mm guide-wire into the suprarenal aorta. Through this catheter exchange the standard guide-wire for a long, super-stiff guide-wire (Amplatz or Schnieder). Remove the catheter and introducer sheath and apply clamps to the artery over the guide-wire or arrest blood flow by snugging the Silastic loops. Make a short transverse arteriotomy in the common femoral artery at the point of entry of the guide-wire. This step is not necessary for some endograft systems that incorporate a long tapering vessel-wall dilator, which can be introduced directly.

6 Under fluoroscopic control introduce the introducer sheath for the endograft over the super-stiff wire and advance it through the aneurysm into the suprarenal aorta.

7 Manoeuvre the X-ray tube to ensure that the origin of the renal arteries is in the centre of the image as viewed on the screen. Especially when the aneurysm is large, the neck including that part of the aorta that gives rise to the origins of the renal arteries tends to be angulated forwards and sometimes laterally as it enters the sac. When this is noted on preoperative CT scans, measure the angles and position the X-ray tube with the same degree of craniocaudal and/or lateral tilt. This step is essential to avoid error when positioning the stent/graft. Lock the X-ray tube securely in position.

8 Via the angiography catheter on the contralateral side obtain an angiogram and mark the position of the lowest renal artery on the screen with a marker pen.

9 Carefully adjust the position of the endograft within its introducer sheath so that the upper margin of the fabric of the graft is aligned with the lower border of the lowest renal artery.

10 Under fluoroscopic control deploy the body of the graft according to the procedure specified by the manufacturer. Usually, fine adjustment of the position of the device is possible after deployment of the upper one or two rows of the stent and another angiogram may be obtained at this stage. However, remember to withdraw the angiography catheter into the sac of the aneurysm before deploying the device fully. Following complete deployment of the body of the device and the ipsilateral limb it is recommended for most devices that gentle pressure is applied on the inside of the graft with a soft Silastic balloon that is incorporated in the system for this purpose. It presses the stent against the wall of the neck of the aneurysm and smoothes out any wrinkles that may be present in the fabric.

11 Obtain an angiogram at this stage to ascertain that the internal iliac artery on the access side has not been crossed and occluded by the fabric of the graft. If this has occurred special care must be taken not to cross the internal iliac artery on the other side when deploying the second limb.

12 Withdraw the sheath from the common femoral artery and, after closing the arteriotomy with interrupted 5/0 polypropylene sutures around the guide-wire, remove the clamps to allow blood flow into the limb.

13 It is now necessary to pass a guide-wire into the short leg on the body of the graft from the opposite groin. Radio-opaque markers are located at strategic points on the device for guidance. Withdraw the angiography catheter from the sheath in the common femoral artery and replace it with a catheter with a shaped end (e.g. cobra) or multipurpose-angled to assist manipulation of the wire into the limb under fluoroscopic control.

14 Check that the guide-wire has been advanced into the lumen of the device by (a) passing a pigtail catheter over the wire and observing that it can be rotated within the device without catching or deforming, and (b) inflating an angiography balloon catheter passed over the wire with dilute contrast medium and observing that it is within the bounds of the metal stent when imaged in both anteroposterior and lateral planes.

15 Exchange the standard 0.35-mm guide-wire for a super-stiff wire advanced well above the renal arteries.

16 Advance the second limb within its introducer system over the super-stiff wire and position it within the short limb on the body of the device under fluoroscopic control using, as a guide, the radio-opaque markers provided for this purpose. When you are satisfied with the position deploy the second limb in accordance with the manufacturer's instructions.

17 It is important to 'cover' the whole of the common iliac artery with the stent/graft if possible and this requires that the intraluminal device is positioned accurately so that the fabric terminates just proximal to the iliac bifurcation. To achieve the necessary precision, insert an angiography catheter and the endograft introducer system through separate puncture sites in the 'contralateral' common femoral artery (opposite side to that through which the main body of the endograft is to be introduced) . Use this catheter to obtain images, and mark the position, of the orifices of the internal iliac arteries prior to deployment of the modular limbs. Modern modular stent grafts are provided with a choice of limbs of different lengths and diameters.

18 Use a Silastic balloon matched to gently mould it and eliminate any wrinkles in the cloth.

19 The basic procedure is now completed (Fig. 29.33) but it is essential to obtain a completion angiogram to ascertain that the position of the device is satisfactory and especially to identify 'endoleaks'.

20 When satisfied with the angiographic appearances remove all sheaths, catheters and guide-wires, close the second arteriotomy with 5/0 polypropylene sutures and restore blood flow to both limbs.

21 Close the groin incisions and check to ensure that the peripheral circulation is satisfactory.

? DIFFICULTY

1. Tortuous or calcified iliac arteries may obstruct access of the introducer sheath carrying the device. It is often possible to straighten the iliac arteries by applying gentle traction upon the external iliac artery from the groin. Dilate any focal stenoses with a balloon catheter. Consider deployment of a Wallstent. Large flexible sheaths with long tapered 'nosecones' are available (Cook) and these can often be negotiated through access vessels that will not permit passage of the device. The introducer system for the device may then be advanced through the sheath. If the external iliac arteries are too small to permit passage of an introducer sheath of sufficient size, take one of the following three actions: (a) expose one common iliac artery through an oblique incision in the iliac fossa and an extraperitoneal approach and suture to it a Dacron tube graft (8 or 10 mm) to function as a 'conduit' through which the larger component (main body) of the device is introduced into the aorta; (b) 'convert' to open repair of the aneurysm; (c) abandon the procedure altogether.
2. It may be impossible to manipulate a guide-wire into the short leg from the second groin. Pass a wire over the bifurcation of the graft from the first groin using a specially shaped, Soss-Omni, catheter and catch the end within the iliac artery using a 'goose-neck' snare to withdraw it through the sheath in the second groin. Advance catheters over the wire from both groins to push the loop well up before carefully withdrawing it to position the end within the aorta. Alternatively, use a brachial approach to advance a wire through the device to the second groin. Again, use a goose-neck snare to capture the wire and withdraw it through the sheath in the groin.
3. *Completion angiography demonstrates an 'endoleak'.* This is defined as 'persistence of blood flow outside the lumen of the endoluminal graft but within the aneurysm sac or adjacent vascular segment'. The presence of an endoleak indicates that the sac is still pressurized and therefore that a risk of rupture persists. Flow in the aneurysm sac visualized on completion angiography may originate from: (a) one or more of the anastomoses (type 1 endoleak); (b) retrograde perfusion from patent lumbar or inferior mesenteric arteries (type 2 endoleak); (c) incomplete seal between the modular parts (type 3 endoleak); or (d) graft porosity (type 4 endoleak). Of these, types 1 and 3 are the most important and should be corrected either by balloon dilatation of the 'anastomosis' or, if this fails, by insertion of a Palmaz stent or an 'extender cuff'. The patient must not be allowed to leave the operating table with a large proximal type 1 endoleak because these are the most dangerous of all. Anecdotal evidence indicates that an unresolved proximal type 1 endoleak is associated with a higher risk of rupture than an untreated aneurysm. If the measures described are ineffective, conversion to open repair must be considered. Most type 2 endoleaks resolve spontaneously due to thrombosis of the vessel. Furthermore, clinical studies have demonstrated that they are rarely the cause of adverse postoperative events. Therefore no further intervention is required if type 2 endoleak is diagnosed from the postoperative angiogram.
4. If, for any reason the endograft cannot be deployed or it is found to be grossly malpositioned, convert the procedure to open repair.

REFERENCE

1. Parodi JC, Palmaz JC, Barone HD 1991 Transfemoral intraluminal graft implantation for abdominal aortic aneurysms. Annals of Vascular Surgery 5:491–499

REPAIR OF POPLITEAL ANEURYSM

Appraise

- After the abdominal aorta, the popliteal artery is the second most common place for aneurysms to occur. Sixty percent are bilateral.
- They are dangerous lesions because of their tendency to thrombosis, with peripheral embolization. Initially, mural thrombus develops within the aneurysm and, possibly because of repeated flexion of the knee joint, fragments break away and embolize into the distal vessels. Because the emboli are small this process can occur insidiously so that the peripheral vascular bed gradually silts up until the aneurysm itself suddenly thromboses completely. Reconstructive surgery is often impossible because of the absence of patent vessels distally to receive a graft. Acute ischaemia from thrombosis of a popliteal aneurysm frequently results in loss of the limb. It has been suggested that thrombolytic therapy prior to operation may give better results than surgery alone. There is also a risk of haemorrhage from rupture of popliteal aneurysms but this is much less common.
- Most popliteal aneurysms should be operated upon electively even if asymptomatic, especially when they contain intraluminal thrombus. (This can be identified by ultrasound scan.)
- Endovascular repair of popliteal aneurysms with a covered endoluminal stent or endograft is an option that is likely to be employed with increasing frequency in the future as devices with sufficient flexibility to cross the knee joint safely become available. At the time of writing, this approach is still regarded as experimental and is not recommended for routine application.

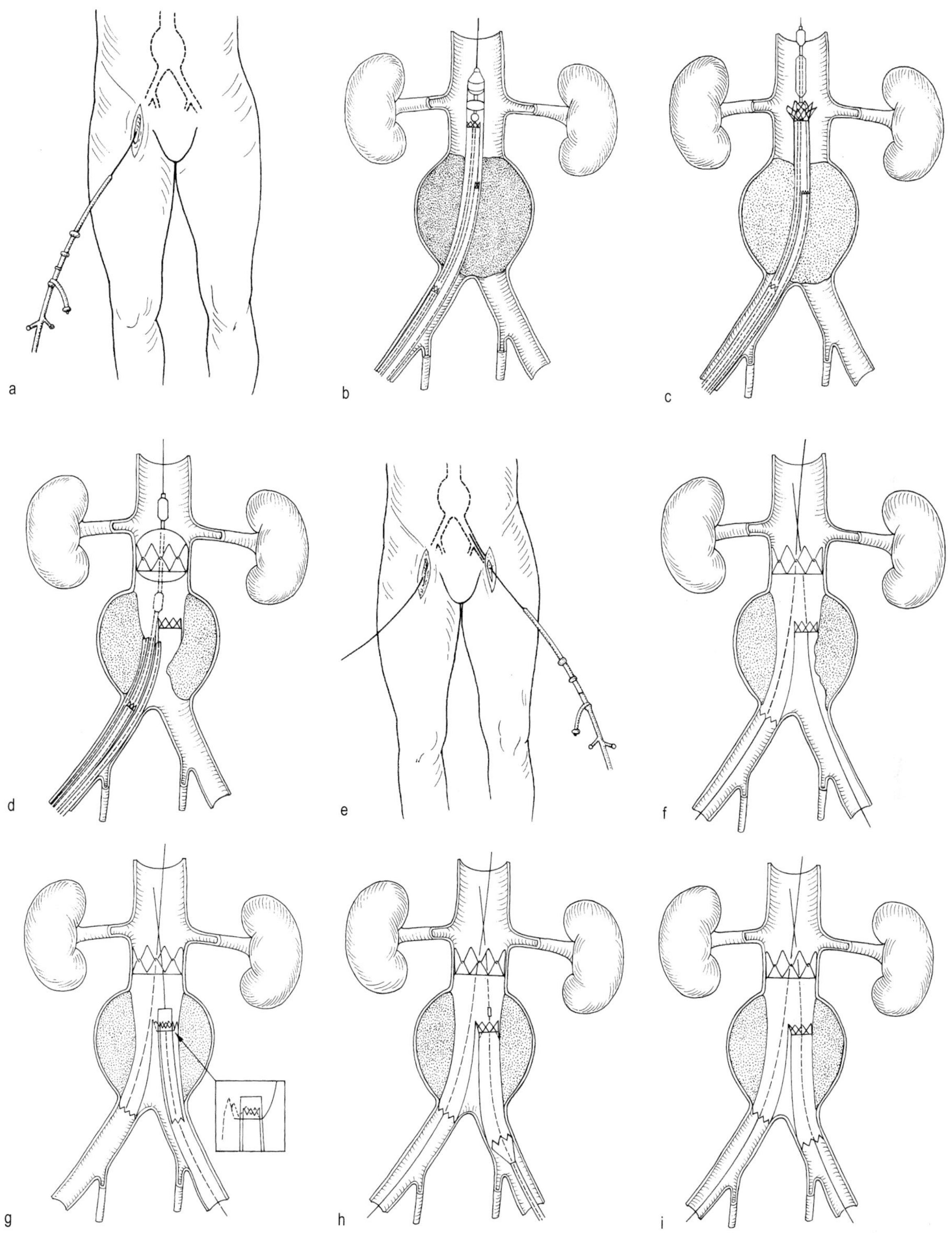

Fig. 29.33 Endovascular repair of abdominal aortic aneurysm with a modular endograft.

- Proximal and distal ligation of the aneurysm in combination with a bypass graft, by a medial approach, has been the most popular operative procedure for many years. However, recent studies have shown that a third of aneurysms treated by this method continue to expand due to pressurization of the sac by geniculate collateral arteries. Therefore, a direct posterior approach with insertion of an inlay graft is to be preferred.

Prepare

Position the patient prone on the operating table. The short saphenous vein can be harvested for use as a bypass with the patient in this position. But, if the long saphenous vein in the thigh is to be used, first excise and prepare it with the patient supine.

Access

1 Make a vertical 'lazy-S' incision over the popliteal fossa. Incise the popliteal fascia and fat pad in the same line to expose the 'diamond' defined by the hamstring muscles above and the two bellies of the gastrocnemius muscle below (see Exposure of the major peripheral arteries, Popliteal artery, above).

2 The popliteal artery lies medial and deep to the popliteal vein. Most aneurysms originate a centimetre or two distal to the adductor opening and terminate proximal to the anterior tibial branch. Divide any veins draining the gastrocnemius muscle which may be found crossing the distal popliteal artery to gain access to the popliteal vein. Take care to protect the sural, lateral popliteal and common peroneal nerves, all of which are particularly vulnerable.

3 Pass silastic loops around the popliteal artery proximal and distal to the aneurysm.

KEY POINT Control

- Note that the principle has been observed of obtaining control of the artery above and below the lesion.

4 The short saphenous vein arises behind the lateral malleolus at the ankle and takes a posterolateral course to enter the popliteal vein at a variable point above the level of the knee joint. In its distal half it is subcutaneous but penetrates the deep fascia to become subfascial proximally. Identify it in the distal popliteal fossa and trace it distally by incising the skin and deep fascia overlying it. Take great care to avoid injury to the sural nerve that runs alongside it. Excise an adequate length and prepare it for use as a reversed vain graft (see Basic principles).

Action

1 Heparinize the patient.

2 Apply clamps proximal and distal to the aneurysm.

3 Incise the aneurysm longitudinally along its whole extent. Oversew vessels that are back-bleeding into the sac using 4/0 figure-of-eight sutures placed across their orifices.

4 Inlay a reversed autologous vein graft with end-to-end anastomoses by the parachute method using 4/0 or 5/0 Prolene sutures. The distal limit of the aneurysm may be obscured by the nerves crossing it making an inlay anastomosis difficult and therefore unsafe. In this case transect the popliteal artery distal to the aneurysm and construct a direct end-to-end anastomosis.

5 Close the wound in layers with a suction drain to the popliteal fossa.

? DIFFICULTY

1. Peripheral embolization from the aneurysm may have occluded the distal vessels.
2. Make an anastomosis to the distal popliteal artery or the tibioperoneal trunk if at all possible. Otherwise, surgical exploration of the tibial arteries and an on-table angiogram may be required to identify the optimal site to receive the bypass.

CAROTID ENDARTERECTOMY

Appraise

- Controversy surrounding this operation was dispelled by the publication of two randomized clinical trials in the early 1980s—one from Europe[1] and the other from America.[2] Both trials showed a significant benefit from surgery for patients with transient cerebral ischaemic attacks and a stenosis at the origin of the internal carotid artery of greater than 70%. Those with a mild stenosis of less than 30% fared better with medical therapy than with surgery, while no clear-cut conclusions could be drawn regarding those with a moderate stenosis of between 30% and 70%.
- The main indication for carotid endarterectomy is therefore transient cerebral ischaemic attacks associated with a stenosis greater than 70%.
- Asymptomatic carotid stenosis is associated with a much lower risk of stroke. But, the Asymptomatic Carotid Surgery Trial has demonstrated benefit in terms of reduction in the stroke rate in patients with the most severe stenoses (>85%).
- Patients who have suffered a complete stroke may be made worse by carotid endarterectomy if operated upon within 3 months of the event. But there may be an indication for operation after this period in those who make a good recovery with limited residual disability; otherwise they will remain at risk from another stroke.
- Surgical intervention for 'strokes in evolution' has potential to prevent or limit the effects of completed stroke in some patients. But there is also a risk of aggravating the condition and this indication is therefore controversial.
- There is little convincing evidence that patients with symptoms of vertebrobasilar insufficiency benefit from carotid endarterectomy.
- Total occlusion of the internal carotid artery is a contraindication to surgery.
- It must be remembered that carotid endarterectomy is a prophylactic operation. It will not improve symptoms due to a previous stroke but, in patients with symptomatic lesions of greater than 70%, it will reduce the risk of the patient suffering another ipsilateral stroke from approximately 20% within 3 years to 2% in the same period.
- Because it is a prophylactic procedure, the complication rate associated with the operation must be extremely low. The justification for carotid endarterectomy is based on the assumption of a combined operative mortality and stroke rate of under 6%. It is therefore essential that those undertaking this operation should maintain an accurate audit of their results and be prepared to refer their patients elsewhere if they cannot achieve this level of performance.
- Endovascular approaches to the treatment of carotid artery disease are currently under investigation. Balloon angioplasty alone is associated with an unacceptably high stroke rate and has been abandoned. However, the results of primary stenting rival those of open surgery, and randomized studies are in progress to determine the relative value of these two

approaches. At the time of writing carotid endarterectomy remains the 'gold standard'. Emboli of thrombotic and atheromatous material are released from the lesion during the course endoluminal interventions and are a potential cause of cerebral injury. This problem is minimized by the use of protective devices including filters and small balloons that are advanced through the lesion on very fine guide-wires prior to any therapeutic manipulation being undertaken The debris that collects behind them is either trapped and withdrawn with the protection device or aspirated. One type of device incorporates occlusion balloons that are placed in the common and external carotid arteries. Continuous aspiration of blood to reverse flow in the internal carotid artery obviates the risk of cerebral embolism without the lesion having to be crossed by a wire first. However, there must be adequate flow via the other cerebral arteries and the circle of Willis to maintain perfusion of the ipsilateral hemisphere for this method to be applicable.

Prepare

1 Duplex scanning accurately diagnoses the presence of internal carotid artery stenosis. Conventional carotid angiography carries a risk of stroke of approximately 1% and is normally to be avoided. Most vascular surgeons are now prepared to accept patients for operation without angiography. If detailed imaging of the carotid artery and intracranial vessels is required use CT or magnetic resonance angiography.

2 CT scanning of the brain confirms whether or not the patient has suffered infarction prior to his operation.

3 Aspirin antiplatelet therapy should be commenced at least 48 hours before operation and should be continued indefinitely after operation.

4 Under general anaesthesia the patient is placed supine on an operating table and the head of the table is raised slightly in order to reduce pressure in the neck veins. The patient's head, supported on a head ring, is turned slightly to the opposite side with the neck extended. The preparation and towelling include the pinna, which is bent forwards and supported in this position by an adhesive drape. This is to allow access for the sternomastoid muscle to be raised from the mastoid process should exposure of the artery be required at a high level.

5 Local anaesthesia in the form of regional, cervical plexus block has the advantage that the patient is able to co-operate in order to identify impaired cerebral perfusion and the need for a cerebral protection shunt (see below). However, general anaesthesia is preferred by many surgeons and patients. A randomized trial (GALA Trial) is being undertaken to determine whether there is any advantage in terms of clinical outcome for either method.

Access

1 Make an oblique skin incision along the anterior border of the sternomastoid muscle extending from the mastoid process to the sternoclavicular joint (Fig. 29.34). Divide all subcutaneous tissue and the platysma muscle in the same line. Cutaneous nerves crossing the line of the incision must be sacrificed and this will leave an area of permanent numbness beneath the line of the jaw. The great auricular nerve should, however, be preserved.

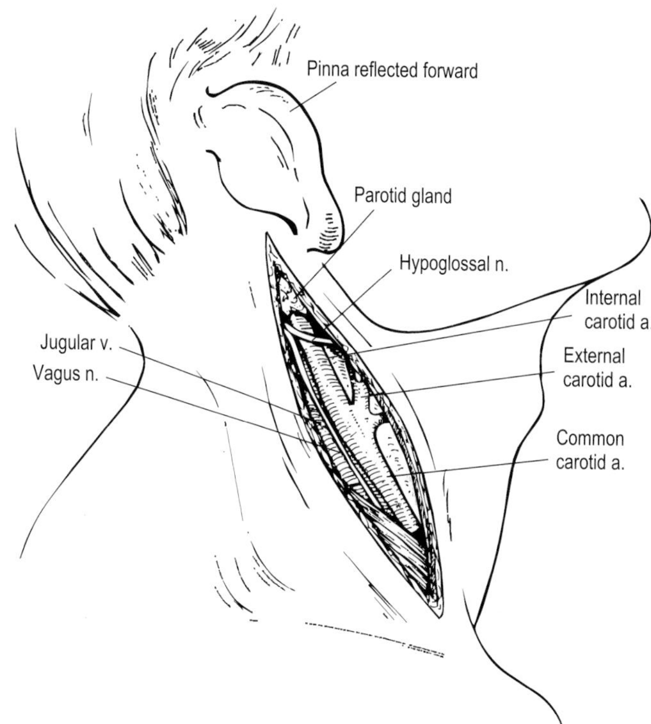

Fig. 29.34 Exposure of the carotid arteries.

2 Mobilize the anterior border of sternomastoid muscle and retract it posteriorly.

3 Identify the facial vein and divide it between ligatures. This allows the internal jugular vein to be displaced posteriorly. There may be additional venous tributaries that need to be divided. In the upper part of the incision mobilize the jugular lymph nodes and retract them posteriorly. Take care to avoid damage to the hypoglossal nerve, which sometimes loops surprisingly low into the neck and may be quite superficial. Find the ansa hypoglossi (also known as the ansa cervicalis) nerve on the surface of the carotid sheath and trace it upwards to locate the hypoglossal nerve. The ansa hypoglossi, which supplies the strap muscles, may be cut without any discernible functional disability. Incision into the lower pole of the parotid gland results in troublesome bleeding, therefore dissect a plane posterior to this structure. The digastric muscle lies beneath it but does not impede access to the artery.

4 Open the carotid sheath initially towards the lower end of the incision to expose the common carotid artery. The vagus nerve lies posteriorly and deep to the artery and is not usually at risk, but its position should be noted so that it can be safeguarded. Pass a rubber sling carefully around the common carotid artery. Expose the carotid bifurcation and trace the internal carotid artery, which lies posterior to the external artery superiorly. It is important to remember that the artery may contain loose thrombotic or atheromatous material, which could be dislodged by rough handling with dire consequences. Therefore use gentle sharp dissection and do not occlude or otherwise

manipulate the vessel until you are ready to apply clamps. Identify and protect the hypoglossal nerve, which sometimes must be lifted off the artery and gently retracted with a soft rubber sling. A small artery and vein loop backwards over the hypoglossal nerve and these should be divided to allow the nerve to be displaced forwards. Clear as much of the artery as possible distal to the bifurcation and very carefully pass a narrow sling around it.

5 Dissect the origin of the external carotid artery and its superior thyroid branch. Pass a single rubber sling around both of these vessels. A single sling used in this way ensures that the ascending pharyngeal artery, which arises from the posterior aspect of the internal carotid artery close to its origin, is controlled also. If slings are placed around the superior thyroid and internal carotid arteries separately, troublesome back-bleeding may be encountered from this vessel following arteriotomy and during dissection of the atheromatous plaque.

6 You are now ready to clamp the arteries, but before proceeding make sure that you know what you are going to do about protecting the brain from ischaemic damage during clamping and that all the necessary instruments are readily to hand.

Cerebral protection

1 The majority of patients will tolerate prolonged clamping of the internal carotid artery without suffering ischaemic damage to the brain. But it is essential to employ a policy that will protect the minority who are at risk.

2 The use of temporary plastic shunts (see General principles) has entirely replaced controlled hypothermia as the method of choice. They are simpler and safer.

3 Shunts may be used routinely or selectively. If used selectively, some test must be employed to identify those in whom they are needed. These include:

- *Internal carotid artery stump pressure measurement*. After the administration of heparin, clamps are applied to the external and common carotid arteries and the pressure in the internal carotid artery is measured with a needle probe connected to a transducer. The pressure measured in this way provides an assessment of the adequacy of the collateral circulation through the circle of Willis. Different criteria have been applied but a mean pressure in excess of 60 mmHg with a good pulsatile pressure wave pattern is often said to indicate adequate perfusion of the relevant hemisphere. If these criteria are met then the operation proceeds without a shunt. If not, a shunt is inserted first.
- *Electroencephalography*. Cerebral function monitoring during clamping permits abnormal patterns to be identified very quickly if cerebral perfusion is inadequate. Action is then taken accordingly as above.
- *Transcranial Doppler*. A substantial reduction in the velocity of blood flow in the middle cerebral artery and loss of 'pulsatility' indicates the need for a shunt. Transcranial Doppler is also very effective for the detection of particulate emboli and can therefore guide the surgeon during his dissection and manipulation of the arteries. A high frequency of emboli detected postoperatively predicts stroke and is an indication for either anticoagulation with low-molecular-weight dextran or, if this should fail to resolve the problem, secondary exploration of the artery.
- *Operate under local anaesthesia*. This is now the preferred method in many centres, local anaesthesia being administered in the form of a regional, cervical plexus block. The patient holds a compressible 'squeeky toy' in his contralateral hand and is asked to squeeze it at intervals. If he is unable to so or if his ability to speak is lost a shunt is inserted to restore adequate perfusion of the ipsilateral cerebral hemisphere.

4 I prefer to use a shunt routinely and this is the method that will be described here. There are small risks associated with shunts related to intimal damage to the artery and air emboli. However, these risks become negligible with familiarity of use.

Action

1 Select the arterial clamps and make sure they are immediately available, together with the Javid shunt and associated large and small ring clamps. Apply a Spencer Wells haemostat to the centre of the shunt.

2 Give heparin intravenously in a dose of 1000 IU for each 10 kg body weight and allow 3 minutes for it to circulate.

3 Apply clamps to the internal carotid, the common carotid and external carotid arteries in that order.

4 Make a longitudinal arteriotomy commencing on the common carotid and extending into the internal carotid beyond the distal limit of the atherosclerotic plaque.

5 Insert the Javid shunt into the common carotid artery and retain it with the larger ring clamp (Fig. 29.35). Temporarily release the Spencer Wells clamp and allow a little bleeding from the

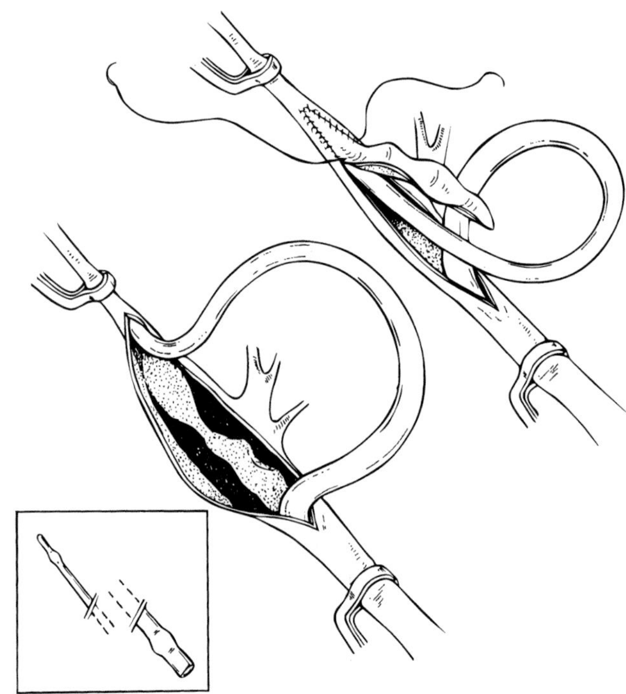

Fig. 29.35 Application of the Javid shunt.

end of the shunt to ensure that it is completely filled and that all air has been ejected. Make a loop with the shunt and insert the other end into the distal internal carotid artery, ensuring that it enters freely without catching and that no air becomes trapped in the process. Apply the ring clamp and, after checking again to ensure there is no air trapped within the shunt, release the Spencer Wells clamp. There are at least 3 or 4 minutes of safe clamping time and without hurrying it usually takes less time than this to initiate flow through the shunt.

6 While an assistant holds open the loop of the shunt, commence the endarterectomy. Using a MacDonald's or Watson–Cheyne blunt dissector, find the plane in the common carotid artery. Develop this around the whole circumference and then cut the 'core' across neatly. Continue the endarterectomy distally and define the ostium of the external carotid artery. It may be best to terminate the endarterectomy here also by cutting across it but the atheroma may extend for only a few millimetres into this vessel, in which case it often lifts out cleanly.

The most important part of the endarterectomy is its termination in the internal carotid artery. In most cases the atheroma 'feathers' away and the plaque lifts out without leaving any edge. If the atheroma does continue distally in this vessel and the plaque must be cut across, place a number of Kunlin sutures across the edge in order to prevent any chance of internal flap dissection (Fig. 29.36). This should rarely be necessary.

7 Once the core has been removed pay meticulous attention to the endarterectomized surface of the artery, recovering all loose flakes and strands, and flush it with heparinized saline (see General principles).

8 Close the arteriotomy with a patch. Simple closure without a patch may be acceptable if the diameter of the internal carotid artery is exceptionally large, which is sometimes the case in male patients. However, there is good scientific evidence to support the routine use of patches and there should, therefore, be few exceptions to this practice. Vein patches are associated with a risk of spontaneous rupture in this situation, with catastrophic consequences. Therefore, patches of prosthetic materials are preferred. These are now manufactured specifically for this purpose. Roll the loop of the shunt towards the proximal end of the arteriotomy and commence the closure in the internal carotid. Use 6/0 polypropylene sutures. Finally, clamp the shunt and remove it. Re-apply clamps to the carotid vessels and complete the closure of the arteriotomy. Flush all vessels before tightening the last stitches.

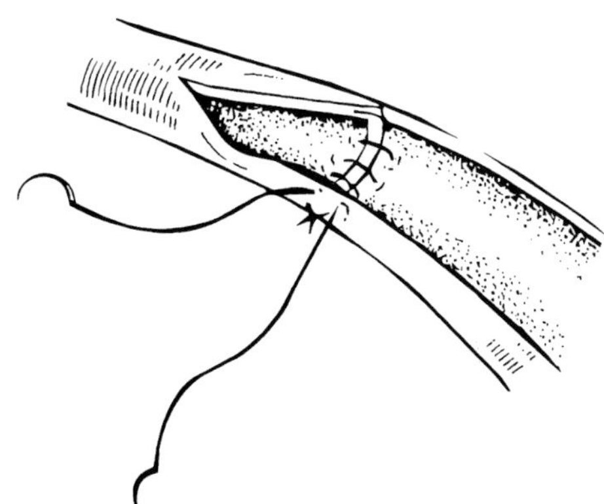

Fig. 29.36 Kunlin sutures to prevent internal flap dissection.

9 *Declamping*. Remove the clamp from the internal carotid artery, allow blood to fill back into the bifurcation, displacing air through the suture line, and then re-apply the clamp to the internal carotid close to the bifurcation. Remove the clamp from the external carotid and then from the common carotid. After three or four heart beats, finally remove the clamp again from the internal carotid artery. The purpose of this declamping procedure is to ensure that any retained air bubbles or small fragments of thrombus pass harmlessly into the external carotid and not into the brain.

? DIFFICULTY

1. The carotid bifurcation is situated high in the neck and it may be difficult to mobilize a sufficient length of the internal carotid artery for satisfactory control.
2. You can expose more of the vessel by extending the incision behind the ear onto the mastoid process. Raise the sternomastoid muscle from its attachment and divide the digastric muscle. If necessary, excise the tip of the styloid process, but avoid damaging the facial nerve.
3. Usually it is sufficient to tunnel beneath the digastric muscle. You may also improve access by using a Pruit–Inahara shunt, which is retained with an intraluminal balloon rather than an external clamp.

Closure

1 Use a continuous suture of 3/0 polyglactin 910 (Vicryl) for the platysma muscle and clips or subcuticular Monocryl for the skin. Insert a small suction drain.

2 Reverse the heparin only if bleeding is excessive.

Aftercare

1 Observe the pulse rate and blood pressure at quarter-hourly intervals for the first hour, half-hourly for 2 hours and then hourly.

2 Observe and chart neurological signs quarter-hourly for the first 3 hours.

3 Remove the drain after 12 hours.

4 Remove the skin clips on the fourth postoperative day.

5 Discharge home on the second or third postoperative day.

6 Continue aspirin antiplatelet therapy indefinitely.

Complications

- *Postoperative bradycardia and hypotension*. This may be associated with stimulation of the nerve to the carotid body. There is, however, no evidence that injecting the nerve with a local anaesthetic agent, as advocated by some surgeons, is of value. Administer atropine at intervals to increase the heart rate and cautiously give more fluid intravenously.

- *Postoperative hypertension.* This must be controlled, if excessive, by the administration of appropriate drugs.
- *Stroke.* If the patient develops a sudden severe neurological defect within the first few hours after operation this may be due to thrombotic occlusion of the artery. Scan the artery with duplex ultrasound. If there is no flow in the artery or the results are equivocal return the patient to theatre immediately and re-explore the vessel. A less-severe neurological defect should simply be observed since it is likely to be transient and due to other causes.
- *Neck haematoma.* A large, tense haematoma is a potential cause of airways obstruction due to a combination of compression and laryngeal oedema and is dangerous. All wound haematomas of any size should be drained by re-opening the wound under local anaesthesia. Do not wait for a stridor or other evidence of airway obstruction before taking action.
- *Cranial nerve lesions.* Temporary dysfunction of the hypoglossal or cervical branch of the facial nerve caused by retraction is common. Trauma to the hypoglossal nerve causes deviation of the protruded tongue to the ipsilateral side. Recovery within a few days is usual but, if permanent, most patients adapt well. Injury to the vagus nerve is manifest by hoarseness. In severe and permanent cases Teflon injections into the vocal cord by an ENT (ear, nose and throat) surgeon may help. The glossopharyngeal nerve is rarely damaged since it lies above and deep to the carotid bifurcation. However, injury to it is potentially troublesome since the patient may have difficulty in swallowing.
- *Late occlusion of the internal carotid artery.* Surveillance by duplex scanning shows that approximately 12% of carotid arteries become occluded within 5 years after endarterectomy. This is due to subintimal fibrous hyperplasia; it occurs slowly and is almost invariably asymptomatic. It must nevertheless be regarded as an undesirable outcome. Antiplatelet agents may help and there is evidence that the incidence is reduced by the routine application of patch closure rather than direct suturing of the arteriotomy. The indication for late surgical re-intervention is re-stenosis without total occlusion accompanied by recurrent transient cerebral ischaemia symptoms. Such a lesion is likely to be due to recurrent atheroma rather than subintimal fibrous hyperplasia.

REFERENCES

1. Kirkpatrick UJ, McWilliams RG, Martin J et al 2004 Late complications after ligation and bypass for popliteal aneurysm. British Journal of Surgery 91:174–178
2. European Carotid Surgery Trial Collaboration Group 1991 MRC European Carotid Surgery Trial: interim results for symptomatic patients with severe (70–90%) or with mild (0–29%) carotid stenosis. Lancet 357:1235–1243

INTESTINAL ISCHAEMIA (ACUTE, MASSIVE ISCHAEMIA)

This may be due to (rarely) a mesenteric embolus, an acute thrombosis or sudden decompensation of an already narrowed mesenteric artery or, in about one-third of cases, the so-called 'non-occlusive infarction', where no arterial blockage is responsible. Acute thrombosis of mesenteric veins is usually present in these circumstances and may be the cause of the infarction.

Appraise

1. Is the gut infarcted or viable? If the former, then the only possible course is resection, which may have to be massive. Make no attempt to construct a primary anastomosis, but exteriorize the ends and close the abdomen. If the patient survives, continuity may be restored at a later date.
2. If the gut appears ischaemic but recoverable, consider vascular reconstruction. If, from the history and antecedents, the case appears to be one of embolism, then open the ileocolic artery at a convenient point and pass a catheter up into the aorta to remove as much of the embolus as possible. If this is successful and pulsation returns to the bowel, the ileocolic artery can be ligated at this point. If not, then a side-to-side anastomosis between ileocolic and right common iliac artery can be carried out and the gut irrigated 'upstream'. This avoids approaching the inaccessible area of the origin of the superior mesenteric artery. If this is unsuccessful it may be necessary to lift the transverse colon upwards and dissect the vascular trunk beneath the neck of the pancreas. The artery can then be opened directly and attempts made to clear it. Successful revascularization usually results in abrupt fall in the blood pressure, due to loss of fluid into the ischaemic loops, and perhaps also 'wash-out' of toxic material from the bowel. Warn the anaesthetist and ask him to transfuse at this stage.
3. Book the theatre for the next day. A 'second-look' operation is always worthwhile and very often you will find ischaemic loops of bowel that were not obvious at the first operation.

CHRONIC INTESTINAL ISCHAEMIA

Appraise

- While genuine cases of 'intestinal angina' due to chronic obstruction of the visceral arteries do certainly exist, they are not easy to define or identify, because there is no exact relationship between arteriographic abnormalities and symptoms.
- Elective reconstruction of the visceral arterial trunks is a highly specialized procedure, which is probably best carried out in centres with a particular interest.
- Endovascular treatment by percutaneous angioplasty with or without stent is the first choice of treatment where technically feasible.
- In practice, most patients with arterial disease and abdominal pain prove to have straightforward organic problems in the gastrointestinal tract, unrelated to the blood supply.

FURTHER READING

National Institute of Neurological Disorders and Stroke 1991 Clinical alert: benefit of carotid endarterectomy for patients with high grade stenosis of the internal artery. Stroke 22:816–817

30

Veins and lymphatics

K.G. Burnand, J. Tan

CONTENTS

VARICOSE VEIN SURGERY

Appraise

- Varicose veins are defined as tortuous dilated superficial veins. Small intradermal subcutaneous veins are excluded.
- Most patients seek treatment for their varicose veins because they dislike the appearance of the large, tortuous veins on their exposed legs. The greater number of varicose vein operations performed in women may reflect the greater importance they attached to attractive legs.
- Many patients complain that their veins ache—a symptom that is often worse at the end of the day or after prolonged standing. Patients also present with ankle swelling, itching, superficial thrombophlebitis and haemorrhage.
- Minor varicose veins and small intradermal subcutaneous veins can be made symptom-free by elastic support stockings.
- Recurrent attacks of superficial thrombophlebitis or severe bleeding from a ruptured varix are clear-cut indications for surgical treatment.
- Surgical ligation and stripping remains the treatment of choice for major incompetence of the long and short saphenous veins, since injection sclerotherapy provides only short-term benefit. Varicose branch veins may be avulsed through local incisions at the time of saphenous vein surgery, but, in the absence of saphenous incompetence, these are equally well treated by injection sclerotherapy. This may be by standard sclerosant such as sodium tetradecyl sulphate or by a foam sclerosant.
- 20–30% of a varicose vein operations are for persistent or recurrent varicosities following saphenous surgery. These recurrent veins can be treated by injection sclerotherapy if there are no residual connections with the femoral or popliteal veins.
- Coincidental varicose veins are often erroneously diagnosed as the cause of painful or swollen legs, which may be the result of arthritis or other causes of leg oedema.
- Most patients with uncomplicated and clear-cut varicose veins require little in the way of investigation beyond a careful history and an examination of the legs to determine the consequence or incompetence of the major sites of communication between the superficial and deep venous systems. Inspection, palpation and the cough, percussion and tourniquet tests provide this information.
- Patients who have lipodermatosclerosis, past ulceration or history of limb fracture or deep vein thrombosis should undergo duplex scanning and bipedal ascending phlebography to enable an accurate assessment of the deep and calf communicating veins to be made.
- Do not carry out varicose vein surgery if the long saphenous vein forms an important collateral channel for obstructed deep veins. Arterial insufficiency is also a relative contraindication to varicose vein surgery.
- Patients with complicated or recurrent varicose veins are more accurately assessed by varicography, in which low-osmolality contrast medium is injected directly into the surface veins to display their course and deep connections. Duplex examination of the reflux in the long and short saphenous trunks provides useful additional information.
- Carefully re-examine patients admitted for varicose vein surgery. Confirm or exclude incompetence in the long and short saphenous veins, and in the calf perforating veins. Mark with an indelible pen, large branch varicosities and the sites of major communicating vein incompetence. Suspect incompetence of calf communicating veins in patients with lipodermatosclerosis. Preoperative marking with duplex scanning may be useful for locating the termination of the short saphenous vein and the sites of incompetent perforating veins.
- A number of new minimally invasive alternatives to ligation and stripping are being assessed, including endoluminal radiofrequency ablation and laser ablation. These cannot be recommended at present until the results of properly conducted clinical trials are available.

HIGH SAPHENOUS VEIN LIGATION (TRENDELENBURG'S OPERATION) AND STRIPPING OF LONG SAPHENOUS VEIN

Appraise

1 Perform the operation, which was described by Friedrich Trendelenburg (1844–1924) of Leipzig in 1890, on patients with varicose veins who have evidence of long saphenous reflux at the groin on clinical, Doppler or duplex examination.

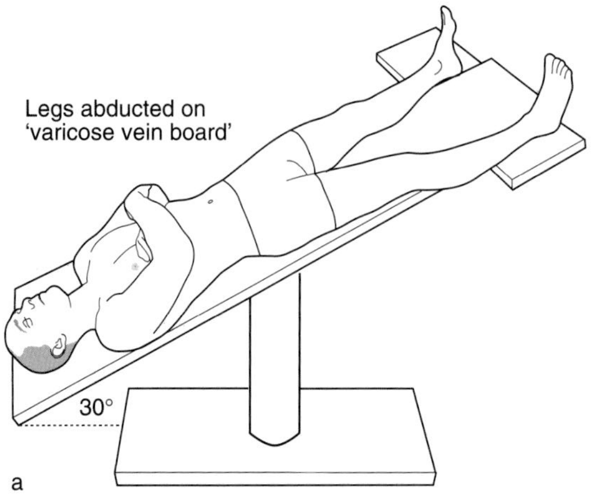

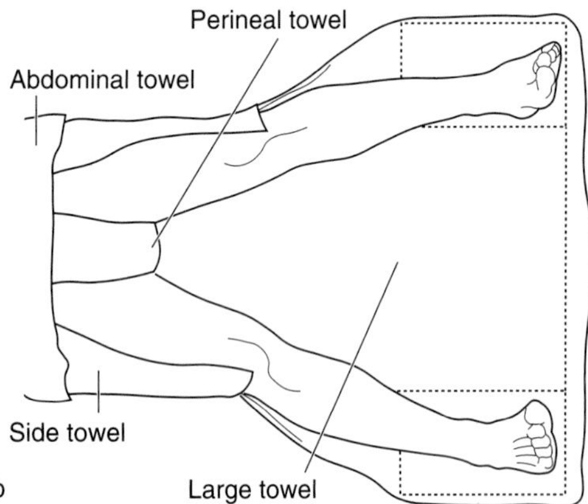

Fig. 30.1 Positioning of patient in venous surgery.

2 Avoid the operation if the long saphenous vein is a collateral channel for obstructed deep veins.

3 Mark all sites of prominent varicosities with indelible pen as 'tram-lines' on either side of the vein to avoid the effect of tattooing.

Prepare

1 Have the skin of the groin and leg shaved before the operation.

2 Place the patient supine in the Trendelenburg position with approximately 30° of head-down tilt with both the legs abducted by 20° from midline and the ankles lying on a padded board. This allows easy access and reduces intraoperative haemorrhage (Fig. 30.1).

3 Prepare all exposed surfaces of the limb from the foot to the groin, up to the level of the umbilicus, with aqueous 0.5% chlorhexidine acetate solution, while an assistant elevates the leg by lifting the patient's foot.

Access

1 Make an oblique incision just below and parallel to the inguinal ligament in the groin crease, over the saphenofemoral junction, which is 2.5 cm lateral to and below the pubic tubercle (Fig. 30.2).

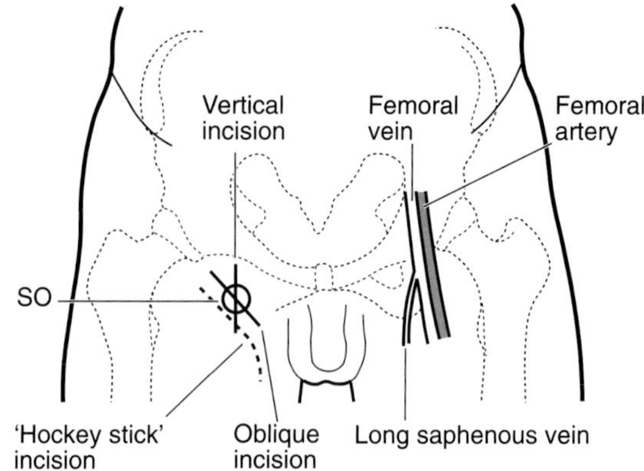

Fig. 30.2 Placing of incisions for access to veins in the groin. Three incisions are shown: vertical, straight oblique, and oblique 'hockey stick' curved. SO, saphenous opening.

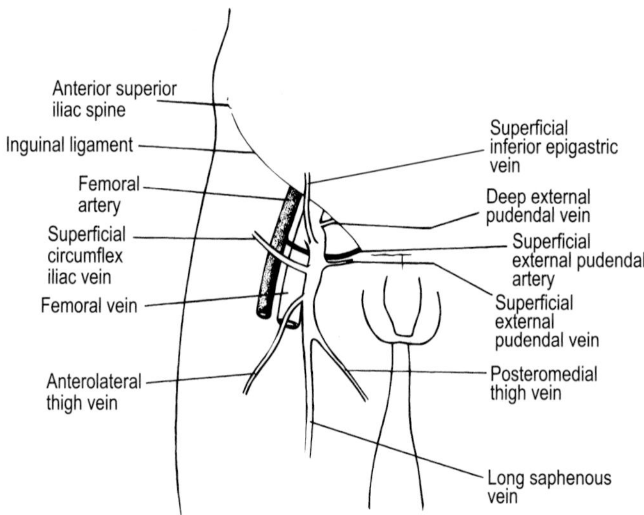

Fig. 30.3 The termination and tributaries of the long saphenous vein in the groin.

2 Deepen the incision through the subcutaneous fat, which is spread by digital retraction and held apart by the insertion of a self-retaining retractor such as Traver's, West's or Cockett's. Modify the length of incision depending on the build of the patient.

Action

1 Bluntly dissect the long saphenous vein out of the surrounding fat and trace it upwards and towards the saphenofemoral junction. The perivenous plane is simple to open and is bloodless when entered.

2 You must dissect out all tributaries that join the long saphenous vein near its termination, ligating them with 2/0 polyglactin before dividing them. The superficial inferior epigastric vein, the superficial circumflex iliac vein, and the superficial and deep external pudendal veins all join the saphenous trunk near its termination. In addition, the posteromedial and anterolateral thigh veins terminate close to the saphenofemoral junction (Fig. 30.3). One or more of these veins may join together before emptying into the saphenous trunk.

? DIFFICULTY

The long saphenous vein normally emerges as a dark-blue tube in the centre of dissection as you free the subcutaneous fat from its surface. Trace a smaller tributary back to the main trunk if it is hard to find.

3 After these tributaries have been divided, approach the saphenofemoral junction. The long saphenous vein dips down through the cribriform fascia over the foramen ovale to join the femoral vein. Carefully separate the subcutaneous fat from the vein by blunt dissection to follow its path. Display the femoral vein for approximately 1 cm above and below the saphenofemoral junction, and clear any small tributaries entering from either side.

▶ KEY POINTS Anatomy

- Do not ligate or divide any large vessel until you have displayed the full anatomy of the long saphenous, its tributaries and its junction with the femoral vein.
- It is easy to mistake the femoral artery for the long saphenous vein, with disastrous consequences if it is inadvertently stripped.

4 Ligate the long saphenous vein in continuity with 0 polyglactin, flush with the saphenofemoral junction and divide it. For greater safety doubly ligate or transfix the saphenous stump. Alternatively, oversew the termination with a 3/0 polypropylene continuous suture.

5 Place a strong ligature around the divided distal end of the long saphenous trunk and hold it up to occlude retrograde blood flow, then make a small transverse venotomy above the ligature through which to introduce the stripper. Use either a flexible intraluminal wire or a disposable plastic stripper with a blunt tip. Gently manipulate the tip of the stripper downwards until it is a hand's breadth below the knee, where it may remain in the saphenous vein or pass into a tributary (Fig. 30.4). If it will not pass, withdraw the stripper and re-insert it with a rotational action. Tie the ligature at the top end to prevent blood from leaking out of the divided long saphenous trunk.

6 Alternatively, use a pin stripper with a small hole at the top to invert and extract the vein. However, this technique has not been shown to have any additional benefit.

7 Be aware of the superficial external pudendal artery, which may pass either anterior or posterior to the saphenous vein. Take care not to damage this vessel; if you inadvertently do so, ligate and divide it with impunity.

8 Make a short oblique incision in one of the skin crease tension lines, 1–2 cm in length, over the palpable tip of the stripper. Ensure that the incision is large enough to allow the head of the stripper to pass. Palpate the vein containing the stripper and dissect it off the saphenous nerve.

9 Make a small side-hole in the vein through which the tip of the stripper can be delivered and attach the T-shaped handle to the stripper.

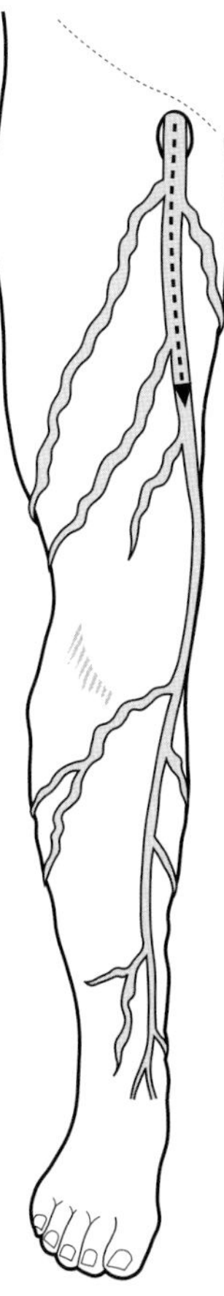

Fig. 30.4 Passage of a flexible intraluminal stripper in the long saphenous vein. Note the tributary below the knee into which the stripper may pass, leaving the main vein.

10 Strip the long saphenous vein from the groin to the knee with steady downward traction. Ease the stripper and the bunched up vein through the lower incision. Clamp the attached long saphenous vein and any tributaries, divide and ligate it with 2/0 polyglactin.

11 Prevent excessive bleeding from the stripper track, either by tightly applying a sterile elasticated bandage while with drawing the stripper, or by gently rolling a swab along the course of the vein before applying bandages. Some surgeons apply a sterile tourniquet to the leg to prevent excessive haemorrhage.

▶ KEY POINTS Anatomical variations at the saphenofemoral junction

- A variable number of tributaries join the long saphenous vein as it approaches the femoral vein.
- Occasionally the anterolateral and posteromedial thigh veins terminate independently into the femoral vein, giving the appearance of a double saphenous vein.
- The long saphenous vein may occasionally be truly bifid with one channel joining the femoral vein below the saphenous opening.

Closure

1 Appose the subcutaneous tissues and fascia with 2/0 polyglactin. Close the skin with 3/0 subcuticular sutures with Monocryl and Steri-Strip tapes.

2 Apply compression bandages to the whole leg to avoid haematoma formation.

Postoperative

1 Keep the leg elevated 15° above the horizontal in bed.

2 Encourage early mobilization after applying additional compression bandages over the bandages put on in the theatre. This reduces the haematoma formation and provides better support when the patient stands. Thromboembolism prophylactic stockings do not provide sufficient compression.

3 Advise the patient to walk rather than stand still or sit with the feet down.

4 Discharge fit patient on the first postoperative day, to re-attend for removal of any non-absorbable sutures a week later.

? DIFFICULTY

1. The passage of the stripper may be impeded by competent valves, varicosity or false passages into small tortuous tributaries. Attempts to forcibly pass the stripper often end in perforation of the vein wall. If you encounter resistance, withdraw the stripper and re-pass it, twisting the free end to rotate the tip facilitate negotiating irregularities in the vein.
2. If there is a hold-up around the knee, try flexing and extending the knee to aid the passage of the stripper, at the same time applying gentle external compression over the tip of the stripper to prevent it from passing into superficial tributaries.
3. If these measures fail, leave the stripper in situ. Pass a second stripper into the long saphenous vein from below the knee, then gradually withdraw the first stripper ahead of the advancing stripper passed from below.
4. If neither stripper will bypass the obstruction, cut down over the tips of both strippers. You may be able to re-direct one stripper through the cut-down incision and passed on down the vein, but if this fails, strip out the two halves of the vein leaving a short residual portion between the two incisions. Alternatively, forcibly avulse this segment of residual vein.
5. Control sudden massive haemorrhage in the groin by applying direct external pressure to the femoral vein above and below the saphenofemoral junction. Summon experienced vascular help. Never attempt to apply an artery forceps blindly.

SAPHENOPOPLITEAL LIGATION AND STRIPPING

Appraise

- This is indicated if there is gross dilatation and reflux in the short saphenous trunk or its tributaries.
- The location of the saphenopopliteal junction is very variable and, in a third of cases, the short saphenous vein enters the popliteal vein above or below the middle of the popliteal fossa.
- Preoperative varicography and duplex scanning or on-table saphenography all provide accurate information about the termination of the short saphenous vein and its proximal tributaries.

▶ KEY POINT Mark the junction

- When you identify the saphenopopliteal junction, mark it on the skin.

- Carry out the short saphenous vein ligation first if you intend to strip the long saphenous vein under the same anaesthetic.

Prepare

1 Place the anaesthetized, intubated patient prone, with pillows under the chest, midriff and pelvis.

2 Place the operating table in 30° of head-down tilt and slightly abduct the legs to ease access.

Access

Make a short transverse incision behind the lateral malleolus at the ankle.

Action

1 Find the short saphenous vein posterior to the lateral malleolus and dissect it from the fat and its accompanying sural nerve.

2 Ligate the vein distally with 2/0 polyglactin. Pass another ligature proximally and use it to elevate the vein in order to create a venotomy to insert a stripper.

3 Having inserted the stripper, pass it up the vein in an identical manner to that described for the long saphenous vein. Tie the ligature at the ankle to prevent blood loss.

4 Make a transverse incision 3–5 cm in length in the popliteal fossa over the saphenopopliteal junction, which was identified and marked by one of the methods described above.

5 Divide the deep fascia in the popliteal fossa vertically and define the short saphenous vein containing the easily palpable stripper. Slightly withdraw the stripper and make sure it is not in the popliteal vein, having entered it through a connecting vein in the lower calf.

6 Gently expose the termination of the vein by blunt dissection, to separate it from the surrounding fat, until you identify the T-junction with the popliteal vein. Apply deep retraction with a Langenbeck's retractor to help display the junction.

7 There is often a tributary joining the short saphenous vein from above, known as the vein of Giacomini, in 2.5–10% of patients; carefully divide it between ligatures.

8 Doubly ligate the stump of the short saphenous vein with 2/0 polyglactin, extract the head of the stripper from the lumen and tie the vein to the stripper.

9 Strip out the vein, and firmly wrap the leg in an elasticated bandage.

Closure

1 Insert continuous 2/0 polyglactin into the subcutaneous tissue and fascia.

2 Close the skin with a 3/0 subcuticular suture and Steri-Strips.

Complications

- These are similar to those of long saphenous vein, but with an additional risk of damage to the popliteal artery, vein and nerve during popliteal dissection.
- The sural nerve is easily damaged unless you gently dissect it free from the vein at the ankle. For this reason, some surgeons never strip the short saphenous vein. There is no controlled trial to settle this controversy and the subject remains a matter of opinion.

INCOMPETENT PERFORATOR OR COMMUNICATING VEINS LIGATION

Appraise

- Communicating veins connect the branches of the saphenous system to the deep veins of the leg by crossing the deep fascia. Blood normally passes from the superficial to the deep veins, but reversal of flow may occur if the valves of the communicating veins become incompetent.
- Three almost constant communicating or perforating veins in the medial calf are particularly important in the development of venous ulceration (Cockett's veins) (Fig. 30.5).
- Ligate these medial calf communicating veins in patients with clinical or duplex scanning evidence of incompetence and who have severe lipodermatosclerosis or healed ulceration.

KEY POINT Contraindication

- Do not ligate the communicating veins in patients with evidence of severe post-thrombotic damage of their deep veins.

- Your objective is to interrupt incompetent medial calf perforating veins, in order to obliterate deep to superficial venous reflux and reduce ambulatory venous hypertension in critical areas above the ankle where venous ulcers are most likely to develop.
- The mechanism of this procedure remains unclear even in patients with venous ulceration, since perforator incompetence may be reversed by the saphenous vein operation of high ligation and stripping.

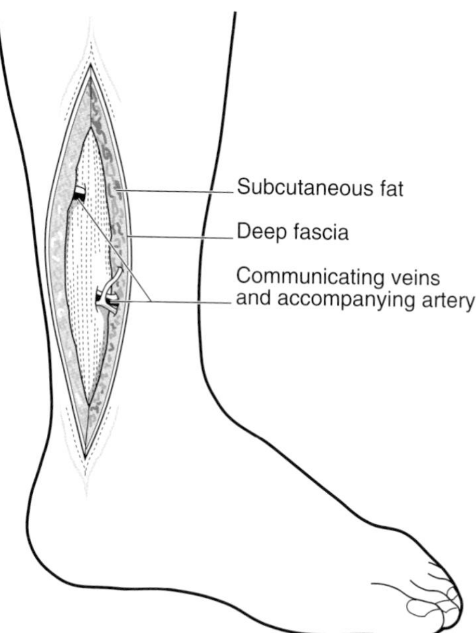

Fig. 30.5 The subfascial operation for ligation of the medial calf communicating vein.

- Perforating veins may be incompetent without causing any skin changes. Failure to ligate these veins may account for recurrence of varicose veins despite satisfactory saphenous vein operations.
- Subfascial endoscopic ligation is a minimally invasive method of interrupting the perforating veins.
- The Cockett's and Linton's procedures of extrafascial or subfascial approaches for the ligation of perforating veins are now of historical importance only. Skin necrosis and poor cosmesis led to them being abandoned.

SUBFASCIAL ENDOSCOPIC PERFORATING VEINS SURGERY

Appraise

1 This is perforator vein interruption performed through an endoscope inserted through small ports placed well away from the active ulcer or area of diseased skin. This avoids making a long and often poorly healing wound (Fig. 30.6). The role of this technique is still to be established.

2 Operating time is saved if the perforators are first mapped out with duplex ultrasound scanning.

3 Perform the operation under tourniquet control.

4 Make a small incision in the upper medial calf and deepen it through the deep fascia. Insert a finger to establish a subfascial plane.

5 Insert the endoscope and advance it along the medial border of the tibia towards the ankle.

6 Bluntly dissect the subfascial space through the endoscope to bring the perforators into view. Clip, avulse or seal these veins using diathermy or a harmonic scalpel inserted through a second port.

7 Suture the wound and bandage the leg.

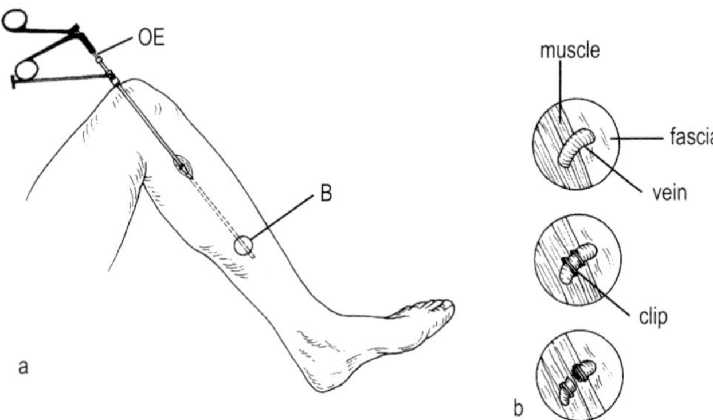

Fig. 30.6 Subfascial endoscopic ligation of communicating veins: (a) the operating endoscope (OE) inserted through a small incision, tissue dissection being achieved using balloon (B) dilatation; (b) the views through the endoscope.

AVULSION OF SUPERFICIAL VARICOSITIES

Appraise

1 Occlude or excise large branch veins that are not in close proximity to the saphenous or perforator systems to prevent unsightly local recurrences and provide a satisfactory cosmetic result.

2 Carefully mark out the superficial varicose veins on either side preoperatively, as varicosities are no longer visible when the patient is anaesthetized and the legs are elevated.

Action

1 Make minute stab incisions over the course of tributaries in the direction of skin tension lines. Draw out a loop of vein by gentle blunt dissection, using specially designed hooks or mosquito artery forceps.

2 Divide the loop between mosquito forceps and tease out the vein in either direction by exerting steady traction and gentle blunt dissection under the skin with fine mosquito forceps.

3 Employ a gentle circular motion on the forceps to help separate the tethering fibrous tissue from the vein.

4 Release traction when the vein starts to stretch, and at this point ligate both ends. Alternatively, continue the traction until the vein breaks, controlling bleeding by local pressure until traumatic venospasm develops.

5 Place incisions 5 cm apart along the course of each tributary. This technique can be used to remove a long segment of varicose vein through 3–5 small incisions.

? DIFFICULTY

- Reduce local blood loss by performing the avulsions after the limb has been exsanguinated with a tourniquet.

Closure

Use interrupted 4/0 nylon mattress sutures or 2/0 polyglactin in the subcutaneous tissues and Steri-Strip tape for the skin.

RECURRENT VARICOSE VEINS

Appraise

1 Recurrent varicose veins are veins that have become varicose after the original treatment. In contrast, residual varicose veins refers to those that were not treated at the original procedure (Fig. 30.7).

2 The causes of recurrent veins include:
- Disease progression, with the development of new venous incompetence between the deep and superficial venous system.
- Inadequate primary procedure, if the tributaries are left unligated, especially in the presence of a dual saphenous system that was not recognized or removed.
- Development of new bridging channels (neovascularization): collaterals may develop following simple ligation, reconnecting the deep veins to the saphenous vein.

3 Diligently examine the varicosities, looking carefully for the scars of a previous operation.

4 Employ duplex scanning to detect reflux in the saphenous veins and in large calf perforators. Varicography also demonstrates communication between varicosities and the deep veins.

Access

1 Operate for recurrent varicose veins under general anaesthesia.

2 Position the patient as for the primary procedure.

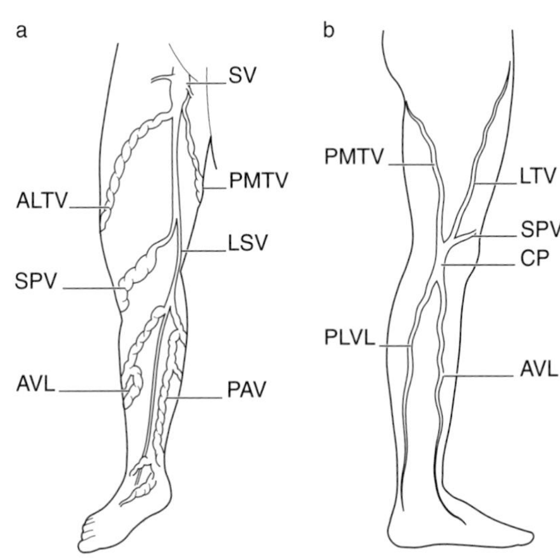

Fig. 30.7 (a) The major superficial tributaries of the long saphenous vein which become varicose. Note that the long saphenous vein itself rarely becomes varicose. (b) The superficial veins on the lateral aspect of the leg. These usually drain into the long saphenous system and are a common site for postoperative recurrences. ALTV, anterolateral thigh vein; AVL, anterior vein of leg (accessory saphenous vein); CP, crossing point; LSV, long saphenous vein; PAV, posterior arch vein; PLVL, posterolateral vein of the leg; PMTV, posteromedial thigh vein; SPV, superior patella vein; SV, saphenous vein.

Action

KEY POINTS Avoid bleeding

- Recurrent varicose veins are often thin-walled, multiple and easily damaged.
- Haemorrhage from torn veins can be severe.

1 Make an adequate incision to ensure good operative access.

2 To reduce the risk of bleeding employ an approach through previously undissected tissue planes, which enables anatomical landmarks and vascular control to be established before tackling the recurrent varices.

Postoperative care

This is the same as for the primary procedure.

GROIN RECURRENCES

Appraise

Control of recurrent varicose veins in the thigh and on the medial side of the leg with an upper thigh tourniquet is suggestive of groin recurrence (recurrent saphenofemoral incompetence).

Varicography or duplex scanning may demonstrate a connection of the varices with the femoral vein in the groin.

Access

1 Make an incision in the groin crease centred on the saphenofemoral junction, 7–10 cm in length, extending laterally over the femoral pulse.

2 Expose the anterior surface of the femoral artery to facilitate access to the femoral vein.

Action

1 Approach the saphenofemoral junction from the lateral side through relatively normal tissues. Open the femoral sheath to expose the anterior surface of the femoral artery.

2 Carefully dissect medially and expose the anterior surface of the femoral vein. Dissect it clean and locate the saphenofemoral junction.

3 Clear the saphenous stump on all sites close to the femoral vein until you can pass a Lahey forceps around it. Ligate it with a 2/0 polyglactin tie before dividing it. For added safety, transfix the stump.

4 Ligate all tributaries individually with 2/0 polyglactin and divide them.

5 Strip the long saphenous vein if it is still present and avulse all superficial varicose veins in the usual manner.

Closure

1 Close the subcutaneous tissue with interrupted 2/0 polyglactin.

2 Close the skin with 3/0 subcuticular suture and Steri-Strip tape.

Complications

1 Second operations are always more difficult than primary. If you do not fully display the anatomy it is easy to damage the major vessels.

2 Take care not to damage the femoral nerve during the lateral approach.

3 Lymphocele or lymph fistula may appear postoperatively, but usually resolves spontaneously.

SAPHENOPOPLITEAL RECURRENCES

Appraise

1 The presence of varices on the posterolateral surface of the lower leg that can be controlled by placing a tourniquet just below the knee joint in a patient who has had previous short saphenous surgery suggests a popliteal recurrence.

2 Because of the variable termination of the short saphenous vein, varicography and duplex scanning are necessary to define the major sites of recurrence.

Access

1 Make a vertical or S-shaped incision across the centre of the popliteal fossa.

2 Enter the popliteal fossa through a posterior approach and identify the popliteal artery and vein before ligating the varices.

Action

1 Deepen the incision through the subcutaneous tissues.

2 Identify the popliteal artery and vein well above the previous scar tissue and trace them down until you are able to identify the stump of the short saphenous vein.

KEY POINT Tibial nerve

- Avoid damaging the nerve, which lies superficial to the popliteal vessels.

2 Divide and ligate all the tributaries entering the popliteal vein, and especially any stump of the short saphenous vein.

3 Strip out any residual short saphenous vein.

Closure

1 Close the subcutaneous tissue with interrupted 2/0 polyglactin.

2 Close the skin with 3/0 subcuticular suture and Steri-Strip tape.

Technical points

- Tourniquets reduce blood loss during varicose vein surgery and so shorten the duration of the operation. There is also a lesser incidence of postoperative haematoma. However, they may cause nerve damage.
- The insertion of autologous or foreign material, such as PTFE (polytetrafluoroethylene), Gore-Tex or Mersilene, as a barrier to reduce recurrence has not so far proved effective.

NEW ALTERNATIVE TREATMENTS

Appraise

Any alternative technique to high ligation and stripping of saphenous vein must produce as good as, or a better, outcome with, ideally, a reduced associated morbidity.

New approaches

1 Endoluminal radiofrequency ablation (VNUS closure system) and endovascular laser treatment have been introduced as minimally invasive alternatives to ligation and stripping of the saphenofemoral or saphenopopliteal veins.

2 Both techniques aim to damage the vessel intima, causing fibrosis and ultimately obliteration of a long segment of the vein trunk.

3 Radiofrequency ablation is performed by inserting a catheter via a small incision in the distal medial thigh to within 1–2 cm of the saphenofemoral junction. The position of the catheter is checked with duplex scanning.

4 High-frequency radio waves are then delivered through the catheter, causing heating of the intima, resulting in damage to the vein wall. The catheter is slowly withdrawn, closing the vein behind it.

5 Laser treatment is performed by threading a bare-tipped laser fibre along the long saphenous vein to the saphenofemoral junction. Check the position with duplex scanning before activating the laser, while slowly withdrawing the fibre.

6 Radiofrequency ablation and laser appear to cause less morbidity than ligation and stripping, but there are no studies that directly compare the long-term recurrence rates of these two techniques.

7 Illuminated powered phlebectomy (TriVex system) uses a suction needle containing a guarded blade which removes veins like a vacuum cleaner. Saline containing local anaesthetic and diluted adrenaline (epinephrine) is instilled around the veins to be removed. These are illuminated by a powerful light source placed next to the varicosities. The varicose veins are sucked into the opening near the needle tip and 'morcellated' by the powered phlebotome. This slices up the veins which have been drawn into the blunt needle.

OPERATIONS FOR DEEP VEIN THROMBOSIS

Appraise

1 Perform duplex scanning to confirm the presence of thrombus.

2 Perform a venogram if you intend to carry out operative treatment.

3 Anticoagulant treatment is commonly used for the treatment of deep vein thrombosis unless anticoagulants are contraindicated.

4 There are two forms of intervention:

- Venous thrombectomy is usually performed to remove a fresh (e.g. less than 5 days), loose and non-adherent thrombus.
- Insertion of filters to 'lock in' thrombus and prevent pulmonary embolism.

5 Operations are not indicated when the thrombus is more than 5 days old, fixed or totally occlusive. Surgery is also inappropriate when the thrombus is confined to the calf. These patients are best treated with anticoagulants.

6 Procedures to lock in the thrombus are indicated if anticoagulation is an unacceptable risk or ineffective, and especially when repeated pulmonary emboli occur despite adequate anticoagulant treatment.

7 Treat the uncommon complications of venous pregangrene (phlegmasia caerulen dolens) and gangrene by catheter-directed thrombolysis or venous thrombectomy.

8 Procedures to lock in the thrombus are thought to lower the mortality from pulmonary embolism in patients with loose propagated thrombus extending into the femoral or abdominal veins, although this has never been tested in a prospective randomized trial.

ILIOFEMORAL VENOUS THROMBECTOMY

Prepare

1 Heparinize the patient before going to theatre.

2 The operation can be performed under regional or spinal anaesthesia. If general anaesthetic is employed, endotracheal intubation and positive-pressure ventilation are preferable to stop any loose thrombi being propagated to the lungs, thus preventing intraoperative embolism.

3 Ensure that the operating table is suitable for taking intraoperative phlebograms.

4 Insert an indwelling urinary catheter to prevent phlebograms from being obscured by the accumulation of dye in the bladder.

5 Position the patient supine with the legs abducted on a radiographic operating table.

Access

1 Make a vertical incision over the femoral vein, extending from the mid-inguinal point to the centre of the thigh for 15–20 cm.

2 Divide the subcutaneous fat down to the deep fascia. The long saphenous vein lies medially, and can be traced up to the saphenofemoral junction.

3 Incise the deep fascia over the femoral vein in a vertical direction and gently dissect the femoral vein from the femoral artery on its lateral border. Use sharp dissection and avoid handling the vein if it contains loose thrombus.

4 Gently pass Silastic slings around the femoral vein above and below the profunda femoris vein, which is also snared.

Assess

1 Confirm the presence of thrombus within the femoral vein by gentle finger palpation.

Action

If the thrombus is present in the iliac vein

1. Tip the operating feet down (30°) to ensure caudal blood flow in the vein to minimize the risk of pulmonary embolism.
2. Administer 5000 units of heparin and make a short transverse venotomy. When the loose thrombus has been flushed out of the venotomy by retrograde flow, pass a large Fogarty venous thrombectomy catheter (size 6–8F) into the inferior vena cava. Inflate the balloon with contrast medium and withdraw it under fluoroscopic control while reducing the balloon diameter until it lies against the orifice of the common iliac vein. Beware of inadvertent insertion into a lumbar vein. Tighten the Silastic tubing around the catheter to prevent troublesome back-bleeding.
3. Pass a second large Fogarty catheter past the iliac thrombus, inflate the balloon and withdraw it to extract the thrombus. Repeat this until no further thrombus is obtained (Fig. 30.8).
4. When all the thrombus appears to have been removed, deflate the caval balloon slightly and withdraw it to remove any loose thrombus that it has trapped.
5. Infuse heparinized saline into the iliac vein and ensure that all the thrombus has been removed. Confirm this using completion phlebography.
6. Residual thrombus may be compressed against the vein wall by deploying a stent.
7. Remove any distal thrombus by the technique described above and close the venotomy with a continuous 6/0 Prolene suture.
8. Create an end-to-side arteriovenous fistula between a tributary of the femoral vein/long saphenous vein to the femoral artery below the venotomy. This ensures higher flow up the vein and reduces the incidence of re-thrombosis. Plan to close the fistula radiologically after 6 weeks.
9. Place a closed suction drain in the wound and close the wound in layers.

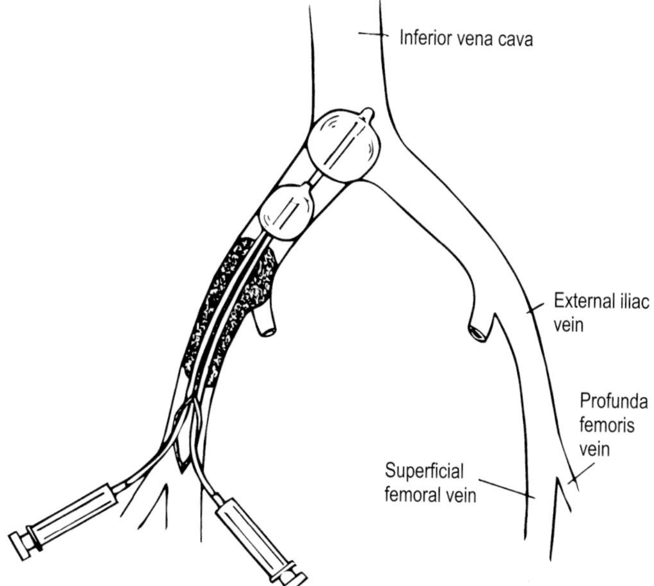

Fig. 30.8 Iliac venous thrombectomy.

If thrombus is present in the femoral vein

1. Give 5000 units of heparin.
2. Apply bulldog clamps on the proximal femoral and superficial femoral veins. Pass a suitable Fogarty venous thrombectomy catheter (4–5F) through a transverse venotomy as far distally as competent valves allow. The catheter rarely passes far down the leg.
3. Pull up the Silastic sling to prevent back-bleeding while the catheter is passed and withdrawn.
4. Inflate the catheter balloon and withdraw it slowly, pulling out the loose thrombus in advance of balloon).
5. Thrombus can be also be removed by manual compression applied along the line of the veins of the calf and thigh muscle or by applying a sterile Esmarch bandage around the limb. Distal thrombus can theoretically be removed using a Fogarty venous thrombectomy catheter passed through a tibial vein.
6. When no more thrombus can be obtained, close the venotomy with 6/0 Prolene suture and the wound in layers with a closed suction drain.

? DIFFICULTY

1. Retrograde passage of the catheter may prove difficult past competent vein valves; a caval filter may be a better option.
2. Loose thrombus trapped by the blocking catheter may be lost when the blocking catheter is withdrawn. A previously placed caval filter prevents this complication.

Postoperative care

1. Keep the patient on subcutaneous, low-molecular-weight heparin and allow mobilization while wearing a compression stocking on the day after surgery.
2. Start an oral anticoagulant on the third or fourth day until therapeutic prothrombin level is reached. Continue this for 3–6 months.
3. Encourage the patient to wear graduated compression stockings to prevent the development of post-thrombotic syndrome in future.

CAVAL CLIPPING

Appraise

This is now indicated only when the abdomen is being explored to remove coincidental pathology such as a malignancy.

The procedure should be avoided whenever possible as it causes significant lower limb oedema in at least 30% of patients.

Action

1. Carefully dissect free and snare a segment of vena cava between two pairs of lumbar veins, using a combination of sharp and blunt dissection.
2. Place a plastic Miles–DeWeese clip around the vena cava and hold it closed with a silk ligature. Alternatively pass three or four

mattress sutures across the vena cava from front to back and tie them down. The vena cava is converted into a number of small channels, preventing large emboli from reaching the lungs (Fig. 30.9).

3 Ensure that you apply the clip above the upper limit of the thrombus. Access may be difficult in a fat patient with a large malignant liver, or with retroperitoneal spread of tumour.

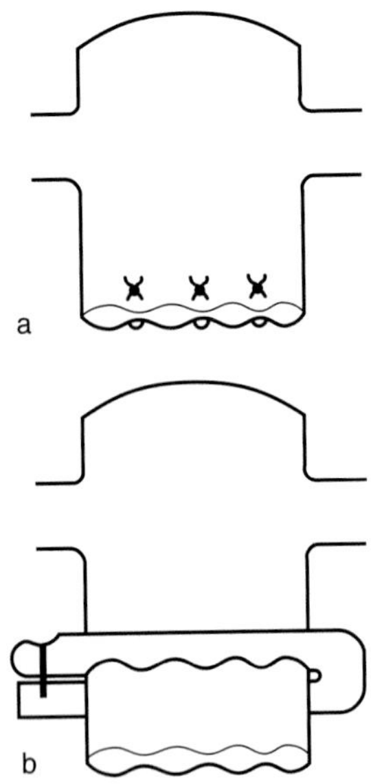

Fig. 30.9 Partial inferior vena cava interruption: (a) the Spencer plication with multiple stitches; (b) the Miles–DeWeese caval clip.

INSERTION OF UMBRELLA FILTER

Appraise

1 Vena cava filters (Fig. 30.10) are now usually inserted by radiologist rather than by surgical insertion.

2 Some filters are removable.

3 The Greenfield–Kimway umbrella filter can be inserted into the inferior vena cava via a venotomy in the internal jugular vein over a guidewire under local anaesthesia.

Access

1 Expose the right internal jugular vein through a transverse incision placed over the sternomastoid muscle, 2 cm above the clavicle.

2 Deepen the incision, dividing the platysma muscle and the clavicular head of the sternocleidomastoid muscle. Alternatively, split and retract the sternal and clavicular heads of the muscle and separate them by retraction to expose the internal jugular vein.

3 Mobilize the vein by blunt dissection and pass a pair of Silastic slings around it.

4 Isolate a 1–2-cm length of vein.

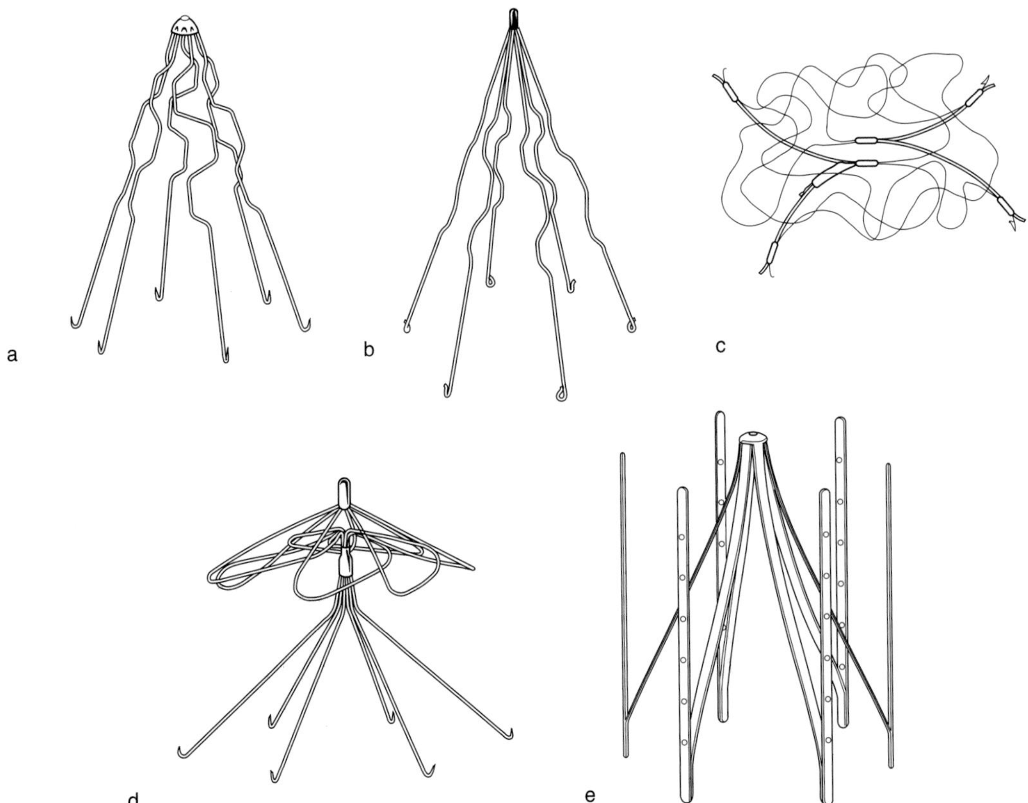

Fig. 30.10 Diagram of the permanent caval filter modules: (a) the stainless steel Greenfield filter; (b) the modified hook titanium Greenfield filter; (c) the birds' nest filter; (d) the Simon nitinol filter; (e) the Venea Tech filter.

5 Make a longitudinal venotomy place two stay sutures into the edges so you can hold it opened, or close it.

6 Dilate the vein with urethral dilators.

7 Insert the catheter containing the filter through the venotomy and screen it into the inferior vena cava using an image intensifier.

8 Prevent continuing blood loss by pulling the edges of the venotomy together with the stay sutures.

9 When you think that the catheter lies in the vena cava below the renal veins, and have confirmed the position using contrast venography, eject the filter, which fixes into the side-wall of the cava by a series of tiny barbs around its periphery. These barbs are designed to prevent the filter from migrating, which is the major complication of the procedure. Incorrect sitting of the filter may also be a problem.

10 Most modern inferior vena cava filters are now inserted percutaneously by a radiologist.

Postoperative

1 Maintain intravenous heparinization for a minimum of 48 hours after the procedure, unless there is a strong contraindication.

2 Encourage all patients who have had a severe deep vein thrombosis to wear graduated compression elastic stockings to prevent the development of the post-thrombotic syndrome and venous ulceration in the future.

▶ KEY POINTS Indications?

- Controlled clinical trials are needed to provide clear guidance on the indications for inserting a venous filter.
- Consider catheter directed thrombolysis and insertion of caval filters in patients with severe leg swelling or a pulmonary embolus.

OPERATIONS FOR VENOUS ULCER AND POST-THROMBOTIC SYNDROME

Appraise

Hopes that operations for saphenous and communicating vein reflux would prevent recurrent venous ulceration in post-thrombotic limbs have not been fulfilled.

A plethora of new operations has been developed in an attempt to improve ulcer prophylaxis. None of them has proved very successful.

Saphenous transposition (Palma operation)

1 This is valuable for symptomatic venous claudication but use it only when the femoral venous pressure rises on exercise (Fig. 30.11).

2 It is valuable only in the absence of naturally developed suprapubic collateral channels, which are often massive.

3 Dissect the contralateral saphenous vein down and mobilize it until you can swing it across in a suprapubic tunnel to anastomose it to the common femoral or profunda femoris vein of the opposite limb, thus providing a collateral channel for a single blocked iliac segment.

4 Patency of bypass may be improved with an arteriovenous fistula.

Valvular repair

1 The valve cusps are tightened using reefing sutures, in an attempt to render incompetent valves competent.

2 It is of value only in the rare condition of primary valve incompetence. It can now be performed angioscopically.

Long saphenous or profunda femoris transposition

1 Divide the femoral vein below the profunda vein and anastomose the distal end, end-to-end to the long saphenous vein below a competent valve (Fig. 30.12).

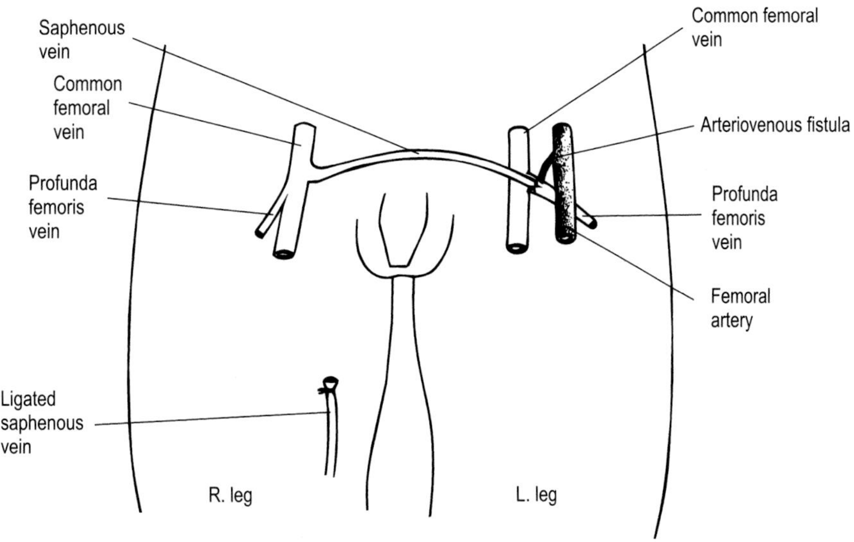

Fig. 30.11 Saphenous transposition bypass.

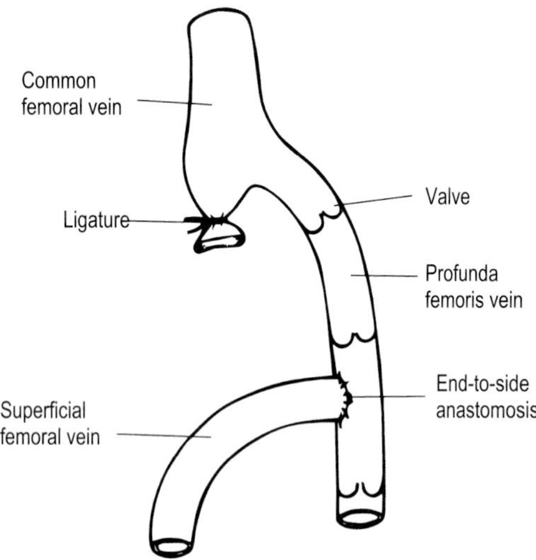

Fig. 30.12 Profunda femoris transposition.

2 Results so far have been disappointing, and the chief protagonists of the operation have abandoned it.

Autograft insertion

Use the opposite saphenous vein to bypass obstructed segments of vein, or transplant a competent valve in a segment of brachial vein into a femoral vein with severe reflux. These transplants rarely retain valvular competence.

Plastic venocuffs

These have been used as a means of external venous support to restore primary valvular competence.

Caval and iliac vein bypass grafting

Complete occlusion of the iliac vein and vena cava can be bypassed with externally supported PTFE as an onlay graft combined with an adjuvant arteriovenous fistula inserted below the graft on each side, and closed at 6 weeks.

Experimental valves

These have been made by intussusception. PTFE or saphenous vein have been used to fill the venous defect caused by the intussusception.

SPLIT SKIN GRAFT FOR VENOUS ULCERATION

Prepare

1 Following bed rest and intensive antiseptic cleaning, the base of the ulcer should improve.

2 Dirty ulcers with poor bases should be excised in theatre down to healthy tissue before attempting skin grafting. Prepare the ulcer by excising the basal tissues with a Humby or Braithwaite knife using tangential excision. This is the best method of preparing almost all ulcers for grafting.

3 Meshed split skin grafts should be applied to the dry base using staples. Postage stamp or pinch graft can be used as an alternative.

Postoperative

1 If investigation shows the deep veins to be normal, surgically treat sites of superficial vein incompetence to provide good ulcer prophylaxis.

2 When the deep veins are shown to have severe post-thrombotic changes on ascending phlebography, prescribe permanent elastic support stockings, and consider one of the operations described above.

LYMPHATIC SURGERY

Appraise

1 If lymphoedema is a likely cause of chronic limb swelling, perform isotope or contrast lymphography to confirm the diagnosis.

2 The majority of the patients with primary and secondary lymphoedema respond readily to active conservative treatment. Regular leg elevation, elastic support and massage are all that is needed to maintain an acceptable level of swelling.

3 If, despite adequate conservative management, a few patients develop severe limb swelling that interferes with mobility, consider operative treatment.

4 Perform bilateral contrast lymphography in most patients considered for lymphatic surgery. This displays anatomical information about the site and cause of the lymphatic impairment and may help to select the appropriate surgical procedure. Most patients with primary lymphoedema have slowly progressive distal lymphatic hypoplasia. A smaller number suffer progressive fibrosis of the proximal lymph nodes, leading to obstruction. The distal lymphatics also slowly disappear in these patients. A few have obstruction of the thoracic duct, and a few have megalymphatics with valvular incompetence.

5 Surgery for lymphoedema can be divided into two broad approaches:

- *Reduction operations*. The lymphoedematous subcutaneous tissue and skin are excised; these procedures can be used to treat all forms of lymphoedema.
- *Bypass operations*. These procedures bypass sites of localized lymphatic obstruction, and are suitable for patients with a proximal occlusion and normal distal lymphatics. The mesenteric bridge operation is applicable for patients with obstruction of the femoral or pelvic lymph nodes. Lymphovenous anastomosis has also been proposed as a means of bypassing lymphatic obstruction. Neither of these procedures has found widespread acceptance in clinical practice.

Prepare

Fully inform the patients about the surgery that is proposed for them. They should have a realistic appreciation of the expected functional and cosmetic results (Fig. 30.13). Patients must understand that lymphatic surgery is palliative, and further surgery may be necessary, later.

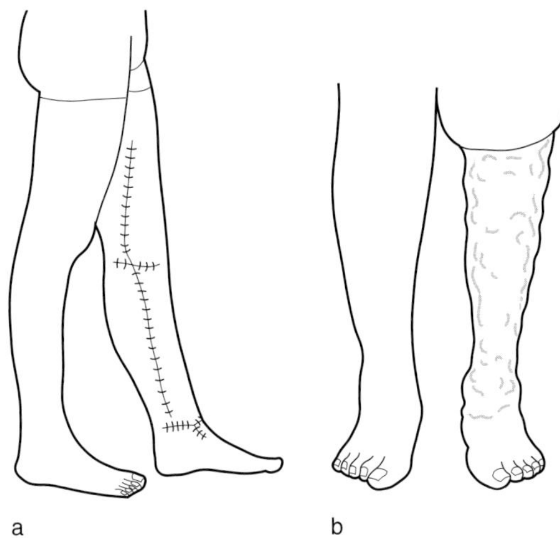

Fig. 30.13 Cosmetic results of reduction operations: (a) Homan's operation; (b) Charles' operation.

REDUCTION OPERATIONS

Prepare

1 Minimize swelling prior to surgery with a period of bed rest and elevation of limb and by compression with a 'lymphopress' machine.

2 Eradicate sepsis prior to surgery. Swab possible sites of infection on admission and send for microscopy and culture. Antibiotics are prescribed selectively. Clean the limb twice daily in an antiseptic bath, paying special attention to the skin creases. Tinea pedis commonly develops between swollen lymphoedematous toes. Take a skin scraping if the diagnosis is suspected and prescribe a suitable antifungal treatment, such as terbinafine.

3 Perform reduction operations under general anaesthesia with the patient in supine position.

4 Position the limb to facilitate operative access. For procedures on the medial side of the leg, elevate the limb to about 30–45° and widely abduct it. This is best achieved by inserting a Kirschner wire through the calcaneum and connecting a metal stirrup to the wire on each side of the foot before elevating the leg with a pulley system. Lower the foot of the operating table and flex the contralateral knee. Stand on the medial side of the leg, between the limb and the operating table.

5 To reduce blood loss, place a tourniquet around the upper thigh and inflate it to 350 mmHg after the limb has been exsanguinated with an Esmarch bandage. Note the time of tourniquet application.

CHARLES' OPERATION

Action

1 This was described by the English surgeon R.H. Charles in 1912. Aim to excise the lymphoedematous skin and subcutaneous tissue between the knee and the ankle, including the dorsum of the foot. This is the procedure of choice when the skin is greatly thickened and abnormal. Preserve skin cover over the knee and the ankle in order to retain the mobility of these joints (Fig. 30.14).

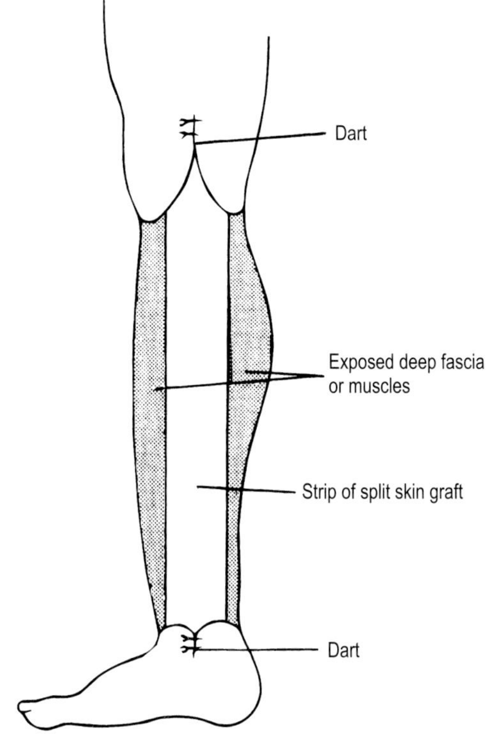

Fig. 30.14 Charles' leg reduction operation.

2 Cover the exposed deep fascia of the leg with split skin grafts taken from the trunk or from the contralateral limb.

3 Take darts of redundant skin and subcutaneous tissue from the medial and lateral sides of the leg at the knee and ankle to prevent a marked 'step' effect and an ugly appearance similar to pantaloons.

4 Staple the skin grafts to the deep fascia and cover them with non-adherent dressings and thick cotton wool held in place with crepe bandages.

5 Plan to maintain elevation of the limb for 1 week, before removing the bandages and inspecting the limb.

Complications

1 Delayed healing may be a problem if the split skin graft fails to take.

KEY POINT Spare skin

- Take spare skin grafts at the initial operation; these can be applied to unhealed areas in the ward at a later stage.

2 Hypertrophic and keloid scars sometimes develop in the grafted skin. Hypertrophic scarring is often associated with chronic infection; treat it by regular cleansing and antibiotics. Prominent tissue can be shaved off with a skin-graft knife. Keloid scar may need to be excised and re-grafted.

3 The Charles' operation is very effective at reducing the excessive bulk of lymphoedematous tissues around the leg, and improving mobility. The final appearance is, however, often bizarre, with swollen feet and thighs joined by a narrow calf.

HOMANS' OPERATION

Appraise

1 John Homans (1877–1954) was Professor of Surgery at Harvard, Boston. Lymphoedematous swelling of the moderate severity in limbs with relatively normal skin is best reduced by the operation described by him.

2 The operation is usually first performed on the medial side of the limb, but the tissues on the lateral side can also be reduced. If you intend to operate on both sides, stage the procedures over 3 months, otherwise skin viability is compromised if the excision extends beyond half the circumference of the limb.

3 Aim to excise lymphoedematous subcutaneous tissues and redundant skin from one side of the limb. When the limb is viewed in cross-section the excised tissues appeared wedge-shaped (Fig. 30.15a).

4 Prefer to raise the skin flaps first, then excise the underlying fat. Overlap the skin flaps to decide how much redundant skin needs to be excised.

Action

1 Make a longitudinal incision from a hand's breadth below the knee to a similar distance above the ankle, beginning just behind the posterior border of the tibia, ending anterior to the medial malleolus. Transverse incisions may also be necessary at each of the longitudinal incision (Fig. 30.15b).

2 Raise skin flaps in an anterior and posterior direction that increase in thickness towards the base of the flap. Extend the flaps for 10–12 cm around the leg or as far as the midline in each direction.

3 Excise all the underlying subcutaneous tissue not included in the skin flaps, down to the deep fascia. Excise any superficial veins and cutaneous nerves with this block of tissue.

4 Overlap the flaps and mark the redundant skin to be excised, allowing for primary closure of the incision. Having excised the skin, if necessary trim the skin flaps in a longitudinal direction. Excise darts at the ankle and knee to avoid dog-ears. The darts should meet the transverse incision at a different point from the longitudinal incision to reduce the chance of wound breakdown. The upper dart may be extended a considerable distance up the limb towards the groin thigh to allow a simple wedge excision of the skin and subcutaneous tissues of the thigh, as shown in Fig. 30.15.

5 Close the skin with interrupted sutures or staples over Redivac drains.

6 Apply a non-adherent dressing to the suture lines and dress the whole limb from the base of the toes with cotton wool and crepe bandages.

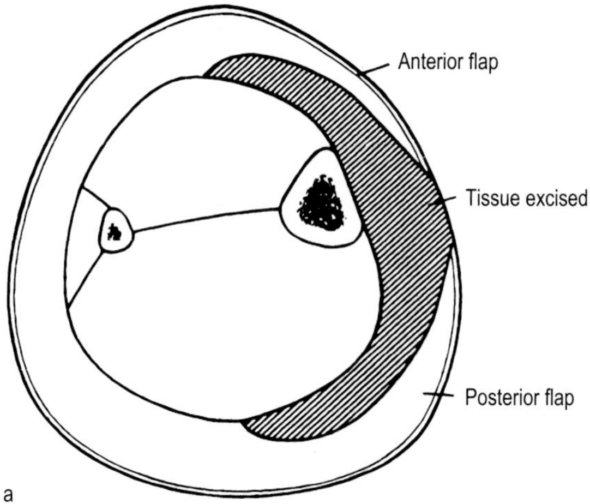

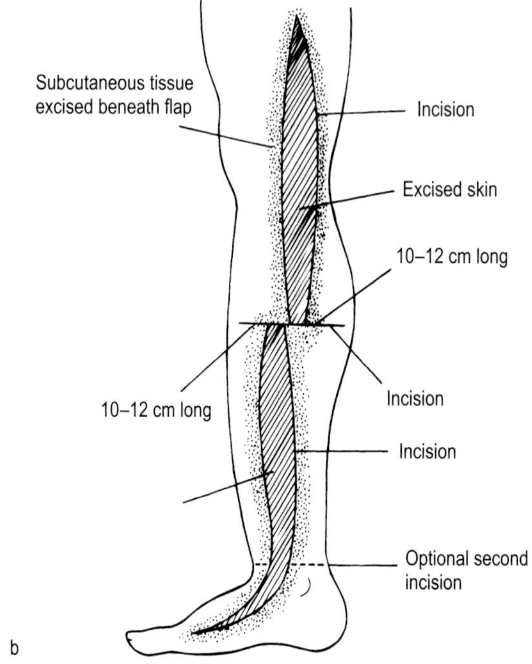

Fig. 30.15 Homan's medial leg reduction operation.

Postoperative care

Nurse the patient with the foot of the bed elevated 10°. Take down the dressing and remove the drains after 1 week, then mobilize the patient.

Complications

1 Although the early results appear good, many patients develop recurrent limb swelling, eventually approaching preoperative dimensions.

2 Repeated reduction surgery may be necessary. Combined with good elastic stocking support, this often produces an acceptable limb, although its size is rarely normal.

3 Skin necrosis, infection and haematoma formation are all recognized problems.

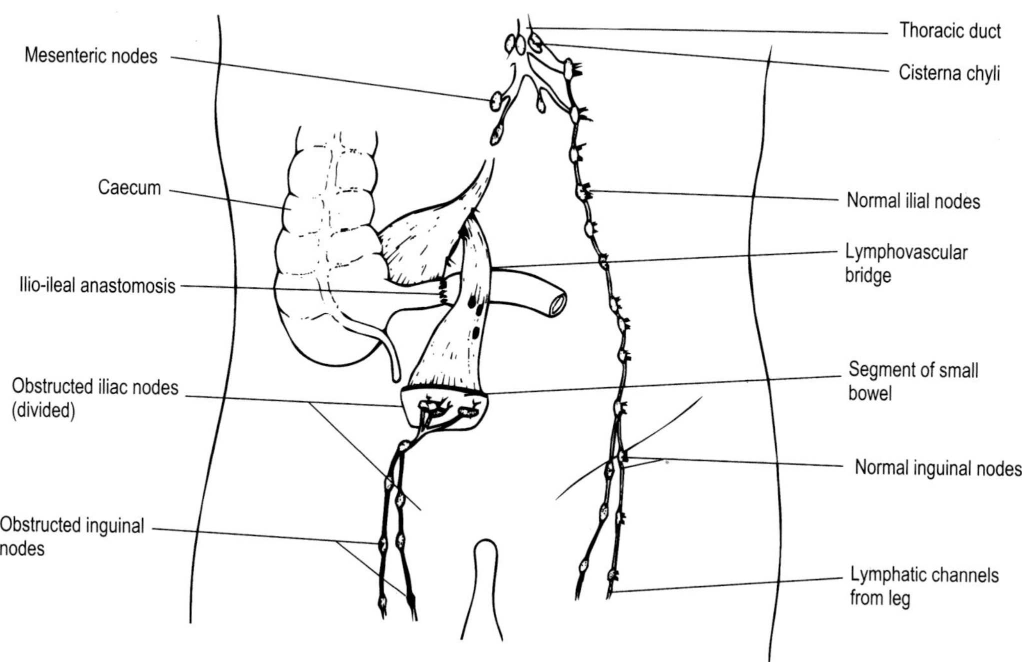

Fig. 30.16 Kinmonth's mesenteric bridge operation.

> **KEY POINTS Skin-flap necrosis**
>
> - Avoid haematoma formation by meticulous haemostasis.
> - Do not risk skin-flap necrosis; avoid cutting the flaps too think or extending the undermining too far.

BYPASS OPERATIONS

KINMONTH'S ENTEROMESENTERIC BRIDGE OPERATION

Appraise

1 Many patients with obstructed femoral or iliac lymphatics may be helped by this operation (Fig. 30.16).

2 An enteromesenteric bridge works only if there are frankly obstructed lymphatics. Demonstrate that the thoracic duct and proximal lymphatic are normal.

3 The operation involves the risks of major abdominal surgery and it has a limited application only.

Prepare

1 Perform the operation under general anaesthesia with the patient supine.

2 Prepare and drape the patient to expose the abdomen and groins.

Action

1 Open the abdomen through a lower midline abdominal incision.

2 If the bridge is to be brought out into apposition with the femoral lymph nodes, make a vertical incision in the groin.

3 Isolate a 5–10-cm length of ileum on its lymphatic and vascular pedicle. Re-anastomose the ileum in one or two layers, in front of, or behind, the pedicle.

4 Make an incision with diathermy along the antemesenteric border of the isolated ileal segment to open it out. Inject 1:400 000 adrenaline (epinephrine) in saline into the submucosal plane and strip away the mucosa by blunt dissection.

5 The contrast lymphangiogram demonstrates the level of obstruction. Confirm the presence of iliac or femoral lymph nodes by palpation at or below the point of obstruction. Select one or more suitably sized lymph nodes and minimally dissect them to expose their proximal surface, taking care to preserve the afferent lymphatics.

6 Incise and bivalve the nodes, using sutures to hold the cut surface open.

7 Bring down the ileal bridge and suture it over the split lymph nodes. You need to create a passage by blunt finger dissection beneath the inguinal ligament, through the femoral canal, to reach the femoral nodes.

Closure

1 Place closed suction drainage in the groin, and close the wound with 2/0 polyglactin to the subcutaneous tissue and interrupted 4/0 nylon to skin.

2 Close the abdomen in the normal manner.

FURTHER READING

Adam DJ, Bello M, Hartshorne T et al 2003 Role of superficial venous surgery in patients with combined superficial and segmental deep venous reflex. European Journal of Vascular and Endovascular Surgery 25:469–472

Amarigi SV, Lees TA 2000 Elastic compression stockings for prevention of deep vein thrombosis. Cochrane Database of Systematic Reviews CD001484

Barwell JR, Davies CE, Deacon J et al 2004 Comparison of surgery and compression with compression alone in chronic venous ulceration (ESCHAR study): randomised controlled trial. Lancet 363:1854–1859

Browse N 1999 Diseases of the veins, 2nd edn. Arnold, London

Burnand K 1998 The new Aird's companion in surgical studies, 2nd edn. Churchill Livingstone, Edinburgh

Campisi C, Boccardo F, Zilli A et al 2001 Long-term results after lymphatic–venous anastomoses for the treatment of obstructive lymphedema. Microsurgery 21:135–139

Corrales NE, Irvine A, McGuiness CL et al 2002 Incidence and pattern of long saphenous vein duplication and its possible implications for recurrence after varicose vein surgery. British Journal of Surgery 89:323–326

Dwerryhouse S, Davies B, Harradine K et al 1999 Stripping the long saphenous vein reduces the rate of reoperation for recurrent varicose veins: five-year results of a randomized trial. Journal of Vascular Surgery 29:589–592

Elias M, Frasier KL 2004 Minimally invasive vein surgery: its role in the treatment of venous stasis ulceration. American Journal of Surgery 188:26–30

Kalra M, Gloviczki P 2003 Surgical treatment of venous ulcers: role of subfascial endoscopic perforator vein ligation. Surgical Clinics of North America 83:671–705

Serror P 2002 Sural nerve lesions: a report of 20 cases. American Journal of Physical Medicine and Rehabilitation 81:876–880

Zamboni P, Cisno C, Marchetti F et al 2003 Minimally invasive surgical management of primary venous ulcers vs. compression treatment: a randomized clinical trial. European Journal of Vascular and Endovascular Surgery 25: 313–318

Zierau UT, Kullmer A, Kunkel HP 1996 Stripping the Giacomini vein: pathophysiologic necessity or phlebosurgical games? Vasa 25:142–147

31

Sympathectomy

J.A. Rennie

CONTENTS

SYMPATHETIC NERVOUS SYSTEM

1 The arteries to the skin and muscle of the limbs have a sympathetic innervation. The sympathetic nerves to the skin of the hands and feet are predominantly vasoconstrictor, but both vasoconstrictor and vasodilator fibres are present to the arteries in muscle. At rest there is a dominant vasoconstrictor tone to skin and muscle. Following sympathetic blockade, skin flow increases markedly and sweating is inhibited, and there is a modest rise in muscle flow. However, the increase in muscle flow during sympathetic blockade is only one-tenth the increase in flow seen during exercise of the muscle. This exercise-induced increase is mediated by the liberation of local metabolites from the contracting muscle fibres.

2 The preganglionic sympathetic fibres, which are myelinated ('white') rami communicantes, pass through the ventral roots of the spinal nerves, travel in the sympathetic chain and synapse in the ganglia. Postganglionic, unmyelinated ('grey') rami communicantes pass from the ganglia to the corresponding spinal nerves to enter the limb in one or other of the major nerve trunks.

3 Hyperhidrosis and facial flushing or blushing are the only absolute indications for thoracic sympathectomy. A relative indication is Raynaud's disease, where a good result can be expected but where a return to the original symptoms can be predicted within 6–12 months.

4 Sympathectomy may also have a role in digital artery thrombosis, secondary to a cervical rib. Reduction in sympathetic tone may reverse pregangrenous changes. Sympathectomy may also benefit patients with post-traumatic pain or causalgia, acrocyanosis and trophic changes following poliomyelitis.

THORACIC SYMPATHECTOMY

Appraise

1 The sympathetic fibres to the arm synapse in ganglia T2–3 (T2 for the hand and T2+3 for the axilla). The upper (T1) ganglion fuses with the inferior cervical ganglion to form the stellate ganglion. Damage to the stellate will produce a Horner's syndrome.

2 There are several approaches to the upper thoracic sympathetic chain: the approaches may be transaxillary or anterior (supraclavicular). However, the thoracoscopic method is well tried and effective and has become the standard against which more complicated procedures must be judged.

THORACOSCOPIC SYMPATHECTOMY

Preparation and consent

1 Order a preoperative chest X-ray for all patients to exclude any pulmonary disease which may make the establishment of a pneumothorax difficult.

2 Obtain fully informed consent for the procedure yourself, ideally at the initial consultation and subsequently in the immediate preoperative period, both verbally and with a patient information sheet.

3 Apart from a clear explanation of the procedure itself, warn all patients about compensatory sweating, Horner's syndrome, postoperative pain in the chest and arms and the occasional need to insert an intercostal underwater chest drain. Finally, advise that there is a 10% failure to resolve facial flushing completely.

Access

1 Perform the procedure under a general anaesthetic, ideally with a double-lumen tube. A standard endotracheal tube is, however, sufficient if the tube cannot be passed successfully.

2 Place the patient in a supine position with both arms abducted to 60°.

3 Once the appropriate lung has been deflated, establish an artificial pneumothorax using a Veress needle inserted through the third intercostal space.

4 Slowly insufflate 1 litre of carbon dioxide into the pleural space.

KEY POINT Be cautious

- Do not introduce the gas rapidly or you may produce a profound bradycardia as the mediastinum shifts away from the needle.

5 Through the same 0.5-cm incision introduce a 5-mm thoracoscope through a cannula, and under direct vision advance it across the pleural cavity until you identify the ribs.

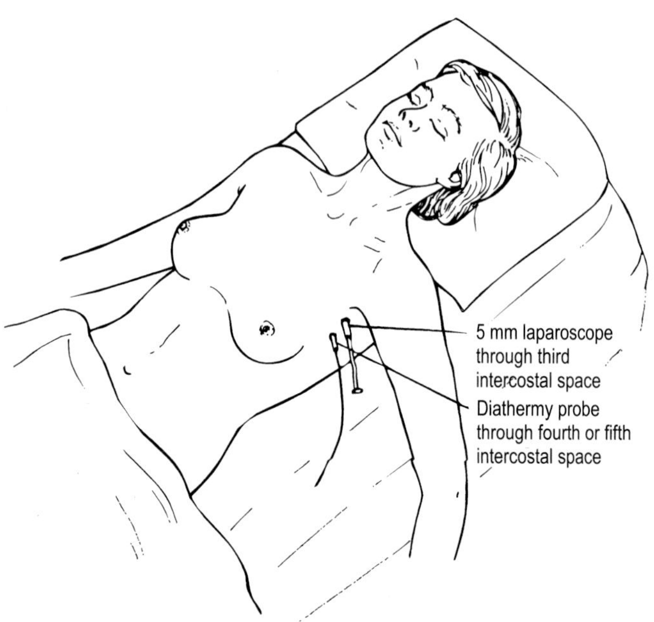

Fig. 31.1 Insert a diathermy probe through an insulated cannula through the fourth or fifth interspace.

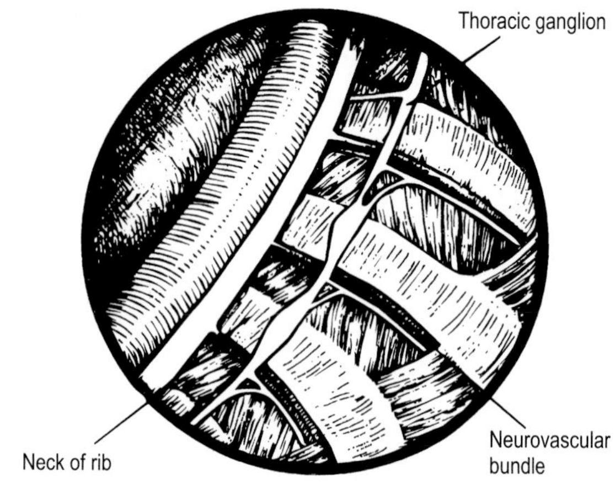

Fig. 31.2 View for left thoracic sympathectomy.

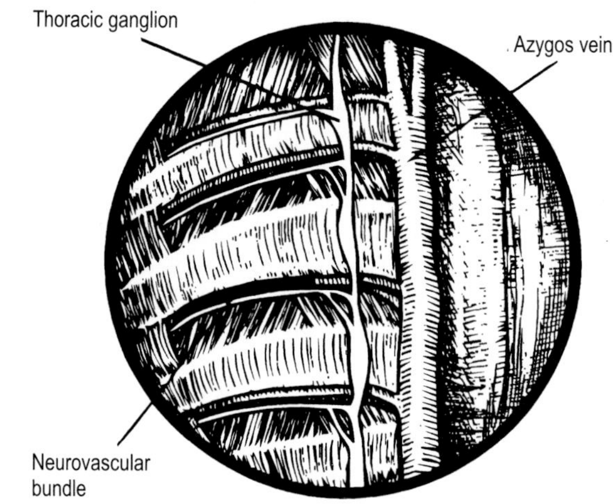

Fig. 31.3 View for right thoracic sympathectomy.

Assess

1 Follow the ribs medially until you see the sympathetic ganglia and chain lying on the necks of the ribs. The highest rib you see on either side is the second, although in the tall, thin patient the first rib may be visible through the thoracoscope.

2 Assess the position of the first rib by asking the anaesthetist to palpate the rib in the supraclavicular fossa. If you see the rib covered by the palpating finger, avoid operating on the chain at that level so as to avoid creating a Horner's syndrome.

3 You may need to divide pleural adhesions to see the ganglia. Slowly introduce carbon dioxide via the cannula at no greater pressure than 10 cmH_2O.

Action

1 Introduce a pair of endoscopic shears via an insulated cannula through a separate stab incision in the anterior axillary line through the fifth intercostal space (Fig. 31.1).

2 Identify the ganglia by pushing against them gently with the scissors to confirm their soft consistency and glistening surface (Fig. 31.2). If adhesions obscure the view over the second rib, you can easily identify the chain by visualizing the fourth or fifth rib and following the chain superiorly.

KEY POINT Anatomy

- In the right chest the azygos vein may lie close to the sympathetic ganglia and it can be of a considerable diameter (Fig. 31.3).

3 If necessary carefully incise the pleura along the lateral border of the azygos vein to expose the sympathetic chain fully. Be willing to rotate the operating table into the 'anti-Trendelenburg' (head-up) position, to decompress the veins and expose the third rib.

4 Carefully dissect the second thoracic ganglia over the second rib using sharp dissection only, to avoid creating a Horner's syndrome. Use the lowest power on the unipolar diathermy current that is necessary to achieve haemostasis. Make a preliminary burn over the rib away from the nerve to select the lowest and most effective power setting. Once you have cleanly dissected the nerve over the second rib, divide it under direct vision. Now place the inferior cut end of the chain below the rib to avoid later regeneration of the sympathetic chain.

KEY POINT Horner's syndrome

- Horner's syndrome should not occur with this thoracoscopic method as the first rib with the T1 ganglion is not visualized.

5 Clipping of the sympathetic chain is possible and is reputed to achieve the same result in both hyperhidrosis and facial flushing. A theoretical advantage is that the clips can be removed later if complicating side-effects are intolerable.

6 Cut or diathermize the chain as it crosses the third rib to isolate the second ganglion.

7 Remove the scissors and cannula. Hold the thoracoscope ready while the lung is re-inflated, with the insertion tube still in place. Finally, check that the lung is fully inflated by re-inserting the thoracoscope and observing the size of any residual pneumothorax.

8 If the lung has re-inflated, remove the thoracoscope and cannula, and close the two small wounds with a stitch or plastic adhesive strip.

Aftercare

1 Have a chest X-ray performed in the recovery area to check for residual pneumothorax. A small pneumothorax is acceptable and is usually re-absorbed within 24 hours. Chest drains are not needed routinely.

2 Return the patient to the ward and discharge the following day as a rule.

3 You can confidently predict the patient's hands will be dry following this procedure. Immediate resolution of facial flushing is noted in 90% of patients, reducing to 85% at 2 years.

4 Compensatory hyperhidrosis, usually on the chest and back, occurs in 50% of patients, whichever method is used.

5 It is safe to operate on both sides of the chest under one anaesthetic.

6 You do not routinely need to insert chest drains.

? DIFFICULTY

1. If the patient becomes bradycardic or hypotensive because of mediastinal shift, or the oxygen tension falls precipitately, stop the surgical procedure, offer to reduce the pneumothorax and allow the anaesthetist to re-inflate the lung. Continue with the procedure once the patient is stabilized.
2. Transient Horner's syndrome may occur if you employ a too high-powered diathermy current, or if you cause damage above the level of the second rib.
3. Haemorrhage may occur as a result of intercostal vessel trauma or damage to the azygos vein during diathermy. Have available a suction device that can pass through the insertion tube and long enough to reach across the hemithorax.
4. Adhesions within the chest may cause you to abandon the procedure. However, most adhesions are amenable to division with a combination of sharp dissection and diathermy.
5. Judicious tipping of the patient in the head-up position may allow you to complete the procedure even though the patient is unable to tolerate one-lung anaesthesia.

TRANSAXILLARY APPROACH

Access

1 Place the patient in a supine position with sandbags under the shoulder and iliac crest. Widely display the axilla by abducting the arm and flexing the forearm, which is then secured to an arm rest by a crepe bandage. Stand behind the patient.

2 The highest rib that can be felt in the axilla is the second. Make an 8-cm oblique incision from latissimus dorsi, running forwards and down across the third rib, roughly in the mid-axilla, as far as the posterior border of pectoralis major.

3 Incise the skin and fatty tissue down to the rib. Divide the periosteum longitudinally with cutting diathermy and reflect it from the superior surface, thereby exposing the costal pleura. It is not necessary to excise a section of rib.

4 Divide the pleura along the upper border of the rib. Insert a rib retractor and open it widely.

5 Displace the apex of the lung downwards with a cloth-covered lung retractor.

6 Always insert a retractor with attached fibreoptic light or a sterile fibre light to illuminate the pleural cavity.

Action

1 Define the ganglia and interconnecting chain as they run beneath the costal pleura over the necks of the corresponding ribs. The neck of the first rib is palpable but the stellate ganglion may be difficult to visualize.

2 Open the pleura over the sympathetic chain on the second rib.

3 Grasp the chain immediately above the second thoracic ganglion with long artery forceps. Divide the chain above the T2 ganglion after clamping the chain above and below with haemostatic clips, such as Ligaclips. Lift the chain forwards to expose the rami communicantes. Divide the rami between haemostatic clips or with diathermy.

4 Do not repair the costal pleura. If you are anxious about the control of bleeding or lung expansion, bring out a chest drain through a separate stab incision in the third intercostal space. Connect the drain to an underwater seal.

5 Perform an intercostal nerve block with bupivacaine (Marcaine) at the end of the operation to reduce the likelihood of intercostal pain.

6 Use strong absorbable sutures around the second and third ribs to close the chest. Ask the anaesthetist to re-expand the lungs. Close the muscle in layers. Close the skin by a standard technique.

7 You may excise the opposite sympathetic chain after re-positioning the patient, provided the lung is fully expanded on the operated side.

Aftercare

1 Order a chest X-ray immediately after the operation to determine whether the lung has re-expanded satisfactorily.

2 Haemothorax may develop following damage to intercostal veins. If there is no intercostal drain, aspirate the blood and insert a drain if blood re-accumulates.

3 Aspirate air from a pneumothorax only if it is symptomatic.

4 There is no treatment for postoperative Horner's syndrome caused by damage to the stellate ganglion, although the majority recover over 6–12 months.

ANTERIOR APPROACH

Access

1 Place the patient supine, with a sandbag under the shoulders, the head turned to the opposite side and the table tilted feet-down to about 30°.

2 Make a 5-cm incision placed 1 cm above the clavicle, so that the medial 1 cm overlies the lateral border of the sternomastoid muscle. Divide the platysma with the skin.

3 Divide the lateral fibres of sternomastoid. Locate and divide any large veins in this area, including the external jugular vein, if they are in the way. Insert a small self-retaining retractor.

4 Locate the scalenus anterior muscle, which runs down the centre of the field to be inserted into the first rib. It is obscured by fatty areolar tissue, which can be teased aside. Carefully avoid the thoracic duct on the left-hand side.

5 Identify the phrenic nerve passing obliquely over the anterior surface of the scalenus muscle (Fig. 31.4). Tape the nerve and gently retract it medially.

6 Transect the scalenus muscle in line with the skin incision, by grasping the muscle bundles with toothed forceps and dividing them with scissors. Divide the posterior surface of the muscle, which is tendinous.

KEY POINT Anatomy

- Avoid damaging the subclavian artery, which lies immediately behind the scalenus anterior.

7 Expose the arch of the subclavian artery. Place a tape around it and mobilize it as far as possible. Gently tear through the suprapleural (Sibson's) fascia immediately below the subclavian artery.

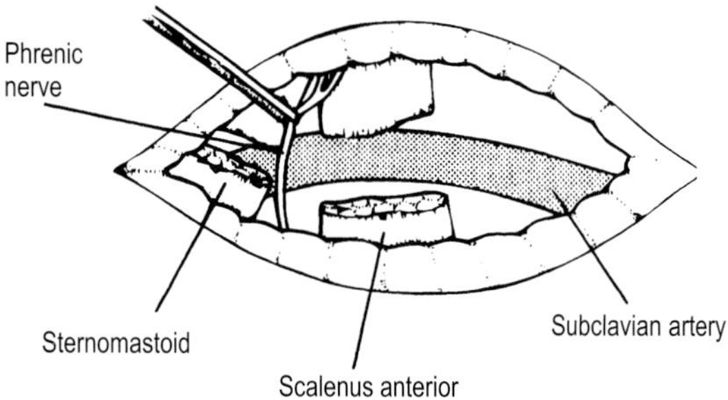

Fig. 31.4 The lateral fibres of sternomastoid have been divided, the phrenic nerve retracted and scalenus anterior divided to expose the subclavian artery.

8 Push the pleura downwards and laterally with swabs, from the neck of the first four ribs. Seal damaged intercostal veins with diathermy or haemostatic clips.

9 Retract the subclavian artery upwards or downwards.

10 The sympathetic chain can now be excised. Identify the stellate ganglion, which lies over the neck of the first rib. The chain runs downwards from this.

Action

1 Pick up the chain with a nerve hook or artery forceps between the stellate ganglion and the second thoracic ganglion. Maintain tension on the chain and divide the rami of the second and subsequent ganglia between haemostatic clips.

2 Divide the chain below the T4 ganglion and below the stellate ganglion. Lift out the chain.

3 Allow the lung to re-expand. Do not repair the scalenus anterior or sternomastoid muscles.

4 Close the subcutaneous tissues with absorbable sutures. Close the skin.

5 If necessary, remove the contralateral sympathetic chain immediately.

? DIFFICULTY

1. If a cervical rib is present, retract the subclavian artery forwards to expose the band or rib. Excise the band or remove the rib with bone-nibbling forceps, until there is no projection left above or at its articulation with the first rib.
2. Avoid injury to the phrenic nerve by ensuring that it is retracted gently.
3. If you recognize that you have injured the thoracic duct, repair it if possible or ligate it.

HORNER'S SYNDROME

1 This is one of the most distressing complications of the open method of sympathectomy. Damage to the stellate ganglion, either by ablation or dissection, may render the patient permanently deformed, although many recover over 6–12 months.

2 Thoracoscopic sympathectomy has virtually abolished this complication. The reason for this is that the highest rib that can be directly viewed intrapleurally via the thoracoscope is the second rib. Avoid using diathermy and employ sharp dissection alone to isolate the ganglion over the neck of the highest, most easily viewed rib. This is safe, and Horner's syndrome should not occur.

3 In a personal series of 440 thoracoscopic sympathectomies, six cases of Horner's syndrome were recorded. Four were transient and resolved over a 1-year period. It is wise to refer these patients to an ophthalmic surgeon.

LUMBAR SYMPATHECTOMY

- Lumbar sympathectomy may be carried out as an open operation or non-operatively by injecting phenol into the lumbar chain. This latter technique has largely superseded the open operation and is particularly suited to the treatment of elderly patients with ischaemic rest pain, as it avoids the postoperative morbidity associated with a surgical sympathectomy.

- Surgical sympathectomy is now reserved for younger patients with hyperhidrosis, intractable vasospastic disease and causalgia, in whom the risk of operation is low and a more complete and permanent interruption of the lumbar sympathetic chain can be secured.
- The number of lumbar ganglia varies, but there are usually four on each side. The second and third ganglia are removed at operation.
- Avoid this technique in males because of the high risk of causing impotence. Some authors claim that to preserve normal ejaculation the first lumbar ganglion on at least one side must be left intact.

Appraise

Peripheral vascular disease

Patients with occlusive atherosclerotic disease of their distal vessels who are consequently unsuitable for vascular reconstruction (absent 'run-off') and have rest pain, pregangrene or dry gangrene of the toes may benefit from a chemical sympathectomy. Its major purpose is the relief of rest pain, which is relieved in 60% of cases for up to 3 years, and further benefit may be obtained by repeated phenol injections depending on the result of testing with galvanometry. The probable mechanism is interference with the afferent sensory pathway.

Sympathectomy does not increase blood flow to the muscle, but causes dilatation of arteriovenous anastomoses. Provided the circulation is relatively stable, it occasionally allows trophic lesions to heal. There is no improvement in the subsequent amputation rate of approximately 50%, and it is not useful if the ankle brachial index is less than 0.35 in non-diabetics, because at this level progressive deterioration is inevitable.[1] Sympathectomy has no place in the treatment of intermittent claudication and is of no proven benefit as an adjunct to aortoiliac bypass grafting. Although there is a transient increase in flow across the graft after sympathectomy from lowering of the peripheral resistance, no long-term improvement in graft patency has been demonstrated. Diabetics often have an autosympathectomy due to peripheral neuropathy and therefore rarely benefit from a sympathetic block.

Thromboangiitis obliterans (Buerger's disease)

This condition, probably of autoimmune origin, affects 30–50-year-old men who are heavy smokers.

Although sympathectomy provides a transient improvement it does not alter the obliterative vasculitis of the distal vessels and progressive gangrene of the toes and foot that occurs if they continue smoking.

Raynaud's syndrome

The primary vasospastic disorder, Raynaud's disease, affects the feet less often than the hands but, if severe and does not respond to precautions against the cold, lumbar sympathectomy tends to give a more lasting improvement than the equivalent procedure in the upper limbs.

Lumbar sympathectomy can be used as a last resort in Raynaud's phenomenon due to scleroderma or haematological disorders such as polycythaemia, cold agglutination, cryoglobulinaemia and sickle-cell disease, where ulceration of the toes has occurred and medical measures have failed.

Hyperhidrosis

Problematic hyperhidrosis of the feet, which is socially embarrassing and causes rotting of socks and shoes, is cured by lumbar sympathectomy.

Causalgia

Also called reflex sympathetic dystrophy, this burning pain associated with hypersensitivity and vasomotor disturbance is usually a consequence of trauma to a somatic nerve, for example from a war injury.

The diagnosis is often difficult and lumbar sympathetic blockade using local anaesthetic can be used to predict which patients will benefit from surgical sympathectomy.[2]

Cold injury

Freezing of the foot at temperatures below −1 °C (frostbite) is associated with arterial spasm and capillary sludging. The resultant tissue loss may be diminished by early sympathetic blockade or sympathectomy. Sympathectomy is not beneficial for feet exposed to the cold at temperatures above freezing (trench foot).

Others

Other indications for lumbar sympathectomy are acrocyanosis and erythromyalgia. It can also be used for the relief of rectal tenesmoid pain from carcinoma of the rectum and other pelvic organs.[3]

SURGICAL LUMBAR SYMPATHECTOMY

Access

1. Place the patient supine with a sandbag beneath the side of the operation to give a 20° tilt.
2. Make an 8–10-cm transverse incision at the level of the umbilicus, starting just medial to the linea semilunaris.
3. Incise the lateral border of the rectus sheath. Split the external oblique muscle and incise internal oblique with cutting diathermy. Carefully separate the transversalis fascia and muscle without entering the peritoneum. Remember that the peritoneum is tougher laterally.

Action

1. Sweep the peritoneum away from the muscle using finger and swab dissection, continuing this mobilization posteriorly and medially until the aorta on the left or the inferior vena cava on the right has been exposed.
2. Repair any holes created in the peritoneum before proceeding further. Place a Deaver retractor over the peritoneum laterally

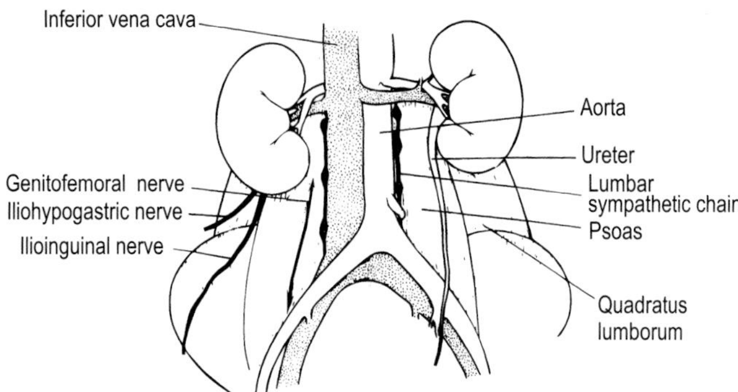

Fig. 31.5 The lumbar sympathetic chain runs down the sides of the bodies of the lumbar vertebrae immediately posterolateral to the inferior vena cava or aorta. The genitofemoral nerve and ureter are important structures that must be avoided.

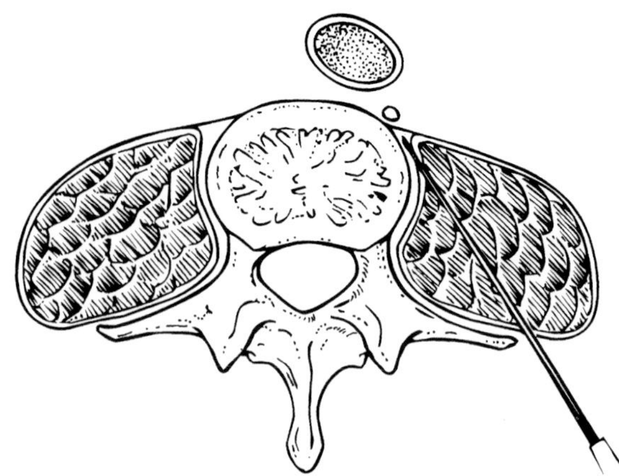

Fig. 31.6 In this posterior approach to chemical lumbar sympathectomy the retroperitoneal space can be located by a sudden loss of resistance to air injection as the needle is advanced through the psoas fascia.

and have it pulled firmly to open the retroperitoneal space in front of quadratus lumborum and psoas, while avoiding entering the wrong plane behind these muscles.

3 Lift the ureter forwards with the peritoneum out of harm's way. Other structures to avoid which may be confused with the sympathetic chain are the genitofemoral nerve, which runs on the anterior aspect of psoas, the psoas minor tendon and para-aortic lymphatics—identifiable because they are more friable than the sympathetic chain (Fig. 31.5).

4 The sympathetic chain on the left is the easiest to approach as it lies on loose areolar tissue alongside the aorta and can be palpated as a ganglionated cord against the vertebral bodies, where it runs just anterior to the insertion of psoas. It passes anterior to the lumbar vessels and posterior to the iliac vessels.

5 On the right side it lies behind the inferior vena cava, which is retracted gently with the tip of the Deaver retractor. Avoid tension and tearing of the lumbar veins, which occasionally pass in front of the sympathetic trunk on this side and can be a source of troublesome bleeding if not recognized and controlled with haemostatic clips.[4]

6 Lift the chain forwards with a nerve hook, diathermize and divide the rami communicantes, then excise the segment containing the second and third ganglia, after applying haemostatic clips, from the lower border of L2 to the lower border of L4.

Closure

1 Check haemostasis and if necessary place a drain in the retroperitoneal space.

2 Repair the muscles in layers with absorbable sutures.

3 Close the skin.

Aftercare

1 Postoperative ileus is brief except if a retroperitoneal haematoma forms, when it may be prolonged. The haematoma may need draining, but usually peristalsis is restored after 48 hours of a conservative regime.

2 Some patients experience post-sympathectomy neuralgia, a burning pain extending into the thigh. The explanation is unknown but it resolves after a few weeks.

3 Men in whom both first lumbar ganglia are inadvertently removed will have a dry orgasm as a result of damage to the ejaculatory mechanism.

4 Some patients suffer from symptoms of orthostatic hypotension following lumbar sympathectomy.

CHEMICAL LUMBAR SYMPATHECTOMIES

Action

1 Position the patient sitting with the legs dependent.

2 Insert a 21G spinal needle at the level of the upper border of L3, a hand's breadth away from the midline. Direct it towards the lumbar vertebral body and reposition as necessary until it just slides off the anterior surface of the vertebra (Fig. 31.6). Aspirate it to ensure that it is not in a blood vessel.

3 Inject radiographic contrast fluid and check the needle position with an image intensifier.

4 If the position is correct, inject 7.5 ml of 7.5% phenol in 50% glycine and nurse the patient sitting for 6 hours to allow the heavy phenol solution to track downwards to bathe the sympathetic trunk, rather than laterally to damage the somatic nerves.

Aftercare

1 Self-limiting post-sympathetic neuralgia may occur, as after surgical sympathectomy.

2 Some patients experience pain down the medial side of the thigh if the phenol tracks laterally around the somatic nerves of the lumbar plexus.

REFERENCES

1. Cotton LJ, Cross FW 1985 Lumbar sympathectomy for arterial disease. British Journal of Surgery 72: 678–683
2. Mockus MB, Rutherford RB, Rosales C et al 1987 Sympathectomy for causalgia. Patient selection and long term results. Archives of Surgery 122:668–672
3. Bristow A, Foster JMG 1988 Lumbar sympathectomy in the management of rectal tenesmoid pain. Annals of the Royal College of Surgeons of England 70:38–39
4. Ellis H 1986 Lumbar sympathectomy. British Journal of Hospital Medicine 35:124–125

32

Transplantation

K. Rolles

CONTENTS

INTRODUCTION

- Solid whole-organ transplantation has been one of the main events in the evolution of 20th-century patient care. Within the field of general surgery a kidney transplant offers a quality of life unattainable by long-term dialysis, and the lack of long-term artificial support for end-stage disease of the liver, heart and lungs makes it likely that there will be a demand for organ transplantation into the foreseeable future.
- Immunosuppressive agents that reduce or abolish graft rejection are vital to the success of organ transplantation. Ciclosporin, acting by calcineurin inhibition within T-cell lymphocytes, blocks progression of the cell cycle from G_0 to G_1 and the production of interleukin 2. In the early 1980s, when used alone or with steroids it improved the 2-year graft survival following kidney transplantation from 50% to 75–80%. Newer drugs include tacrolimus, rapamycin and mycophenolate mofetil. Others in preclinical trials, often differing in their mode of action, are leflunomide, brequinar, mizoribine, deoxyspergualin and FTY 720.

  In addition, a number of biological agents such as antibodies to various antigens present on human lymphocytes are available, although so far they have not proved to be any more efficacious than pharmacological agents. Ciclosporin and tacrolimus given long-term have a tendency to produce nephrotoxicity and neoplasia, especially of the skin and lymphoid tissue, so it is desirable that the dose is progressively reduced. There is evidence that in some cases, unfortunately as yet unpredictably, graft acceptance, without the continued use of immunosuppression, can develop in the long term.
- The donor pool comprises:
  Brain-stem dead: heart-beating 'cadavers'—over 90% of solid-organ donors, usually providing multiple organs.
  Non-heart-beating cadavers, providing suitable organs for kidney and increasingly for liver transplantation, occasionally lung transplants but not for hearts.
  Living related donors, such as identical twins, siblings, parents, children, first-order cousins, providing excellent donor organs for kidney transplants; and, with appropriate techniques, segments of livers, pancreas and lung can be grafted.
  Living unrelated donors: spouses, partners, friends, altruists and paid donors (illegal in the UK).
- The success of organ transplantation has resulted in a shortage of solid organs for transplantation. There are almost 6000 patients waiting in the UK and 50 000 in the USA. The shortfall results in part from cultural, religious, financial, legal and political conditions and varies in different countries. In addition, permission to remove organs after death is usually determined by prior consent of the donor, or of the surviving relatives. In some countries, although not in the UK, people need to 'opt out'—that is, state while alive that they refuse to have organs removed—otherwise it is assumed that they permit it. In the UK this issue is being discussed at present. Other discussions are taking place regarding the practicalities and ethics of xenotransplantation (Greek: *xenos*=strange, foreign)—the use of animal organs—and cloning as a means of providing autotransplantable tissues.
- Brain-stem death must be established before organs are removed from a patient with irreversible cerebral destruction. If the plasma electrolytes or blood gases are abnormal, or if there is suspicion of drug intoxication, organ donation is not pursued. The diagnosis must be made by two independent medical practitioners, each carrying out the examination individually, on two separate occasions.

  The following must be absent:
  Pupillary reflexes.
  Corneal reflex.
  Caloric response.
  Gag reflexes.
  Spontaneous breathing when disconnected from ventilator.
- Tissue transplantation has been successfully practised for many years, including the cornea, which evokes little reaction. Bone and skin are also transplanted, but essentially serve to provide a non-cellular matrix into which recipient cells can grow. The donor cells are destroyed. Immunosuppressive agents are unnecessary.

THE MULTIPLE ORGAN DONOR

Appraise

It is possible to remove both kidneys, the liver, the pancreas, the small bowel, the heart and both lungs for transplantation from a single donor using techniques that will not interfere with the immediate function of the transplant organs in their respective recipients.

Donor screening and exclusions

1 Potential donors must be excluded if there is any possibility of transmitting to potential recipients the following:

- AIDS/HIV.
- Hepatitis B.
- Hepatitis C.
- Malaria.
- Tuberculosis.
- Rabies.
- Creutzfeldt–Jakob disease (CJD).
- Glioblastoma multiforme.
- Other extracerebral malignancy.

All prospective donors must be screened for antibody to HIV-1 and HIV-2, hepatitis C and hepatitis B surface antigen and core antibody. Positive donors must not be used.

2 The social history of the donor must be scrutinized as far as possible; prospective donors with a clear history of intravenous drug abuse, prostitution or homosexuality should be excluded from organ donation.

Prepare

1 The ventilated heart-beating brain-dead donor may be physiologically unstable, requiring inotropes to maintain systemic vascular resistance and other pharmacological agents such as pitressin or desmopressin (des-amino-des-aspartate-arginine vasopressin, DDAVP) to control diabetes insipidus. Carefully maintained fluid balance is important so be willing to institute invasive monitoring such as Swan–Ganz catheterization and direct arterial pressure measurements. Pulse oximetry and cardiac monitoring are essential. Have available body-warming equipment to compensate for hypothermia.

2 Have an anaesthetist in attendance. A general anaesthetic is unnecessary but neuromuscular blocking agents such as curare should be given before the first incision to prevent muscular spasms and spinal reflexes, which may be induced by the surgical procedure.

3 Blood loss during the surgical procedure may profoundly destabilize the donor's cardiovascular status and you must take great care to minimize blood loss at all times. Have available 4–6 units of cross-matched bank blood for use during the surgical procedure.

4 The donor's surgical team must be self-sufficient and provide surgical instruments, cannulas, sterile bags for the excised organs, ice, cooling fluids, preservation fluids and cardioplegic solution.

KEY POINT Avoid blood loss

- Strictly maintain complete haemostasis.

Access

1 Make a midline incision from the jugular notch to the symphysis pubis.

2 Split the sternum longitudinally with a Gigli saw. Leave the pericardium and pleural cavities intact if possible.

3 Retract the sternal edges with a self-retaining retractor after securing haemostasis by liberal application of bone wax.

Assess

1 Perform a detailed inspection of all abdominal contents to exclude unsuspected pathology. The incidence of unsuspected pathology increases in proportion to age. Absolute contraindications to proceeding with organ retrieval are peritoneal contamination due to ruptured bowel and the presence of disseminated intraperitoneal cancer. Cirrhosis of the donor liver excludes subsequent transplantation of that organ.

2 Focal abnormalities found in one or more sites in the abdomen or chest need not prohibit organ retrieval but remove biopsy specimens of all suspicious lesions for histological examination. You must not reimplant retrieved organs before excluding malignancy histologically.

Action

1 Commence careful dissection of the structures in the free edge of the lesser omentum leading to the porta hepatis. Ligate and divide the common bile duct just above the duodenum. Dissect and control with rubber slings. Carefully search for abnormalities of the hepatic arterial supply. Seventeen percent of donors have an accessory or aberrant right hepatic artery passing to the porta hepatis posterior to the portal vein and common bile duct. Twenty-three percent have an accessory left hepatic artery arising from the left gastric artery. Identify these variations early and preserve the vessels.

2 Mobilize the duodenum by Kocher's procedure. Isolate the inferior vena cava above the renal veins and below the liver, and control it with a nylon tape.

3 Divide the peritoneal attachments of the liver, starting with the left triangular ligament and proceeding to the falciform ligament, thus exposing the anterior surface of the suprahepatic vena cava (Fig. 32.1).

4 Divide the right triangular ligament and continue by dividing the upper and lower layers of the coronary ligament while progressively dislocating the liver upwards and to the left, thus separating the liver from the bare area of the diaphragm. Ligate and divide the right adrenal vein, which has now been exposed, and continue dissecting to free the retrohepatic vena cava from the posterior abdominal wall. Achieve complete mobilization of the vena cava by dividing the peritoneum of the right side of the lesser sac. Divide the remnant of the lesser omentum, leaving the liver attached by its blood vessels only.

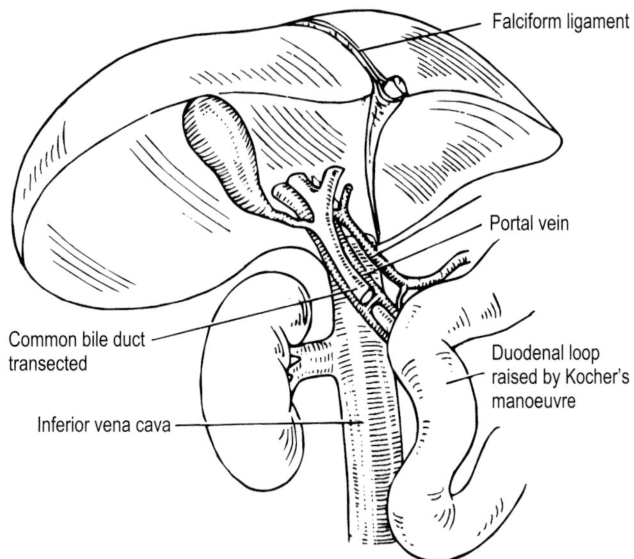

Fig. 32.1 Removal of donor liver. The liver has been dislocated upwards; the common bile duct has been transected low down.

5 Begin mobilization of the right kidney by dissecting the peritoneum from its anterior surface and controlling the right renal vein and vena cava below the renal vein with rubber slings.

6 Gently lift the kidney from the renal fossa and sweep away surrounding fatty tissue to expose the renal artery or arteries and vein, and control them with further rubber slings.

7 Dissect the ureter with plenty of surrounding connecting tissue down as far as the pelvic rim and then divide it (Fig. 32.2).

8 Repeat the procedure for the left kidney. In addition, ligate and divide the left adrenal and gonadal veins. Also identify, ligate and divide the large lumbar vein opening into the posterior aspect of the left renal vein.

9 Expose and control the lower aorta just above the bifurcation, for subsequent cannulation and flush-cooling of the liver and kidneys.

10 Dissect and control the superior mesenteric vein below the transverse mesocolon for later cannulation of the portal vein and flush-cooling of the liver.

11 Mobilize the pancreas at this stage if it is required. Completely divide the gastrocolic and gastrosplenic omentum. Retract the stomach to expose the pancreas. Divide the lienorenal ligament and, using the spleen as a 'handle', carefully mobilize the tail and the body of the pancreas, working towards the midline. Dissect and control with a rubber sling the origin of the splenic artery at the coeliac axis.

12 The cardiac surgical team should now prepare the required thoracic organs for removal. When all the dissections have been completed give 30 000 IU of heparin intravenously. Place a cannula (size 16–20F) in the portal vein via the superior mesenteric vein and place another in the infrarenal abdominal aorta. Place a third cannula in the infrarenal vena cava.

13 Stop mechanical ventilation. Stop circulation with cardioplegic solution infused through the aortic root. Start flush-cooling of abdominal organs via the portal and aortic cannulas using 3–6 litres of Ringer's lactate solution at 4 °C. Simultaneously exsanguinate the donor via the inferior vena caval cannula to ensure venous decompression and thus effective flush-cooling of the abdominal organs.

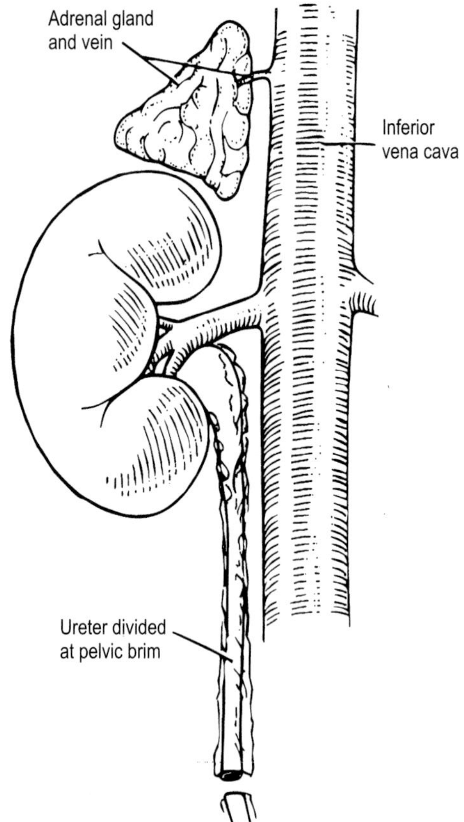

Fig. 32.2 Dissection of the donor kidney on the right.

14 Following removal of the thoracic organs by the cardiac surgical team wait until the abdominal organs are visibly pale and palpably cold before removing them by dividing the remaining vascular connections. Follow the coeliac axis and the renal arteries back to the aorta. In each case excise a rim of aorta—a 'Carrel patch'.

15 Remove all cannulas. Suck out all free fluid and make a careful watertight wound closure using continuous 0 or no. 1 nylon.

ORGAN PRESERVATION

1 Cool the organs in situ by infusing large volumes of isotonic cold crystallized solution such as Ringer's lactate, thus reducing the temperature of the perfused organs to 8–15 °C (as above).

2 Excise the organs when they are visibly pale and palpably cold. Flush them through once more with approximately 1 litre of a preservation solution (University of Wisconsin solution for the liver and hypertonic citrate solution for the kidneys), which will equilibrate throughout the extracellular space of the organ during the preservation period.

3 Double-wrap the organs in sterile bags and place them in boxes of ice where they will remain until reimplantation. Cooling continues to approximately 0 °C in ice over the next few hours.

4 Currently used preservation solutions are hypertonic, contain non-diffusible large anions and usually have a high potassium content corresponding with that of intracellular fluid. These solutions are more effective than physiological saline for cold preservation of organs because they prevent cell swelling and intracellular electrolyte loss during the hypothermic inactivation of the sodium pump.

5 Immediate life-supporting function can be expected from a kidney that has been preserved in one of these solutions for up to 24 hours. Between 24 and 72 hours viability will be preserved but, because of acute tubular necrosis, delayed function is likely.

6 Immediate life-supporting function is an absolute prerequisite for the transplanted liver or heart, thus reducing the safe preservation time dramatically. For the liver, University of Wisconsin solution is clearly the best preservation solution, allowing preservation time for up to 20 hours. For the heart, 4–6 hours is currently the safe limit.

7 Record on forms provided the donor's demographic details, blood group, anatomical abnormalities and time of circulatory arrest. Record the type and volume of preservation solution used. Arrange for samples of donor spleen and lymph node to accompany each organ, together with the copy of the data form to its final destination.

TISSUE TYPING

1 Despite 30 years of clinical organ transplantation, the role of human leucocyte antigen (HLA) matching remains controversial and enigmatic. At least four different gene loci on chromosome 6 code for the human major histocompatibility complex (MHC) and are known as HLA, B, C and D. Currently, antigens that are cell-surface gene products, usually glycoproteins, of the A B and D loci are routinely determined and matched for donor and recipients in renal transplantation.

2 For renal transplantation from closely related donors such as a parent or sibling, graft survival appears to be directly related to the degree of HLA matching, whereas in the unrelated cadaver donor situation, kidneys fully matched at the A, B and D loci (six antigens) enjoy outstandingly good survival, but any lesser degree of matching significantly prejudices survival.

3 In liver transplantation and heart transplantation no convincing relationship has yet been demonstrated between HLA matching and graft survival. Donors and recipients are usually paired on the basis of ABO blood group compatibility only.

KIDNEY TRANSPLANTATION

Appraise

1 Donor kidneys for transplantation may be obtained from:

- *Living related donors.* Usually confined to those with close genetic links such as mothers and fathers, sisters and brothers and occasionally first-order cousins. The results of living related kidney transplantation have always been superior to those of cadaver kidney transplantation. In the UK, the Human Organ Transplant Act 1989 stipulates that for any proposed living related organ donation genetic relationship between the donor and the recipient must be established by DNA fingerprinting before the transplant can legally proceed.
- *Living unrelated donors.* A small but increasing number of transplants have been performed between related but not genetically linked individuals such as husbands and wives and vice versa. Close friends may also donate. Before a living unrelated donation can legally take place in the UK, a dispensation from ULTRA (the Unrelated Liver Transplant Regulatory Authority) must be obtained, and is a statutory requirement.
- *Unrelated brain-stem-dead heart-beating cadaver donors.* Organs are removed immediately following arrest of the circulation. Ninety percent of all kidney transplants occurring in the UK are based on this type of donor.
- *Unrelated non-heart-beating cadaver donors.* Kidneys may be used from a donor following a cardiac standstill as long as the kidneys can be safely removed and cooled within 60 minutes of circulatory arrest. This type of donation is often associated with delayed initial function of the transplant kidney due to acute tubular necrosis.

2 Kidney transplantation currently offers the best chance of long-term survival combined with near-normal quality of life for those suffering from end-stage chronic renal disease.

3 The cost of a well-functioning kidney graft, or any other organ graft, is lifelong treatment with non-specific immunosuppressive agents. Ultimately, the main threat to long-term survival of the kidney graft recipient is likely to be the complications of long-term immunosuppressive therapy in the form of infections and an increased incidence of neoplasia. In addition, hypertension and accelerated cardiovascular disease are commonly seen. After 5 years, recipient death with a functioning graft is the commonest cause of graft loss.

4 End-stage renal disease of all types comprise the indications for renal transplantation. Chronic glomerulonephritis accounts for 60% of all cases of chronic renal failure. Diabetic nephropathy, reflexing pyelonephritis, polycystic disease and previously failed kidney grafts are the other main indications for transplantation.

LIVING RELATED KIDNEY DONATION

Appraise

Remember, the donor has volunteered to undergo a major surgical operation, with all its potential attendant morbidity, which is not of any personal benefit. The altruistic donation of one kidney leaves the kidney donor in a higher risk group for the future with respect to the development of renal failure.

Donor kidneys may be retrieved by the open approach, usually through a muscle-cutting loin incision or, increasingly more frequently, laparoscopically.

THE OPEN APPROACH

Prepare

1 Perform HLA tissue typing and ABO blood grouping. Ensure compatibility with the recipient. Screen for hepatitis B and C and HIV. Demonstrate proof of genetic relationship between

donor and recipient by DNA fingerprinting (restriction fragment length polymorphism).

2 Perform diethylenetriamine penta-acetic acid (DTPA) scan to ensure that each of the potential donor's kidneys contributes 50% to total renal function. Gross functional asymmetry between the two kidneys will prohibit donation.

3 Perform an aortogram with selective views of both renal arteries, or magnetic resonance angiogram. A kidney with a single renal artery is desirable. Multiple renal arteries supplying both kidneys prohibit kidney donation.

4 Ensure that kidney preservation solutions (ice, organ bags, and cannulas) are available for the operative procedure.

Access

1 Place the anaesthetized donor on the operating table in the lateral position.

2 Make a 20-cm muscle-cutting loin incision over the 12th rib. Gain access to the retroperitoneal space through the bed of the 12th rib. Take care to avoid the pleura, which is attached to the medial half of the upper border of the 12th rib. Sweep the peritoneum forward, keeping it intact.

Action

1 Carefully dissect the kidney free of its perirenal fat and the adrenal gland and gently draw it up into the wound to facilitate dissection of the renal pedicles.

2 Dissect both renal vein and renal artery and control each with a soft rubber sling. On the left side divide and ligate the gonadal vein and the adrenal vein. Look for a large lumbar vein entering the posterior aspect of the renal vein. Ligate and divide it. Mobilize the renal vein fully to its confluence with the inferior vena cava.

3 Dissect the renal artery to the aorta. On the right side this requires elevation and retraction of the inferior vena cava and necessitates ligation and division of one or more lumbar veins.

4 Dissect the ureter to the pelvic brim. Ligate it distally at this point and divide it.

5 When attached by its blood vessels only, confirm that the kidney is undergoing diuresis. Give 30 g of mannitol intravenously. Apply vascular clamps to the renal vessels and rapidly excise the kidney. Take it to a side trolley and rapidly flush-cool via the renal artery using a kidney preservation solution at 4 °C. Continue perfusion of the kidney until the effluent from the renal vein is clear and the kidney is palpably cold.

6 Double-wrap the kidney in sterile polythene bags and place it in a bag of ice until the time for reimplantation.

7 Carefully ligate the cut donor renal vessels and close the loin incision in layers over a large silicone tube drain.

THE LAPAROSCOPIC APPROACH

This may be performed extraperitoneally through the loin or more usually transperitoneally through an anterior approach. Four or five ports are used and the excised kidney is delivered through a 6-cm Pfannenstiel incision. The procedure may be conducted entirely laparoscopically or 'hand-assisted' by inserting a hand through the suprapubic incision.

TRANSPLANTATION OF THE DONOR KIDNEY

Appraise

- Ninety percent of renal transplants performed in the UK use unrelated 'cadaver' donor kidneys. Less than 10% of kidney transplants are donated by a close living relative.
- 'Cadaver' kidneys are exchanged between transplant centres on the basis of clinical need and tissue matching.
- Organ exchange and transport are arranged by a central distribution agency, the UK Transplant Support Services Authority (UKTSSA).
- Organs are transported in boxes of crushed ice by special courier.

Prepare

1 Before commencing the recipient operation carefully check the information sheet accompanying the donor kidney, paying particular attention to ABO blood group compatibility and any anatomical abnormality recorded.

2 Ensure that an immunological cross-match is negative between recipient serum and donor lymphocytes from the spleen and lymph node samples accompanying the kidney. A positive cross-match absolutely prohibits transplantation as it demonstrates preformed antibodies in the recipient's serum that are capable of killing donor lymphocytes. If the transplant were to proceed in the face of a positive cross-match, the kidney would be hyperacutely rejected.

3 Remove the kidney from its box of ice and check its anatomical details. Some dissection of excess donor tissues may be necessary. Perform this on a sterile trolley. Ensure that you have an adequate source of light and an assistant. When the dissection is completed replace the kidney in sterile bags and pack it away once again in the box of ice.

KIDNEY TRANSPLANT OPERATION

Appraise

1 The donor kidney is reimplanted into the right or left iliac fossa and vascularized from the iliac vessels. This is an example of heterotopic (Greek: *heteros*=other+*topos*=a place) transplantation, as the kidney is not reimplanted into its normal anatomical—orthotopic (Greek: *orthos*=straight, right)—position.

2 The reasons why this heterotopic position is most appropriate are:

- It provides easy access to the iliac vessels.
- The blood supply of the donor ureter is entirely derived from the renal vessels and so should be kept short.
- The implanted kidney is usually easily palpable and amenable to percutaneous procedures such as biopsy with relatively low risk.

Prepare

1 Ensure the prospective recipient is normokalaemic (*kalium*, modified Latin from Arabic *quail*=potash, potassium).

2 Have a central venous pressure line inserted and cautiously rehydrate the recipient. Most chronically dialysed patients are under-hydrated and hyperkalaemic.

Access

1 Place the patient on the operating table in the supine position.

2 Pass a urinary catheter and attach it to a 1-litre bag of saline via an infusion line.

3 Make a 'hockey-stick' incision starting 1 cm above the symphysis pubis and curving laterally to the pararectal line. Proceed vertically up the pararectal line to just above the level of the umbilicus. Incise the abdominal wall along the pararectal line and make an extraperitoneal approach to the external iliac vessels. Ligate and divide the inferior epigastric vessels. Control the spermatic cord with a nylon tape.

4 Insert a self-retaining ring retractor such as Denis Browne's and adjust it to provide full access to the operative field.

Action

1 Mobilize both the external iliac artery and vein and control them with nylon tapes. Carefully ligate and seal the perivascular lymphatic vessels with diathermy.

2 Remove the prepared donor kidney from ice.

3 Perform an end-to-side anastomosis between the renal vein and the external iliac vein using continuous 5/0 polypropylene or PDS (polydioxane sulphate).

4 Perform an end-to-side anastomosis between the donor renal artery and the external iliac artery using similar suture materials.

5 Remove the clamps from the iliac vessels, thus perfusing the graft, and secure haemostasis.

6 Fill the bladder with physiological saline from the previously attached infusion line to distend it and help identify the bladder in the pelvis.

7 Spatulate the end of the ureter, pass below the spermatic cord and perform an anastomosis to the dome of the bladder using continuous 4/0 synthetic absorbable suture such as PDS. Fashion a submucosal tunnel by incising the bladder muscle down to the mucosa over a 2-cm distance in line with the ureter. Lay the distal ureter in the groove created and close the bladder muscle loosely over the top of the ureter using interrupted absorbable sutures. Test the anastomosis by refilling the bladder with saline (Fig. 32.3).

8 Take a renal biopsy before closing the wound in layers over a large silicone tube drain.

Postoperative

1 Leave the urethral catheter in situ for a minimum of 5 days.

2 Ensure meticulous fluid replacement to maintain a urine output of more than 100 ml/hour.

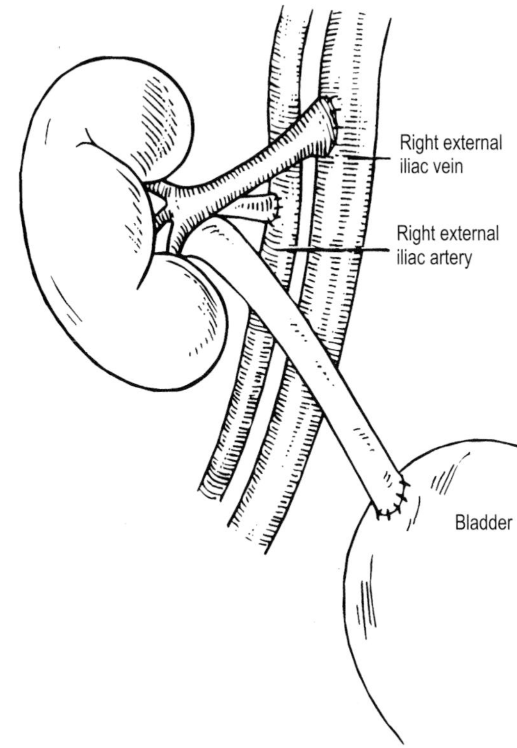

Fig. 32.3 Renal transplantation. The renal vessels have been united end-to-side to the external iliac vessels. The ureter is joined to the dome of the bladder.

3 Perform daily full blood count, blood urea, electrolyte and creatinine estimations.

4 Record the patient's weight and fluid balance accurately.

Complications

- *Delayed function* of cadaver grafts occurs in up to 40%, due to acute tubular necrosis. Acute tubular necrosis results from ischaemic injury to the kidney graft, which may occur in the donor before removal, during the preservation period, if it is excessively long, or during the implantation period, if this is excessively long. Acute tubular necrosis is confirmed on DTPA scan and renal biopsy and usually resolves within 6 weeks.
- *Vascular thrombosis* may occur rarely, approximately 5%, leading to infarction and loss of the graft, which must then be removed. A transplant nephrectomy requires removal of all donor tissue, reconstitution of iliac vessels by vein patch if necessary and oversewing of the bladder.
- *Urinary leakage* may occur as a result of terminal ischaemic necrosis of the donor ureter. Operative intervention is almost always necessary. Reimplant the ureter into the dome of the bladder or perform uretero-ureterostomy to the recipient's own ureter.
- *Acute cellular rejection* is seen in up to 80% of cases within 1 week of transplantation. Clinically there is oliguria, pyrexia and a rising creatinine and blood urea. You should obtain histological confirmation by percutaneous biopsy. Give antirejection therapy, usually high-dose steroids, to suppress the immune

response. In a small minority of cases rejection is uncontrollable and results in infarction of the graft leading to the need to remove the graft.

Results

1 For living related donor kidneys, graft survival is over 90% at 1 year and 80% at 5 years.

2 Cadaver kidney graft survival is 80% at 1 year and 65–70% at 5 years.

LIVER TRANSPLANTATION

Appraise

1 More than 125 000 liver transplants have been performed in over 200 liver transplant centres worldwide since Starzl reported the first liver graft in 1963. The introduction of cyclosporin in 1979 was associated with a significant improvement in both short-term and long-term survival following liver grafting. The longest surviving recipient of a liver graft is now more than 35 years post-transplant.

2 Auxiliary transplantation of the liver, heterotopic, for non-malignant cases of liver disease has had its proponents from time to time. The problems of creating sufficient space for an extra liver, or part of a liver, kinking of the vascular anastomoses and the development of malignancy in the recipient's own liver have precluded its widespread adoption. Auxiliary partial orthotopic liver transplantation, described by Gubernatis,[1] is an interesting technical variant where a donor right or left lobar graft is implanted orthotopically following resection of the same lobe of the recipient's own acutely failing liver. The expectation here is that full recovery of the recipient's native liver will occur so that the grafted lobe may subsequently be removed or abandoned and immunosuppression withdrawn. This expectation is not always achieved.

3 Orthotopic liver transplantation as originally described and practised required the removal of the recipient's own liver together with the retrohepatic inferior vena cava between the renal veins and the diaphragm. For very small recipients, usually children, transplantation of a part of a larger liver obtained either by splitting a cadaver graft or by left hemihepatectomy of a living related donor requires the recipient's own retrohepatic vena cava to be left in situ. For children, the partial liver graft usually consists of segments 2 and 3 and possibly 4 of the donor organ. For adults, a partial graft consisting of segments of 5, 6, 7 and 8, whether obtained from a 'split' cadaver graft or from a living related donor, usually provides sufficient functional liver cell mass. A graft weight to recipient body weight ratio of 0.8–1% is essential to immediately sustain life. Alternatively, using volumetry based on three-dimensional computed tomography (CT) or magnetic resonance imaging (MRI), the living donor graft should be 40% of the recipient's calculated standard liver volume. Leaving the recipient's own vena cava in situ also allows the option of a single cavocaval side-to-side anastomosis (the so-called piggy-back technique). Several large series of living related donor liver transplants have recently been reported demonstrating excellent outcomes for both adult and paediatric recipients but also showing significant early morbidity for both donor and recipient. Biliary tract complications currently occur in up to 36% of recipients and 20% of donors. Donor mortality appears to be just under 1% at present, an unacceptably high figure in the view of many surgeons. I shall describe the original orthotopic liver transplant procedure.

4 In 70% of cases transplantation is for end-stage chronic liver disease due to cirrhosis arising from a variety of different causes such as primary biliary cirrhosis, primary sclerosing cholangitis, post-hepatitic cirrhosis, autoimmune chronic active hepatitis and alcohol-related liver disease. In approximately 12% it is for primary hepatic malignancy and in another 10% for acute liver failure resulting from fulminant hepatitis acute (drug) poisoning or idiosyncratic drug reactions. Metabolic diseases account for 6% of cases, including:

- Where the liver is itself a target organ of the metabolic abnormality such as Wilson's disease and α_1-antitrypsin deficiency and tyrosinosis.
- Where a hepatic enzyme defect leads to damage and failure to other organs such as primary hyperoxaluria, familial hypercholesterolaemia and some forms of familial amyloidosis. Here, liver transplantation is used as a highly effective form of gene therapy.

Prepare

1 Carry out a full biochemical haematological, bacteriological and virological screening including hepatitis viruses A–G. Replicating HBV must be suppressed by antiviral treatment with lamuvidine or adefovir, to prevent post-transplant recurrence in the graft which may cause its rapid destruction. Similarly, HCV may be treated to suppress or eliminate it preoperatively with interferon and ribavirin, if time and liver function permit.

2 Magnetic resonance angiography and cholangiography are required to assess the vasculature and biliary tract of the recipient liver. An occluded portal vein may be a relative contraindication to transplantation. In the presence of an occluded portal vein, transplantation may still be possible if the splenic vein or the superior mesenteric vein are patent and accessible.

3 Perform lung function tests and carefully evaluate cardiac function. Measure pulmonary artery pressure and perform cardiac output studies followed by a detailed anaesthetic assessment.

4 Assess the neuropsychiatric state, including CT scans of the brain.

5 Control ascites, oesophageal varices and encephalopathy by maximizing medical treatment.

6 Immediately before operation have 20 units of blood, fresh-frozen plasma and platelets cross-matched. Give prophylactic broad-spectrum antibiotics at the induction of anaesthesia.

7 Inspect the donor liver graft before starting the recipient operation.

Access

1 Make a bilateral subcostal incision with upward extension to the xiphoid. Pin back the abdominal wall flaps so created, to the lower chest wall.

2 Insert a Thompson retractor system to elevate the lower costal margin.

Assess

KEY POINTS Unsuspected co-existent disease?

- Examine the intraperitoneal contents carefully.
- Do not proceed if you discover extrahepatic tumour.
- Remove a biopsy section of suspect tissue for frozen-section histology.

Resect

1 Dissect the structures in the free edge of the lesser omentum leading to the porta hepatis.

2 Ligate and divide the common bile duct as close as possible to the porta hepatis.

3 Dissect and control the common hepatic artery and portal vein with rubber slings.

4 Dissect the infrahepatic vena cava above the renal veins and control it with a nylon tape.

5 Divide the peritoneal attachments of the liver starting with the left triangular ligament and proceeding to the falciform ligament thus exposing the anterior surface of the suprahepatic vena cava.

6 Progressively dislocate the liver from the hepatic fossa while dissecting the liver from the bare area of the diaphragm.

7 Completely mobilize the retrohepatic vena cava from the posterior abdominal wall, ligating and dividing the right adrenal vein.

8 Apply vascular clamps to the vascular connections of the liver and excise it, maximizing the length of vessels for the subsequent reimplantation of the new graft (Fig. 32.4).

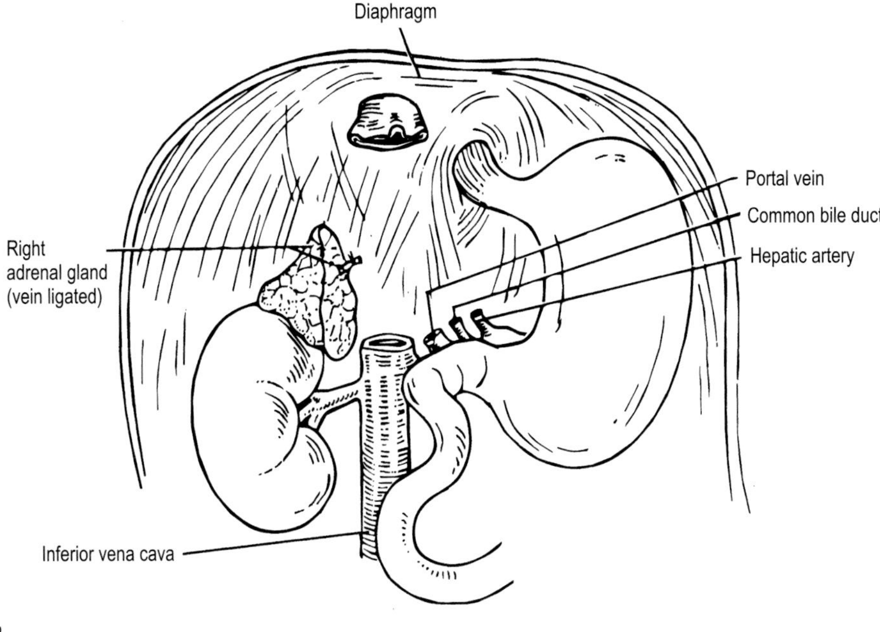

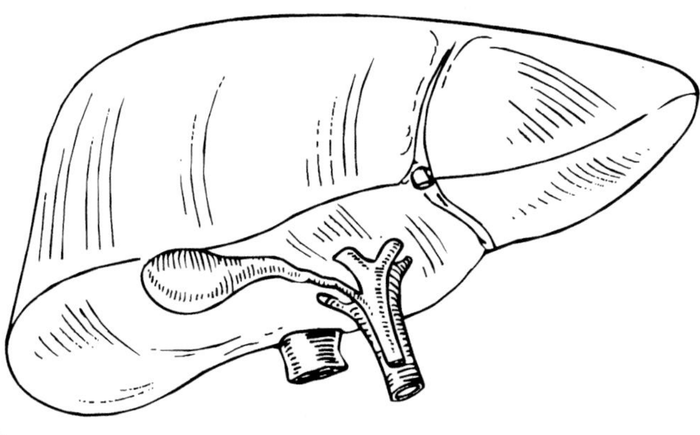

Fig. 32.4 Diagram of recipient liver resection: (a) the removed liver with divided common bile duct, portal vein, hepatic artery and inferior vena cava; (b) the bed for the donor liver. The duodenal loop is mobilized by Kocher's manoeuvre.

KEY POINTS Cirrhotic liver fracture?

- Liver fracture during the mobilization of the liver causes rapid blood loss.
- Clamp the portal vein, hepatic artery and infrahepatic vena cava to reduce blood loss.
- You can now divide the clamped structures and complete the retrohepatic dissection in a bloodless field.

9 In recipients with borderline renal or cardiac function institute venovenous bypass during the anhepatic period, inserting percutaneously placed cannulas in the left femoral vein and left internal jugular vein. Flows of up to 3 litres/minute are observed, which support cardiac output and effective renal perfusion during the anhepatic period.

Replace

1 Remove the new liver from ice.

2 Begin the reimplantation with the suprahepatic vena caval anastomosis using a continuous 2/0 polypropylene (Prolene) or polydioxanone (PDS) or polyester (Merseline) suture. Follow this with the infrahepatic vena caval anastomosis using a continuous 3/0 polypropylene suture. Before completing the infrahepatic anastomosis insert a 16F flexible cannula into the retrohepatic vena cava for subsequent flushing of the liver.

3 Anastomose the donor and recipient portal veins end-to-end using 5/0 polypropylene. Before completing this anastomosis flush out the graft via the portal vein with 500 ml of 5% human albumin solution at room temperature. This removes air and preservation fluid from the liver, which escapes through the retrohepatic caval vent.

4 Complete the anastomoses of the portal vein and infrahepatic vena cava and remove clamps from the infrahepatic vena cava, suprahepatic vena cava and portal vein in that order, thus perfusing the new graft with portal-venous blood (Fig. 32.5).

5 Reconstruct the hepatic arterial supply as an end-to-end anastomosis between the donor and recipient common hepatic arteries using interrupted 6/0 polypropylene.

6 Reconstruct the biliary tract as an end-to-end, duct-to-duct anastomosis using interrupted 5/0 PDS. Splinting is not necessary. Use a 50-cm Roux loop of upper jejunum if there is no recipient common bile duct, as in biliary atresia or primary sclerosing cholangitis.

7 Perform a donor cholecystectomy and a liver biopsy.

8 Check thoroughly for haemostasis, inspecting all anastomoses and placing extra sutures when necessary, and then close the abdomen in layers over two large silicone tube drains.

Postoperative

1 Transfer the patient to the intensive care unit.

2 Continue ventilation until the patient's cardiovascular condition is stable.

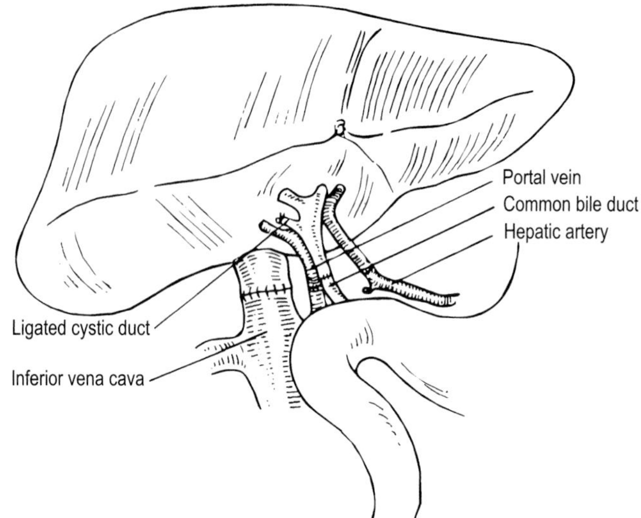

Fig. 32.5 Diagrammatic appearance of donor liver in situ after completing the anastomosis; the first anastomosis, of the superior cut end of the recipient vena cava to the upper end of the donor intrahepatic cava, is not visible. The gallbladder of the donor liver has been removed.

3 Carefully monitor temperature, blood pressure, pulse, central venous pressure (CVP), ECG, pulmonary artery wedge pressure, cardiac output and systemic vascular resistance.

4 Monitor haemoglobin, haematocrit (maintaining at 30%), potassium, calcium and magnesium, blood gases, blood lactate and pH.

KEY POINT Graft function?

- Increasing blood lactate levels and acidosis are indicative of poor early graft function.

5 Measure and replace fluid losses, including urine output, abdominal drainage and nasogastric losses.

6 Begin immunosuppressive therapy immediately.

7 Cover with broad-spectrum antibiotics for at least 48 hours.

8 Check liver function tests and coagulation profiles twice daily.

Complications

1 Bleeding may occur within the first 24 hours resulting from vasodilatation as the patient warms up. Bleeding may also occur as a result of poor synthesis of clotting factors by the new graft. Correct any coagulation abnormalities with fresh-frozen plasma, platelets and cryoprecipitate as necessary. If bleeding continues, intra-abdominal haematoma may accumulate sufficiently to cause tamponade resulting in hypotension and anuria. Re-explore the abdomen to evacuate haematoma and improve haemostasis as much as possible. The retrohepatic area, particularly in the region of the right adrenal, is a common site for postoperative bleeding.

2 A right pleural effusion develops in nearly all patients during the first postoperative week. Treat it expectantly unless it rapidly increases in size or causes compression or collapse of the underlying lung. In this case aspirate it or insert an underwater seal drain.

3 Vascular occlusion is a rare (5–10%) but serious complication, particularly in the first few postoperative weeks. Hepatic arterial thrombosis may lead to extensive patchy infarction of the graft or acute liver failure, requiring urgent re-transplantation. Portal vein thrombosis may be clinically silent. Hepatic arterial thrombectomy or thrombolysis is rarely of benefit, but portal vein thrombectomy is frequently effective.

4 Diagnose acute rejection on biopsy in up to 80% of grafts within the first postoperative week. Treat it by increasing immunosuppression, for example giving 1 g of methylprednisolone (Solu-Medrone) intravenously once daily for 3 days. Repeat the biopsy to assess the response.

5 Send samples of urine, saliva, faeces, blood and appropriate skin swabs every 48 hours for bacteriological and virological surveillance.

KEY POINT Infection?

- Infection under high-dose immunosuppressive cover is serious and could be fatal.

6 Perform a HIDA (hepatobiliary imidodiacetic acid) scan 10–14 days postoperatively to assess the integrity of the biliary tract. Proceed to ERCP (endoscopic retrograde cholangiopancreatography) or transhepatic percutaneous cholangiography if the HIDA scan is equivocal. If there is a small leak at the anastomosis it may heal following careful stenting or nasobiliary drainage inserted endoscopically. Large biliary leaks are usually associated with a substantial infrahepatic bile collection and may signify donor duct necrosis. Reconstructive surgery using a Roux loop is usually the best approach. For an obstruction of the anastomosis, once again temporary stenting may suffice if it is possible to pass a stent across the obstruction; otherwise proceed to reconstructive surgery, performing a choledochojejunostomy using a 50-cm Roux loop.

Results

1 An 85% 1-year patient survival and 65% 5-year patient survival are currently being achieved by most major liver transplant centres. A recurrence rate of about 65% at 5 years for those transplanted for malignant disease of the liver underscores the poor long-term prognosis of transplantation for malignant disease, but still compares well with resectional surgery for primary liver cancer.

2 Chronic rejection of the graft occurs in up to 10% of liver transplant recipients, appearing histologically as progressive dropout of liver parenchymal cells and loss of portal tract bile ducts. These changes are due to a progressive obliterative arteriopathy, where the lumina of the major arteries of the graft become progressively obstructed by the accumulation of foamy macrophages of recipient origin. Re-transplantation is the only solution. The falling incidence of chronic rejection seen in recent years has been attributed to more effective immunosuppressive drugs and a more proactive approach to liver graft dysfunction through biopsy.

REFERENCE

1. Gubernatis G, Pichlmayr R, Kemnitz J et al 1991 Auxiliary partial orthotopic liver transplantation (APOLT) for fulminant hepatic failure: first successful case report. World Journal of Surgery 15:660–666

PANCREAS TRANSPLANTATION

Appraise

The development of microangiopathy, nephropathy and neuropathy appears not to be inevitable among diabetic patients, but may occur in individuals despite ostensibly good blood sugar control by exogenous insulin. Against this backdrop the rationale for pancreatic transplantation has been as an approach to the treatment of diabetes mellitus whereby prevention, arrest or reversal of the long-term complications of diabetes may be achieved.

Transplantation of pancreatic tissue has been performed both clinically and experimentally by two different approaches:

- Transplantation of the whole or part of the pancreas as a solid vascularized organ graft, which includes both endocrine and exocrine components of the gland.
- Transplantation of the insulin-producing tissue only—the islets of Langerhans.

VASCULARIZED GRAFTS

Appraise

1 No single technique has been universally adopted in the 40 years since Kelly performed the first vascularized graft in the 1966.[1] The question of whether it is better to graft the whole pancreas or a segment comprising the body and the tail of the organ is still unresolved, but the balance of opinion now favours the whole-organ graft. Those who advocate the whole-organ preparation claim that it is beneficial to engraft as much of the donor endocrine mass as possible, thus minimizing islet exhaustion due to too small a graft, as in the segmental technique. Those advocating the simpler segmental graft claim that it is a lower-morbidity, lower-mortality procedure for the recipient. Other controversial areas include:

- Thrombosis of the graft.
- Drainage of exocrine secretion.
- The diagnosis and treatment of rejection.

2 Despite these technical difficulties the results of pancreas transplantation have improved substantially over the last decade. In recent years, the most favoured technique is that of transplanting the whole pancreas of the donor into the left or right iliac fossa of the recipient, draining the pancreatic exocrine secretion directly into the bladder, as described by Sollinger et al.[2] These authors also found that a fall in the urinary amylase output from the graft was an early marker of impending graft rejection, indicating the need for antirejection therapy. More recently,

because of sometimes insurmountable bladder problems with frequency, dysuria and cystitis, many surgeons have reverted to pancreatic duct drainage into a Roux-en-Y loop of jejunum.

Achievements

1 A well-functioning pancreas graft exerts good control of blood glucose excursions without dietary restrictions and 24-hour blood glucose profiles are normal or near normal.

2 Glucose-tolerance curves show an abnormal pattern of insulin release leading to a slower return of blood glucose to basal levels.

3 Glucose-tolerance curves are similar whether the pancreatic graft venous effluent is drained into the systemic circulation or into the portal circulation, but plasma insulin levels are at least twice as high in those with a systemic venous drainage. Glycosylated haemoglobin values (HbA_{1C}) are maintained within the normal range.

4 Evidence for pancreas transplantation altering the natural history of the secondary complications of diabetes is slowly emerging. Diabetic nephropathy in transplanted kidneys appears to be prevented by a well-functioning pancreas graft. There are also some reports of improved peripheral nerve conduction time following pancreas transplantation. In general, retinopathy is not objectively improved but many patients with diabetic eye problems have found an improvement in acuity.

Techniques

1 The artery and vein of the pancreas graft are anastomosed end-to-side to the common iliac artery and vein of the recipient.

2 For the whole-organ graft some 'bench' surgery is required; that is, at a separate sterile work table.

3 An interposition graft comprising the donor common iliac artery bifurcation is anastomosed to the splenic artery and the superior mesenteric artery of the graft so that only a single anastomosis to the recipient artery is required. In addition, a 6-cm length of donor duodenum is retained and anastomosed to either the dome of the bladder or a loop of jejunum to provide exocrine drainage. The graft is placed intraperitoneally. In contrast, the segmental graft requires no bench procedure and is usually placed extraperitoneally. Exocrine drainage is into a Roux loop or obturated by duct injection with Neoprene.

Results

1 More than 20 000 pancreas grafts have now been reported worldwide; 94% of these have been associated with a kidney graft. In 80%, the pancreas is transplanted simultaneously with a kidney from the same donor. In 14%, a successful pancreas transplant is followed some months later by a kidney transplant usually from a third-party donor. Only 6% of pancreas transplants are performed alone.

2 1-year patient survival is currently 95% with a graft survival of over 80%. The use of the new immunosuppressants, such as tacrolimus and mycophenolate mofetil, appears to have significantly improved outcome in recent years.

ISLET CELL TRANSPLANTATION

Avoidance of major surgery, graft thrombosis and pancreatic exocrine secretion management difficulties readily makes islet transplantation an attractive option. Islet grafting can be accomplished by percutaneous placement, and purified islets are in theory more amenable to immunological modulation prior to transplant. In practice, however, islet cell transplantation has its own major difficulties. Specifically these include:

- Efficient separation of islet tissue from the whole pancreas.
- Preservation of the islet tissue.
- The most appropriate site for islet implantation.
- The rejection of the islet graft.

Nevertheless, as a result of much experimental work performed over the last two decades, the techniques of islet separation and preservation are much improved. It is estimated that, to render an insulin-dependent diabetic normoglycaemic by means of an islet graft, approximately 10 000 islets per kilogram of recipient's body weight are necessary. The efficiency of current separation techniques is such that more than one donor is usually necessary for each islet cell transplant. Intraportal or intrasplenic injection appear to be the favoured sites of placement for islet grafts at present, but excellent islet survival has been reported in rodents by placement beneath the renal capsule. Islet rejection remains a problem. In addition to T- and B-cell-mediated immunological mechanisms, it is likely that scavenging mechanisms, such as phagocytosis by macrophages, assume an important role in islet graft destruction.

Several hundred attempts at human islet cell grafting have been reported over the years with insulin independence achieved for a few days only. However, a clinical programme of islet transplants using intraportal injection and achieving excellent insulin independence rates at up to 5 years has been reported recently by workers at Edmonton, Alberta. Highly efficient islet separation techniques, immediate transplantation of the prepared islets into the portal vein by transhepatic or transjugular injection, and the use of the powerful immunosuppressive drugs tacrolimus and sirolimus have been the main factors underpinning this remarkable success.

REFERENCES

1. Kelly WD, Lillehei RC, Merkel FK et al 1967 Allotransplantation of pancreas and duodenum along with the kidney in diabetic nephropathy. Surgery 61:827–833
2. Sollinger HW, Kalayoglu M, Hoffman RM et al 1985 Results of segmental and pancreaticosplenic transplantation with pancreaticocystostomy. Transplantation Proceedings 17:360–362

SMALL-BOWEL TRANSPLANTATION

Appraise

- Transplantation of the small bowel may be indicated for small numbers of adults and children who have suffered massive small-bowel loss and are unable to sustain body weight by either enteric feeding or total parental nutrition. In most countries the demand for small-bowel transplantation to date has been low. In small children, transplantation of the liver together with the small bowel has produced better results than transplantation of the small bowel alone.

- Lillehei was the first to report the technical feasibility of small-bowel transplantation in the dog. Several attempts at human small-bowel transplantation followed, with extremely poor results. The introduction of cyclosporin A in 1978 revived interest in clinical small-bowel transplantation and this has been reinforced by the development of new agents such as tacrolimus and mycophenolate mofetil. Many major transplant centres now have modest series of small-bowel grafts, but graft survival longer than 3 years remains a rare event.

  Major clinical problems are:

  Immunological rejection of the graft.

  Septicaemia due to bacteriological translocation across the graft during rejection episodes.

  Fluid and electrolyte losses from the graft.

  Graft-versus-host disease, which may be fatal.

  Technical problems, including vascular thrombosis and torsion of the graft pedicle.
- Small-bowel grafts can be obtained from cadaveric donors or from living related donors. The potential of careful and close HLA matching in grafts taken from living related donors may prove critical for the long-term survival of the small-bowel graft.
- Access to the recipient's major abdominal blood vessels may be very difficult as candidates for small-bowel transplantation have invariably undergone numerous previous surgical procedures.
- Implantation of the graft is straightforward, with the superior mesenteric artery of the graft anastomosed end-to-side to the recipient abdominal aorta and the vein anastomosed to the inferior vena cava, or the portal vein if available.

REFERENCE

1. Lillehei RC, Goott B, Miller FA 1958 The physiological response of the small bowel of the dog to ischaemia including prolonged in vitro preservation of the bowel with successful replacement survival. Annals of Surgery 150:43–54

HEART TRANSPLANTATION

Appraise

- Eight years after the first successful series of orthotopic heart transplants in dogs, carried out by Lower and Shumway,[1] Barnard,[2] using the same technique, performed the first human heart transplant in 1967. The wave of worldwide enthusiasm for human heart grafting that followed Barnard's contribution was almost totally dissipated by 1970, when it had become clear that the development of a successful surgical technique had preceded the development of suitable immunological means and immunosuppressive agents to monitor and prevent graft rejection.
- Heart transplantation continued in a very few centres over the following decade. The introduction in 1980 of ciclosporin A, a potent new non-steroidal immunosuppressant, sparked a second wave of worldwide enthusiasm, which has been sustained and has established heart transplantation as an extremely effective therapy for various types of end-stage heart disease. More than 50 000 transplants have now been performed.

Indications

- Ischaemic heart disease and its complications, due to coronary artery insufficiency.
- Cardiomyopathy of various types.
- Some cases of congenital heart disease.

Contraindications

- Pulmonary hypertension.
- Other systemic disease or infection.
- Age greater than 55 years.

Donor and recipient matching criteria

- ABO compatibility.
- Negative direct lymphocytotoxic cross-match, that is donor cells not killed by recipient serum.
- Body weight of donor and recipient within 10% of each other.
- Cold preservation time of donor heart not exceeding 4 hours.

Technique

1. Perform a median sternotomy.
2. Establish full cardiopulmonary bypass, placing cannulas in the superior and inferior vena cava transatrially and a return cannula in the ascending aorta.
3. Apply aortic and pulmonary artery clamps and excise the recipient's heart across a transatrial plane just dorsal to the atrial appendages. Leave the posterior atrial wall with the orifices of the systemic and pulmonary veins intact. Divide the aorta and pulmonary trunk just distal to their respective valves.
4. Insert a cannula (12–14F) in the left ventricle, through the apex of the myocardium, to act as a vent.
5. Implant the new heart, which consists of more of the donor atria in order to preserve the sinoatrial node.
6. Perform left and right atrial anastomoses, followed by aortic and pulmonary artery anastomoses, using continuous polypropylene sutures.
7. On completion of the anastomoses, release the aortic clamp and allow the heart to fill via the coronary circulation, displacing air through the left ventricular vent.
8. When all air is displaced, clamp and remove the vent, release all other clamps and snuggers and reduce bypass flow rate. If the heart does not restart spontaneously, apply a direct current (DC) shock if necessary.
9. Place temporary pacing wires in the donor right atrial wall and stop bypass. Remove cannulas.
10. Repair the pericardium and close the chest with pericardial drainage.

Rejection

Perform transjugular endomyocardial biopsies regularly—initially every 3–5 days to detect and treat rejection as early as possible.

Results

One-year survival is 85–90% in most large centres; 5-year survival is currently 75%.

REFERENCES

1. Lower RR, Shumway NE 1960 Studies on orthotopic transplantation of the canine heart. Surgical Forum 11:9–18
2. Barnard CN 1967 The operation. South African Medical Journal 41:1271–1274

HEART–LUNG TRANSPLANTATION

The first reported human heart–lung transplant was performed by Cooley in 1968.[1] The recipient survived only 4 hours after surgery. Further attempts were reported by Lillehei in 1969 and Barnard in 1971, with similar short-term survival.

Reitz, working at Stanford, California, performed the first heart–lung transplant under ciclosporin immunosuppression in 1981.[2] This patient survived 5 years. Heart–lung transplantation is now a well-established therapy for certain cardiopulmonary disorders.

Indications

- Primary pulmonary hypertension.
- Pulmonary hypertension secondary to Eisenmenger's syndrome.
- Cystic fibrosis.
- Emphysema.

Whether heart–lung transplantation will be succeeded by single or double lung transplants for cystic fibrosis and emphysema remains to be seen. The potentially serious disadvantage of heart–lung grafting for end-stage lung disease is that a healthy, well-functioning recipient heart is excised (and used for another heart recipient) to be replaced by an allograft that is susceptible to the many complications of allotransplantation, including the risk of both acute and chronic graft rejection.

Donor and recipient matching

1. This is similar to that for heart transplantation. Size matching of the donor lungs to the recipient thoracic cage is very important, as over-inflation occurs if the lungs are relatively too small and inadequate ventilation occurs if the lungs are too large.
2. Donor organs are much more difficult to obtain than hearts alone. Many potential donors are precluded on account of pulmonary infection due to mechanical ventilation. Thus, in view of size matching and scarcity of suitable uninfected donors, a potential heart–lung recipient may need to wait a long time before transplantation.

Technique

1. Make a median sternotomy.
2. Establish full cardiopulmonary bypass as described for heart transplantation.
3. Excise both lungs and heart of the recipient, separately if necessary.
4. Take care not to damage the phrenic nerves or the vagal trunks.
5. Leave the posterior wall of the right atrium intact and in continuity with the superior and inferior vena cavae.
6. Carefully insert the donor heart–lung block.
7. Anastomose right atrium, trachea and aorta in that order, using polypropylene sutures and venting the right and left ventricles as described for the heart graft.
8. On filling the heart by releasing the aortic clamp, the cardiac cycle usually starts spontaneously.
9. Remove vents and withdraw bypass.
10. Close the chest with appropriate pericardial and pleural drainage.

Results

Currently, 1-year patient survival is 78%, with a 5-year survival of 50%. These results are the same for patients undergoing transplantation for cystic fibrosis and for the other indications.

REFERENCES

1. Cooley DA, Bloodwell RD, Hallman GL et al 1969 Organ transplantation for advanced cardiopulmonary disease. Annals of Thoracic Surgery 8:30–46
2. Reitz BA, Burton NA, Jamieson SW et al 1980 Heart and lung transplantation. Autotransplantation and allotransplantation in primates with extended survival. Journal of Thoracic and Cardiovascular Surgery 80:360–371

FURTHER READING

Advisory Group on the Ethics of Xenotransplantation 1996 Animal tissues into humans: recommendations and report. Department of Health, London

Bismuth H, Houssin D 1984 Reduced size orthotopic liver transplantation in children. Surgery 95:367–370

Campbell KWS, McWeir J, Ritchie WA et al 1996 Sheep cloned by nuclear transfer from a cultured cell line. Nature 280:54–66

Couinaud C 1981 Controlled hepatectomies and exposure of the intrahepatic bile ducts. Couinaud, Paris

Lancet 1976 Diagnosis of brain death (editorial). Lancet ii:1069–1070

Medawar PB 1944 The behaviour and fate of skin autografts and skin homografts in rabbits. Journal of Anatomy, London 78:176–199

Michels NA 1951 The hepatic, cystic and retroduodenal arteries and their relations to the biliary ducts. Annals of Surgery 133:503–523

National Institutes of Health Consensus Development Conference 1984 Statement: liver transplantation 1983. Hepatology 4 (Suppl 1):1075–1105

Starzl TE 1969 Experience in hepatic transplantation. Saunders, Philadelphia

Strong RW, Lynch SV, Ong TH et al 1990 Successful liver transplantation from a living donor to her son. New England Journal of Medicine 322:1505–1507

Warnock GL, Kneteman NM, Ryan EA et al 1992 Long term follow-up after transplantation of insulin producing pancreatic islets into patients with type I (insulin dependent) diabetes mellitus. Diabetologia 35:89–95

33

Thorax

T. Treasure, R.R. Kanagasabay

CONTENTS

INTRODUCTION

KEY POINTS Anatomy

- Acquire an intimate three-dimensional knowledge of the thorax and its contents.
- You will be dissecting within and around vital structures.

Thoracic and cardiac surgery are highly specialized and depend heavily not only on your competence but also on the supporting team and facilities. If a patient is stable for a while, or can be stabilized, prefer to arrange transfer to an expert centre as the best way to save life and preserve function. That must be understood; however, any surgeon who has to deal with trauma should be able to open the chest safely, through an appropriate incision, and perform well-judged surgery.

In this chapter we aim to guide both your judgement that something surgical needs to be done, and, once embarked upon, how to do it. We also wish to instruct aspiring surgeon and assistants, who wish to understand how and why operations are performed.

Technical principles: some reminders:

1. The safety margin during intrathoracic dissection is small. The bronchi and vessels are short, their branches close together and they are therefore vulnerable
2. In addition, the respiratory reserve of the patient is often compromised. The main pulmonary veins have strong walls but pulmonary arteries have fragile walls, at risk of rupture, with sudden heavy loss of blood.
3. Remember the principles of proximal control; if dissection is difficult it may be wise to encircle the more proximal pulmonary artery. Do not rely on simple ligatures; rely instead on secure suture or stapling of the main vessels.
4. Accurate bronchial closure is perhaps the most vital step in pulmonary resection in order to avoid the risk of breakdown of the suture line. Many surgeons use staplers.
5. Well sited chest tubes allow full re-expansion of the lung and drain fluid and air in the postoperative period.

KEY POINTS Cardiac function

- Learn how to avoid the formation of air embolism.
- Familiarize yourself with the speedy, effective management of cardiac arrest.

DIAGNOSTIC BRONCHOSCOPY

Appraise

- Diagnostic fibreoptic bronchoscopy is widely used by chest physicians and intensivists; rigid bronchoscopy is mainly used by surgeons who also use fibreoptic instruments to extend the range of observation.
- It is used to obtain tissue for histology, samples for microbiology and to assess the operability of tumours, and the scale of operation needed for their attempted cure.
- There are almost no contraindications, since fibreoptic bronchoscopy can be carried out under local anaesthesia augmented with intravenous benzodiazepine sedation. General anaesthesia is the norm for rigid bronchoscopy.
- Be wary of using the fibrescope to take biopsies of very vascular lesions, or in patients taking anticoagulants. Have available a rigid bronchoscope in case major or intractable bleeding occurs. Also have to hand adrenaline-soaked swabs and a bronchial blocker.
- Rigid bronchoscopy allows straight- and angled-view rigid telescopes to be passed in order to visualize in particular the

upper lobe orifices. Suckers and biopsy forceps may also be passed through the rigid bronchoscope.

Prepare

1 *Adults* are usually given general anaesthetic for rigid bronchoscopy. If a relaxant is given, oxygen is ideally supplied through a Venturi jet on the bronchoscope.

2 *Children* should be given general anaesthesia.

3 *Infants* are best given inhalation anaesthesia rather than using a relaxant.

4 Make sure you have good suction available.

Action

1 Pass the bronchoscope with the bevel facing posteriorly over the middle of the tongue until you see the tip of the epiglottis.

2 Elevate the epiglottis so that the cords come into view, then rotate the instrument 90° and pass the tip through the vocal cords.

3 Insert a moist swab or guard between the instrument and the gums and teeth to protect them from pressure and support the bronchoscope with your left thumb while manipulating it with your right hand. Take care not to catch the lips between the teeth and the bronchoscope.

? DIFFICULTY

1. If you pass the bronchoscope too far posteriorly, it enters the postcricoid region and oesophagus instead of the larynx (Fig. 33.1).
2. In difficult cases try using a long-bladed laryngoscope.

4 The fibrescope may be passed through the rigid endoscope in order to visualize the more distal airways.

Assess

1 Note the presence of:

- Endobronchial tumour and its site.
- Stenosis, which may be circular, oval or irregular, and is due to extrinsic compression.

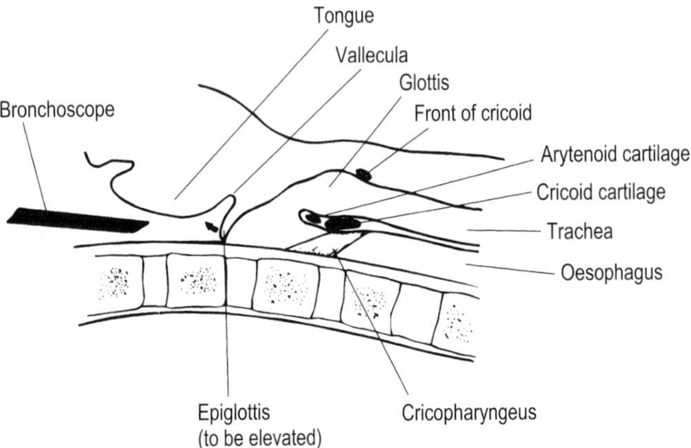

Fig. 33.1 Passage of the rigid bronchoscope.

- Vocal cord paralysis.
- Incursion of the lower tracheal wall, usually on the right side.
- Evidence of subcarinal widening.

2 Evidence of the last three indicates extensive disease and probable inoperability.

? DIFFICULTY

1. Haemorrhage is the most important and dangerous complication. It is due to bleeding from a vascular tumour or a vascular area of diseased bronchial wall. Rarely it is due to biopsy of a branch of the pulmonary artery lying adjacent to a segmental bronchus. Keep the bronchoscope in position and suck out the blood. Apply through the bronchoscope a swab soaked in 1:1000 adrenaline solution. Place the patient in the head-down position. Keep the bronchoscope in place until the patient is coughing again. Then remove the bronchoscope and place the patient in the lateral position with the bleeding side underneath. If there is severe bleeding from the pulmonary artery, pass a Thompson blocker or Fogarty catheter into the bronchus. If the bleeding continues when the blocker is released after 10–15 minutes, perform a thoracotomy.
2. Cardiac arrest may occur due to anoxia in elderly patients or those with cardiac disease. Premedication with atropine may act as a preventive. Always employ cardiac monitoring in such patients. The arrest can usually be treated successfully in routine fashion.
3. Laryngeal oedema usually occurs in children. Never force too large a bronchoscope through the small larynx.

FLEXIBLE BRONCHOSCOPY

Appraise

- This can be performed in conscious patients. It can be passed directly via the nose, through a rigid bronchoscope or through a single-lumen endotracheal tube in ventilated patients. Paediatric or intubating bronchoscopes can be passed through double-lumen tubes and are especially useful in assessing the correct positioning of these. The endoscope can be passed distally into the bronchial tree, allowing selective bronchial sampling and biopsy, and allows the upper lobe orifices to be well visualized. Its main disadvantage is its limited capacity for suction, making it difficult to remove viscid secretions and deal with significant bleeding after biopsy. However, it can be passed in patients with jaw deformities or rigid cervical spine in whom the rigid endoscope cannot be used (Fig. 33.2).
- *Intensive care unit.* Pass the endoscope through an endobronchial tube using a bronchoscopy adapter, which allows you to pass the bronchoscope without loss of gas pressure within the ventilator circuit. Apply suction for short periods only, since there is a risk of hypoxia developing.

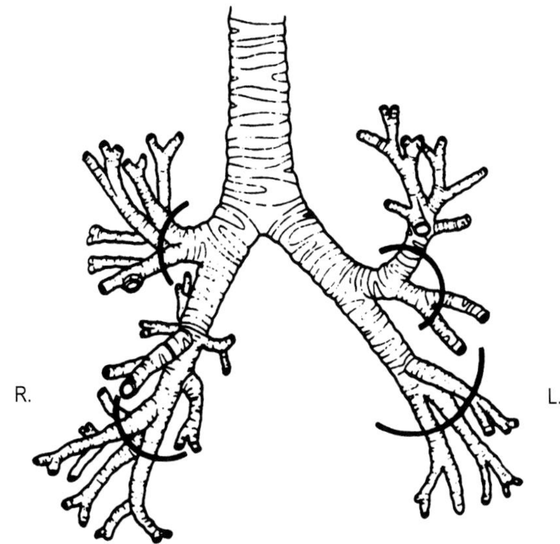

Fig. 33.2 Increased range of the fibrescope over the rigid scope plus telescopes.

- Transbronchial biopsy of lung parenchyma can be obtained and is valuable in the diagnosis of interstitial lung diseases, and distal sputum specimens can be aspirated, sometimes requiring the use of bronchoalveolar lavage. Perform a chest radiograph following transbronchial biopsy to exclude pneumothorax.
- Unless you are expert, avoid using the fibreoptic bronchoscope in children, where the small-calibre airway creates difficulty.
- The rigid bronchoscope is better for removing a foreign body and for larger biopsies when fibreoptic biopsies are negative, and especially in cases of very vascular tumours or patients taking anticoagulants.
- Prefer the rigid instrument when investigating active bleeding, because it offers more effective suction and also when dealing with tracheal strictures and obstructing neoplasms.
- The fibrescope can be used to aid the introduction of anaesthetic tubes in difficult cases.
- When performing bronchoscopy as part of a combined diagnostic procedure such as bronchoscopy plus mediastinoscopy, prefer to perform the bronchoscopy last, so that, if bleeding is caused during the bronchoscopy, the patient can be placed in the lateral position so that you do not need to abandon the mediastinal part of the operation.

Prepare

1. Use local anaesthesia and intravenous diazepam sedation.
2. Pass the fibrescope through an endotracheal tube during general anaesthesia.
3. Always employ an oxygen saturation monitor when performing bronchoscopy under local anaesthesia with sedation.
4. Closely observe the respiratory rate or use a capnograph (Greek: *kapnos* = smoke, carbon dioxide + *graphein* = to write).

Action

1. Pass the fibrescope through the nostril or the mouth.
2. Examine the bronchial tree systematically, including all the segmental orifices and their branches.
3. During rigid bronchoscopy the fibreoptic instrument can be passed through it to view the more peripheral bronchi.
4. Remove biopsies, cytology brushings or carry out bronchial washing to obtain histological or cytological diagnosis.

Complications

The risk of haemorrhage is very small as the biopsies are tiny.

THERAPEUTIC BRONCHOSCOPY

FOREIGN BODY IN THE BRONCHIAL TREE

Appraise

1. If you suspect that a foreign body has been inhaled, perform bronchoscopy at once to prevent complications such as bronchiectasis, lung abscess and empyema.
2. Infants commonly inhale peanuts. You need special forceps because the nuts tend to fragment. It may be valuable to withdraw the bronchoscope and the foreign body together because the calibre of the bronchoscope is so small.
3. Proceed to thoracotomy and bronchotomy when the foreign body is stuck and you cannot extract it with special grasping forceps.
4. Lobectomy or segmental resection is required if the foreign body is out of reach of the bronchoscope and if intensive physiotherapy fails to expel it.
5. Long-standing foreign bodies may become incorporated into dense granulation tissue. They can be very vascular and may also resemble endobronchial malignancy.

PULMONARY ATELECTASIS

Appraise

1. If physiotherapy and transnasal or per-oral suction have failed to clear the retained secretions, perform bronchoscopy.
2. Inhalation of vomit warrants immediate bronchoscopy. You may need to carry out lavage with saline or sodium bicarbonate solution, 1.4%.
3. Bronchoscopy often aids the placement of minitracheostomy catheters to facilitate postoperative physiotherapy.

Prepare

1. For adults, prefer local anaesthesia. Give a benzocaine lozenge to suck, or lidocaine 2% viscous solution to anaesthetize the mouth and pharynx. Instil 2 ml of 4% lidocaine into the larynx through a special curved cannula, while holding the tongue forward.

2 Have available oxygen and resuscitation facilities, especially when you bronchoscope cardiac-compromised patients who may develop sudden cardiac arrest.

3 Prefer general anaesthesia for children.

4 Preferably sit the patient up.

OTHER INDICATIONS

- Bronchoscopy may be used when dilating tracheal or bronchial strictures.
- Excess granulation tissue can be removed, and obstructing tumour palliated using endobronchial lasers, cryotherapy, diathermy or piecemeal resection with biopsy forceps.

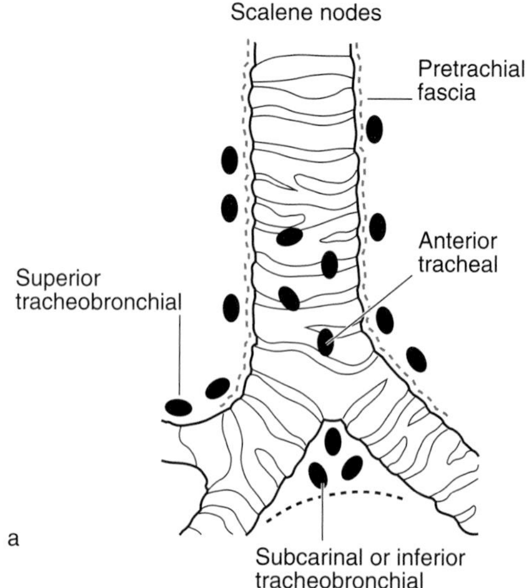

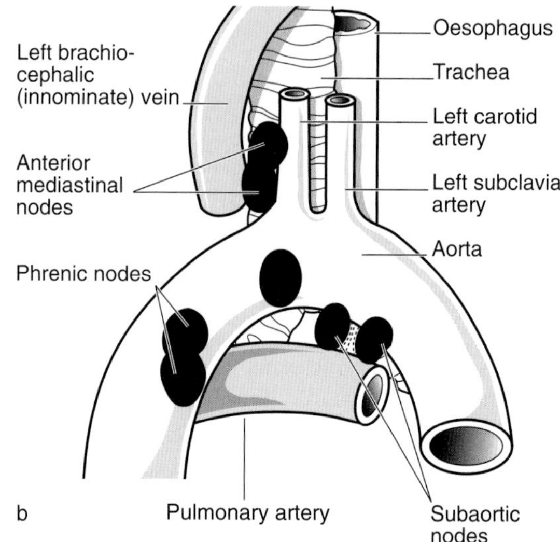

Fig. 33.3 Mediastinal lymph nodes.

MEDIASTINOSCOPY

Appraise

- This is valuable in the preoperative assessment and staging of carcinoma of the bronchus. Patients with involved mediastinal node disease N2 and N3 in the TNM (tumour, node, metastasis) classification, are usually deemed inoperable.
- Mediastinoscopy permits the investigation and assessment of a mediastinal mass or a mass due to lymph node pathology in the mediastinum. A diagnosis of tuberculosis, lymphoma or sarcoidosis may readily be made.
- Anterior mediastinal pathology lies anterior to the vessels and the plane of dissection, so is not amenable to mediastinoscopy. Subaortic and left anterior hilar nodes are also inaccessible (Fig. 33.3).

? DIFFICULTY

1. Mediastinoscopy increases the risk of haemorrhage in the presence of superior vena caval obstruction.
2. A large goitre interferes with access.
3. Beware patients with relatively short necks. The brachiocephalic artery may cross anterior to the trachea, quite high up, and so is at risk during the dissection.
4. In children and young adults beware, the innominate vein may be suprasternal in position.

- When performing bronchoscopy as part of a combined diagnostic procedure such as bronchoscopy plus mediastinoscopy, prefer to perform the bronchoscopy last, so that, if bleeding is caused during the bronchoscopy, the patient can be placed in the lateral position so that you do not need to abandon the mediastinal part of the operation.

Prepare

1 Lay the patient supine with a pad under the shoulders. Tilt the table head-up.

2 Make a short transverse incision in the suprasternal notch, at least two finger-breadths above the sternum.

Action

1 Use scissors to dissect down to and through the raphe between the strap muscles to reach the pretracheal fascia and then open it. Avoid the thyroid isthmus and thyroid veins. If you encounter bleeding at this stage, apply pressure with a swab for a short time to produce a dry field and then continue the dissection.

2 Dissect with your finger inside the pretracheal fascia down to the level of the upper lobe bronchus on the right and behind the aorta on the left to the same level (Fig. 33.4).

3 Introduce the mediastinoscope into the created space and use blunt dissection with a pledget or blunt sucker end to visualize the gland masses previously palpated, which are outside the fascia. These are usually the right paratracheal and superior tracheobronchial glands. The subcarinal nodes can be found by dissecting distal to and over the carinal region but this is more difficult.

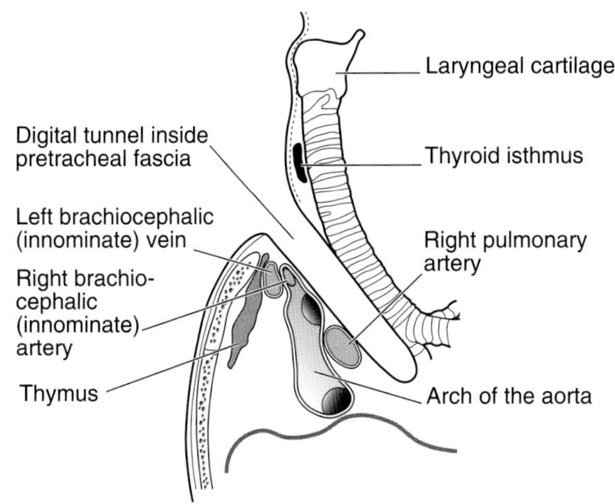

Fig. 33.4 Mediastinoscopy.

> **KEY POINT Tissue planes**
>
> - Stay close to the trachea and deep to the vessels, especially the innominate artery.

4 Aspirate before taking a biopsy and observe the proposed biopsy site as you withdraw the needle for signs of pulsatile bleeding, even if you have not been able to aspirate blood.

5 Very hard masses, although in themselves not particularly vascular, may be fixed to vascular structures posteriorly. Avoid very vigorous pulling on biopsy specimens; make sure you completely detach them before removing them.

6 By instilling local anaesthetic, and infiltrating the wound at the end, you can make this relatively painless and suitable as a day-case procedure.

> **KEY POINTS Inadvertent damage**
>
> - Do not damage the pulmonary artery, especially the right upper lobe branch, the superior vena cava or the azygos vein. There is less risk of damage to the innominate artery unless it is densely hidden in a gland mass and not palpable. If bleeding occurs, try inserting gauze packing. It is very rarely necessary to have to open the chest to control bleeding.
> - You may open the pleural cavity anteriorly to produce a pneumothorax. Detect it with postoperative routine chest X-ray. Insert a tube connected to an underwater seal drain.

ANTERIOR OR PARASTERNAL MEDIASTINOTOMY

Appraise

1 This allows you to diagnose an anterior mediastinal or lymph node mass in the mediastinum. It is particularly valuable for investigating and staging of tumours of the left upper lobe, which spreads initially to the nodes in the subaortic fossa.

2 If you are inexperienced this is safer and easier than mediastinoscopy. You can remove large biopsy specimens under direct vision, palpate the upper lobe and remove biopsies if indicated. Major venous bleeding is probably less easy to control than during mediastinoscopy, where packing alone may suffice.

Access

Make a short incision over the second interspace or as indicated by the position of the mass on CT (computed tomography) scan and X-ray.

Action

1 Deepen the incision and divide the intercostal muscles of the space.

2 Some approach the mediastinum by resecting a cartilage but I avoid this because of the risk of tearing the internal thoracic artery.

3 Avoid, or ligate, the internal thoracic vessels. Dissect off the parietal pleura to expose the mediastinum and lung root extrapleurally.

4 Biopsy the mediastinal mass or mediastinal and hilar nodes.

5 If necessary, open the pleura to inspect the lung or obtain a further biopsy.

6 If a thoracoscope or laparoscope is available, you can introduce it through the incision to obtain an improved view.

Closure

1 Insert a drainage tube into the extrapleural space through a lower anterior intercostal space, or a pleural drain if the pleura is opened.

2 Routinely close the wound in layers.

PREOPERATIVE MANAGEMENT

Appraise

1 Carefully assess patients with carcinoma by history and examination, looking for evidence of metastatic disease. Re-examine the posteroanterior chest X-rays.

2 Check the haemoglobin, blood film and establish the blood group. Exclude platelet abnormalities and the presence of hepatitis B antigen.

3 Order liver function tests in patients with carcinoma.

4 Exclude diabetes or other general disease.

5 If it is available, order a CT scan of the chest and upper abdomen with contrast to assess the tumour and related hilar and mediastinal nodes and to exclude adrenal metastases.

6 Be willing to repeat the physician's diagnostic bronchoscopy if you retain any doubt.

7 If there is possibility of spread to the mediastinal lymph glands (N2), perform mediastinoscopy or anterior mediastinotomy for left upper lobe lesions.

8 If it is available, order CT scan of the brain or obtain bone scans if you suspect spread.

9 Assess respiratory function clinically, including exercise tolerance, which is often adequate. Note the presence of obesity, body build, blood pressure and evidence of coronary artery disease. Radiological evidence of lung or lobar collapse suggests shunting may be present. The simple measurement of forced vital capacity and forced expiratory volume in 1 second (FEV_1) provides evidence of airways obstruction.

10 Order electrocardiography (ECG).

11 Carry out needle biopsy of suspicious peripheral lesions, using fine-needle and cytological examination or a Tru-cut needle biopsy. Ultrasound or CT scanning aid localization.

12 Pleural effusions on the side of a malignancy are suggestive of spread. Perform pleural aspiration and cytology, together with pleural biopsy prior to embarking upon lung resection.

Prepare

1 Smoking must stop.

2 Physiotherapy is particularly vital for the postoperative care of the patient. Order breathing exercises to be taught beforehand to improve lung function and increase diaphragmatic movement. Aim to reduce sputum, aided by starting an antibiotic after sputum culture. Bronchodilators may also be helpful to relieve bronchospasm, such as salbutamol.

3 Prescribe subcutaneous heparin, continued until the patient is fully mobile as prophylaxis against deep venous thrombosis and pulmonary embolism.

POSTOPERATIVE MANAGEMENT

Aims

1 Restore full expansion of the residual lung or ipsilateral residual lobes.

2 Clear bronchial secretions and prevent infection.

3 Prevent pneumothorax.

Action

1 Order X-rays to assess progress, usually on days 1, 3, and 5.

2 For pain relief we routinely use:

- an extrapleural paravertebral catheter to infuse local anaesthetic to the intercostal nerves from above to below the thoracotomy.
- patient-controlled analgesia (PCA).
- regular background oral analgesia such as paracetamol.
- other additional measures as required.

3 *Chest drainage*. We use basal and apical under water seal drains following lobectomy with optional suction of 10–15 mmHg or cmH_2O. Measure the volume of fluid and record any air leak. The drains can be removed once drainage and air leaks stop. Occasionally air leaks continue for up to 2 weeks. A small residual air space is acceptable but do not accept persisting leaks, likely to result from 1–2-mm calibre bronchi on the raw surface of the lung.

4 Physiotherapy aims to help remove sputum and so maintain full lung expansion. Tipping, and routine use of the incentive spirometer can be helpful. Minitracheostomy may also be indicated.

5 Early ambulation is possible even when the patient is still connected to a drainage tube. We get patients out of bed the next day and walking as soon as possible. Encourage active breathing exercises and leg exercises.

6 Monitor for and treat, cardiac arrhythmia.

KEY POINTS Arrhythmia

- Be aware that atrial fibrillation may reflect hypoxia.
- Arrhythmias after pneumonectomy may herald a problem of mediastinal shift or pneumonectomy space infection and bronchopleural fistula.

7 Continue antibiotic prophylaxis for several days, changing it if there is clinical evidence of failure to improve, and if X-rays display pulmonary consolidation.

8 Minimal surgical emphysema is common following pneumonectomy. More marked emphysema may result from a blocked drainage tube, or a delayed air leak after the tube has been removed. The lung is often adherent and does not collapse fully, while pressure in the space builds up rapidly. Unblock an existing tube or insert a new one following radiological assessment. Sudden early appearance of surgical emphysema following pneumonectomy may indicate a significant bleed into the space, forcing the air into the surrounding tissues.

Complications

- *Bleeding*. If more than 200–300 ml of blood per hour drains during the first 2–3 hours, check the blood coagulation for platelet or clotting factor deficiency. Replace the blood loss and consider exploring the chest if the bleeding continues and there is no apparent haematological cause. The bleeding is usually from a bronchial artery or pulmonary venous branch.
- *Empyema*. This is due to infection of retained pleural fluid, serous or blood, and the presence of organisms unresponsive to the prophylactic antibiotic. Full re-expansion of the lung obliterates the space and is usually sufficient. This is a major complication following pneumonectomy; treat it by emptying the space, instilling appropriate antibiotics and lavage. If these simple measures fail, institute open drainage by rib resection. Alternatively perform fenestration by resecting short lengths of three ribs anterolaterally over the base of the space. Suture the skin margins to the pleural edge, creating a permanent window that will not close in the absence of a tube. After some months it may be possible to close the window. Exclude the presence of a small bronchopleural fistula.
- *Bronchopleural fistula* is a rare complication after segmental or lobar resection and is now very uncommon following pneumonectomy. Treat by draining the space and re-suture the

bronchus stump. Small fistulae may heal with continued drainage.

- *Atelectasis* (Greek: *ateles* = incomplete + *ektasis* = stretching out; incomplete expansion) should respond to physiotherapy.
- *Respiratory failure* is more likely in elderly chronic bronchitics, the emphysematous and heavy smokers. It may result from spill of blood or infected sputum into the lower lung at operation. Monitor for clinical evidence of carbon dioxide retention, such as tiredness, sweating or rising blood pressure, and check progress with blood gas estimation. If you confirm respiratory failure, move the patient to a high-dependency or intensive care unit. Continuous positive airways pressure (CPAP) administered via a face-mask may help but often temporary ventilation is needed if the patient is becoming exhausted. Avoid continuous positive-pressure ventilation, which interferes with bronchial stump healing.

CHEST DRAINS

Appraise

1 Inappropriate, imperfect insertion of chest drains causes morbidity.

2 Drains are usually inserted to drain air or fluid (blood, effusion, pus, chyle). Air is customarily drained by placing the tube in the apex and fluid is drained basally. Provided the pleural space is not loculated the actual position is probably not important. To avoid injury to underlying structures, insert drains into the 'triangle of safety', bounded by the anterior axillary line, the mid-axillary line and the level of the nipple. Remember how high the diaphragm rises.

3 Lie the patient back on a pillow with the arm abducted, providing access to the target triangle. Clean the skin, infiltrate local anaesthetic generously but within the limits imposed by the patient's weight. Wait for at least 10 minutes. Make a short skin incision sufficient to admit a finger. Using a blunt dissector or artery forceps, dissect down to the pleura immediately above a rib and enter the chest by blunt dissection. Feel the pleura 'give' as a distinct 'pop'. Insert a finger to confirm that you are safely in the chest. Place a simple suture across the midpoint of the incision to close the wound when the drain is removed and tie a knot in the end. Place another suture at the corner of the incision to secure the drain. Now insert the drain, with the aid of a Roberts clamp if necessary.

UNDERWATER SEAL DRAINAGE

1 Connect the outer end of the drainage tube to a long tube passing well below the level of a measured amount of water in the bottle so that the fluid provides a seal preventing entry of air into the chest.

2 Check that drainage is free by noting the fluid swing in the long tube on inspiration, provided no suction is connected.

3 If necessary, connect the short tube, which allows escape of air, to a source of suction; this can be increased up to a negative pressure of 20 cmH_2O or 20 mmHg (3–5 kPa; Fig. 33.5).

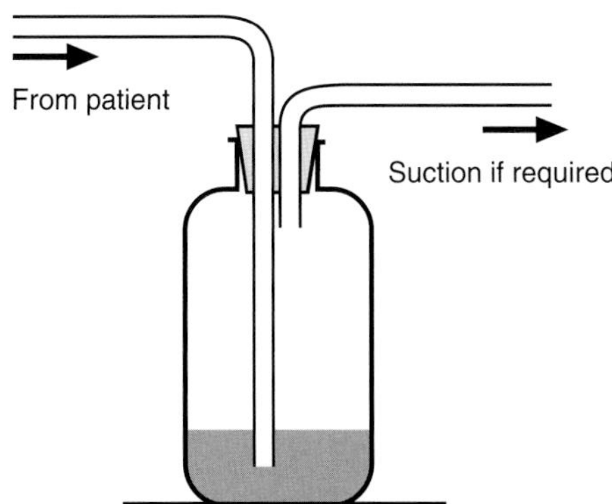

Fig. 33.5 Underwater seal drainage.

Suction is never important in immediate management and has its own dangers. Never turn off suction while leaving the apparatus connected to the bottle, since the drain is effectively blocked. Ensure that the suction device is low-pressure, high-volume to prevent obstruction. Wall suction with a regulated adapter is ideal. Never apply suction to drains inserted following pneumonectomy since it produces mediastinal shift.

4 Clamping a chest drain is almost never indicated and is potentially dangerous. Never clamp drains while patients are being transferred. Never raise the drainage bottle above the patient or fluid may enter the chest.

5 Suction may be helpful in the following situations:

- Where there is a pneumothorax and the lung does not inflate with simple drainage.
- After performing a pleurodesis (Greek: *desis* = a binding together).
- When draining a haemothorax or empyema, to help avoid the drains blocking.

KEY POINT Danger with drains

- Never apply suction to chest drains following pneumonectomy.

6 If suction is not used, resistance to drainage increases as the bottle fills with fluid. Change the bottle once it is more than half full to ensure good continued drainage.

POSTEROLATERAL THORACOTOMY

Appraise

This is the usual route of access for:

- Pulmonary operations.
- Some oesophageal operations.
- Posterior, middle mediastinal and mainly unilateral anterior mediastinal lesions.
- Repair of coarctation, division of patent ductus arteriosus, and thoracic aneurysms.

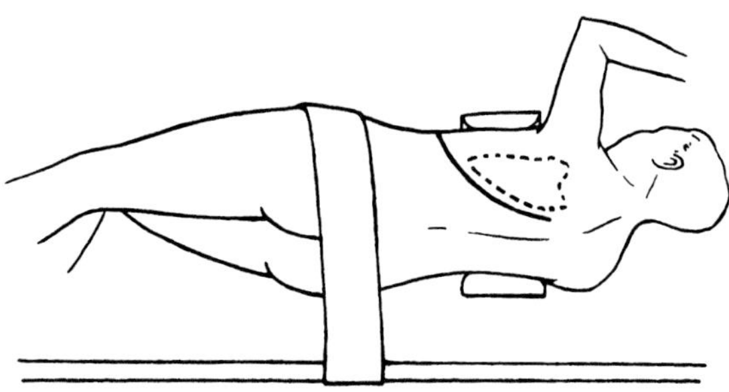

Fig. 33.6 Position for posterolateral thoracotomy.

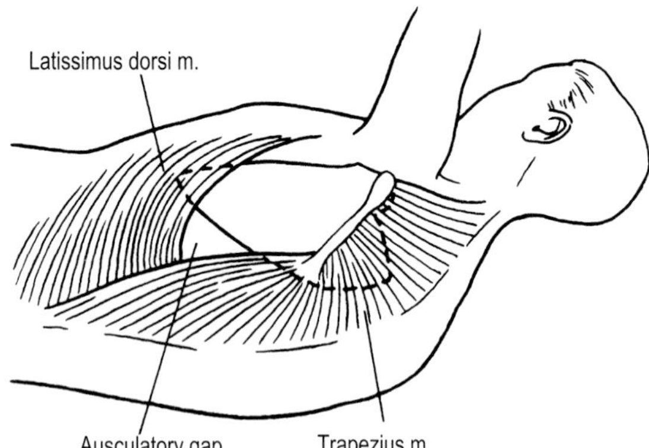

Fig. 33.7 Arrangement of superficial muscle layers.

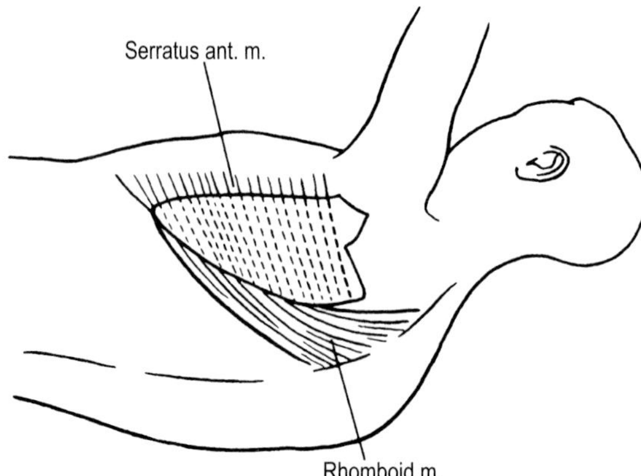

Fig. 33.8 Arrangement of deep muscle layers.

Access

1 Place the patient in the lateral position with the chest arched over a soft pad, such as a Holmes Sellors support. Position the arms and legs as in Figure 33.6.

2 Approach all standard lobectomies through the fifth interspace. Modify the approach if you predict specific problems such as pleural involvement or adhesions at the apex.

3 Cut the skin in a smooth curve, running from midway between the midline and medial border of the scapula posteriorly, skirting the angle of the scapula by 2.5 cm, and passing forward to the anterior axillary line.

Action

1 Divide the muscles using the diathermy point, coagulating cut vessels. The muscles are arranged in two layers: the superficial layer of trapezius and latissimus dorsi, the deeper layer of the rhomboid and serratus anterior. Preserve the serratus anterior muscle almost intact by dividing this layer through the aponeurosis below the muscle fibres, right to the anterior extent of the wound (Figs 33.7, 33.8). We usually leave it completely intact.

2 Count the ribs from the apex by passing a hand up under the scapula. It is difficult to identify the first rib and the uppermost rib you can feel is usually the second. The third rib has a characteristically flatter, broader shape.

3 Divide the periosteum of the upper border of the sixth rib with the diathermy point.

4 Strip the periosteum from its upper border, using a curved rougine, working posteroanteriorly. Alternatively divide the intercostal muscle above the rib using diathermy without stripping the periosteum.

5 Rib resection or division is rarely necessary provided you free the costotransverse ligament posteriorly using a notched chisel and then open the retractor gradually and gently.

6 Open the pleura along the length of the wound after warning the anaesthetist to allow the lung to fall away. The periosteal separation may be extended anteriorly deep to the wound.

7 Insert a rib spreader.

8 Divide light or filmy adhesions with scissors or diathermy.

9 Use a mounted gauze swab and blunt dissection to strip the lung in the extrapleural plane when widespread marked adhesions are present.

KEY POINT Tissue planes

- Do not wander. Having found the plane of dissection, stay in it.

10 A hot pack controls diffuse oozing; coagulate bleeding points with diathermy. The extrapleural strip need be over an area of dense localized adherence only if the rest of the lung is free.

Closure

1 Insert apical and basal drains anterolaterally two or three spaces below the wound. with the skin and pleural holes off-set to direct the drain and create a tunnel for a better seal. Pass the apical tube up the apex of the chest, usually sited anteriorly to the basal drain (Fig. 33.9).

KEY POINTS *Aide-mémoire*

- Anterior apical drain for air.
- Big-back basal drain for blood.

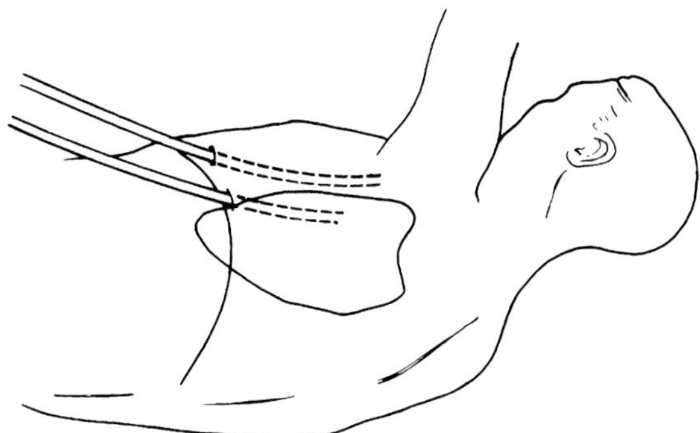

Fig. 33.9 Siting of drainage tubes.

2 Position the drain exit sites sufficiently far anterior so that the patient will not lie in discomfort on them.

3 Use a Holmes Sellors approximator to draw the ribs together and close the intercostal layer with a continuous suture of absorbable synthetic suture, approximating the edge of the stripped intercostal layer above to the intercostal muscle below the rib that has been stripped. This intercostal closure is usually sufficient, avoiding the need for pericostal sutures which often causes chronic post-thoracotomy pain from nerve entrapment.

4 Unite each muscle layer with a continuous absorbable suture.

ANTEROLATERAL THORACOTOMY

Appraise

1 This provides access to the heart, pericardium and lung, previously but now rarely used for closed mitral valvotomy. Median sternotomy is used for most cardiac operations performed with cardiopulmonary bypass.

2 It may be used for open cardiac massage in cardiac arrest and for pericardial drainage.

3 Use a shorter version for open-lung biopsy in diffuse pulmonary disease.

Access

1 Lay the patient rotated obliquely with the ipsilateral (Latin: *ipse* = self, same) hip and shoulder supported on pillows or sandbags. Elevate the ipsilateral arm, carefully avoiding nerve traction.

2 Usually employ the fifth intercostal space and follow the line of the appropriate rib which can readily be counted anteriorly. In the female, curve the incision below the breast.

3 Start the incision close to the midline and extend it to the axilla, passing 2.5 cm below the angle of the scapula if you need additional length.

Action

1 Divide the pectoralis major muscle in the line of the incision and split the serratus anterior muscle along the line of the rib selected.

2 Divide the periosteum using the diathermy point and strip it from the upper border of the rib posteroanteriorly.

3 Open the pleura in the depth of this layer. Take care to avoid the internal mammary vessels close to the sternum.

4 Open the pericardium anteriorly to the phrenic nerve, as this gives better access.

Closure

1 Suture the intercostal layer with an absorbable suture. The medial portion is difficult to close because the muscle layers are thin and attenuated at this site.

2 If the costal cartilage fracture when the spreader is opened, resect a small portion to avoid local friction.

3 Close the muscle layers with continuous sutures. Insert a drainage tube through a separate incision laterally below the level of the main wound.

MEDIAN STERNOTOMY

Appraise

1 This usually provides best access for cardiac operations using cardiopulmonary bypass. It produces less postoperative pain and respiratory upset.

2 A shorter version of this incision allows exposure of the trachea for resection of a stricture or tumour.

3 Use it to remove anterior mediastinal tumours such as thymomata, germ cell tumours and rarely for retrosternal goitre.

4 Bilateral bullous lung disease and pulmonary metastases may be approached but access to the left lower lobe is limited by the heart.

5 The incision can be performed rapidly using appropriate equipment. In an emergency if a sternal saw is unavailable, prefer an anterior thoracotomy.

Prepare

1 Place the patient supine with the arms by the side. For cardiac surgery attach ECG electrodes to shoulders and chest wall, percutaneously insert a radial artery catheter for arterial pressure monitoring and a central venous pressure line via the internal jugular vein.

2 Insert a urinary catheter, rectal and nasopharyngeal temperature probes.

3 Prepare the skin to allow access to groins and also to the leg in coronary artery bypass operations.

4 In a patient with a stocky neck place a sandbag under the shoulder blades and extend the neck to improve exposure.

Action

1 Incise from the lower margin of the suprasternal notch to the xiphoid process.

2 Divide the subcutaneous tissue with the diathermy point down to the sternal periosteum to maintain haemostasis. Keep

between the pectoralis major muscles and precisely mark the midline of the sternum with the diathermy. The sternum is least wide at the second space.

3 Carefully avoid veins that lie in the immediate suprasternal region by keeping close to the upper border of the bone. There is also a large vein frequently crossing the xiphisternal junction; control it with diathermy.

4 Free tissues from the deep surface of the xiphisternum by passing a finger up from below, avoiding the danger of catching a fold of pericardium in the saw with risk of injury to the heart.

5 Divide the sternum longitudinally using a reciprocating saw, hugging the posterior surface to avoid damaging the heart, ascending aorta or left innominate vein. You may use a Gigli saw, drawing it down from above after passing up extra-long Roberts forceps behind the sternum hugging its posterior surface. You may also use an oscillating saw.

6 Seal periosteal vessels on both aspects of the sternum with diathermy. If possible, avoid pressing in bone wax to control bleeding from exposed marrow.

7 Insert a self-retaining retractor, dissect between the lobes of the thymus and incise the pericardium in the midline.

? DIFFICULTY

1. If the heart is not visible, moving freely behind the pericardium, suspect pericardial adhesions.
2. Take great care in opening the pericardium.

8 Extend the incision up to the reflection on the aorta, avoiding the left innominate vein, and down to the diaphragm. Sew the pericardial edges to the skin to form a well and improve the exposure of the heart.

Closure

1 If you opened the pericardium, introduce pericardial and anterior mediastinal drains (24–28F catheter) through separate skin incisions below the xiphoid process and through separate openings in the rectus sheath.

2 Using a heavy trocar-pointed needle, or awl if the specialized sutures are not available, pass non-ferrous wire sutures through each side of the sternum. Firmly close the sternum by twisting the wire. Alternatively, pass the needle close to the edge of the sternum, from the second space caudally, avoiding the internal mammary vessels.

3 Approximate the muscle and the subcutaneous layers with polyglactin 910 (Vicryl) sutures, 1 and 00, respectively. Suture the linea alba accurately to avoid an incisional hernia.

PNEUMONECTOMY

Appraise

1 This is commonly performed for carcinoma involving upper and lower lobes, either because it crosses the fissure or impinges on both lobar bronchi.

2 It is rarely necessary nowadays for destruction of a lung by tuberculosis, other infections or bronchiectasis.

Access

1 Employ a posterolateral thoracotomy through the fifth space.

2 If the chest wall is fixed, be prepared to excise the pleura to free the lung. Rarely you need to resect a portion of the chest wall.

Assess

1 Inspect the site and note the local extent of the tumour, including the attachment to or involvement of the chest wall.

2 Check especially for involvement of the main pulmonary artery, either pulmonary vein or even the left atrium by direct tumour extension or involved lymph nodes.

3 You may be able to establish resectability only after opening the pericardium to ascertain that you can obtain proximal control of the main vessels.

4 Check for involvement of the oesophagus posteriorly by infiltrated nodes or direct tumour extension.

5 Look for infiltrated subcarinal nodes involving the origin of the opposite bronchus.

6 Check for involved right paratracheal nodes with secondary involvement of the superior vena cava and right phrenic nerve.

7 Palpate for enlarged nodes in the aortic hollow involving the recurrent laryngeal nerve or the aortic wall on the left side.

Action

1 Dissect inside the adventitia and divide the pulmonary artery between ligatures or preferably oversew with 4/0 vascular suture. We recommend using a vascular clamp such as a Satinsky. If necessary, divide the left artery close to the main trunk after dividing the ligamentum arteriosum while preserving the recurrent laryngeal nerve.

▶ KEY POINT Care

- Beware! The left pulmonary artery is very short.

2 You may divide the pulmonary veins extrapericardially; alternatively, open the pericardium for easier access to the veins as they enter the left atrium (Fig. 33.10).

3 Divide the veins between ligatures. If the tumour extends proximally, divide the veins after applying a vascular clamp, such as a Satinski, to the left atrium, then suture this with 3/0 non-absorbable suture.

4 Isolate and divide the bronchus close to the carina. Stapling is now the standard method but alternatively use a bronchus clamp or open division with direct suture.

5 Divide the inferior pulmonary ligament.

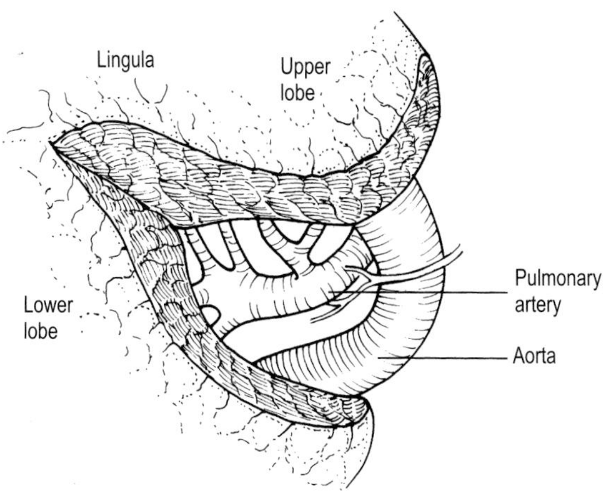

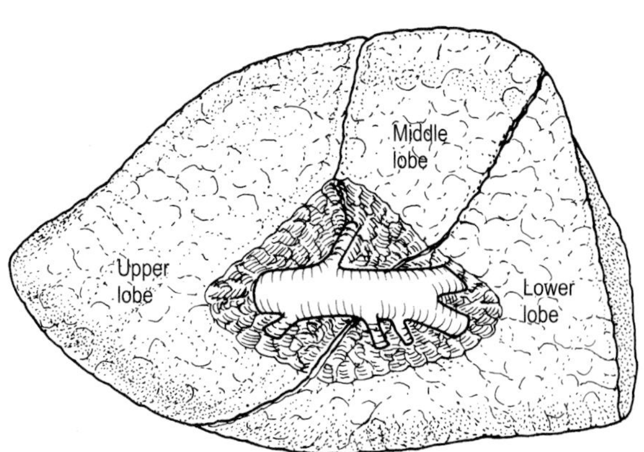

Fig. 33.10 Anatomical relations of the hila of the lungs.

Closure

1 Do not routinely insert a drain. Some surgeons insert a drain, clamp it (one of the few indications for clamping a chest drain), and release it for a few seconds every half-hour to allow graduated drainage.

> **KEY POINT Drains**
>
> - Never apply suction to a chest drain inserted following pneumonectomy.

2 Carefully close the intercostal layer to avoid leakage of fluid into the muscle layers.

3 Routinely examine the patient to assess the position of the mediastinum and order a postoperative chest X-ray to confirm your findings. If there is gross shift towards the operated side, instil air under strict aseptic precautions, using a syringe, filter and three-way tap.

4 If you insert a drain remove it on the first postoperative morning.

LOBECTOMY

Appraise

1 This is the preferred operation for:
- Bronchial carcinoma, ideally when the lesion is sited peripherally in the lobe.
- The resection of localized bronchiectasis not controlled by conservative measures.
- The resection of tuberculous disease which has not responded fully to antituberculous chemotherapy.

2 Each lobectomy has individual variations dependent upon the relevant anatomical features. The principles of the operation can best be illustrated by a description of a right upper lobectomy, followed by a brief description of resection of the other lobes.

RIGHT UPPER LOBECTOMY

Access

With the patient in the lateral position, perform a right posterolateral thoracotomy through the fifth intercostal space.

Assess

1 Check the paratracheal area and lobar hilum for enlarged nodes.

2 Assess whether there is tumour crossing the fissure, necessitating a bilobectomy or pneumonectomy. If you have embarked on exploratory thoracotomy on a patient deemed by preoperative respiratory function tests to be suitable for lobectomy, but not pneumonectomy, be particularly thorough in your assessment before dividing any vessels.

Action

1 If the disease is adherent to the chest wall, be prepared to carry out local extrapleural separation.

2 Dissect the hilum anteriorly and expose the superior pulmonary vein. Find the middle lobe vein inferiorly and isolate the main portion of the upper lobe vein superiorly for ligation. Ligate the segmental branches distally and divide the vein. Take care posteriorly in the dissection as the main right pulmonary artery trunk lies deep to the vein (Fig. 33.11).

3 Display the upper branch of the right pulmonary artery superiorly to the vein and separate it from the superior vena cava anteriorly. Dissect the artery in the subadventitial plane and divide it between ligatures; this branch supplies the apical and anterior segments. Display the main trunk. Look for the recurrent branch to the posterior segment and, if you see it, divide it between ligatures. If you do not see it now, secure it after dividing the right upper lobe bronchus.

4 Rotate the lung anteriorly and expose the right upper lobe bronchus by dissecting the pleura over its posterior aspect. Divide the bronchial artery branch to the upper lobe bronchus and ligate it or seal it with diathermy.

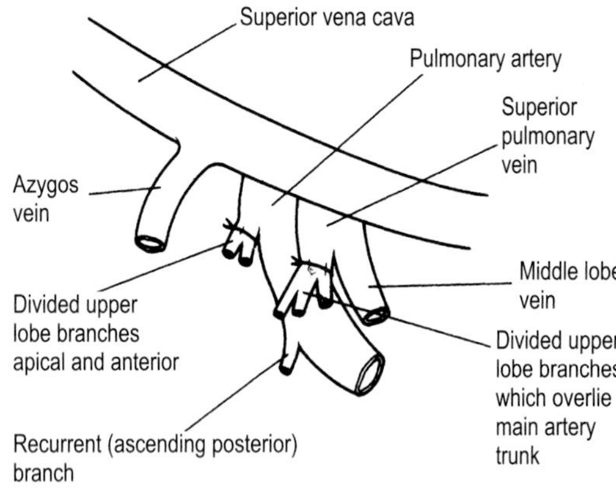

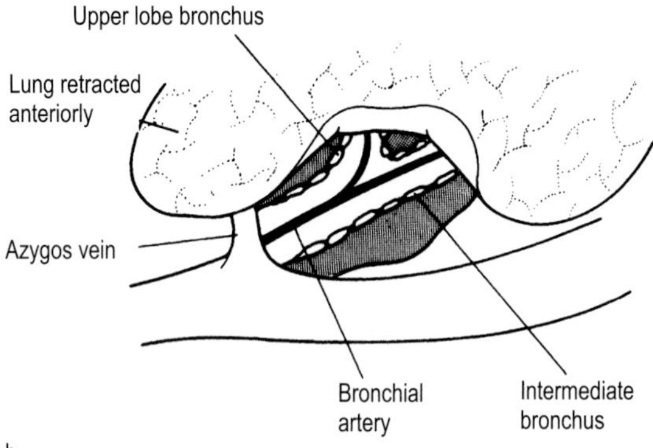

Fig. 33.11 Right upper lobectomy.

5 Pass an O'Shaughnessey forceps around the upper lobe bronchus as close to the main bronchus as possible. The bronchus is usually stapled but alternatively divide and suture it.

6 Separate the lobe from the lower lobe posteriorly and the middle lobe anteriorly. The ease of separation depends on the degree of development of the fissures. This is most easily done by having the anaesthetist lightly inflate the remaining lobes while you apply light traction on the distal bronchus clamp and at the same time separate the lobes. Keep in the correct plane and pick up minor venous or arterial branches that cross the lobar plane.

7 Remove the lobar and anterior hilar lymph nodes for biopsy. Remove the paratracheal nodes also if a preliminary mediastinoscopy was not performed. Divide the inferior pulmonary ligament if necessary to allow easy upward rotation of the remaining lobes. Lightly suture the middle lobe, if it is freely mobile, to the lower lobe to prevent it from becoming rotated and necrotic.

DETAILS OF THE OTHER LOBECTOMIES

Left upper lobectomy

1 Retract the upper lobe inferiorly and then anteriorly as you work your way down the main pulmonary artery as it lies in the oblique fissure. Between three and five arterial branches will be found going to the upper lobe. Divide these between ties.

2 Divide the superior pulmonary vein from in front of the hilum, having first checked that there is a normally situated inferior vein to drain the lower lobe. Note that the lingular artery may arise from the lower lobe artery and not the main pulmonary artery.

3 Dividing the arterial branches exposes the upper lobe bronchus which may then be divided.

4 Complete the dissection of the fissure with diathermy or staples.

5 Divide the inferior pulmonary ligament as before.

6 Achieve perfect haemostasis, since there is often a sizeable artery within it.

Right lower lobectomy

1 Dissect in the fissure between the three lobes to expose the arterial branches. Beware that the middle lobe artery(s) may arise opposite the apical lower lobe branch and must not be inadvertently ligated.

2 After dividing the arterial branches divide the inferior pulmonary vein. Now expose the bronchus. The apical segmental bronchus may arise opposite the middle lobe bronchus. In this case it is safer to divide the apical bronchus separately from the main lower lobe bronchial closure, to avoid compromising the middle lobe airways.

3 Complete the dissection of the fissure with diathermy or staples as before. If the middle lobe has a narrow pedicle, tether it to the upper lobe to avoid potential postoperative torsion with a couple of 4/0 polypropylene sutures.

Left lower lobectomy

1 This is very similar to the dissection for right lower lobectomy with the exception that the arterial branches usually need to be divided individually in order to preserve the lingular arteries.

2 Beware of dividing the bronchus too proximally and narrowing the upper lobe airway.

Middle lobectomy

Divide the middle lobe venous branches from the front. Next retract the middle lobe anteriorly and dissect the horizontal and oblique fissures. Identify the branches carefully and divide only those to the middle lobe—usually two. The bronchus lies behind. The horizontal fissure is often incomplete and requires further dissection, using diathermy. Avoid using staples in the horizontal fissure as they will distort the geometry of the remaining upper lobe.

Sleeve resection or sleeve lobectomy

1 This usefully extends the scope of lobectomy, so avoiding pneumonectomy, especially if lung function is compromised.

2 It is indicated for carcinoma of the right or the left upper lobe that is too close to the main bronchus to permit the 1.5-cm bronchial clearance necessary for lobectomy (Fig. 33.12). It may

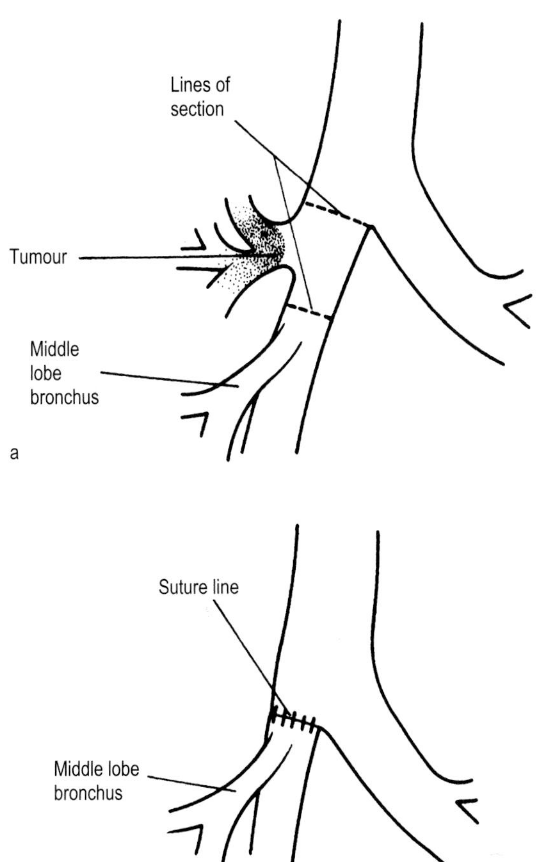

Fig. 33.12 Sleeve lobectomy.

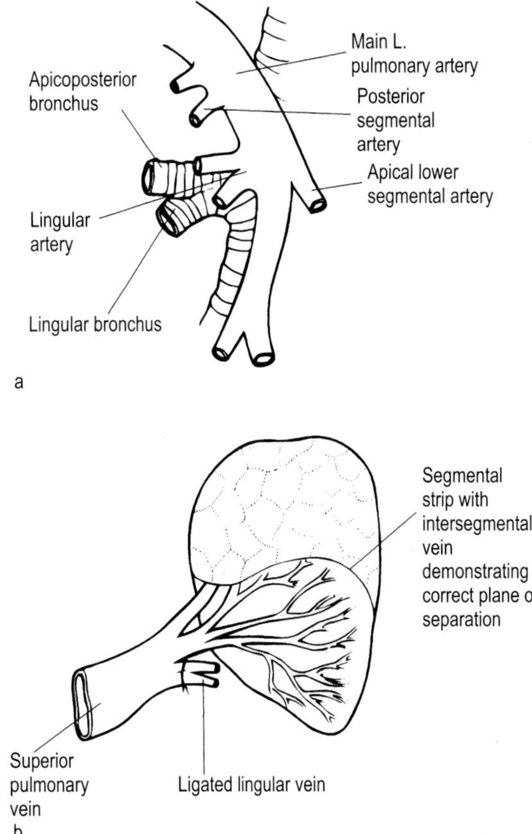

Fig. 33.13 Dissection of lingular segmental resection.

also allow the removal of bronchial carcinoids or a tuberculous stricture.

SEGMENTAL RESECTION

Appraise

1 This operation is less frequently performed now that resections for tuberculous disease have become rare. It is now more usual to remove wedges of parenchyma with modern stapling devices.

2 Small (1–2 cm) peripheral bronchial carcinomas may be satisfactorily removed by this operation in elderly patients with reduced respiratory reserve. The lesion should be in the centre of the segment.

3 Occasionally metastatic lesions may be removed in this manner.

4 Bronchiectatic disease may be localized to segments, as, for example, the lingula.

5 Chronic inflammatory disease, such as an abscess, may be resected.

KEY POINT Anatomy

- Do not embark on this procedure without an intimate knowledge of the segmental bronchi and arterial branches.

Action

1 Isolate and divide the relevant segmental pulmonary artery branches and the segmental bronchus. Segmental veins course between the segments, so control them as you encounter them.

2 The operation is easier if the segmental bronchus can be isolated first; the corresponding arteries can then be found and confirmed while the segment is being stripped out.

3 In the left upper lobe segments you need to ligate the arterial branches in order to obtain access to the corresponding segmental bronchi.

4 Preserve any doubtful arterial branch until it is clear that it is passing to the relevant segment, to avoid causing pulmonary infarction.

5 Treat the apical lower and lingular segments exceptionally as a lobe with division of the corresponding segmental vein (Fig. 33.13).

6 Strip the segment while exerting traction on the distal bronchus with the lung gently inflated. The intersegmental vein acts as a good guide to the correct plane.

7 Deal with the raw lung surface as described in lobectomy.

COMPLICATIONS OF CHEST TRAUMA

Patients with chest injuries frequently have multiple injuries that all require treatment. Immediately decide the correct priority for treating multiple injuries. A valuable system is the acute trauma life support (ATLS) protocol.

RIB FRACTURE

Appraise

Rib fractures of themselves are of only limited significance and rarely require special treatment other than adequate analgesia. They may result in bleeding, lung laceration and pneumothorax. Injuries to the first and second ribs imply a greater force of injury; suspect major vascular injury.

Action

1 Do not attempt fracture fixation.

2 Ensure that the patient's pain is well controlled to allow early chest physiotherapy and so prevent sputum retention with consequent chest infection.

3 Patient-controlled intravenous analgesia or intercostal nerve blocks are occasionally required.

FLAIL SEGMENT

Appraise

Multiple fractures may result in a flail or paradoxical segment. A portion of chest wall becomes completely mobile, embarrassing respiration, often associated with underlying pulmonary contusion. There are few early radiographic features of pulmonary contusion, but later appearance of diffuse pulmonary infiltrates, together with progressively rising oxygen requirements and hypoxia, signal the condition. As the injured lung becomes less compliant, the effects of the paradoxical segment become more severe.

Action

1 Fracture fixation and chest strapping do not help.

2 Treatment of the flail segment and the underlying contusion are supportive.

3 Ventilation is often required.

SUCKING CHEST WOUNDS AND PNEUMOTHORAX

Appraise

A breach of integrity of the chest wall producing a sucking wound leads to a pneumothorax.

Tension pneumothorax is signalled by absence of air entry, shift of the mediastinum to the contralateral side, raised jugular venous pressure and incipient circulatory collapse. Be aware that the jugular venous pressure is not raised in the presence of hypovolaemia.

Action

1 Immediately insert an intercostal chest drain. In extremis, an intravenous cannula is a quicker life-saving manoeuvre.

2 Cover any sucking chest wound with an airtight dressing once you have established adequate intercostal chest drainage.

LUNG INJURY

Appraise

1 Lung lacerations may be caused by fractured ribs protruding into the chest cavity. The resulting pneumothorax often responds to simple drainage, but large air leaks may require open repair, particularly if the lung remains collapsed.

2 Repair the laceration with a running 4/0 polypropylene suture or with a stapling device.

3 Severely injured or 'burst' lung may require more major formal resection.

4 If there is a large air leak, perform bronchoscopy to specifically exclude a tracheal or proximal bronchial injury.

DIAPHRAGMATIC INJURY

Appraise

Suspect this often overlooked injury in any patient presenting with major chest trauma who has a poorly defined hemidiaphragm, or basal chest shadowing, particularly on the left side.

Plain chest X-ray and CT scanning may be helpful, but the most helpful investigations are diaphragmatic ultrasound and/or barium studies of the small bowel.

Action

1 Repair using direct suture, augmented if necessary with polypropylene mesh.

2 Delayed operation is often complicated by adhesions.

MAJOR VASCULAR INJURY

Appraise

1 Injuries to the great vessels are usually associated with multiple injuries. The most serious is aortic transaction with circumferential disruption of the vessel wall, usually just distal to the origin of the left subclavian artery. The tear is contained by the adventitial layer only and is associated with a number of characteristic radiographic features:

- Mediastinal haematoma (wide mediastinum).
- Left pleural effusion.
- Distortion of the left main bronchus, being pushed down into a more horizontal configuration by the expanding periaortic mass.
- Extrapleural apical 'cap' of blood.

2 Distinguish this condition from aortic dissection—pathological separation of the layers of the aorta—extending usually over some length. Aortic dissection occurs spontaneously in hypertensive patients, and is usually unrelated to trauma.

3 Suspect aortic transection when there has been a violent acceleration/deceleration injury. It is difficult to assess the size of the mediastinum in multiply injured patients, when it may not be possible to perform an erect posteroanterior chest film. The most sensitive investigation is aortography, although transoesophageal echocardiography and contrast spiral CT scanning may also be used.

Action

1 Employ left thoracotomy.

2 If you do not work in a cardiothoracic unit and are without access to cardiopulmonary bypass or a shunt, all you can do is clamp above and below the transection. Carry out direct repair, or more usually, interpose a short tube graft. This is associated with a high risk of paraplegia, which is time-related.

3 The aim of operation is to establish control above and below the site of the transection before dissecting the region of the injury so that, if the aorta ruptures, clamps can be swiftly applied.

PENETRATING STAB WOUNDS OR PERFORATING WOUNDS

Action

1 Such wounds may not necessarily demand a thoracotomy. Treat the patient conservatively and deal with the wounds locally if there is no clinical evidence of serious internal damage or bleeding and the chest X-ray is satisfactory. Note the direction of the wound to estimate which structures are at risk.

2 Remember that stab wounds in the lower half of the chest may be associated with diaphragmatic puncture and intra-abdominal injury to the spleen, liver or hollow viscera.

3 Undertake thoracolaparotomy if you remain in doubt following careful assessment. Overlooked diaphragmatic penetration may result in fatal strangulation of an incisional hernia after a long delay.

4 Transthoracic echocardiogram may demonstrate a pericardial effusion, highly suggestive of a cardiac injury. Explore it, provided you have adequate facilities available.

WOUNDS OF THE HEART AND PERICARDIUM

Appraise

1 Many gunshot wounds are rapidly fatal but some patients, especially those with stab or knife wounds, reach you with a haemopericardium and evidence of cardiac tamponade.

2 Clinical features are of falling cardiac output: peripheral vasoconstriction, tachycardia and low blood pressure associated with rising venous pressure. Intravenous resuscitation increases the venous pressure further. If the patient has survived with a cardiac wound, it is likely to be atrial or a minor ventricular injury.

3 Confirm the clinical diagnosis with X-ray and ultrasonography.

Prepare

Establish a good intravenous infusion and order adequate blood replacement. This is mandatory because, on opening the pericardium, rapid and profuse bleeding is likely.

Action

1 Aspirate the pericardium to confirm the diagnosis. This may temporarily relieve tamponade.

2 Expose the heart through a left anterolateral thoracotomy via the fifth space if bleeding persists, recurs or is obviously severe and requires emergency operation. Median sternotomy may be preferable for central or right-sided penetrating wounds, especially if bypass is available and indicated. If there are wounds on both sides, a clamshell incision may be fashioned by performing bilateral anterior thoracotomies through the fourth space and joining them by dividing the sternum transversely.

3 Control atrial wounds with finger pressure or an appropriate atraumatic clamp such as a Satinski clamp or, occasionally, a Duval forceps. Suture with 3/0 or 4/0 vascular sutures. Restore adequate blood volume once bleeding is under control.

4 Control ventricular wounds with finger pressure and then insert 2/0 sutures. Use a pad of Dacron, Teflon or pericardium to reinforce the closure if the muscle is friable.

5 Some penetrating wounds may be associated with valvular damage requiring investigation and subsequent treatment.

6 Drain the pericardium adequately and close the chest routinely.

ASPIRATION OF THE PERICARDIUM

Perform this for cardiac tamponade resulting from the accumulation of blood following trauma, or fluid developing as a result of pericardial inflammation.

Prepare

1 Sit the patient up at 45° (Fig. 33.14).

2 Confirm the clinical diagnosis with echocardiography.

Action

1 This is best done in the catheter laboratory, the X-ray department under screening or with ultrasound.

2 Infiltrate the skin below the xiphisternum and to the left of the midline with local anaesthetic.

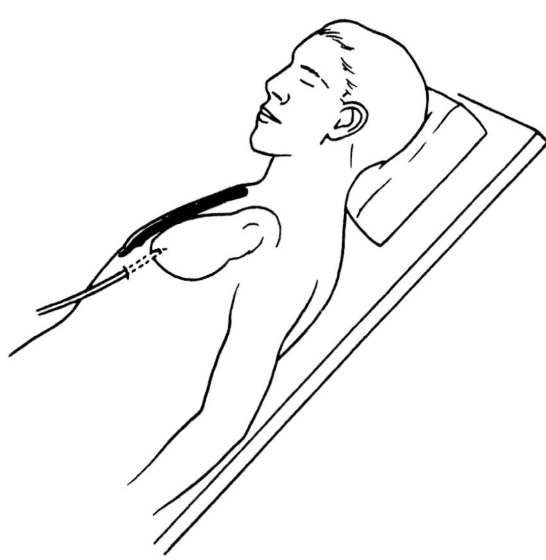

Fig. 33.14 Technique of aspiration of the pericardium.

3 Advance the needle towards the right shoulder; the inferior aspect of the pericardium has a definite resistance.

4 Push the needle through the pericardium and aspirate the fluid.

5 It is possible to introduce a plastic catheter such as Intracath through a larger-bore needle or a small cannula if aspiration needs to be maintained.

6 Leave a pericardial drain in situ for at least 24 hours to limit further re-accumulation, and to encourage obliteration of the space.

EMPYEMA THORACIS

Appraise

1 Pus may collect in the pleural cavity following pneumonia, oesophageal perforation or thoracic operations. Antibiotic therapy has modified the presentation of this condition. Confirm the diagnosis radiologically, by ultrasound and by aspiration.

2 An intercostal catheter may effectively drain thin pus, as is often the case in postoperative patients.

INSERTION OF INTERCOSTAL CATHETER

Action

1 Use the chest X-ray, ultrasound or CT scan to establish the most dependent point of the cavity to be drained.

2 Have the patient semirecumbent and rolled a little away from the affected side.

3 Make every effort to have the skin entry of the tube anterior to the mid-axillary line and tunnelled into the bottom of the cavity which is usually more posterior.

4 Use 0.5% or 1% lidocaine local anaesthesia. Raise a skin weal then infiltrate the subcutaneous tissue, muscle and especially the pleural layer.

5 Make a 1.5-cm transverse incision over the lower portion of the cavity.

6 Insert a chest drain. Prefer blunt dissection with artery forceps and finger pressure. If the ribs are too closely crowded to admit a drain then you will need to perform a rib resection. Secure the drain with a stitch.

7 Connect the catheter to the drainage bottle and underwater seal. Suction may be used if thought beneficial (see p. 489).

OPEN DRAINAGE BY RIB RESECTION

This has largely be replaced by the use of modern tube drains and antibiotics. You must be sure that the lung is adherent to the chest wall around the cavity.

Action

1 Use a double-lumen endotracheal tube if there is any chance of communication with the airway or a pulmonary abscess.

2 Make 5-cm incision in the line of a rib, insert a self-retaining retractor and divide the muscles with diathermy to expose the ribs.

3 Resect the lowest appropriate rib after checking by aspiration.

4 Divide the periosteum with diathermy and strip it from the rib, working forwards along the upper border and backwards along the lower edge of the rib.

5 Excise approximately 2–3 cm of rib.

6 Open into the cavity and remove the coagulum and thickened pleura for histological examination and pus for bacteriological culture.

7 Suck out the pocket and remove any large fibrin masses using sponge-holders and swabs.

8 Insert the multiply fenestrated drainage tube at the base of the cavity.

9 Tunnel the tube subcutaneously so that the point of entry into the skin is anterior so the patient will not lie on the tube. Fix the drain securely and close the wound in layers. A purse-string suture is not needed as the drain will be withdrawn slowly.

10 Apply suction initially and then use a valved bag. Institute intensive physiotherapy to aid rapid re-expansion of the lung and quick obliteration of the cavity.

EXCISION OF THE EMPYEMA AND PULMONARY DECORTICATION

This operation is an alternative to open drainage. Prefer it if the lung is very trapped and the patient is young and fit. However, the degree of healing and re-expansion that can occur with conservative management is impressive.

Action

1 Perform a posterolateral thoracotomy.

2 Free the lung and empyema in the extrapleural plane. This may be a very difficult procedure if the empyema has been present for some weeks or months.

3 Stripping is difficult to achieve and often incomplete over the diaphragm.

KEY POINTS Dangers

- There is risk of damage to the superior vena cava on the right and the aorta on the left.
- Take care stripping the apex of the thorax.

4 Remove the organized fibrin overlying the visceral pleura linking with the outer wall of the empyema cavity, which has been freed by the extrapleural strip. You must achieve complete decortication to obtain full expansion of the lung (Fig. 33.15).

5 Institute adequate drainage of the pleural space and intensive physiotherapy, since air leak from the lung surface may be considerable.

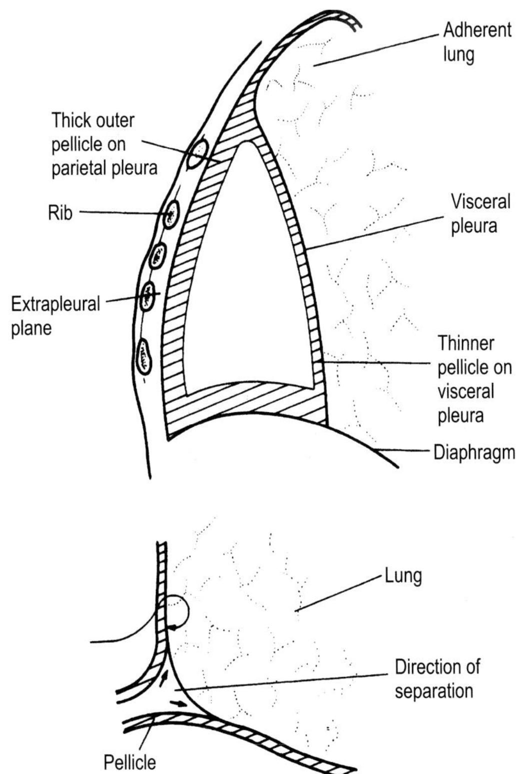

Fig. 33.15 Excision of empyema and decortication.

SPONTANEOUS PNEUMOTHORAX

Appraise

1 This is commonly seen in young adults with a typically tall, thin body habitus. The usual cause is rupture of apical bullae in the upper lobe, although sometimes the apex of the lower lobe or other areas are affected. It presents with chest pain or shortness of breath or occasionally with tension pneumothorax.

2 The cause in older patients is bullous emphysema.

Assess

1 The majority of cases respond to medical management by either aspiration or chest drainage, and surgery is not indicated for a first episode. The chance of further pneumothoraces after two episodes exceeds 50% and so surgery is then warranted.

2 If the lung remains deflated, or there is a persistent air leak for more than 5 days even on a first episode, then surgery is indicated. A single episode on both sides of the chest or a single episode of tension pneumothorax are also indications for surgery.

Action

1 The mainstays of treatment are closure of the air leak or the creation of pleural adhesions to prevent further collapse. This is performed by video-assisted thoracic surgery (VATS) in thoracic units and thoracotomy is rarely needed for this condition.

2 Closure of the air leak is performed by stapling, depending on the size of the bullae or with sutures or ties if VATS cannot be used or is unavailable.

3 Pleural adhesions are formed either by performing a parietal pleurectomy, abrasion of the pericardium with a rough swab, or a chemical pleurodesis with talc. Pleurectomy is done by gently stripping the parietal pleura away from the chest wall. A dissecting pledget mounted on a Roberts clamp can be helpful.

> **KEY POINTS Dangers to extrapleural structures**
>
> - Superior vena cava.
> - Azygos venous arch.
> - Sympathetic chain.
> - Aorta and recurrent laryngeal nerve.

5 It is not necessary to extend the pleural strip over the danger areas. Also, stop the pleural strip above the hilum.

6 Occasionally spontaneous pneumothorax is accompanied by significant bleeding into the chest. The usual cause for this is tearing of an apical adhesion at the site of a previously ruptured bulla. The bleeding can sometimes be brisk enough to require urgent surgery, but in any case can be controlled by clips or diathermy. Minor bleeding stops without surgery if the lung can be made to inflate by insertion of a chest drain. After pleurectomy or pleurodesis, leave both apical and basal drains in situ, on suction, for at least 48 hours, or until any air leak ceases.

LUNG BIOPSY

Appraise

1 Lung biopsy is often useful in cases of suspected interstitial lung disease where there is doubt about the diagnosis. Patients with atypical chest infections sometimes require lung biopsy also.

2 Inspect preoperative chest X-ray and CT scan to identify the affected areas to biopsy.

Assess

Patients referred for this procedure are sometimes severely compromised by their respiratory disease but usually they have chronic lung disease and management depends on histological information.

Access

1 Video-assisted thoracic surgery (VATS) with anaesthesia by a double-lumen tube is best, performed in a specialist unit.

2 An open procedure may be carried out by the posterior approach through the auscultatory triangle.

3 The submammary approach is appropriate in a very sick patient in the intensive care unit on a ventilator. If circumstances justify it, this is within the competence of a non-specialist surgeon.

PULMONARY EMBOLECTOMY

Appraise

1 Pulmonary embolism is a relatively common diagnosis in most hospitals, although massive pulmonary embolism requiring surgical treatment is uncommon.

2 It is usually seen in patients who have multiple risk factors for deep venous thrombosis such as immobility, malignancy, pelvic or orthopaedic surgery.

3 Presentation is with hypoxia, chest pain and signs of right heart strain both clinically and on ECG. At its most extreme patients may develop acute circulatory collapse.

4 The role of surgery is in patients with incipient or established circulatory collapse. If facilities for interventional radiology and catheter disobliteration of emboli are available, this can be considered as an alternative.

Action

1 Aggressively replace circulating volume, achieve adequate oxygenation and anticoagulation.

2 If the patient is pulseless a period of cardiac massage may help to break up and disperse the clot in the main pulmonary artery and improve the haemodynamics.

3 If there is no response to these measures, consider surgical embolectomy through a median sternotomy. The right heart is distended. Place two stay stitches side by side on the main pulmonary artery. Make a vertical incision between the stay stitches. Clot is seen in the main pulmonary artery. Extract it using sponge-holding forceps; there is then brisk back-bleeding. The pulmonary artery can be controlled by use of the stay stitches while the incision is closed.

4 This is the classical operation but it is very infrequently indicated and much less often successful.

THORACOSCOPY

Appraise

1 Endoscopic performance of minimally invasive procedures in the chest has become routine since high-quality video systems and dedicated instruments became available. Outside the setting of a cardiothoracic unit, it may still be possible to perform basic thoracoscopic procedures using a standard laparoscope. More complex procedures require dedicated staplers and instruments, which may not be widely available.

2 Procedures that can be performed in this manner include diagnostic pleural biopsy, drainage of pleural effusion and pleurodesis, lung biopsy, evacuation of a haemothorax and drainage of an empyema. Sympathectomy is described in Chapter 31.

Action

1 Use double-lumen anaesthesia and let the lung down before starting. If there is fluid present, use a needle and syringe to locate a safe entry point into the effusion.

2 Safe insertion of the thoracoscope is as important in the chest as in the abdomen, and parallels insertion of chest drains. Make a short skin incision sufficient to admit a finger.

3 Using a blunt artery forceps, dissect down to the pleura immediately above a rib and enter the chest by blunt dissection. The pleura 'gives' as a distinct 'pop'. Insert a finger to confirm that you are safely in the chest.

4 Insert the port and thoracoscope.

5 The safest site is where the fluid can be aspirated. In case of doubt go no lower than one space below the tip of the scapula to avoid injury to the diaphragm.

6 Insert further ports under direct vision. Suckers and other instruments can be inserted directly through incisions without the need for more ports.

7 Drain pleural effusions, breaking down thin loculae or adhesions with the sucker tip. Take pleural biopsies. If the diagnosis of malignancy is obvious from the macroscopic appearance then a pleurodesis can be performed by insufflating talc at the same operation.

34

Head and neck

M.P. Stearns, R.W.R. Farrell, M. Hobsley

CONTENTS

GENERAL PRINCIPLES

- Details of anatomy tend to be more important in the head and neck than in other regions. Numerous structures are crowded into a small volume and many of them, such as the facial nerve, perform important functions—some are vital to life itself, such as the recurrent laryngeal nerve and the internal carotid artery. Refresh your memory of the local and neighbouring anatomy before performing a new or unfamiliar operation. Before embarking on any major procedure consider seeking advice from, or collaborating with, a plastic, thoracic, dental or neurosurgeon or otolaryngologist.
- The airway may be threatened by the accumulation of blood, by laryngospasm, etc., so insist on endotracheal intubation for all but the simplest procedures.
- Gastrointestinal complications such as peritonitis, paralytic ileus and disturbances of water and electrolyte balance are rare, as is thromboembolism.
- Postoperative chest complications occur following direct interference with respiratory passages or after long operations but are less common than following abdominal or thoracic surgery.
- Even massive resections of tissues are therefore well tolerated. Infection is uncommon and healing is usually by first intention. When skin grafting is necessary to repair a defect, the grafts take well. Good healing is evidence of the good blood supply enjoyed by the territory. The good blood supply determines that the principal operative hazard, after damage to important anatomical structures, is primary haemorrhage.

MINIMIZE BLOOD LOSS

1 Discuss likely blood loss with the anaesthetist, who may decide to use hypotensive anaesthesia, lowering the arterial blood pressure by such agents as ganglion blockers. If you do operate under hypotension, remember the increased risk of reactionary haemorrhage shortly after the wound has been closed, so delay closure until you are certain that the blood pressure has been restored to normal.

2 Venous bleeding is more difficult to control than arterial. Venous pressure, and therefore venous bleeding, can be minimized by paying careful attention to posture. Position the patient so that the area being operated on is at a higher level than the heart. Carefully protect local veins from direct pressure resulting from clumsy positioning of the head, neck or shoulders, and the presence of supports or towels, etc. If it is necessary to divide a large vein draining the operative area, postpone this step in the operation to the latest possible moment. The anaesthetist helps to reduce venous pressure by maintaining the clearest possible airway and by keeping arterial carbon dioxide tension normal or below normal.

3 Control blood vessels before dividing them; in this way you obviate excessive blood loss from, for example, a haemostat slipping off the cut vessel. For sizeable vessels, pass two ligatures with an aneurysm and tie them around the vessel before dividing the vessel between them.

KEY POINT Anatomy

- Acquire a detailed knowledge of the anatomy, in order to anticipate encountering vessels so that you can control them before cutting them.

4 Many surgeons infiltrate the skin and subcutaneous tissues with a solution of 1/200000 adrenaline (epinephrine) in normal saline, thereby producing vasospasm and reducing bleeding.

5 Diathermy is a valuable aid to haemostasis, but use it carefully. It stops bleeding by coagulating the tissues at more than 1000°C, potentially causing extensive destruction. Cutting diathermy produces high-intensity energy over a small sphere from the active electrode; coagulating current produces a lower intensity over a larger sphere. It is traditional to use the cutting current to incise tissues and the coagulating for producing haemostasis, on the principle that the larger zone of action of

the coagulating current compensates for any small inaccuracy in identifying the bleeding point. Prefer to use the cutting current for haemostasis, having first made sure that each bleeding point has been accurately identified; this discipline reduces unnecessary tissue destruction to a minimum.

6 After the operation, use suction drainage to obliterate the dead space under the skin flaps, thereby reducing the risk of reactionary haemorrhage and haematomas. Note that in the neck a haematoma is a potentially lethal complication, because of its possible effect upon the patency of the airway.

KEY POINTS Threats to the airway

- After any extensive procedures, especially those involving resection of the lower jaw, ask yourself whether such factors as an unstable tongue or laryngeal oedema might be a particular threat to the maintenance of the airway in the postoperative period.
- Be prepared to perform a temporary tracheostomy in such circumstances.

REPLACE BLOOD LOSS

1 Before operation, ensure that every patient has been asked about any history of a bleeding tendency, that a haemoglobin estimation has been performed and that blood has been taken for grouping and serum saved in case cross-matching becomes necessary.

2 With regard to which cases require blood to be cross-matched before the operation, it is difficult to lay down rules. Much depends upon your experience and that of the anaesthetist. Blood transfusion is rarely necessary for conservative parotidectomy under good hypotensive anaesthesia, but, if you are inexperienced operator, working with normotensive anaesthesia, have 2 units of blood cross-matched and have 4 units cross-matched before an extensive resection involving bone and/or block dissection of the cervical lymph nodes.

3 Normally the anaesthetist controls blood replacement during the operation. The principles are accurate measurement of the blood loss by weighing swabs and measuring the volume of the contents of the sucker bottle, with prompt and complete replacement, preferably monitored by the measurement of central venous pressure or of urine output.

PAROTIDECTOMY[1]

Appraise

1 Assess a parotid lump before operation by careful clinical examination. Pain and facial nerve palsy are diagnostic of malignancy apart from tuberculosis. Fine-needle aspiration cytology is accurate in about 85% of cases,[2] but the role of needle biopsy is debatable. Small discrete masses usually require surgical rather than conservative management.[3] Most parotid neoplasms are benign.[4]

2 The facial nerve and its five main branches run through the substance of the parotid salivary gland and are at risk in any operation designed to remove parotid tissue (parotidectomy).

3 Plan to expose the facial nerve and its branches at an earlystage of any parotidectomy and over a sufficiently wide area to ensure that the required resection of parotid tissue is done without cutting the nerve (conservative parotidectomy). However, if the object of your operation is to remove a lump in the parotid with a wide margin of normal tissue, you will sometimes find that this condition is impossible to fulfil; an adequate margin cannot be achieved unless you sacrifice the whole nerve (radical parotidectomy) or one or more of its branches (semi-conservative parotidectomy).[5]

4 If the decision is not clear-cut whether to sacrifice the main nerve, lean towards radicalism in elderly males, conservatism in young females. Biopsy the lump, and ask for an immediate histological opinion on frozen sections, provided:

- You take extreme precautions against spreading the tumour in taking the biopsy; parotid tumours are notorious for their tendency to implant.
- Your pathologist is an expert in the histopathology of parotid lesions.[6]

5 Repair any gap you produce in the facial nerve system by immediate primary suture, if possible, or by bridging the defect with a free cable graft taken as a routine from the great auricular nerve at the beginning of the operation. Ignore any damage to the fifth (cervical) branch.

6 Operations for recurrent parotitis that is not due to parotid calculus (i.e. the group of conditions known as Sjögren's syndrome or keratoconjunctivitis sicca) require total conservative parotidectomy.

Prepare

1 If you confirm a malignant tumour, discuss the implications with the patient, especially if there is a prospect of sacrificing part or all of the facial nerve.

2 Check that male patients are clean-shaven on the side of the tumour and ensure that all patients are shaved for 5 cm around the external ear in all directions.

3 Have the patient lying near your side of the operating table. Tilt the top half of the operating table upwards until the external jugular vein collapses. Extend the patient's head on the neck, turn it away from you and place it on a head-ring to stabilize it.

4 To protect the patient, and protect yourself from charges of negligence, monitor the facial nerve. Insert needle electrodes into the ipsilateral frontalis and mentalis muscles to record electromyographic signals from them, producing audible and visual signals when the facial nerves supplying them are stimulated. They can also be used to apply electrical stimulation as an aid to identifying a doubtful nerve fibre.

5 Ensure that the patient's eyes are protected from possible damage by lotions used in the skin preparation. Clean the skin over the area shown in Figure 34.1.

6 Sew the towels in place to leave exposed only the area shown in Figure 34.1. Push a twist of cotton wool (which is added to the swab count) into the external auditory meatus with a pair of artery forceps and then discard them.

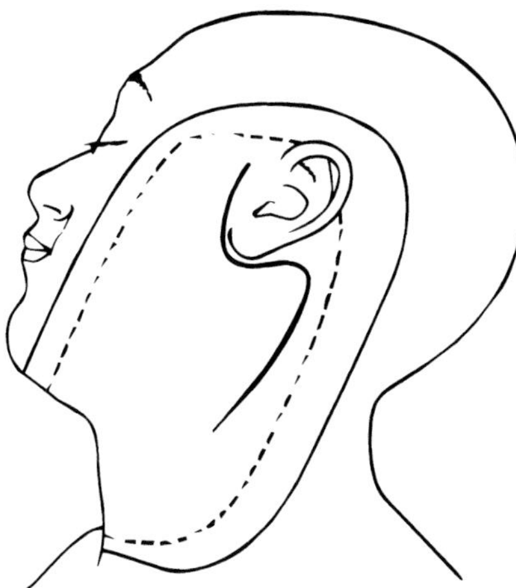

Fig. 34.1 The standard S-shaped cervicofacial incision for parotidectomy. Clean the skin of the area enclosed in the continuous line and towel up so as to leave exposed the area enclosed by the dotted line.

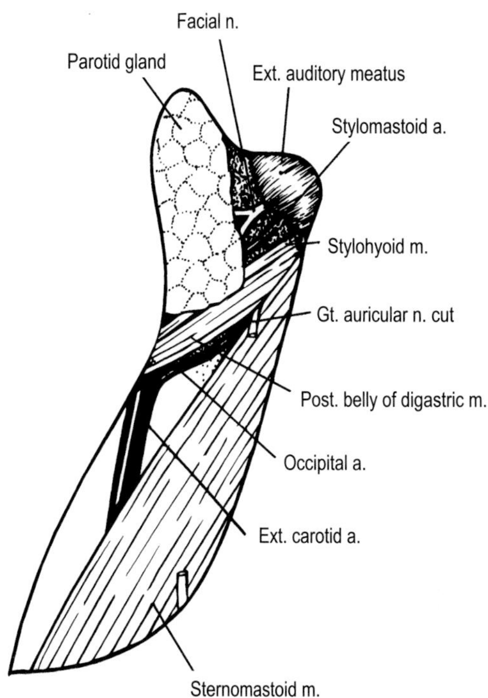

Fig. 34.2 The S-shaped incision has been deepened in the upper third (in front of the ear) to the bony external auditory meatus, and in its lower third to the stylohyoid muscle. This leaves a bridge of tissues in front of the mastoid that must be whittled away to expose first the stylomastoid artery, then the facial nerve.

7 Ask the anaesthetist to maintain the patient in hypotension if possible.

Access

1 Follow the standard S-shaped cervicomastoid–facial incision (Fig. 34.1). The lower, cervical, part lies in the upper skin crease of the neck, extending forwards to the external jugular vein. The upper, facial, part lies in the skin crease at the anterior margin of the auricle, extending upwards to the zygoma. Between these two parts, the mastoid part of the incision curves gently backwards over the mastoid process. If you intend to remove a lump in this area, exaggerate the posterior curve to encompass the lump.

2 Start by making the cervical part of the incision. Make the incision in three parts from below upwards, stopping all bleeding before proceeding to the next part. In this way you avoid bleeding from the upper part of the wound obscuring your field lower down. Incise skin, fat and platysma.

3 Identify the external jugular vein near the anterior end of the wound, and two branches of the great auricular nerve vertically below the anterior margin of the auricle (Fig. 34.2). Preserve the vein but sacrifice the thinner, usually more anterior, branch of the nerve. Dissect free but do not yet excise, about 4 cm of the thicker branch of the nerve.[7] The nerve runs upwards towards the ear and breaks up into two or three branches; if possible, include a centimetre of each branch with the segment of stem excised.

4 Facilitate the dissection by placing a row of artery forceps on the subcutaneous fat of the upper margin of the wound. Have your first assistant, standing opposite you, to lift the forceps. Identify the anterior border of the sternomastoid muscle. Follow the border upwards and posteriorly towards the mastoid process, as far as the incision permits. Deepen the dissection to expose in turn the posterior belly of the digastric and the stylohyoid muscles, proceeding at this stage only as far as is convenient.

5 Perform the mastoid part of the incision and deepen it on to the sternomastoid muscle. Continue to expose the anterior border of the muscle right up to the mastoid process. Place more artery forceps on the upper subcutaneous border of the wound and have your assistant pull the superficial part of the lower pole of the parotid gland forwards from the anterior border of the sternomastoid. Friable, yellow parotid tissue forms the visible aspect of the anterior margin of the incision.

6 Continue to expose the posterior belly of the digastric and the stylohyoid muscles upwards towards the mastoid process as far as is convenient at this stage.

7 Create the facial part of the incision and deepen it along the anterior surface of the cartilaginous external auditory meatus by pushing in an artery forceps and opening the blades in an anteroposterior plane. Deepen this plane until you can feel the junction between the cartilaginous and bony external auditory meatus (Fig. 34.2).

8 You now have a large S-shaped incision in which two deep cavities, one in the neck and one in front of the ear, are separated by a bridge of tissues where the dissection has not been deepened to the same extent, in the region of the front of the mastoid process. Whittle away these tissues piecemeal; push a closed, curved artery forceps from the upper cavity downwards at 45° towards the lower cavity so that the tips emerge. Separate the tips of the artery forceps and cut the tissue between them. Concentrate on defining the region where the anterior border of the sternomastoid and the two deeper muscles reach the anterior surface of the mastoid process. The dissection approaches the

region of the facial nerve, so take increasing care. Remove smaller bites of tissue. Have the diathermy apparatus turned to the lowest mark.

9 The signal that you are close to the facial nerve is to see the stylomastoid artery, running downwards and forwards in the same general direction as the facial nerve. Control it with ligatures or with diathermy coagulation and divide it. Continue the dissection and about 3 mm deeper you find the facial nerve trunk. It is 3–6 mm in diameter, white but with fine red vessels visible on its surface, and it bifurcates 1–2.5 cm below the base of the skull.

10 Further steps depend upon the exact operation you wish to perform.

SUPERFICIAL PAROTIDECTOMY

Appraise

1 You cannot determine clinically that a lump in the parotid gland is confined to the superficial part, so cannot determine beforehand to perform a superficial parotidectomy.

2 The definite indication for superficial parotidectomy is therefore recurrent parotitis from a stone in the parotid duct at a site inaccessible from the mouth.[8]

3 You must remove as much parotid tissue and as long a length of parotid duct as you can reasonably achieve, otherwise there is a risk of recurrent flare-up of the residual infected tissues.

Access

1 Perform the cervicomastoid–facial S-shaped incision.

2 Expose the main trunk of the facial nerve and its primary bifurcation.

Action

1 Choose either the upper or the lower main division of the nerve to start the dissection, whichever seems the most convenient. Aim to reflect forwards the parotid tissue superficial to the facial nerve and its five branches until you reach the anterior margin of the gland.

2 Place the closed blades of fine, gently curved mosquito forceps, concavity superficial, along the exposed division of the nerve and in contact with the nerve.

3 Push the forceps points along the surface of the nerve for about 5–10 mm into the region where the nerve is still unexposed and use the curve of the blades to make the points emerge through the parotid tissue (Fig. 34.3).

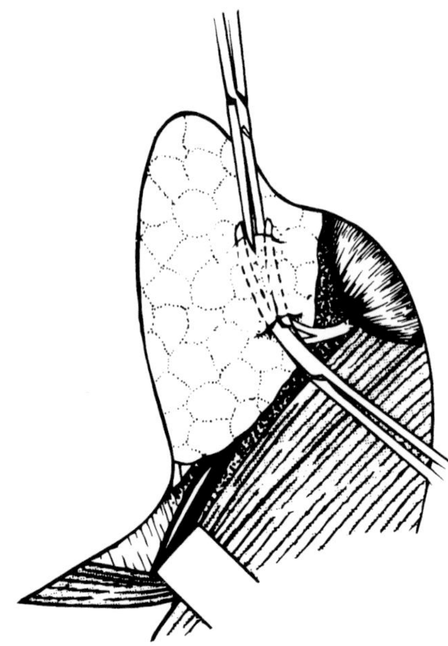

Fig. 34.3 The trunk of the facial nerve and its primary bifurcation have been exposed. When the scissors divide the bridge of tissue covering the blades of the forceps, a further segment of the upper division of the nerve will become visible.

4 Parotid tissue is tough, requiring a surprising amount of force to split it. Separate the points of the artery forceps, elevate the whole instrument to tauten the overlying tissue bridge. Divide the bridge with scissors, exposing a further few millimetres of the nerve.

5 Repeat the manoeuvre, following the more posterior nerve at any bifurcation. You eventually reach beyond the margins of the parotid gland—at the zygoma if you have followed the upper division, beyond the external jugular vein if you have followed the lower division.

6 Repeat the process with the other main division of the facial nerve and its most posterior branch. You have now exposed the facial nerve trunk and its temporal and cervical branches.

7 The zygomatic branch arises from the upper division, the mandibular from the lower division, and there are at least two buccal branches, one from each division, and sometimes a third, usually from the lower division.. Working from the periphery towards the centre of the gland, follow the other main nerve branches forwards to the anterior margin of the parotid gland, that is along a vertical line halfway between the anterior and posterior borders of the masseter muscle.

8 Reflect the skin from the anterior flap until you reach the superior and anterior margins of the gland. With a little more dissection along the nerve branches you free the gland except for the parotid duct.

KEY POINTS Caution

- Do not reflect the anterior skin flap at an earlier stage than this.
- A deeply placed, growing tumour may, by the pressure of its expansion, cause atrophy of the superficial glandular tissue, so that the facial nerve lies close to the skin.
- In these circumstances the nerve is in danger of being cut during too early skin flap reflection.
- This caution does not apply when operating on an inflamed gland.

9 Dissect the parotid duct forwards to the anterior border of the masseter muscle, where it turns medially to perforate the cheek and reach the mouth. Free from it the closely applied buccal nerve branches, then tie the duct at the anterior border of the masseter with an absorbable suture and cut the duct. The excision is complete.

KEY POINTS Pay attention to the nerves

- If there is a bleeding point so close to the facial nerve that you are afraid that an attempt at stopping the bleeding with artery forceps or diathermy may injure the nerve, ask your assistant to press on the point with a swab and turn your attention to dissecting another part of the facial nerve system. When you return to the original spot the bleeding will probably have stopped.
- The fifth, cervical, branch is not cosmetically important as it supplies only a part of the platysma. However, do not be tempted to sacrifice it at an early stage of the operation; the fourth, mandibular, branch often arises very far forwards from the fifth branch. Make quite certain that you have identified and preserved the fourth branch before you can consider sacrificing the fifth. The fourth branch takes a very long route, dipping behind the angle of the jaw into the submandibular region of the neck before turning upwards and medially to reach the lower lip. Damage to this branch produces the ugly deformity of loss of the Cupid's bow of the lower lip.
- You encounter several cross-communications between the five branches of the nerves. Preserve these if you find it easy to do so, but otherwise do not hesitate to cut them.
- Two of the buccal branches are intimately related to the parotid duct. Carefully separate and preserve them before you dissect the duct.

Checklist

1 Has the anaesthetist raised the blood pressure to normal for the patient or at least greater than 100 mmHg? If not, you risk a high incidence of reactionary haemorrhage. Restore the table to the horizontal position to ensure that any tendency to bleeding becomes immediately manifest.

2 Have you removed the cotton wool from the external auditory meatus?

Closure

1 Close the skin with a continuous blanket suture. There is no need for a subcutaneous stitch.

2 Always insert a suction drain via a stab incision 5 cm below the cervical end of the incision.

PAROTIDECTOMY FOR A LUMP IN THE PAROTID REGION

Appraise

1 Most lumps in the parotid region are parotid tumours, and most of the tumours are benign adenomas.[9] Also, most lumps are clinically unremarkable, that is they present no features that enable you to distinguish between non-neoplastic, neoplastic benign and neoplastic malignant lumps.[10] The well-recognized ability of adenoma cells to implant if shed into the wound renders a preliminary open biopsy inadvisable. However, fine-needle aspiration cytology does not seem carry an associated risk of implantation.

2 Controversy besets the decision as to whether to remove the lump with a wide margin ofs normal tissue after exposing and protecting the facial nerve, or whether to enucleate the lump in the hope of preserving the nerve. Enucleation is well known to carry an unacceptable incidence of recurrence. The available evidence suggests that enucleation does not reduce the incidence of permanent damage to the facial nerve and that the incidence of recurrence after enucleation and radiotherapy is unacceptably high.[1] Standard management in the UK, the universal management in the USA, is for excision of an unremarkable lump with the widest possible margin of normal tissue, with exposure and preservation of the facial nerve unless the tumour is invading it, or a branch of it. In this case the lump is malignant, so sacrifice the nerve element.

Access

1 Employ the cervicomastoid–facial S-shaped incision.

2 Expose the main trunk of the facial nerve and, if possible, its primary bifurcation. Dissect forwards along the nerve or along its upper and lower divisions. It is soon evident whether the lump is in the part superficial to the facial nerve, or deep to the nerve, and whether the nerve trunk or main divisions run into the lesion rather than being pushed aside by it.

Assess

1 Perform superficial, conservative, parotidectomy, as previously described, if the lump is superficial to the facial nerve.

2 Perform total conservative parotidectomy if the lump is deep to the facial nerve.

Action

1 Dissect under the trunk, divisions and branches of the facial nerve. With your fingers, gently lift the nerves off the underlying deep part of the parotid gland until there is clear space between the nerves and the whole of the deep part of the gland.

2 Identify the external carotid artery and companion vein if there is one, at the upper border of the stylohyoid muscle. Ligate and divide the artery and companion vein.

KEY POINTS Anatomy

- Ensure the artery is the external, not the internal, carotid artery.
- Identify the occipital branch that arises from the external carotid artery at this level running backwards and upwards along the lower border of the stylohyoid muscle
- Confirm that the artery enters the lower pole of the deep part of the parotid gland.

3 Mobilize the deep part of the parotid and its contained lump by working from the anterior and posterior parts of the gland towards the centre and from its lower pole upwards. Aim to mobilize the deep part so as to remove it above or below the facial nerve system, or between the two main divisions in the region of the bifurcation, whichever is most convenient (Fig. 34.4).

4 Facilitate mobilization of a lower pole containing a large tumour by dividing the stylomandibular ligament, of which the anterior insertion is into the angle of the jaw. If necessary, fracture the styloid process to gain more room.

5 Continue to mobilize the deep parotid off the masseter muscle and mandible anteriorly, and the bony external auditory meatus posteriorly. As you approach the upper part of the gland, identify the termination of the external carotid artery at the upper pole where it bifurcates into the superficial temporal artery and the maxillary artery. Tie and divided these arteries and their accompanying veins. The deep parotid is now free and you can remove it.

RADICAL PAROTIDECTOMY

Perform it with sacrifice of the facial nerve if this, or its main divisions, are surrounded by tumour.

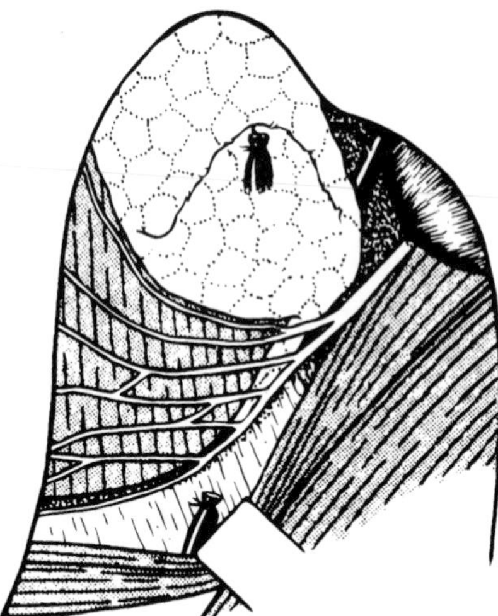

Fig. 34.4 Mobilization of the deep lobe of the parotid gland. The external carotid artery (and companion veins, not shown) have been divided at the lower pole of the gland, and the latter has been turned upwards to be delivered (in this case) above the main trunk of the facial nerve.

Action

1 Reflect the skin forwards to the anterior margin of the gland.

2 Find the external carotid artery at the lower pole of the gland and divide this and its companion vein between ligatures.

3 Divide the trunk of the facial nerve and mobilize the posterior aspect of the whole gland off the cartilaginous and bony external auditory meatus.

4 Divide the facial nerve branches at the anterior border of the gland and mobilize the whole gland backwards off the masseter muscle and the posterior border of the mandible.

5 Mobilize the whole gland from below upwards. Doubly ligate and divide the superficial temporal and maxillary arteries at the upper pole of the gland and remove the freed whole gland with its contained facial nerve system.

6 Perform semiconservative parotidectomy, sacrificing one or more branches of the facial nerve but preserving at least one of the upper four branches, if necessary, to preserve an adequate margin round the lump. Repair the cut branches end-to-end if the cut ends will meet; otherwise bridge the gap or gaps using the segment of greater auricular nerve you obtained earlier, with the finest available suture material.

? DIFFICULTY

1. The intention is to remove the lump with an adequate margin of normal tissue and this demands constant concentration.
2. Frequently feel the parotid and intended specimen to ensure that you are not too close to the lump.
3. To assist in preserving the margin, modify the incision as necessary to avoid cutting directly through skin onto the swelling. In case of doubt, be willing to include a layer of extraparotid tissues such as sternomastoid or other muscles, a slice of cartilage or a sliver of bone from the external auditory meatus.
4. If you are unable to control the maxillary veins before dividing them they retract under cover of the zygoma and bleeding may troublesome. Insert deep sutures to obliterate this plexus of veins.

REFERENCES

1. Hobsley M 1983 A colour atlas of parotidectomy. Wolfe Medical Publications, London
2. Al-Khafaji BM, Nestok BR, Katz RL 1998 Fine-needle aspiration of 154 parotid masses with histologic correlation: a 10 year experience at the University of Texas MD Anderson Cancer Center. Cancer 84:153–159
3. McGurk M, Hussain K 1997 The role of fine needle aspiration cytology in the management of the discrete parotid lump. Annals of the Royal College of Surgeons of England 79:198–202
4. Hibbert J (ed.) 1997 Scott Brown's otolaryngology, Vol 5. Laryngology and head and neck surgery. Oxford University Press, Oxford, p 5/20/6
5. Stevens KL, Hobsley M 1982 The treatment of pleomorphic adenomas by formal parotidectomy. British Journal of Surgery 69:1–3

6. Hobsley M, Thackray AC 1985 Salivary glands. In: Hadfield JG, Hobsley M, Morson BC (eds) Pathology in surgical practice. Edward Arnold, London, pp 22–34
7. Christensen NR, Jacobsen SD 1997 Parotidectomy: preserving the posterior branch of the greater auricular nerve. Journal of Laryngology and Otology 111:556–559
8. Suleiman SI, Thomson JPS, Hobsley M 1979 Recurrent unilateral swelling of the parotid gland. Gut 20:1102–1108
9. Hobsley M 1973 Salivary tumours. British Journal of Hospital Medicine 10:553–562
10. Hobsley M 1981 Sir Gordon Gordon-Taylor: two themes illustrated by the surgery of the parotid gland. Annals of the Royal College of Surgeons of England 63:264–269

EXPLORATION OF THE LOWER POLE OF THE PAROTID

Appraise

1 The exploration may be used to determine if a lump in the neck is or is not in the lower pole of the parotid gland. The lower pole of the gland extends well down into the neck behind the angle of the jaw and is separated anteriorly from the submandibular salivary gland only by a thickened sheet of fascia, the stylomandibular ligament

2 The procedure can be employed to obtain a large piece of tissue from the gland for histological examination.

Access

1 Make the incision in the upper skin crease of the neck, starting just in front of the external jugular vein, extending backwards to a point vertically below the lowermost tip of the mastoid process.

2 Identify the external jugular vein and expose the two divisions of the greater auricular nerve. Sacrifice the thinner division of the nerve. Mobilize the thicker division but preserve it for the moment; you may sacrifice the thicker division later.

3 Define the anterior border of the sternomastoid muscle. Place a row of artery forceps on the subcutaneous fat of the upper margin of the wound and have your assistant raise this edge off the muscle.

Assess

If you are exploring for a lump that may be in the lower pole, you can now determine whether the lump moves upwards with the parotid in the upper leaf of the incision, or whether it lies on a deeper plane between the sternomastoid and the posterior belly of the digastric, or deeper, muscles.

? DIFFICULTY

If you are still unable to decide on the location of the lump, extend the incision upwards, with a curve convex posteriorly, across the mastoid process to reach the point where the anterior margin of the lobule of the auricle reaches the face (see Fig. 34.2). Continue raising the flap of skin and superficial parotid forwards off the anterior border of the sternomastoid muscle. The greater exposure enables you to decide the position of the lump.

Action

1 If the lump is in the parotid, continue the operation as a parotidectomy for a lump. Even if the lump seems very superficial, do not be tempted to excise it locally. To safeguard the facial nerve and ensure complete removal of the lump, you must carry out a formal parotidectomy after exposing the trunk of the facial nerve.

2 If the lump is not in the parotid, remove the lump, leaving the parotid untouched.

3 If you aim to take a generous biopsy of the parotid, undertake step 1 in Access above. Deepen this cervical part of the dissection to expose the posterior belly of the digastric and the stylohyoid muscle. Define these muscles up to the region of the mastoid process.

4 You will find that a large portion of the lower pole of the parotid gland is now elevated with the anterior skin flap. You can remove a large biopsy of this mobilized portion without risk to the facial nerve.

Closure

1 Ensure that haemostasis is complete.

2 Close the skin only.

3 Always insert a suction drain through a separate stab incision 5 cm below the midpoint of the cervical part of the incision.

OPERATIONS ON THE PAROTID DUCT ORIFICE IN THE MOUTH

Appraise

1 Stomatoplasty (Greek: *stoma*=mouth+*plassein*=to form or reform) is used to enlarge the parotid duct orifice,[1] either to enable a calculus in the parotid duct to be passed more easily or to prevent a stricture forming at the orifice after the duct has been explored, for example to remove a stone from the duct.

2 Two branches of the facial nerve are closely applied to the parotid duct in the cheek and may even wind around the duct. Therefore, do not pass ligatures round the duct to prevent a stone from escaping or to assist retraction; contrast this with the procedure for removal of stone from the submandibular duct.

Access

1 Ask the anaesthetist to use a per-nasal endotracheal tube, thereby leaving the mouth free for your manipulations. Also ask him to pack the pharynx around his tube, as a precaution against blood from the mouth being aspirated into the lungs.

2 Fix the patient's mouth open with a dental prop or Ferguson's forceps inserted between the teeth or gums of the jaws on the side opposite to your operation. Insert a towel clip with its jaws in the horizontal plane, into the tip of the tongue and have your assistant retract the tongue towards the opposite side also.

3 Identify the papilla on which the parotid duct opens on the inside of the cheek, immediately opposite the second upper molar tooth. Take an atraumatic 2/0 absorbable synthetic stitch on a half-circle (30 mm) cutting needle and put a stitch into the

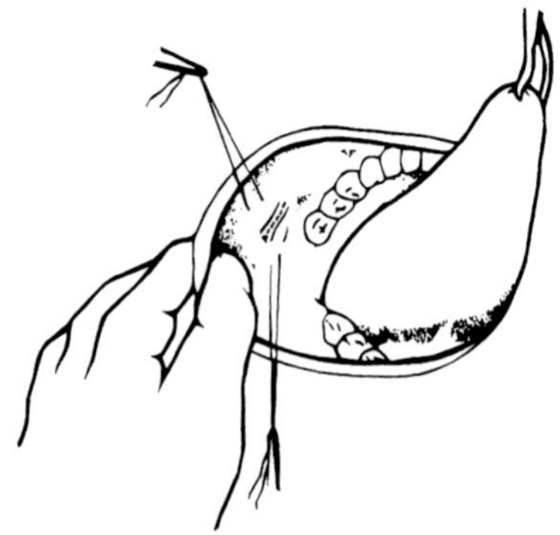

Fig. 34.5 The approach to the right parotid duct orifice. The dental prop in the left side of the mouth is not shown. The tongue is retracted to the opposite side with the towel clip. The operator pulls the angle of the mouth towards himself and at the same time pushes the cheek inwards to make the papillary region prominent inside the mouth; the assistant helps in achieving the latter effect by pulling on the two stay sutures. The dotted line indicates the incision to be made through the mucosa of the cheek and the mucosa of the wall of the duct.

mucosa and underlying muscle of the cheek, about 5 mm above the papilla. Do not tie this stitch; cut it so that each end is 15 cm long, and grip the ends of the stitch with a pair of artery forceps (Fig. 34.5).

4 Insert a similar stitch about 5 mm below the papilla. Have your assistant pull on the two stitches, thereby elevating the region of the papilla towards you.

Access

1 Feel the region of the papilla with two fingers of one hand, exerting counter-pressure with the fingers of the other hand applied to the external aspect of the cheek. Can you feel a stone?

2 Identify the parotid duct orifice using a lacrimal duct dilator, which is a fine probe with a slight bend at each end in the shape of an elongated letter 'S'. To facilitate this manoeuvre, use one hand to guide the dilator and, with the other, pull the angle of the mouth forwards towards you with your thumb working against the metacarpophalangeal joint of your index finger, and push the cheek inwards with the fingertips.

3 At this stage, you are ready to remove a stone from the parotid duct, or to proceed immediately to stomatoplasty, as indicated by your findings.

REMOVAL OF STONE FROM THE PAROTID DUCT: INTRAORAL APPROACH

Action

1 If you can feel the stone at the orifice, keep the papillary region pushed inwards into the mouth by the manoeuvre just described and cut down on the stone with a short-bladed, long-handled scalpel. Start the incision at the orifice of the duct and carry it horizontally backwards for 1 cm.

2 When you have deepened the incision sufficiently, the stone becomes visible. Grasp it with fine-toothed dissecting forceps, and lift it out of the duct. You will find that your incision has divided two layers of mucosa, the lining of the inside of the cheek and the inner lining of the wall of the parotid duct.

3 If you cannot feel a stone in the duct, pass the lacrimal duct dilator into the orifice and along the duct for 2 cm. Get your assistant to hold the dilator steady, keep the papillary region of the cheek pushed inwards into the mouth with your other hand and cut down on the dilator, carrying the incision from the orifice of the duct horizontally backwards for 1 cm.

4 Explore the duct as far back as possible by passing the lacrimal duct dilator. You may be able to feel a stone grating on the tip of the probe. If you do, try milking the stone forward by digital pressure on the parotid gland and duct from outside. This manoeuvre is not often successful, but is worth trying.

5 Whether or not you found and removed the stone, complete the operation by fashioning a large parotid duct orifice.

PAROTID DUCT STOMATOPLASTY

Action

Enlarge the orifice of the parotid duct. To do this, pass a lacrimal duct dilator into the duct for 1–2 cm, get your assistant to hold it steady, keep the papillary region of the cheek pushed inwards into the mouth with your other hand and cut down on the dilator. Take the incision from the orifice of the duct horizontally backwards for 1 cm. Remove the dilator.

Closure

You will find that your incision has divided two layers of mucosa, the lining of the inside of the cheek and the inner lining of the wall of the parotid duct. Unite these two layers with a series of interrupted, 3/0 absorbable synthetic sutures around the margins of the incision (Fig. 34.6).

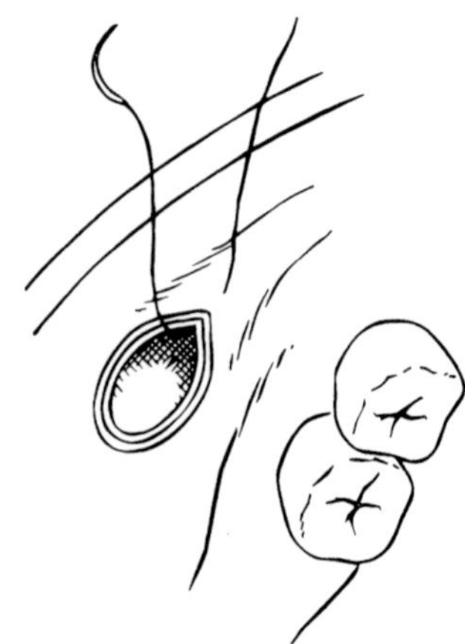

Fig. 34.6 Sewing together the two layers of the mucosa, of the cheek and of the duct. The stitch shown is the first of six or eight that will be inserted at intervals all round the periphery of the now enlarged stoma of the parotid duct.

Checklist

1 Make sure all bleeding has stopped.

2 Remove the stay sutures above and below the duct orifice and the towel clip from the tongue, and check that bleeding does not continue from the puncture wounds.

3 Ask the anaesthetist to remove the pharyngeal pack. If the pack has been effective, there will be no blood on the deeper part of the pack.

4 Remove the dental prop or Ferguson's forceps.

REFERENCE

1. Suleiman SI, Thomson JPS, Hobsley M 1979 Recurrent unilateral swelling of the parotid gland. Gut 20:1102–1108

REMOVAL OF STONE FROM THE SUBMANDIBULAR DUCT

Appraise

1 Do not attempt this operation unless the stone is easily palpable well forward in the floor of the mouth and its presence has been confirmed by radiological investigation.

2 If the stone is more posterior and can only just be felt in the floor of the mouth, or if the submandibular salivary gland is clearly chronically infected, then remove the whole gland together with the stone and as much duct as possible (see the description of excision of submandibular salivary gland for calculous disease, below). If there is any possibility of this situation arising, obtain the patient's informed consent.

3 A stone easily accessible in the anterior part of the duct may slip back into the gland during manipulations in the region of the duct. To prevent this happening, gain control of the duct behind the stone with a ligature under-running the duct at an early stage of the operation.

Access

1 Ask the anaesthetist to pass a nasal endotracheal tube and to pack off the pharynx.

2 Keep the patient's mouth open with a dental prop or Ferguson's forceps inserted between the teeth or gums of the molar region of the contralateral side of the mouth.

3 Grasp the tip of the tongue with a towel clip, closed with the jaws in a horizontal plane, and have your assistant retract the tongue towards the contralateral side.

Assess

1 Inspect and feel the submandibular duct in the floor of the mouth. Make sure that the stone is present and where you expect it to be, well forward in the duct.

2 If you cannot feel the stone, do not explore the sub-mandibular duct. Either the stone has passed spontaneously or it has fallen back along the duct into the gland. In the latter circumstance, you should be able to feel it by bimanual palpation via the neck and the floor of the mouth simultaneously. If you can feel the stone in the gland, try to milk it forwards into the duct. If you fail to milk it forwards, the only method of removing the stone safely is to remove the whole salivary gland with it, by the cervical route.

▶ KEY POINTS Check before proceeding

- Is this larger operation justified by the duration and severity of the patient's symptoms?
- Did you obtain the patient's signed consent for the larger operation?
- If the answer to both these questions is 'yes', proceed to submandibular sialoadenectomy for calculous disease.

3 If the stone is probably, and maybe visibly, situated well forward in the submandibular duct, proceed as below.

Action (Fig. 34.7)

1 Insert an atraumatic 0 monofilament nylon stitch on a 30-mm half-circle cutting needle under-running the submandibular duct, immediately proximal to the stone. Do not tie it. Cut it so that each end is 15 cm long, grasp the two ends in the jaws of a pair of artery forceps, to be drawn upwards and proximally along the duct by your assistant. This kinks and obliterates the lumen, preventing the stone from slipping backwards into the gland.

2 Insert a similar stitch, with a deep bite, vertically into the floor of the mouth in the midline between the terminations of the ridges marking the right and left submandibular ducts for your assistant to pull towards you and to the contralateral side.

3 Identify the orifice of the ipsilateral submandibular duct by passing a fine lacrimal duct dilator through the orifice. With the

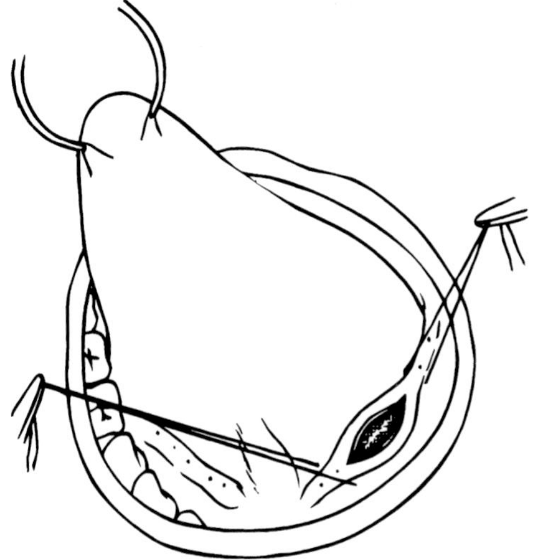

Fig. 34.7 Cutting down on the stone through the mucosa of the floor of the mouth and the muscle and mucosa of the wall of the duct. The duct is steadied, and counter-pressure exerted against the scalpel blade by the two stay sutures, while traction on the proximal one prevents the stone slipping proximally into the gland.

dilator in place, attempt to leave the terminal 0.5 cm of the duct intact.

4 With a small-bladed, long-handled scalpel, cut boldly down on to the stone along the length of the duct.

5 Lift out the stone with fine-toothed dissecting forceps.

6 Leave open the linear incision in the anterior wall of the duct.

7 If the stone is impacted at the orifice of the duct, try milking it backwards along the duct, so preserving the integrity of the duct orifice. If you are forced to slit open the orifice, complete the operation by performing a stomatoplasty, sewing the duct lining to the mucosa of the floor of the mouth to leave an enlarged (0.5 cm) orifice, exactly as in the operation of parotid duct stomatoplasty.

Checklist

1 Make sure all bleeding has stopped.

2 Remove the two stay sutures, and the towel clip from the tongue, and check that bleeding does not continue from the puncture wounds.

3 Ask the anaesthetist to remove the pharyngeal pack. If this has been effective, there will be no blood on the deeper part of the pack.

4 Remove the dental prop or Ferguson's forceps.

SUBMANDIBULAR SIALOADENECTOMY

SUBMANDIBULAR SIALOADENECTOMY FOR CALCULOUS DISEASE

Appraise

1 The mandibular, fourth, branch of the facial nerve dips down into the neck behind the angle of the jaw and then curves upwards and medially to cross superficial to the posterior part of the submandibular salivary gland on its way to the angle of the mouth. This branch is therefore at risk during submandibular sialoadenectomy.

2 The facial artery and vein lie in a groove on the deep aspect of the posterior pole of the superficial lobe of the gland. The vessels are so intimately bound to the gland that you should not attempt to dissect them away from it.

3 The gland has a superficial and a deep lobe; the separation is not complete, the two portions being continuous around the posterior edge of the mylohyoid muscle.

Access

1 Ask the anaesthetist to provide hypotension if possible.

2 Lay the patient close to your side of the table, positioned with head-up tilt from the waist, sufficiently steep to cause collapse of the external jugular vein. Turn the patient's head away from you, with the head extended on the neck, stabilized on a head ring.

3 After cleaning the skin and applying towels, make an incision through skin and platysma in the upper skin crease of the neck, about 5 cm below the lower border of the mandible, extending from a point 2 cm lateral to the anterior midline of the neck to a point vertically below the angle of the jaw.

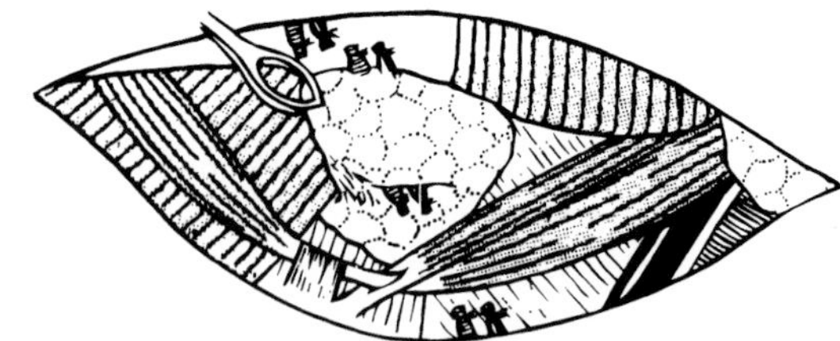

Fig. 34.8 Excision of submandibular gland for calculous disease. The superficial lobe of the submandibular salivary gland has been mobilized by dividing the facial vessels above and below the gland (they are adherent to the deep aspect), and the beginning of the deep lobe can be seen. The deep lobe extends forwards deep to the mylohyoid muscle, and the duct starts at the anterior end of the lobe. Deep to the deep lobe lies the lingual nerve.

Action

1 Identify by palpation the inferior border of the submandibular salivary gland.

2 Deepen the cervical incision in the direction of the inferior border of the gland until you expose the border.

3 Keeping as closely as possible to the surface of the gland, dissect all round the superficial lobe until it is free except for the area where it becomes continuous with the deep lobe. During the course of this dissection, you meet the facial artery and vein both at the lower and upper borders of the posterior pole of the superficial lobe (Fig. 34.8).

4 Preferably ligate and divide the artery and vein separately, at both the upper and the lower borders, leaving a segment of each vessel remaining attached to the gland. If you keep very close to the superficial surface of the gland, you stand little chance of injuring the mandibular branch of the facial nerve, which is retracted upwards by your assistant within the superficial flap of tissues.

5 Apply a pair of tissue forceps to the gland as it dips deep to the posterior border of the mylohyoid muscle. Have your assistant pull the gland laterally and retract the posterior border of the mylohyoid medially while you free the deep part of the gland from the deep surface of the mylohyoid by blunt dissection. At this stage you may be able to feel the stone stuck in the duct at the point where the duct leaves the anterior pole of the deep lobe.

KEY POINTS Caution

- Do not dissect further forwards at this stage, even if it seems technically easy.
- If you do you may damage the lingual nerve where it crosses the lateral–superficial–aspect of the duct.

6 Now have your assistant retract the deep portion of the gland medially, that is round the edge of the mylohyoid muscle. Dissect by blunt dissection along the deep surface of the deep

lobe, separating it from the hyoglossus muscle on which it lies. Keep very closely to the gland, because it also lies in contact with the lingual nerve. You can recognize the nerve as a rather broad (7.5 mm) thin band of white tissue, running forwards and medially on the hyoglossus and a little above the level of the submandibular duct.

7 At the anterior pole of the gland you may again feel the calculus, since this is the most common site, and see the commencement of the duct. Now dissect forwards along the duct, taking special care not to damage the lingual nerve as it crosses the superficial aspect of the duct from above downwards, and then winds right round the lower border of the duct to cross its medial aspect from below upwards.

8 Free the duct as far forwards as possible, nearly to its termination in the mouth. Tie the duct distally with an absorbable synthetic ligature, and cut it across. Remove the duct and gland with the contained stone.

Closure

1 Check that haemostasis is perfect when the anaesthetist has raised the blood pressure sufficiently.

2 Close the wound in two layers, with 4/0 absorbable synthetic for the platysma, 6/0 nylon for the skin.

3 Insert a suction drain through a separate stab incision 5 cm below the middle of the wound.

SUBMANDIBULAR SIALOADENECTOMY FOR TUMOUR

Appraise

1 If a submandibular salivary gland swelling is not due to a calculus, assume it to be due to a tumour. Fine-needle aspiration cytology may aid the diagnosis.

2 With clear-cut evidence that the tumour is malignant, a radical submandibular sialoadenectomy with resection of a segment of the mandible (a 'commando' operation) may be performed, outlined at the end of the chapter.

3 If there is no evidence of malignancy, assume that the tumour is a mixed salivary tumour and aim to remove the submandibular salivary gland with a wide margin of normal tissue, so as to ensure completeness of the excision and to guard against any implantation recurrence.

4 Warn the patient of possible weakness of the angle of the mouth and the lower lip, loss of general sensation and taste from the ipsilateral half of the anterior two-thirds of the tongue and subsequent development of wasting and paralysis of the ipsilateral half of the tongue.

Access

1 Make a skin crease incision through skin and platysma in the upper skin crease of the neck, extending from 2 cm lateral to the anterior midline of the neck to a point vertically below the angle of the jaw. Do not hesitate to extend this incision in either direction to facilitate removing a large tumour.

2 Deepen the incision towards the lower border of the submandibular salivary gland, but stop a few millimetres short of actually exposing the gland.

Assess

By palpation, bimanually if necessary, determine the exact site and extent of the tumour in the gland. In particular, decide whether the tumour reaches the superficial aspect of the superficial lobe, because if it does you may need to modify the plane of your dissection.

Action

1 Dissect free the superficial aspect of the superficial lobe. If the tumour does not reach this aspect, it is acceptable to dissect close to the gland, preserving the mandibular branch of the facial nerve in the overlying platysmal flap as described in the similar operation for calculous disease. If the tumour does reach this superficial aspect, perform the mobilization in a plane more remote from the gland. Try to identify the mandibular branch of the facial nerve and preserve it, provided that this does not jeopardize your margin around the tumour. Divide the facial vessels between ligatures, well above and below the posterior pole of the gland.

2 Continue the mobilization of the superficial and deep lobes as described in the corresponding operation for calculous disease, but wherever the tumour reaches the surface of the salivary gland make certain of your margin by excising the neighbouring normal tissue. This policy usually only entails the sacrifice of fibres from such muscles as the anterior belly of the digastric anteriorly, the intermediate tendon of the digastric and the stylohyoid muscle inferiorly, the stylomandibular ligament posteriorly and the mylohyoid, stylohyoid, hyoglossus and posterior belly of the digastric medially.

KEY POINTS Fate of the nerves

- The lingual nerve is an intimate relation of the deep portion of the submandibular gland.
- If possible preserve all or part of the nerve, but occasionally it must be sacrificed to ensure complete tumour excision.
- If the hypoglossal nerve is intimately related to the inferior border of the gland it may also need to be sacrificed.

3 Dissect the submandibular duct forwards as far as possible, tie and divide it, and lift out the block of tissue.

Closure

1 Check that the anaesthetist has restored the blood pressure to an acceptable level while you ensure that haemostasis is perfect

2 Close the wound with one layer of skin sutures.

3 Insert a suction drain via a separate stab incision 5 cm below the middle of the wound.

EXCISION BIOPSY OF A BASAL CELL CARCINOMA OF THE FACE

Appraise

1 A basal cell carcinoma (rodent ulcer) may be treated by operation or by radiotherapy. If you choose to resect it you must excise it with a wide margin of normal tissue, both around the lesion and deep to it. A 'wide margin' means preferably 1 cm, but in regions where skin is precious, for example near the eye, 0.5 cm is acceptable.

2 If the ulcer is small, in a region where there is plenty of redundant skin, excision and primary closure may be possible. Otherwise you may need to apply a skin graft, preferably full-thickness graft. The cosmetic result following split skin grafting on the face is unacceptable. There are two suitable free full-thickness donor sites. Facial surgeons can rotate flaps to cover large defects, but do not attempt these unless you are experienced with the techniques.

Assess

1 Carefully assess by inspection and palpation the extent of the lesion and the required area of excision. It is not yet possible to determine required depth of excision.

2 Plan the excision taking into account the relaxed skin tension lines.[1] After the excision, you may then be able to close the defect by primary suture with the scar lying in the skin crease.

KEY POINTS Lesions near eyes and nose

- Take care when excising tumours near the eyes and nostrils.
- Excisions in these areas often result in cosmetic and functional defects.
- If possible refer such tumour resections to specialists.

Action

1 Mark out the oval of skin that you intend to excise.

2 Cut vertically through the skin along the oval line, until superficial fat is clearly visible everywhere in the wound. It is not possible to make a curved incision with a straight knife-blade, but a series of short linear incisions permits your incision to follow the marked oval closely.

3 Deepen the incision at one end of the oval. Raise the skin at one end with toothed forceps, using a clean scalpel or scissors including some subcutaneous tissue near the lesion.

4 At this stage you will find it easier to decide by palpation how deeply the lesion extends. Make sure that your plane of cutting is sufficiently deep to give a wide margin of normal tissue below, as well as all round, the tumour.

5 Complete the excision by starting again at the opposite end, meeting the other excision deep to the lesion.

6 Inspect the wound for bleeding and stop it with diathermy.

7 Take a single sheet of petroleum jelly (Vaseline) gauze, lay it on the wound and cut out a piece the shape and size of the wound as a pattern for cutting a full-thickness (Wolfe) graft of skin.

8 Lay the pattern on the chosen donor site. The loose skin immediately below the clavicle and the groove between the side of the head and the medial aspect of the posterior part of the pinna make suitable donor sites. Cut out a full-thickness area of skin corresponding in size and shape to the pattern, with minimal subcutaneous fat. Cut off any remaining fat using a sharp scalpel. Sew up the defect in the donor area.

9 After ensuring there is no residual bleeding following ulcer excision, lay in the graft. Stitch in the graft using interrupted non-absorbable sutures, tying the knots so that they lie on the surrounding intact skin rather than on the skin graft. You should produce sufficient tension in the graft to discourage haematoma without an excess that would produce a strangulation effect on the graft with consequent necrosis.

10 After protecting the patient's eyes, nostrils, mouth and hair, spray the grafted area with a artificial skin preparation such as Nobecutane, used sparingly. As the film hardens, repeat the procedure several times to produce a firm dressing.

Checklist

1 Dress the donor site.

2 Check that the specimen, properly labelled and accompanied by the appropriate request forms, is sent to the histopathologist.

REFERENCE

1. Borges F 1973 Elective incisions and scar revision. Little Brown, Boston

LOCAL EXCISION OR BIOPSY OF AN INTRAORAL LESION

Appraise

1 Small lesions in the surface of the oral mucosa, whether on cheek, tongue, palate, floor of mouth or inner surface of the lips, are best dealt with by excision biopsy, removing a sufficiently wide margin of normal tissue to ensure that excision is complete.

2 Make sure, however, by careful palpation beforehand, how deeply the lesion penetrates beneath the mucosa. Remember that you must achieve an adequate margin of normal tissue on the deep aspect of the lesion as well as around it.

3 The oral tissues are very vascular, so take special precautions to minimize haemorrhage and so prevent aspiration of blood into the lungs.

Access

1 Ask the anaesthetist to pass a per-nasal endotracheal cuffed tube and to inflate the cuff. A further precaution against aspiration of blood is to have the pharynx packed with 2.5-cm ribbon gauze.

2 Fix the patient's mouth open with a dental prop or Ferguson's forceps inserted between the teeth or gums of the molar region on the side opposite to the lesion.

3 Position the patient with a head-up tilt of about 15°, sufficient to cause the external jugular vein to collapse. Use a head-ring to stabilize the position of the head.

Assess

1 Palpate the lesion carefully again to assess its depth. Tissues often feel different when the patient is anaesthetized, making you change your decision about the depth of penetration of the lesion.

2 If you are still sure that you can remove the lesion with a wide margin of normal tissue on all aspects, and without producing deformity or serious loss of function, proceed to excision biopsy (see below). If you are doubtful, biopsy the lesion (see below).

EXCISION BIOPSY

Action

1 Form a mental picture of the exact position and shape of your incision.

2 Using a 3/0 absorbable suture on a half-circle 30-mm or 50-mm cutting needle, according to the depth of bite required, insert a stitch through the tissues near each end of your proposed incision. The stitches must traverse the tissues far enough from the incision that they will not be cut when you make the incision. Match the depth of stitch to the required depth of excision. Leave the two ends of each untied but held in four artery forceps.

3 Excise the lesion with at least a 5-mm margin in all directions. Make the wound roughly oval, the direction of the long axis of the oval being dictated by the need to minimize damage to neighbouring structures. Do this as speedily as possible, as you cannot control bleeding until the excision is complete.

4 Pull each stitch end across the wound towards the opposite end of the other stitch, forming a cross. This controls the worst of the bleeding if your assistant maintains traction on the stitch ends.

5 Inspect the excised specimen with the naked eye. Does the excision appear complete? Excise more if necessary

6 If excision appears complete, tie the stitches in the form of the cross, as your assistant has been holding them.

7 Complete haemostasis using diathermy and further sutures if necessary while maintaining a clear field with the sucker.

BIOPSY

Appraise

Decide where you will take your biopsy. Plan to excise the rim of the lesion in continuity with a generous portion of the neighbouring normal tissue. In general, the excised piece is oval with its long axis at right angles to the margin of the lesion.

Action

1 Insert one or two deep sutures of 3/0 absorbable material through normal tissues on either side of your proposed excision, and leave the ends untied. Do not insert sutures into the lesion itself, since this may spread neoplasm.

2 Excise the specimen, taking care not to cut your sutures.

3 Tie the suture or sutures. Usually this stops all bleeding, but if it fails to do so, use diathermy or insert more sutures.

Checklist

1 Was there any blood on the deeper parts of the pharyngeal pack? If there was, monitor the possibility of chest complications later.

2 Are you sure that the specimen has been correctly bottled and labelled, that the request form for the pathology department has been accurately filled out and that you are satisfied with the arrangements for conveying the specimen to the laboratory?

3 Should you send part of the specimen for bacteriological examination, if the lesion could be tuberculous? Remember that any such sample must be sent in a sterile container without formalin.

PARTIAL GLOSSECTOMY

Appraise

1 Excise small lesions of the anterior two-thirds of the tongue with laser-cutting.

2 Excise larger lesions with a wide margin, since tumour planes in the tongue are indiscrete and a 0.8-mm margin is required.

KEY POINTS Preserve tongue functions?

- The tongue's important functions include speaking, mastication and deglutition.
- Preserve mobility as far as possible.
- Preserve length, especially of the tip, in preference to width or thickness.

3 We shall describe a wedge excision of the tip of the tongue.

Access

Prepare the patient as for a local excision biopsy of an intraoral lesion.

Assess

1 Palpate the lesion and its surroundings carefully. Do not forget the neck and postnasal space.

2 Decide the width and length of wedge that you need to remove to ensure a wide margin of normal tissue around the lesion.

Action

1 Use a dental prop to keep the mouth open. If you are right-handed, stand on the patient's right. If you are left-handed, reverse all references to side in these instructions.

2 Lay your left index finger along the dorsum of the tongue, your thumb along the ventral aspect, to the right of the

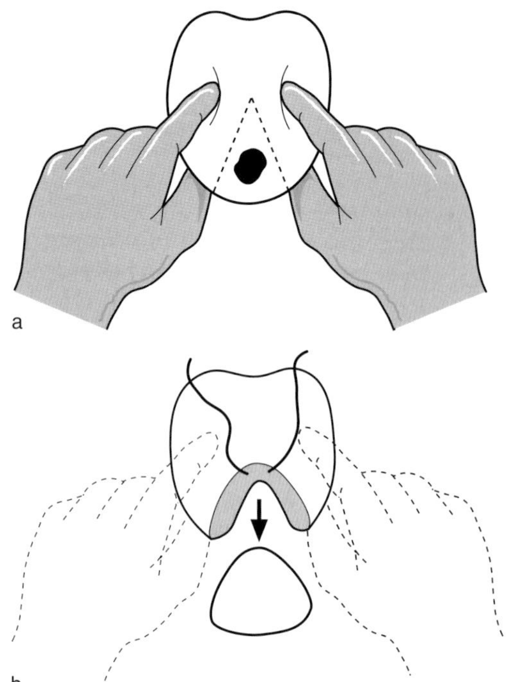

Fig. 34.9 Digital pressure method for controlling bleeding: (a) the index finger and thumb on each side are applied just outside the margins of the proposed excision (indicated by the lines); (b) the start of the repair—the deepest suture has been inserted.

right-hand margin of your proposed excision. Squeeze the tongue (Fig. 34.9a).

3 Have your assistant, standing on the patient's left, squeeze the tongue between the index finger and thumb, to the left of the left-hand margin of your proposed excision.

4 Excise the wedge carrying the lesion, using a hand-held carbon dioxide laser if available. If you use a knife, the digital pressure of your assistant and yourself minimizes bleeding.

5 Insert a series of interrupted absorbable 3/0 sutures to approximate the muscles in the deeper parts of the defect (Fig. 34.9b). Temporarily relax the fingers, first on one side and then on the other, to assess the efficacy of these sutures in stopping bleeding from the deeper parts of the wound. Insert further sutures to close the mucosa along the dorsal and ventral surface of the tongue, and to stop bleeding from the superficial layers.

WEDGE EXCISION OF THE LIP

Appraise

1 Early tumours of the lip can be removed with a wide margin by this operation.

2 Particularly in elderly people, up to one-third of the length of the lip can be removed in this way with an acceptable functional and cosmetic result.

3 In a young patient, or if the length of lip to be excised exceeds one-third, various plastic operations are available (see Ch. 39); these are more difficult than they appear, so attempt them only if you are expert.

Assess

1 Inspect and palpate the lesion and its surroundings with care.

2 Decide on the width and length of wedge necessary to remove the lesion with a clear margin of 0.5–1.0 cm of normal tissue.

Action

1 Cut out the wedge, taking the full thickness of the lip, using bipolar diathermy to control the bleeding, if it is available. Alternatively control bleeding with finger pressure or use non-crushing intestinal clamps.

2 Close the defect with three layers of interrupted sutures: 3/0 absorbable sutures for the muscle and for the mucosa, and very fine non-absorbable sutures for the skin and the vermilion border.

KEY POINTS Appearance of the lip

- Pay especial attention to the accuracy with which you join the two edges of the vermilion border and the mucocutaneous junctions.
- It is useful to 'tack' these first.

EXCISION OF SUPRAHYOID (SUBMENTAL) CYST

Appraise

1 A cystic, subcutaneous swelling in the midline of the neck above the level of the hyoid bone may be a thyroglossal cyst or a simple lesion such as a dermoid cyst. If the lump moves on swallowing and on protrusion of the tongue, it is thyroglossal; if it does not, it is a dermoid cyst. Of course lymph nodes can occur in this area.

2 The distinction between the two types can be difficult. Therefore, when operating on a lump you have diagnosed as a dermoid cyst, always look for evidence of a track upwards towards the tongue or downwards towards the hyoid. If you find such evidence, you must alter your diagnosis to thyroglossal cyst and change your operation accordingly.

Access

1 The patient lies supine, with the upper half of the table angled sufficiently upwards to cause the external jugular veins to collapse. Extend the head on the neck but flex the cervical spine on the thoracic spine. Achieve this by placing a sandbag under the shoulders and use a head ring. This position facilitates access to the front of the neck, without putting the strap muscles and the superficial tissues on stretch.

2 Clean the skin from the level of the mouth to the clavicles, and laterally from the anterior midline of the neck to the posterior border of each sternomastoid muscle. Tuck a pad of sterile wool beneath the neck and scapular regions.

3 Towel up to expose the lesion and a surrounding margin of 5 cm in all directions. Stick the disposable drapes to the skin of the neck around the exposed area.

4 Make a transverse, skin crease, incision centred over the lump and extending 2–3 cm past its borders on either side. Deepen this through the skin and superficial fascia, and achieve haemostasis using diathermy.

5 With a clean knife-blade, deepen the incision through the platysma and then through the fascial layers until you reach the surface of the lesion.

6 Raise flaps of skin and the other superficial tissues upwards and downwards using a combination of sharp and blunt dissection, to expose the whole of the superficial aspect of the lump.

Action

1 Using fine, curved artery forceps, open up the plane between the surface of the lump and the surrounding fascia. Continue what should prove a relatively bloodless dissection in all directions until you expose the deep aspect of the lesion.

2 In the region of the deep aspect, be particularly careful not to miss any fibrous extension of the wall of the cyst, either penetrating the median raphe between the underlying right and left mylohyoid muscles on its way to the tongue, or passing downwards towards the hyoid bone.

3 Assuming that you find no such extensions, complete the dissection of the deep aspect to free the lump.

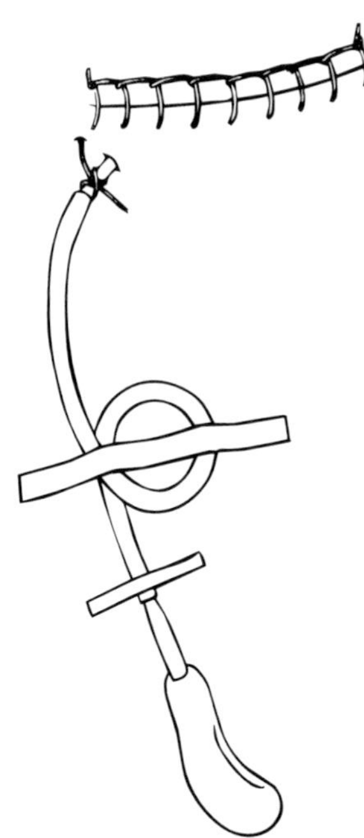

Fig. 34.10 Some details of the closure. Blanket stitch gives firm, side-to-side apposition along every millimetre of the incision, ensuring that the incision is airtight. The suction/drain tubing is stitched to the skin using a clove hitch to ensure that the tube cannot slip in or out. Two strips of Elastoplast strapping or paper tape are used to fix the tubing. The first fixes a loop so that pulling on the end of the apparatus does not pull the tube out of the wound. The drainage tube is connected to a vacuum system such as Redivac.

Closure

1 Check haemostasis. Have the table flattened so that bleeding points manifest themselves and can be sealed rather than bleed after the skin is closed.

2 Insert a suction drain 2.5 cm below the incision near either the right or the left extremity of the wound and arrange the tube to lie along the length of the wound. Make sure that there are several side-holes in the part of the tube that is left lying within the wound and that there are no side-holes in the external part. Stitch the tube to the skin to maintain the optimal position. Tie the ends of the stitch around the tube as a clove hitch, firmly anchoring the tube. Ask the anaesthetist to remove the sandbag.

3 Close the skin with a continuous blanket or subcuticular stitch (Fig. 34.10). Skin apposition must be perfect along the whole length of the wound to promote healing but also to create an airtight wound so that the suction drainage can work efficiently.

4 Connect the drainage tubing to the suction bottle (Fig. 34.10). Check that after the air has been evacuated from the wound the system is airtight.

EXCISION OF THYROGLOSSAL CYST, SINUS AND FISTULA

Appraise

1 The isthmus and part of the lateral lobes of the thyroid gland originate at the foramen caecum (Latin: *caecus*=blind), at the junction of the posterior third and anterior two-thirds of the tongue, and during fetal life migrate downwards to reach their definitive position anterior to the thyroid cartilage and overlapping the upper end of the trachea. The course of this migration is midline, first through the tongue itself and between the muscles of the submental region, then closely applied to the hyoid bone, or even through it; at this stage the tract loops upwards and backwards for a short distance before again turning downwards to the isthmus of the thyroid gland (Fig. 34.11).

2 Any part or all of this thyroglossal tract may persist. Persistence of the whole tract produces a fistula between the mouth and the neck, but this is rare. The sinus, which is more common, is an opening in the skin near the level of the thyroid isthmus connecting with a track that proceeds upwards for a variable distance towards the foramen caecum. The most common lesion is the cyst, which may lie at any point in the track but most often in the region of the hyoid bone, and which may have associated with it a variable stretch of persistent track both upwards and downwards.

KEY POINT Complete excision

- Whatever the exact lesions, ensure that all persistent portions of the track are excised, otherwise recurrence is inevitable.

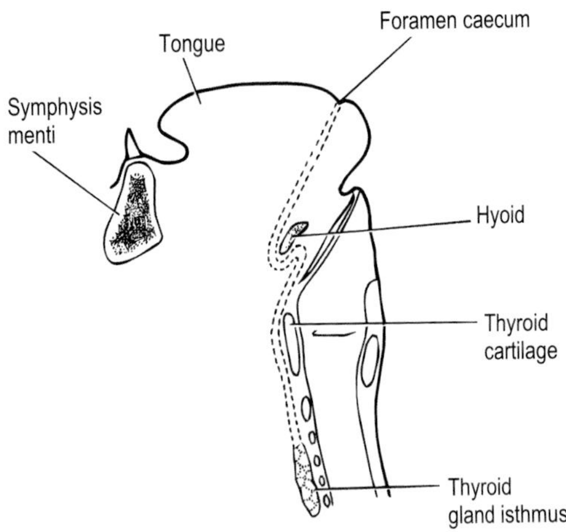

Fig. 34.11 Midline sagittal section through the mouth and neck to show the path taken by the thyroid between the foramen caecum at the base of the tongue and the definitive position of the gland. Note the intimate relationship between the track and the posterior aspect of the body of the hyoid, and the angle at which the suprahyoid portion of the track inclines.

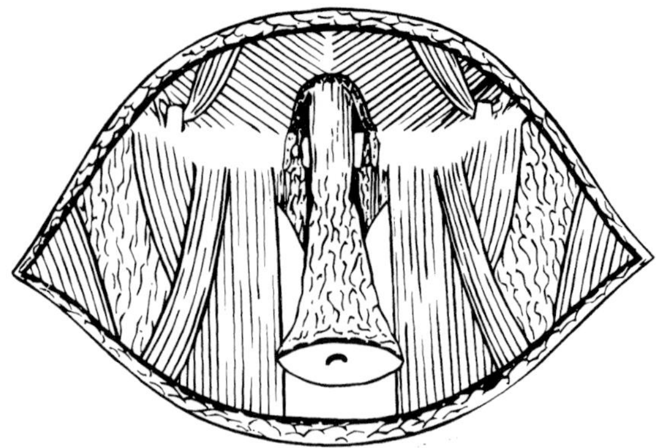

Fig. 34.12 Flaps of skin with platysma have been raised, leaving the opening of the sinus surrounded with an ellipse of skin. The track has been cored out to the body of the hyoid, the central portion of the bone has been detached in continuity with the track, and a cylinder of muscle is cored out in the midline from the submental muscles in a direction backwards and upwards at 45° (see Fig. 34.11).

3 The intimate relationship between the track and the back of the body of the hyoid necessitates excision of a segment of the bone from the midline to make sure that this portion of the track has been excised.

4 Operations are described separately for (a) a thyroglossal sinus and (b) a thyroglossal cyst lying just below the body of the hyoid.

EXCISION OF THYROGLOSSAL SINUS

Access

1 Make a symmetrical elliptical collar incision at the level of the opening of the sinus, circumcising the sinus with an oval of skin and also excising any skin scarred by infections of the track.

2 Raise flaps of skin and platysma together; the lower flap need be raised for only 2–3 cm, but the upper flap must be raised in the midline to a level at least halfway between the hyoid and the symphysis menti (Fig. 34.12).

Action

1 Dissect the oval of skin and superficial fascia and the fibrous tissue around the upward track from the sinus opening, raising a tube of tissues containing the track. At this and every subsequent stage, be careful to keep a margin of tissue between your instruments and the track itself.

2 The opening of the sinus may be situated above the thyroid isthmus, in which case you may be able to feel a fibrous cord, representing the lowest part of the track, running downwards from your dissected tube. Dissect this cord and follow its lower end downwards to the thyroid isthmus to include it in your specimen.

3 Continue coring out the upper part of the track upwards until you reach the level of the hyoid bone. Pass a blunt dissector, such as Macdonald's, deep to the body of the hyoid and gently separate the bone from the attached muscles and the underlying thyrohyoid membrane for a distance of about 1 cm, centred on the midline. Use bone-cutting forceps to excise this segment of bone, leaving it in continuity with the track.

4 Above the hyoid, the track plunges through the median raphe of the mylohyoid muscles in a direction sloping at 45° backwards and upwards. It traverses the deeper submental muscles to reach the foramen caecum. Have your assistant put an index finger in the mouth and push the base of the tongue downwards towards you. Core out a cylinder of muscle in the direction described to complete the dissection of the track.

5 The uppermost part of the track is practically never patent, and indeed may not be palpable even as a fibrous cord, but it is wise to extend this procedure for 2 cm deep to the mylohyoid. If necessary be prepared to continue until you are separated from the mouth and your assistant's finger by only the mucous membrane covering the tongue. Cut across the core of muscle and remove the whole dissected track.

Closure

1 Achieve haemostasis.

2 Suture the defect in the submental muscles in one or more layers. Repair any midline defect in the strap muscles produced by coring out the track.

3 Insert a suction drain via a separate stab incision in the lower flap.

4 Close the skin.

EXCISION OF THYROGLOSSAL CYST

Access

1 Make a symmetrical collar incision, centred over the cyst.

2 Raise flaps of skin including platysma muscle, downwards to the lower margin of the cyst and upwards to a point in the midline,

halfway between the body of the hyoid and the symphysis menti.

Action

1 Dissect all round the superficial aspects of the cyst. As you approach the deep aspect, separate the sternohyoid muscles in the midline to facilitate the view of the deep aspect.

2 Search for any downward extension of the track as a fibrous cord in the midline. If you find one, follow it as far downwards as you can feel it, or to the isthmus of the thyroid gland, and excise it separately.

3 Mobilize the cyst upwards on its deep surface. You will find that it is intimately adherent to the body of the hyoid bone in the midline.

4 Resect 1 cm of the body of the hyoid as described above, in continuity with the cyst.

5 Complete the excision by the coring-out procedure of the muscles of the submental region as described above.

Closure

This is the same as after the excision of a thyroglossal sinus.

OPERATIONS FOR BRANCHIAL CYST, SINUS AND FISTULA

Appraise

1 Portions of the first or second branchial (Greek: *branchion*=a gill) clefts may remain patent, usually the second cleft. The complete lesion is a fistula with one opening in the pharynx near the posterior pillar of the fauces and the other in the skin at the junction of middle and lower thirds of the anterior border of the sternomastoid muscle. The complete fistula is not as common as a branchial sinus, where the lower opening and the main track are present but the track does not communicate at its upper end with the pharynx.

2 The branchial cyst occurs when the central portion only of the second cleft remains patent. There is then a cystic spherical swelling deep to the junction of the upper and middle thirds of the sternomastoid muscle and becoming superficial at the anterior border of the muscle. A large branchial cyst encroaches on what is clinically the parotid region. In such case, be careful to proceed in a manner that enables you to carry out a formal parotidectomy if necessary (see Exploration of the lower pole of the parotid). The description given in this section assumes that the clinical diagnosis of branchial cyst is straightforward and that there is no possibility that the swelling is a parotid tumour.

3 Finally, the first arch remnant may give rise to a cyst in the parotid region, or the cyst may communicate as a sinus posteriorly with the cartilaginous external auditory meatus or anteriorly with an opening in the skin of the submandibular region, or there may be a complete fistula between the submandibular region and the external auditory meatus. The simple cyst cannot be distinguished clinically from other lumps in the parotid region, and you will remove it by a conservative parotidectomy, with full exposure and identification of the facial nerve. If the cyst communicates with the external auditory meatus, you may find during the parotidectomy that a cartilaginous extension from the external auditory meatus runs into the cyst. You can cut across this funnel of cartilage and leave the resulting defect open, then proceed with the parotidectomy; after the facial nerve is well exposed you can close the cartilaginous defect by sewing soft tissues together over it without danger to the facial nerve.

4 The operations described in detail in this section are those for a typical (second cleft) branchial sinus or fistula and branchial cyst.

EXCISION OF BRANCHIAL SINUS OR FISTULA

Access

1 Position the patient supine, with the upper half of the operating table tilted upwards sufficiently to cause the external jugular vein to collapse. Turn the patient's head to the opposite side.

2 Clean the skin from the level of the mouth to the clavicle and from the anterior midline of the neck to as far posteriorly as can be reached. Tuck a pad of sterile wool beneath the neck and scapular regions.

3 Towel up to leave exposed an area from the jaw above to 5 cm below the opening of the sinus below and from the anterior midline of the neck to the anterior border of the trapezius posteriorly.

4 Make an elliptical incision (Fig. 34.13) in the skin around the opening of the sinus; the long axis of the incision should be horizontal, in the skin crease, and about 5 cm long, while the short axis should give sufficient clearance above and below the margins of the opening.

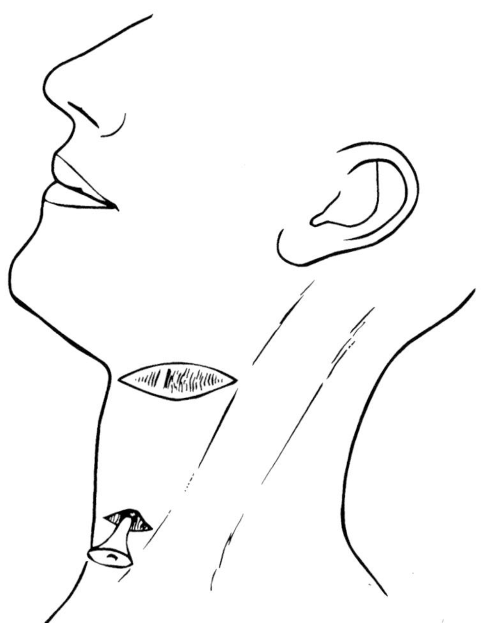

Fig. 34.13 The opening of the sinus or fistula low in the neck is circumcised with an elliptical incision and the track is cored out upwards by incising the deep fascia. At the level of the hyoid, a second incision is made and the mobilized track is drawn upwards through the second incision.

5 With a clean knife-blade, deepen the incision through the subcutaneous tissue and the platysma. Exert traction on the skin ellipse with tissue forceps or a stitch, and you should be able to feel the track from the lower aspect of the wound as a fibrous cord running upwards along the anterior border of the sternomastoid, deep to the deep, investing cervical, fascia.

6 Dissect upwards on all aspects of the track, coring it out from the fascial planes of the neck. To facilitate this dissection, raise the upper skin flap in the plane deep to the platysma and incise the deep fascia upwards along the anterior border of the sternomastoid, superficial to the track.

7 If the track can be palpated to ascend higher in the neck than you can comfortably expose through your incision, make a further horizontal skin crease incision with the skin knife at the level of the hyoid bone, extending from 2 cm short of the anterior midline of the neck to the anterior border of the sternomastoid—a step incision. Use the clean knife to deepen this incision through subcutaneous tissue and platysma, and then elevate the lower flap in the plane deep to the platysma until you can pass a pair of long curved artery forceps downwards through the upper incision to grasp the skin ellipse at the lower end of the track. Pull the skin ellipse upwards under the skin-bridge between the two incisions so that it presents at the upper incision. You now have comfortable access to complete the dissection.

Action

1 Continue the dissection of the track upwards. Remember that the most efficient way of finding the direction of the track is to feel the fibrous cord with your fingers.

2 The usual course of the track is between the external and internal carotid arteries and then deep to the posterior belly of the digastric muscle. Divide the digastric at its intermediate tendon anteriorly and 2 cm behind the track posteriorly. When you have excised the segment of muscle between these points, it is easy to follow the track upwards to its termination.

3 Deep to the posterior belly of the digastric, the track lies superficial to the middle constrictor muscle of the pharynx (Fig. 34.14).

▶ KEY POINTS Anatomy

- Avoid damaging the hypoglossal nerve, running forwards between the track and the middle constrictor at the level of the lower border of the digastric.
- Look out for, and preserve, the glossopharyngeal nerve, which runs a similar course about 1 cm higher up.

4 Immediately above the glossopharyngeal nerve, the track swings forwards and its fibrous sheath blends with the aponeurosis covering the middle constrictor. At this point there may be a connection between the interior of the track and the lumen of the pharynx, but it is not important to discover whether such a connection exists. Simply apply two pairs of artery forceps to the track where it blends with the muscle, cut between the forceps, and tie off the pharyngeal end.

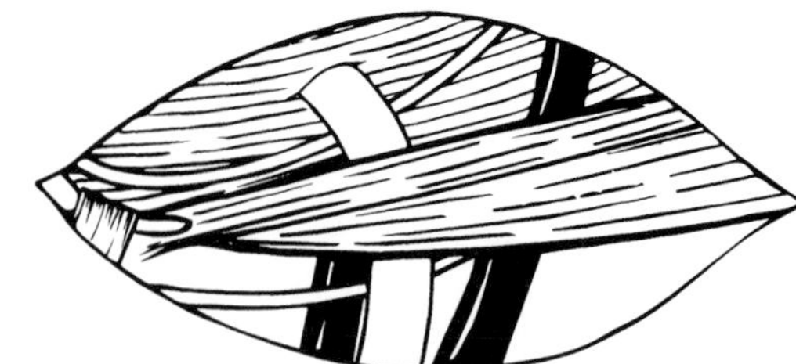

Fig. 34.14 The track is now followed further upwards, passing between external and internal carotid arteries deep to the posterior belly of the digastric, to merge with the fascia covering the middle constrictor. The glossopharyngeal and hypoglossal nerves run between the track and the middle constrictor.

? DIFFICULTY

The really difficult technical problem is the sinus in the submandibular region with a track extending into the parotid region, with or without a palpable cyst in the parotid region. If you operate only occasionally in the parotid region do not lightly attempt to operate on this condition. For this reason the procedure will be described in principle only:

1. Commence as for a superficial parotidectomy and take it to the stage where the cervical and mandibular branches of the facial nerve have been exposed well forwards along their course, at least to the anterior border of the parotid gland itself.
2. Circumcise the submandibular sinus and dissect the track backwards into the parotid region.
3. If, as is usual, the track is superficial to the facial nerve, complete the operation by performing the superficial parotidectomy. Occasionally, however, as you dissect the track backwards you see it run into the deep part of the parotid, and you must perform a deep or total conservative parotidectomy.

Closure

1 Insert a drain through skin and platysma via a point just below the lower incision, and lay the part of the tube within the wound up through the bed of the track to the middle constrictor.

2 Repair the vertical incision in the deep fascia with fine silk or absorbable synthetic ligature. Check haemostasis carefully, especially in the tunnel between the upper and lower incisions.

3 Close the skin incisions, fix the tube to the skin and attach the tube to suction as described for the excision of suprahyoid, submental, cyst.

EXCISION OF BRANCHIAL CYST

Access

1 Make a horizontal, skin crease, incision at the level of the lesion, that is, at the junction of upper and middle thirds of the sternomastoid, extending from 1 cm anterior to the anterior margin

of the lesion to halfway between the anterior and posterior borders of the sternomastoid.

2 Deepen the incision through subcutaneous tissue and platysma, and reflect the flaps upwards and downwards in the plane deep to the platysma, to the upper and lower margins of the lump.

3 Incise the deep, investing cervical, fascia over the lump in a direction parallel to the anterior border of the sternomastoid.

4 Use a self-retaining retractor to separate the upper and lower flaps of skin and platysma. Have your assistant retract the anterior border of the sternomastoid posteriorly. You now have excellent access to the swelling.

Action

1 Using careful blunt dissection, wipe away the intervening areolar tissue to display the wall of the cyst. Continue the dissection around the superficial aspect of the cyst and then proceed around the deep aspect of its lower pole.

2 Immediately deep to the cyst lies the beginning of the external and internal carotid arteries. Be careful not to damage these or the vagus nerve lying behind the internal carotid artery.

3 The cyst wall is often very thin; try not to damage it, as it is easier to be certain that you have removed the whole cyst if it remains intact throughout the operation. If you leave fragments of the wall behind, the lesion may recur.

4 Continue the dissection upwards behind the cyst mobilizing it from the middle constrictor muscle. Note and preserve the hypoglossal nerve, running forwards between the cyst and the middle constrictor at the level of the lower border of the posterior belly of the digastric, and 1 cm higher up the glossopharyngeal nerve, running in the same direction and in the same plane (Fig. 34.14 shows the relevant anatomy of this area).

5 Sometimes the cyst does not extend much above the level of the posterior belly of the digastric, but often it does extend considerably upwards, deep to the posterior belly. In such a case, excise a segment of the posterior belly, from the middle tendon in front to the posterior margin of the cyst behind, so that the dissection can proceed safely upwards on both superficial and deep aspects of the cyst.

6 Occasionally, at the deep aspect of the cyst above the level of the glossopharyngeal nerve, you find a fibrous track arising from the cyst and blending with the fascia covering the middle constrictor, rather like the top end of a branchial fistula. Divide this track between two pairs of curved artery forceps and tie the end attached to the muscle. Usually, you will find no evidence of this track and the simple blunt dissection around the cyst is sufficient to free it. Remove the cyst.

Closure

1 Check for bleeding. Use diathermy to stop bleeding points, with special care not to damage the nerves you have demonstrated during the dissection. Insert a drainage tube via a skin puncture 5 cm below the incision.

2 Repair the deep fascia along the anterior border of the sternomastoid with absorbable sutures, such as Vicryl.

3 Close the skin and apply suction to the drain.

EXCISION BIOPSY OF CERVICAL LYMPH NODE

Appraise

1 Never attempt this operation under local anaesthesia if general anaesthesia is available. Cervical lymph nodes may feel superficial yet lie deeply in the neck, and the dissection to remove them may be much more difficult than you expect.

2 Depending on the position of the lymph node, neighbouring structures may be at risk during the operation. An example commonly encountered is the accessory nerve, either in the anterior triangle of the neck at the junction of upper and middle thirds of the anterior border of the sternomastoid muscle, or in the posterior triangle at the junction of the middle and lower thirds of the sternomastoid.

3 Handle lymph glands very gently during dissection. Rough handling is likely to distort the internal structure of the node and make histological interpretation difficult.

4 The operation described here is for a lymph node lying under cover of the anterior border of the sternomastoid muscle near the junction of its upper and middle thirds. The principles illustrated can be applied to an operation on a lymph node anywhere else in the neck.

Access

1 Position the patient supine with the upper half of the operating table tilted upwards sufficiently to cause the external jugular vein to collapse. Turn the patient's head to the opposite side.

2 Clean the skin from the level of the mouth to the clavicle and from the anterior midline of the neck to as far posteriorly as can be reached. Tuck a pad of sterile wool beneath the neck and scapular regions.

3 Towel up to leave exposed a circular area of radius about 5 cm around the palpable lymph node.

4 Make an incision across the palpable lump and extended for 1 cm beyond its margins in both directions, in the direction of the lines of skin tension, in this case roughly horizontally, with a slight convex curve downwards. Deepen this incision through skin and platysma.

5 Achieve haemostasis with diathermy coagulation.

Assess

1 Feel the lump carefully again. Is it covered only with fascia or is any other structure between your fingers and the swelling?

2 If the intervening tissues are fascia only, deepen your incision through these tissues with a clean scalpel until you can see the surface of the lymph node itself.

3 If there is some structure other than fascia in the way, you must move it out of the way, excise it or cut through it so as to reach the surface of the lymph node. Exactly what you do depends upon the nature of the structure. The commonest in this particular site is the anterior border of the sternomastoid muscle.

Usually it is easy to spread apart the edges of the wound in the skin and platysma with retractors, to divide the fascia where it joins the anterior border of the muscle over a distance of about 3 cm and retract the anterior border of the muscle laterally. The fascia overlying the lymph node can now be incised.

Action

1 Dissect the lymph node free from its surroundings. A good way to do this is to lay a small, curved artery forceps along the surface of the node, with the curve of the forceps corresponding with the curvature of the surface. Insert the tips of the blades of the forceps between the gland and the free edge of investing fascia where you have cut it in order to reach the swelling. Gently push the forceps further along this plane and then separate the blades, thereby stripping the fascia off the lymph node. Cut the fascia with scissors between the separated blades of the forceps, so as to increase the exposure.

2 Repeat this process of combined blunt and sharp dissection all over the superficial aspect of the lymph node. Minimize bleeding by sealing the vessels using diathermy before you cut them. A dry field facilitates the dissection.

3 During this superficial clearance, there is no need to handle the lymph node at all. As you approach the deep aspect, it becomes necessary to push the gland in one direction so that you can free it in that area of its bed from which you are displacing it. This manipulation is likely to damage the gland; be very gentle, and use a finger rather than a metal instrument.

4 Somewhere in this deep aspect you will nearly always find a fairly large feeding artery to the gland. In this region also it is easy to damage neighbouring important structures such as the accessory nerve, because the exposure is limited by the overhanging gland. The safe rule is to cut only tissues that you can see perfectly.

5 When you have completed the dissection deep to the lymph node, it lies free. Remove the node, cut it into two equal parts, put one into a container that will later be filled with formol saline and sent for histological examination, and put the other into a sterile empty container so that it can be sent for culture, including for tuberculosis.

Closure

1 Ensure complete haemostasis. Ask the anaesthetist to flatten the operating table; this change of posture raises venous pressure and sometimes starts bleeding, and it is better that this should happen while you have the wound still open rather than after you have sewn up.

2 Sew up any deep muscle that you have had to divide and platysma, using 2/0 absorbable sutures.

3 Close the skin wound using a subcuticular polypropylene or a blanket stitch using nylon.

Postoperative

1 Is there any sign of a haematoma forming?

2 Are the two portions of the specimen being properly dealt with?

SCALENE NODE BIOPSY

Appraise

1 The pad of fat lying superficial to the lower end of the scalenus (Greek: *skalenos*=uneven; usually a triangle with unequal sides) anterior muscle contains a number of small lymph nodes that are often involved, even if they are not palpably enlarged, by diseases of the lungs or mediastinum.

2 If the nodes on the left side are palpable, or if the intrathoracic disease being investigated involves only the upper lobe of the left lung, perform the biopsy on the left side. In all other circumstances perform the biopsy on the right side, since the glands on the right side are much more likely to be involved.

Access

1 Position the patient and drape as for cervical lymph node biopsy.

2 Make a 5-cm horizontal skin-crease incision 2.5 cm above the clavicle, extending from the anterior border of the trapezius muscle to the posterior, lateral, border of the sternal head of the sternomastoid muscle. Deepen the incision through the platysma muscle.

3 Divide between ligatures the external jugular vein and its tributaries. The main vein runs vertically just deep to the platysma, about the middle of the incision.

4 Divide the clavicular head of sternomastoid by gently passing a blunt dissector, such as Watson–Cheyne's, deep to the muscle and cutting down upon the dissector. Make the cuts in successive small portions, so that you can prevent troublesome bleeding from veins within the muscle. Remember also that your dissector is close to the internal jugular vein, and accordingly take care over this manoeuvre.

Action

1 Retract the margins of the wound with a self-retaining retractor. The fat pad lying superficial to the scalenus anterior muscle is now visible, but it may be overlain by the transverse cervical vessels just above the clavicle. Push these vessels downwards, grasp the fat pad with plain dissecting forceps immediately above the vessels and cut horizontally into the fat pad until the fascia covering the scalenus anterior becomes visible. Lift the fat pad upwards and with scissors or knife elevate the fat pad off the fascia from below upwards (Fig. 34.15).

2 Important structures form the bed of the fat pad and you must take care not to damage them. Lying on the anterior surface of the scalenus anterior muscle, but deep to the fascia, is the phrenic nerve, running more or less vertically downwards but with a trend from lateral to medial. Medial to the scalenus anterior is the internal jugular vein, lateral to the muscle lies the brachial plexus.

3 As the elevation continues, retract the omohyoid muscle upwards; the muscle crosses the upper part of the field obliquely, running in a superomedial direction.

4 When you have freed the fat pad as far as you can conveniently push the omohyoid, cut through the upper end of the pad to remove it completely.

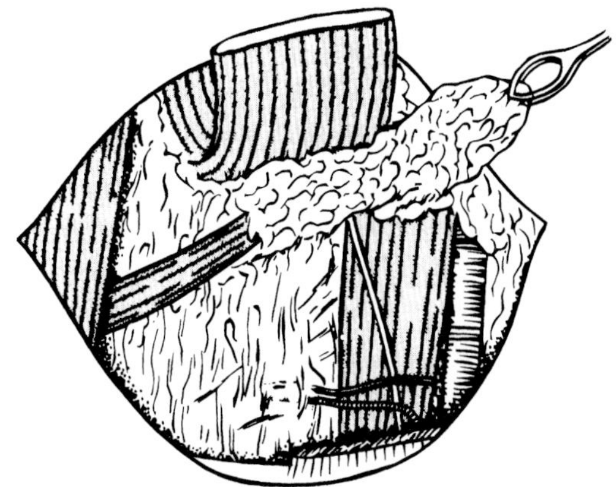

Fig. 34.15 Scalene node biopsy. Flaps of skin with platysma have been raised, the clavicular head of sternomastoid divided. The fat pad covering the scalenus anterior is excised between the transverse cervical vessels below and the omohyoid muscle above. Damage to the brachial plexus, phrenic nerve and internal jugular vein must be avoided.

5 Check haemostasis. Note whether lymph is accumulating in the wound. This complication is of course more likely on the left side. Try to find the damaged lymphatic duct or thoracic duct and tie it off.

Closure

1 Repair the clavicular head of sternomastoid with fine sutures.

2 Drain the wound by a suction drain via a separate stab incision.

3 Sew up the skin.

OPERATIONS ON TUBERCULOUS CERVICAL LYMPH NODES

Appraise

1 You may encounter tuberculous cervical lymph nodes in three main surgical situations:

- An undiagnosed lump.
- A mass that is biopsied to establish the diagnosis but does not disappear with chemotherapy.
- A *cold* abscess.

2 The removal of an enlarged, undiagnosed lymph node in the neck has been described. Remember to send half of the specimen for culture, including culture for acid-fast organisms, as well as the other half for histology. If the histology demonstrates tuberculosis, consult a physician regarding chemotherapy or, if one is not available, start triple therapy, combining three common drugs such as streptomycin, isoniazid and rifampicin, while awaiting the reports on culture of the organisms and sensitivity tests upon them.

3 Biopsy a larger mass of lymph nodes. When a histological report of tuberculosis has been received, start chemotherapy. Usually its influence the mass shrinks and disappears. If not, suspect that the organisms are not sensitive to the combination of drug that you are using.

Operate if:

- The mass of infected glands becomes larger.
- The centre of the mass becomes fluctuant, indicating a cold abscess.
- The skin becomes involved and threatens to break down.

4 Aspirate a cold abscess, inserting a hypodermic needle through uninvolved skin at some distance from the lesion so as to produce a long oblique track with a valvular effect that should minimize the risk of sinus formation. Send the material for culture and sensitivity tests. However, if all or most of the lesion is solid, embark on open operation as described later.

5 Sometimes, though not often now in countries with a high standard of primary health care, you may see a lesion that has already progressed to the stage of a cold abscess, or skin involvement with inflammatory changes and scar formation or even sinuses.

KEY POINTS Confirm the diagnosis before treating

- No matter how typical the clinical picture, confirm the diagnosis of tuberculosis by biopsy.
- It is unthinkable to subject a patient to several months of chemotherapy without a definite diagnosis.

6 In these circumstances, since the material obtained by aspiration of a cold abscess often fails to clinch the diagnosis, carry out open operation.

Principles of open operation

1 Make a horizontal skin-crease incision over the swelling, of a generous length to provide adequate exposure.

2 Modify the incision where necessary to excise all affected skin.

3 Reflect flaps of skin and platysma upwards and downwards to the limits of the involved lymph nodes.

4 Divide the investing fascia of the neck in the region of any fluctuant area or areas, entering the abscesses and evacuating their contents.

5 If the main purpose of the operation is to confirm the clinical diagnosis, scrape the walls of the abscess cavity with a curette to obtain generous portions of the granulation tissue for culture and histology.

6 If the main purpose of the operation is to excise infected glands that have proved resistant to chemotherapy, dissect out as many of the involved lymph nodes as is technically possible. This is a difficult operation, because the lymph nodes tend to be adherent to neighbouring structures that are functionally important and must be preserved.

7 It is not possible to specify more than the principles rather than detail all the difficulties and dangers that you may encounter. These depend on the exact site of the involved lymph nodes. For example, the lymph nodes of the anterior triangle may be adherent to the jugular vein, the common carotid artery and its two branches, and the vagus nerve. The jugulodigastric group may be adherent to the hypoglossal, accessory and glossopharyngeal nerves. Involved lymph nodes in the posterior triangle may lie around the lower part of the accessory nerve.

8 When you have completed the excision, ensure that you have achieved meticulous haemostasis and then close the skin, if possible without drainage. If much skin has been excised, some rearrangement of the skin flaps may be necessary to achieve primary closure.

BLOCK DISSECTION OF CERVICAL LYMPH NODES

Appraise

1 Many carcinomas of the head and neck metastasize to the cervical lymph nodes. Whatever the best mode of treatment for the primary, whether surgery or radiotherapy, control of affected cervical lymph nodes is best obtained by excising them.

2 Your intention is to remove a block of connective tissue containing the nodes from the anterior and posterior triangles, extending from the clavicle below to the base of skull above.

KEY POINTS Operation is futile unless:

- The primary growth is cured or curable.
- There are no metastases at more distant sites.

Access

1 If you are removing the primary growth at the same time, extend the standard approach for parotidectomy, glossectomy, mandibulectomy, laryngectomy appropriately, to create flaps that lay open the neck on the side of the growth.

2 If you are performing the block dissection as a separate procedure following apparent cure of the primary tumour, create a modified Y-shaped incision with equal limbs (Fig. 34.16).

3 Reflect the flaps to expose the entire neck from clavicle to mandible and mastoid, and from midline backwards to trapezius. There are many different incisions available, all of which give good exposure and closure. The MacFee incision of two parallel transverse incisions gives limited exposure, and trauma to the flap outweighs any potential advantage.

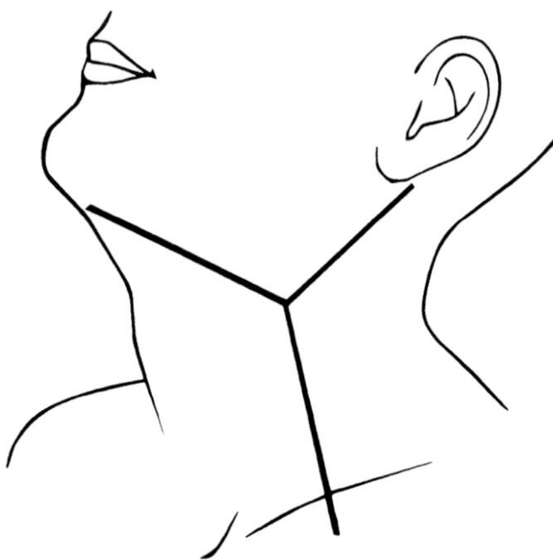

Fig. 34.16 Block dissection of the neck. The incision.

Action

1 Divide the clavicular and sternal heads of the sternomastoid just above their insertions. Gently dissect the lower end of the internal jugular vein, separating it from the common carotid artery and, deep to that, the vagus nerve. Be careful on the left side not to damage the thoracic duct. Ligate and divide the vein, placing two stout non-absorbable ligatures on the lower stump.

2 Divide the inferior belly of omohyoid and extend the dissection laterally just above the clavicle to the anterior border of trapezius.

KEY POINT Caution

- Beware an unusually high subclavian vein.

3 Deepen the dissection to the prevertebral fascia covering the scalenus muscles and brachial plexus. Find the plane by blunt dissection.

4 In front of the trachea divide the thyroid isthmus and inferior thyroid veins, so that the hemithyroid gland and strap muscles, first divided above the clavicle and sternum, can be stripped upwards. Ligate and divide the inferior thyroid vessels, preserving the recurrent laryngeal nerve unless a laryngectomy has already been carried out. Head and neck surgeons do not perform hemithyroidectomy unless the primary tumour lies close by, such as laryngeal carcinoma, or the tumour arises in the thyroid.

5 Now dissect the block upwards, taking the hemithyroid gland, sternomastoid, internal jugular vein and all connective and lymphoid tissues from the anterior and posterior triangles. Clean the tissues off the trapezius border and leave the brachial plexus, prevertebral fascia, scaleni, vagus and phrenic nerves, thoracic duct, carotid vessels, trachea and oesophagus intact. Divide the accessory nerve as it enters the trapezius. At the top of the wound divide the sternomastoid again and carefully cut the deeper fascial planes until, drawing the specimen forwards, you can find and dissect again the upper end of the internal jugular vein. Ligate and divide it as near as can be carried out at the skull base.

6 Cut the deep fascia close to the lower border of the mandible and clear the contents of the submental and submandibular triangles. Divide Wharton's duct so that the submandibular gland can be removed as part of the block excision. If necessary, be prepared to take the lower pole of the parotid gland, remembering you will probably sacrifice the cervical branch of the facial nerve. Leave intact the lingual and hypoglossal nerves.

7 You need to ligate sundry large veins such as the common and posterior facial, and, as you work downwards, the remaining vascular attachments near the external carotid artery that must be doubly ligated and divided are the facial and sternomastoid arteries. Divide the upper attachments of the sternohyoid and sternothyroid muscles, and the accessory nerve at its entry into the sternomastoid. Divide a few residual shreds of carotid sheath and the specimen is free (Fig. 34.17). Occasionally, you must sacrifice the external carotid artery in the same block.

Technical

1 If it is not necessary to remove the thyroid gland, preserve the sternothyroid and sternohyoid muscles.

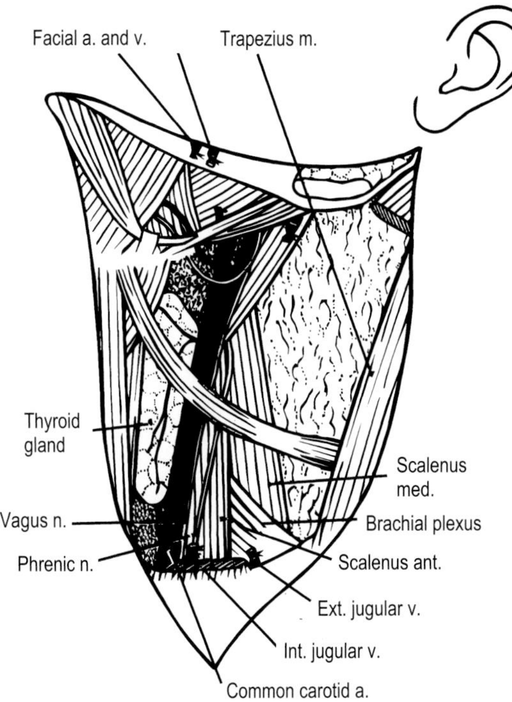

Fig. 34.17 Neck dissection completed.

2 In selected cases of 'floor of mouth' cancer, clearance may be limited to the upper half of the neck.

3 If there are bilateral metastases, preserve the internal jugular vein on one side if possible. Separate the two block dissections by a period of not less than 6 weeks.

4 Modified radical neck dissection preserves the sternomastoid muscle, accessory nerve and internal jugular vein. It is now the usual mode of treatment for metastatic neck disease.

Closure

1 Ensure complete haemostasis.

2 Ensure the adhesion of the skin flaps by meticulous skin closure and use continuous vacuum drainage to encourage primary healing.

RADICAL PAROTIDECTOMY WITH BLOCK DISSECTION

1 Patients with proven malignant disease of the parotid gland require a formal block dissection in continuity with the parotidectomy. The posterior end of the upper skin flap is modified by prolonging it as the mastoid–facial part of the standard parotidectomy incision (Fig. 34.18a).

2 Frequently the disease spreads posteriorly to involve the external ear, and anteriorly to involve the mandible in the region of the angle. Remove the pinna and the posterior part of the mandible, including the ramus and the body as far forwards as the second molar tooth, in continuity with the rest of the excised tissue. The modification of the skin incisions is shown in Figure 34.18b.

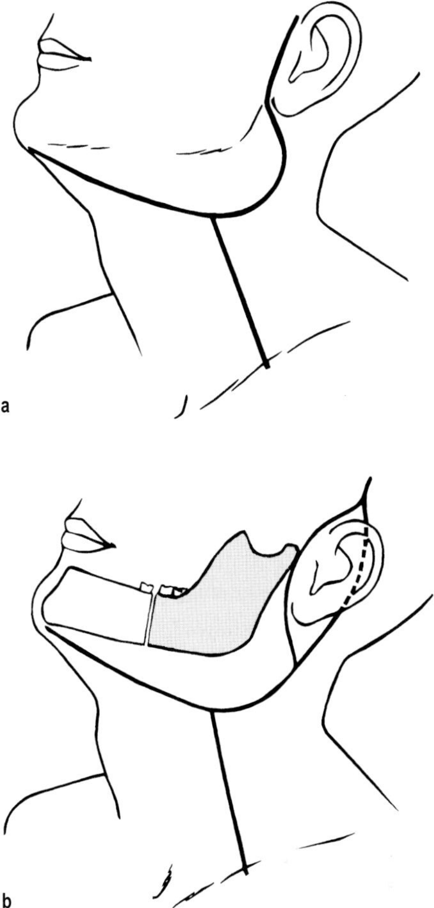

Fig. 34.18 (a) Modified Y-incision for block dissection to include radical parotidectomy. The posterior limb becomes prolonged as the upper two-thirds of a formal parotidectomy incision (see Fig. 34.1). This incision is also suitable for the 'commando' operation, provided that the anterior limb is extended fully to the symphysis menti. (b) Modified Y-incision for block dissection with excision of the pinna and radical parotidectomy. The portion of the mandible to be removed if the tumour extends close to that bone is indicated.

3 Widely sacrifice any area of skin infiltrated by the tumour. Reflect the upper flap well forwards to expose the masseter muscle and clear the mandible of the buccinator muscle, forwards to the second molar socket.

4 If the patient is edentulous, now clear the medial aspect of the body without opening the oral mucosa. If the molars are present, cut the mucosa in their vicinity to free them from the mouth. Divide the body through the socket of the second molar tooth.

5 Now free the inner aspect of the ramus from the temporalis muscle, which is attached to the coronoid process, and the pterygoid muscles—the lateral attached to the mandibular condyle, the medial to the mandibular angle. Divide the masseter from the zygoma at the upper border of the coronoid and condylar processes to free the bone and attached lower portion of the masseter, and then continue the dissection posteriorly to remove the whole parotid. If indicated, also resect the zygomatic

arch. Closure of the skin flaps can be difficult after this operation, if you need to sacrifice much infiltrated skin. A better option is to accept inevitable skin loss and replace skin and subcutaneous soft tissues with a free vascularized or pedicled myocutaneous flap.[1]

RADICAL SUBMANDIBULAR SIALOADENECTOMY WITH RESECTION OF SEGMENT OF MANDIBLE AND BLOCK DISSECTION ('COMMANDO' OPERATION)

1 An operation involving resection of a segment of the body of the mandible in continuity with a block dissection of the cervical lymph nodes is often called a 'commando' operation—a military term for a highly trained and ruthless service group.

2 Proven malignant disease of the submandibular gland requires resection of the neighbouring segment of mandibular body to achieve a wide clearance. Another indication is carcinoma of the floor of the mouth or of the tongue adjacent to the mandible.

3 The incision is of the type shown in Figure 34.18a, without the posterior parotid extension and with the anterior end of the upper incision prolonged to reach the symphysis menti. Obtain good exposure with wide elevation of the upper flap to the upper border of the body of the mandible.

4 After the excision, repair the mucosa and muscles of the floor of the mouth and submandibular region. The defect in the body of the mandible can be immediately repaired with a titanium prosthesis provided that the area has not been X-irradiated. Alternatively, accept the defect. Provided that the region of the symphysis menti is intact, a gap in the body does not produce a severe deformity or instability of the lower jaw.

REFERENCE

1. Gallegos NC, Watkin G, Cook HP et al 1991 Further evaluation of radical surgery following radiotherapy for advanced parotid carcinoma. British Journal of Surgery 78:97–100

FURTHER READING

Fleming WB 1988 Infections in branchial cysts. Australian and New Zealand Journal of Surgery 58:481–483

Freidberg J 1989 Pharyngeal cleft sinuses and cysts and other benign neck lesions. Pediatric Clinics of North America 36:1451–1469

Jesse RH, Ballantyne AJ, Larson D 1978 Radical or modified radical neck dissection: a therapeutic dilemma. American Journal of Surgery 136:516–519

Jones AS, Cook JA, Phillips DE 1993 Squamous cell carcinoma presenting as an enlarged cervical lymph node: the occult primary. Cancer 72:1756–1761

Micheau C, Klijanienko J, Luboinski B et al 1990 So called branchiogenic carcinoma is actually cystic metastases in the neck from tonsillar primary. Laryngoscope 100:878–883

Radkowski D, Arnold J, Healy GB 1991 Thyroglossal duct remnants: preoperative evaluation and management. Archives of Otolaryngology Head and Neck Surgery 117:1378–1381

Razack M 1977 Influence of initial neck node biopsy on the incidence of recurrence in the neck and survival in patients who subsequently undergo curative resectional surgery. Journal of Surgery and Oncology 9:347–352

35

Orthopaedics and trauma: amputations

N. Goddard, G. Harper

CONTENTS

INTRODUCTION

Approximately 5500 amputations are performed each year in England. The number steadily increases as the population ages; 75% of the patients are over 60 years of age, and 65% are men.

KEY POINTS Aims of amputation

- The prime intention is to excise all pathology.
- The second aim is to restore maximal limb function.

Appraise

1 The main indications for amputation are:
- Vascular disease—arterial or venous.
- Diabetes (diabetes and vascular disease together account for about 85% of amputations).
- Trauma (10%).
- Tumours (3%).
- Infection (now only responsible for 1.5% of amputations).
- Neurological causes such as nerve injury and its secondary effects.
- Congenital problems.

2 Major upper limb amputations are rarely required (only 3% of the total).

GENERAL PRINCIPLES

Appraise

1 If you are in any doubt about the necessity for amputation obtain a second opinion from a senior colleague.

KEY POINTS Anticipate

- Before elective operations contact the regional limb-fitting centre, when possible, for advice on the best level and type of procedure.
- Remember, you will obtain the best results by drawing in the informed involvement of a trained team, including nurses, physiotherapists, occupational therapists, prosthetists and social workers.

2 Operate using general anaesthesia whenever possible.

3 Level of amputation and the type of prosthesis are influenced by:
- Viability of soft tissues.
- Underlying pathology.
- Functional requirements.
- Comfort.
- Cosmetic appearance.

4 Energy conservation is an important consideration when planning lower-limb amputation and the chosen level is crucial. Energy expenditure following bilateral below-knee amputation is still less than that of a unilateral above-knee amputation. Plan to preserve every possible dynamic structure, including the knee joint and the epiphysis in children.

5 Appraise the blood supply of the limb clinically by looking for skin colour changes, shiny atrophic appearance and lack of hair growth. Feel for skin temperature changes. Be willing to order transcutaneous Doppler recordings and measurement of the ankle–brachial index, thermography, radioactive xenon clearance, transcutaneous PO_2 measurement

6 Assess the bone by taking plain radiographs in two planes: tomograms or a radioisotope bone scan. In the presence of bone or soft-tissue malignancy, ensure that the lesion has a confirmed diagnosis with a biopsy. Computed tomography (CT) and magnetic resonance imaging (MRI) are essential in fully staging the lesion and assessing the necessity for amputation. Limb-sparing surgery has recently become more feasible provided the correct

indications are followed under guidance from expert tumour surgeons.

Prepare

1 As the surgeon performing the operation it is your personal responsibility to obtain consent and explain possible complications. Fully inform the patient of the proposed operation. Obtain consent to amputate, if necessary, more proximally than you intend.

2 Give prophylactic antibiotics: penicillin (or erythromycin) plus one other broad-spectrum antibiotic. Swab and culture any wounds preoperatively.

2 Clean the limb and seal off the infected or necrotic areas.

3 Arrange for the disposal of the limb after amputation to the pathology department or straight to the incinerator.

4 Clearly mark the limb with indelible marker.

Action

General techniques

1 Use a tourniquet except in peripheral vascular disease. Exsanguinate the limb by elevation for 2–4 minutes rather than an Esmarch bandage.

2 Prepare the skin and apply the drapes.

KEY POINTS Skin flaps

- Mark the proposed skin flaps preoperatively.
- They should be approximately as long as the base is wide at the level of bone section.
- Leave them too long rather than too short.
- If amputation follows traumatic injury, preserve all viable skin to create an adequate stump.
- In the presence of vascular disease do not undermine the edges of the flaps.
- Handle the flaps gently.

3 Wherever possible include underlying muscles in the flap (myoplastic flap) since this greatly improves the skin blood supply and covers and protects the stump. Muscles provide power, stabilization and proprioception to the stump. In emergency cases remove all dead muscle (this avoids gas gangrene) and leave viable muscle (red, bleeding and contracting). In elective cases cut the muscle with a raked incision angled towards the level of bone section.

4 Double-ligate major vessels with strong silk or linen thread. Ligate other vessels with absorbable material such as polyglycolic acid (Dexon).

5 Gently pull down nerves, divide them cleanly and allow them to retract into soft tissue envelopes. Ligate major nerves with a fine suture prior to and just above the site of division. This stops bleeding from accompanying vessels and decreases neuroma formation.

6 Prepare to cut the bone at the appropriate level. Remember that the stump must be long enough to gain secure attachment to the prosthesis and to act as a useful level but short enough to accommodate the prosthesis and its hinge or joint mechanism. Divide the periosteum and cut the bone with a Gigli or power saw. During bone section, cover the soft tissues with a moist pack and irrigate afterwards to remove bone dust and particles from the soft tissues. Round-off sharp bone edges with a rasp.

7 Check that the flaps will approximate easily.

8 Release the tourniquet and secure haemostasis.

9 Insert a suction drain.

10 Suture the flaps together without tension, starting with the muscle. Handle the skin carefully and close it with staples if available, or interrupted nylon sutures.

11 In the presence of infection or if you have any doubt about the viability of the flaps, approximate the muscles loosely over gauze soaked in saline or proflavine to prevent them from contracting. Do not close the skin. Plan delayed primary closure at 5–7 days.

Aftercare

1 Apply a well-padded compressible but not crushing dressing, using either cotton wool or latex foam. Hold this in place with crepe bandage taking care to avoid fixed flexion or other deformity of neighbouring joints.

2 Except in cases with infection or doubtful flap viability, apply a *light* shell, maximum four layers, of plaster of Paris over the dressing. This makes the patient more comfortable and able to be more mobile in bed. In specialist centres a prosthetist can apply a rigid dressing to which a temporary pylon can be attached, allowing early ambulation.

3 Leave the dressing undisturbed if possible for 10 days.

KEY POINTS Inspect the wound if there is:

- Increasing pain.
- Seepage of blood or pus through the dressing.
- Rising temperature and pulse.

4 Order regular physiotherapy to prevent joint contractures.

5 Encourage mobilization and use of the stump as soon as the patient is comfortable.

6 When the wound has healed and sutures have been removed, apply regular stump bandaging to maintain the shape of the stump.

7 As soon as possible refer the patient to the local limb-fitting centre if you had not already done so before operation.

Special situations

Amputations in children

Children's amputations present their own special problems:

- Growing bones at the site of amputation will overgrow by apposition, not related to growth at the proximal growth plate. You may need to revise the bone to prevent skin problems.
- If possible, always preserve epiphyseal growth plates.

- Perform a disarticulation more distally rather than an amputation through a long bone at a more proximal level if at all possible. The disarticulation prevents terminal overgrowth of the bone.
- Children suffer less than adults from the complications of amputation such as phantom pain, neuroma, etc. They adapt amazingly well to prostheses if fitted correctly at an early age.

Decision-making for amputations in major trauma

1. Objective criteria help predict amputation following lower extremity trauma. The Mangled Extremity Score (MESS) is one such system. It uses four significant criteria of skeletal/soft-tissue injury, limb ischaemia, shock, and patient age.
2. Such systems help you to discriminate between salvageable limbs and those better managed by primary amputation.

Complications

Haematoma

KEY POINTS Prevention of haematoma

- Avoid by meticulous haemostasis at the time of amputation.
- Double-ligate major vessels.
- Prevent infection, which may cause secondary haemorrhage.
- Never close the stump before releasing the tourniquet.

- Haematoma in the stump predisposes to infection and greatly delays prosthetic fitting.
- Drain collections of blood by aspiration or a small incision. Perform this in the operating theatre under sterile conditions, not on the ward. Local anaesthesia is usually sufficient.
- If there is clearly uncontrolled haemorrhage, apply firm compression and elevate the limb while you make arrangements to explore the stump under a general anaesthetic.

Infection

- Amputation stumps are more at risk of infection than most other surgical wounds. The stump tissues are often poorly vascularized, there are often infected lesions in the distal extremity, and patients are often frail, elderly, with poor resistance to infection.
- Give prophylactic antibiotics to all lower-limb amputees. Choose antibiotics that are active against gas gangrene organisms, *Escherichia coli* and staphylococci.
- Handle all soft tissues with care and avoid leaving dead muscle and long sections of denuded cortical bone in the stump.
- Treat wound infections promptly with antibiotics. Incise and drain any collection of pus.
- If a chronic sinus fails to dry up with a course of antibiotics lasting up to 6 weeks, explore the stump under general anaesthesia. You usually find a focus of infection such as a small bony sequestrum or a lump of infected suture material..

Flap necrosis

1. Prevent this complication by carefully assessing skin viability prior to amputation and by handling all skin edges and flaps with the utmost care. Use a myoplastic flap wherever possible as this always has a better blood supply.
2. Treat small areas of wound necrosis conservatively. The wound often granulates beneath the patch of blackened, sloughing skin, which eventually separates spontaneously.
3. Major flap necrosis requires either a wedge resection down to and including bone or re-amputation to a higher level.

Joint contractures

KEY POINTS Susceptibility to joint contractures

- The hip and knee joint are particularly prone to contractures.
- Among patients, the elderly and immobile, and those with serious head injuries, prolonged coma or chronic pain are most at risk.

1. Treat or prevent mild contractures by early active and passive exercises, place the joints in a corrective posture, fit a prosthesis that retains the position, and encourage mobilization. For example, regularly lying the patient prone discourages hip contractures.
2. Severe contractures may require serial plasters or surgical release; otherwise applying a prosthesis is likely to be impossible and useless.

Neuroma

1. All cut ends of nerves form neuromata but they are painful only if trapped in scar tissue or exposed to repeated trauma. Ensure that transected nerves lie deep within the normal tissues of the limb proximal to the end of the stump.
2. Treat painful neuromata by resecting the neuroma together with a length of the affected nerve, well away from the area of scar tissue.

Phantom limb sensation

1. Always warn the patient before amputation about the likelihood of still feeling that the missing part of the limb is present. Do not introduce the concept of phantom pain, however.
2. After amputation, reassure the patient that this feeling will gradually fade away. Meanwhile warn against attempting to use a limb that is not present.

Phantom pain

1. This complication is most common with proximal rather than distal amputations, in patients who had severe pain before amputation and in those who have been in contact with other patients with phantom pain.
2. The cause is unknown and the pain is untreatable even by nerve section or cordotomy. Be continually optimistic and supportive and remember that this distressing symptom occasionally leads

to suicide. Involve the whole team in giving the patient support and encouragement.

Failure to use a prosthesis

1 Patients most likely to adapt to a prosthesis are those who have the physical ability, mental capability and the determination to do so. The most adaptable are those who were able to stand and walk, with or without aids, shortly before operation.

2 In both the upper and lower limbs, the higher the amputation the less likely it is that a prosthesis will be used. If the energy expenditure in a wheelchair is less than on a prosthesis, it requires a determined patient to get out of the wheelchair.

KEY POINTS Facilitating the use of a prosthesis

- The earlier a prosthesis is applied, the more likely it is to be used.
- In specialist centres, rigid casts are applied to the stump to which a prosthesis can be attached. Patients are mobilized within 48 hours of operation.
- Advantages of early application are reduced postoperative oedema, considerably reduced pain, profound psychological benefits, fewer complications of immobility such as joint contracture and osteoporosis, shorter hospital stay, earlier maturation of the stump and earlier return to full social activities.

HINDQUARTER AMPUTATION

Appraise

1 This radical operation is usually performed for malignant disease of bone or soft tissue of the pelvis or upper thigh. It is beyond the scope of anyone except a skilled and specially experienced expert.

2 It is included to demonstrate the principles if you are an assistant. The detailed steps were described by Gordon-Taylor and Monro.[1]

3 The incision is shown in Fig. 35.1. The external iliac, deep epigastric and internal iliac branch vessels are divided, as are the femoral, obturator and sciatic nerves. The pelvis is sectioned at the symphysis pubis and upwards from the greater sciatic notch to the iliac rim. The anterior portion of the pelvis is freed and removed with the hindquarter, and the wound is closed.

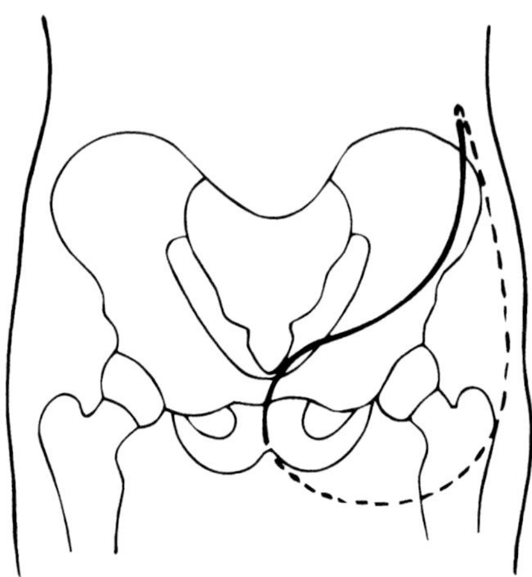

Fig. 35.1 Incision for hindquarter amputation.

REFERENCE

1. Gordon-Taylor G, Monro R 1952 The technique and management of hindquarter amputation. British Journal of Surgery 39:536–541

ABOVE-KNEE AMPUTATION

Appraise

Decide on the level of the amputation bearing in mind the following considerations:

- The longer the femoral stump the better the control of the prosthesis.
- Do not transect the femur lower than 15 cm above the knee joint; this allows room for the hinge mechanism of the prosthesis. If the stump is longer, the artificial knee joint is lower than on the normal leg. This is most marked when the patient sits.
- Always perform a myodesis (Greek: *desis*=a binding together), anchoring a muscle group to the femur. This prevents the femur from migrating through the stump, resulting in skin necrosis; it also makes it difficult for the patient to control the prosthesis during walking.
- If there is fixed flexion deformity at the hip, fashion a shorter stump in order to fit into a prosthesis.
- If the patient is unlikely to walk after amputation, leave a short stump if the hip is stiff.

If possible, do not amputate through the femur in children, since this removes the lower, growing end of the bone.

Action

1 Place the patient supine with a sandbag beneath the buttock.

2 Use a tourniquet if there is room for it without interfering with the operative area.

KEY POINT Your position

- Operate from the opposite side of the table from the affected leg. This gives you better access to, and elevation of, the stump during the operation.

3 Mark out equal anterior and posterior flaps, their bases sited at the proposed level of bone section.

4 Deepen the incision to the deep fascia, allowing the skin to retract slightly. From this level divide the anterior muscles with a raking cut aimed at the level of bone section.

5 Identify the femoral vessels beneath the sartorius muscle and doubly ligate them. Pull down the femoral nerve, ligate it with a fine suture and then cut it cleanly, allowing it to retract.

6 Divide the periosteum around the whole femur at the level of proposed section. Cut through the bone with a Gigli or amputation saw, protecting the soft tissues as previously described.

7 Now retract the distal femoral fragment and locate the profunda femoris vessels in the tissues behind the femur. Ligate them, then identify the sciatic nerve. Pull it down gently, ligate it and then divide it cleanly, allowing it to retract.

8 Complete the division of the posterior muscles using a raking cut to match the anterior flap.

9 Remove the limb.

10 Secure haemostasis.

Close

1 Round off the end of the bone with a rasp.

2 Now turn your attention to the flaps, which should be roughly equal in size and thickness. They are composed of muscle and skin and are called myoplastic flaps. Perform a myodesis after drilling a small hole in the posterior cortex of the femoral stump. Draw and fix the quadriceps muscle over the end of the bone with a stitches of the same type of thread. Stitch the remaining muscles to the quadriceps, attempting to retain roughly equal tension in all the muscle groups.

3 Insert a suction drain.

4 Close the skin with interrupted nylon stitches plus adhesive such as Steri-Strip tapes.

5 Apply a well-padded compression dressing and hold it in place by taking two or three turns of crepe bandage round the waist. Be careful, however, to avoid pulling the stump into a position of flexion with the dressing.

Aftercare

1 Remove the drain at 48 hours.

2 Encourage maximum mobility as soon as the patient is comfortable. Ensure regular physiotherapy is given, including prone lying to prevent a flexion contracture at the hip.

3 Inspect the wound at 10 days and remove the sutures when healed.

4 Apply a firm stump bandage daily thereafter to mould the stump into a roughly conical shape.

5 Arrange for the fitting of a temporary pylon by the third or fourth week and plan for definitive limb-fitting between the sixth and twelfth week.

BELOW-KNEE AMPUTATION

Appraise

1 Carefully assess the viability of the soft tissues of the lower leg when considering amputation at this level, looking for evidence of peripheral vascular disease, diabetic gangrene or trauma.

KEY POINTS Flap lengths?

- Use a long posterior flap, or a skew flap, in peripheral vascular disease, diabetes and trauma.
- Equal flaps are suitable for amputating tumours or for severe acute infection.

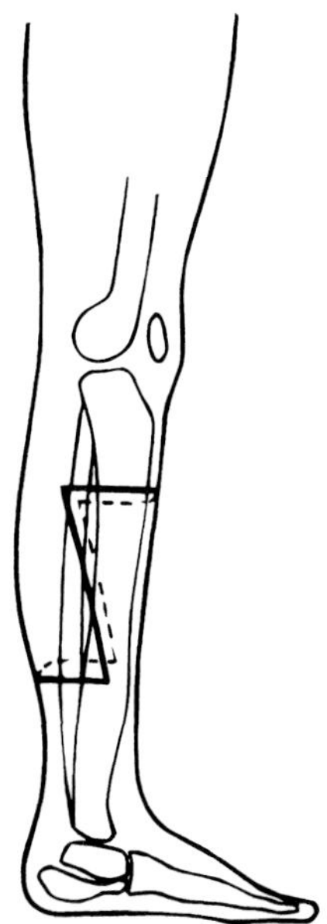

Fig. 35.2 Incision for below-knee amputation.

Table 35.1 Required tibial length for below-knee amputation in cases of fixed flexion deformity of the knee

Fixed flexion deformity	Tibial length
35°	6–10 cm
15°	10–15 cm
5°	>20 cm

2 Do not consider this amputation in the non-ambulant patient but otherwise always try to preserve the knee.

3 A third of its length is the optimal level for tibial section. Do not make it longer than this or the resulting flaps will not contain sufficient muscle to maintain its viability. The minimum length is 6 cm. If there is a fixed flexion deformity of the knee then the required tibial lengths are as indicated in Table 35.1.

Access

1 Seal off any infected, gangrenous areas by enclosing them in a polyethylene bag.

2 Employ general or epidural anaesthesia.

3 Apply a tourniquet to the thigh unless the amputation is for peripheral vascular disease.

4 Place the patient supine on the operating table with a padded, inverted bowl underneath the proximal tibia.

5 Mark the skin flaps (Fig. 35.2).

Action

1 Start the anterior incision at the base of proposed bone section, cutting transversely round each side of the leg to a point two-thirds of the way down each side. Then take the incisions

distally on each side, passing slightly anteriorly to a point well below the length that is likely to be required.

2 Join the two incisions posteriorly.

3 Deepen the longitudinal incisions down to deep fascia. Anteriorly incise straight down to bone and then on to the interosseous membrane. Ligate the anterior tibial vessels at this point.

4 Elevate the periosteum of the tibia for 1 cm proximal to the level of section. Divide the tibia using a Gigli or amputation saw. Bevel the anterior half of the tibial stump with the saw and a rasp. Divide the fibula 1 cm proximally and bevel the bone laterally.

5 Use a bone hook to distract the distal part of the tibia. Divide the deep posterior muscles of the calf at the same level as the tibia. At this stage identify and ligate the posterior tibial and peroneal vessels. Cleanly divide the posterior tibial nerve, allowing it to retract.

6 Use a raking cut through the soleus and gastrocnemius muscles down to the end of the posterior flap. Remove the limb.

Close

1 Complete the smoothing and bevelling of the tibia and fibula using bone nibblers and a rasp.

2 Bevel gastrocnemius and soleus medially and laterally, and trim the excess skin to fashion a rounded, slightly bulbous stump.

3 Release the tourniquet and secure haemostasis.

4 Insert a suction drain brought out medially through the wound.

5 Bring the posterior flap forwards over the bone and suture it anteriorly to the deep fascia of the anterolateral group of muscles, using a strong absorbable suture.

6 Close the skin, preferably with closely placed staples, or with interrupted nylon sutures and adhesive strip such as Steri-Strip tapes. Do not leave any 'dog ears' laterally.

7 Apply a dressing of gauze and sterile plaster wool, then apply gentle compression of the stump with a crepe bandage. Apply a further layer of plaster wool and then a light plaster cast to mid-thigh level. Mould the plaster over the femoral condyles to prevent it from slipping down. Do not use plaster if there is any infection.

Aftercare

1 Elevate the leg.

2 Remove the drain at 48 hours by gently pulling it out of the top of the plaster cast.

3 Mobilize the patient early but retain the plaster cast undisturbed for at least 10 days.

4 Remove the sutures at 14 days.

5 Apply a daily stump bandage.

6 Arrange for daily hip and knee physiotherapy.

7 As soon as the wound has fully healed arrange for the fitting of a temporary pylon, either patellar-tendon-bearing or ischial-bearing, depending on the quality of the stump. Now arrange for definitive limb-fitting.

SYME'S AMPUTATION

Appraise

1 This was described by James Symes (1799–1870), Professor of Surgery in Edinburgh, in 1842 as an alternative to below-knee amputation. Transmetatarsal and tarsometatarsal amputation is occasionally required for severe trauma. For elective amputation, Syme's amputation is functionally superior.

KEY POINTS Benefits of Syme's amputation

- Properly performed, Syme's is the best amputation of the lower limb.
- The stump is end-bearing with good proprioception and the modern cosmetic prostheses are very light and comfortable.

2 Ensure that there is adequate circulation in the foot. The posterior tibial pulse must be palpable. The skin of the heel must be of good quality.

Action

1 Place the patient supine with the foot extending beyond the end of the table.

2 Apply a tourniquet to the thigh.

3 With the foot and ankle in a neutral position, mark the skin flaps (Fig. 35.3). The plantar flap runs from the tip of the lateral malleolus across the sole (curving slightly forward) to a point just below the medial malleolus. The dorsal flap joins the ends of the plantar incision at an angle of 45° from the line of the tibia.

4 Deepen the incision in the plantar flap down to the bone. On the dorsum divide the extensor retinaculum and pull down the extensor tendons, dividing them as high as possible.

5 Open the ankle joint, plantar-flex the foot and divide the medial and lateral collateral ligaments from within. Take care to avoid the posterior tibial nerve and artery on the medial side.

6 Dislocate the talus downwards and open the posterior capsule of the ankle, exposing the posterosuperior surface of the os calcis and the anterior surface of the tendo achilles.

7 With a periosteal elevator, reflect periosteum and soft tissue from the medial and lateral sides of the os calcis down to the

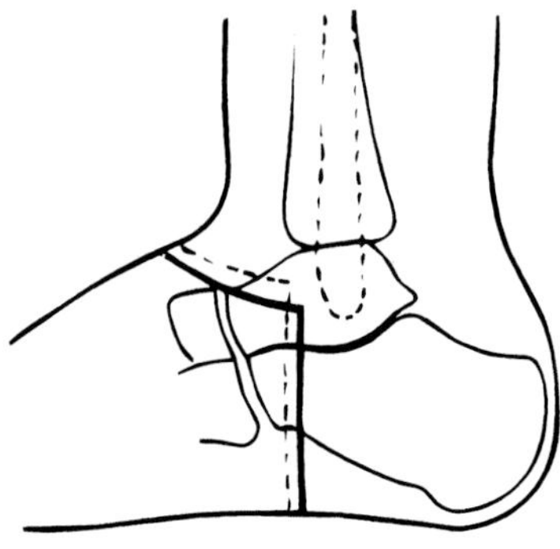

Fig. 35.3 Incision for Syme's amputation.

inferior surface of the bone. Continue this dissection so as to free the inferior surface.

8 Detach the long plantar ligament from the tuberosity of the os calcis and continue until you reach the plantar incision. The proximal end of the bone is now free except for the insertion of the tendo achilles. Carefully divide this from above downwards, keeping close to the bone. Avoid buttonholing the skin flap behind the tendon.

9 Now remove the foot.

Close

1 Turn the heel flap backwards and upwards and free the malleoli and distal centimetre of tibia. Remove the malleoli and a thin slice of tibia with a saw.

KEY POINT Ensure a flat platform

- Make sure your tibial cut is at right-angles to the line of the bone and that you leave the subarticular bone intact.

2 Round off the bone edges.

3 Release the tourniquet and secure haemostasis.

4 Insert a suction drain.

5 Suture the heel flap to the margin of the dorsal incision in two layers with subcutaneous synthetic absorbable material such as polyglycolic acid (Dexon) and interrupted nylon to skin. Begin skin closure in the middle and continue to each end.

6 Ensure that the heel flap remains centred over the cut end of the tibia. The flap may be secured with adhesive such as Steri-Strip tapes.

7 If the heel flap is very unstable, transfix it percutaneously with a Kirschner wire or Steinmann pin passed up into the tibia.

8 Apply a well-padded pressure dressing and retain this either with adhesive strapping to the upper calf or a lightweight above-knee plaster cast.

Aftercare

1 Elevate the leg.

2 Remove the drain at 48 hours but do not disturb the dressing.

3 If you have not transfixed the heel flap, inspect the wound at 5 days to check the position of the flap. Otherwise, inspect the wound at 14 days, when the sutures and the percutaneous pin may be removed.

4 Carefully apply a stump bandage thereafter and arrange the fitting of a prosthesis as soon as the swelling has subsided, usually at 2–4 weeks.

AMPUTATION OF THE TOES

Appraise

1 Avoid amputating single toes if possible. Neighbouring toes tend to develop secondary deformity and take more weight.

2 Remove all the toes (the 'Pobble' operation) if there are multiple painful, fixed deformities or if several toes are gangrenous.

3 Ray resection of toes may be required for gangrene or diabetes.

4 If you need to amputate the great toe, try to preserve the attachments of the short flexor and extensor tendons on the proximal phalanx.

Action

1 Use a tourniquet after exsanguination.

2 Mark out a racquet incision for amputation of individual toes. For amputation of all the toes use a transverse incision, passing across the root of the toes on the plantar aspect, that is overlying the proximal phalanx, and across the metatarsophalangeal joints on the dorsum. The eventual scar should lie dorsally.

3 Take the flaps straight down to bone and dissect off the proximal phalanx.

4 Preserve the base of the proximal phalanx if possible, dividing the bone just distal to the insertion of the capsule. This creates a small wound cavity, which heals quickly, and the amputation does not damage the transverse metatarsal ligaments. Alternatively, perform a careful disarticulation.

5 Secure haemostasis.

6 Close the skin with interrupted nylon sutures.

7 Apply a bulky compression dressing, passing a few turns of crepe bandage round the ankle to hold the dressing in position.

Aftercare

1 Elevate the leg.

2 Remove the sutures at 10 days and mobilize the patient.

3 Where individual toes have been amputated, ask the chiropodist to supply a toe spacer.

4 Where all the toes have been amputated, order a special insole that incorporates a combined metatarsal and cavus support, together with a cork toe-block faced with sponge rubber.

THE UPPER LIMB

1 Many of the indications for amputation in the hand have changed in recent times as a result of improvements in surgical method, prosthetics and plastic surgery. These techniques require special expertise.

2 Some of the operations are suitable for semi-elective use, provided you adhere to the principles of soft-tissue and wound management.

3 Here we shall consider only some of the common and simpler procedures.

AMPUTATION OF FINGERS

Action

1 Use an exsanguinating tourniquet.

2 Place the arm on a side table.

3 Mark the incision, which should be placed so that the scar will lie on the dorsal aspect and the stump will be covered by volar skin.

4 Do not suture together the ends of the extensor and flexor tendons over the end of the bone.

5 Identify the digital nerves and isolate them from the vessels before dividing them cleanly, 1 cm proximal to the stump.

6 Round off the end of the bone and remove the articular cartilage and prominent condyles when performing a disarticulation.

7 Reduce the bulk of the fibrofatty subcutaneous tissue to allow the skin edges to be brought together without difficulty.

8 Release the tourniquet and secure haemostasis before closure.

9 Avoid tight skin closure, otherwise painful and ischaemic torsion may develop as a result of postoperative swelling. Some soft tissue retraction occurs during the first 2 months but do not, on this account, leave excessive slackness of the stump; this causes an unsightly, unsupported soft-tissue mass.

10 Apply a compression dressing of gauze and narrow crepe bandage.

AMPUTATION THROUGH THE DISTAL PHALANX

If less than one-quarter of the length of the nail remains, the patient may be troubled later by an irregular hooked nail remnant. Therefore ablate the nail bed and excise the lateral angles as completely as possible.

DISARTICULATION THROUGH THE DISTAL INTERPHALANGEAL JOINT

1 Incise the skin in the midlateral line on either side of the neck of the middle phalanx. Join these two incisions across the dorsum at the level of the joint and across the volar pulp 1 cm distal to the flexor crease (Fig. 35.4).

2 Dissect back the fibrofatty tissue to reveal the digital vessels and nerves, the extensor expansion and the flexor tendon in its sheath.

3 Divide the extensor and flexor tendons at the level of the neck of the middle phalanx and allow them to retract.

4 Ligate the digital vessels and divide the nerves proximally.

5 Divide the capsule and collateral ligaments to complete the amputation.

6 Shape the head of the middle phalanx using bone nibblers and close the wound as described above.

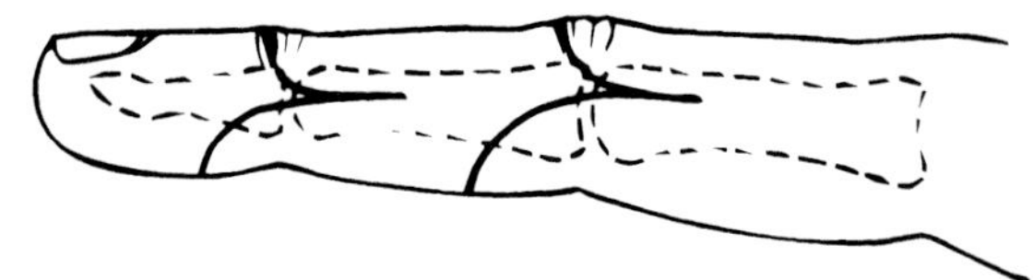

Fig. 35.4 Incision for disarticulation through interphalangeal joints.

AMPUTATION THROUGH THE MIDDLE PHALANX

Proceed as above but retain the attachment of flexor digitorum superficialis to bone.

DISARTICULATION THROUGH THE PROXIMAL INTERPHALANGEAL JOINT

Proceed as above but fashion a volar flap 1.5–2 cm long.

AMPUTATION THROUGH THE PROXIMAL PHALANX

We do not advise amputation of a single digit at this level. Disarticulation at the metacarpophalangeal joint is preferable except in special circumstances, such as multiple amputations.

DISARTICULATION THROUGH THE METACARPOPHALANGEAL JOINT

Assess

1 As a rule, employ this operation only for the middle and ring fingers. It is particularly suitable for the hand of a man doing manual labour, since a powerful grip can be retained.

2 The two disadvantages are the obvious deformity and a gap between the fingers through which small objects in the hand may fall.

3 Disarticulation of the index or little fingers at this level leaves the metarcarpal head projecting and unprotected. Oblique amputation through the metacarpal shaft is preferable.

Action

1 Mark the skin incisions, which should lie over the proximal part of the proximal phalanx on each side, leaving sufficient skin to permit full abduction of the other fingers without tension in the cleft.

2 Join the incisions anteriorly just distal to the flexor crease and posteriorly over the metacarpal head with an extension along the line of the metacarpal (Fig. 35.5).

3 Complete the amputation as described above.

AMPUTATION THROUGH THE SHAFT OF THE METACARPAL

Action

1 Use the same skin incision as for a disarticulation in the middle and ring fingers.

2 For the index and little finger use an incision along the midlateral aspect of the radial, or ulnar, border of the hand from the junction of the proximal and middle thirds of the metacarpal to the metacarpophalangeal joint (Fig. 35.5). Fashion a larger palmar flap and a smaller dorsal flap and joint the incisions in the cleft at the level of the web.

3 Amputate the middle and ring fingers by dividing the metacarpal cleanly through the neck, taking care not to splinter the bone.

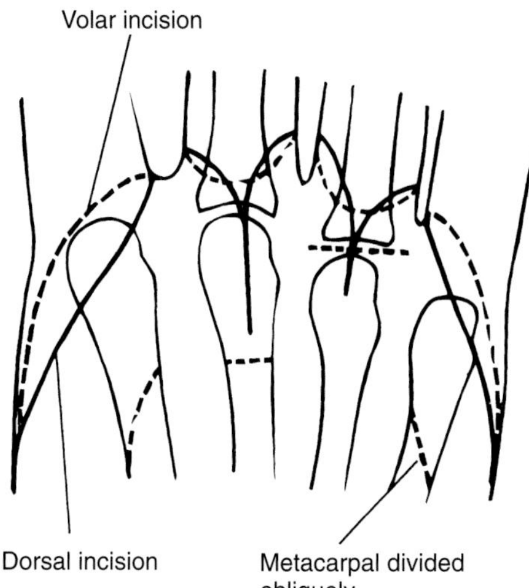

Fig. 35.5 Incision for disarticulation through a metacarpophalangeal joint and for amputation through a metacarpal.

4 Amputate the index and little fingers by exposing the middle third of the metacarpal, stripping the muscular attachments and dividing the bone obliquely with a power saw. Smooth the edges of the bone and allow the muscles to fall back over the stump. Divide the digital nerves to the radial border of the index or the ulnar border of the little finger in the proximal part of the wound.

MAJOR UPPER-LIMB AMPUTATIONS

Appraise

These are fortunately rarely required, usually for trauma, occasionally for malignancy, severe infection and congenital abnormalities or deformities. Except in an emergency, obtain a second opinion.

KEY POINTS Forearm amputations in childen

- Following forearm amputation in children, the bone will not grow in proportion to the rest of the body.
- Following above-elbow amputation, the humerus continues to grow and indeed may require revision with time.

Prepare

1 Whenever possible operate using general anaesthesia and an exsanguinating tourniquet.

2 Place the patient supine with the arm on a side table.

3 Rest the arm on an inverted bowl just proximal to the site of the amputation.

Aftercare

1 Remove the drain at 48 hours.

2 Start physiotherapy to the remaining joints in the limb at 48 hours.

3 Remove the sutures at 10 days.

4 Refer to the local limb-fitting centre as soon as the wound has healed.

BELOW-ELBOW AMPUTATION

1 Mark out equal dorsal and volar skin flaps with their bases at the junction of the middle and lower third of the ulna, approximately 17 cm distal to the olecranon process.

2 Ensure that the arm is supinated on the table without any torsional strain below the elbow. If you do not avoid this, the cut flaps will be drawn into an oblique position by the elasticity of the skin.

3 Reflect the flaps deep to the deep fascia. Cut the muscles and tendons with a slightly raked incision aimed at the level of bone section.

4 Incise the periosteum circumferentially at the level of section and divide the bones with a Gigli or a power saw.

5 Identify and ligate the main vessels. Gently pull down the nerves and divide them cleanly as high as possible.

6 Release the tourniquet and secure haemostasis.

7 Insert a suction drain.

8 Close the deep fascia over the bone ends using interrupted synthetic absorbable material such as Dexon. Close the skin with interrupted fine nylon sutures plus Steri-Strip tapes.

ABOVE-ELBOW AMPUTATION

1 Mark out equal anterior and posterior flaps with their bases 20 cm from the tip of the acromion process of the scapula.

2 Reflect the flaps deep to the deep fascia.

3 Divide the muscles with a raking incision down to bone.

4 Divide the bone with a Gigli or power saw.

5 Ligate the main vessels. Pull down the nerves and shorten them by about 2.5 cm so that they retract into the depths of the wound.

6 Release the tourniquet if present and secure haemostasis.

7 Insert a suction drain.

8 Close the deep fascia over the bone using synthetic absorbable material such as Dexon. Close the skin and apply a compression dressing.

FOREQUARTER AMPUTATION

Appraise

1 This is beyond the scope of all but highly skilled, specially experienced surgeons. It is included merely to demonstrate the extent of the excision, usually for extensive tumour, if you are an assistant. There are two methods available: the posterior approach described by Littlewood (Fig. 35.6) and the anterior approach of Berger (1887), which is preferred.

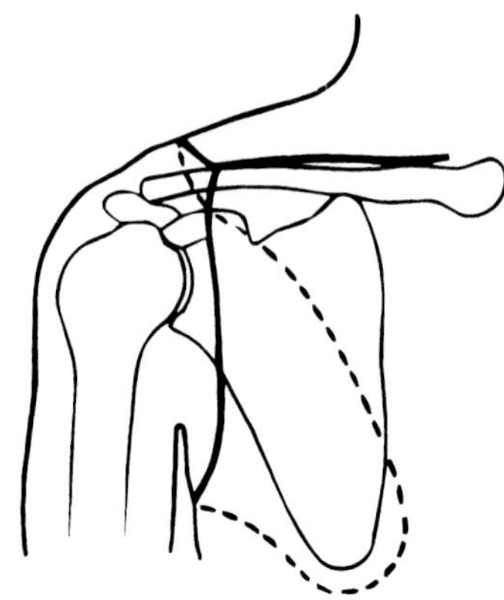

Fig. 35.6 Incision for forequarter amputation.

2 The clavicle is divided, the vessels including the subclavian artery and axillary vein are divided as are the trunks of the brachial plexus. The attaching muscles are divided, including pectoralis major and minor, trapezius, latissimus dorsi, levator scapula rhomboids and serratus anterior.

3 The forequarter, including the scapula is removed and the wound closed.

FURTHER READING

Angel JC, Weaver PC 1979 Amputations. In: Bentley G, Greer RB III (eds) Rob and Smith's operative surgery, 4th edn. Orthopaedics Part 1. Butterworths, London

Gerhardt JJ, King PS, Zettl JH 1982 Amputations. Immediate and early prosthetic management. Hans Huber, Bern

Helfet DL, Howey T, Sanders R et al 1990 Preliminary results of the Mangled Extremity Severity Score. Clinical Orthopaedics 256:80–86

Anonymous 1991 Symposium on Amputations. Annals of the Royal College of Surgeons of England 73:133–176

Thompson RG 1972 Complications of lower extremity amputation. Orthopedic Clinics of North America 3:323

Tooms RE 1987 Amputations. In: Crenshaw AH (ed.) Campbell's operative orthopedics. Mosby, St Louis, pp 597–646

36

Orthopaedics and trauma: general principles

N. Goddard

CONTENTS

PREOPERATIVE PREPARATION

Appraise

1 Most elective orthopaedic operations are carried out on otherwise healthy patients, but always assess the patient's fitness for operation beforehand. When operating for trauma ensure that the patient is adequately resuscitated.

2 Postpone elective operations until any concomitant illness such as a chest or urinary infection or hypertension has been corrected. This is especially so if one is contemplating implanting a prosthetic device (e.g. a total joint replacement).

3 Correct blood loss and dehydration before emergency operations.

4 *Antibiotics*. It is recommended practice usually to administer an antibiotic intravenously at the time of induction of anaesthesia, followed up by two further doses at 8-hourly intervals, making three doses in all. The choice of antibiotic depends upon the nature of the operation, the likely infecting organism and the patient's potential sensitivity. It is usual to use a broad-spectrum antibiotic (cefradine 500 mg t.d.s.) or an agent that has a potent anti-staphylococcal activity.

> **KEY POINTS Avoid bone infection at all costs**
>
> - Infection of bone and non-living implants is a potentially catastrophic complication.
> - Give prophylactic antibiotics for all but the most minor operations on bone, when an implant is used, and if there is an open wound.

5 *Anticoagulation*. The routine use of prophylactic anticoagulants for major orthopaedic operations, particularly on the hip joint, is controversial. The current consensus from the British Orthopaedic Association[1] is that, while chemical agents (e.g. heparin and warfarin) may reduce the incidence of deep venous thrombosis, death from other causes may be increased and there is no reduction in the rate of fatal pulmonary embolism. Anticoagulant therapy itself may also lead to excessive intra- or postoperative bleeding complications and ultimately jeopardize a total joint replacement. However, where there is a previous history of thromboembolic disease it is advisable to give heparin 5000 IU subcutaneously twice daily. If the patient is already fully anticoagulated, aim to reduce the international normalized ratio (INR) to less than 2 over the course of the operation, maintaining the patient on intravenous heparin infusion and reverting to oral anticoagulation commenced when the patient is mobile—hopefully within 24–48 hours.

6 *Anaesthesia*. General anaesthetic is appropriate for most orthopaedic procedures, especially for prolonged operations when a tourniquet is used. Under some circumstances (e.g. a patient with rheumatoid arthritis), it may be preferable to operate under a regional block (spinal, epidural, axillary). Some procedures (e.g. carpal tunnel decompression) may be performed using a local anaesthetic wound infiltration. In addition, local anaesthetic is a useful adjunct in postoperative pain relief. In my opinion Bier's blocks, while theoretically safe, provide an unsatisfactory operative field for anything but the simplest of procedures.

TOURNIQUETS

Appraise

1 Most orthopaedic operations on the limbs, especially the hand, are facilitated if performed in a bloodless field using a pneumatic tourniquet. It has been said that attempting to operate on a hand without a tourniquet is akin to trying to repair a watch at the bottom of an inkwell!

2 Use a tourniquet with caution if the patient suffers from peripheral vascular disease or if the blood supply to damaged tissues is poor. Peripheral vascular disease, however, is not an absolute contraindication to the use of a tourniquet.

KEY POINTS Dangers of exsanguination

- Do not exsanguinate the limb in the presence of distal infection, suspected calf vein thrombosis or foreign bodies, so as to avoid propagating the infection, dislodging any blood clot or shifting the foreign body.
- Take care when exsanguinating an injured limb or a limb that is fractured.

Action

1 Apply a pneumatic tourniquet of appropriate size over a few turns of orthopaedic wool around the proximal part of the upper arm or thigh.

2 Exsanguinate the limb either by elevation (Bier's method) or with a soft rubber exsanguinator (Rhys-Davies). If the latter is not available, use an Esmarch bandage, but take particular care if the skin is friable, as in a patient with rheumatoid disease. A stockinette applied over the skin prior to exsanguination reduces the likelihood of shear stresses and potential skin damage.

3 Secure the cuff and inflate until the pressure just exceeds the systolic blood pressure for tourniquets on the upper limb, and to twice the systolic blood pressure for tourniquets on the lower limb. In practice, 200 mmHg is appropriate for the upper limb and 350 mmHg for the leg. Higher pressures are unnecessary and may cause soft-tissue damage by direct compression, especially in thin patients. Never allow the pressure to exceed 250 mmHg in the arm or 450 mmHg in the leg.

4 If the tourniquet is accidentally deflated or slips during the operation, allowing partial or complete return of the circulation, deflate the cuff completely, re-position and re-fasten it and elevate the limb before re-inflating the cuff.

KEY POINTS Precautions with tourniquets

- Record the time of inflation of the tourniquet and the duration of its application, which must be kept to a minimum by careful planning of the operation.
- Exsanguination after preparing the skin can save 5 minutes or more of ischaemic time.
- 60–90 minutes is usually regarded as a safe period for an arm.
- Up to 3 hours is acceptable, but not desirable, for the leg.
- If necessary, temporarily release and then re-inflate the tourniquet, but be prepared for a poorer operative field.

5 I prefer to release the tourniquet and achieve satisfactory haemostasis before closing the wound. Some surgeons, however, prefer to close and dress the wound prior to tourniquet release. Under these circumstances a drain is usually necessary and any plaster must be split.

Aftercare

1 On completion of the operation always ensure that the circulation has returned to the limb. Locate and mark the position of the peripheral pulses to facilitate subsequent postoperative observations.

2 Reduce the likelihood of swelling by applying bulky cotton wool and crepe bandage dressing for at least 24 hours after the operation. Encourage and supervise active exercises. A good orthopaedic maxim is 'Don't just lie there—do something!'.

SKIN PREPARATION

Elective surgery

1 There should be no break or superficial infection in the skin of a limb or the area of the trunk that is to be operated on. If necessary postpone the operation until any wound has healed or infection eradicated.

2 Instruct the patient to bathe or shower within 12 hours of the operation using an antiseptic soap. Preoperative shaving is a matter of personal preference, but should be performed as late as possible and by an expert. Poor preoperative shaving may result in multiple skin nicks, which in turn become colonized with bacteria, increasing the risk of postoperative infection.

3 Mark the limb or digit to be operated on with an indelible marker. Give instructions to re-mark it if the mark is accidentally erased before the operation.

4 Prepare the skin with either iodine or chlorhexidine in spirit or aqueous solution. Iodine solutions are more effective skin antiseptics but are also the most irritant. Avoid pooling of alcohol-based solutions beneath a tourniquet or diathermy pad, with an attendant risk of explosions!

Emergency surgery

1 Prepare the skin in the anaesthetic room after induction of anaesthesia.

2 Cover open wounds with a sterile dressing held in place by an assistant.

3 Clean the surrounding skin with a soft nail brush and warm cetrimide (Savlon) solution, removing ingrained dirt and debris.

4 Remove the dressing and clean the wound itself in similar fashion to remove all dirt and debris, controlling bleeding by local digital pressure.

5 Irrigate the wound with copious volumes of physiological saline. A pulsed lavage system may be extremely helpful in this regard.

6 Complete the cleansing and irrigation of the wound in the theatre as part of the definitive surgical treatment.

REFERENCE

1. British Orthopaedic Association 1999 Total hip replacement: a guide to best practice. BOA, London

OPEN WOUNDS

1 Resuscitate the patient, if necessary, according to ATLS (advanced trauma life support) principles and guidelines before dealing with an open wound.

2 Take a culture swab from the wound and send it for culture and sensitivities. This may be useful in the management of later infection.

KEY POINTS Initial management

- Clean open wounds in the accident and emergency department and cover them with an iodine-soaked dressing.
- Leave this dressing undisturbed and do not repeatedly uncover the wound to inspect it until the patient is in theatre.
- This will significantly reduce the rate of wound infection.

3 If possible take a Polaroid or digital photograph of the wound prior to the dressing being applied to give you (or the treating surgeons) an idea of the extent and configuration of the underlying wound and to avoid disturbing the dressings unnecessarily.

4 Stop the bleeding by applying local pressure. Elevate the limb if necessary. Do not attempt blind clamping of any bleeding vessels, to avoid damaging adjacent structures.

Appraise

1 Determine how the wound was sustained and whether it is recent and clean, or long-standing and dirty, and superficial or deep. The longer the period since the injury, the deeper and dirtier the wound, the greater the need for antibiotics and tetanus prophylaxis.

2 Consider what structures may have been damaged and test for the integrity of arteries, nerves, tendons and bones.

3 Make an initial assessment of skin loss or damage and look for exit wounds following penetrating injuries.

4 An X-ray will show the extent of bone damage and the presence of radio-opaque foreign bodies (remember that not all foreign bodies are radio-opaque).

5 Always request X-rays of the skull, lateral cervical spine, chest and anteroposterior views of the pelvis in multiply injured patients, but do not let this delay treatment.

6 Depending on the extent of the wound, carry out further assessment and treatment without anaesthesia or with regional or general anaesthetic. Avoid local infiltration anaesthesia.

Prepare

1 Give a broad-spectrum antibiotic, unless the wound is clean, superficial and recent in origin.

2 If the wound is dirty, deep and more than 6 hours old, give 1 g of benzylpenicillin, and 0.5 ml of tetanus toxoid intramuscularly if the patient has been actively immunized in the past 10 years.

3 If the patient has not been actively immunized, give 1 vial (250 units) of human tetanus immunoglobulin in addition to the toxoid. Ensure that further toxoid is given 6 weeks and 6 months later.

4 Clean the wound and prepare the skin, as described above.

5 Apply a proximal tourniquet when appropriate.

Assess

1 Gently explore the wound, examining the skin, subcutaneous tissues and deeper structures. Follow the track of a penetrating wound with a finger or a probe to determine its direction and to judge the possibility of damage to vessels, nerves, tendons, bone and muscle. If you suspect muscle damage, slit open the investing fascia and take swabs for an anaerobic bacterial culture. Decide into which category the wound falls, since this determines the subsequent management.

2 Simple clean wounds have no tissue loss, although all wounds are contaminated with microorganisms, which may already be dividing. In clean wounds seen within 8 hours of injury, the bacteria will not have yet invaded the tissues.

3 Simple contaminated wounds have no tissue loss. However, they may be heavily contaminated and if you see them more than 8 hours after the injury, they can be assumed to be infected. Late wounds show signs of bacterial invasion, with pus and slough covering the raw surfaces, and redness and swelling of the surrounding skin. Although there is no loss of tissue from the injury, the infection will result in later soft-tissue destruction.

4 Complicated contaminated wounds result when tissue destruction (e.g. loss of skin, muscle or damage to blood vessels, nerves or bone) has occurred, or foreign bodies are present in the wound. Recently acquired low-velocity missile wounds fall into this category since there is insufficient kinetic energy to carry particles of clothing and dirt into the wound.

5 Complicated dirty wounds are seen after heavy contamination in the presence of tissue destruction or implantation of foreign material, especially if the wound is not seen until more than 12 hours have elapsed.

6 High-velocity missile wounds deserve to be placed in a category of their own. For instance, when a bullet from a high-powered rifle strikes the body it is likely to lose its high kinetic energy to the soft tissues as it passes through, resulting in extensive cavitation. Although the entry and exit wounds may be small, structures within the wound are often severely damaged. Muscle is particularly susceptible to the passage of high-velocity missiles and becomes devitalized. It takes on a 'mushy' appearance and consistency and fails to contract when pinched or to bleed when cut. If the bullet breaks into fragments or hits bone, breaking it into fragments, the spreading particles of bullet and bone also behave as high-energy particles. The whole effect is of an internal explosion. In addition, the high-velocity missile carries foreign material (bacteria and clothing) deeply into the tissues, causing heavy contamination.

The risk of tetanus and gas gangrene is increased when the wound is sustained over heavily cultivated ground in which the organisms abound. Devitalized ischaemic muscle makes an excellent culture medium. As haematoma and oedema formation develop within the investing fascia, tissue tension rises, further embarrassing the circulation and causing progressive tissue death. Although handgun bullets, shotgun pellets, shrapnel from shells and fragments from mine, grenade and bomb explosions have a relatively low velocity, they behave as high-velocity missiles when projected into the tissues from nearby. When a shotgun is fired from close to the body, the wad and the pellets are carried in as a single missile.

7 Open fractures can be classified in a variety of ways. Probably the most widely accepted is the Gustilo classification, which is particularly useful in discussing soft-tissue reconstruction:

- Type I: an open fracture with a cutaneous wound <1 cm.
- Type II: an open fracture with extensive soft-tissue damage.
- Type IIIA: high-energy trauma irrespective of the size of the wound. There is adequate soft-tissue coverage of the fractured bone, despite extensive soft-tissue lacerations or flaps.
- Type IIIB: there is an extensive soft-tissue injury with loss of tissue, accompanied by periosteal stripping and bone exposure. These wounds are usually associated with massive contamination.
- Type IIIC are open fractures associated with vascular and/or neurological injury requiring repair.

Action

1 Stop all bleeding. Pick up small vessels with fine artery forceps and cauterize or ligate them with fine absorbable sutures. Control damage of major arteries and veins with pressure, tapes or non-crushing clamps, so as to permit later repair.

2 Irrigate clean simple wounds with copious volumes of sterile saline solution without drainage. Do not attempt to repair cleanly divided muscle with stitches but simply suture the investing fascia. Close the skin accurately.

KEY POINTS Infected wounds

- Never close an apparently simple infected wound immediately.
- Take a swab for culture.
- Remove any retained foreign material, radically excise and debride any dead or devitalized tissue and drain any potential pockets of infection.
- Systemic antibiotic or local instillations may be started but will not make up for poor technique.
- Pack the wound with gauze soaked in sterile isotonic saline solution and cover with an occlusive dressing. Plan to renew the packing daily until the wound is clean and produces no further discharge.
- Provided there is no redness or oedema of the surrounding skin, close the wound by delayed primary suture, usually after 3–7 days.

3 Complicated contaminated wounds can be partially repaired after excising the devitalized tissue. Once bone stability has been achieved, damaged segments of major arteries and veins should be repaired by an experienced surgeon using grafts where appropriate. Loosely appose the ends of divided nerves with one or two stitches in the perineurium, so that they can be readily identified and repaired later when the wound is healed and all signs of inflammation have disappeared. Similarly, identify and appose the ends of divided tendons in preparation for definitive repair at a later date. Do not remove small fragments of bone that retain a periosteal attachment, or large fragments whether they are attached or unattached. Excise devitalized muscle, especially the major muscle masses of the thigh and buttock. Remove foreign material when possible. Some penetrating low-velocity missiles are better left if they lie deeply, provided damage to important structures has been excluded. Remove superficial shotgun pellets. Low-velocity missile tracks do not normally require to be laid open or excised, but do not close the wound. Excise damaged skin when the deep flap can be easily closed, if necessary by making a relaxing incision or applying a skin graft. Do not lightly excise specialized skin from the hands; instead leave doubtful skin and excise it later, if necessary, on expert advice.

4 Stabilize any associated fracture. It may be possible merely to immobilize the limb in a plaster cast, cutting a window into it so that the wound can be dressed. An open fracture, however, is not an absolute contraindication to surgical stabilization using the appropriate device (plates and screws, intramedullary nails), but such should be undertaken only by an experienced trauma or orthopaedic surgeon. In an emergency situation it is preferable to use temporary skeletal traction and external fixator.

5 Complicated dirty wounds require similar treatment of damaged tissues such as nerves and tendons, but do not attempt to repair damaged structures other than major blood vessels. Pack the wound and change the dressing daily until there is no sign of infection, then close the skin by suture or by skin grafting.

6 Lay open high-velocity missile wounds extensively. Foreign matter, including missile fragments, dirt and clothing, is carried deeply into the wound, so contamination is inevitable. Explore and excise the track, since the tissue along the track is devitalized, lay open the investing fascia over disrupted muscle to evacuate the muscle haematoma and excise the pulped muscle, leaving healthy contractile muscle that bleeds when cut. This leaves a cavity in the track of the missile.

7 Mark divided nerves and tendons for definitive treatment later. Excise the skin edges and pack the wound with saline-soaked gauze. Treat any associated fracture as described above. Change the packs daily until infection is controlled and all dead tissue has been excised. Only then can skin closure be completed and the repair of damaged structures be planned.

EXTERNAL FIXATION

There are many types of external fixator, ranging from the simple unilateral frame (Denham, Orthofix), multilateral frames (Hoffman) through to the more complicated circular frames (Ilizarov) and hybrid devices. The essential feature of the external fixator is that it provides a stable reduction of any fracture by using percutaneously introduced wires or pins into the bone, which are then attached to an external frame.

The Ilizarov and similar circular frames are beyond the scope of this chapter, but in an emergency you should be familiar with the principles involved, and the techniques of applying a simple unilateral frame. Such a frame is constructed from one or more rigid bars, which are aligned parallel to the limb, to which the threaded

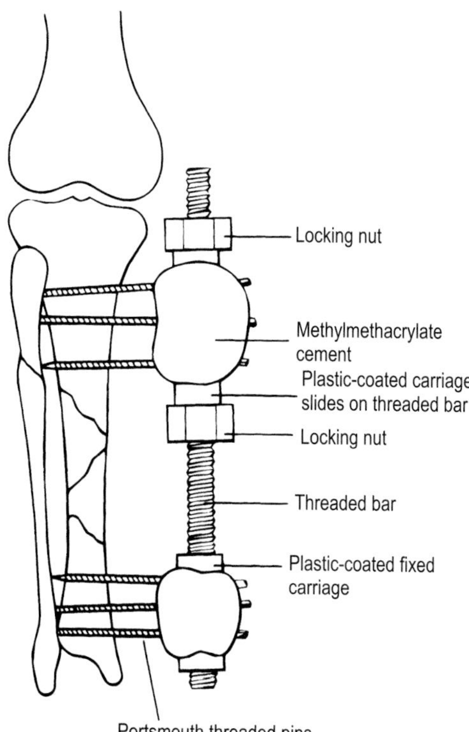

Fig. 36.1 The Denham external fixator.

pins that are drilled into the fragments of bone are attached. In the more sophisticated devices (Orthofix, AO, Monotube, Hoffman) this is done by clamping the pins to universal joints, which allow the position of the fragments to be adjusted before the clamps are finally tightened. In the simplest form, here described, the pins are held to the bar with acrylic cement (Denham type; Fig. 36.1).

Prepare

1. Treat the wound as outlined above.
2. Reduce the fracture, either open under direct vision, or closed using an image intensifier.
3. Maintain the reduction using bone clamps, traction or temporary wires.

Action

1. Make a stab wound through healthy skin proximal to the fracture site, bearing in mind the possible need for subsequent skin flaps.
2. Drill a hole through both cortices of the bone approximately at right-angles to the bone with a sharp 3.6-mm drill. Take care in drilling the bone that the drill bit does not overheat, which may in turn cause local bone necrosis leading to the formation of ring sequestra with subsequent loosening and infection of the pins. Measure the depth of the distal cortex from the skin surface.
3. Insert a threaded Schantz pin into the drill hole so that both cortices are penetrated.
4. If possible insert two more pins approximately 3–4 cm apart into the proximal fragment and three pins into the distal fragment in similar fashion. Biomechanically the stability of the fixator is enhanced if there are three pins in each of the major fragments with the nearest pin being close to the fracture line.
5. Loosen the locking nuts that hold the carriages on to the rigid bar and hold the bar parallel to the limb and 4–5 cm away from the skin.
6. Place one carriage opposite the protruding ends of each set of three pins and adjust the locking nuts to hold the carriages in position.
7. Fix the pins to the carriages with two mixes of acrylic cement for each carriage, moulding the cement around the pins and the carriage, maintaining the position until it is set.
8. Remove any temporary reduction device and carry out the final adjustment on the locking nuts to compress the bone ends together.
9. Dress the wound.

Aftercare

1. Keep the pin tracks clean and free of scabs and incrustations by daily cleaning with sterile saline or a mild antiseptic solution. A rigorous regime will minimize the risk of pin-tract infection and premature pin loosening.
2. An external fixator is essentially only a temporary measure before definitive treatment can be carried out. It is seldom used as the sole method of fracture management and should therefore be removed at a time when the wound is healthy, at which time it may be possible to definitively stabilize the fracture.
3. Fixator removal is simple. Cut the pins with a hacksaw or bolt cutters and then unscrew them. The acrylic cement can be removed from the carriages, which may be used again.

OPEN (COMPOUND) FRACTURES

Appraise

1. Assess the patient according to ATLS principles and resuscitate as necessary.
2. Manage the wound as outlined above.
3. X-ray the bone to determine the pattern of the fracture and to decide on the appropriate method of reduction and fixation.

Prepare

1. Anaesthetize the patient.
2. Prepare the skin.
3. Clean the wound.

Action

1. Explore and reassess the wound.
2. Expose and assess the fracture. Remove only small and completely unattached fragments of bone. Retain any bone that has a remaining periosteal attachment, as this bone is potentially still viable.

3 Free the bone ends from any adjacent fascia and muscle through which they may have buttonholed.

4 Wash away any blood clot and other debris.

5 Strip the periosteum for 1–2 mm only from the bone ends to allow accurate reduction without the interposition of soft tissues.

6 Using a combination of traction, bone clamps, levers and hooks, reduce the major fragments into an anatomical position. If necessary, extend the original wound to improve access.

7 If the fracture is stable, immobilize in a plaster cast after definitive treatment of the wound. Leave a window in the cast to permit wound inspection and changes of dressings.

8 Apply an external fixator when the wound is contaminated or there is extensive skin loss.

KEY POINTS Fixation?

- If the fracture is unstable and there is a simple, clean wound, then it may be appropriate to internally fix the fracture.
- If there are multiple injuries or if the wound is contaminated an external fixator may be more appropriate.
- Do not forget the possibility of immediate amputation if the limb is severely mutilated with associated neurovascular injuries (Gustilo grade IIIB or C).

SKELETAL TRACTION

Appraise

1 Temporary skeletal traction can be applied using skin traction, and indeed this is the method of choice when using a Thomas splint for immobilization of a femoral fracture as a first aid measure. For prolonged treatment insert a traction pin through the tibia or calcaneus. Other sites such as the olecranon or metacarpals are occasionally used.

2 Skeletal traction is a simple and safe method of immobilizing a limb after injury or operation. It may be seen as a temporary measure, as definitive treatment, or as a supplement to treatment. With the more widespread use of increasingly sophisticated internal fixation devices skeletal traction is less frequently employed as a definitive method of treating long-bone fractures. Skeletal traction requires careful supervision and adjustments to remain effective.

3 There are two types of pin in common usage (Fig. 36.2). Each has a triangular or square butt, which inserts into a chuck, and a trocar point. The Steinmann pin is uniform throughout but the Denham pin has a short length of screw thread wider than the main shaft near its centre, which screws into one cortex of the bone and minimizes sideways slip during traction.

Prepare

1 Clean the skin and drape the limb, leaving about 10 cm exposed on either side of the site of entry.

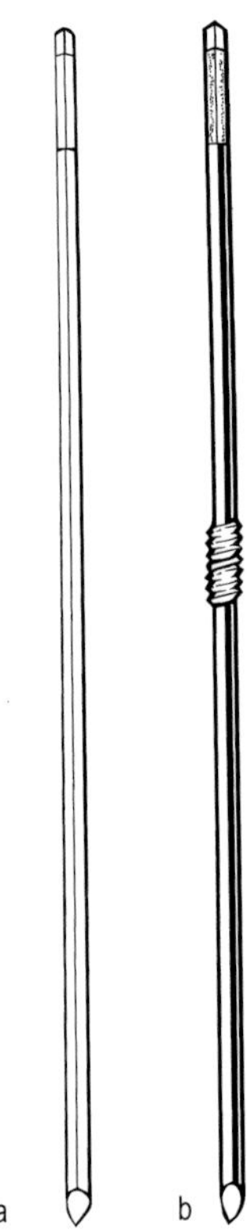

Fig. 36.2 (a) Steinmann pin; (b) Denham pin.

2 Anaesthetize the skin, subcutaneous tissue and periosteum on both sides of the bone at site of entry and exit of the pin with 1% lidocaine.

3 Make sure that the pin selected fits the sockets in the stirrup.

Action

1 To insert the pin through the upper tibia, make a 5-mm stab incision in the skin on the lateral side of the bone 2.5 cm posterior to the summit of the tibial tuberosity; this avoids damage to the common peroneal nerve when a medial approach is used. If the tibial plateau is fractured, make the nick and insert the pin 2.5–5.0 cm distally.

2 To insert the pin through the calcaneus, make a 5-mm stab incision in the skin on the lateral side of the heel 2.5 cm distal to the tip of the lateral malleolus.

3 Introduce the point of the pin through the nick at right-angles to the long axis of the limb and parallel to the floor with the limb in the anatomical position. Avoid obliquity in either plane.

KEY POINTS Care inserting pins

- Drill the pin through both cortices of the bone with a hand drill until the point just bulges under the skin on the opposite side of the limb.
- Take care that the pin does not suddenly penetrate the skin to impale your hand or the opposite limb. This is particularly likely if the bone is thin and porotic.

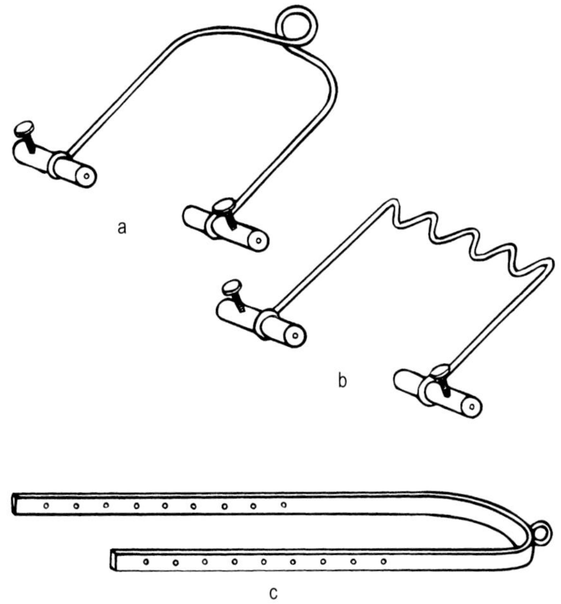

Fig. 36.3 Traction loops: (a) the Bohler stirrup; (b) the Nissen stirrup; (c) the Tulloch-Brown 'U' loop.

4 Incise the skin over the exit point and gently push the pin through until equal lengths are protruding on either side. When using the Denham pin the threaded section should be screwed into the cortex a further 6–8 mm so that the thread engages the bone.

5 Make sure that the skin is not distorted where the pin passes through. Make tiny relieving incisions if necessary.

6 Dress the punctures with small squares of gauze soaked in tincture of benzoin.

7 Attach traction cords or a traction stirrup to the pin. Three types of stirrup are available (Fig. 36.3):
- The Bohler stirrup, for general use
- The Nissen stirrup, for more accurate control of rotation
- The Tulloch-Brown 'U'-loop for Hamilton Russell traction.

8 Put guards on the ends of the pin.

9 Attach a length of cord to the centre of the stirrup through which the traction will be applied.

Aftercare

1 Keep the pin tracks clean and free of scabbing and incrustation as described above.

2 Continually monitor the position of the fracture and adjust the traction as necessary so as to maintain an accurate reduction.

3 Monitor the condition of the patient as the enforced prolonged period of recumbence predisposes them to chest infection and pressure sores.

SIMPLE SKELETAL TRACTION

1 Simple skeletal traction over a pulley fixed to the end of the bed usually suffices for relatively stable fractures (e.g. of the tibial plateau).

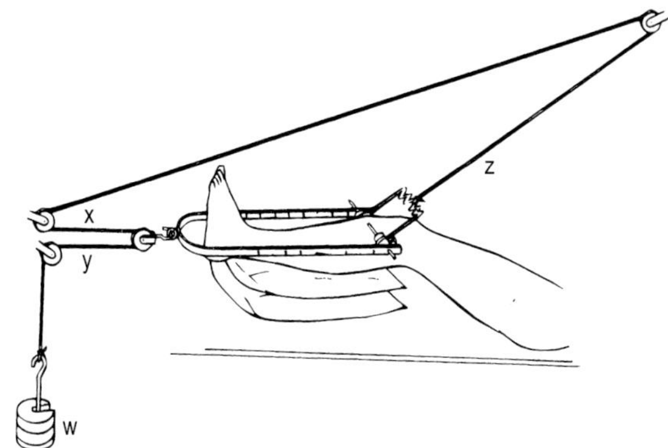

Fig. 36.4 Hamilton Russell skeletal traction.

2 Unstable fractures need the support of a splint. Support the calf on two or three pillows with the point of the heel clear of the bed. Have the traction string horizontal and apply sufficient traction weights so as to reduce the fracture and restore alignment and length of the bone. Usually 4–5 kg is sufficient depending upon the weight of the patient.

HAMILTON RUSSELL TRACTION

This is a convenient method for fractures and other conditions around the hip (e.g. dislocation or acetabular fractures). It controls the natural tendency of the leg to roll into external rotation and avoids the use of a Thomas splint, the ring of which causes discomfort if the hip is tender.

Action

1 Set up the apparatus as in Figure 36.4, passing the cord through the pulleys as indicated. The sections of string 'x' and 'y' must be parallel to the horizontal and the section 'z' must lead in a cephalic direction. Support the calf either on two ordinary pillows or on slings of Domette bandage attached to the 'U'-loop with safety pins.

2 Attach between 2 and 5 kg of weight to the end of the cord and make sure that it is clear of the floor. Remember that the effective traction is doubled as a result of the pulley arrangement.

3 Keep the point of the heel clear of the bed to avoid pressure sores.

4 Place a foot rest between the bars of the loop to maintain the foot at a right-angle to the leg.

5 A separate cord running from the Nissen stirrup through the more proximal pulley can be attached to a handle so facilitating knee flexion exercises.

SLIDING SKELETAL TRACTION

Sliding skeletal traction with the leg supported on a Thomas or similar splint is a standard method of conservative treatment for femoral shaft or supracondylar fractures.

Action

1 Set up the apparatus as shown in the diagram in Figure 36.5. Apply 4–8 kg of weight for traction ('W').

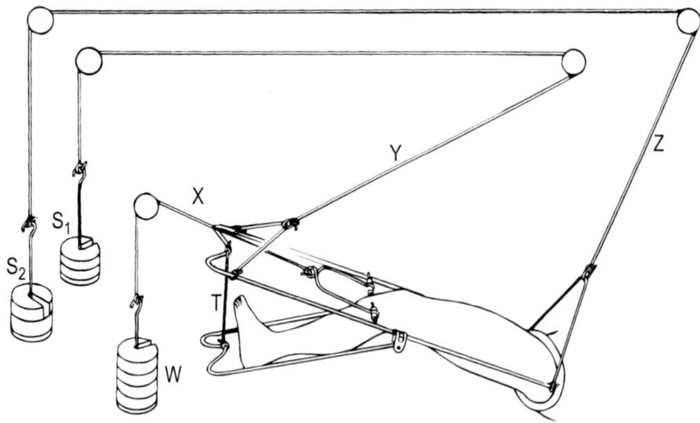

Fig. 36.5 Sliding skeletal traction with a Thomas splint.

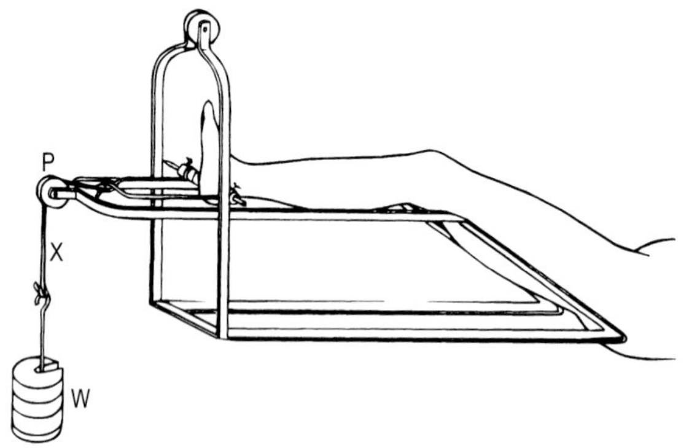

Fig. 36.6 Calcaneal skeletal traction with a Bohler–Braun frame.

2 The splint should have a Pearson's or equivalent knee attachment so that the knee may be flexed (20° for shaft fractures and 40° or more for supracondylar fractures). Tie the distal end of this attachment to that of the main splint with traction cord. Only the cord 'X' is concerned with traction. Cords 'Y' and 'Z' and weights 'S_1' and 'S_2' merely suspend the splint to aid nursing.

3 Support the limb from the sides of the splint with Domette bandage held in place with safety pins. Pad the underside of the limb with sheets of cotton wool.

CALCANEAL TRACTION

1 Use calcaneal traction with the leg supported on a Bohler–Braun frame in the conservative treatment of unstable fractures of the tibia.

2 It may be combined with a padded plaster cast to provide more lateral stability.

3 Set up the apparatus as shown in the diagram in Figure 36.6.

4 Apply 2–4 kg of weight ('W'). Support the calf and thigh from the side-bars of the frame with slings of Domette bandage. Pad under the limb with cotton wool.

Aftercare

As above, but with any tibial fracture constantly check on the neurovascular status of the limb looking for compartment syndrome.

SKULL TRACTION

Appraise

1 Skull traction is often employed to immobilize the cervical spine after injury (fracture, subluxation or dislocation) and sometimes after operations on the neck.

2 The traction is applied through skull tongs inserted under local anaesthetic prior to the administration of any general anaesthetic. The anaesthetist then has the benefit of the added security of the traction.

3 The common devices available for skull traction are either the Crutchfield tongs or a Cone skull caliper. I have found the Cone caliper easier to apply and less likely to slip than the Crutchfield device.

Access

1 The patient lies supine with the head carefully supported so as to avoid sudden and unexpected movement.

2 Establish the insertion point for the caliper, which is at the point of maximal diameter of the skull in a line running across the vertex of the skull from one mastoid process to the other. In practice this is usually 2–3 cm above the top of the ear.

3 Shave a small area of the scalp at the proposed insertion points and moisten the surrounding hair to keep it flat.

4 Place a waterproof layer and sterile towel under the head and drape off the bared area. Prepare the skin with a suitable antiseptic agent. Leave the face of the conscious patient uncovered.

5 Infiltrate the scalp down to the pericranium with 5 ml of 1% lidocaine and 1:200 000 adrenaline (epinephrine) on each side, anaesthetizing an area about 1.5 cm in diameter.

6 Open the Cone calipers to their fullest extent and place the points symmetrically on either side of the midline of the scalp. Mark the position of the points with a skin marker.

7 Make a stab incision down to the pericranium on either side. Bring the caliper back into position and introduce the pin through the conical end of the caliper.

8 The caliper is the tightened such that the tips of the cones abut the outer table of the skull. The pins are then tightened down through the outer table to a predetermined depth.

Aftercare

1 Usually no dressing is required, but keep the pin sites clean.

2 Apply traction or proceed to manipulation as desired. Tie the traction cord to the ring on the caliper and not to the screw.

PERIPHERAL NERVE REPAIR

1 Complete disruption of a peripheral nerve may be associated with both open and closed injuries and recovery will not take place unless continuity is re-established surgically.

2 Peripheral nerve repair (Fig. 36.7) is a specialist technique but, faced with it in the field, you should be aware of the

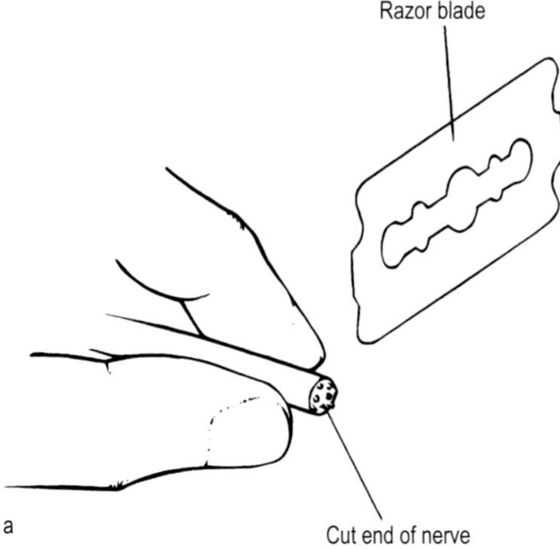

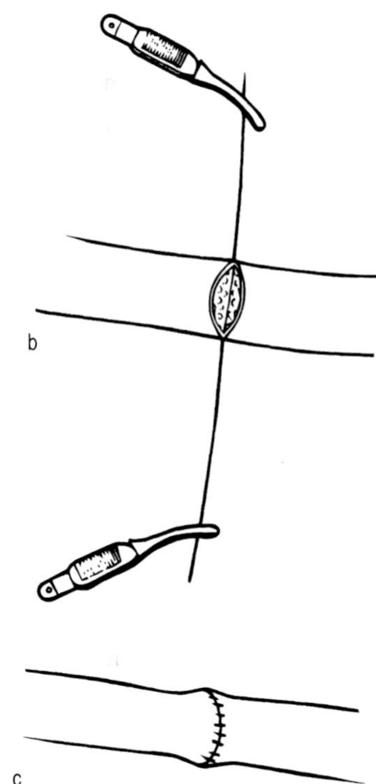

Fig. 36.7 Nerve suture: (a) cutting back to pouting fibres with a razor blade; (b) first and second sutures in place; (c) sutures completed.

principles. If you feel unable to attempt a primary repair then mark the nerve ends with a non-absorbable suture to assist their location at the time of the definitive operation.

Appraise

1 Always assume that a peripheral nerve injury in the presence of an open wound is the result of a complete division of the nerve fibres (neurotmesis). You must therefore identify the nerve when the wound is treated and satisfy yourself as to its integrity. If it is divided, either mark or appose the ends in their correct orientation for secondary repair later.

2 Some form of magnification is essential in repairing a peripheral nerve. While an operating microscope may not be available, simple magnifying loupes will usually suffice.

3 It is entirely acceptable to treat a peripheral nerve injury conservatively in the absence of an open wound. A neurapraxia (block to conduction of nerve impulses without disruption of the axon or its supporting cells) will usually recover spontaneously in days or weeks, and an axonotmesis (the axon undergoes Wallerian degeneration) in the time it takes for the axons to regenerate. This is calculated by measuring the distance from the site of injury (e.g. a fracture) to the point at which the motor nerve enters the first muscle innervated distal to the lesion. Axons regenerate at a rate of 1 mm/day and so it will take approximately 90 days, for example, for reinnervation of the brachioradialis to occur following an injury to the radial nerve at the distal end of the spiral groove of the humerus. Electrophysiological studies (EMG, nerve conduction) may give some pointers as to the likely nerve lesion and will help in documenting recovery.

4 If recovery fails to occur in the predicted time and if the nerve conduction studies show no improvement then explore the course of nerve and treat any lesion appropriately.

KEY POINTS When to repair?

- Primary repair undoubtedly gives the best results and may sometimes be undertaken in specialist centres.
- If the patient is stable and fit for transfer, then do so.
- Secondary repair is safer and sometimes easier when the wound is soundly healed and the danger of infection has passed.

Prepare

1 Do not attempt immediate primary nerve repair unless you have adequate magnification (loupes or operating microscope) and are sufficiently experienced in the techniques involved. If there is any doubt it is safer to mark or appose the nerve ends for later exploration and repair.

2 Prepare the skin.

3 Apply a tourniquet.

Access

1 Clean and explore the wound.

2 If there is a previous wound that has healed, excise the previous scar if necessary, and extend the wound proximally and distally along the course of the nerve.

3 If there was no wound, make an incision 15 cm long along the course of the nerve centred at the site of injury. Use a 'lazy-S' incision if the incision crosses the flexor crease of a joint.

4 Always begin by exposing the nerve in normal tissue on either side of the site of injury and then work towards the site of the injury, carefully dissecting along the course of the nerve. In the case of an open wound there may be extensive scar tissue and adhesions.

Assess

1 Decide whether repair is possible or not.

2 If repair is possible but beyond your competence, what action should you take?

KEY POINTS Repair not possible, or beyond your competence?

- Free the ends of the nerve from the surrounding soft tissues and place a marker suture of 4/0 nylon or other non-absorbable material, through the perineurium 2–3 cm proximally and distally from the site of injury to facilitate later alignment of the ends.
- If possible, appose the ends now, with two or three stitches for ease of later identification.
- If the ends cannot be apposed without tension, tack them to the underlying soft tissues to prevent retraction until definitive repair can be undertaken.

Action

1 If this is a delayed repair there may be fibrous scar tissue at the cut ends, or joining the ends.

2 If necessary, cut transversely across fibrous scar tissue that may be joining the ends together.

3 Hold one end of the nerve firmly using a special nerve-holding clamp (a finger and thumb will suffice in extremis) and carefully cut thin slices of tissue from the exposed end with a sharp razor blade at right-angles to the long axis of the nerve until all the scar tissue has been excised and the nerve bundles can be seen pouting from the cut surface (Fig. 36.7a).

4 Repeat the procedure on the other end of the nerve. It may be necessary to resect a centimetre or more from each end of the nerve because of the intraneural fibrosis (neuroma) caused by the initial injury.

5 If this is a primary closure place the nerve ends in their correct rotational orientation. If this is delayed closure similarly identify the correct rotational alignment.

6 Mobilize the nerve from the surrounding soft tissues proximally and distally as far as is necessary to bring the ends together without tension, carefully preserving and dissecting out the main branches. Flex a neighbouring joint if necessary. If it proves impossible to appose the nerve ends then an interposition graft may be necessary.

7 Release the tourniquet and achieve perfect haemostasis.

8 Ensure again that the ends of the nerve are correctly orientated

9 Place an 8/0 nylon stitch through the perineurium on one side of the nerve. Cut the suture 3 cm from the knot and hold the ends in a small bulldog clip (Fig. 36.7b).

10 Place a second suture directly opposite the first and place another bulldog clip on the ends. These act as stay sutures and facilitate rotation of the nerve while placing further sutures.

11 Place further sutures through the perineurium, 1.5 mm or so apart, around the circumference of the nerve.

12 After completing the repair of the superficial surface, turn the nerve over by passing one bulldog clip suture under and the other over the nerve.

13 Complete the repair. Cut the first pair of sutures and turn the nerve back to the correct position (Fig. 36.7c).

14 Close the soft tissues and skin without altering the position of the limb if there is any danger of putting tension on the suture line.

15 Apply a padded plaster without increasing the tension on the repair.

16 Remove plaster and skin sutures after 3 weeks and gently mobilize the limb. If joints were flexed to avoid tension they must only be extended gradually over the next 3 weeks, if necessary by applying serial plasters at weekly intervals, or by incorporating a hinge with a locking device to allow flexion but no more than the set amount of joint extension.

TENDON SUTURE

Appraise

Tendons are relatively avascular structures and heal by the ingrowth of connective tissue from the epitenon. When the tendon is divided within a fibrous sheath on the flexor surface of the hand, for example, the sheath is also damaged and the connective tissue from the healing sheath grows into the healing tendon, causing adhesions. For this reason injuries to the digital flexor tendons within the sheath should preferably be treated by experienced hand surgeons. Tendons may also require suturing as part of another procedure such as tendon transfer.

KEY POINT Delayed repair?

- It is entirely safe to perform a delayed primary repair of a divided flexor tendon up to 14 days post-injury without adversely affecting the final outcome.

Assess

1 Examine the wound. As with nerve injuries, if it is in the vicinity of a tendon and there is no distal action, assume that the tendon is divided until it is shown to be intact on clinical examination.

2 If no action is demonstrated or if there is doubt, explore the wound.

Action

1 Prepare the skin.

2 Apply the tourniquet.

3 Explore the wound and extend it if necessary in order to identify any divided tendons.

4 If the wound is suitable for primary closure then proceed to repair the tendons. If not, delay the repair until the wound is healed and is no longer indurated, maintaining full mobility of the joints in the meantime by physiotherapy.

5 When several tendons are divided (e.g. at the wrist), make sure that the cut ends are correctly paired. It is not unheard of to suture the proximal end of one tendon to the distal end of another or even to the cut end of a nerve!

6 Draw the cut ends together after picking up the paratenon round each end of the tendon with fine mosquito forceps, flexing neighbouring joints if necessary.

7 Secure the cut ends of the tendon by passing one needle into an exposed tendon end and bring it out of the side of the tendon about 1.5 cm from the cut end. Now pass this needle transversely through the tendon 3–4 mm nearer to the cut end. Re-insert this needle on the other side of the tendon to create a mirror image and bring it out through the cut end (Fig. 36.8a).

8 Freshen the ends of the tendon by cutting them with a no. 15 blade.

9 Use a 3/0 braided non-absorbable (Ethibond) suture with a 15-mm straight needle at both ends using a modified Kessler core stitch (Fig. 36.8a). Repeat this process using the second needle on the other tendon end.

10 Make a half-hitch and approximate the tendon ends till they just meet. Complete the knot with at least six throws. Cut the knot flush; this should now have been buried within the tendon (Fig. 36.8b).

11 Complete the repair with a simple running suture of 6/0 monofilament nylon with a small curved needle. It is helpful to begin the running stitch on the posterior face, leaving the cut end of the suture long with which to turn the tendon through 180° for ease of access. The final repair must be smooth, with no bunching at the repair site.

12 Release the tourniquet and secure haemostasis.

13 Close the wound with suction drainage if necessary.

14 Apply a padded plaster so that the suture line is not under tension and remove after 3 weeks in the upper limb and 6 weeks in the lower limb.

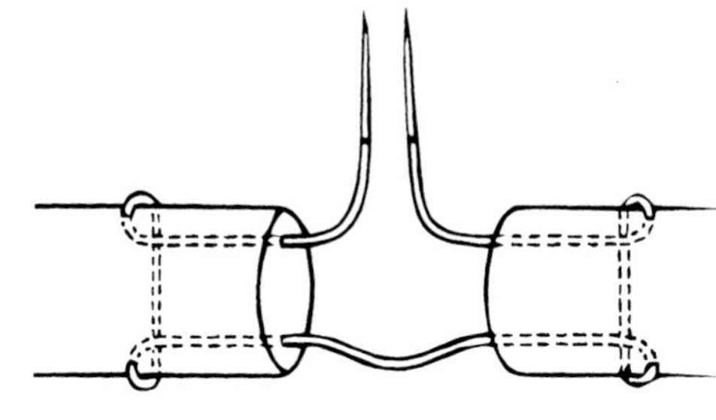

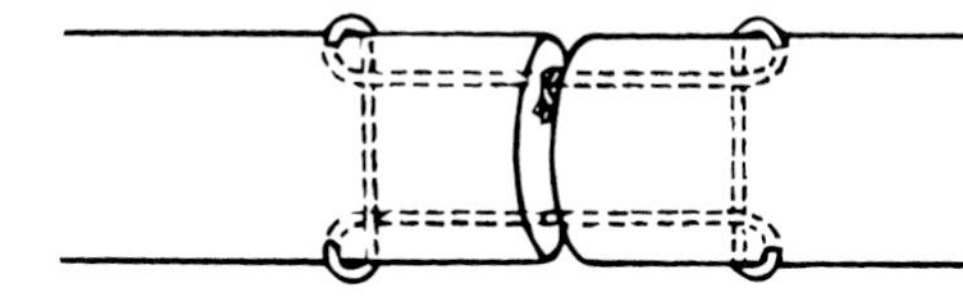

Fig. 36.8 End-to-end suture of a tendon.

BIOPSY

Biopsy of bone or soft tissue may be taken at an open operation or by aspirating material through a needle (closed biopsy). Closed biopsy is now usually performed by interventional radiologists, who are able to take specimens with extreme accuracy aided by the modern imaging techniques at their disposal. In both cases material is taken from the margin of the lesion, for the tissue in the centre is often necrotic and difficult to identify. Take at least two specimens—one for culture and the other for histological examination.

OPEN BIOPSY

Appraise

Bone biopsy is indicated in order to investigate a potential bone tumour (benign or malignant) or where infection is suspected.

KEY POINT Advice on technique and siting

- In the case of a potential malignant tumour ask the advice of a surgeon experienced in bone tumour management on the technique and also the siting of the biopsy and scars so that it will not interfere with any later surgery.

Action

1 Apply a pneumatic tourniquet if possible. In the case of possible infection, do not exsanguinate the limb.

2 Incise the skin over the most superficial aspect of the lesion, taking care to place the incision in such a way that it will be excised if later surgery is required.

3 Incise the deep fascia and split the muscle in the line of its fibres until the margin of the lesion or the bone is reached.

4 Take a wedge-shaped piece of tissue from the margin of the lesion approximately 1 cm long by 0.5 cm thick and 0.5 cm deep. Place it in formal saline unless specific staining techniques are required. Consult the pathologist beforehand if in doubt.

5 Take a further similar specimen for immediate culture.

6 If pus is present, aspirate as much as possible and take a swab for culture.

7 Take a further specimen for microscopic examination and a further specimen for culture from a different part of the lesion if it is large enough.

8 If the lesion is in bone, remove the specimen with a sharp osteotome and include the periosteum.

9 If the lesion is not obvious, drill a Kirschner wire or a thin twist drill into the suspected site and examine the area under the image intensifier, or take plain X-rays in two planes at right-angles. Note the relationship of the lesion to the marker before taking the specimens.

10 Examine radiologically once more to ensure that the specimen has indeed been removed from the lesion.

11 Label each specimen immediately and accurately.

12 Release the tourniquet and secure haemostasis.

13 Close the wound and apply a pressure dressing.

14 Ensure that the specimens are sent to the pathological laboratory.

DRAINAGE OF ACUTE OSTEOMYELITIS

Appraise

1 Assume that any unwell infant or child with an area of local bone tenderness has osteomyelitis until proved otherwise and treat as such. For drainage of joints in the case of septic arthritis see the appropriate chapter.

2 If an abscess is present on initial clinical examination, or if pain, temperature, local swelling and tenderness fail to improve within 12 hours of starting antibiotic therapy, undertake operative treatment immediately.

3 Do not wait until there is radiological (X-ray) evidence of infection. It is then too late. However, an isotope bone scan may be helpful in determining the site of infection. Magnetic resonance imaging (MRI) can show the extent of the problem.

Prepare

1 Take blood for culture, haemoglobin, ESR (erythrocyte sedimentation rate), CRP (C-reactive protein), WBC (white blood cell count) and differential white cell count.

2 Give cloxacillin 100–200 mg/kg of body weight daily in divided doses intravenously until there is clinical improvement, usually apparent within 24 hours. If the patient is intolerant of penicillins give cefradine 100 mg/kg of body weight daily.

3 Change antibiotic as necessary when sensitivities are known, as a result of blood culture or operation. Otherwise continue with oral flucloxacillin 50–100 mg/kg, when there is clinical improvement.

4 If operation proves to be necessary (see above), perform it under a general anaesthetic. Mark the most tender point on the limb before premedication.

Action

KEY POINT Tourniquet?

- Apply a tourniquet if possible but do not exsanguinate the limb for fear of propagating the infection.

1 Prepare the skin and apply the drapes.

2 Centre the skin incision over the most tender point on the bone and extend proximally and distally for 2.5–3.0 cm.

3 Incise the deep fascia and retract the soft tissues until the periosteum is exposed.

4 Pus may already have escaped into the soft tissues but, if not, incise the periosteum and take specimens for culture. Excise obvious dead tissue.

5 If frank pus is not visible, swab the bone surface.

6 Drill a single hole with a 2-mm twist drill, 5 mm proximal to the epiphyseal line which is easily identified under the periosteum. If pus emerges, drill a second and, if necessary, a third hole 5 mm proximal to the preceding hole. Usually, a single drill hole is sufficient to ensure that there is no pus in the medullary cavity.

7 Irrigate the wound with saline and insert a suction drain through normal skin. Plan to remove the drain after 24 hours or when drainage ceases.

8 Close the skin and apply a padded back splint so that the limb is immobilized and the wound can be inspected. Remove the slab when the wound is healed.

Aftercare

Continue antibiotics for 10 days or longer if necessary, until the clinical signs of infection subside and the inflammatory markers (ESR, CRP) fall.

CHRONIC OSTEOMYELITIS

Appraise

Chronic pyogenic infection of bone may give rise to a recurrently discharging or permanent sinus and be associated with an underlying sequestrum. Identify a sequestrum radiologically by tomography, CT scanning or MRI. In the case of a chronically discharging wound a sinogram may determine the extent of the sinus. It is the sequestrum (a piece of dead bone) that is generally the source of the chronic infection. Therefore operative treatment is not indicated in the absence of a sequestrum or sinus.

Action

1 Under general anaesthetic apply a tourniquet to the elevated limb but do not exsanguinate it.

2 Prepare the skin and apply the drapes.

3 It is helpful to identify the extent of the sinus by injecting methylthioninium chloride (methylene blue) solution into its opening until it oozes from the sinus. Express excess dye with a swab, but it is still very messy!

4 Centre the skin incision on the mouth of the sinus and excise it. Extend the incision in the direction of any sequestrum, excising any previous scars.

5 Carefully dissect around the track of the sinus down to the bone. The sinus track is usually visible through the surrounding cuff of normal tissue. Excise the sinus track.

6 The entrance of the sinus into the bone will be stained blue. Strip the periosteum proximally and distally to expose any dead underlying bone, which has a white appearance.

7 Remove dead bone with an osteotome and/or bone nibblers and open the medullary cavity.

8 Remove the sequestrum if present, and unroof the part of the cavity stained blue. Curette out all granulation tissue that has been stained by the dye.

9 Irrigate the cavity thoroughly, with a mixture of half-strength hydrogen peroxide and alcoholic Betadine and then physiological saline.

10 Place one or more chains of gentamicin-impregnated methyl methacrylate beads into the cavity so that it is completely filled. The chains must not be kinked or intertwined, which would make their subsequent removal difficult. Leave the last bead of each chain protruding above skin level to facilitate later removal

11 Place a perforated drain under the skin before closure, and connect it to a non-evacuated suction bottle.

12 Close the skin, leaving the terminal bead of each chain protruding from the wound, and dress the wound.

Aftercare

1 Remove the drain after 24–48 hours, or when the discharge ceases.

2 Remove beads by gentle traction on the protruding bead after 10–14 days. An anaesthetic is not usually required.

3 If the chain breaks, leave the beads in situ and remove them subsequently under a general anaesthetic or sedation when the wound is well healed.

ACUTE SEPTIC (PYOGENIC) ARTHRITIS

Appraise

1 In all cases of acute arthralgia, especially in children who are systemically unwell, suspect septic arthritis.

2 If possible, attempt to aspirate the joint (it may be difficult to aspirate a hip) when the signs and symptoms of infection are present in association with a leucocytosis or a raised ESR. A negative aspiration, however, does not exclude infection.

Prepare

1 Take blood for culture, haemoglobin, CRP, WBC count and ESR.

2 X-ray the joint, but remember that these are generally normal in the presence of acute infection.

3 Give cloxacillin and methicillin intravenously.

4 Administer a general anaesthetic.

5 Clean and drape the skin.

Action

1 Insert a wide-bore needle attached to a syringe into the joint through the site of easiest access, maximum tenderness or fluctuation. Do not pass needles through an area of cellulitis because of the risk of infecting a sterile effusion.

2 Aspirate any fluid present for culture, cell counts, Gram stain and an immediate microscopy. If the aspirate is free from pus and no organisms are seen on the smear, treat by antibiotics and immobilization alone, until the results of cultures and all cell counts are available. Do not be confused by a report of 'pus cells' being present—these are merely inflammatory cells and are themselves diagnostic of infection.

3 Open the joint in all doubtful cases involving the hip, if the aspirate is obvious pus, if organisms are visible on the smear or are subsequently grown and if the cell counts exceed 100 000/mm^3.

4 Make an incision 2.5–3.5 cm long at the site of aspiration and approach the joint, if possible through a standard approach (see sections on individual joints).

5 Make a cruciate incision in the capsule and irrigate the joint thoroughly with physiological saline, removing all pus, fibrin or other debris.

6 Insert a suction drain and close the skin only.

Aftercare

1 Immobilize the joint in a stable position in a padded plaster with access to the wound, or skin traction for the hip.

2 Change the antibiotic if necessary when the cultures of the blood or aspirate are available. Change from intravenous to oral administration after 24–48 hours in the light of clinical improvement.

3 Remove the suction drain after 24–48 hours or when drainage ceases.

4 Continue antibiotics and immobilization for 6 weeks.

FURTHER READING

Brown KLB, Cruess RL 1982 Bone and cartilage transplantation in orthopaedic surgery. Journal of Bone and Joint Surgery 64A:270–279

Dixon RA 1978 Nerve repair. British Journal of Hospital Medicine 20:295–305

Gelberman RH, Berg JSV, Lundborg GN et al 1983 Flexor tendon healing and restoration of the gliding surface. Journal of Bone and Joint Surgery 65A:70–79

Johnson KD, Cadambi A, Seibert GB 1985 Incidence of adult respiratory distress syndrome in patients with multiple musculoskeletal injuries: effect of early operative stabilization of fractures. Journal of Trauma 25:375–384

Klenerman L, Miswas M, Hughland GH et al 1980 Systemic and local effects of the application of a tourniquet. Journal of Bone and Joint Surgery 62B:385–388

Lowbury EJL, Lillie HA, Bull JP 1960 Disinfection of the skin of operative sites. British Medical Journal 2:1039–1044

Müller ME, Allgöwer M, Schneider R et al 1979 Manual of internal fixation. Techniques recommended by the AO group, 2nd edn. Springer-Verlag, Berlin

Nade S 1979 Clinical implications of cell function in osteogenesis. Annals of the Royal College of Surgeons of England 61: 189–194

Nade S 1983 Acute haematogenous osteomyelitis in infancy and childhood. Journal of Bone and Joint Surgery 65B:109–120

Nade S 1983 Acute septic arthritis in infancy and childhood. Journal of Bone and Joint Surgery 65B:234–242

Patzakis MK, Gustilo RV, Chapman MW 1982 Management of open fractures and complications. In: Frankel VH (ed.) Instructional course lectures. American Academy of Orthopaedic Surgeons, Vol 31. Mosby, St Louis, pp 62–88

Seddon H 1975 Surgical disorders of the peripheral nerves, 2nd edn. Churchill Livingstone, Edinburgh

Shipley JA, van Meerdervoort HF, van den Endej 1981 Gentamicin polymethyl methacrylate beads in the treatment of chronic bone sepsis. South African Medical Journal 59:905–907

Stewart JDM, Hallet JP 1983 Traction and orthopaedic appliances. Churchill Livingstone, Edinburgh

37

Orthopaedics and trauma: upper limb

N. Goddard

CONTENTS

THE ANTERIOR (DELTOPECTORAL) APPROACH TO THE SHOULDER

Appraise

1 The glenohumeral joint may be exposed through anterior, posterior or transacromial approaches, but most procedures can be carried out satisfactorily through the anterior approach (Fig. 37.1).

2 This is a straightforward approach through muscle planes and is truly 'extensile' in the manner described by Henry. It is particularly suited for exposure of the upper humerus for internal fixation or draining a potentially infected joint.

Prepare

1 Operate under a general anaesthetic.

2 Place the patient supine on the operating table in a semi-reclining (beach chair) position with a long narrow sandbag between the shoulder blades or alternatively with the head supported in a neurosurgical head ring.

3 Have your unscrubbed assistant elevate the arm.

4 Clean the skin from the scapula posteriorly, round the axilla and over the chest wall to the midline anteriorly, and from the angle of the jaw to the costal margin and down the arm to the elbow.

5 Towel the head separately (see Ch. 26).

6 Tuck a large drape, backed by a waterproof sheet, carefully between the table and the trunk. Cover the trunk with another large sheet, the upper edge of which reaches the lower margin of the head towels. Wrap the arm in a medium-sized towel, from the fingertips to the mid-point of the upper arm, and secure this towel firmly with an open-weave bandage or stockinette.

7 Cover the exposed skin with a transparent adhesive skin drape, taking care to seal the axilla.

Access

1 Incise the skin and subcutaneous fat in an arc from the clavicle above, downwards over the tip of the coracoid process to the anterior axillary fold following the anterior border of the deltoid muscle. Raise the flaps of skin and fat medially and laterally to expose the deltopectoral groove running obliquely across the wound (Fig. 37.1a).

2 Identify the cephalic vein in the deltopectoral groove and incise the investing fascia throughout the length of the vein.

KEY POINTS Cephalic vein

- While it may be possible to preserve the vein by retracting it medially it is often damaged during the course of an operation.
- It is therefore preferable to ligate the cephalic vein.
- Take care at the lower end where the vein is often duplicated, and then ligate it proximally before it penetrates the clavipectoral fascia immediately below the clavicle.

3 It is not necessary to remove the ligated segment of vein, but cauterize its tributaries as you encounter them.

4 Separate the deltoid from the pectoralis major by blunt dissection and retract the muscles with a large self-retaining retractor, exposing the coracoid process and the underlying short head of biceps and coracobrachialis (Fig. 37.1b).

5 In a simple operation for drainage of the joint it is not necessary to divide the coracoid process but be willing to do so if you require more extensive exposure.

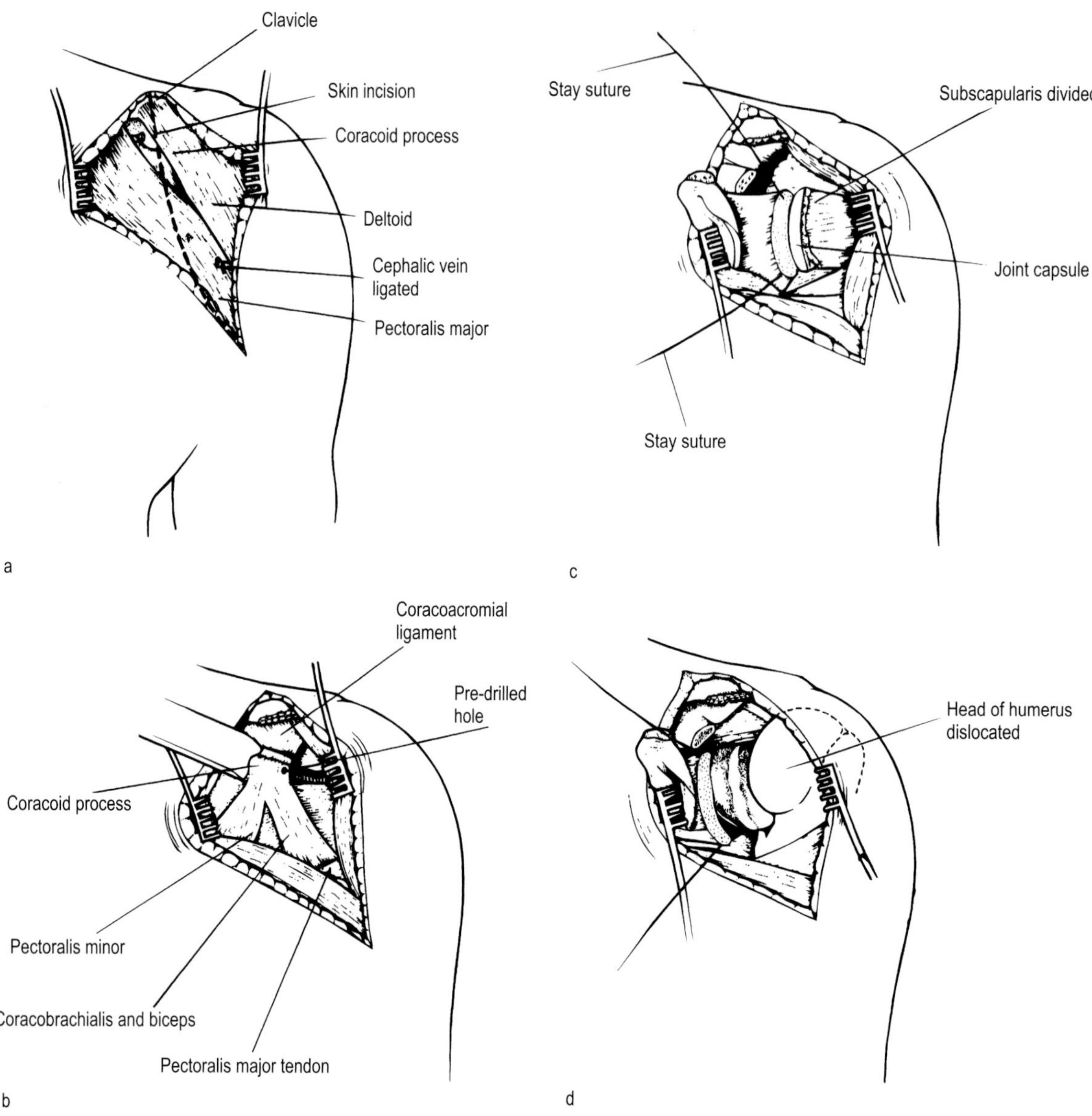

Fig. 37.1 Anterior exposure to the shoulder joint: (a) the skin incision—location of the deltopectoral groove and coracoid process; (b) division of the coracoid process with its attached muscle; (c) division and retraction of the subscapularis and the capsule; (d) dislocation of the head of the humerus.

6 Retract the bulk of the coracobrachialis and short head of biceps medially, so exposing the underlying subscapularis. It is possible to extend the approach distally along the lateral border of the biceps so exposing the entire humeral shaft (see below).

7 Externally rotate the arm and identify the lower border of subscapularis by seeing the branches of the anterior circumflex humeral vessels lying on its surface. Divide these between ligatures.

8 Identify the upper margin of subscapularis and place stay sutures at the upper and lower margins at the musculotendinous junction. Divide the muscle just lateral to the stay sutures (Fig. 37.1c).

9 The underlying capsule is usually adherent to the deep surface and is frequently divided at the same time, opening the joint as the subscapularis is retracted medially.

10 If necessary now dislocate the head of the humerus by external rotation and extension of the arm.

Closure

1 Internally rotate the arm. Apply gentle traction on the stay sutures to draw together the divided subscapularis muscle. Suture the muscle with 2/0 synthetic absorbable sutures.

2 Insert a suction drain.

3 Draw the margins of the deltoid and pectoralis major muscles together with two or three absorbable sutures.

4 Close the skin and dress the wound.

Aftercare

1 A simple dressing usually suffices, with the arm supported in a collar-and-cuff-type sling.

2 Remove the drain at 24 hours and begin early assisted motion of the shoulder.

APPROACHES TO THE UPPER ARM

Orthopaedic operations on the upper arm are infrequent but access to the humerus is occasionally required for internal fixation of fractures or exposure of the radial nerve.

ANTEROLATERAL APPROACH

Appraise

This approach to the humeral shaft avoids the major neuromuscular structures.

KEY POINTS Anatomy: radial nerve

- The radial nerve is still susceptible to damage as it passes laterally in the spiral groove around the posterior aspect of the humerus.
- Take great care to protect it.

Prepare

1 Have 2 units of cross-matched blood available.

2 Operate under general anaesthesia.

3 Place the patient supine on the operating table with a large arm table in place.

4 An unscrubbed assistant elevates the arm so that it can be cleaned from the neck to the wrist.

5 Place a small triangular towel or split sheet in the axilla and take it over the tip of the shoulder. Fasten with a towel clip.

6 Place a waterproof sheet and covering towel over the arm board and tuck under the trunk.

7 Place a large sheet over the trunk and head.

8 Wrap the forearm and hand in a small towel and bandage firmly to the forearm with an open-weave bandage or stockinette.

9 Cover the exposed upper arm with a large transparent adhesive drape.

Access

1 Palpate the moveable mass of the biceps muscle overlying the fixed mass of the brachialis.

2 Make a longitudinal skin incision along the lateral border of the biceps from the deltoid above to the elbow below. Note that the upper part of the incision takes in the inferior limit of the anterior approach to the shoulder. Once again this is an extensile approach.

3 In the proximal part of the wound retract the deltoid laterally and the biceps and cephalic vein medially, dividing the lateral tributaries to expose the shaft of the humerus.

4 Distal to the insertion of the deltoid expose the brachialis muscle and split it longitudinally down to bone with the scalpel directed obliquely towards the midline of the humerus anteriorly (Fig. 37.2).

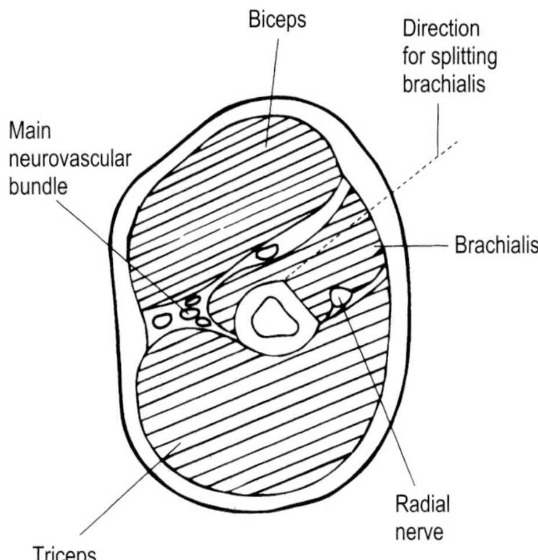

Fig. 37.2 Cross-section through the middle third of the arm showing the lateral part of the brachialis that is not covered by the biceps. This is split in the direction of the dotted line to expose the front of the distal half of the humerus. The cut slopes in to reach the midline of the shaft.

KEY POINTS Protect the radial nerve

- Strip the muscle off the bone with a periosteal elevator.
- The outer strip of the brachialis protects the radial nerve from direct damage, but avoid forceful retraction.

5 If necessary extend the wound proximally by incising the skin in the line of the deltopectoral groove to the clavicle.

6 Detach the deltoid from its origin to the clavicle as far laterally as the acromioclavicular joint with the cutting diathermy. Leave sufficient tissue attached to the clavicle to take the sutures when closing.

7 Turn back the detached deltoid laterally to expose the tendon of pectoralis major. This may then be cut to allow retraction of the muscle medially, exposing the long and short heads of biceps and the neurovascular bundle.

8 The anterior surface of the lower third of the humerus can be exposed by extending the skin incision distally along the lateral border of the biceps, curling medially and then distally again, to cross the elbow crease in the midline of the forearm (Fig. 37.3).

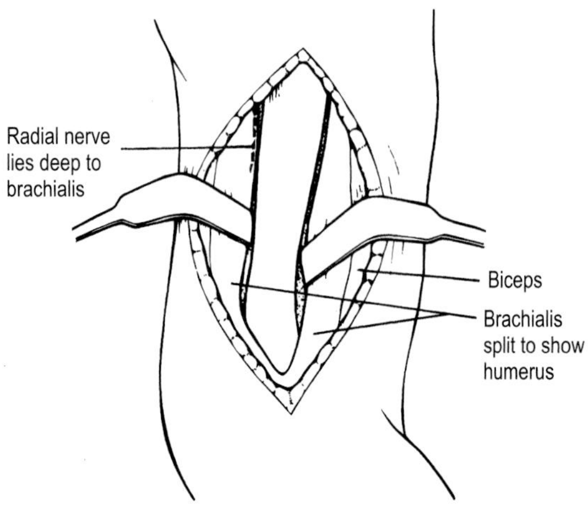

Fig. 37.3 The distal exposure of the humerus.

9 Split the brachialis as far as the elbow joint and flex the elbow to open the wound.

Closure

1 Re-attach the deltoid and approximate the margins of the brachialis with 2/0 absorbable sutures.

2 Place a suction drain in a subcutaneous layer.

3 Suture the skin.

Aftercare

1 Apply a firm dressing and elevate the arm for 24 hours.

2 Use a sling until the wound has healed.

3 Encourage the patient to exercise the fingers, elbow and shoulder as soon as postoperative pain permits.

APPROACHES TO THE ELBOW

Appraise

1 The elbow joint may be exposed from the anterior, posterior, medial or lateral aspects.

2 Avoid the anterior approach except for very special circumstances.

3 The posterior approach gives access to the whole of the lower end of the humerus, while the medial and lateral approaches give a more limited access to the corresponding side of the joint, which is sufficient for more limited procedures.

KEY POINTS Anatomy: avoid nerve damage

- For simple drainage of a joint the posterolateral approach is the most straightforward.
- But take care to avoid damaging the posterior interosseous branch of the radial nerve.

POSTEROLATERAL APPROACH (Fig. 37.4)

Appraise

This approach is particularly suitable for draining the elbow or for exposing the head of the radius. If necessary it can be extended distally to expose the upper proximal third of the radius and adjoining ulna.

Prepare

1 With the patient under general anaesthetic, apply a pneumatic tourniquet high on the upper arm.

2 Position and prepare the arm as if the humerus were to be exposed (see p. 549), leaving 12 cm of skin exposed above and below the tip of the olecranon.

3 Have an assistant flex the elbow and hold the arm across the chest.

Access

KEY POINT Again, protect the nerve

- Pronate the forearm so as to move the posterior interosseous nerve away from the operative field and to minimize the risk of accidental injury.

1 Begin the skin incision 3 cm proximal to the tip of the olecranon and continue distally between the olecranon and the lateral epicondyle down to the subcutaneous border of the ulna.

2 Divide the subcutaneous tissue and cut the deep fascia between the ulna and the anconeus and the extensor carpi ulnaris muscles (the Kocher interval).

3 Strip the anconeus from the ulna subperiosteally. Retract it laterally to expose the capsule covering the radial head and in the distal part of the wound the supinator muscle.

4 Incise the capsule over the radial head, so entering the joint. Extend this down to the annular ligament if you require greater access.

5 If necessary irrigate the joint with physiological saline.

Closure

1 Release the tourniquet.

2 Secure haemostasis.

3 Re-attach the anconeus.

4 Close the skin.

Aftercare

Support the arm in a collar-and-cuff sling.

SUPRACONDYLAR FRACTURES

Appraise

No matter how experienced you are, be circumspect when treating a displaced supracondylar fracture, especially in a child. It

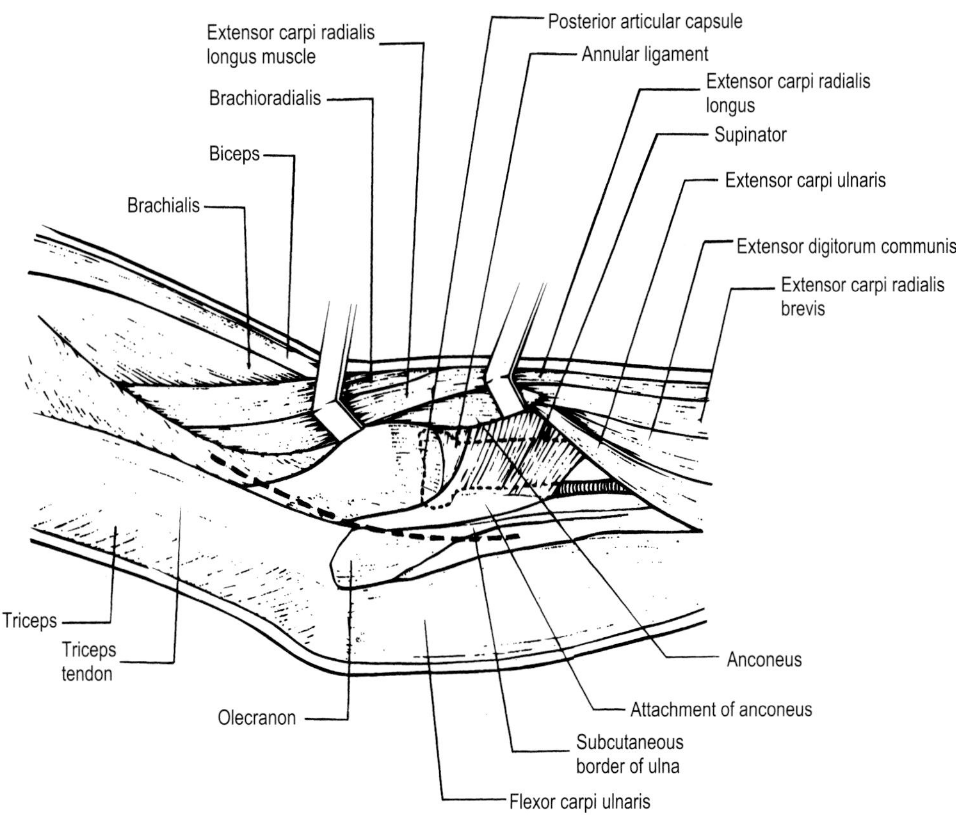

Fig. 37.4 Exposure of the head of the radius.

always remains a cause for concern and anxiety because of the potential for damage to the adjacent neurovascular structures and consequent long-term complications.

KEY POINTS Treatment options

- Look for signs of ischaemia and then for nerve damage.
- There is no optimal treatment for this injury in children. Cast immobilization is appropriate for an undisplaced fracture, but continually monitor the position lest it drifts into varus.
- Traction is very safe but requires hospitalization.
- Do not attempt percutaneous pinning unless you are very experienced, and have access to an image intensifier.
- Open reduction is occasionally indicated when the fracture is seemingly irreducible by closed means.

In the presence of potential ischaemia splint the arm in extension to avoid further compressing the brachial artery.

CONSERVATIVE TREATMENT

1. This fracture can be treated conservatively by manipulation or olecranon traction in children.
2. Take anteroposterior radiographs of both elbows in a comparable position, usually acutely flexed, after closed reduction.
3. Draw a line along the epiphyseal surface of the lower humeral metaphysis and measure the angle between this and a line perpendicular to the long axis of the humerus. Compare this angle (Baumann's angle) on the two sides (Fig. 37.5).
4. Residual varus (Latin: =bent, towards the midline) or valgus (Latin: =originally meant bow-legged; now means bent away from the midline) tilt of more than 10° requires operative correction.
5. Circulatory impairment, either before or after closed reduction, demands immediate exploration of the brachial artery if the circulation cannot be restored by allowing the elbow to extend. Unless you are experienced, seek advice if at all possible (see Ch. 29).

POSTERIOR APPROACH

This gives the widest access to the lower end of the humerus and the elbow joint.

Prepare

1. With the patient under general anaesthetic, apply a pneumatic tourniquet high on the upper arm.
2. Position and prepare the arm as if exposing the humerus, leaving 12 cm of skin exposed above and below the tip of the olecranon.
3. Have an assistant flex the elbow and hold the arm across the chest.

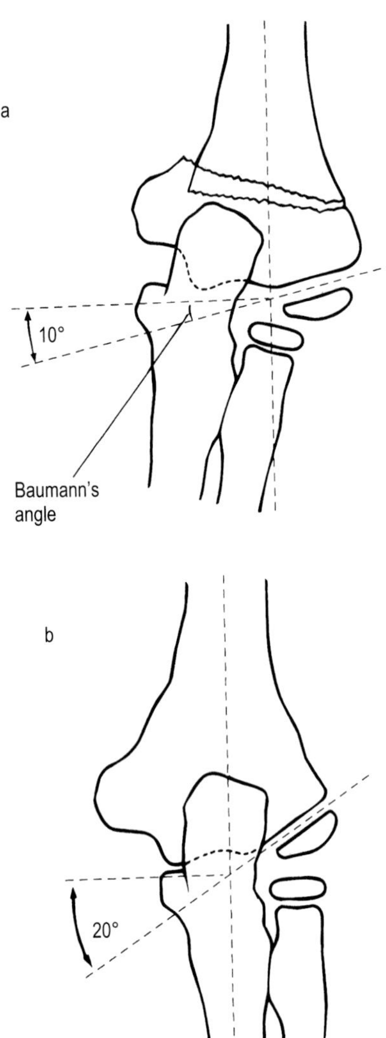

Fig. 37.5 Measurement of Baumann's angle.

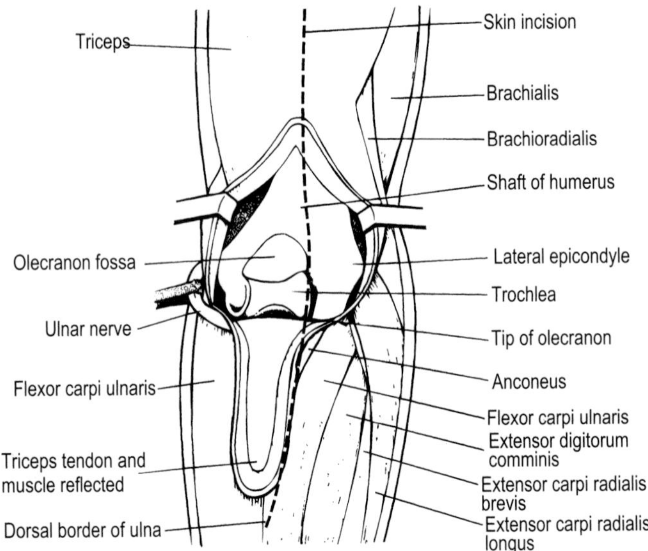

Fig. 37.6 Posterior approach to the elbow joint.

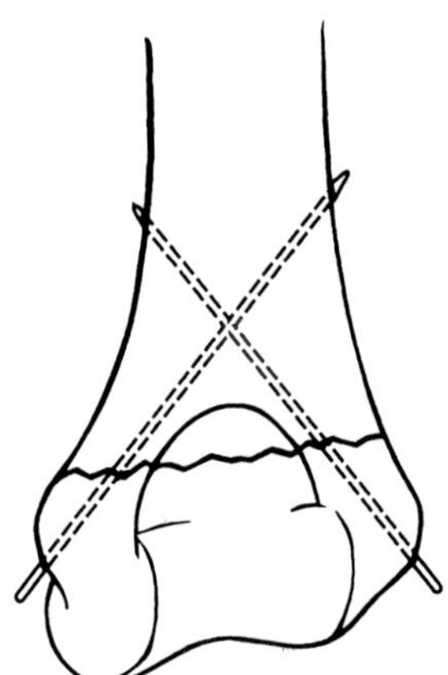

Fig. 37.7 Supracondylar fracture of the humerus held by crossed Kirschner wires.

Access

1 Start the skin incision in the midline 10 cm proximal to the tip of the olecranon and extend it distally in a gentle curve to pass just lateral to the tip of the olecranon, ending 5 cm distal to it over the subcutaneous border of the ulna.

2 Dissect the skin and subcutaneous tissues medially and laterally as far as the epicondyles and hold the edges apart with a self-retaining retractor.

3 Identify but do not disturb the ulnar nerve as it lies in its groove on the posterior surface of the medial epicondyle.

4 Identify the attachment of the central portion of the triceps tendon to the olecranon. Turn down a tongue-shaped flap, 7 cm long, based on the olecranon attachment by incising the tendon and the underlying muscle down to the bone (Fig. 37.6).

5 Sweep the residual attachments of the triceps muscle medially and laterally off the posterior surface of the condyles in continuity with the common flexor and extensor attachments, so exposing the distal humerus.

Action

1 Drill a 1-mm Kirschner wire (K-wire) through the fracture surface of the distal fragment at approximately 45° to the long axis of the humerus, so that it emerges through the medial epicondyle and the overlying skin. Take care to avoid the ulnar nerve.

2 Withdraw the wire until only 1–2 mm protrudes from the fracture.

3 Reduce the fracture under direct vision, freeing any interposed soft tissue.

4 Flex the elbow to 90° and drill the K-wire back across the fracture to engage the lateral cortex of the shaft of the humerus (Fig. 37.7).

5 Through a small stab wound over the lateral condyle, drill a second wire across the fracture site to engage the medial cortex of the shaft.

6 Occasionally, a third wire needs to be introduced from either the medial or lateral side, if the fixation is not stable.

7 Confirm the accuracy of the reduction and the position of the wires by X-rays to check the accuracy of the reduction. Do not accept any position that is less than perfect.

8 If satisfactory, cut the wires leaving the ends just beneath the skin.

Closure

1 Suture the long head of triceps back into place with interrupted absorbable sutures through the aponeurosis.

> **KEY POINT Is the circulation intact?**
>
> - Check the circulation and leave instructions that the radial pulse is to be taken every hour for the next 12 hours.

2 Release the tourniquet and stop the bleeding.

3 If necessary, place a suction drain under the skin before closing it.

Aftercare

1 If the fixation is stable immobilize the arm in a collar-and-cuff sling. If you are doubtful, apply a padded plaster back slab.

2 Remove the Kirschner wires at 3–4 weeks.

DECOMPRESSION OF THE ULNAR NERVE

Appraise

1 Decompression of the ulnar nerve may be carried out for relieving ulnar neuritis or nerve entrapment. Occasionally it needs to be transposed anteriorly so as to gain length to repair the nerve following injury, or as part of another procedure.

2 If operating for a compression neuropathy, it is advisable to obtain preoperative nerve-conduction studies.

Action

1 Position the patient supine with a tourniquet applied to the upper arm as high as possible.

> **KEY POINT Sufficient access?**
>
> - Check that the shoulder will externally rotate sufficiently to allow access to the medial aspect of the elbow.

2 Attach an arm table to the side of the operating table. If the shoulder is stiff, place the patient in a lateral position, or alternatively prone with the arm behind the back in a 'half-Nelson' position.

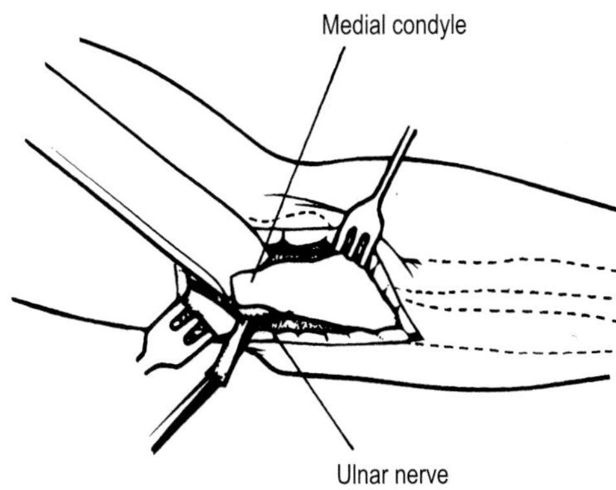

Fig. 37.8 Medial approach to the elbow joint.

3 Use a medial approach (Fig. 37.8), regardless of the position of the patient.

4 Flex the elbow to a right angle. Begin the skin incision 3 cm proximal to the medial epicondyle and carry it just anterior to the epicondyle for a further 3 cm.

5 Identify the ulnar nerve in the groove on the posterior aspect of the medial epicondyle. It is usually easier to find the nerve at the proximal end of the incision. Incise the investing fascia in the line of the nerve, preserving its blood supply.

6 Place a saline-soaked tape around the nerve and gently lift it from its bed.

7 Free the nerve proximally up to the medial intermuscular septum, where there may be a tight band, which you should release.

8 Decompress the nerve distally as it passes between the two heads of flexor carpi ulnaris. Several short small articular branches may be divided, but preserve the branch to flexor carpi ulnaris. This is usually sufficient in the majority of cases of ulnar neuritis, so that transposition is not necessary.

9 If the nerve is unstable (dislocatable) or if additional length is required, then transpose it anteriorly and proceed as follows:

10 Divide the common flexor origin anterior to the ulnar nerve, leaving a cuff of tissue attached to the bone for later re-attachment.

11 Place the nerve deep to the common flexor muscle mass and ensure there are no kinks in its course.

Closure

1 Re-attach the common flexor muscles with three or four absorbable mattress sutures.

2 Release the tourniquet and close the wound.

Aftercare

1 Immobilize the elbow in a collar-and-cuff sling until the patient is comfortable.

2 Remove the stitches and mobilize the elbow at 10–12 days.

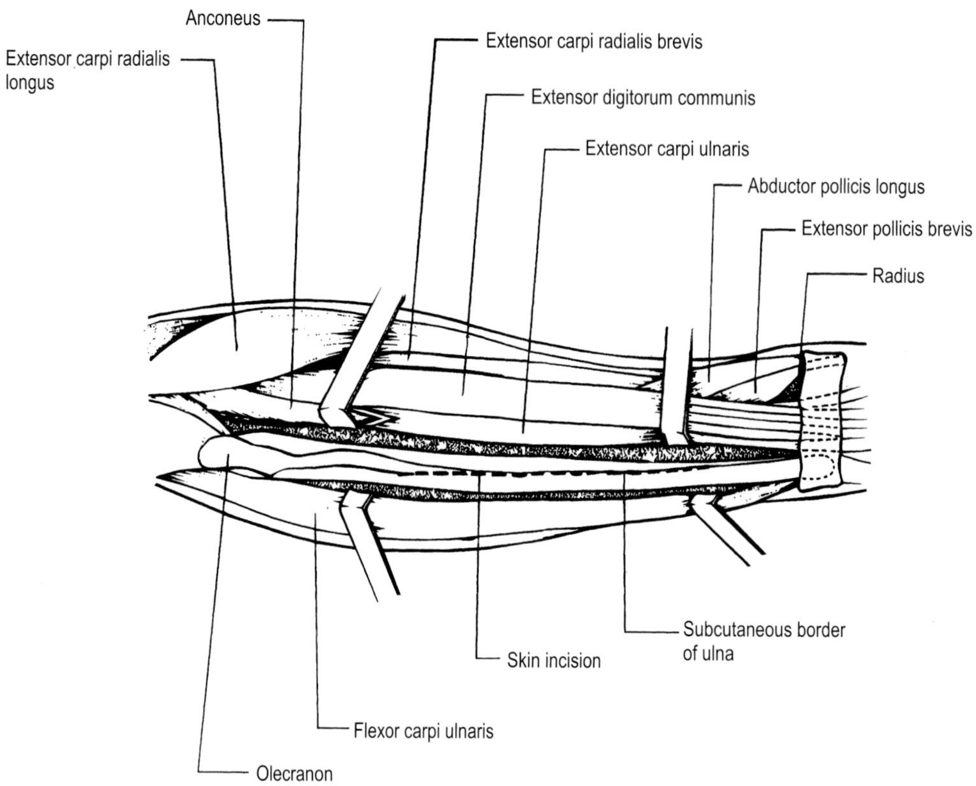

Fig. 37.9 Exposure of the shaft of the ulna.

APPROACHES TO THE FOREARM

Preferably approach the shafts of the radius and ulna through separate incisions—the ulna from behind and the radius from the front.

POSTERIOR APPROACH TO THE ULNA (Fig. 37.9)

Prepare

1 The patient, under general anaesthesia, lies supine. Have a large arm table attached to the operating table.

2 Apply a pneumatic tourniquet around the upper arm.

3 Prepare the skin from above the elbow to the fingertips.

4 Cover the arm board with a waterproof sheet and towel.

5 Drape off the arm just proximal to the elbow with a triangular towel.

6 Cover the head and trunk with a large sheet.

7 Cover the fingers and hand with stockinette that can be extended up to the tourniquet if necessary.

8 Pass the arm through a large sheet with a hole in the centre.

Action

1 Much of the ulna, like the tibia, is immediately subcutaneous, so exposure is generally simple, straightforward and safe. Incise the skin along the subcutaneous border of the ulnar over that part of the forearm to be exposed.

2 Divide the common aponeurosis, which attaches to the bone the flexor carpi ulnaris and flexor digitorum profundus medially, and the extensor carpi ulnaris laterally.

3 Separate the muscles from the bone with a periosteal elevator to expose the shaft of the ulna.

THE ANTERIOR (HENRY) APPROACH TO THE RADIUS (Fig. 37.10)

Prepare

1 Prepare the arm as above.

2 Supinate the forearm.

Access

1 Incise the skin, beginning at the radial styloid in the interval between the brachioradialis and the flexor carpi radialis muscles, and extend this proximally in a straight line as far as the lateral side of the biceps tendon, to expose the whole radial shaft. More limited exposure to any part of the radius is gained by using an appropriate part of this incision.

2 Starting at the distal end of the incision, identify and protect the sensory branch of the radial nerve as it lies beneath the brachioradialis.

3 Mobilize flexor carpi radialis and the radial artery and vein. Retract them medially to expose flexor digitorum superficialis, flexor pollicis longus and pronator quadratus in the floor of the wound.

4 Pronate the forearm and elevate flexor pollicis longus and pronator quadratus subperiosteally from the outer edge of the radius. Strip them medially to expose the distal two-thirds of the anterior aspect of the radius.

5 To expose the proximal third of the radius, supinate the forearm and extend the incision proximally. Divide and tie the large superficial vein crossing the middle part of the wound.

6 Expose the biceps tendon and divide the deep fascia on its lateral side with blunt-nosed scissors.

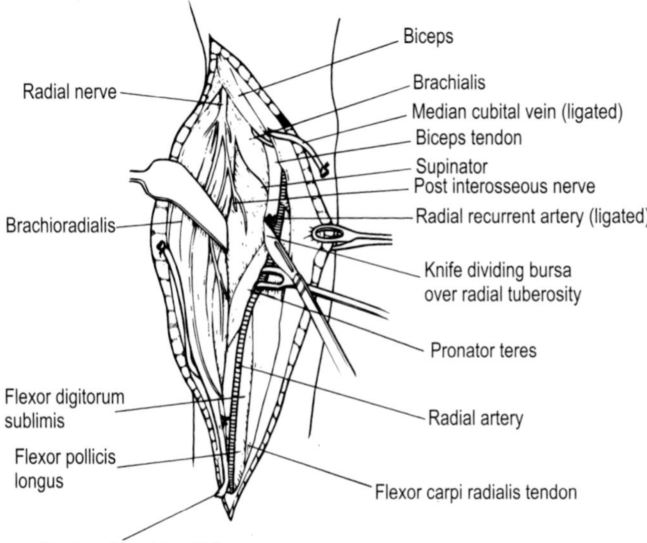

Fig. 37.10 Anterior approach to elbow and proximal radial shaft.

7 Retract the belly of brachioradialis and the long and short radial extensors of the wrist laterally, and the flexors medially, to expose the radial artery. Divide and carefully ligate the fan-shaped leash of vessels passing laterally from the artery (Fig. 37.11).

8 Flex the elbow to 90° to expose the belly of the supinator.

9 Cut down to the tuberosity of the radius immediately lateral to the attachment of the biceps tendon.

KEY POINTS Protect the nerve

- From this point sweep the supinator laterally off the bone with a periosteal elevator.
- Supination of the forearm protects the posterior interosseous nerve which lies within its substance.

10 Pronate the forearm to expose the lateral aspect of the radius.

Closure

1 Replace the muscles that have been stripped from the bone and tack them into place with absorbable sutures as appropriate.

2 Release the tourniquet and stop the bleeding.

3 Insert a suction drain if necessary.

4 Close the skin.

APPROACHES TO THE WRIST

ANTERIOR (VOLAR) APPROACH (Fig. 37.12)

Prepare

1 Position the anaesthetized patient with the affected limb on a large arm table.

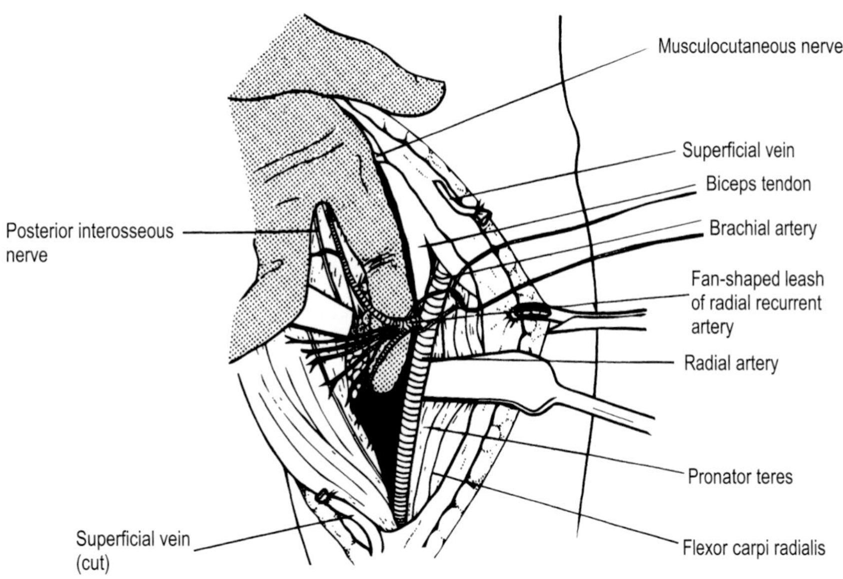

Fig. 37.11 Division of the branches of the radial artery.

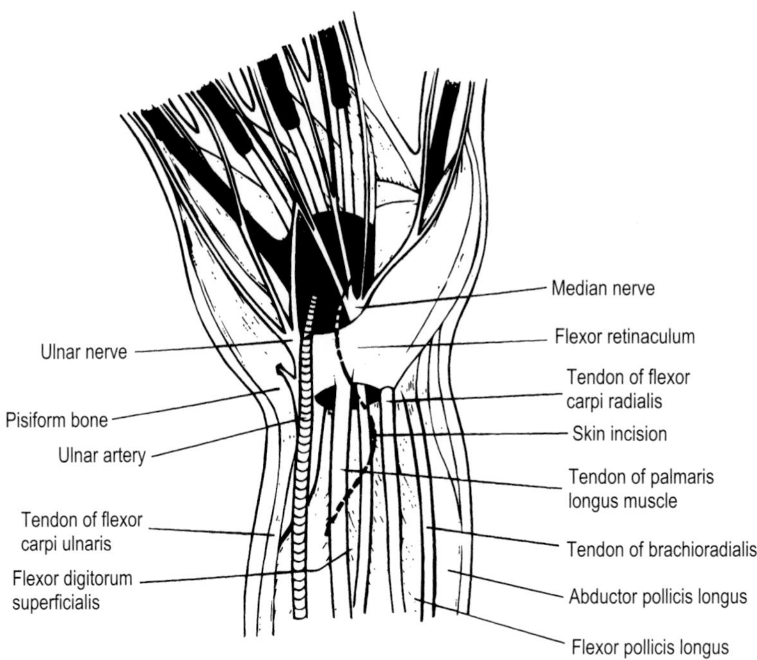

Fig. 37.12 Anterior approach to the wrist.

2 Use a pneumatic tourniquet on the upper arm.

3 Clean the forearm and fingers and drape the limb as described for the upper arm, but leave the fingers and hand exposed.

Access

1 Incise the skin in line with the radial border of the ring finger as far as the midpoint of the transverse palmar crease. Cross the wrist crease either transversely in the skin crease for 1 cm or with a small zigzag incision, and then extend the incision proximally along the radial side of the flexor carpi radialis tendon for 3–4 cm.

2 Retract the skin edges with skin hooks exposing the palmar aponeurosis. The transverse carpal ligament is exposed in the distal part of the wound and is continuous proximally with the deep fascia of the forearm.

3 Carefully incise the palmar fascia, further exposing the transverse carpal ligament (flexor retinaculum) between palmaris longus and flexor carpi radialis. Incise the transverse carpal ligament to expose the median nerve and its recurrent branch, which is motor to the muscles of the thenar eminence.

4 Retract the median nerve and palmaris longus towards the ulnar side to expose the tendon of flexor pollicis longus, and have this retracted medially.

5 The pronator quadratus lies in the floor of the wound. Carefully elevate this from its radial border to expose the lower end of the radius and the radiocarpal joint.

Closure

1 Remove the tourniquet and stop bleeding.

2 Close the skin only.

POSTERIOR (DORSAL) APPROACH

Prepare

As for anterior approach.

Access

1 Pronate the forearm.

2 Make a straight incision 10 cm long on the dorsum of the wrist centred on Lister's tubercle (the bony prominence on the dorsum of the distal radius).

3 Retract the skin edges with skin hooks and expose the extensor retinaculum. Divide this along the line of the sheath of the extensor carpi ulnaris tendon (ECU) and turn it towards the radial side of the wound to sequentially expose the extensor tendons in their respective compartments (Fig. 37.13).

4 Continue elevating the extensor retinaculum as far as Lister's tubercle. This provides access to the distal and radio-ulnar joint, radiocarpal joint and carpal bones.

Closure

1 Pass the extensor retinaculum deep to the extensor tendons and suture it back to the ECU sheath.

2 Release the tourniquet and stop the bleeding.

3 Close the skin.

LATERAL APPROACH (Fig. 37.14)

This is a particularly useful approach to the distal radius especially for internal fixation or decompression of the first extensor compartment (De Quervain's tenosynovitis).

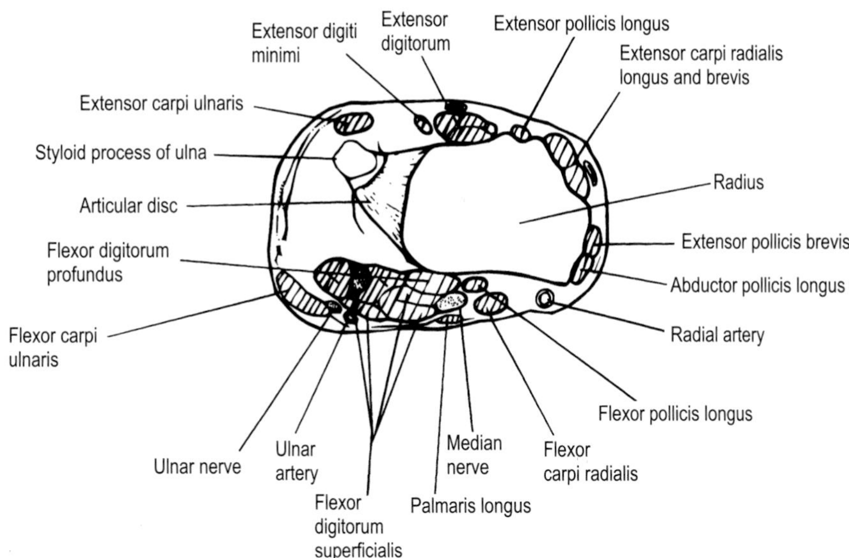

Fig. 37.13 Cross-section through the distal end of the right radius and the styloid process of the right ulna.

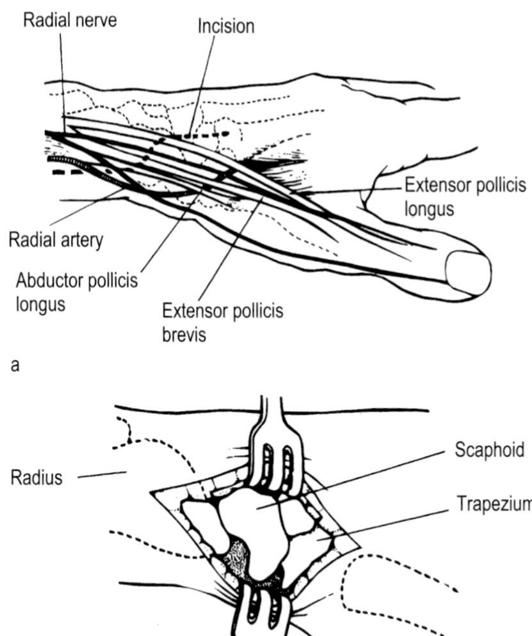

Fig. 37.14 Lateral approach to the wrist: (a) skin incision; (b) approach completed.

Prepare

As for anterior approach.

Access

1 Make a longitudinal oblique incision 5 cm long centred on the tip of the radial styloid.

2 Extend the incision in a palmar direction towards the tendons of extensor pollicis brevis and abductor pollicis longus and then proximally, parallel to the radius. Curve the distal limb towards the extensor pollicis longus and then parallel to it.

KEY POINTS Anatomy: dorsal radial nerve branches

- Identify the dorsal branches of the radial nerve immediately deep to the skin.
- Protect them throughout to avoid causing a painful neuroma.

3 Retract extensor pollicis brevis and abductor pollicis longus, the radial artery and the dorsal branch of the radial nerve towards the palm. The tubercle of the scaphoid and the lateral capsule of the wrist joint are exposed distally and the lower end of the lateral aspect of the radius proximally.

Closure

1 Close the capsule with interrupted absorbable sutures.

2 Release the tourniquet and stop the bleeding.

3 Close the skin.

DECOMPRESSION OF THE EXTENSOR POLLICIS BREVIS AND ABDUCTOR POLLICIS LONGUS TENDONS

Appraise

Described by the Swiss surgeon (1868–1940), tenosynovitis of extensor pollicis brevis and abductor pollicis longus tendons (De Quervain's syndrome) usually resolves following local steroid injections or immobilization of the wrist and thumb. When conservative treatment fails, operation is required.

Action

1 Use the lateral (radial) incision, taking great care to avoid damage to the superficial branches of the radial nerve.

2 Divide the extensor retinaculum covering the tendons on the lateral aspect of the radius—first extensor compartment.

3 Open the tendon sheaths of abductor pollicis longus and extensor pollicis brevis in the line of the tendon and lift each tendon in turn from its bed with a small, blunt tendon hook. It is not unusual to find an accessory tendon lying in a third compartment; if you miss this it will cause persistent symptoms.

4 Remove as much of the inflamed synovium as possible from the surface of the tendon using a small pair of curved scissors or fine bone nibbler.

Closure

1 Release the tourniquet and stop bleeding.

2 Close the subcutaneous fat and skin.

3 Immobilize the thumb and wrist in a padded plaster until the sutures are removed at 10 days.

GANGLION OF THE DORSUM OF THE WRIST

Appraise

1 A simple ganglion is the result of cystic degeneration of fibrous tissue. They commonly arise from a synovial joint or less frequently from a tendon sheath.

2 The commonest site is on the dorsal aspect of the wrist where they nearly always originate from the scapholunate joint.

3 Recurrence is common unless you carefully remove the ganglion.

Prepare

1 As for anterior approach. There are advocates for performing this operation under purely local anaesthetic, but this does not really permit the use of a tourniquet.

2 My preference therefore is to perform the operation under either a regional block or general anaesthetic, which allows a tourniquet to be used and permits a better exposure of the neck of the ganglion, so theoretically reducing the risk of recurrence.

Action

1 Make a transverse incision in a skin crease over the apex of the swelling.

2 Deepen it carefully until you see the bluish-grey surface of the ganglion.

3 Carefully dissect around the ganglion with small curved scissors.

4 Do not grasp it with toothed forceps, to avoid puncturing it.

5 The swelling is often multilocular and passes between the tendons. Carefully identify its attachment to the capsule of the joint.

6 Trace the ganglion down to its origin and remove the small portion of the capsule (or tendon sheath) to which the ganglion is attached, as well as the ganglion itself.

7 Remove the tourniquet and close the skin.

Aftercare

1 Apply a compression dressing for 24 hours and then replace this with a small adhesive dressing.

2 Remove the stitches at 10 days.

MEDIAN NERVE DECOMPRESSION IN THE CARPAL TUNNEL

Appraise

1 Decompress the median nerve if conservative treatment with night splints, steroid injections and diuretics fails to relieve the symptoms of carpal tunnel syndrome, or if abnormal neurological signs are present. Look in particular for wasting and weakness of the thenar muscles and dryness of the skin over the radial two-thirds of the hand.

2 I always advise preoperative nerve conduction studies prior to surgical decompression.

3 Combine decompression with flexor tendon synovectomy in rheumatoid arthritis when the proliferating synovium is the cause of nerve compression.

Prepare

As for anterior approach.

Action

KEY POINT Preserve the palmar cutaneous branch of the median nerve

- Incise the skin in line with the radial border of the ring finger as far as the midpoint of the transverse palmar crease. This avoids potential damage to the palmar cutaneous branch of the median nerve.

1 Deepen the incision down through the longitudinal fibres of the palmar aponeurosis to expose the transverse fibres of the flexor retinaculum.

2 Insert a small self-retaining retractor.

3 Incise the flexor retinaculum longitudinally with a scalpel to expose the median nerve. Pass a McDonald's dissector deep to the retinaculum to protect the nerve while the remaining transverse fibres are divided.

4 Ensure that the proximal part of the retinaculum has been adequately released where it disappears under the skin at the proximal end of the wound, by passing a dissector along the surface of the median nerve. This is a common site of inadequate decompression, which can result in persistent symptoms.

5 Take care not to damage the transverse palmar arch at the distal end of the incision.

6 If there is an associated hypertrophic synovitis affecting the flexor tendons, as in rheumatoid disease, perform a flexor synovectomy by stripping the synovium with a fine pair of bone nibblers.

Closure

1 Release the tourniquet; the nerve will 'blush' at the site of compression.
2 Stop any bleeding.
3 Close the skin.

Aftercare

1 Apply a firm compression dressing and then replace it with an adhesive dressing after 24 hours.
2 Instruct the patient to exercise the fingers immediately after the operation.
3 Remove the stitches at 10 days.

APPROACHES TO THE HAND AND FINGERS

The unique sensibility and mobility of the hand and fingers call for special care whenever surgical treatment is contemplated.

PALMAR APPROACH (Fig. 37.15)

Appraise

KEY POINTS Palmar skin creases

- Incisions may be made anywhere in the palm of the hand provided that they do not cross the skin creases at right-angles.
- Cross skin creases obliquely (Brunner incisions) or, as far as possible, parallel to but not within the creases (Fig. 37.15).
- Take the creases into account with any pre-existing lacerations or injuries.

Prepare

1 Use a general anaesthetic or regional block.
2 Attach the arm table to the operating table.
3 Apply a pneumatic tourniquet to the upper arm.
4 Have an unscrubbed assistant grasp the forearm immediately below the elbow while you clean the skin from the assistant's forearm to the patient's fingertips.
5 Place the towels as if the operation were to be on the wrist.

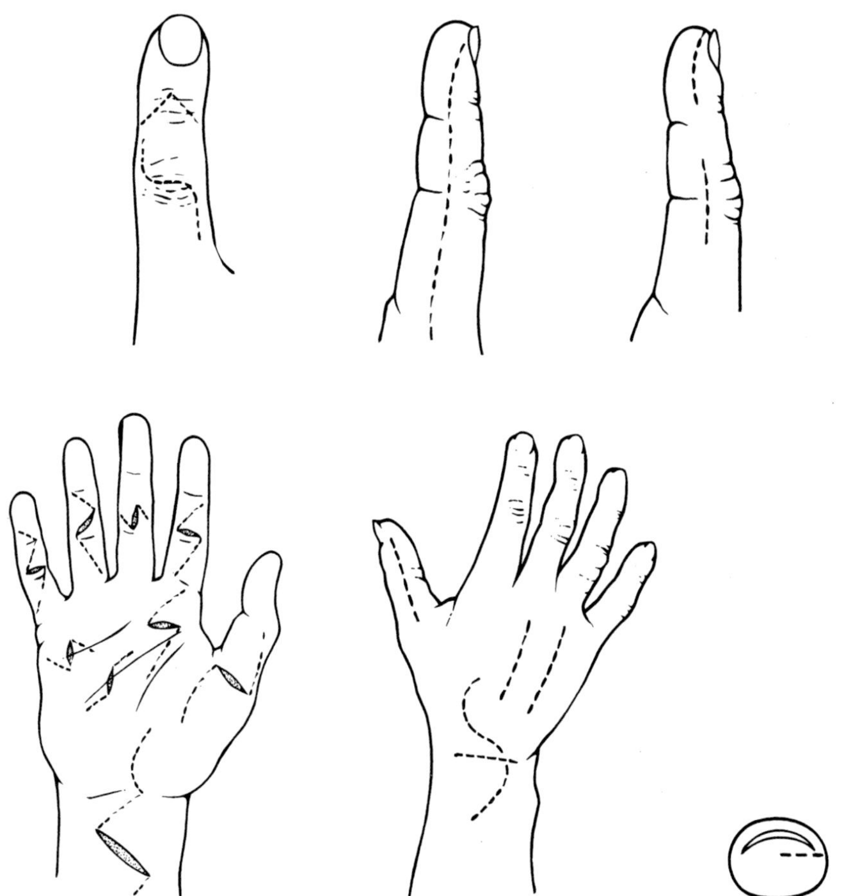

Fig. 37.15 Skin incisions in the hand and fingers.

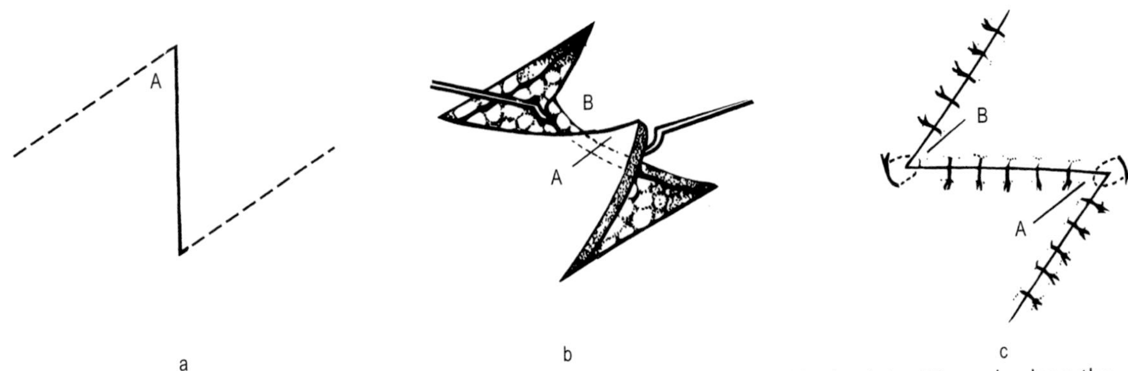

Fig. 37.16 Simple Z-plasty to release a long narrow contracture: (a) the central limb of the Z is made along the line of the contracture, and the other two limbs (broken lines) are made as shown; (b) the flaps are shifted; (c) the flaps are sutured in their new positions.

6 Place the hand on the hand table in a supinated position and secure the fingers and thumb with a 'lead hand'.

Action

1 Incise the skin and subcutaneous tissue, obliquely crossing the skin creases at their apices. Extend the incision proximally and distally over the structure to be exposed.

2 Carefully dissect the skin and subcutaneous tissue from the underlying fascia and retract the edges with skin hooks.

3 Expose the deeper structures with incisions made according to anatomical considerations and not necessarily following the skin incisions.

? DIFFICULTY

If there is a pre-existing contracted scar, or if additional length is required, consider inserting a Z-plasty of the skin (Fig. 37.16).

Closure

1 Release the tourniquet and control bleeding.

2 Close the skin.

3 Apply a non-adherent dressing such as tulle gras or Jelonet, and padded dressing, leaving the fingers mobile.

Aftercare

1 Reduce the dressing as soon as is practical and commence early mobilization.

2 Remove the sutures at 7–10 days.

DORSAL APPROACH TO THE HAND

Appraise

1 The direction and placement of incisions on the dorsum of the hand is not so critical as those on the palm. They may be longitudinal or transverse, whichever is most appropriate (see Fig. 37.15).

2 Take care, though, to preserve the veins, which are predominantly dorsal. If you damage them you risk causing excessive swelling of the fingers.

Prepare

As for the palmar approach.

Access

1 Incise the skin over the structure to be exposed.

2 Retract the skin edges.

3 Avoid damaging the superficial nerves and veins.

4 Employ simple periosteal dissection to expose the underlying bone.

Closure

1 Release the tourniquet.

2 Close the skin.

Aftercare

1 Apply a non-adherent and padded dressing. Elevate the arm in the roller towel if the patient is in hospital, or in a sling for 24 hours.

2 Instruct the patient to move the fingers as soon as possible after the operation, even though this may be painful.

Mid-lateral incisions on the digits

Appraise

You may create a mid-lateral incision (Fig. 37.17) on either the radial or ulnar side of the digit, giving access not only to the corresponding side but also to the palmar and dorsal aspects of the fingers or thumb. In general, incisions on the radial side are more convenient.

Prepare

1 As for approaches on the hand and wrist.

2 Place the hand on the arm table with the forearm in mid-rotation and the thumb uppermost.

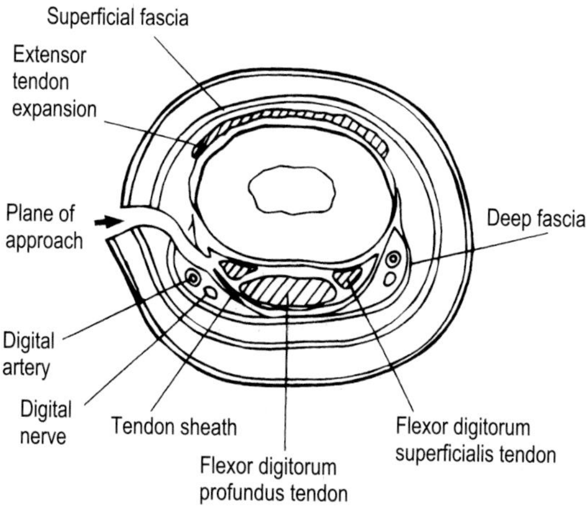

Fig. 37.17 Lateral approach to expose the flexor tendons and phalanges.

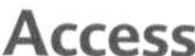

Access

1 Flex the interphalangeal joints to 45°.

2 Incise the skin longitudinally on the radial side of the digit from the apex of the proximal interphalangeal joint skin crease to the apex of the distal interphalangeal skin crease.

3 Extend the incisions proximally or distally in the same lateral line as required.

4 Carefully deepen the incision towards the shaft of the phalanx between the dorsal and palmar neurovascular bundles, which are in the respective flaps.

5 Deepen the wound towards the anterior or posterior aspect of the phalanges as required.

Closure

1 Release the tourniquet.

2 Suture the skin only.

Aftercare

1 Apply a pressure dressing.

2 Mobilize the fingers as soon as the underlying condition will allow.

RELEASE OF TRIGGER FINGER OR THUMB (Fig. 37.18)

Appraise

The thickening in the tendon and the flexor sheath usually lies deep to the distal palmar crease or over the metacarpophalangeal joint of the thumb and is easily palpable. This represents the opening of the flexor tendon sheath (the A1 pulley).

Prepare

1 As for any hand procedure.

2 A tourniquet is desirable for this operation.

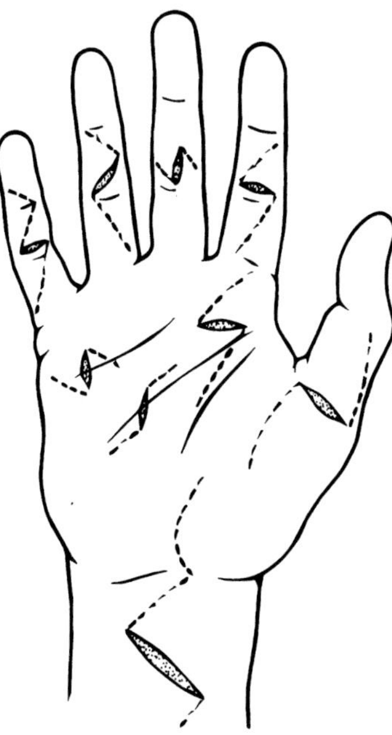

Fig. 37.18 Exposures for the suture of divided flexor tendons. Lacerations (solid lines) may be extended along the dotted lines to provide additional exposure.

3 It may be possible to perform this procedure using a local anaesthetic infiltration, provided that you are reasonably quick and that the patient can tolerate the discomfort of the tourniquet for the 5–7 minutes of the operation.

4 If you are performing the operation under pure local anaesthesia, delay inflating the tourniquet until the skin is prepared and drapes are in place.

KEY POINT Diabetic?

- A significant proportion of patients with trigger fingers have diabetes mellitus, which may complicate the perioperative management.

Action

1 Make a transverse or short oblique incision in the skin over the thickened tendon sheath 1.5 cm long.

KEY POINTS Trigger thumb? Preserve the radial digital nerve

- Take particular care when releasing a trigger thumb as the radial digital nerve has a tendency to lie immediately subcutaneously.
- This is not the case with trigger fingers.

2 Deepen the incision down through the palmar fascia using blunt dissection to avoid damaging the digital nerves and vessels.

3 You immediately encounter the flexor tendon sheath. Incise the thickened portion of the A1 pulley longitudinally.

4 Deliver both flexor tendons into the wound with a tendon hook and ensure that they both move freely. If there is any residual tightness it may be necessary to excise a small portion of the sheath.

Closure

1 Release the tourniquet and secure haemostasis.

2 Suture the skin.

Aftercare

1 Apply a non-adherent dressing and elevate the hand for 24 hours.

2 Reduce the dressing after 24 hours and commence active mobilization of the fingers.

3 Remove the sutures after 10 days.

PYOGENIC INFECTIONS OF THE HAND (Fig. 37.19)

Appraise

1 Pyogenic infections of the hand are common and present with cellulitis alone. Most resolve with antibiotics, elevation and rest.

2 Incise and drain as soon as an abscess develops or you detected the presence of pus, either visually or because of increasing pain and tenderness.

3 Open subcuticular, intracutaneous and subcutaneous infections where they are most superficial.

4 Take a swab for bacteriological analysis.

5 Local anaesthetic is not always necessary and many abscesses can be incised using a freezing spray of ethyl chloride, or no anaesthetic at all.

6 Web and palmar space infections are rare. Very little swelling is obvious in the palm, but the back of the hand is oedematous and pain is severe.

7 Tendon sheath infections cause swelling and tenderness along the line of the sheath, and the finger cannot be extended passively because of excruciating pain.

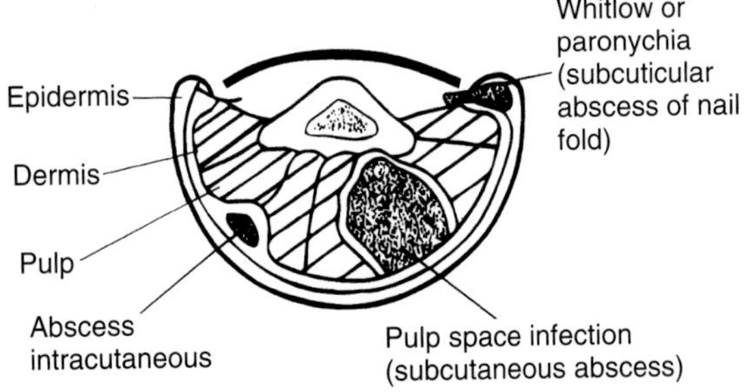

Fig. 37.19 Superficial and deep infections of the digits.

Action

Superficial infections

1 Accurately localize the most tender point with the tip of an orange stick before inducing anaesthesia.

2 Prepare the hand for a palmar approach but do not exsanguinate the limb.

3 When the infection is superficial, make a cruciate incision over the most tender point and cut away the corners of the skin to saucerize the lesion. Take a swab for bacteriological analysis.

4 If pus extends under the nail, remove only that portion of the nail that has been raised from the nail bed.

5 Incise in the line of the skin crease over the most tender part when a web or palmar space is infected. Do not incise the web itself.

6 Carefully explore between the deeper structures (Fig. 37.20) by blunt dissection and follow the track to the abscess cavity.

7 Insert a small latex drain.

8 Cut back the skin edges to ensure adequate drainage but do not insert a drain.

9 Leave the incision open to ensure drainage.

Tendon sheath infections

1 Drain tendon sheath infections through transverse incisions at either end of the sheath (Fig. 37.21).

2 Irrigate the sheath with antibiotic solution through a fine ureteric catheter until the effluent is clear.

3 Leave the catheter in place for subsequent irrigation if necessary. Local anaesthetic can also be instilled for postoperative pain relief.

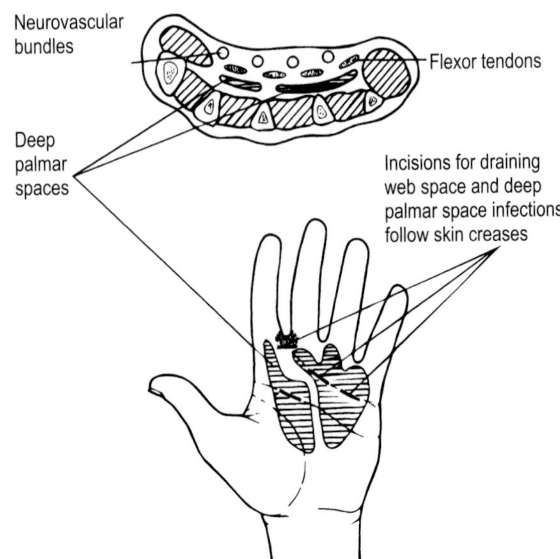

Fig. 37.20 Incisions for the drainage of web and deep palmar space infections.

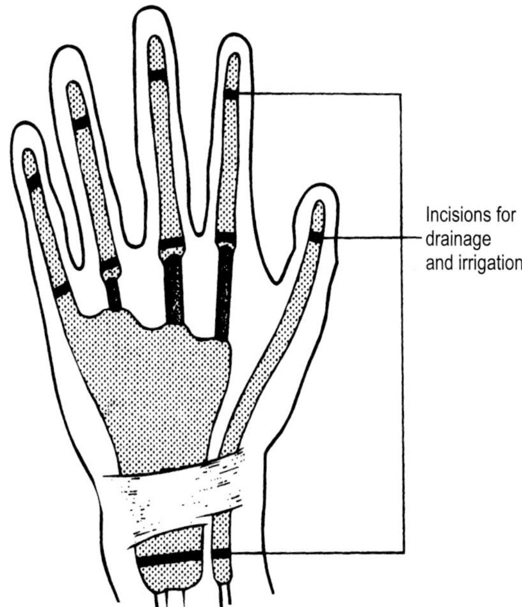

Fig. 37.21 Drainage of tendon sheath infections.

Palmar space infections

1 When the infection is superficial, make a cruciate incision over the most tender point and cut away the corners of the skin to saucerize the lesion. Take a swab for bacteriological analysis.

> **KEY POINTS Dorsal approach?**
>
> - Deep palmar space infections can be drained through a dorsal approach between the first and second metacarpals.
> - Make a small stab incision and simply bluntly dissect with a clip or curved scissors to open the deep palmar space.

2 Leave a soft latex drain in situ until the drainage ceases.

Aftercare

1 Place the corner of a gauze dressing in the wound to keep it open.

2 Apply Tubigrip to the fingers or a fluffed-up pressure dressing to the palm as appropriate and immobilize the hand with a plaster-of-Paris back slab with the fingers in semiflexion.

3 Elevate the hand and re-dress it daily so long as the wound is draining and then leave the dressings until epithelialization is complete.

OPERATIONS ON THE NAILS

PARTIAL AVULSION OF A NAIL

Appraise

1 It may be necessary to remove a portion of the nail in the presence of infection or trauma.

2 Preserve as much of the nail as possible to splint any associated soft tissue or bony injury.

Action

1 Remove only that part of the nail that is separated from the nail bed, using fine scissors.

2 Apply a non-adherent dressing and Tubigrip.

EVACUATION OF A SUBUNGUAL HAEMATOMA

Appraise

1 The diagnosis is usually obvious, generally the result of a crushing injury to the fingertip.

2 It is frequently associated with a fracture of the distal phalanx, which in theory renders this an open fracture, so you should prescribe antibiotics.

3 Check that the nail is not dislocated from the nail bed; if it is, it should be reduced.

Prepare

No specific preparation is necessary.

Action

1 Although there are more sophisticated devices available it is a simple matter to trephine the nail.

2 Use a red-hot needle or paper clip and the blood spurts out under pressure.

3 Cover the hole with a sterile dressing.

FURTHER READING

Bailey DA 1963 The infected hand. HK Lewis, London.
Barton NJ 1984 Review article. Fractures of the hand. Journal of Bone and Joint Surgery 66B:159–167
Fisk GR 1984 Review article. The wrist. Journal of Bone and Joint Surgery 66B:396–407
Grace TG, Eversmann WW 1980 Forearm fractures. Treatment by rigid fixation with early motion. Journal of Bone and Joint Surgery 62B:396–407
Henry AK 1957 Extensile exposure applied to limb surgery, 2nd edn. E&S Livingstone, Edinburgh
Keon-Cohen BT 1966 Fractures at the elbow. Journal of Bone and Joint Surgery 48A:1623–1639
Macnicol MF 1979 The results of operation for ulnar neuritis. Journal of Bone and Joint Surgery 61B:159–164

38

Orthopaedics and trauma: lower limb

N. Goddard

CONTENTS

APPROACHES TO THE HIP AND PROXIMAL FEMUR

1 The hip joint is deeply placed and relatively inaccessible.

2 It may be exposed by several routes that are variations of the anterior, posterior and lateral approaches, which themselves afford good access for most purposes.

3 The anterolateral approach is an extensile approach and provides adequate access for drainage of a potentially septic hip as well as more complex procedures such as total hip arthroplasty.

4 The lateral approach is usually used for open reduction and internal fixation of femoral fractures.

ANTEROLATERAL APPROACH

Prepare

1 Order 2 units of cross-matched blood.

2 A general anaesthetic is preferable, especially in a child. However, if the general condition of the patient precludes it, use an epidural or spinal anaesthetic.

3 Place the patient supine on the operating table with a sandbag under the buttock of the side to be operated on.

4 Have an unscrubbed assistant elevate the leg.

5 Clean the skin distally from the umbilicus to the knee, including the anterior abdominal wall, perineum and as much of the buttock as possible.

6 Place a waterproof sheet under the affected leg and over the opposite leg, tucking it under the buttock.

7 Place a large drape over the waterproof sheet so that the whole of the unaffected leg and foot and the lower part of the operating table are covered. Pull the top edge firmly into the groin to exclude the genitalia from the field.

8 If possible, use a split sheet to shut off the groin. If this is not possible, fold a medium-sized towel corner-to-corner and place the centre of the long side firmly in the groin. Take one corner under the leg and the other over the iliac crest, and clip the corners together onto the skin at the posterior end of the iliac crest.

9 With the scrubbed assistant, hold a medium towel outstretched by the corners under the leg from the lower third of the thigh to beyond the foot. Direct that the leg be lowered carefully into it and turn the bottom end over the foot before carefully wrapping the lower thigh, leg and foot in the towel. Bandage the towel firmly on to the leg with an open-weave bandage or stockinette.

10 Cover the patient's head and trunk with a large drape.

11 Place the leg through the hole in a large split sheet. Pull the sheet firmly into the groin and around the buttock but leaving the anterolateral aspect of the thigh exposed from the iliac crest distally.

12 Cover the exposed skin with a large adhesive drape wrapped around the thigh.

Access (Fig. 38.1)

1 Make a straight incision extending from the anterior superior iliac spine directed towards the tip of the greater trochanter. This follows the junction between gluteus medius and tensor fascia lata.

2 Incise the fascia overlying the interval between the two muscles and develop the plane proximally towards the anterior superior iliac spine. Insert a self-retaining retractor, such as the Norfolk and Norwich type, between the two.

KEY POINT Anatomy

- Identify the interval between the gluteus medius posteriorly and tensor fascia lata muscle anteriorly. It is often easier to separate the two muscles immediately proximal to the anterosuperior corner of the greater trochanter.

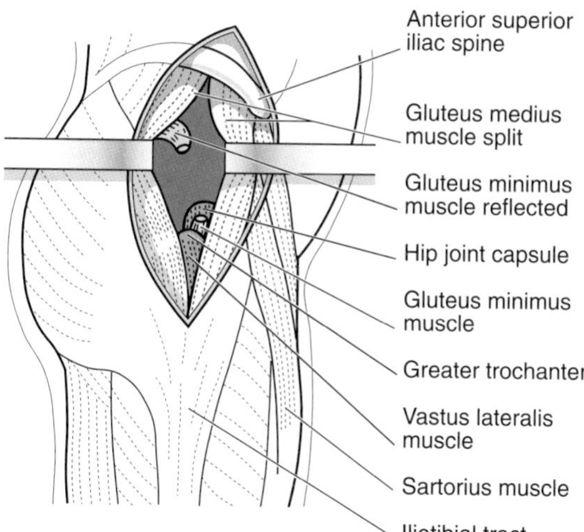

Fig. 38.1 Diagrammatic view of anterolateral approach to the right hip, viewed from the patient's right side. After identifying the opening up of the interval between the tensor fascia lata and gluteus medius muscles, retract them. You may not see the gluteus minimus muscle beneath the gluteus medius but if you do, you may retract it posteriorly. Below is the joint capsule and greater trochanter.

3 It should now be possible to see the tendon of the gluteus minimus and the capsule of the hip joint.

4 Retract the gluteus minimus posteriorly and incise the capsule of the hip joint, draining any accumulated intra-articular fluid. Send a sample for bacteriological analysis.

Closure

1 Remove the self-retaining retractor, allowing the gluteus medius and tensor fascia lata muscles to fall back into place, requiring only a few interrupted absorbable sutures to appose the edges.

2 Insert a suction drain.

3 Suture the subcutaneous fat and skin.

LATERAL APPROACH TO THE PROXIMAL FEMUR

1 This exposure may be carried proximally to expose the hip joint if required.

2 Use the distal part of the approach alone for access to the proximal part of the femur and the femoral neck, when treating fractures in this region.

Prepare

1 Cross-match 2 units of blood.

2 Operate with a general anaesthetic if possible, or with epidural or spinal anaesthesia.

3 If you are operating for fixation of a femoral neck fracture, place the patient supine on the orthopaedic operating table with a radiolucent perineal post to allow access for an image intensifier or portable X-ray machine. Operative fixation of femoral neck fractures is, however, beyond the scope of this chapter.

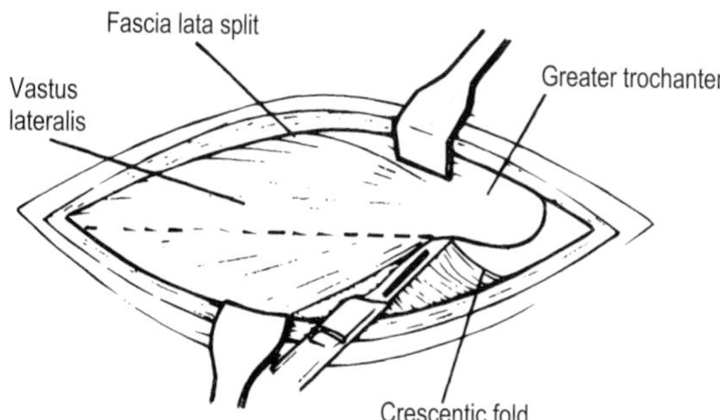

Fig. 38.2 Cutting down on to the femoral shaft.

4 Straightforward exposure of the femur is usually carried out with the patient in the lateral position. A traction table and X-ray control are not necessary.

5 Clean the skin from the level of the umbilicus to the knee, including the perineum and buttock and the circumference of the thigh.

6 Hang a large drape over the sound side from the groin to beyond the toes.

7 Hang another large drape over the affected leg from the mid-thigh to beyond the toes.

8 Cover the trunk above the iliac crest with a third large sheet.

9 Cover the remaining part of the thigh with two small towels, leaving only a rectangle of skin 30 cm long by 20 cm wide exposed on the lateral side of the thigh. The anterior superior iliac spine is situated at the top corner of this rectangle.

10 Hold the towels in place with a transparent adhesive drape.

Access (Fig. 38.2)

1 Palpate the posterosuperior corner of the greater trochanter and make a straight longitudinal incision from that point for 15 cm distally, through the skin and subcutaneous fat.

2 Split the fascia lata longitudinally, posterior to the insetion of the tensor fascia lata muscle, in the line of the incision. Insert a self-retaining retractor to expose the vastus lateralis.

3 Identify the aponeurotic attachment of the vastus lateralis to the anterolateral surfaces of the femur, just below the greater trochanter.

4 Identify the posterior attachment of the vastus lateralis. Insert two Trethowan bone spikes and lift the body of the vastus lateralis forwards, releasing it from its attachment to the linea aspera (Latin: *asper*=rough), cauterizing vessels as you go.

5 Reflect the muscle subperiosteally from the anterolateral aspect of the femur and strip the muscle from the anterior and lateral aspects of the femur with a periosteal elevator. Insert the tip of your index finger between the vastus lateralis and the anterior surface of the femur and palpate the lesser trochanter on the posteromedial aspect of the bone.

6 Pass a Lane's lever carefully around the femoral shaft with the tip absolutely in contact with the bone, so that it lies between the lesser trochanter and the femoral neck. This exposes the

anterior and lateral surface of the upper femoral shaft and the base of the femoral neck.

7 Strip the posterior portion of the muscle from the bone in similar fashion and insert a second Lane's lever around the underside of the femoral shaft.

Closure

1 Insert a suction drain.

2 Allow the vastus lateralis to fall back into its resting position; it is not necessary to insert any sutures at this point.

3 Repair the fascia lata with a continuous absorbable suture.

4 Close the subcutaneous fat and skin.

APPROACHES TO THE UPPER LEG

1 The femoral shaft may be approached from the anterior, medial or lateral aspects.

2 The posterolateral approach is the most convenient and most commonly used.

POSTEROLATERAL APPROACH (Fig. 38.3)

Appraise

1 Use the posterolateral approach to the femoral shaft unless you specifically require access to the medial side of the femur.

2 The approach may be extended proximally and distally if necessary and is most commonly employed to reduce and internally fix fractures of the femoral shaft.

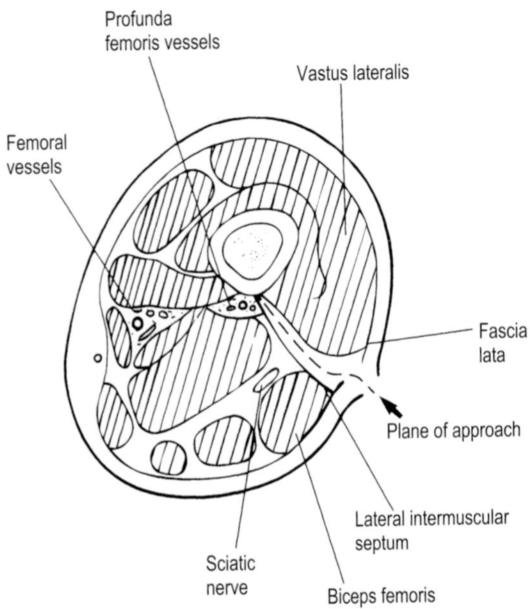

Fig. 38.3 Transverse section of the mid-thigh showing the posterolateral approach to the femoral shaft along the dotted line.

Prepare

1 Have 2 units of cross-matched blood available.

2 Use a general anaesthetic.

3 For operations on the distal two-thirds of the thigh, it may be possible to use a tourniquet but this may compromise the exposure.

4 Place the patient supine on the operating table with a sandbag under the buttock of the affected side.

5 Elevate the leg and clean the skin from the iliac crest and buttock—or the tourniquet, when used, to the upper tibia.

6 Place a large sheet across the operating table and over the sound leg, and pull the upper edge firmly into the groin to cover the genitalia.

7 Place the long edge of the 'shut-off' towel in the groin, or immediately below the tourniquet, and pull it firmly round the thigh; fasten it with a towel clip on the lateral side.

8 Place a medium-sized drape on the table with its upper edge at the level of the knee joint and carefully lower the leg on to the towel.

9 Fold the distal edge of the towel proximally over the foot and then wrap the towel around the leg.

10 Bandage the towel firmly to the leg with an open-weave bandage or stockinette.

11 Cover the trunk with a large sheet and clip it to the underlying sheet on either side of the thigh.

12 Pass the leg through the hole in a split sheet. Clip the margins of the split to the skin at the upper limit of the operating field.

13 Wrap a large transparent adhesive drape round the thigh to cover the exposed skin.

Access

1 Palpate the tendon of the biceps femoris at the level of the lateral femoral condyle and also the posterior margin of the greater trochanter.

2 Incise the skin along the whole or part of the line joining these two points to gain access to the appropriate part of the thigh.

3 Incise the fascia lata in the line of the incision and locate the lateral intermuscular septum immediately anterior to the biceps femoris.

4 Insert a finger between the septum and the bulk of the vastus lateralis lying anteriorly and continue the dissection down to the bone in this plane with a knife.

5 Ligate the perforating branches of the profunda femoris vessels as you encounter them.

Closure

1 Insert a suction drain.

2 Close the fascia lata with 0 absorbable sutures.

3 Close the skin, dress and bandage the wound.

APPROACHES TO THE KNEE

1 Most operations on the knee joint are carried out from the front, but many do not require a full and formal exposure of the whole joint, and a more limited exposure is adequate.

2 The posterior approach is used to gain access to the popliteal fossa and occasionally to the posterior part of the knee joint.

ANTERIOR APPROACH (Fig. 38.4)

Appraise

1 Use this approach for operations on the extensor mechanism of the knee joint and to gain wide access to the inside of the joint itself.

2 Use the anterolateral and anteromedial approaches when you require limited access, for example to carry out meniscectomy or removal of loose bodies.

Prepare

1 Use a general anaesthetic.

2 Apply a tourniquet to the mid-thigh.

3 Place the patient supine on the operating table.

4 Drape the leg as if the distal femoral shaft were being exposed, leaving the skin exposed from the tibial tubercle to the tourniquet.

5 Cover the exposed skin with a transparent adhesive drape.

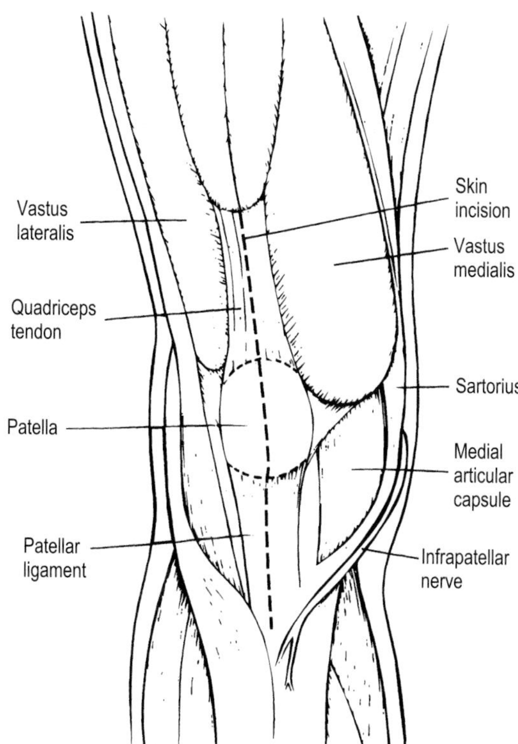

Fig. 38.4 Anterior approach to the knee joint.

Access

1 Make a straight incision 15 cm long in the midline, extending proximally from the upper margin of the tibial tubercle.

2 Deepen the incision to expose the patellar ligament, the anterior surface of the patella and the quadriceps tendon, and the distal fibres of the rectus femoris (Fig. 38.4).

3 Reflect the skin and subcutaneous fat as a single layer medially to expose the junction of the quadriceps tendon and the vastus medialis, the medial border of the patella and the patellar ligament.

4 Make an incision along the medial edge of the quadriceps tendon and through the capsule along the medial margin of the patella and medial edge of the patellar ligament into the joint.

5 If required, evert the patella, retract it laterally, and flex the knee at the same time (Fig. 38.5). Extend the incision proximally into the rectus femoris if this proves to be difficult.

Closure

1 Extend the knee and return the patella to its normal position.

2 Close the incision in the capsule and the quadriceps tendon with interrupted absorbable synthetic sutures.

3 Close the subcutaneous fat and skin.

POSTERIOR APPROACH (Fig. 38.6)

Appraise

1 Use this approach to gain access to the popliteal fossa.

2 Use it to gain access to the posterior compartment of the knee joint, for example to repair the torn posterior cruciate ligament or to expose the popliteal vessels.

3 Use the medial or lateral part of the full approach for more limited exposure.

Prepare

1 Use a general anaesthetic.

2 Apply a mid-thigh tourniquet.

3 Place the patient prone on the operating table.

4 Have an assistant flex the knee to 90° and raise the thigh off the table.

5 Place the drapes as described for the anterior approach.

Access

1 Start the skin incision 7 cm proximal to the medial femoral condyle and extend it distally to the transverse skin crease; then curve it laterally and distally again, along the medial side of the head of the fibula.

2 Reflect the skin and subcutaneous tissue to expose the popliteal fascia.

3 Identify the posterior cutaneous nerve of the calf (Latin: *sural* = calf), lying beneath the fascia between the two heads of the gastrocnemius muscle.

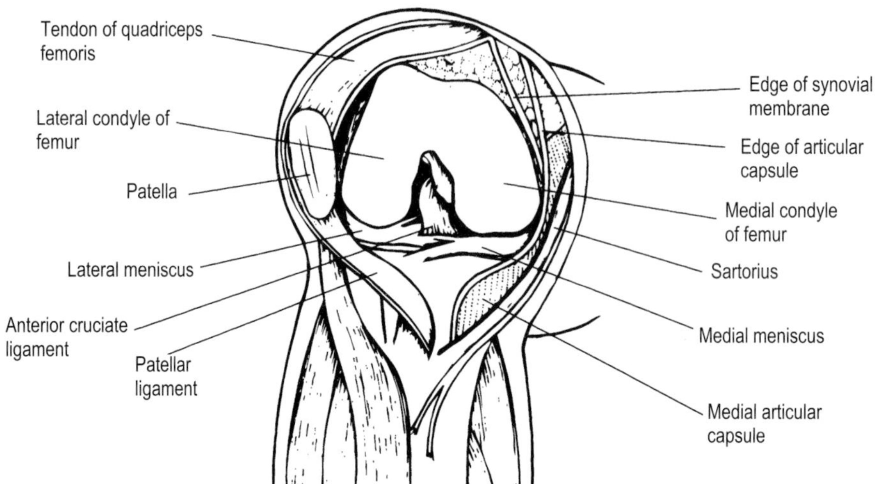

Fig. 38.5 The knee exposed through the anterior approach and flexed.

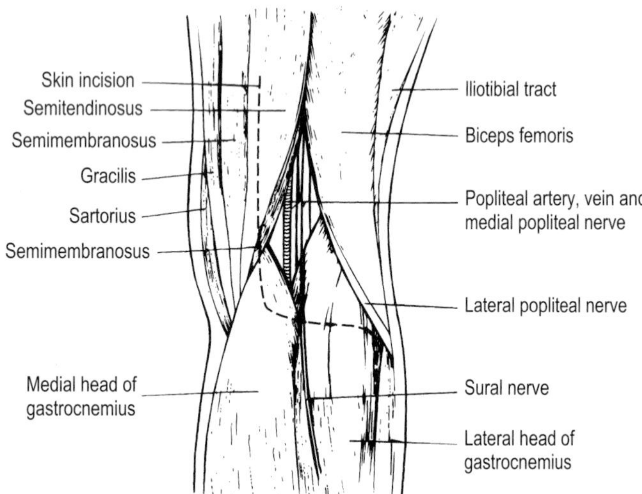

Fig. 38.6 The posterior approach to the knee joint.

4 Incise the fascia and trace the nerve proximally to its origin from the posterior tibial nerve.

5 Trace the posterior tibial nerve distally and identify its branches to the calf muscles; then trace it proximally to the apex of the popliteal fossa where it joins the common peroneal nerve.

6 Follow the common peroneal (Greek: *perone*=fibula) nerve distally along the medial border of the biceps tendon.

7 Expose the popliteal artery and vein lying anteriorly and medially to the posterior tibial nerve. Gently retract them to expose the superior lateral and superior medial genicular vessels passing beneath the muscles just proximal to the origin of the two heads of gastrocnemius.

8 If you require access to the knee, then retract the semitendinosus medially and expose the attachment of the medial head of gastrocnemius to the joint capsule, incising it longitudinally at this point.

9 Retract the gastrocnemius laterally, using it to protect the nerves and vessels, and enter the posteromedial compartment of the joint.

10 Approach the posterolateral compartment between the tendon of biceps femoris and the lateral head of gastrocnemius.

Closure

1 Release the tourniquet.

2 Suture the capsule with interrupted synthetic absorbable sutures.

3 Close the deep fascia and the skin.

SIMPLE KNEE ARTHROTOMY

Appraise

1 If it becomes necessary to open a knee for drainage of a possible infection, carry out open meniscectomy, or remove a loose body.

2 It is not necessary to perform a full approach. All that is required is a limited anterolateral or anteromedial approach.

Prepare

1 Use a general anaesthetic.

2 Apply a tourniquet to the exsanguinated limb.

3 Drape the leg for the anterior approach.

Access

1 It is easier to use an anterolateral incision for ease of access. Incise the skin on the lateral side of the knee from the lateral margin of the patella, downwards and slightly

backwards to a point 1 cm below the articular margin of the tibia.

2 Incise the capsule in the line of the incision.

3 Pick up the synovium with forceps and nick it with a knife. In the presence of an effusion it bulges forwards into the wound.

4 Obtain a specimen for bacteriology and irrigate the joint.

Closure

1 Retract the edges of the capsule and pick up each end of the synovium with fine curved artery forceps.

2 Close the synovium with a continuous 2/0 absorbable synthetic suture on a round-bodied needle.

3 Extend the knee and close the capsule with 0 interrupted absorbable synthetic sutures.

4 Close the subcutaneous tissue and skin.

5 Apply a compression bandage from the ankle to the lower thigh. Extend the bandage to the upper thigh after removing the tourniquet.

Aftercare

1 Begin static quadriceps exercises immediately the patient recovers from the anaesthetic and progress to straight leg raising exercises as soon as possible. Allow weight-bearing as tolerated by the patient.

2 Remove the sutures at 7–10 days.

3 Bandage the knee so long as there is any tendency to swell, usually 3–4 weeks, and continue quadriceps exercises until the bulk of the muscle recovers.

APPROACHES TO THE LOWER LEG

The shafts of the tibia and fibula are subcutaneous and may therefore be exposed by incisions through the overlying skin.

ANTERIOR APPROACH (Fig. 38.7)

Appraise

1 Use the anterior approach for access to the shaft of the tibia and the anterior compartment of the lower leg.

2 Expose the fibula through a separate lateral incision if required.

Prepare

1 Cross-match 2 units of blood.

2 Use a general anaesthetic.

3 Exsanguinate the leg and apply a pneumatic tourniquet to the thigh.

4 Place the patient supine on the operating table.

5 The unscrubbed assistant grasps the calf and elevates the leg.

6 Clean the skin from the ankle proximally.

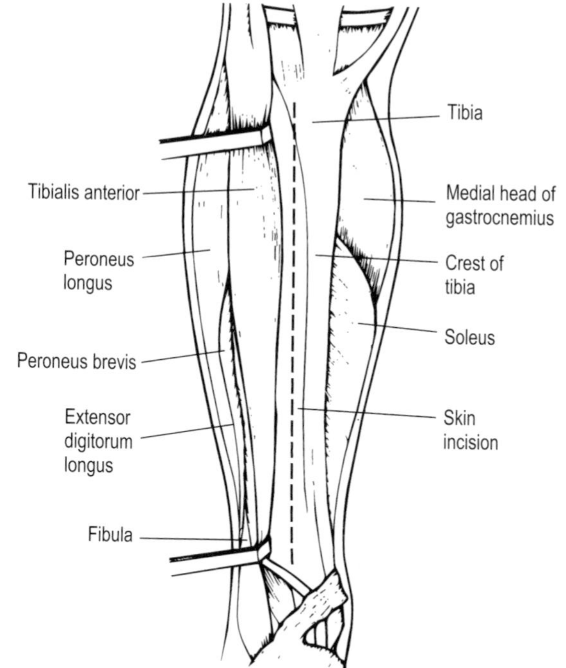

Fig. 38.7 The anterior approach to the shaft of the tibia.

7 Have a scrubbed assistant apply a stockinette to the foot and continue to support the leg while it is further prepared as far as the tourniquet.

8 Place a large sheet across the operating table and over the sound leg.

9 Place the shut-off towel or split sheet immediately distal to the tourniquet.

10 Continue to drape the leg as described above.

Access

1 Incise the skin longitudinally 1 cm lateral to the crest of the tibia, from the tibial tubercle to the ankle.

2 Reflect skin flaps medially and laterally to expose the subcutaneous surface of the tibia and the tibialis anterior muscle.

Closure

1 Release the tourniquet.

2 Insert a suction drain.

3 Close the skin with 2/0 interrupted sutures.

TIBIAL COMPARTMENT FASCIOTOMY

Appraise

1 Decompression of the fascial compartments of the leg may be indicated in the following circumstances:
- After extensive closed soft-tissue injuries of the lower leg.
- After proximal vascular reconstruction following arterial injury.
- For chronic exertional compartment syndrome.

KEY POINTS Compartment pressures

- Measure the individual compartment pressures prior to operation.
- Suspect impending ischaemia when the compartment pressure reaches 10–30 mmHg below the diastolic pressure.
- Higher pressures indicate an urgent need for fasciotomy.
- Impending or established compartment syndrome is a surgical emergency.

2 To measure the compartment pressure, you require a slit catheter (14G intravenous cannula), a length of plastic manometer tubing connected to a pressure transducer (a sphygmomanometer suffices if necessary). Prepare and sterilize the skin. Instil 2 ml of 1% lidocaine into the skin and insert the catheter into the anterior compartment. When it is satisfactorily positioned withdraw the trocar. Inject a small quantity of saline into the catheter to fill the dead space. Prefill the manometer tubing with saline and connect this via a three-way tap to the slit catheter and the pressure monitor, ensuring that there are no air bubbles in the system. Now connect the three-way tap to the pressure recorder and measure the compartment pressure.

Prepare

Prepare as for the anterior approach.

Access

1 The anterior and lateral compartments can be decompressed through a full-length longitudinal anterolateral skin incision lateral to the crest of the mid-tibia extending from the level of the tibial tuberosity to just proximal to the ankle.

2 Incise the fascia covering the tibialis anterior muscle and extend the incision in the fascia subcutaneously both proximally and distally so completely decompressing the anterior muscle group. By slightly undermining the skin it is also possible to decompress the lateral compartment, avoiding damage to the superficial peroneal nerve. In cases of exertional compartment syndrome only, it may be possible to perform a limited decompression through a short skin incision and then extend the fascial incision with a Smillie meniscectomy knife.

3 The superficial and deep posterior compartments can be decompressed in a similar fashion using a single longitudinal posteromedial incision made just medial to the posteromedial border of the tibia.

4 Incise the deep fascia and extend the incision proximally to the level of the tibial tuberosity and distally to a point 5 cm proximal to the medial malleolus, using the same technique.

KEY POINT Emergency decompression

- In an emergency excise the middle half of the fibula; this provides decompression of all compartments.

Closure

1 It is possible to close the skin only following release of chronic exertional compartment syndrome.

2 In acute compartment syndrome leave the wounds open and plan to suture the skin 3–5 days later when the swelling has subsided. If necessary apply a split skin graft.

3 Be willing to inspect the wound in the interim period.

Aftercare

1 Apply a compression dressing.

2 Elevate the leg.

3 Ability to mobilize the patient depends on the underlying reason for the fasciotomy.

APPROACHES TO THE ANKLE

1 Operations on the ankle joint itself can usually be accomplished through an anterior approach.

2 Separate incisions are required to gain access to the malleoli and to the posterior aspect of the joint.

ANTERIOR APPROACH (Fig. 38.8)

Appraise

Use this approach to gain access to the ankle joint itself and for arthrodesis or arthroplasty.

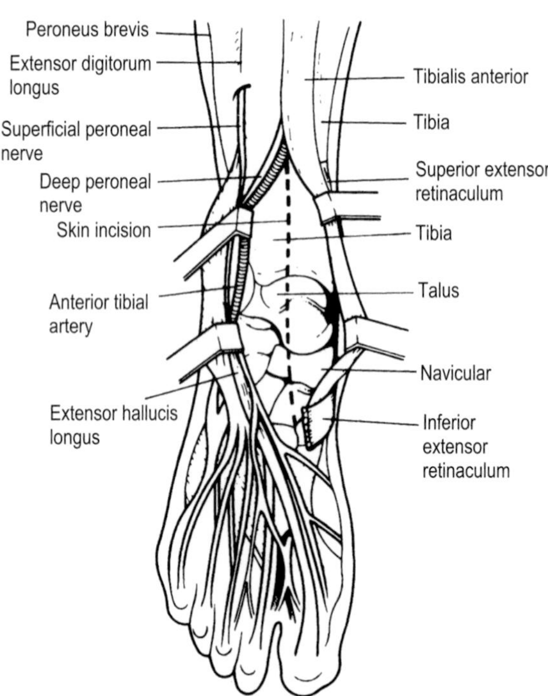

Fig. 38.8 The anterior approach to the ankle joint.

Prepare

1. Use a general anaesthetic.
2. Exsanguinate the leg and apply a pneumatic tourniquet to the thigh.
3. Have an unscrubbed assistant hold the leg just below the knee joint and elevate it.
4. Clean the skin from the assistant's hands to the tip of the toes, paying particular attention to the skin between them.
5. Grasp the foot in a stockinette and then drape the limb as described above.

Access

1. Make an incision in the skin 10 cm long in the midline, centred over the middle of the ankle joint.
2. Incise the superficial fascia, avoiding the superficial peroneal nerve, which crosses the wound diagonally. Retract it laterally.
3. Incise the deep fascia and the extensor retinaculum and identify the anterior tibial artery and the deep peroneal nerve between the tendons of tibialis anterior and extensor hallucis longus.
4. Retract the neurovascular bundle, extensor hallucis longus and extensor digitorum laterally and the tibialis anterior medially.
5. A pad of fat frequently obscures the anterior capsule of the ankle joint. Excise it.
6. Incise the joint capsule longitudinally and open the ankle joint.

▶ KEY POINT Anatomy

- Do not confuse the ankle joint with the talonavicular joint, which is unexpectedly close to it.

Closure

1. Release the tourniquet and stop the bleeding.
2. Insert a suction drain.
3. Close the deep fascia.
4. Close the skin.

POSTERIOR APPROACH (Fig. 38.9)

Appraise

Use the posterior approach to gain access to the Achilles tendon and the posterior aspect of the ankle joint and distal end of the tibia.

Prepare

1. Use a general anaesthetic.
2. Exsanguinate the leg and apply a pneumatic tourniquet to the thigh.

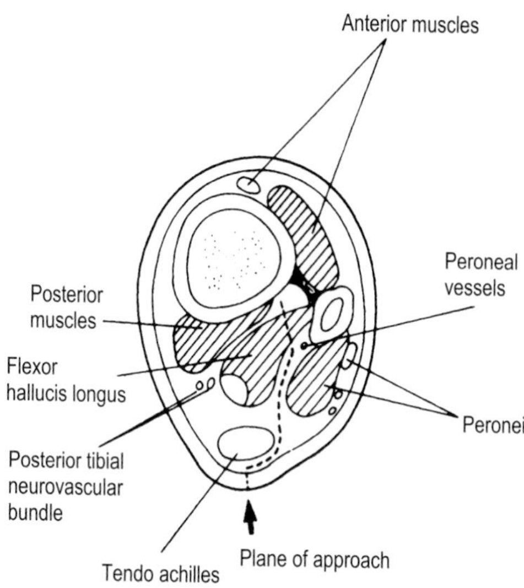

Fig. 38.9 Transverse section of the lower leg just above the ankle joint showing the posterolateral approach to the lower tibia along the dotted line.

3. Place the patient prone on the operating table with the foot hanging over the end.
4. Have an unscrubbed assistant hold the leg just distal to the flexed knee.
5. Clean the leg from the toes to the assistant's hands.
6. Grasp the foot in a stockinette and then drape the limb as described above.
7. Extend the knee and cover the trunk and thighs with a large sheet.

Access

1. Make an incision 15–20 cm long in the midline of the calf, ending at the calcaneum.
2. Expose the lateral side of the Achilles tendon, retracting the sural nerve and short saphenous vein laterally with the skin flap.
3. Deepen the incision through the fascia into a fat-filled space crossed by a branch of the peroneal artery; identify, doubly ligate and divide it.
4. Locate peroneus brevis laterally and flexor hallucis longus medially. Separate these muscles proximally, dividing part of the fibular attachment of flexor hallucis longus if necessary, taking care to preserve the peroneal vessels running down the back of the fibula.
5. Retract peroneus brevis laterally and flexor hallucis longus medially to expose the posterior aspect of the ankle joint and the distal tibia.

Closure

1. Release the tourniquet and stop the bleeding.
2. Insert a suction drain.

3 Close the deep fascia.

4 Close the skin.

REPAIR OF RUPTURED ACHILLES TENDON (Fig. 38.10)

Appraise

Ruptures of the Achilles tendon are frequently missed.

KEY POINTS Decisions

- There is a debate as to whether surgical repair of ruptured Achilles tendon is preferable to plaster immobilization.
- There is probably very little to choose between the two as far as the end result and re-rupture rate are concerned.
- Surgical repair may be preferable in young patients with sporting aspirations.
- If you decide on operation do not delay.
- If the diagnosis is delayed, wait to allow swelling and bruising to subside.
- If you have any doubt about the diagnosis, prefer to plaster the leg with the foot in full equinus for 8–10 weeks.

Prepare

1 Operate using general anaesthesia.

2 Exsanguinate the leg by elevation only, and apply a pneumatic tourniquet to the thigh.

3 Clean and drape the ankle for the posterior approach.

Action

1 Incise the skin in the midline from the mid-calf to the proximal transverse skin crease. Never use curved or flapped incisions (Fig. 38.10).

2 Carefully elevate the skin for 2 cm on either side of the midline and retract the skin gently with skin hooks.

3 Identify and retract the sural nerve and the short saphenous vein laterally.

4 Open the paratenon and expose the ends of the ruptured tendon, which are usually very ragged, like a shaving brush.

5 Plantar-flex the foot and insert an absorbable size 0 core suture in a modified Kessler pattern, as described in Chapter 36 for tendon suture (see also Fig. 36.8a). Pull the suture tight to close the gap in the tendon.

6 Insert a 4/0 running suture around the ragged ends of the repaired tendon and then suture the paratenon.

Closure

1 Release the tourniquet and stop the bleeding.

2 Insert a suction drain.

3 Suture the skin with fine interrupted subcuticular sutures and Steri-Strip tapes.

Aftercare

1 Apply a padded compression dressing with the ankle in full plantar flexion.

2 Apply a plaster-of-Paris slab to the front of the ankle from the upper tibia of the toes and bandage it in place. Elevate the leg.

3 Remove the drain and inspect the wound after 24–36 hours.

4 The skin overlying the tendo achilles has a tendency to heal badly and to slough. Avoid pressure over the wound by nursing the patient on the side.

5 Change the plaster at 10–14 days and inspect the wound. By this stage the skin should have healed; apply a below-knee plaster with the foot in full plantar flexion. Allow up non-weight-bearing.

6 At 2 weeks replaster the leg with the foot in 50% plantar flexion and again 2 weeks later with the foot in neutral position. Encourage full weight-bearing at this stage. Remove the plaster after a further 2 weeks and encourage ankle mobility.

7 Do not allow full sporting activities for at least 3 months after the repair.

RADICAL RESECTION OF THE NAIL BED (ZADEK'S OPERATION) (Fig. 38.11)

Appraise

1 This operation is suitable for chronic ingrowing toenails.

2 Do not undertake the operation in the presence of sepsis but merely remove the nail and wait for about 2 months until the sepsis has subsided.

3 Do not perform the operation in the presence of peripheral vascular disease.

Prepare

1 The operation may be performed under local ring-block anaesthesia with a rubber band as a digital tourniquet.

2 Clean and drape the lower leg and foot as described above, placing a shut-off towel around the instep.

Action

1 Remove the nail, if present, by separating it from the underlying nail bed with a MacDonald's elevator.

2 Make two incisions, 1 cm long, extending proximally from each corner of the nail to the transverse skin crease just distal to the interphalangeal joint.

3 Lift the skin and subcutaneous tissue as a flap and dissect this proximally.

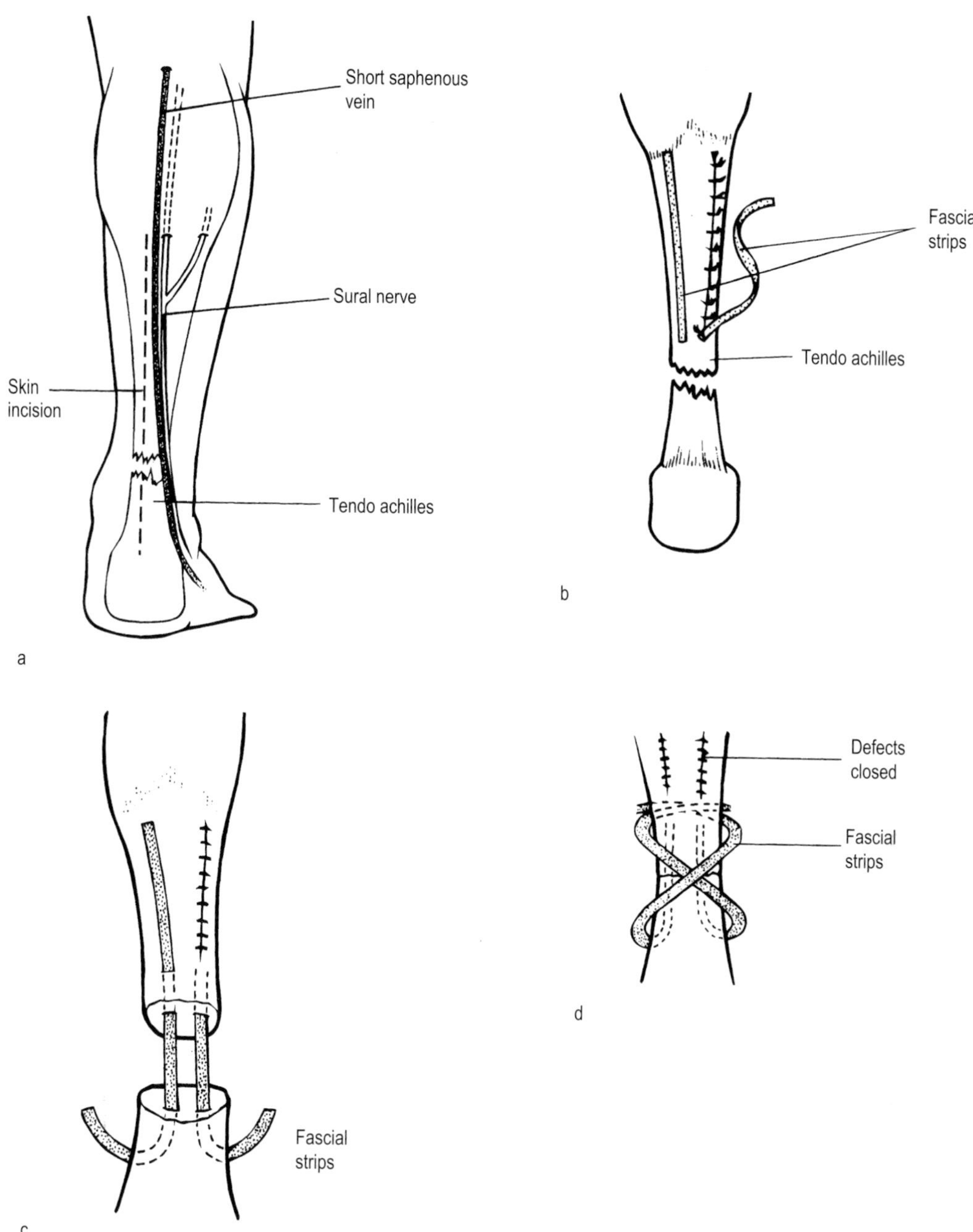

Fig. 38.10 Repair of ruptured Achilles tendon: (a) exposure; (b) turning down of fascial strips; (c) and (d) fascial darn.

4 Carry the dissection under the edges of the skin incisions on either side of the terminal phalanx to the midlateral line to complete the clearance of the germinal matrix of the nail.

5 Cut across the nail bed transversely at the site of the lunula (Latin: diminutive of *luna*=moon; the opaque whitish half-moon at the root of the nail) and join this transverse incision to the dissections under the nail folds.

6 Remove the block of nail bed from the surface of the proximal phalanx as far back as the insertion of the extensor tendon.

7 Check that you have not left behind any fragments of germinal matrix.

Closure

1 Draw the skin flap distally and carefully insert and tie one or two stitches to attach it to the nail bed. The tissues are fragile and the sutures easily cut out.

2 Close the incisions on either side.

Aftercare

1 Dress the wound with a non-adherent dressing.

2 Apply pressure with Tubigrip bandage.

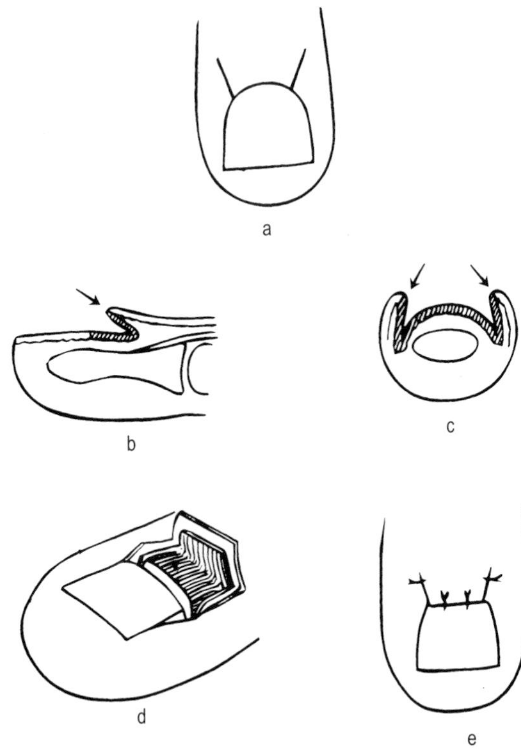

Fig. 38.11 Radical resection of the nail bed.

3 Release the tourniquet.

4 Elevate the foot for 24 hours.

5 Allow weight-bearing with or without crutches as pain permits.

6 Remove the dressings and the stitches after 12–14 days.

FURTHER READING

Antrum RN 1984 Radical excision of the nail fold for ingrowing toenails. Journal of Bone and Joint Surgery 6B:63–65

Henry AK 1957 Extensile exposure applied to limb surgery, 2nd edn. E&S Livingstone, Edinburgh

Müller ME, Allgöwer M, Schneider R et al 1979 Manual of internal fixation. Techniques recommended by the AO group, 2nd edn. Springer-Verlag, Berlin

Nistor L 1981 Surgical and non-surgical treatment of Achilles tendon rupture. Journal of Bone and Joint Surgery 63A:394–399

Rorabeck CH, Bourne RB, Fowler PJ 1983 The surgical treatment of exertional compartment syndrome in athletes. Journal of Bone and Joint Surgery 65A:1245–1251

Zadik FR 1950 Obliteration of the nail bed of the great toe without shortening the terminal phalanx. Journal of Bone and Joint Surgery 32B:66–67

Plastic surgery

M.D. Brough, P. Butler

CONTENTS

GENERAL PRINCIPLES

Plastic surgery (Greek: *plassein* = to mould) is concerned with the restoration of form and function of the human body. It is used in the repair and reconstruction of defects following damage or loss of tissue from injury or disease or from their treatment. It is used in the correction of congenital deformities. It also includes aesthetic or cosmetic surgery, which involves the treatment of developmental or naturally acquired changes in the body.

There have been many advances in plastic surgery in recent years, giving rise to a multitude of new methods of reconstruction. These include improved techniques in microsurgery, tissue expansion, liposuction and craniofacial surgery. The most important development has been the recognition and application of axial pattern flaps. Several hundred cutaneous, myocutaneous and other flaps have now been identified but only those used more commonly will be described in this chapter.

Prepare

KEY POINTS Planning repair

- Plan for repair and reconstruction of tissue defects well in advance of operation.
- Carry out the simplest procedure to achieve wound healing.
- If you need to reconstruct a defect in stages ensure that one stage does not jeopardize a subsequent one.

1 In the region of the proposed operation, identify the lines of tension within the skin described by the Professor of Anatomy in Vienna, Carl Ritter von Langer (1819–1887). Try to make all incisions parallel to these lines. When this is not possible, consider using a Z-plasty or local flap in closing the wound to help prevent the formation of scar contracture postoperatively.

2 When planning a large flap or a sophisticated reconstruction, mark out a plan of the flap on the patient with a skin marker the day before operation. For smaller flaps and simple incisions, mark out the area of incision on the patient after preparing the area, before incising the skin. Use a fine pen and ink for marking out the lines of incisions on the face. Use a broad proprietary marking pen in other areas. Try to follow these lines, as they provide a useful guide once the skin has been incised and tension in the surrounding skin has changed. Be prepared, however, to make adjustments on occasions according to the circumstances.

3 While general anaesthesia is now very safe, do not forget that many operations can be carried out under regional anaesthesia or local anaesthesia (see Ch. 2). Many operations on the hand, for example, can be performed under regional anaesthesia, including cases of replantation. Large areas of split skin graft can be taken from the lateral aspect of the thigh by infiltrating the lateral cutaneous nerve of the thigh in the region of the inguinal ligament with local anaesthetic. Many other procedures can be carried out under regional anaesthesia, if necessary with the assistance of a sedative. Many simple skin lesions can be excised under local anaesthesia with 1% lidocaine. To excise small lesions in the head and neck region, where the skin is highly vascular, use 2% lidocaine with 1:80000 adrenaline (epinephrine). Wait 5 minutes after injecting the mixture, to provide a relatively avascular field as well as anaesthesia. When carrying out extensive excisions of the face or scalp under

general anaesthesia, inject a dilute solution of 0.5% lidocaine with 1:200000 adrenaline (epinephrine).

Technique

Sutures

1 On the face, approximate the deep dermis of the skin edges with interrupted 5/0 polyglactin 910 sutures. Accurately appose the skin edges with 6/0 interrupted nylon sutures. Remove them on the third or fourth postoperative day. If they remain longer, suture marks form which may prove impossible to remove without producing a more ugly scar.

2 Elsewhere on the body, approximate the deep dermis of the wound edges with 3/0 polyglactin 910 sutures and use subcuticular polypropylene sutures whenever possible, tying a knot at either end to prevent slipping. Leave these sutures in for 10 days or longer if there is a tendency for the scar to stretch because of its site.

Instruments

1 Respect tissues and their viability by handling them with care and using the appropriate instruments. Control and steady the skin with skin hooks or fine-toothed forceps. Do not crush it by grasping it with non-toothed forceps.

2 For accurate suturing, use a fine needle-holder with a clasp that feels comfortable. Practise using needle-holders with their own cutting edges for cutting sutures so you can use them effectively. They are particularly useful when you are inserting many interrupted sutures, the accuracy of which is not crucial to the overall result.

3 Microvascular surgery requires specialized instruments.

Drains

1 For general principles see Chapter 1.

2 When moving large flaps introduce large suction drains at the donor site, which has a large potential cavity.

Diathermy

1 Beware of unipolar diathermy when coagulating vessels near the skin. The burnt tissue may be visible and painful.

2 Always use a bipolar coagulator for fine work and flaps. The current from a unipolar machine could destroy the vessels in the base of a flap as it is being raised.

SKIN COVER

1 Close skin wounds primarily to provide ideal skin cover following incisions of the skin, excisions of skin lesions and simple lacerations.

2 Use split skin grafts to repair wounds with significant skin loss, to avoid skin closure with tension, or following trauma with an appreciable degree of crush injury to the local tissues. Skin graft survival depends on adequate vascularity of the base of the wound.

3 Use skin flaps, which carry their own blood supply and are temporarily self-sufficient, in primary or secondary repair or reconstruction. Use them as primary cover for vital structures such as exposed neurovascular bundles or for structures that have an inadequate blood supply to support a graft, such as bare bone, bare cartilage, bare tendons and exposed joints.

SKIN CLOSURE

Appraise

1 Employ primary skin closure following simple skin incisions, surgical excision of small skin lesions and to repair simple lacerations.

2 Do not carry out primary closure if the tension in closing the wound causes blanching of the skin.

Action

1 Whenever possible, make incisions following the direction of the tension lines, particularly on the face.

2 For excisions, mark the skin in ink, planning to excise the minimal necessary amount of tissue. Draw an ellipse with pointed ends around this mark, parallel to the tension lines (Fig. 39.1a).

3 On the face, inject the surrounding tissue with 2% lidocaine and 1:80000 adrenaline (epinephrine), and wait 5 minutes for both components to take effect.

4 Make a vertical cut through the skin along the lines of the ellipse. Ensure that you adequately clear the lesion in depth.

5 Undermine the skin edges beneath the layer of subcutaneous fat to facilitate approximating the edges without tension (Fig. 39.1b).

KEY POINTS Skin viable?

- If the skin edges have been crushed, do not further insult them by inserting sutures, but carefully trim away dead skin and apply a simple dressing. Close the skin after a delay of 24-48 hours.
- Beware of skin that has been degloved or torn from its fascial base. Resect it primarily.
- If damaged skin is possibly viable, replace it, re-examine it at 48 hours, and then resect it if it does not bleed when it is cut.

6 Place a skin hook in each end of the wound and ask your assistant to draw them apart. This manoeuvre approximates the edges (Fig. 39.1c).

7 Close the wound in layers.

8 Apply a small dressing, or use no dressing at all if practical.

SKIN GRAFTS

Appraise

1 A skin graft (Greek: *graphion*=a style; something inserted) is a piece of skin detached from its donor site and transferred to a recipient site. It may contain part of the thickness of the skin

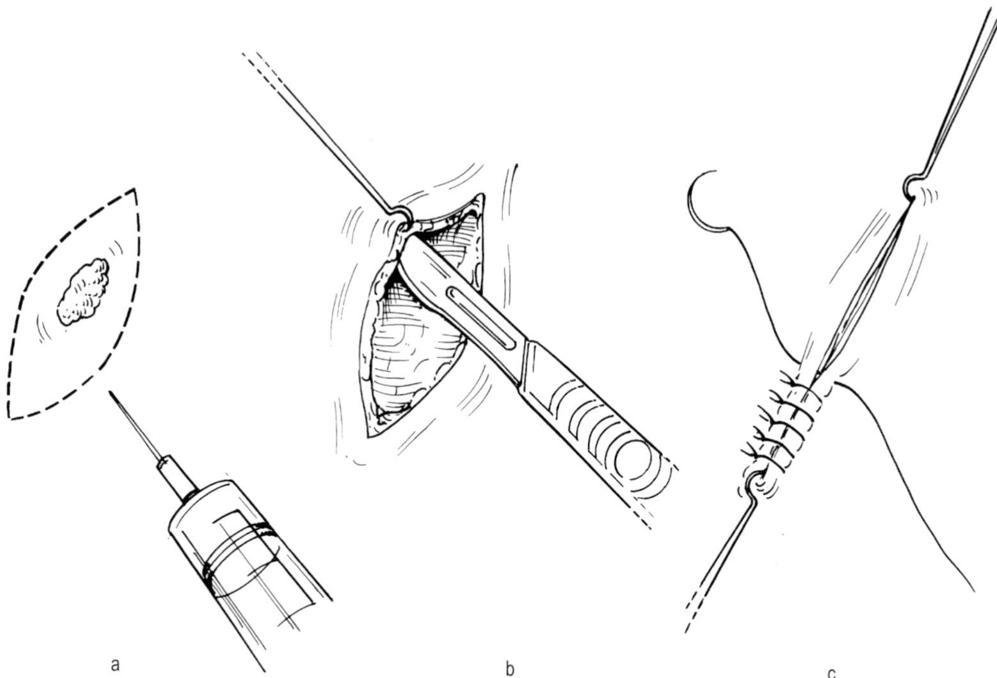

Fig. 39.1 Simple excision of skin lesion: (a) the skin is marked and surrounding skin infiltrated with local anaesthetic; (b) undermining the lateral skin margin; (c) the wound ends are distracted with skin hooks to help approximate the edges of the wound.

(a split skin graft described by the German surgeon Karl Thiersch in 1874) or the full-thickness graft of skin, described in 1874 by the Austrian ophthalmologist John Wolfe, who settled in Glasgow.

2 A skin graft depends for its survival on receiving adequate nutrition from the recipient bed. Thus, thin split skin grafts survive more readily than thick split skin grafts or full-thickness grafts.

3 If there is a poor vascular bed, or infection, no graft will survive. In these cases prepare the graft bed appropriately with dressings (see below), or consider using a flap.

4 Choose an appropriate donor site for each individual patient.

SMALL SPLIT SKIN GRAFT

Appraise

1 A split skin graft is a sheet of tissue containing epidermis and some dermis taken from a donor site. It is obtained by shaving the skin with an appropriate knife or blade. A layer of deep dermis is preserved at the donor site and, when dressed appropriately, this is re-epithelialized from residual skin adnexae.

2 Use a small split skin graft to repair traumatic loss of small areas of skin from the hand or fingers, and occasionally in other parts of the body. Avoid using them on the tips of the thumb and index fingers since they tend to become hyperaesthetic.

3 Choose the donor site carefully. On the upper limb prefer skin from the medial aspect of the arm where the donor site is inconspicuous; on the forearm an ugly resultant scar may be visible.

Action

1 Mark out on the medial aspect of the arm an area of skin which is more than sufficient to cover the recipient site.

2 Inject 2% lidocaine and 1:80 000 adrenaline (epinephrine) intradermally into and beyond the marked area and wait for 5 minutes.

3 Lubricate the marked area with liquid paraffin.

4 Grip the arm on the lateral aspect with your left hand so that the skin which is marked out becomes tense, with a convex surface.

5 Cut the graft from the marked area using a Da Silva knife (Fig. 39.2).

6 Dress the donor site with a calcium alginate dressing, one layer of paraffin gauze, several layers of dressing gauze and a crepe bandage.

7 Apply the split skin graft directly on to the recipient site, spread it and anchor it using a minimal number of sutures.

8 Apply paraffin gauze, dressing gauze and a crepe bandage.

9 Re-dress the graft at 5 days.

10 Re-dress the graft donor site at 10 days.

LARGE SPLIT SKIN GRAFT

Appraise

1 Use these grafts following extensive skin loss from burns, trauma or radical excisional surgery.

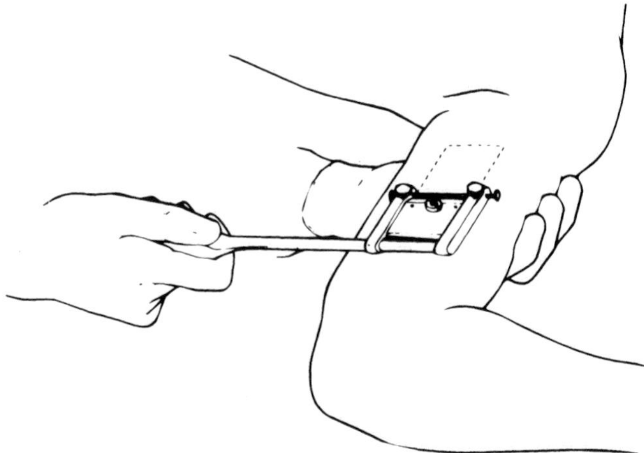

Fig. 39.2 Taking a small split skin graft with a Da Silva knife.

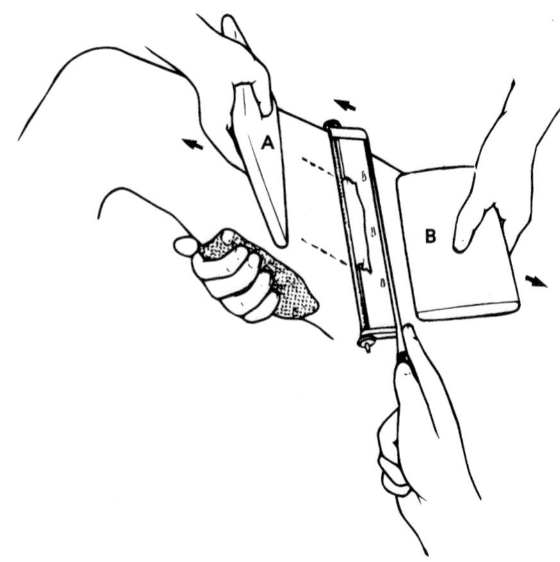

Fig. 39.3 Taking a large split skin graft from the thigh, the surgeon advances board A in front of the knife as it progresses along the thigh. The assistant tenses the skin of the thigh in his right hand, using a large swab to prevent his hand from slipping, and tenses the skin behind the knife using board B.

2 Adequately prepare the recipient site to ensure a good 'take' of the graft. Grafts take best on exposed muscle or well-prepared granulation tissue. They do not reliably survive on exposed fat where there is a poor vascular supply.

3 The take of a graft can be improved in certain circumstances by meshing it, quilting it, or by delaying its application and then exposing it. These are described below.

4 Use an electric dermatome, if available, to harvest the graft using the same principles outlined below.

Prepare

1 Following 'cold' surgical excisions apply pressure to obtain haemostasis. Avoid diathermy if possible since skin grafts do not take over diathermy burns.

2 Where subcutaneous fat is exposed, suture the overlying skin down to the muscle or deep fascia to cover it.

3 For infected wounds, take swabs for bacterial culture and prepare the recipient site with dressings of Eusol (Edinburgh University solution of lime) and paraffin. Change them 3–4 times a day. The recipient site is ready to receive a graft when it appears healthy and compact and has red granulation tissue with minimal exudate.

KEY POINTS Haemolytic streptococci

- Do not apply grafts in the presence of beta-haemolytic streptococci, group A.
- First eradicate the infection with regular dressing changes and appropriate systemic antibiotics.

4 Choose the donor site most readily available to provide a large area of skin graft; this is usually the thigh. In young people, use the inner aspect of the thigh, where the donor site will be hidden. In elderly people, use the outer aspect of the thigh, where the skin is slightly thicker, so that if healing is delayed the wound is accessible and is easily managed.

Action

1 Prepare both recipient and donor sites by applying skin antiseptic.

2 Have your assistant spread a large swab on the side of the thigh opposite to the proposed donor site. With a hand on the swab it is possible to support the thigh and tense the skin at the donor site by gripping the skin firmly with the swab.

3 Set the blade on the Watson knife to take the appropriate thickness of skin graft. Use a medium setting at first and then adjust it accordingly.

4 Apply liquid paraffin on a swab to the donor site and along the knife blade.

5 Ask your assistant to hold the edge of a graft board at the starting point with the other hand (Fig. 39.3).

6 Cut a skin graft with the Watson knife, holding a board in your non-cutting hand and advancing this a few centimetres in front of the knife. Start with the knife at 45° to the skin and once the blade has entered the dermis rotate it axially so that it runs just parallel with the skin surface. Use a 'sawing' action with the knife, advancing the blade only a few millimetres at a time. When you have harvested an adequate length of skin, turn the blade upwards and cut the graft off with one firm movement. If the graft is not detached with this movement, cut along its base with a pair of scissors.

7 Place the skin graft, outer surface downwards, on a damp saline swab and make sure that you have obtained sufficient skin; in case of doubt, take another strip of split skin.

8 Dress the donor site with calcium alginate dressing, one layer of paraffin gauze, dressing gauze, cotton wool and a crepe bandage.

9 Apply the skin graft to the recipient defect, ensuring that it is placed with its cut surface applied to the wound. The outer surface is opaque, the inner surface is shiny. Spread it, using two pairs of closed non-toothed forceps.

10 Cut off the surplus skin at the wound edge, leaving a margin of 3 mm around the periphery.

11 If the skin has been applied on a site to which you can apply a satisfactory compression dressing, do not use sutures.

12 Dress with several layers of paraffin gauze, dressing gauze, wool and crepe bandage, immobilizing the joints above and below the graft with a bulky dressing.

13 In areas where it is difficult to apply a compression dressing, immobilize the graft with interrupted sutures at the edge or insert a circumferential continuous suture around the graft.

14 Dress with paraffin gauze, dressing gauze, wool and strips of adhesive dressing.

15 Keep the graft site elevated postoperatively.

16 For grafts on the lower limb below the knee, do not allow the grafted area to be dependent for 7 days; fluid will collect between the graft and the base unless the graft is meshed. Then arrange progressive mobilization with compression support to the leg and foot including the graft.

DELAYED EXPOSED GRAFTS

Appraise

1 Use a delayed graft when the graft in its recipient site can be exposed indefinitely by the patient without being disturbed.

2 Apply a delayed graft to surgical wounds when haemostasis is difficult to establish peroperatively. Since the graft is exposed, it can be monitored regularly to ensure that it has taken.

Action

1 Prepare the recipient site during the operation to excise all dead or doubtful tissue and any foreign material, after achieving haemostasis.

2 Dress with several layers of paraffin gauze, dressing gauze, wool and a crepe bandage.

3 Harvest large split skin grafts adequate to cover the defect and dress the donor site (see below).

4 Spread the split skin graft on paraffin gauze with the external opaque surface on the gauze. Fold and wrap this in a saline-soaked swab and place it in a sterile jar to be stored in a refrigerator at 4°C.

5 On the following day, remove the dressing from the recipient site.

6 Apply the skin graft to the defect and spread it to cover all areas. Trim and store any excess skin at the margin.

7 Remove the paraffin gauze and leave the skin graft exposed.

8 Observe the graft at regular intervals. If serum collects beneath it, roll this out with cotton wool budded sticks soaked in saline, either to the edge or through a small incision made in the graft.

9 Be sure that the exposed area is well protected from any injury, particularly while the patient is asleep.

MESHED GRAFTS

Appraise

1 Meshed grafts are useful for providing skin cover to large areas, particularly when there is limited availability of donor skin, as often occurs in extensive burns.

2 They survive more reliably, as any underlying seroma that collects escapes through the interstices of the graft, leaving the graft elements intact.

3 They are effective in covering irregular surfaces as they can be moulded to these.

4 Unfortunately the resultant appearance is less satisfactory than a sheet graft.

Action

1 Prepare the donor site in the usual way.

2 Harvest long, thin strips of split skin graft, as described above.

3 Dress the donor site.

4 Pass the skin graft through the skin mesher. It may need to be placed on a carrier for this, depending on the type of instrument (Fig. 39.4).

5 Apply the mesh graft directly on to the recipient site using two pairs of non-toothed forceps.

6 Spread the skin out appropriately to cover all suitable recipient areas.

7 Suture the graft with continuous sutures at the periphery only if the area is difficult to dress.

8 Dress the area with a calcium alginate dressing, one layer of paraffin gauze, dressing gauze, cotton wool and crepe bandage.

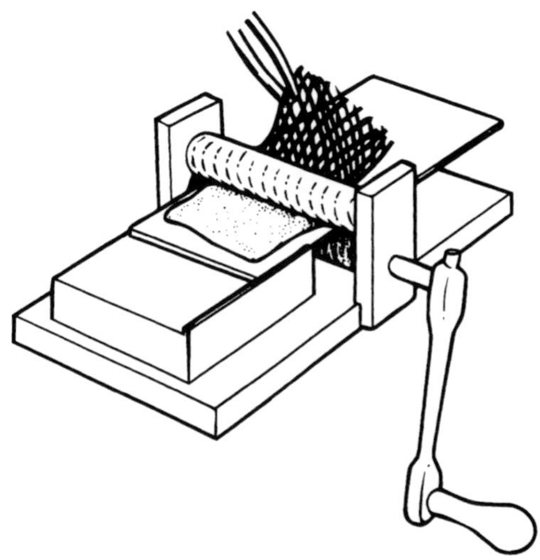

Fig. 39.4 Meshing a split skin graft. The skin graft has been placed on a plastic carrier and is being passed through the skin mesher. The cut skin, elevated at one corner by a pair of forceps, can be stretched to three times its original size or more, depending on the carrier used.

9 Re-dress at 4 or 5 days.

10 Continue to re-dress at approximately 3-day intervals until the interstices have epithelialized.

QUILTED GRAFTS

Appraise

These are most usefully applied to large areas of the tongue or any other highly vascular area. Any method of graft fixation is liable to cause bleeding beneath the graft. However, at each suture site a small area of graft take is ensured, and epithelialization subsequently spreads out from each of these.

Action

1 Prepare the donor site.

2 Harvest the skin graft.

3 Put two large sutures in the anterior aspect of the tongue and pull it forwards.

4 Apply the skin graft to the tongue and trim the excess at the edges.

5 Place multiple 3/0 absorbable sutures at the edge of the graft and throughout its surface (Fig. 39.5).

6 No dressing is required.

7 Remove the traction sutures.

FULL-THICKNESS GRAFTS

Appraise

1 These give better cosmetic results than split thickness grafts as they contract less. The quality of the skin is better but they need a very good vascular bed in order to survive.

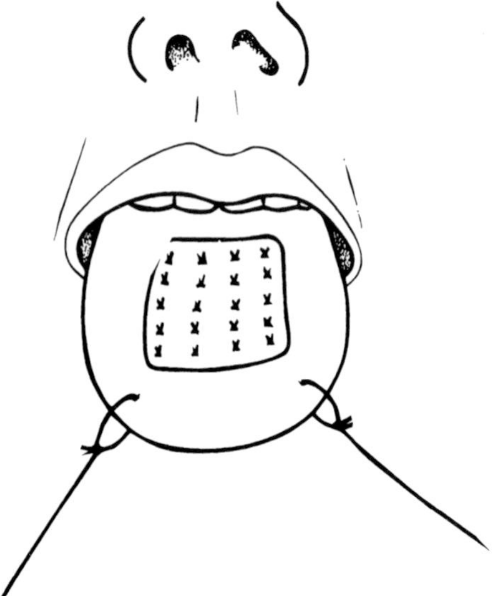

Fig. 39.5 Quilted graft. The graft is fixed to a defect on the dorsum of the tongue with multiple sutures.

2 Their most common application is on the face following excision of small lesions, and the best results are achieved in the eyelid region and around the medial canthus.

3 They can occasionally be used on the hand, but are not generally used elsewhere, as large grafts leave a large primary defect.

4 The best donor sites are those with surplus skin so that the skin can be closed primarily with an insignificant scar. The most common donor areas are post-auricular, pre-auricular, upper eyelid, nasolabial and supraclavicular skin.

Action

1 Mark the area of skin to be removed and measure it.

2 Mark out a similar area in the donor site, allowing an extra 2.5 mm or more at each margin for the contour difference that will be present at the recipient site.

3 Plan an ellipse at the donor site around the proposed graft to allow primary closure.

4 Inject local anaesthetic at the excision and donor sites.

5 Create the defect at the recipient site.

6 With a size 15 blade, cut around the margins of the planned donor skin.

7 Raise the full ellipse of skin and subcutaneous tissue.

8 Undermine the skin edges at the donor defect and close this primarily.

9 Place the skin graft on to a wet saline swab, skin surface down.

10 Using small, curved scissors, cut the subcutaneous fat off the skin graft and excise the redundant skin.

11 Place the skin graft into the defect and suture the edges at the periphery. Leave the suture ends long.

12 Use tie-over sutures to fix the dressing of paraffin gauze and proflavine wool.

13 Apply a pressure dressing for 24 hours, if possible.

14 Dress the donor site.

15 Plan to re-dress the recipient site at 1 week.

COMPOSITE GRAFTS

Appraise

1 Composite grafts consist of skin and other tissue, usually subcutaneous fat and some underlying cartilage.

2 They are most commonly used where there is significant loss of a nostril rim.

3 Occasionally, they are used for defects at the periphery of the pinna.

Action

1 Mark out the defect that will be left after excision of diseased or damaged skin, with if necessary excision of traumatized or contaminated wound edges.

2 Identify a site on either pinna that corresponds in both size and shape to the planned defect.

3 Mark out this area with ink.

4 Prepare both ears.

5 Plan the reconstruction of the donor defect.

6 Inject 0.5% lidocaine and 1:200 000 adrenaline (epinephrine) into both sites and wait for 5 minutes.

RANDOM PATTERN SKIN FLAPS

Introduction

1 Skin flaps are used to repair or reconstruct defects where there is an inadequate blood supply to support a skin graft. They survive on their own blood supply which they bring with them and this may be beneficial to the recipient site. It may help by introducing a new blood supply to an avascular area following irradiation, or to a fracture site where there is delayed union.

2 The quality of the skin in a skin flap is almost normal and its texture and cosmetic appearance are much better than a graft. A skin flap may, however, lose its nerve supply and have its vascular supply and lymphatic drainage partly compromised in the transfer.

3 Until relatively recently, all skin flaps were based on a random vascular pattern. It was recognized that flaps with a length greater than their base would survive in certain areas. It is now realized that the reason for this survival is that these flaps had, unknowingly, been based on an axial pattern basis. If a flap is designed around a recognized artery and vein, with these vessels passing down its central axis, it may be safely transferred with a very large length-to-breadth ratio. Indeed, the breadth need be the artery and vein alone, providing they remain patent.

4 Many of the superficial muscles of the body have one principal vascular hilum, and these muscles can be rotated about the hilum on a single pedicle. It has further been realized that the skin overlying these superficial muscles receives its vascular supply from them. Consequently the muscle with its overlying skin can be transposed as a single unit, forming a myocutaneous flap. A large number of these flaps have been described, but the more commonly used ones alone will be described below.

5 Special terms are traditionally used in relation to flaps. Delay indicates partial division of a flap at its base and re-suturing. This procedure encourages an improved blood supply to the flap from the opposite attachment. Complete division at the base carried out a few days later is then usually safe. After a flap has been transferred safely, the bridging portion may be divided. The two ends are trimmed and one is sutured into the new recipient area while the other is replaced in the donor site. This is referred to as in-setting.

6 When planning a flap, it is useful to employ a sheet of sterile paper or other similar material to act as a template. This can be cut to shape and used as a trial flap.

Z-PLASTY

Appraise

1 Z-plasties are used for releasing linear contractions. These usually develop along linear scars that traverse Langer's lines.

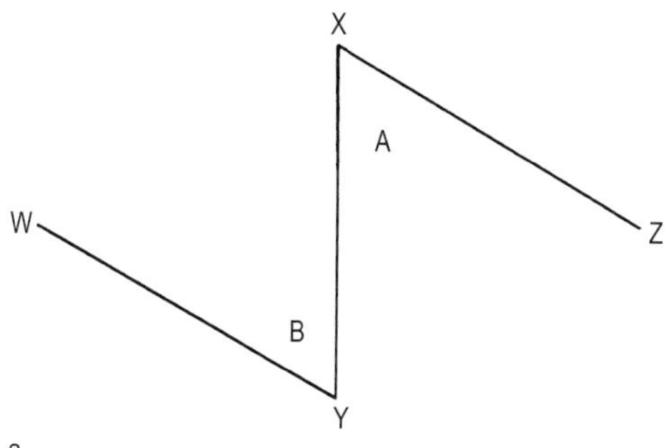

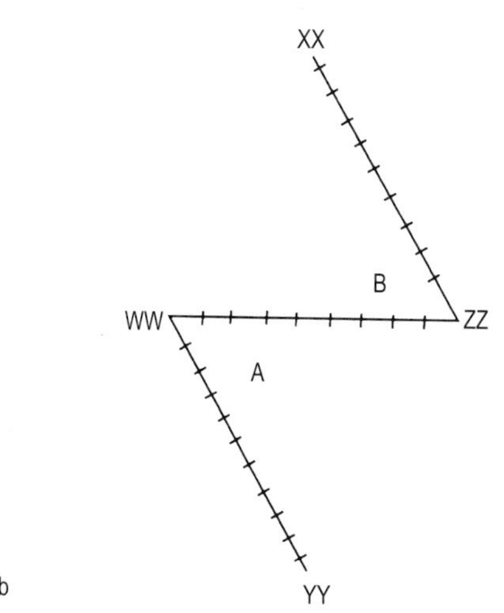

Fig. 39.6 Z-plasty. Contracture along X–Y is released to XX–YY by raising and interchanging flaps A and B. The distance W–Z is shortened to WW–ZZ.

2 These linear contractions are often most evident when crossing the concavity of the flexor aspect of a joint, but they can occur on extensor surfaces and in other areas unrelated to joints.

KEY POINT Breadth taken into length

- In effect, skin is drawn in from the sides to increase the length.

Action

1 Draw a line along the full extent of the contracture (Fig. 39.6).

2 From one end, draw a line at 60° to the first line and of the same length.

3 From the opposite end, draw a line at 60° on the opposite side of the line for the same length.

4 Incise along the central line and excise any scar tissue.

5 Incise along the two lateral lines through the full thickness of skin and subcutaneous tissue.

6 Raise the flaps so formed, lifting the skin and subcutaneous tissue as one, holding the tip of each flap with a skin hook.

7 Interchange the two skin flaps.

8 If the flaps do not meet comfortably, undermine the skin and subcutaneous tissue around the periphery of the wound to allow them to lie correctly.

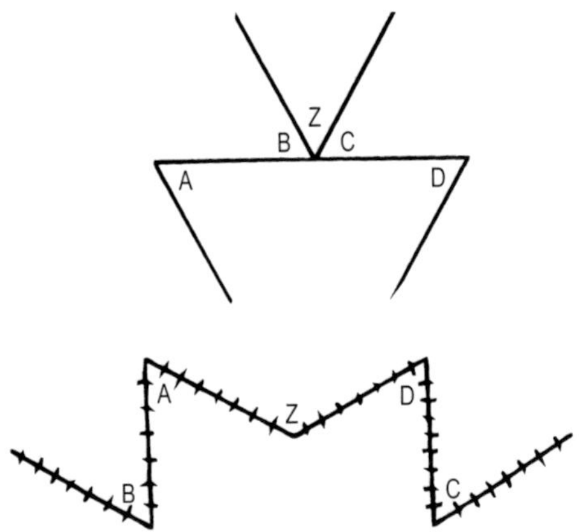

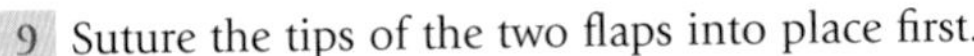

Fig. 39.7 W-plasty. This consists of two Z-plasties along the same contracture placed in reverse direction and meeting at the central point. Flaps A and B are interposed and flaps C and D are interposed. Flap Z stays in the same place but is raised during surgery to permit undermining at its base to allow it to stretch.

9. Suture the tips of the two flaps into place first.
10. Suture the remaining edges of the flaps.
11. Dress the wound.

Technical points

1. The angle of the Z-plasty can be varied according to circumstances.
2. If the scar contracture is particularly long, use two or more Z-plasties, either in series or at intervals along the length of the contracture.
3. For scar contractures across a web space, use a W-plasty (Fig. 39.7). This consists of two Z-plasties, placed in reverse direction to each other, meeting at the base of the web space.

TRANSPOSITION FLAP

Appraise

1. Small transposition flaps on the face have long been used. It is well recognized, that in this region, because of the vascularity of the skin, flaps with a large length-to-breadth ratio can be used safely.
2. Transposition flaps allow skin from an area of abundance to be moved to a defect where primary closure is inappropriate.
3. On the face, there is an abundance of skin appropriate for transposition flaps in the nasolabial area, the glabellar area and the upper eyelid.
4. In other parts of the body, many axial pattern flaps are used as transposition flaps.

Action

1. Mark out the defect in ink.
2. Plan the transposition flap in an adjacent area with superfluous skin and mark this out (Fig. 39.8).

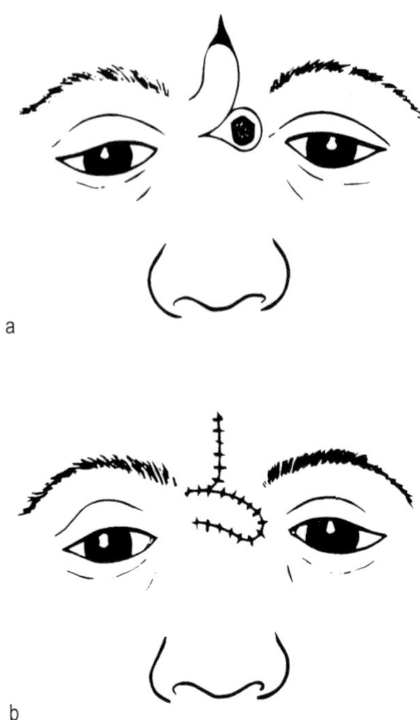

Fig. 39.8 Transposition flap. A lesion in the region of the medial canthus is excised and a transposition flap from the glabellar region is used to reconstruct the defect. A small triangle of skin at the apex of the flap is discarded and the donor site is closed primarily.

3. Check that the margin of the flap most distal from the defect is long enough from the fulcrum at its base to reach the most distal part of the defect. This is the limiting factor of the flap.
4. Excise the lesion to create the defect.
5. Raise the flap, including skin and subcutaneous tissue, and support the tip of the flap on a skin hook.
6. Transpose the flap into the defect and check that it fits.
7. Undermine the edges of the donor site defect and also the edges of the excision area to allow the flap to sit more comfortably in the defect.
8. Close the donor defect in layers.
9. Suture the flap in place.
10. Leave the flap exposed if possible, so you can monitor it.

Rhomboid flap

Appraise

1. A rhomboid flap is, as its name suggests, a flap with the shape of an equilateral parallelogram—a lozenge shape.
2. The rhomboid flap is most useful when the appropriate ellipse for excision of a defect is at right-angles to Langer's lines. It has a similar effect to a transposition flap carried through 90°.

Action

1. Mark out the area of the defect.
2. Around this, draw the smallest possible rhomboid with equal sides.

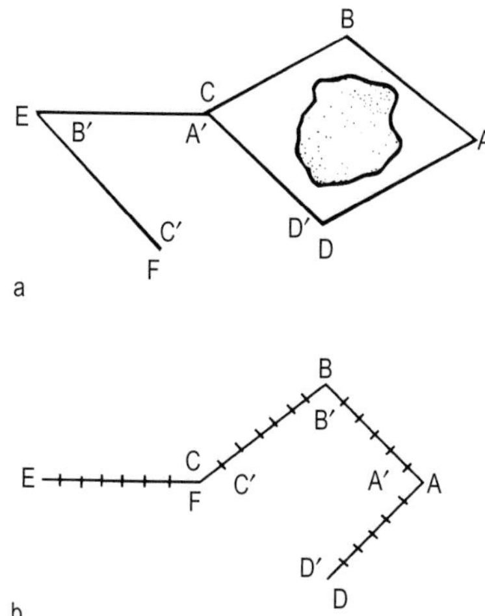

Fig. 39.9 Rhomboid flap. A rhomboid defect is created: ABCD. CE and EF are drawn with equal length, making a smaller rhomboid: A′B′C′D′. After transposition of the flap to the defect, the donor defect is closed primarily by approximating F to C.

3 Draw two further lines of equal length as shown in Fig. 39.9.

4 Excise the lesion.

5 Transpose the flap, as shown in the diagram.

6 Undermine the edges.

7 Close the donor defect.

8 Suture the flap in place.

ROTATION FLAP

Appraise

1 These are large flaps used to close relatively small defects.

2 They use excess skin at a distance from the defect and borrow small amounts of skin from a large area.

3 They are principally used to borrow skin from the neck to take up to the face. They can be used on the scalp and for treating sacral pressure sores.

Action

1 Mark out the skin defect.

2 Draw an isosceles triangle around the defect, with the apex of the triangle at or pointing towards the centre of the arc of rotation of the flap (Fig. 39.10).

3 Draw the arc of the rotation flap.

4 Raise the skin and subcutaneous tissue of the flap.

5 Undermine the skin at the edge of the defect and along the skin margin opposite the flap.

6 Rotate the flap into the defect.

7 Suture the flap.

8 If necessary, excise a wedge of tissue along the skin edge opposite the flap to assist rotation. If necessary, 'cut-back' into the flap at the opposite end of the arc of the flap from the defect, to create a better fit.

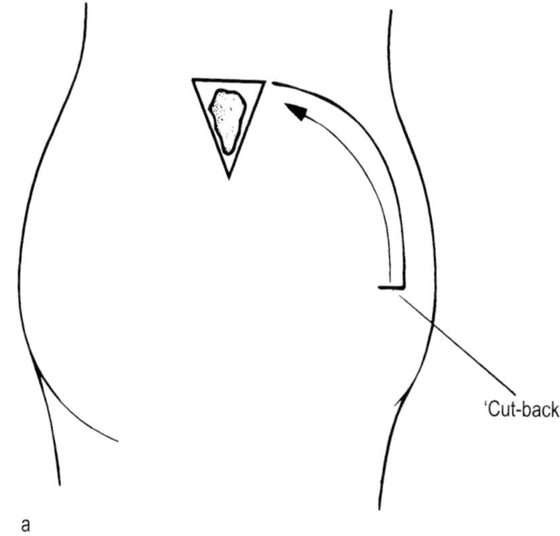

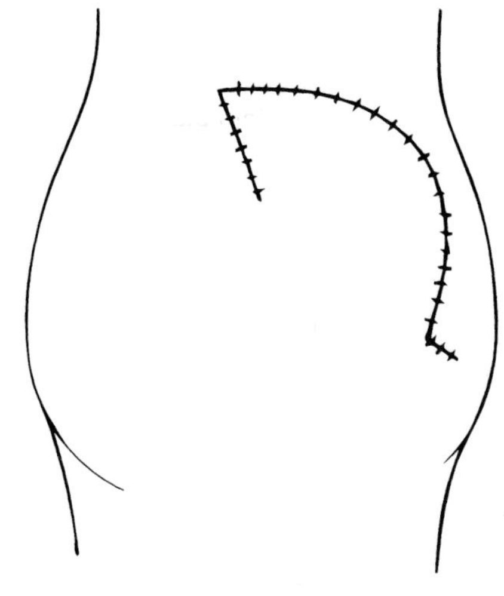

Fig. 39.10 Rotation flap. A sacral ulcer is created into a triangular defect and a flap from the buttock is rotated into this. A small cut-back allows greater mobility in rotation.

ADVANCEMENT FLAP

Appraise

1 Advancement flaps are most commonly used on the face to preserve feature lines or structures of the face.

2 They can be used on the forehead or for defects of the eyebrow. Frequently, in these situations, bilateral advancement flaps are used simultaneously to reconstruct one defect.

Action

1 Mark out the defect.

2 Mark out the smallest possible square or rectangle enclosing this defect, with lines parallel and at right-angles to Langer's lines.

3 Extend the marks of the sides running parallel to Langer's lines in each direction from the defect, thus delineating two flaps (Fig. 39.11).

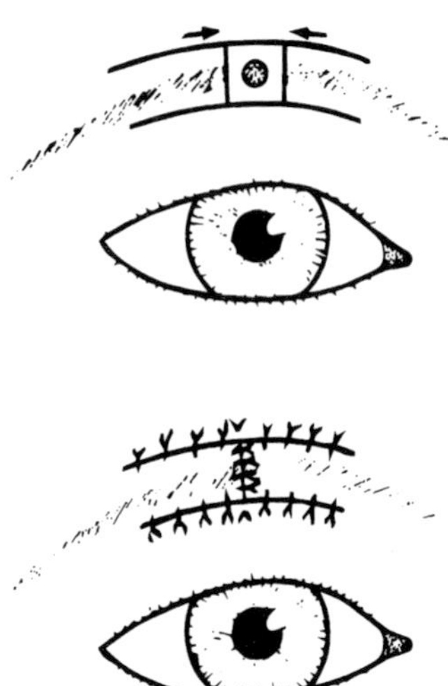

Fig. 39.11 Advancement flap. A defect in the eyebrow is excised and two advancement flaps, one from each side, are raised and advanced to meet each other over the defect. The natural lines of the eyebrow are preserved.

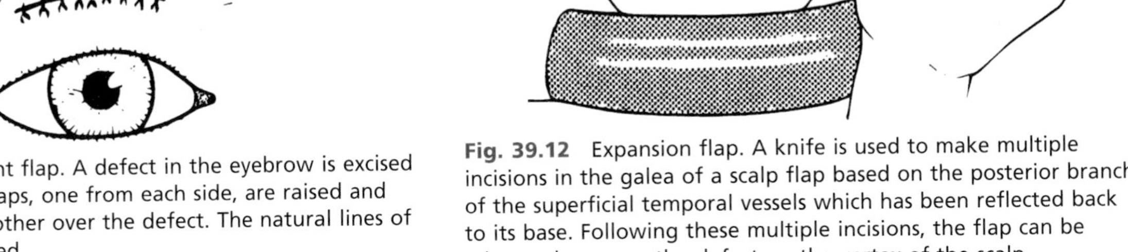

Fig. 39.12 Expansion flap. A knife is used to make multiple incisions in the galea of a scalp flap based on the posterior branch of the superficial temporal vessels which has been reflected back to its base. Following these multiple incisions, the flap can be advanced to cover the defect on the vertex of the scalp.

4 Create the defect.

5 Elevate the flaps and advance them towards each other.

6 Suture them together.

7 Suture their sides.

EXPANSION FLAP

Appraise

1 These flaps are used specifically for repairing and reconstructing defects of the scalp.

2 Flaps on the scalp are notorious for their inability to stretch because of the inelasticity of the galea (Latin: =a helmet).

3 Division of the galea allows some stretching of the skin to take place, especially in younger patients.

Prepare

1 Pay particular attention to the preoperative planning of the flap. Remember that the scalp flap will move in three dimensions.

2 Shave the patient's hair over the whole scalp to a length of 1 cm. Leave long locks of hair only if you can confidently cope with these during the operation.

3 Make a careful plan of the flap to be used, and mark the outline of this.

4 Completely shave the hair for 1 cm on either side of this line and for 1 cm around the outline of the defect.

5 Wash the hair thoroughly to remove all cut and shaved hairs.

Action

1 Place the patient, face downwards, on the operating table. Use a neurosurgical head-rest to support the head, if this is available.

2 Mark out the defect on the scalp.

3 Mark out the flap as previously planned. The flap may be of transposition, rotational or advancement design.

4 Plan a wide base to the flap around the periphery of the scalp to ensure that at least one principal vascular system enters its base.

5 Inject the planned outline of the flap with 0.5% lidocaine and 1:200000 adrenaline (epinephrine) and wait at least for 5 minutes.

6 Excise the lesion and create the defect.

7 Incise along the margins of the flap to elevate it with the underlying galea so that this is included with the flap.

8 Reflect the flap backwards, exposing the galea.

9 Support the flap on the palm of the hand and make multiple incisions just through the galea with a no. 15 blade across the full width of the flap (Fig. 39.12).

10 Identify the principal vessels beneath the surface of the galea and avoid dividing them.

11 Make multiple transverse incisions at right-angles to the first set along the whole length of the flap.

12 Reflect the flap back into the defect.

13 Suture the flap into place with one layer of 3/0 silk or nylon.

14 Always insert suction drains under the flap.

15 Dress with paraffin gauze, dressing gauze, cotton wool and crepe bandages.

16 Re-dress after 48 hours and, if possible, leave exposed.

CROSS-LEG FLAP

Appraise

1 This used to be the most commonly used flap to cover fractures of the tibia and fibula with extensive overlying skin loss.

2 There are now many fasciocutaneous and free flaps described that are more suitable but, on rare occasions, cross-leg flaps may be useful.

3 Cross-arm flaps and cross-thigh flaps can be created using the same principle.

Prepare

1 Mark out the minimal defect on the leg.

KEY POINT Pre-plan the procedure

- Plan the whole operation meticulously 24 hours beforehand.

2 Plan a flap from the calf of the donor leg, based medially, preserving the long saphenous vein superiorly. Do not exceed a 1 : 1 length-to-breadth ratio.

3 Enlarge the defect to a size that will receive a safe flap; that is, make the defect fit the flap.

4 Using tapes, ensure that with the legs kept closely together, the flap when hinged on its medial axis will stretch to the distal part of the defect, allowing enough tissue to create a bridge between the two legs.

5 Place the patient's legs on top of a bead bag and apply vacuum so the patient's legs are fixed in what will be their postoperative position.

6 Maintain the patient's legs in this bead bag for as much of the next 24 hours as is practical so that he becomes used to the position preoperatively.

Action

1 With the patient under general anaesthesia, apply a tourniquet to reduce bleeding.

2 Create the planned defect, obtain haemostasis, then remove the tourniquet from the leg.

3 Elevate the planned flap from the opposite leg, raising the deep fascia with the flap.

4 Check that with the legs in the appropriate position, the flap fits the defect.

5 Take a split skin graft from the thigh of the recipient leg and dress the donor area.

6 Apply and suture the split skin graft to the flap donor site and to the back of that part of the flap which will form a skin bridge between the two legs (Fig. 39.13).

7 Suture the four corners of the flap into place and subsequently suture the edges.

8 Dress the skin graft at the flap donor site and use minimal other dressings.

9 Splint the two legs in the bead bag and apply vacuum.

10 Ensure that there is no tension or torsion on the flap and that it is viable.

11 Monitor the flap postoperatively for any changes.

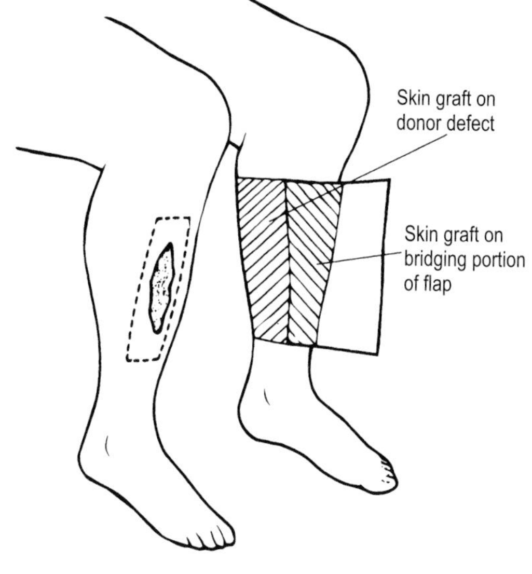

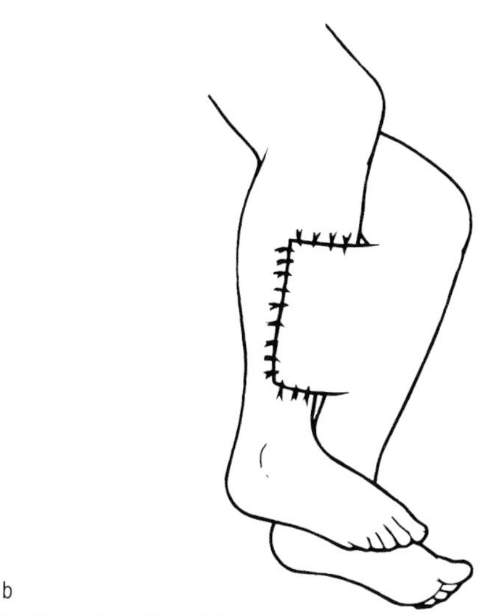

Fig. 39.13 Cross-leg flap. (a) A skin defect on the front of the right leg is enlarged to accommodate the flap from the calf of the left leg. After the flap has been raised from the left leg, the donor defect and a portion of the bridging part of the flap are grafted before suturing the flap in place. (b) The cross-leg flap is sutured in place.

Complete

1 Perform a 'delay' procedure after 2 weeks using local anaesthesia only, partially dividing the base and then re-suturing this wound.

2 Take the patient back to the operating theatre after the third week and divide the flap completely under general anaesthesia, allowing a generous portion to be in-set at the recipient site.

3 Suture the flap into place avoiding tension.

4 Suture the proximal portion to its donor site.

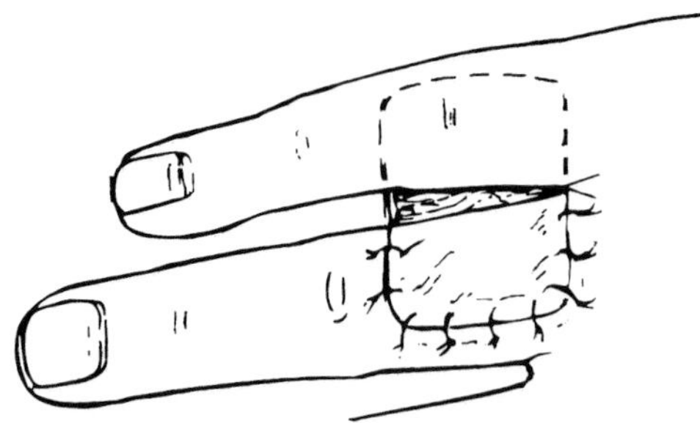

Fig. 39.14 Cross-finger flap. A flap from the dorsum of the ring finger is used to cover a defect on the flexor aspect of the proximal interphalangeal joint of the little finger. The donor site is repaired with a split skin graft sutured in place.

CROSS-FINGER FLAP

Appraise

1 Cross-finger flaps are a convenient means of obtaining good-quality skin cover for defects on the flexor aspects of the fingers, where split skin grafts would contract.

2 Take them from the dorsum of an adjacent finger.

Action

1 Mark out the defect on the flexor aspect of the finger.

2 Apply a tourniquet and create the defect.

3 Mark out a flap on the dorsum of the adjacent finger opposite the defect, or as near as possible, avoiding the skin over the joints.

4 Elevate the rectangular flap with its base adjacent to the injured finger.

5 Place the flap over the defect (Fig. 39.14).

6 Increase the size of the defect to fit the flap.

7 Remove the tourniquet and achieve haemostasis.

8 Take a small split skin graft with a Da Silva knife.

9 Apply the skin graft to the donor defect.

10 Suture the flap into the defect.

11 Dress the wounds and splint the two fingers together after inserting some dressing gauze between the fingers.

12 Plan to divide the flap at 2 weeks, in-setting the skin bridge at both recipient and donor sites, and re-dress the wounds.

13 Remove all sutures 1 week later.

REVERSE DERMIS FLAP

Appraise

1 This flap is similar to the cross-finger flap but is used for defects on the dorsum of the finger.

Action

1 Mark out the defect.

2 Use a tourniquet to control bleeding and create the defect.

3 Mark out an appropriate flap on the dorsum of an adjacent finger, as with a cross-finger flap.

4 Shave the planned flap with a Da Silva knife, removing a thin sheet of epidermis and superficial dermis.

5 Elevate the rectangular flap with subcutaneous tissue, leaving it attached at its base adjacent to the finger with the defect.

6 Increase the size of the defect to fit the flap.

7 Remove the tourniquet and achieve haemostasis.

8 Suture the flap in place.

9 Take a small split skin graft and apply this to the donor site and the flap.

10 Splint the two fingers together with some gauze dressing between the fingers.

11 Plan to divide the flap at 2 weeks, and in-set the bridge portion of the flap at both donor and recipient sites.

12 Remove all sutures 7 days later.

ABDOMINAL TUBE PEDICLE FLAP

Appraise

1 These flaps were formerly used as the standard technique for transferring a large amount of skin and subcutaneous tissue from the abdomen to a distant site such as the foot, the face, or elsewhere where there was extensive loss of tissue. They have been superseded almost totally by the introduction of axial pattern flaps, applied either as pedicle flaps or transferred as free flaps using microvascular surgical techniques. However, they may be useful in a few isolated situations.

2 Raise a planned rectangular area of abdominal skin and subcutaneous tissue by dividing along each side and, while still attached at each end, form the middle part into a tube. After a delay procedure, detach one end and transfer it to a wrist. When it has established a local blood supply, detach the other end and transfer it to the side of the defect. In further stages the whole flap is transferred to the defect and spread over it.

3 The patient requires approximately 5 months of hospitalization, with many operations, and failure is not uncommon at some stage.

4 Tube pedicle flaps can be raised from other sites, including the back and thigh.

Action

Raising the tube pedicle

1 Mark out a rectangular area 20 cm × 8 cm obliquely on the lower abdomen.

2 Incise along the long edges down to the deep fascia.

3 Dissect along the deep fascia between the two edges to elevate a bridge of skin and subcutaneous tissue.

4 Approximate the two skin edges of the bridge beneath the subcutaneous tissue to form a tube, and suture as far as possible in each direction.

5 At either end suture the skin down to the base to create a closed tube (Fig. 39.15a).

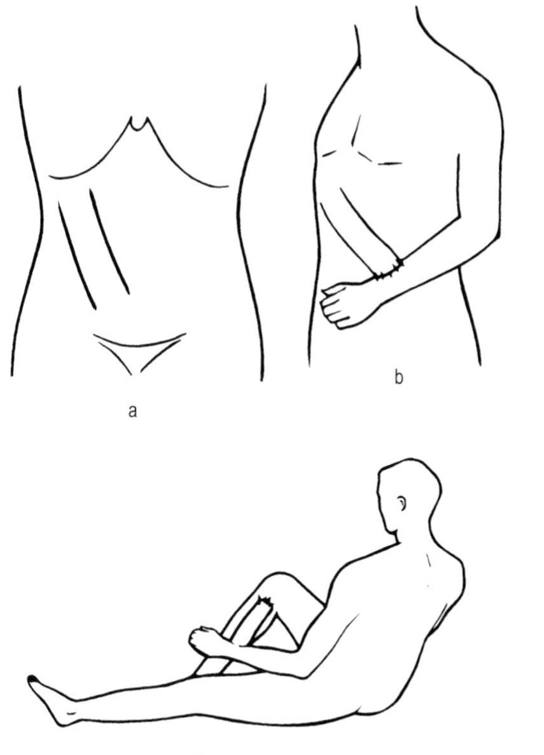

Fig. 39.15 Abdominal tube pedicle flap: (a) the flap is raised on the abdomen; (b) the lower end is transferred to the wrist; (c) after 3 weeks the abdominal end is detached and sutured around the defect on the contralateral leg.

6 Apply a large split skin graft to the residual raw area beneath the skin tube if this defect cannot be closed primarily.

Delay of the flap

1 At 2 weeks, under local anaesthesia, partially divide the base of the flap at one end, dividing through three-quarters of the skin and subcutaneous tissue, ligating and dividing the underlying vessels.

2 Re-suture the wound and apply a small dressing.

Division of the tube

1 3 weeks after raising the tube, divide the base of the tube completely, passing through the delay incision.

2 Close the residual defect on the abdomen using a split skin graft if necessary.

3 Place the patient's contralateral arm on to the abdominal wall and find a suitable recipient site at the level of the wrist to insert the tube pedicle.

4 Mark out an appropriate sized circle on the wrist.

5 Elevate the skin and subcutaneous tissue from half of this circle and reflect it backwards as a flap. This produces a circular defect.

6 Suture the free end of the abdominal tube pedicle to the circular defect (Fig. 39.15b).

7 Splint the arm to the chest wall after applying plenty of padding beneath the axilla.

Delay of abdominal tube pedicle

1 This is carried out under local anaesthesia 2 weeks after insertion to the wrist.

2 Make an incision at the base of the flap still attached to the abdominal wall.

3 The technique is the same as that used in the first delay procedure.

Transfer of flap to defect

1 Free the abdominal tube flap from the abdominal wall by dividing the tube at its residual attachment to the abdomen, passing through the delaying incision.

2 Close the donor defect with a split skin graft if necessary, and dress the wound.

3 Transfer the arm with its attached pedicle to the site of the defect.

4 Mark out a recipient site for the tube pedicle, preferably on the distal side of the defect, so that the seam of the flap overlies the defect.

5 Create a circular defect with a healthy skin margin at the edge of the main defect.

6 Excise any scar tissue from the end of the tube pedicle, and insert the tube pedicle into the skin defect (Fig. 39.15c).

7 Immobilize the limbs appropriately.

Delay of tube pedicle

Carry out a delay of the tube pedicle at the wrist end using the same technique as before.

Transfer of whole flap to defect

1 Divide the flap from the wrist, incising through the site of the delay incision.

2 Return the original skin flap from the wrist to its former site, thus leaving a residual semicircular wound, and suture this.

3 Mark out a circular area on the opposite side of the defect from the initial attachment of the tube pedicle.

4 Create a circular defect with healthy skin margins at this site.

5 Insert the free end of the tube pedicle into this defect, keeping the seam over the defect.

Insert the flap

1 Allow the flap to 'soften' before in-setting. This may involve waiting for 4 or 5 weeks or more.

2 Excise any doubtful tissue in the base to ensure that it is healthy.

3 Excise the seam of the tube pedicle and spread the skin of the tube pedicle over the defect.

4 Suture the edges into the edge of the defect.

5 Do not carry out any further revisions of the flap until it has been allowed to settle for at least several weeks and preferably for several months.

AXIAL PATTERN SKIN FLAPS

SCALP FLAP

Appraise

1 Scalp flaps are most commonly used for reconstructing defects of the hair-bearing skin on the face. They are usually used for reconstructing the upper lip, lower lip and chin areas in males, but there are many other occasional applications.

2 The flap is based on the posterior branch of the superficial temporal artery.

Prepare

1 Plan the flap on the day before operation.

2 Cut all the hair in the area of the operation to less than 1 cm in length.

3 Shave the hair completely in the area of the planned incisions.

4 Check that the posterior branch of the superficial temporal artery is palpable and that there are no significant scars on the scalp, suggesting previous damage to this vessel.

5 Wash the head thoroughly to remove all cut and shaved hair.

Action

1 Mark out the defect.

2 If appropriate, increase the defect to the shape of a whole cosmetic unit.

3 If appropriate, increase the defect to make it symmetrical on either side of the midline.

4 Make a template of the defect with sterile paper.

5 With one end of a tape attached to the template, and a second fixed on the zygomatic arch below the point where the artery was palpated, swing the template up on to the vertex of the scalp using the point on the zygomatic arch as the pivot.

6 Mark out an appropriate area on the scalp behind the anterior hairline around the template.

7 Infiltrate the scalp along the marked line with 0.5% lidocaine and 1:200000 adrenaline (epinephrine), and wait for 5 minutes.

8 Elevate the flap together with the underlying galea, starting at its distal extremity.

9 Identify the posterior branch of the superficial temporal vessels in the pedicle of the flap as it is raised, and adjust the shape of the pedicle if necessary to include these vessels (Fig. 39.16).

10 Taper the pedicle to 2 cm at its base, so that it can be rotated.

11 Transpose the flap into the defect, and in-set.

12 Cover the posterior aspect of the flap with paraffin gauze.

13 Close the donor defect primarily if possible. If it is too large, cover it with a split skin graft.

14 Plan to divide the flap at 2 weeks, providing there is a large in-set. If you are in doubt, divide the flap at 3 weeks and return the pedicle.

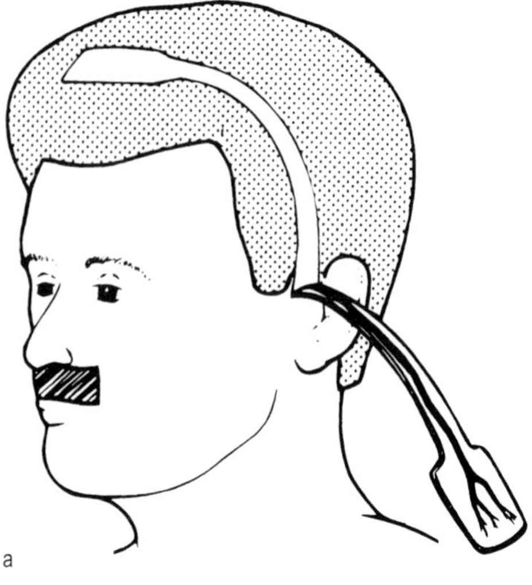
a

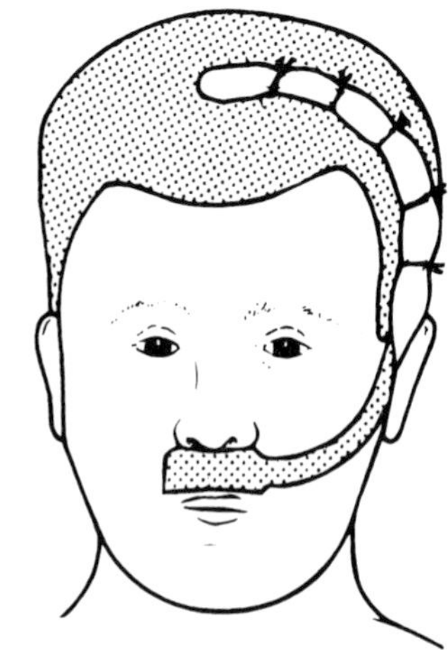
b

Fig. 39.16 Scalp flap. A defect of the upper lip is created and a matching area from the vertex is swung down on a pedicle based on the posterior branch of the superficial temporal artery. (a) The flap is pivoted above the zygomatic arch and turned to fill the defect. (b) A split graft is applied to the donor defect with a tie-over dressing.

FOREHEAD FLAP

Appraise

1 The forehead flap has been used extensively in the past to provide lining of the oral cavity after major resections for tumour. It is occasionally used for resurfacing defects of the scalp and of the cheek. It is the best flap available for total nasal reconstruction.

2 It has been largely superseded by other myocutaneous and free flaps in its use for oral lining but it remains an easy, safe and reliable flap to use, especially in the elderly and debilitated patient.

3 Its main disadvantage is the relatively poor cosmetic defect of its donor site.

4 It is not a true axial pattern flap, but it simulates one, surviving on the anterior branch of one superficial temporal artery and its

accompanying vein. The distal part of the flap normally acquires its vascular supply from the opposite anterior branch of the superficial temporal artery and the supraorbital and supratrochlear vessels. When these vessels to the flap are divided, the vascular network between the branches of the various vessels is adequate to allow the flap to survive on the supply from the single vascular pedicle.

Action

1 Create the defect and measure its dimensions.

2 Mark out the flap on the forehead, making this symmetrical and preferably including the whole of the forehead skin as a cosmetic unit.

3 Increase the defect to accommodate the flap.

4 If the flap is to be used for intraoral lining, excise the coronoid process of the mandible to allow the flap to pass inside the zygomatic arch.

5 Elevate the flap, commencing at the margin distal to the flap pedicle.

6 Identify and ligate the anterior branch of the contralateral superficial temporal artery and the supraorbital and supratrochlear vessels on both sides.

7 Lift the flap in the plane beneath the frontalis muscle.

8 Identify the anterior branch of the superficial temporal artery and its accompanying veins on the undersurface of the flap, and taper the pedicle to a 2-cm margin, including these vessels (Fig. 39.17).

9 If the flap is to be used intraorally, pass this through to the mouth beneath the zygoma.

10 If there is inadequate space to carry this out, excise a segment of the zygomatic arch.

11 To avoid a further operation some 2 weeks later, shave the epidermis and superficial dermis from that part of the pedicle that will remain buried between the skin surface and the intraoral surface.

12 Suture the flap in place.

13 Use 3/0 polyglactin 910 sutures to elevate the skin of the eyebrows on either side symmetrically.

14 Lay several layers of paraffin gauze on the donor site.

15 Harvest a large split skin graft to cover the defect in one sheet. In a young person, use the inner aspect of the arm in preference to the thigh as this gives a better colour match.

16 Store the skin.

17 Apply this skin as a delayed graft 24 hours later.

18 After 2 weeks, divide the pedicle and return it, to provide symmetry to the face.

TONGUE FLAP

Appraise

1 Tongue flaps are used for repairing large palatal fistulae, providing mucosa in lip reconstruction and reconstructing defects of the pharynx and oral cavity.

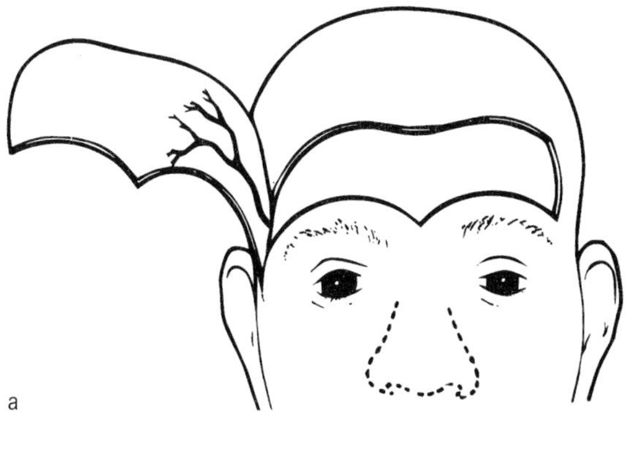

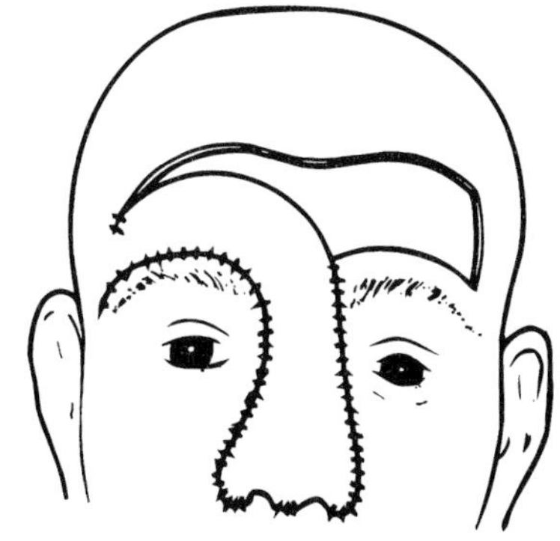

Fig. 39.17 Forehead flap: (a) the forehead skin elevated on the anterior branch of the superficial temporal vessels of one side; (b) forehead flap being used for total nasal reconstruction. The flap is divided and in-set at 3 weeks.

> **KEY POINT Take care**
>
> ■ Suture these flaps very carefully otherwise they readily dehisce. This is because of the difficulty in splinting them.

2 They are not easily tolerated by young children since they are unable to co-operate. Tongue flaps are, therefore, rarely useful below the age of 6 years.

3 Most tongue flaps are not true axial pattern flaps but rely on the rich vascular network within the muscles of the tongue.

4 Flaps for palatal fistulae are taken from the dorsum, those for lining the oral cavity or the pharynx are taken from the lateral aspect, and those providing a vermilion border are taken from the anterior part. In all cases close the defect primarily.

Action

1 Create the defect and measure the dimensions.

2 Insert a large stay suture in the tip of the tongue and pull it forwards.

3 Place two large stay sutures as far to the back of the tongue as possible and use these as the principal stay sutures.

4 Plan and mark out the flap on the tongue. Flaps for palatal fistulae can be based anteriorly or posteriorly, but this depends on the position of the defect.

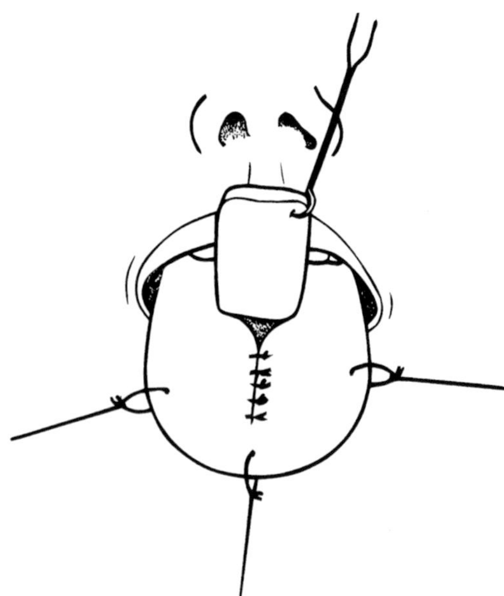

Fig. 39.18 Tongue flap. A posteriorly based tongue flap from the dorsum has been raised for closing a palatal fistula. The donor defect has been closed primarily.

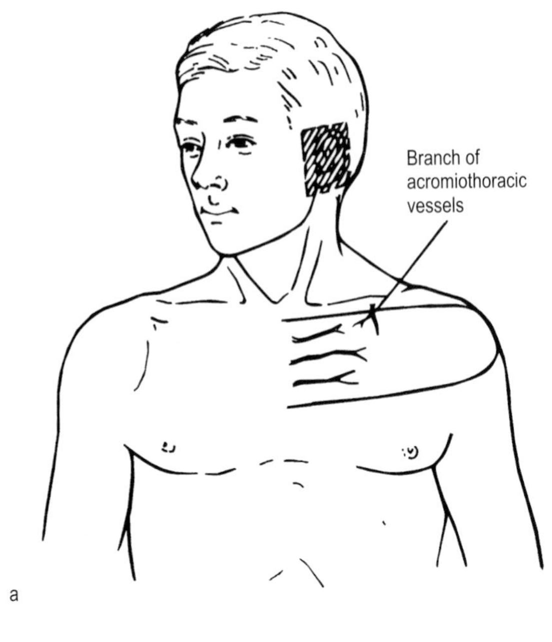

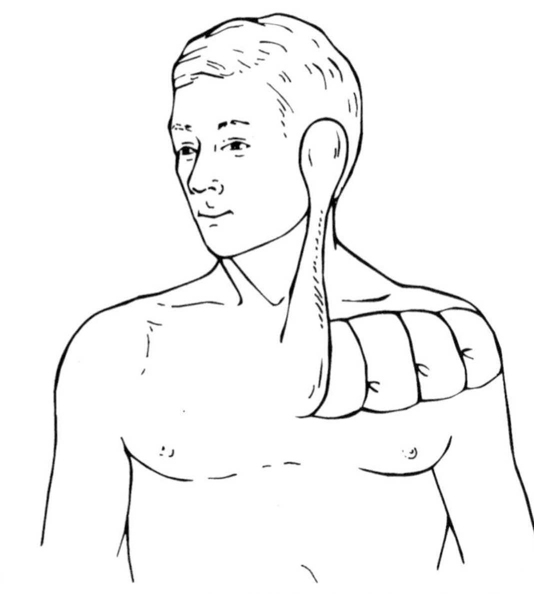

Fig. 39.19 Deltopectoral flap: (a) the flap is based on the second, third and fourth branches of the internal thoracic artery; (b) the flap being used to reconstruct the skin in the region of the pinna after a pinnectomy. The donor defect in this case is covered with a split skin graft and a tie-over dressing. The pedicle is divided and returned at 3 weeks.

5 Elevate the flap of mucosa together with a sheet of muscle approximately 4–5 mm thick.

6 Check that the flap fits the defect.

7 Close the donor defect primarily (Fig. 39.18).

8 Suture the most inaccessible part of the flap into the defect first with interrupted sutures.

9 Work proximally, leaving the easiest, most anterior, suture until last.

10 Observe the flap carefully; it may require re-suturing at any time.

11 Divide the flap at 2 weeks, and in-set.

DELTOPECTORAL FLAP

Appraise

1 This flap, sometimes known as a Bakamjian flap after its innovator, is used for providing skin flap cover to the chin, the cheek, the region of the pinna and the neck. It can be used to provide lining to the oral cavity and pharynx but may require the development of a temporary oral or pharyngeal fistula, which is unsatisfactory.

2 When raised conventionally there is necrosis of the tip in approximately 15% of cases. Because of this and its unsightly donor defect, it has been superseded by other flaps for mucosal replacement but is occasionally useful for large skin defects.

Action

1 Create the defect.

2 Mark out the flap based on the second, third and fourth perforating branches of the internal thoracic artery (Fig. 39.19).

3 Mark the upper margin of the flap along a line parallel with the clavicle, along its inferior margin. Use a line along the superior margin if a block dissection of the neck has been carried out with a McPhee incision.

4 Mark the inferior border of the flap parallel to and 10 cm below the upper border.

5 Mark the distal end of the flap as a semicircle extending to the midlateral line over the deltoid muscle.

6 Elevate the flap from its lateral margin including the fascia overlying the deltoid and pectoralis muscle.

7 Divide the branch from the acromiothoracic artery, as this perforates the clavipectoral fascia.

8 Divide and ligate the cephalic vein at the margin of the flap.

9 Reflect the flap medially to within 4 cm of the midline.

10 Dissect further medially, very carefully, to avoid dividing the perforating branches on which the flap survives.

11 Pass the flap up to the defect.

12 If the flap passes directly to the defect on the external surface, tube the intervening bridge over the neck.

13 If a block dissection has been carried out and the flap is for intraoral use, shave the epidermis from the central portion of the flap and pass the flap subcutaneously up to the defect. This manoeuvre converts the reconstruction into a one-stage operation.

14 Suture the flap into the defect.

15 Establish haemostasis on the donor site and cover it with paraffin gauze.

16 Take a split skin graft, store it and apply it to the donor site at 24 hours as a delayed graft.

17 At 3 weeks, divide the pedicle if exposed and in-set the flap.

18 Return the remainder of the pedicle to the donor site after excising the split skin graft in the appropriate area.

PECTORALIS FLAP

Appraise

1 This is a versatile flap for reconstruction following excision of tumours in the head and neck region. It will reach the pharynx, the lower cheek, the neck and shoulder and will just reach the floor and lateral walls of the oral cavity as well as the area of the pinna.

2 It is a myocutaneous flap based on the pectoral vessels supplying the pectoralis major muscle. These in turn supply skin overlying the muscle.

3 Its most useful application is for intraoral reconstruction, where an island or paddle of skin the size of the defect is transferred from the lower chest wall on the distal part of the flap. The muscle is transposed subcutaneously with this island of skin and protects the carotid vessels when a block dissection has been carried out. The donor site can be closed primarily.

4 Web contractures may develop in the neck postoperatively when the flap is used in the anterior part of the oral cavity.

KEY POINTS Caveats

- Hesitate to use this flap in hirsute males, where transposing hairy skin to the oral cavity may prove disadvantageous.
- In addition, the skin island is cumbersome and less reliable in obese individuals and in women with large breasts.

Action

1 Create the defect.

2 Measure the size of the defect.

3 Measure and mark an appropriate area of skin overlying the distal inferior portion of the pectoralis major muscle just above the costal margin (Fig. 39.20). Do not include skin across the midline or skin more than 2 cm below the lower margin of the pectoralis muscle.

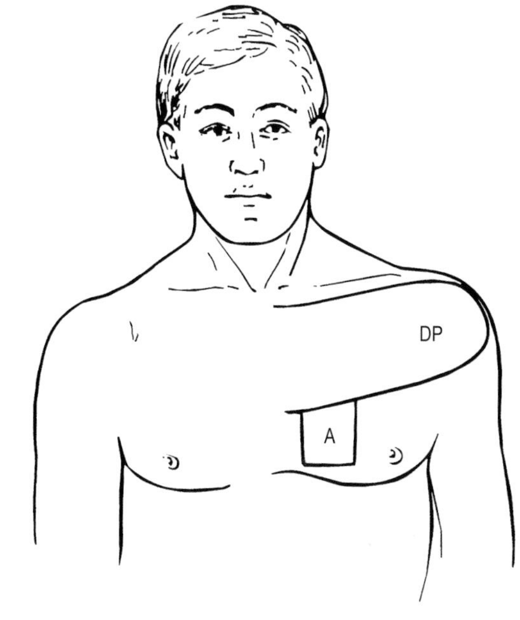

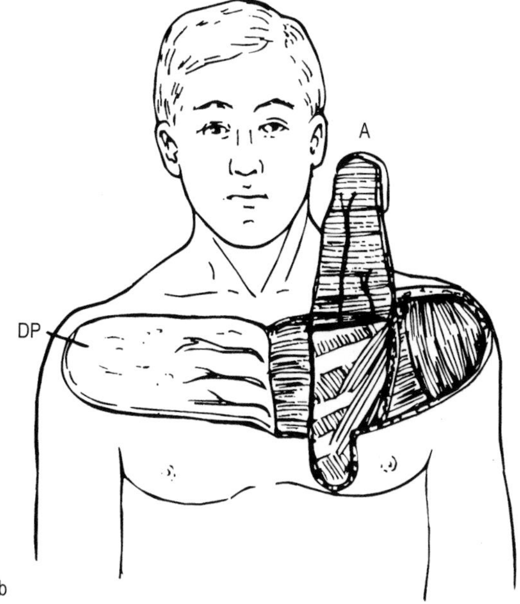

Fig. 39.20 Pectoralis flap: (a) the pectoralis muscle is used to transfer a cutaneous island of skin (A) from the chest wall into the neck; (b) to help exposure, a deltopectoral flap (DP) is reflected medially. The pectoralis muscle with its attached paddle of skin (A) is dissected free to the clavicle where it can be passed directly or subcutaneously to a defect above this level.

4 Mark out a deltopectoral flap (see above) above the skin paddle.

5 Elevate the deltopectoral flap medially; you can omit this step if you are experienced, by passing the pectoralis flap under the deltopectoral flap.

6 Identify the lateral margin of the pectoralis muscle and elevate its border.

7 Dissect this distally to the sternal attachment, freeing the muscle from its attachments to the chest wall.

8 Dissect the distal element free from the midline.

9 Elevate the muscle with its attached skin island up to the clavicle. In doing this, look for and protect the two vascular pedicles on the undersurface.

10 Divide the attachment of the muscle to the humerus at the margin of the deltoid muscle.

11 Pass the flap subcutaneously beneath the neck skin if a block dissection has been carried out and pass the island of skin into the defect. Some rotation of the muscle pedicle may be necessary. Make sure the flap sits comfortably in place, and suture the skin paddle into the defect.

12 Suture the edges of the muscle to adjacent tissue to support it when the patient sits up.

13 If neck skin has been incised or excised to accommodate the muscle pedicle, take a split skin graft and apply this to the exposed muscle.

14 Close the donor defect primarily. This may require wide undermining to allow approximation of the skin edges.

15 Return and suture the deltopectoral flap.

LATISSIMUS DORSI FLAP

Appraise

1 The most useful application of this flap is as a myocutaneous flap in breast reconstruction and reconstruction of chest wall defects. It can be used in pharyngeal reconstruction and for defects of the back up to and just above the nape of the neck.

2 It can be used as a muscle flap alone to cover a large defect, or the muscle can be used to transfer a small island of skin, as in breast reconstruction, or a large island of skin. If a large island is transferred, primary closure of the donor site is not possible.

3 The flap has wide application in free tissue transfer (see below).

4 The flap is based on the thoracodorsal vessels, and these enter the muscle just below its insertion into the humerus.

Action

1 For an anterior chest wall defect, lay the patient on the table in the lateral position.

2 Create and measure the defect on the anterior chest wall.

3 Mark out the island of skin on the back overlying the latissimus dorsi muscle appropriate to the defect (Fig. 39.21).

4 Check that the island will reach the defect, using a tape based in the region of the vascular hilum at the lower margin of the posterior axillary fold. Remember, the most posterior

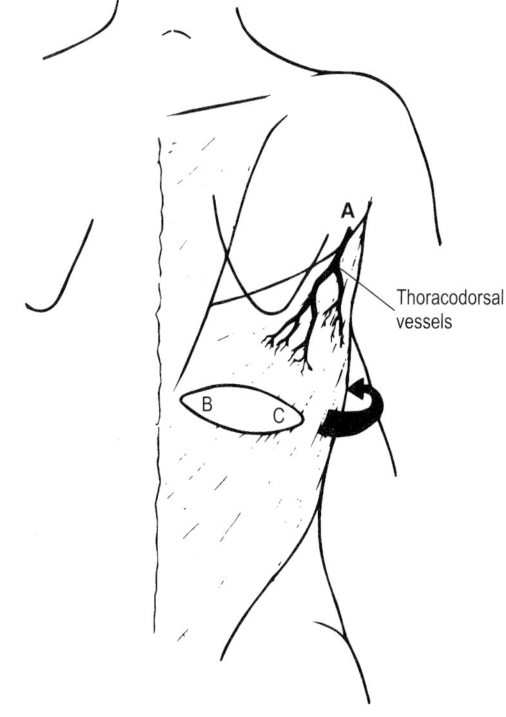

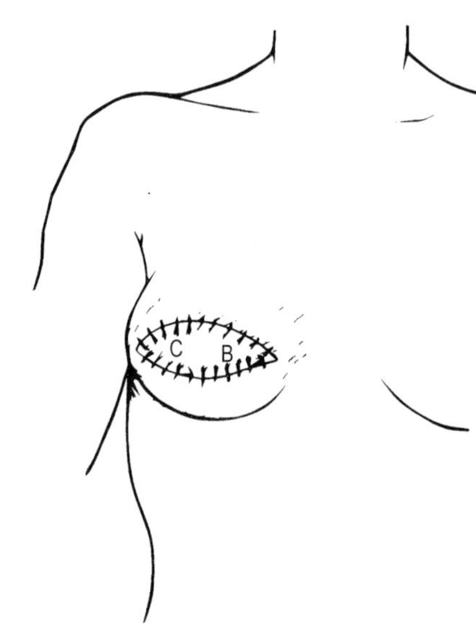

Fig. 39.21 Latissimus dorsi flap. The skin overlying the right latissimus dorsi flap is elevated from the muscle, leaving a central elliptiform island of skin attached to the muscle. The muscle is freed from its peripheral and underlying attachments and passed subcutaneously to the defect on the anterior chest wall, pivoted on its insertion (A) where the thoracodorsal vessels enter the muscle (a). In breast reconstruction, the muscle is sutured into the region of the reconstructed breast and the island of skin inserted into the mastectomy scar. A prosthesis is inserted beneath the flap (b).

point of the flap has to reach the most anterior point of the defect.

5 Incise the skin along the marked lines around the island down to the muscle.

6 Dissect the skin and fascia off the upper surface of the whole muscle proximal and distal to the skin paddle.

7 Identify the anterior border of the muscle.

8 Separate the muscle from the underlying serratus muscles and ribs.

9 Divide the muscle from its attachment, distally and posteriorly.

10 Separate the muscle up to its pedicle, identifying and preserving the principal vessels on the underlying surface.

11 Dissect gently at the hilum to avoid damaging the principal vessels.

12 Identify the vessels to the serratus anterior muscle arising from the thoracodorsal vessels, and divide them.

13 Develop a subcutaneous tunnel between the defect of the flap and the anterior chest wall defect.

14 Pass the flap subcutaneously through this tunnel into the anterior wall defect.

15 Close the donor site defect primarily, if possible, even if this means extensive undermining. Insert a large suction drain.

16 Change the patient to the supine position, re-towelling if necessary.

17 Undermine the skin edges of the defect where appropriate.

18 Suture the latissimus dorsi muscle to the chest wall.

19 If this is a breast reconstruction, insert a prosthesis beneath the latissimus dorsi muscle.

20 Suture the skin paddle of the flap to the skin defect.

TRAM FLAP

Appraise

1 The transverse rectus abdominis muscle (TRAM) provides an alternative flap for breast reconstruction to the latissimus dorsi muscle. It has the advantage that it can normally transfer sufficient autologous tissue to avoid the necessity of using an implant.

2 The flap can also be used for reconstructing chest wall defects and defects of the perineum. In either of these circumstances the skin paddle may be taken in the vertical plane (a vertical rectus abdominis muscle or VRAM flap), with the skin paddle lying completely over the muscle.

3 The flap may be used as a pedicled flap based either on the superior deep epigastric vessels for breast reconstruction or chest wall defects, or on the inferior deep epigastric vessels for perineal defects.

4 When used as a free flap, most commonly for breast reconstruction, prefer to use the inferior deep epigastric vessels, which are larger and more reliable. These vessels can be dissected through the muscle, avoiding harvesting of the muscle to raise a deep inferior epigastric perforator (DIEP) flap.

5 The abdominal skin wound closure is similar to that of an abdominoplasty (see below).

▶ KEY POINTS Two disadvantages

- The first is the loss of muscle and usual need to replace this with a prosthetic mesh.
- The second is the unreliability of survival of the skin paddle beyond the muscle boundaries.

Action

1 Mark the patient preoperatively in the standing position.

2 For breast reconstruction plan to excise the mastectomy scar if possible.

3 Avoid large skin flaps if the patient has been treated by radiotherapy.

4 Mark the midline and edges of the recti abdominis muscles.

5 Plan and mark the skin island to be transferred centrally over the contralateral muscle just below the level of the umbilicus. If you are an experienced surgeon, you will centre the flap in the midline.

6 Mark a symmetrical ellipse to be excised that includes the planned skin island of the flap.

7 In the operating theatre, excise the mastectomy scar and raise the adjacent skin flaps to accommodate the flap.

8 Shave the epidermis off the skin adjacent to the planned skin island but within the marked outer ellipse. The residual dermis protects the subdermal pedicle, which in turn contributes to the viability of the subcutaneous flap beyond the boundaries of the skin paddle. Excise the residual skin of the symmetrical ellipse, the skin paddle and the subcutaneous fat (Fig. 39.22).

9 Cut through the deep fascia around the base of the subcutaneous fat to be included on the flap. Include in this the perforating vessels close to the midline both below and just above the umbilicus.

10 Gently pass your finger around the rectus abdominis muscle distal to the flap until the whole muscle is isolated. Cut through it with a cutting diathermy, identifying and ligating the inferior epigastric vessels when you encounter them on the undersurface.

11 Cut vertically through the middle of the anterior sheath of the muscle superiorly.

12 Elevate the muscle with the overlying subcutaneous fat and skin up to the costal margin.

13 Create a subcutaneous tunnel from the abdominal wall cavity through to the mastectomy wound and pass the skin paddle through this.

14 Orientate the skin paddle and fat and tack the base into place checking there is no tension on the pedicle.

15 Suture the flap into place in layers and insert a Redivac drain.

16 Close the donor defect by suturing the upper part of the anterior rectus sheath first with a continuous 1 polypropylene suture.

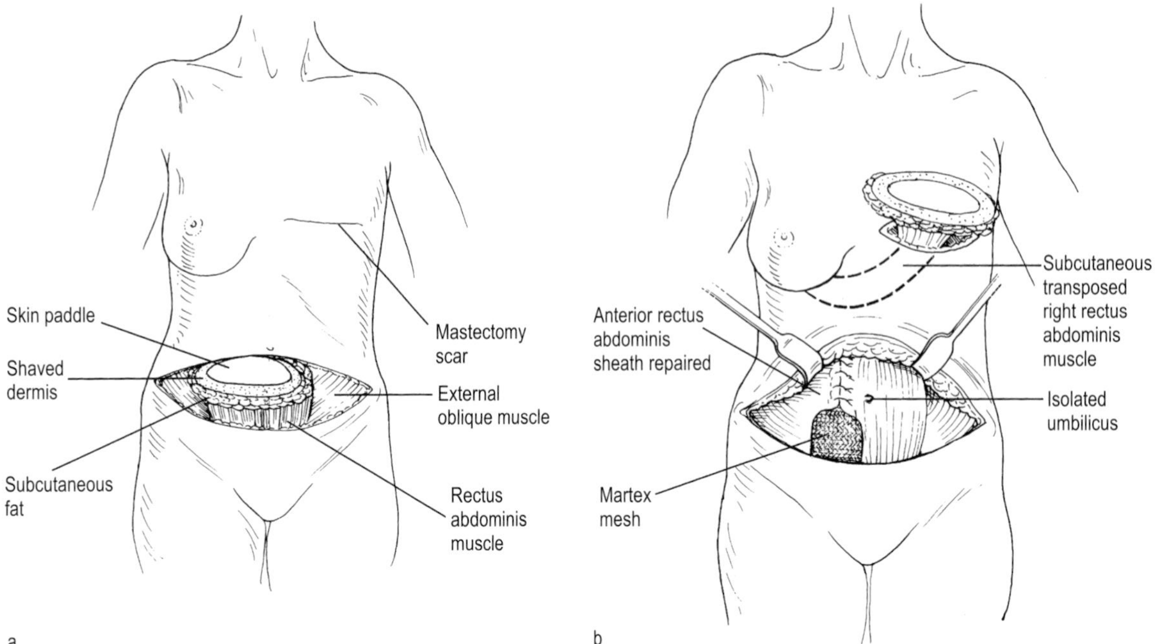

Fig. 39.22 TRAM flap. Being used for a left breast reconstruction, the flap is isolated in the abdomen with a skin paddle, a surrounding area of shaved dermis and subcutaneous fat lying over and adjacent to the right rectus abdominis muscle. The remaining skin and subcutaneous fat from the larger ellipse is excised (a). After division of the lower part of the right rectus abdominis muscle, the flap is transferred on the upper part of the muscle and passed subcutaneously into the opened mastectomy wound. The anterior rectus sheath of the upper part of the muscle is closed and the defect of the anterior sheath below this is repaired with Marlex mesh (b).

17 Repair the residual defect in the anterior sheath with Marlex mesh sutured firmly in place with a continuous 1 polypropylene suture.

18 Close the abdominal wall in layers transposing the umbilicus to its new site as appropriate. Insert two Redivac drains.

19 Support the abdomen with a pressure garment and lightly dress the breast wounds.

20 Remove the drains when the drainage has diminished and remove the sutures at 3 weeks.

GROIN FLAP

Appraise

This can be used for defects of the lower abdominal wall, but its greatest application is providing skin cover for severe injuries to the hand or wrist. It is therefore most useful when the skin over the iliac crest is relatively thin.

KEY POINTS Study the vascular patterns

- The groin flap is an unusual axial pattern flap as the vascular pattern is variable.
- The flap is based on either the superficial circumflex iliac vessels or the superficial epigastric vessels or a combination of the two. Details of these variations need to be known only if the flap is to be used as a free flap.

Action

1 Create the defect on the hand.

2 Identify the femoral artery by palpation.

3 Mark a point over this 2 cm beneath the inguinal ligament.

4 Draw a line from this point to the anterior superior iliac spine which acts as the axis of the flap.

5 Mark an area over the iliac crest close to the mid-axillary line, which is to be used for the definitive skin cover.

6 Mark the flap to include this with parallel lines on either side of the central axis at an equal distance from it (Fig. 39.23).

7 First incise the skin laterally down to the deep fascia and include the fascia with the flap.

8 Reflect the flap medially.

9 At the edge of the sartorius muscle include the fascia, overlaying it with the flap, and so ensure that the superficial circumflex vessels are retained within the flap.

10 Dissect the flap free to within 3 cm of the femoral vessels.

11 Check that the defect on the hand will accommodate the flap.

12 Close the donor defect primarily up to the pedicle of the flap, if necessary flexing the knee and hip.

13 Tube the portion of the flap that will bridge the gap between groin and hand by suturing the two skin edges together.

14 Suture the distal part of the flap into the defect.

15 Immobilize the limb against the trunk after placing padding between the limb and the trunk.

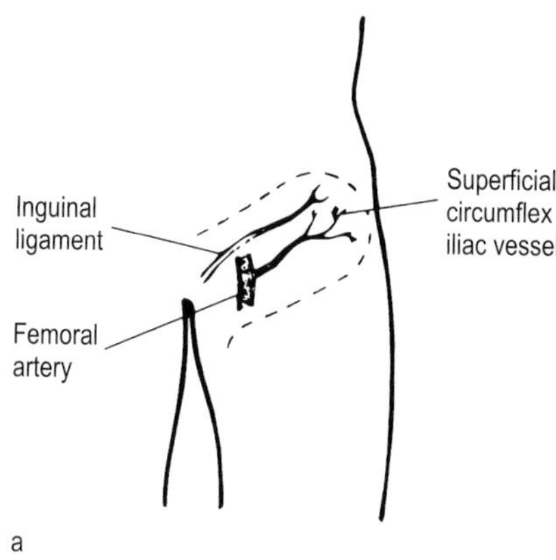

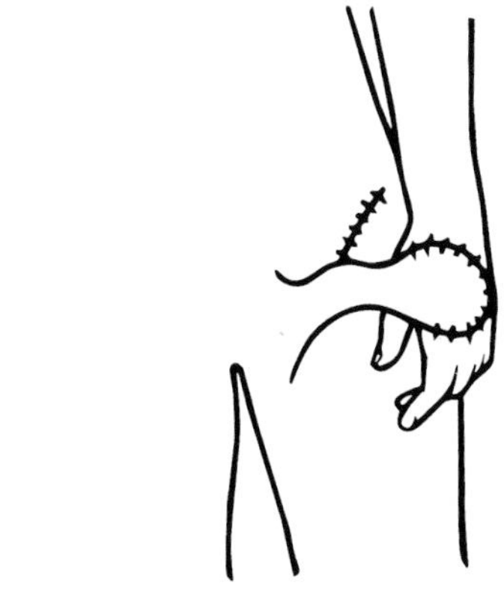

Fig. 39.23 Superficial groin flap. The inguinal ligament is marked in the groin and the position of the projected line of the superficial circumflex iliac vessels is also drawn. This line acts as the axis of the groin flap to be raised (a). After raising the flap the distal portion is sutured into the defect on the hand and the proximal portion is tubed (b). The donor defect is closed primarily.

16 Perform a delay procedure at 2 weeks by incising half of the skin at the base of the pedicle opposite the suture line.

17 Identify the axial vessels; ligate and divide them.

18 Re-suture the wound.

19 3 weeks after the initial procedure, divide the pedicle completely at its base and in-set it into the groin wound.

20 In-set the flap into the hand defect with a few sutures. If tension is apparent in the skin, do not suture it at all but cover the exposed part of the flap with a paraffin gauze dressing.

21 Insert the flap 2 days later.

22 Thin the flap 3 months later, if necessary, by excising the subcutaneous tissue in stages.

TENSOR FASCIA LATA FLAP

Appraise

1 This flap is useful in treating trochanteric pressure sores and defects of the groin, particularly when the femoral vessels are exposed.

2 It can also be used for ischial pressure sores and defects of the upper thigh and lower abdominal wall.

3 It is a myofasciocutaneous flap and is based on the vessels to the tensor fascia lata muscle.

4 Inclusion of the lateral cutaneous nerve of the thigh within the flap allows it to be used as a sensory flap.

Action

1 Place the patient supine on the table, rotate the pelvis through 30° and support this and the leg on the side of the defect.

2 Create and measure the defect in the groin.

3 Identify the site of entry into the muscle of its vascular pedicle, the transverse branch of the lateral femoral circumflex artery. This point is 8 cm distal and just lateral to the anterior superior iliac spine.

4 Keep this point in the base of the flap.

5 Draw a line from the anterior superior iliac spine to the lateral margin of the patella and use this as the anterior margin of the flap.

6 Mark the posterior margin of the flap using a width of 6–10 cm (Fig. 39.24).

7 Mark the distal extremity of the flap so that it is not more than two-thirds of the length of the thigh. Check that the flap will reach the defect.

8 Incise the skin distally down to the deep fascia.

9 Incise the skin on the anterior and posterior margins and elevate the flap together with the fascia lata.

10 As the flap is reflected proximally, the tensor fascia lata muscle comes into view. If necessary, divide any small distal vascular pedicle into the muscle after first identifying the large vascular pedicle proximally.

11 Check that the flap will rotate into the defect.

12 Incise the skin between the flap and the defect, and undermine it on either side, allowing the flap to lie in this defect.

13 Excise any excess thigh skin to allow the flap to sit comfortably.

14 Suture the flap into place.

15 Close the donor defect primarily as far as possible.

16 Take a skin graft from the opposite thigh and apply it to the residual flap donor defect.

17 Dress the graft and its donor site with paraffin gauze, dressing gauze, cotton wool and crepe bandage.

18 Leave the flap exposed and nurse the patient on his contralateral side.

BICEPS FEMORIS FLAP

Appraise

1 This flap is particularly useful for ischial pressure sores.

2 It is a myocutaneous flap but can be used as a simple muscle flap.

3 The biceps femoris muscle receives a segmental blood supply from several vessels which are branches of the profunda femoris

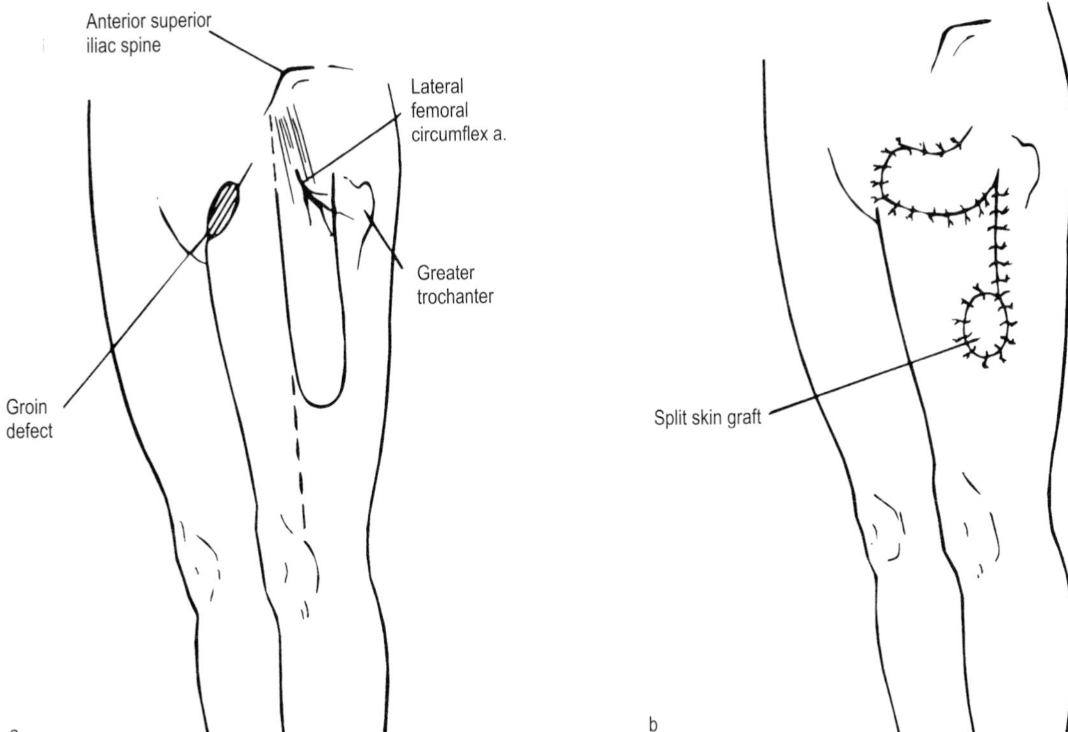

Fig. 39.24 Tensor fascia lata flap. Used to repair a groin defect, the anterior margin of the flap is marked on a line from the anterior superior iliac spine to the lateral border of the patella (a). After transposition of the flap, the donor site is closed primarily although the distal portion may require a split skin graft (b).

artery. In order to preserve all these vessels the flap is transferred as an advancement flap.

4 An advantage of this flap is that it can be advanced more than once.

Action

1 Place the patient prone on the table.

2 Create the defect by excising the whole lining to the ischial pressure sore cavity. With an osteotome reduce the prominence of the ischial tuberosity.

3 Draw a line from the ischial tuberosity to the head of the fibula. Use this as the axis of the flap and mark an elliptiform flap, 8–10 cm broad around this, extending proximally to the defect and distally to within 5 cm of the crease of the knee joint (Fig. 39.25).

4 Incise along the lines down to the margins of the biceps femoris muscle.

5 Divide the origins of the biceps femoris, semitendinosus and semimembranosus muscles at the ischial tuberosity.

6 Divide the biceps femoris tendon at the distal margin of the flap. Divide semimembranosus and semitendinosus distally if necessary to provide greater mobility of the flap.

7 Advance the flap into the defect and suture the muscle to obliterate the dead space.

8 Suture the skin of the flap into the skin defect after inserting a large suction drain.

9 Suture the distal portion of the flap defect primarily and apply minimal dressings.

10 Nurse the patient on the contralateral side.

11 Leave the sutures in place for at least 3 weeks.

GASTROCNEMIUS FLAP

Appraise

1 Both heads of the gastrocnemius muscle can be used separately for covering defects on the anterior aspect of the leg.

2 They can be used as simple muscle flaps or as myocutaneous flaps.

3 The flaps are used for covering exposed bone in the upper third of the tibia and for covering the exposed knee joint, sometimes even in the presence of a metal prosthesis.

4 The muscle flap alone is more malleable and versatile than a myocutaneous flap.

5 Although the lateral head is slightly longer, use the nearest muscle head to the defect. Do not use both heads simultaneously.

Action

1 Place the patient in the lateral position with the affected leg uppermost.

2 Mark out and create the defect.

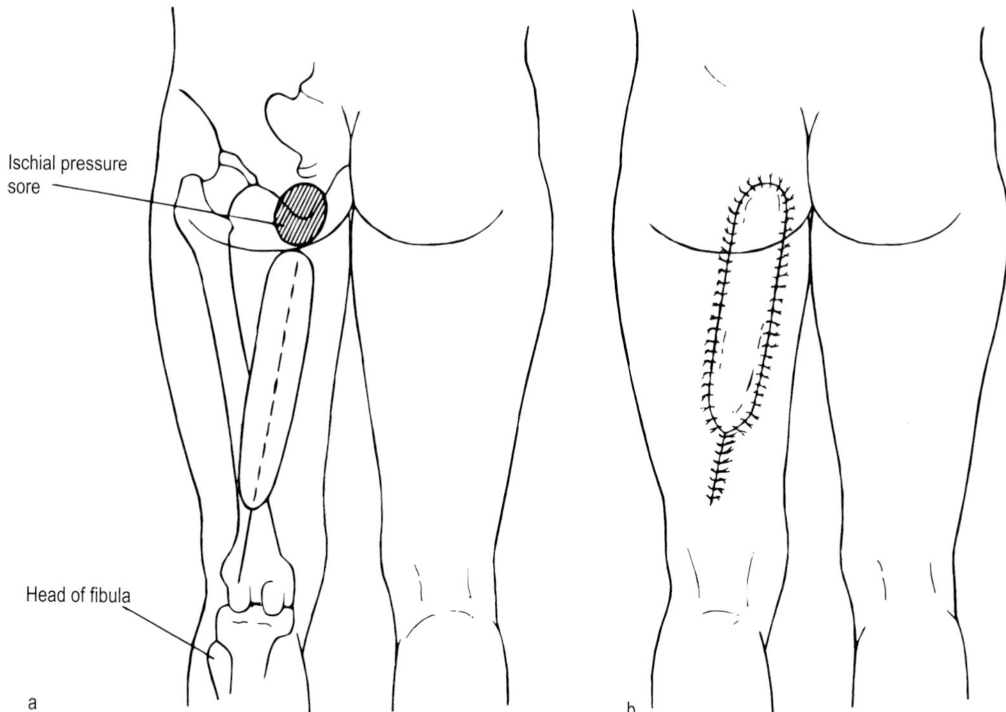

Fig. 39.25 Biceps femoris flap. The flap is drawn with its axis on a line between the ischial tuberosity and the head of the fibula (a). After excising the pressure sore and trimming the bone, the origins and insertion of the long head of biceps femoris, semitendinosus and semimembranosus are divided. The skin and underlying muscle are advanced into the defect, closing the distant donor site primarily (b).

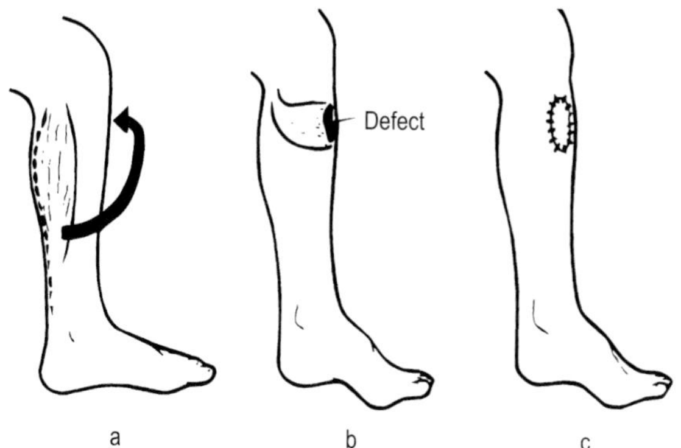

Fig. 39.26 Gastrocnemius flap: (a) a defect in the region of the tibial tuberosity can be covered with the medial head of gastrocnemius; (b) the flap is raised through a posterior midline incision and passed subcutaneously into the defect; (c) a split skin graft is placed over the muscle within the defect.

3 Make a vertical incision through skin and subcutaneous tissue down the midline of the calf, posteriorly.

4 Identify the muscle bellies of gastrocnemius and their relevant attachments to the tendo calcaneus (Fig. 39.26).

5 Separate the fascia overlying the respective belly of the muscle to be used.

6 Incise the tendon just distal to the muscle attachment.

7 Elevate the muscle belly proximally by dissecting laterally and medially, dividing its attachment to the opposite belly.

8 Free the muscle belly to the level of the popliteal fossa, preserving the vascular pedicle passing into it.

9 Create a subcutaneous tunnel from the base of the muscle belly to the defect and enlarge to accommodate the muscle flap.

10 Pass the muscle belly through this tunnel into the defect.

11 Suture the muscle to the edges of the defect.

12 Close the donor defect in layers and insert a suction drain.

13 Take a thick split skin graft from the thigh and apply it to the exposed muscle in the defect.

14 Splint the leg for 10 days.

15 Allow weight-bearing at 10 days and mobilize progressively. Fit an elastic support stocking to cover the graft overlying the muscle. This should be worn for 3 months.

FASCIOCUTANEOUS FLAP

Appraise

1 These flaps have their greatest use in providing skin cover to exposed bone in the middle third of the leg.

2 When based proximally, they may not be true axial pattern flaps but depend on preserving the rich vascular network lying superficial to the deep fascia.

3 You may use flaps with a 3 : 1 or more length-to-breadth ratio.

4 With intimate knowledge of the anatomy of the vessels which perforate the deep fascia, long flaps based distally can be

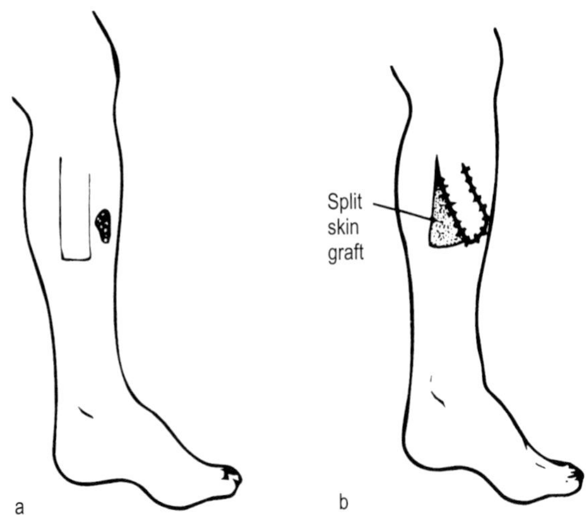

Fig. 39.27 Fasciocutaneous flap: (a) a small defect on the anterior aspect of the leg can be covered with a medially based fasciocutaneous flap; (b) the flap is transposed into the defect and a split skin graft is placed on the donor defect.

designed and may be useful in covering the exposed distal third of the tibia.

Action

1 Mark out and create the defect.
2 Mark out the flap based proximally with a 2:1 ratio.
3 Check that the flap will reach the defect when transposed (Fig. 39.27).
4 Incise the flap distally, passing through skin, subcutaneous tissue and deep fascia.
5 Elevate the flap proximally, incising along the lateral margins and preserving the deep fascia with the flap.
6 Transpose the flap into the defect.
7 Suture the flap into the defect in layers.
8 Take a split graft from the opposite thigh.
9 Apply the split skin graft to the flap donor defect. Dress with paraffin gauze and dressing gauze and retain with tie-over sutures.
10 Leave the flap exposed so that it can be monitored.

TISSUE EXPANSION

Appraise

1 The principle of tissue expansion is exemplified by the stretched abdominal wall resulting from pregnancy.
2 A tissue expander (Fig. 39.28) is inserted beneath the deep fascia or superficial muscle and expanded serially by injections of saline into an attached reservoir to stretch the overlying skin.
3 Following expansion the expander is removed and the surplus skin used to cover the adjacent defect.
4 Expanders are most effective when placed on a bone base. They are particularly effective when placed on the calvaria (Latin: = skull) to expand scalp, and on the chest wall to expand skin for breast reconstruction. They have limited value in limbs.

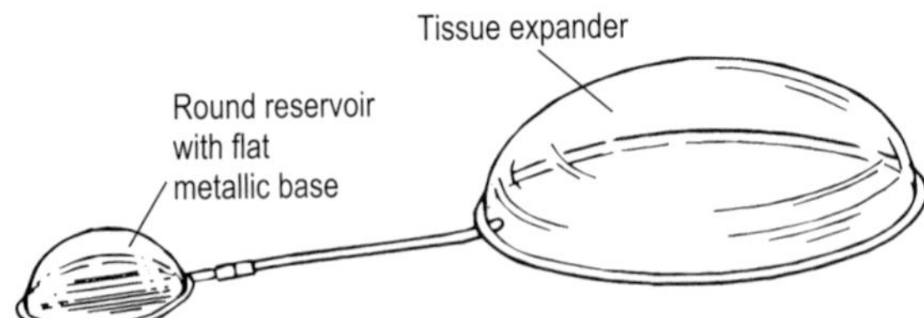

Fig. 39.28 Tissue expander and reservoir.

KEY POINT Is the skin healthy and normal?

- Do not use tissue expanders under badly scarred or irradiated skin.

5 There are some more sophisticated tissue expanders available specifically designed for breast reconstruction. Some of these have a double lumen, one of which is filled with silicone. Others have a reservoir that can be detached from a valve linking it to the expander, allowing the expander to be left in situ.

Action

1 Identify an area of normal skin to be expanded which is adjacent to the defect.
2 Choose an appropriate tissue expander whose base will lie within the boundaries defined.
3 Make an incision beyond the chosen area in a radial direction.
4 Attach the reservoir to the expander and insert saline. Remove air from the system and check its patency.
5 Make an appropriate pocket for the expander and insert it. This pocket should be submuscular or subfascial but may be subcutaneous.
6 Make a separate pocket for the reservoir in a suitable accessible adjacent subcutaneous area and insert it.
7 Recheck the patency of the system and close the wound.
8 Serially inject saline into the reservoir as an outpatient procedure.
9 When sufficient expansion or more has been achieved, re-admit the patient for the second stage.
10 Remove the expander and stretch the expanded skin over the defect.

GRAFTS OF OTHER TISSUES

CARTILAGE GRAFTS

1 Cartilage grafts are used in reconstructing cartilaginous defects of the nose, large defects of the lower eyelids and major defects of the ear.
2 Total reconstruction of an ear is technically extremely challenging. Do not attempt it if you are not experienced in this form of operation.

NOSE

1 Composite defects of skin and cartilage at the nostril margin can be reconstructed using composite grafts from the ear, as described under composite skin grafts (see above).

2 Most other small cartilaginous defects of the nose can be reconstructed using cartilage from other parts of the nose during a corrective rhinoplasty.

3 If there is extensive cartilaginous loss and the nasal tip requires support, take an L-shaped bone graft from the iliac crest and insert it through a mid-columellar incision.

4 More sophisticated techniques include the insertion of homograft cartilage (see below) or calvarial bone graft inserted from above after reflecting a bicoronal scalp flap.

EYELIDS

1 You rarely need to provide cartilage support for the upper eyelid.

2 Large defects of the lower eyelid often require the introduction of cartilage for support and the best donor site for this is the septum of the nose. This provides a composite graft of cartilage and mucous membrane. The latter is used to reconstruct the conjunctival surface.

Action

1 Create the defect and measure it.

2 Mark an appropriate area of the septum using a nasal speculum, commencing at least 3 mm behind the anterior limit of the septum.

3 Infiltrate the marked area with 0.5% lidocaine and 1 : 200 000 adrenaline.

4 Infiltrate the septum on the opposite side with the same preparation.

5 After allowing at least 7 minutes for the adrenaline to take effect, incise the mucosa, passing through this and the underlying cartilage but avoid penetrating the nasal mucosa on the contralateral side.

6 Separate the contralateral nasal mucosa from the cartilage using a mucosal elevator.

7 Cut around the full margin of the graft and remove it.

8 Stop the bleeding with pressure for 5 minutes timed by the clock.

> **KEY POINT Risks of diathermy**
>
> - Avoid diathermy; it can cause necrosis and subsequent perforation in the residual mucosal surface.

9 Insert the graft into the defect and stabilize it with an absorbable suture through the cartilage at each margin.

10 Suture the conjunctival surface with 6/0 absorbable suture.

11 Suture the skin with 6/0 nylon.

EAR

1 Costal cartilage is used for total ear reconstruction.

2 Reconstruction of a major portion of the ear may be difficult. It is sometimes justifiable to discard those cartilaginous segments already present and perform a total ear reconstruction.

3 If there is inadequate skin available, you must employ preoperative tissue expansion (see above), or use a temporoparietal flap.

Action

1 Measure the normal ear and make a template for the new ear.

2 Make a straight, oblique incision over the medial end of the seventh and eighth costal cartilages.

3 Retract the skin and subcutaneous tissue and expose an area of cartilage equivalent to the size and shape of the ear.

4 Mark out an outline of cartilage from the template using the seventh and eighth costal cartilages and excise this.

5 Close the donor defect in layers.

6 Place the graft on a wooden board on a table and carefully shape the cartilage, creating a well-defined helical rim and an antihelical fold.

7 Make an incision along the hairline of the posterior margin of the auricular skin where it meets hair-bearing scalp skin.

8 Create a subcutaneous pocket beneath the auricular skin to accommodate the cartilage graft.

9 Insert the graft and close the skin.

10 Insert sutures through the skin in the region of the scaphoid fossa and concha, to highlight the contour of the grafts.

11 After 6 months, reflect forwards the cartilage graft together with the underlying subcutaneous tissue and insert a split skin graft on to the posterior surface of the reconstructed ear and the postauricular region to create a postauricular sulcus.

VASCULAR GRAFTS

Appraise

1 Large vascular grafts are described in Chapter 29. Employ small-vessel grafts for replanting and free-flap transfer. They are occasionally used when limb vessels have been injured.

2 Vein grafts are used to replace both damaged arteries and veins.

3 Choose a vein graft that matches the vessel that has been destroyed.

4 Use magnification for the repair and a microscope when repairing grafts under 2 mm in diameter.

Action

1 Identify the length of vessel that has been damaged.

2 Place an appropriate size clamp on normal vessel on either side of the damaged section and resect this damaged section.

3 Inspect the cut ends under magnification and check that the endothelium is normal. If it is not, resect further.

4 Check that there is good flow of blood from the cut proximal arterial stump, or the cut distal venous stump, by holding the adventitia of the vessel with jeweller's forceps, and temporarily releasing the clamp.

5 Select a superficial vein of appropriate size and length for insertion as a graft into the defect. For vessels greater than 2 mm diameter, use the long saphenous vein, which is the best available vein graft for both arteries and veins. For vessels smaller than this, use veins from the dorsum of the foot or from the flexor aspect of the forearm.

6 Make an incision through the skin directly over the full length of the chosen vein.

7 By blunt dissection, isolate the full length of the vein to be used.

8 Ligate all branches of the vein graft or use the bipolar coagulator to seal minute branches. Do not use unipolar diathermy, which will damage the graft.

9 Isolate a segment of vein graft longer than that required. Ligate and divide the vessel proximally and distally.

10 Remove the graft and irrigate it gently with warm heparinized Hartmann's solution or saline to exclude leaks.

11 Place the graft in the site of the defect, ensuring that the blood flow in the graft will be in the usual direction.

12 Choose an appropriate double clamp. Place one portion of this clamp on the proximal end of the divided normal vessel and the other on the vein graft.

13 Under magnification, clean the adventitia from the vessel walls of both stumps using small scissors.

14 Flush the stumps with heparinized Hartmann's solution, being careful not to grasp the endothelium with forceps.

15 Dilate the vessel with vessel dilators and approximate the ends.

16 Suture the anterior wall with interrupted 8/0 or 10/0 nylon sutures. Turn the clamp over and suture the opposite wall.

17 Before inserting the final two sutures, check that the anastomosis is patent.

18 Carry out a similar anastomosis at the distal end, checking that the graft has been stretched to its original length and that there is no torsion.

19 Remove the distal clamps first and then remove the proximal clamps.

20 If there is small leak at either anastomosis, cover it with a warm swab but do not occlude the vessel.

21 If there is a gross leak, reapply a single clamp to obstruct the flow and insert extra sutures. Remove the clamp and observe.

22 If flow is not established, resect the anastomosis and repeat.

OTHER GRAFTS

1 Nerve grafts, tendon grafts and bone grafts are described in Chapter 36.

2 Homograft (Greek: *homos*=same; from the same species) bone, xenograft (Greek: *xenos*=strange, foreign; from a different species) cartilage and xenograft collagen are all used, after appropriate preparation, in reconstruction. Theoretically, they act as a scaffold into which the patient's own tissue grows. The benefit with xenograft cartilage and xenograft collagen may be only temporary as the graft tends to be absorbed.

3 Homograft and xenograft skin may be used as temporary biological dressings in burns but they are eventually rejected.

MICROVASCULAR SURGERY

1 Microvascular surgery involves the anastomosis and repair of small vessels.

2 It has clinical application in cases of replantation and free tissue transfer.

3 The surgery is highly specialized. Operations may take many hours and require special instruments in addition to an appropriate microscope.

4 This type of operation should be carried out only in specialized units.

REPLANTATION

Appraise

Consider replantation following accidental amputation or devascularization of any of the following parts:

- Limbs proximal to the ankle or wrist joints: this is called macroreplantation.
- Parts of limbs distal to the ankle or wrist joint: this is called microreplantation.
- The ear.
- The scalp.
- The penis.
- Composite pieces of facial tissue.

Action

1 Control bleeding from the amputation stump by simple pressure and elevation.

2 Avoid clamping vessels to stop haemorrhage unless essential, as this may cause unnecessary damage.

KEY POINTS Care of the amputated part to be replanted

- The part to be re-implanted should have been placed in a polythene bag, which is laid on ice.
- Cool but do not freeze the amputated part since freezing prevents successful replantation.
- If a part is devascularized and not fully amputated, cool this part by placing polythene bags containing ice around it.

3 Contact the nearest microvascular surgery unit and take advice.

4 Prepare the patient and amputated part for urgent transfer.

MACROREPLANTATION

Appraise

1 The force required to sever a major portion of a limb is considerable and patients who have suffered such an injury may have other injuries to their body which may take priority in treatment.

2 Criteria for attempting replantation are:
- The patient should be relatively fit.
- The amputated portion should not be too severely damaged.
- The 'warm ischaemic time' of the amputated part should not exceed 6 hours. Muscle is unlikely to recover after this period and if it is revascularized it could infuse a fatal dose of nephrotoxic substances, including myoglobin, into the circulation.
- There should be a reasonable prospect of some functional recovery.

Action

1 Debride and clean both the proximal stump and the wound of the amputated part.

2 Shorten the skeletal structures and fix these. This should allow primary anastomosis of vessels and nerves.

3 Revascularize the amputated part by anastomosing the appropriate artery, or arteries, using vein grafts if necessary.

4 If the warm ischaemic time has been relatively long, revascularize the part prior to skeletal fixation. Allow perfusion of the amputated part for several minutes, discarding the venous blood. Transfuse the patient appropriately. Revise the anastomoses after skeletal fixation if necessary.

5 Anastomose twice the number of veins as the number of arteries repaired, again using vein grafts if necessary.

6 Repair the tendons and muscles.

7 Repair the nerves.

8 Carry out extensive fasciotomies, incising through skin, subcutaneous tissue and deep fascia on the proximal stump and on the amputated part.

9 Harvest a split skin graft and apply this to the fasciotomy sites and any other residual raw areas where there has been skin loss.

10 Monitor the limb carefully postoperatively, and be prepared to return the patient to theatre at any time if there is doubt about viability of the replanted or revascularized part.

FREE TISSUE TRANSFER

Appraise

1 Free tissue transfer is used in many forms of reconstruction. It consists of transferring tissue from one part of the body to another.

2 Isolate the tissue on a recognized vascular pedicle and, after transfer to its distant site, anastomose the vessels of the vascular pedicle to appropriate nearby vessels, either directly or with vein grafts.

3 The arterial supply to the tissue is usually established with an end-to-side anastomosis to an adjacent artery, so that the distal flow of this artery is not terminated.

4 The venous drainage of the tissue is usually established via end-to-end anastomoses to superficial veins or to venae comitantes of a nearby artery. Occasionally, if the venous drainage is inadequate, you can apply leeches to the compromised tissue temporarily until adequate venous drainage is established.

5 Most free flaps currently used in reconstruction consist of cutaneous or myocutaneous flaps. Apart from the flaps described above there are many other cutaneous and myocutaneous flaps which are occasionally used.

6 Other free tissue transfers include the following:
- Vascularized bone grafts from rib, iliac crest, fibula, radius and metatarsal.
- Osseocutaneous flaps from the iliac crest, fibula, radius or metatarsal with overlying skin.
- Sensory cutaneous flaps.
- Muscle flaps with motor innervation.
- Fascial flaps.
- Small bowel, for oesophageal reconstruction.
- Omentum, for soft tissue defects.
- Testis, re-siting a high undescended testicle in the scrotum.
- Digits or parts of digits from toe to hand.

7 One of the most common free flaps used in reconstruction is the radial forearm flap. It is based on the radial artery and either the venae comitantes or superficial veins, usually the cephalic, can be used for venous drainage.

8 The flap can be raised as a fasciocutaneous flap providing a small, thin, pliable flap useful in intraoral reconstruction, as an osseocutaneous flap for bone reconstruction, or simply as a fascial flap with a skin graft for covering small soft tissue defects on the limbs.

9 It is only occasionally used as a pedicled flap, although in these circumstances it may be based distally for use in the hand. Its elevation for use as a free flap is described below (Fig. 39.29).

Action

1 Perform an Allen's test prior to surgery to confirm that the ulnar artery alone will provide sufficient blood flow to the hand. The

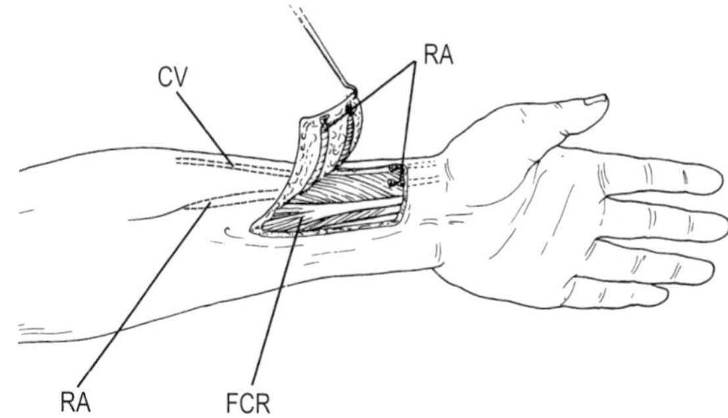

Fig. 39.29 Radial forearm flap. In elevating the flap from the medial aspect, the radial artery (RA) is identified distally, lateral to the flexor carpi radialis muscle (FCR) and divided. As the flap is raised the cephalic vein (CV) is also divided distally.

radial and ulnar arteries are occluded to the raised, fisted hand, which then appears pale on opening it if either artery is released. The whole hand should flush within 10 seconds.

2 Use a template of the defect to determine the size and shape of the flap to be harvested. Mark this out on the ventral aspect of the forearm with the distal limit extending to within 2 cm of the wrist joint. Check that the flap overlies the radial artery which can be palpated. Confirm that the distal end of the cephalic artery also lies within the area of the flap.

3 Exsanguinate the limb with elevation alone and apply the tourniquet.

4 Raise the flap from the medial side first and include the underlying fascia.

5 Dissect laterally raising the fascia but being careful not to remove the paratenon of the flexor tendons.

6 Beyond flexor carpi radialis retain the loose areolar tissue passing down to the radial artery and its accompanying venae comitantes and include these with the flap.

7 Isolate and divide these vessels distally beyond the distal limit of the flap.

8 Continue the dissection laterally by dividing the flap at its distal and then its lateral border preserving, if possible, the branches of the radial nerve by dissecting these out from the under surface of the flap.

9 Identify the radial artery and cephalic vein in the proximal attachment of the flap. Divide the skin proximally with one longitudinal incision keeping these in sight.

10 Dissect the cephalic vein up to the cubital fossa.

11 Dissect the radial artery up to its origin from the brachial artery if this length of artery is required.

12 When appropriate, divide and clamp the artery and vein and transfer the flap.

13 Ligate the stumps of the two vessels.

14 Repair the donor defect with a split skin graft and immobilize.

15 If you are experienced you may wish to use a transposition, rotation or other local flap to close the donor defect primarily.

16 Dress the donor site and subsequently remove sutures as appropriate.

BURNS

Appraise

KEY POINTS Special circumstances

- Treat patients with burns involving 15% of the body surface area (10% in children), or severe burns of the face or hands in a specialized burns unit.
- Treat patients with any significant inhalation burn in a specialized unit.

1 The treatment of patients with extensive burns is complex and ideally these patients should also be treated initially in an intensive care unit.

2 Either colloid or crystalloid can be used in fluid replacement but the principle of using the former is described below.

Assess

1 Take a careful history, paying attention to the time and nature of the accident. Was smoke was present and did the accident occur in an enclosed space? Note what kind of clothes were worn by the patient and what first aid was given.

2 Find out the patient's normal medication.

3 Examine, looking for signs of an inhalation burn. Record the extent and distribution of superficial and full-thickness burns. Pinprick sensation is usually preserved in superficial burns but do not rely on it.

4 The best guide to the depth of burn is found by taking an accurate history of the mechanism of the burn.

- Thermal burns with gases usually cause superficial burns.
- Thermal burns with liquids usually cause deep dermal burns. Boiling water and fat cause full-thickness burns. Boiling water that has cooled for 5 minutes causes superficial burns.
- Contact with hot solids and flames usually cause full-thickness burns.
- Electrical burns usually cause full-thickness skin loss.
- Radiation burns are usually superficial.
- Chemical burns are usually superficial.

5 Estimate the area of the burn using a Lund and Browder chart or 'the rule of nines'.

6 Examine the patient to exclude other injuries.

7 Weigh the patient.

Action

1 Give oxygen if you suspect an inhalation burn. Consider ventilation, particularly if the blood PO_2 is low (normal range 10.5–13.5 kPa).

2 Set up a reliable intravenous line after taking blood for a full blood count and biochemical profile.

3 Catheterize and record the urine output hourly.

4 Give PPF (plasma protein fraction) using a Muir and Barclay formula as a guide to the volume to give to replace plasma lost through the burn. This involves giving a volume in millilitres of half the weight in kilograms multiplied by the percentage burn in each of six periods. These periods start at the time of the burn and include three of 4 hours, two of 6 hours and one of 12 hours. Use the packed cell volume (PCV), urinary output and clinical state of the patient to adjust the volume of PPF given.

5 Prescribe appropriate medication, including:

- Adequate analgesia.
- Adequate anti-emetics.
- H_2-receptor antagonists.
- Adjust the doses of insulin, steroids or anticonvulsants if given previously.

6 Do not give antibiotics for the burn per se but reserve these for use later.

7 Treat the burn wounds according to their depth.

SUPERFICIAL BURNS

Action

1 Clean the burn wound and remove the roof of all blisters.

2 Expose superficial burns of the face but apply sterile liquid paraffin to reduce crusting.

3 For burns of the perineum, clean these and expose but apply silver sulfadiazine (Flamazine) cream. Nurse the patient without dressings on a sterile sheet on a low-air-loss or water bed but keep him warm.

4 Cover superficial burns of other areas with two layers of paraffin gauze and a bulky absorptive dressing. Leave this dressing for 1 week unless it becomes soaked, whereupon you should change it. Change the dressing at 1 week and subsequently twice per week until the wound is healed.

DEEP DERMAL BURNS

1 Tangentially shave with a graft knife between the second and fifth day.

2 Continue to shave until you observe punctate bleeding from the surface.

3 Achieve haemostasis with pressure and apply a split skin graft.

4 Re-dress at 4 days.

5 When fully healed, measure and apply a pressure garment. This is an elasticated garment specifically measured for the individual to cover the area of the burn wound. Advise the patient to wear this for 6 months or longer if necessary to minimize hypertrophy and contracture of the resulting scars.

6 If you do not have facilities or expertise for this management, treat the burn conservatively and re-dress twice each week.

7 Treat areas that are not healed at 3 weeks as full-thickness burns.

EXTENSIVE FULL-THICKNESS BURNS

ESCHAROTOMY

1 Note the areas of full-thickness burns that are circumferential around digit, limb or trunk. If the viability of the distal part is jeopardized, or if respiration is hindered as with partial circumferential burns of the chest wall, carry out an escharotomy (Greek: *eschara*=a hearth; the mark of a burn).

2 Give an appropriate intravenous dose of diazepam.

3 Take a scalpel and incise along the full length of the full-thickness burn, allowing subcutaneous fat to bulge out of the escharotomy wound.

4 Repeat the longitudinal escharotomy at different sites of the circumference until you have restored satisfactory perfusion of the distal part.

5 Dress the wounds with paraffin gauze or silver sulfadiazine (Flamazine).

Action

1 Identify a suitable area, not exceeding 20% of the body area, to treat primarily.

2 Identify a suitable donor site for the skin graft.

3 Excise the chosen area of full-thickness burn with a scalpel and be sure that the resultant bed consists of viable tissue. It is often safer to excise all subcutaneous fat to leave a graft bed of deep fascia. Achieve haemostasis.

4 Harvest a split skin graft and mesh this (see above).

5 Apply the mesh graft to the burn wound site and dress with several layers of paraffin gauze and an absorbent dressing.

6 Re-dress after 4 days.

KEY POINT Importance of timing

- Do not excise burn tissue between the fifth and the twelfth day post-burn, as the patient may be in an unsuitable catabolic state.

7 Do not excise further burn until the donor site has healed and is ready for reharvesting, or another donor site is available.

Small areas

1 Operate between the second and fifth day.

2 Excise all burn tissue and apply a split skin graft.

3 If the viability of subcutaneous fat is in doubt, excise this down to the deep fascia.

4 If the viability of the tissue is still in doubt, dress the wound and bring the patient back to the theatre 48 hours later. Re-assess viability at this second operation. Excise further if necessary and graft.

5 Re-dress after 4 days.

OTHER WOUNDS

1 Do not close infected wounds primarily. They arise in a multitude of different situations.

2 Two common causes presenting to plastic surgeons include pressure sores and necrotizing fasciitis. Their management is described below.

WOUNDS FROM PRESSURE INJURIES

Appraise

1 Pressure injuries are common and difficult to detect in the early stages of development. The tissues between the skeleton and an external surface are compressed, causing a variable degree of ischaemia, which may be sufficient to cause necrosis. Necrosis may involve the superficial skin, the full thickness of skin or all the tissues overlying the skeleton.

2 Pressure injuries can occur in many sites but are most frequently found in well-recognized 'pressure areas' over the backs of the heels and around the pelvis, over the ischial tuberosity, the sacrum and the greater trochanter.

3 They result from the patient lying on or against a hard surface for a prolonged period. They may occur when the patient is comatose or under general anaesthesia or when the area is

insensate, as in diabetic neuropathy or paraplegia. They are more likely to occur in these circumstances if the patient is thin, poorly nourished, cachectic and relatively immobile. Some surgical patients are therefore at particular risk.

4 There may be no significant evidence of the injury for some time after the event. Usually the first sign is erythema in the damaged area. Blistering usually indicates a superficial injury only. If the damage is deep the skin colour changes to blue and then to black as a thick eschar develops over a period of many days. This remains dry for several weeks before the necrotic tissue starts to separate.

5 Spontaneous separation of the underlying necrotic tissue may take many weeks or even months. When the necrotic tissue has separated, the wound will heal by secondary intention. A residual sinus will persist if necrotic tissue remains buried or if the underlying bone becomes infected.

6 As many patients with these injuries are debilitated, the above process may take many months and treatment is aimed at accelerating the healing process without insulting the patient further with unnecessary surgery.

Action

1 Avoid these injuries by identifying those patients particularly at risk.

2 Attend to their general health, specifically their nutrition and other medical disorders.

3 Take appropriate precautions when they are on the operating table and when in bed on the ward. Use one of the many specialized mattresses or beds to distribute the weight of the patient where possible. If these are not available the nursing staff may need to assist a change of position of the patient at least every 2 hours.

4 Cover superficial wounds with non-adherent dressings such as paraffin gauze and change on alternate days until healed.

5 Cover hard eschar with simple protective dressings only, or leave exposed if appropriate.

6 When the eschar starts to separate use a debriding agent such as Eusol and paraffin dressings changed daily.

7 Assist separation of the eschar by using a forceps and scissors during a dressing change. Repeat this with every change of dressing and avoid formal debridement in theatre and an unnecessary general anaesthetic.

8 Take wound swabs at regular intervals to monitor the organisms present but use antibiotics sparingly, for example if there is evidence of surrounding cellulitis.

9 Advise the patient to have a regular bath or shower, if appropriate, to help clean the wound and improve the patient's morale.

10 When a cavity is established use a vacuum dressing. After irrigating and cleaning the wound with saline, insert the foam dressing, introduce the drain and cover with an occlusive dressing. Apply negative pressure to the drain via the pump and leave for 2–3 days before repeating.

11 If a vacuum pump is not available, change the dressings to calcium alginate when the necrotic tissue has separated and a surface layer of red granulation tissue is evident. Change this daily.

12 If a large cavity persists consider introducing a large cutaneous or myocutaneous flap (see above, Rotation flap, Biceps femoris flap, Tensor fascia lata flap).

13 Also consider continuing with dressings until healed, avoiding surgery and allowing uninterrupted mobilization.

NECROTIZING FASCIITIS

Appraise

KEY POINT Recognize and act

- If the patient is to survive you must make an early diagnosis and act immediately.

1 This is a rare condition but you must recognize it immediately as serious and life-threatening.

2 There is a focal point where the infection commences, and this often arises from a surgical intervention.

3 The condition results usually from the symbiotic effect of the coincidental occurrence of an aerobic staphylococcus and an anaerobic streptococcus.

4 The bacteria appear to spread initially and preferentially along fascial planes. The overlying subcutaneous fat and skin are subsequently rendered ischaemic and necrotic.

Action

1 Look out for:
- Unexpected local cellulitis.
- Rapidly expanding cellulitis.
- Deteriorating general condition.

2 Take wound swabs and blood specimens for culture of organism and sensitivities.

3 Commence on appropriate antibiotics.

4 Mark the edge of the area of erythema on the skin.

5 If the area of erythema is seen to progress beyond the marked line within a few hours, take the patient to theatre immediately.

6 Use a cutting diathermy to remove all skin showing erythema as well as underlying subcutaneous fat and deep fascia.

7 Remove any tissue suspicious of being involved in the infective process.

8 Dress the wound with gauze soaked in saline and further absorbent dressings, leaving the skin adjacent to the wound available for inspection.

9 Take the patient back to theatre after 24 hours or earlier if there are signs of progression of the disease.

10 Carry out further debridement of infected tissue.

11 Repeat this after a further 24 hours, remaining vigilant until all signs of infection have been eradicated.

12 When the patient is stable, consider covering the residual defect with split skin grafts or skin flaps or a combination of these.

FACIAL CLEFTS

KEY POINTS Inexpert?

- These descriptions are reminders for surgeons working in isolation but who have been trained in the procedures. They are also included for trainees helping at operations who can offer intelligent and effective assistance at these highly skilled procedures.
- Do not attempt them if you are inexpert because you may create disastrous results.

CLEFT LIP

Appraise

1. The treatment of clefts of the lip and palate may be very complex. Refer patients for treatment at specialist centres with a paediatrician, a paediatric anaesthetist, an orthodontist, an ENT surgeon, an oral surgeon, a dentist, an audiologist and a speech therapist as well as the plastic surgeon.
2. The extent of the cleft of the lip is variable and ranges from a slight notch in the vermilion border to a complete cleft of the whole lip.
3. The cleft may be bilateral and there may be an associated cleft of the palate.
4. Midline clefts of the lip, with absence of philtrum (Greek: *philtron*=love potion; median groove of upper lip) and columella (Latin: = a little column) and associated hypoteleorism, are rare. Refer patients to a specialized unit, as should those with rare oblique clefts of the face involving the lip.
5. Repair clefts of the lip at 3 months of age or soon after birth.
6. If the cleft is bilateral, repair the two sides separately with a 1-month interval between operations. Repair the more severe cleft first.
7. A prominent philtrum, particularly obvious in bilateral cleft lips, can be corrected preoperatively with orthodontic appliances. If these are not available, apply simple Elastoplast strapping from cheek to cheek across the prominent philtrum, to help reduce it before operation.
8. There are many techniques for repairing a cleft of the lip, but the Millard repair as described below is popular. The steps are outlined.

Prepare

1. Identify the midpoint of the philtrum on its vermilion border, and mark (Fig. 39.30, point 1).
2. Identify the vermilion border at the base of the normal philtral column and mark (point 2).
3. Mark the corresponding point on the vermilion border at the base of the projected contralateral philtral column (point 3).
4. Mark the midpoint of the junction of the columella with the philtrum (point 4).

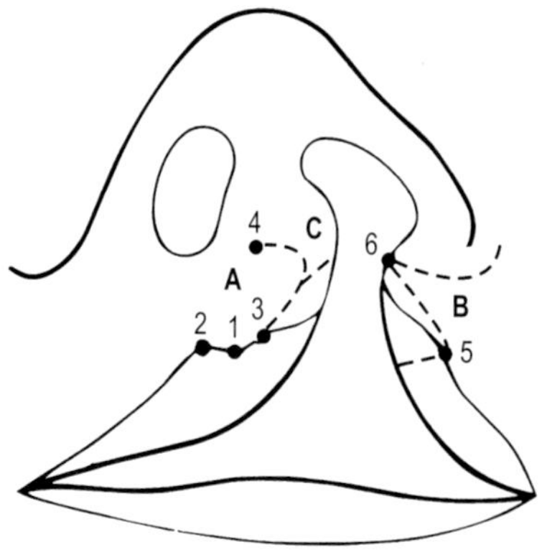

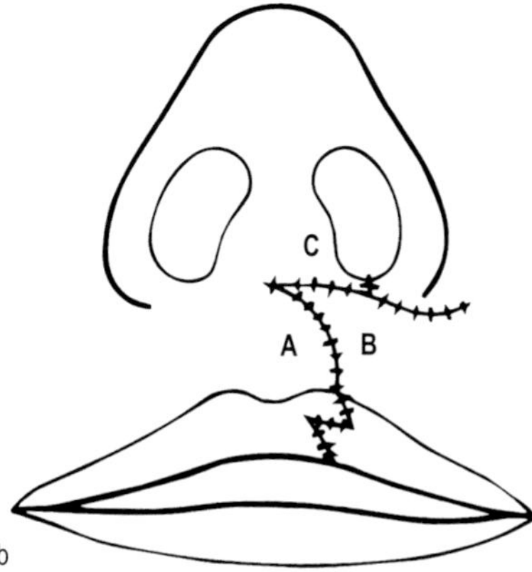

Fig. 39.30 Cleft lip—the Millard repair: point 1 is the centre of the Cupid's bow; point 2 is the peak of the Cupid's bow on the normal side; point 3 is the projected point of the peak of the Cupid's bow on the cleft side; point 4 is the junction of the midpoint of the philtrum and columella; point 5 is the start of the mucosal thickening of the cleft side; point 6 is the medial extremity of the alar base on the cleft side. The dashed lines indicate the incisions (a). Flaps A and B have been sutured into place and flap C is used to create the nostril sill. A Z-plasty has been introduced into the vermilion mucosa (b).

5. On the lateral segment of the lip, mark the vermilion border at a point where the white roll disappears (point 5).
6. On the lateral segment, mark the most medial point of normal skin, horizontally level with the base of the nostril (point 6).
7. Draw a straight line between points 5 and 6 and a curved line between points 3 and 4 of equal length.
8. Infiltrate the area with local anaesthesia using 0.5% lidocaine and 1 : 200 000 adrenaline (epinephrine).

Action

1. With a size no. 11 blade, cut through the full thickness of the lip along the curved line of the medial segment.
2. Excise the mucosal surface lateral to this, preserving a small triangular flap of normal skin (the 'C' flap).
3. Excise the mucosa medial to the straight line on the lateral segment.

4 Incise the lateral segment from point 6 laterally around the base of the ala.

5 Reflect back the skin and identify the muscles inserted into the alar base.

6 Divide these muscles and dissect them free from their attachment to the alar base.

7 Identify and dissect free the muscle in the medial segment.

8 Suture together the orbicularis oris muscle from each segment with 4/0 absorbable suture.

9 Approximate the skin using 6/0 polyglactin 910 as a subcutaneous suture.

10 Approximate point 6 to point 4.

11 Approximate point 5 to point 3.

12 Use the 'C' flap to create a nostril sill.

13 Suture the skin with 6/0 nylon.

14 Suture the skin and mucosa within the nostril with 6/0 polyglactin 910.

15 Adjust the mucosa of the lip and suture. If necessary incorporate a small Z-plasty.

16 Remove sutures at 3–4 days.

CLEFT PALATE

Appraise

1 A cleft palate often occurs in conjunction with a cleft lip, but may occur separately.

2 The extent of the cleft palate varies from a complete cleft to a submucous cleft, where the palate is apparently intact but there has been failure of fusion of the levator palati muscles across the midline.

3 Repair the muscle in submucous clefts of the palate to ensure satisfactory function of the palate during speech.

4 Repair clefts of the palate at about 6 months of age to restore the speech mechanism to normal as early as is practical.

5 The bone defect may be constructed with a bone graft after the secondary dentition has erupted.

Prepare

1 Insert a suitable mouth gag such as the Dingman.

2 Pack the pharynx with ribbon gauze.

3 Mark out bilateral flaps on the palate passing from the uvula along the side of the cleft to its apex and anteriorly along the midline to within 3 mm of the alveolus (Fig. 39.31).

4 Continue marking laterally, keeping just within the margin of the alveolus and passing backwards behind the hamulus to the anterior pillar of the fauces.

5 Infiltrate the flaps with 0.5% lidocaine and 1:200 000 adrenaline (epinephrine).

Action

1 Incise along the marked edges of one flap, commencing at the tip of the split uvula.

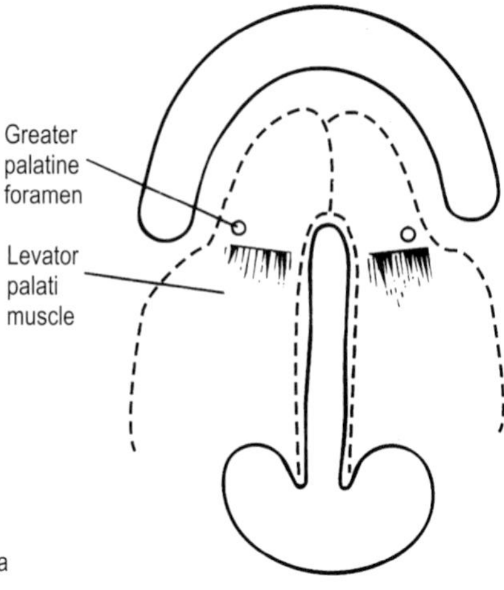

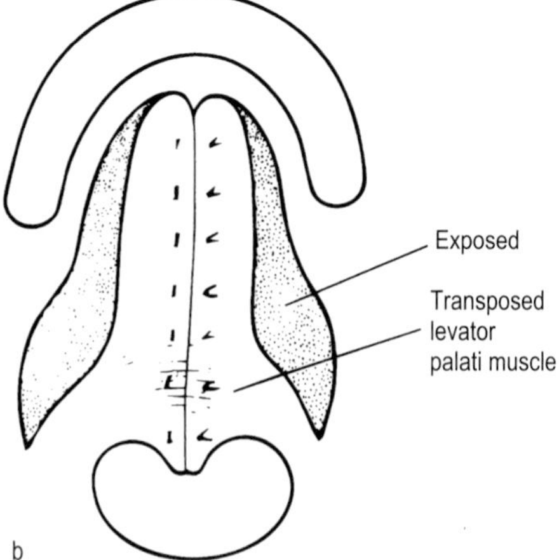

Fig. 39.31 Cleft palate repair. (a) The flaps of the two-flap repair. Note the attachment of the levator palati into the hard palate. This muscle should be dissected off the hard palate and sutured together in the midline. The subsequent repair of the mucosa of the soft palate leaves a residual exposed area laterally which epithelializes spontaneously during the first postoperative week (b).

2 Elevate the flap from its anterior margin as a mucoperiosteal flap.

3 Scrape the periosteum off the palate using a Mitchell trimmer.

4 On approaching the greater palatine artery, identify this as it emerges through its foramen and dissect the flap away from the bone around its perimeter.

5 Using the Mitchell trimmer, separate the nasal mucosa from the palatal bones.

6 Identify the levator palati muscle inserted into the posterior margin of the hard palate and place a spatula between this attachment and the nasal mucosa.

7 Cut down through this attachment on to the spatula, freeing the levator palati muscle completely from the hard palate.

8 Dissect the levator palati free from both underlying nasal mucosa and its covering palatal mucosa.

9 Repeat the dissection on the opposite side.

10 Repair the nasal mucosa with 4/0 polyglactin 910, commencing anteriorly and work posteriorly to reconstruct the uvula.

11 Suture the two ends of the levator palati together in the midline with 4/0 polyglactin 910 sutures.

12 Repair the oral mucosa in the midline using 4/0 polyglactin 910 sutures. Use deep mattress sutures in the central portion.

13 The anterior tip of the two flaps when sutured together may protrude into the mouth. They need not be sutured down as they adhere to the palate very early in the postoperative phase if left free.

ANTERIOR CLEFT PALATE

Appraise

1 A cleft of the anterior palate coexists with a cleft of the lip.

2 It can be partially closed at the time of the lip repair but is usually closed at the time of the palate repair when this is also present.

3 Repair in specialized centres is usually achieved in layers by mobilizing the nasal mucosa on the cleft side first and suturing this to the vomerine mucosa. The lateral and medial mucoperiosteal flaps are closed over this.

4 For the inexperienced or isolated surgeon a more reliable closure is achieved by overlapping and suturing the mucoperiosteal flap of the cleft side to the vomerine flap.

Action

1 Insert a Dingman gag.

2 Mark out a flap on the vomer with its base at the vomerine margin (Fig. 39.32).

3 Mark out a lateral flap as for repair of a cleft palate. Infiltrate both flaps with 0.5% lidocaine and 1:200 000 adrenaline (epinephrine).

4 Elevate both flaps.

5 Oppose and suture the raw surface of the two flaps together.

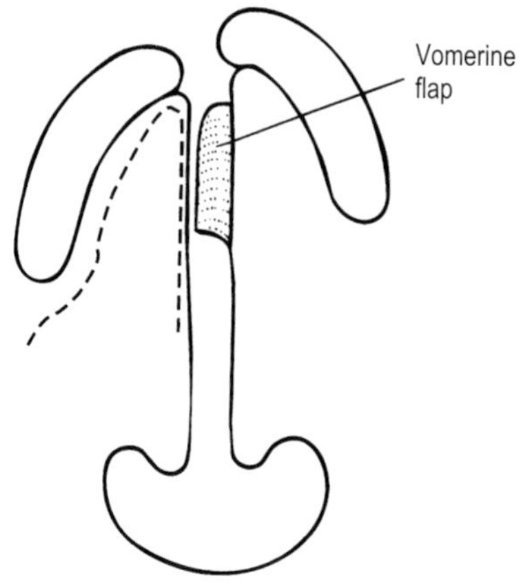

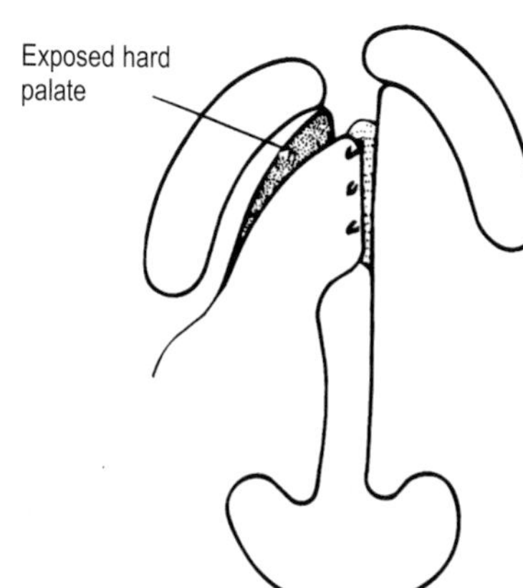

Fig. 39.32 Anterior palate repair. A superiorly based vomerine flap is raised off the septum (a). A palatal flap is raised laterally and mobilized. The two flaps are sutured raw surface to raw surface using mattress sutures (b).

PHARYNGOPLASTY

Appraise

1 A pharyngoplasty is necessary to reduce the velopharyngeal space when this is responsible for nasal escape during speech. This is usually due to the soft palate being too short to reach the posterior pharyngeal wall.

2 Carry out preoperative assessment with a nasendoscope wherever possible.

3 There are many different kinds of pharyngoplasty. Most provide a reduction in the anatomical size of the velopharyngeal space.

4 A few, including the Ortichochea repair described below, attempt not only to reduce the anatomical size of this space but also to provide a dynamic sphincter, which helps closure during speech.

Action

1 Insert a Dingman gag.

2 Mark a rectangular pharyngeal flap, based inferiorly and reaching as high as can be visualized on the posterior pharyngeal wall.

3 Infiltrate the flap with 0.5% lidocaine and 1:200 000 adrenaline (epinephrine).

4 Identify the palatopharyngeus muscle within the posterior pillar of the fauces, and insert a McIndoe scissors behind this after penetrating the mucosa.

5 Separate the blades of the scissors and dissect free the muscle along its length. Dissect it free to its lower limit and divide it at this point.

6 Dissect the opposite muscle free in the same manner, preserving some overlying mucosa.

7 Raise the posterior pharyngeal flap down to its base and achieve haemostasis of its bed.

8 Suture the muscle belly of each of the two flaps to the raw surface of the pharyngeal flap with 4/0 polyglactin 910 sutures.

9 Improve the attachment by suturing the mucosa of the muscle flap to the mucosa of the pharyngeal flap along the various attachments with 6/0 polyglactin 910.

CRANIOFACIAL SURGERY

Appraise

1 Craniofacial surgery involves correction of abnormalities of the facial and cranial bones and overlying soft tissues.

2 Many cranial abnormalities occur as part of well-recognized syndromes. Others result from premature fusion of one or more of the cranial sutures.

3 This surgery was pioneered by Tessier, who has classified the different types of facial cleft.

4 Craniofacial surgery is now recognized as a specialty in its own right. It often involves combined expertise from several specialists, including a neurosurgeon, ophthalmic surgeon, maxillofacial surgeon, ENT surgeon and paediatric surgeon as well as the plastic surgeon.

5 These cases are rare but often much can be done to help these patients in specialized centres where this surgery is carried out.

LYMPHOEDEMA

Appraise

1 There are many operations described to treat lymphoedema but the cosmetic result of these is uniformly disappointing.

2 The application of microlymphatic surgery, anastomosing lymphatic vessels in cases of obstructive lymphoedema, has not produced the dramatic results initially anticipated.

3 Use pressure garments and other conservative measures before considering surgery.

4 Surgical intervention of the upper limb is rarely indicated.

5 In moderate cases of lymphoedema of the lower limb, where cosmesis is important, excise longitudinal wedges of skin and underlying fat serially, avoiding the necessity to graft the limb, as first described by Homan (Fig. 39.33).

6 In very severe cases of lymphoedema of the limb use the Charles operation.

7 Lymphoedema of the genitalia of men and women is treated with wedge excisions of the tissue involved and primary closure.

8 Localized areas of lymphoedema around the eyelids can be reduced using local excision and closure, preferably with a blepharoplasty technique (see below).

MODERATE LYMPHOEDEMA

1 When operating on the lower limb, insert a Steinmann pin through the calcaneum, apply a metal stirrup and support the limb from above for the duration of the procedure.

2 Exsanguinate the limb and apply a tourniquet proximally on the thigh as high as possible.

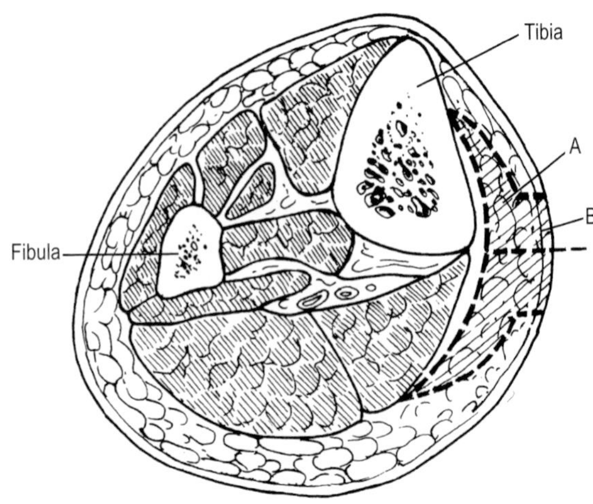

Fig. 39.33 Homan's operation for reduction of moderate degree of lymphoedema. Transverse section of mid-calf showing incisions (dotted line) on medial aspect. Fat (A) is excised first followed by excision of redundant skin (B) before wound closure.

3 Mark a line from the medial aspect of the thigh passing over the medial part of the knee joint to a point 1 cm posterior to the medial malleolus.

4 Incise down this line to the deep fascia leaving this intact.

5 Dissect in the plane just superficial to the deep fascia raising flaps anteriorly and posteriorly, being careful to seal all vessels perforating the deep fascia using diathermy current or ligatures.

6 Thin the flaps by removing fat from their deep surface leaving the flaps at least 1 cm thick, constantly checking the viability of the edge as you resect.

7 Remove less fat as you progress anteriorly and posteriorly as well as at each end of the incision.

8 Allow the skin flaps to overlap and excise the excess skin to allow them, after excision, to meet along the original incision line without tension.

9 Be meticulous with haemostasis.

10 Close the wound with mattress sutures over two large Redivac drains.

11 Dress with dressing gauze cotton wool and a firm crepe bandage and keep the leg elevated.

12 Mobilize slowly after 10 days but defer removing the sutures for at least 14 days.

13 Measure and apply a pressure garment as soon as possible to be worn for at least 3 months or longer.

14 Consider repeating this procedure on the lateral side after 3 months.

15 You may consider further surgery with liposuction (see below) or repeating the excision on the medial aspect raising the flaps more extensively in anterior and posterior directions.

SEVERE LYMPHOEDEMA

1 Insert a Steinmann pin through the calcaneum to support the limb from above for both the operation and the early post-operative phase.

2 Exsanguinate the limb and apply a tourniquet proximally.

3 Take split skin grafts from the surface of the limb to be treated if this is suitable. If it is not, take split skin grafts from another donor area and dress the donor site. Store the skin grafts.

4 Excise all skin and subcutaneous tissue down to the deep fascia, from the limb.

5 Preserve the skin of the sole of the foot and the toes, and leave skin to cover the malleoli.

6 Preserve enough skin to flute into the defect at the upper margin of excision.

7 Achieve haemostasis and dress the limb with several layers of paraffin gauze, dressing gauze, absorbent dressings and bandage.

8 Remove the dressings after 24 hours and apply the stored skin while the limb remains elevated by traction on the Steinmann pin. This manoeuvre allows exposure of the skin grafts circumferentially on the limb.

9 Mobilize the limb when the skin grafts are stable, between 10 and 14 days.

10 Order pressure garments to be worn for at least 3 months postoperatively and in most cases indefinitely.

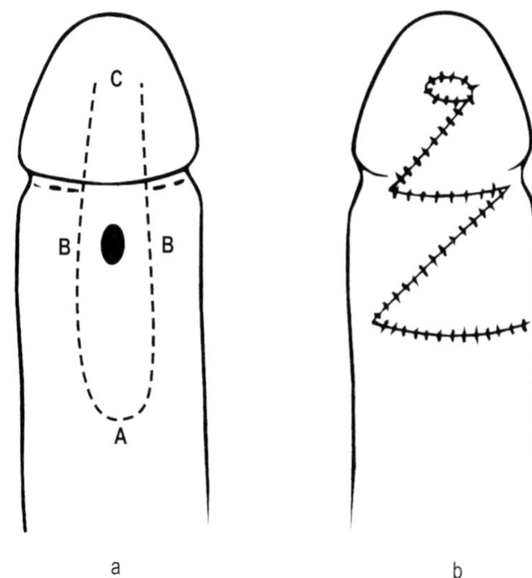

Fig. 39.34 Distal hypospadias repair. A plan of the incisions should be marked preoperatively. The proximal flap must have adequate length for A to reach C when hinged at point B adjacent to the external meatus (a). After suturing the lateral margins of this flap, lateral flaps are mobilized using the redundant preputial skin and closed in a Z-plasty fashion (b).

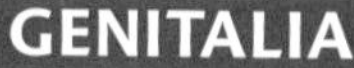

GENITALIA

HYPOSPADIAS

Appraise

1 The male urethral meatus may appear on the surface at any point in the midline between its normal position at the tip of the glans penis and the perineum.

2 In many cases of hypospadias (Greek: *hypos*=under+*span*=to draw), a tight fibrous band, the chordee, is evident distal to the ectopic meatus, which causes curvature of the penis when in the erect position.

3 Reconstructive surgery to place the meatus in its normal position at the tip of the glans is intended to produce an apparently normal penis without urethral fistula.

4 Many operations have been designed to treat the condition but none consistently fulfils the above criteria.

5 Experienced surgeons advocate a one-stage procedure, but if your are an inexperienced surgeon, proceed with a staged reconstruction.

6 Ideally, carry out operation in infancy. Some surgeons prefer to wait until the child is continent of urine to release the chordee and then reconstruct the urethra just before the child starts school.

Release of chordee

1 Under general anaesthesia carry out a Horton test. Place some rubber tubing around the base of the penis and pull it tight. Inject the corpora with physiological saline to produce an erect penis and note the extent of chordee. Release the rubber tubing.

2 Mark the extent of the chordee in ink. Mark out a Z-plasty for reconstruction following excision of the chordee.

3 Incise down the central line overlying the chordee.

4 Excise all underlying fibrous tissue.

5 Use a bipolar coagulator to achieve haemostasis.

6 Raise the flaps of the Z-plasty, transpose them and suture them with 6/0 polyglactin 910. Do not dress the wound.

Distal shaft correction

1 Under general anaesthesia carry out a Horton test as above.

2 If any chordee is still evident, excise this and defer reconstruction for a further 6 months.

3 If no chordee is apparent, mark out a rectangular flap proximal to the meatus with its base at the meatus. The flap should be 1 cm broad and long enough to reach the glans when turned distally (Fig. 39.34).

4 Mark out a strip of skin distal to the meatus from the meatus to the glans.

5 Catheterize the urethra with a small Foley catheter.

6 Elevate the flap and reflect it distally.

7 Cut along the margins of the strip of skin and elevate the edges.

8 Suture the flap to the cut edges of the strip of skin using 6/0 absorbable suture.

9 Elevate lateral flaps of skin by incising around the attachment of preputial skin to the glans. Mobilize the flaps round to the dorsal surface.

10 Suture the flaps across the reconstructed urethra, so that the suture line between the two flaps traverses the reconstructed urethra. Use 6/0 polyglactin 910.

11 Suture a foam dressing around the reconstructed penis. This prevents interference from the patient. Suture or strap the catheter to the upper thigh.

12 Remove the dressing and catheter at 10 days.

Proximal shaft, scrotal and perineal hypospadias

1 As with distal shaft hypospadias, there are many operations to correct these deformities. Reconstruct the urethra with flaps of preputial skin from the redundant foreskin or use a free graft of preputial skin.

2 Use local skin flaps to cover the reconstructed urethra.

3 In perineal hypospadias, use the hairless strip of skin in the middle of the scrotum for the urethral reconstruction in this region.

EPISPADIAS AND ECTOPIA OF THE BLADDER

Appraise

1 Epispadias and ectopia of the bladder represent different expressions of the same basic embryological defect.

2 These rare conditions require highly specialized treatment, where one-stage correction is advocated.

Action

1 If specialized treatment is not available do not carry out a pelvic osteotomy.

2 Close the bladder wall with abdominal flaps.

3 Tighten the bladder neck at a second stage.

4 In a third stage, close the residual epispadias by passing a funnel of mucosa through the base of the penis to the ventral surface and reconstruct the resultant hypospadias.

PHALLOPLASTY

Appraise

1 Construction of a penis in gender reassignment or total reconstruction in the rare cases of amputation where replantation is not possible or not successful is technically challenging and should only be done by those specialized in this field.

2 A common principle is to use a tubed free radial forearm flap. A lateral longitudinal element is turned inside and tubed to reconstruct the urethra.

3 An inflatable stent can be inserted into the reconstructed organ to allow simulation of an erection.

4 The development of fistulae and damage to the insensate skin are common complications.

VAGINAL ATRESIA

Appraise

1 In a few patients with vaginal atresia it is possible to stretch the small dimple at the site of the vaginal orifice with graded dilators and operation surgery. Advocate this treatment whenever possible.

2 Failure of conservative treatment is an indication for surgery.

3 The success of surgery, providing there is a satisfactory take of graft, will depend much on the perseverance of the patient with regular dilatation after surgery, particularly during the first 6 months.

4 Vaginal reconstruction after major trauma, treatment for tumour or previous surgery requires the introduction of a pedicled or free flap such as a gracilis myocutaneous flap.

Action

1 Make a cruciate incision at the vault of the vaginal dimple.

2 Use sharp dissection to open a space up to the perineal membrane.

3 Use blunt dissection above this to create the full vaginal space.

4 Take a large split skin graft from the thigh and mesh it.

5 Apply the meshed graft to a stent the size of the vagina and suture the edges over the stent.

6 Insert the graft on the stent and then remove the stent.

7 Pack tightly the reconstructed vagina with multiple pieces of sponge foam dressings.

8 Suture the labia together with three sutures of 0/0 nylon to retain the foam dressings in place.

9 Re-dress under general anaesthesia 2 weeks later.

10 Prevent contraction of the graft by retaining a vaginal dilator in place at night and encourage regular dilatation during the day.

SCARS

HYPERTROPHIC SCARS

Appraise

1 These present as red, raised, broad, hard, itchy scars that are unsightly and uncomfortable. They develop a few months after the wound has healed.

2 Beware of excising or revising them unless there was failure of primary healing or unless a marked contraction has developed. Simple excision of the scar alone will probably cause a larger one to develop.

Action

1 Inject the scar tissue only with triamcinolone.

2 Repeat the injections at monthly intervals for 3–6 months or longer if necessary until the scar is soft.

3 Avoid excessive injections and avoid injecting the triamcinolone into the surrounding skin. This may cause skin atrophy.

4 If the scars are extensive, fit and apply a pressure garment as early as possible. Advise the patient to wear this garment for 6–12 months.

Pressure garments

1 A pressure garment is a synthetic elastic garment that is specifically measured to fit part of an individual.

2 In applying pressure to a scar, it modifies the maturation and limits hypertrophic scar formation, provided it is applied early.

3 Pressure garments are most useful in reducing hypertrophic scar formation and preventing the development of contractures, particularly from burn wounds.

4 They are also used in controlling progressive lymphoedema.

KELOIDS

Appraise

1 Keloids (Greek: *kelis*=scar+*eidos*=like) have a different histological appearance from hypertrophic scars.

2 They are most commonly found in patients of African origin but can be found in all races.

3 Excision of keloids, like excision of hypertrophic scars, only temporarily cures the problem. A larger lesion will develop in its place and this treatment is to be condemned.

4 Treatment with triamcinolone, as used for hypertrophic scars (see above), reduces the size of most keloids but does not eliminate them. This may, however, be the best treatment.

5 Excision of the whole keloid followed by radiotherapy to the resultant scar can be very effective. This requires expertise in radiotherapy but may not be suitable for young patients.

Action

1 Identify the boundaries of the keloid.

2 Excise its central bulk, keeping the margin of excision at the lateral borders and in depth within the keloid tissue. Close the wound primarily, preserving a rim of keloid tissue at all margins. Keep all sutures within this rim.

3 Give monthly injections of triamcinolone into the residual scar as for a hypertrophic scar (see above).

4 Apply pressure to the area for at least 3 months afterwards with a pressure garment specifically fitted for the patient if appropriate.

5 If the keloid is extensive, take a split skin graft from the surface of the keloid and apply to the raw surface after removing the major bulk of the keloid. Again, keep all sutures within the keloid tissue and apply pressure postoperatively.

AESTHETIC SURGERY

1 You should undertake these operations only if you are an expert. Aesthetic (Greek: *aisthanesthai*=to feel, perceive) operations demand specialist management, since they are intended to be pleasing to the patient.

2 These operations can nearly always be deferred until specialist treatment is available, but a brief outline of the more common operations is given below.

3 Careful preoperative assessment and full explanation of the expectation of the results of surgery and all potential complications are vital parts of management of patients in this field of surgery.

FACELIFT

Appraise

1 The principal aim of a facelift is to resuspend the soft tissues of the face, which have fallen as a result of gravity and other factors. This may involve tightening or reducing muscles and removal or replacement of subcutaneous fat and skin.

2 There are many different types of facelift, some involving the use of an endoscope.

3 There are also many associated procedures that can be carried out at the same time, such as an endoscopic brow lift to elevate and stretch the forehead skin and a platysmaplasty to increase the cervicomental angle.

4 In the cheek the skin may be elevated by dissecting in the subcutaneous plane or in the plane of the superficial musculoaponeurotic system (SMAS) or in both.

Action

1 Make a vertical incision in the temple hairline down to the pinna. Extend this around the lower two-thirds of the pinna and backwards horizontally into the lateral occipital hairline (Fig. 39.35).

2 Raise the skin anterior to this incision and undermine it halfway to the nasolabial fold and an equivalent distance towards the chin and the neck. Avoid dividing branches of the facial nerves.

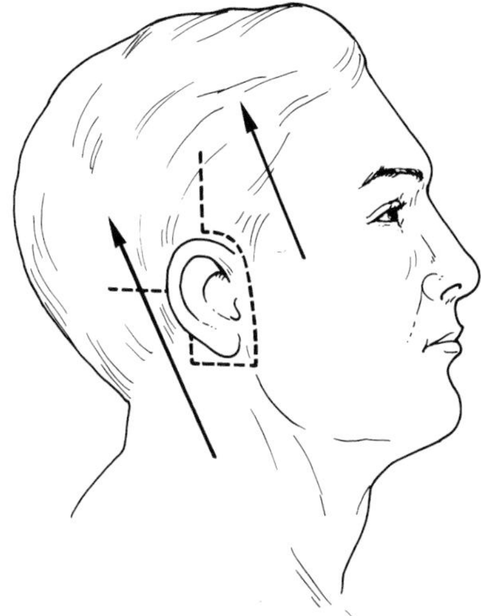

Fig. 39.35 Facelift. The skin incision is marked by the dotted line. After undermining and SMAS plication, the skin is pulled in the direction of the arrows and, after excision of excess skin, the wound is closed.

3 Plicate the superficial fascia (the SMAS layer) to reduce subsequent tension on the skin.
4 Retract the skin flap towards the incision line and excise the excess tissue.
5 Suture the flap into place along the original incision margin.
6 Insert a small corrugated drain beneath the postauricular skin.
7 Repeat the process on the opposite side to produce symmetry.

RHINOPLASTY

Appraise

1 Compare and contrast the patient's assessment of his or her nose with your own assessment of the nose.
2 Establish exactly what the patient wants.

Action

1 Shave or cut the vibrissae in the nostrils.
2 Make an intercartilaginous incision on each side through mucosa between the alar and lateral cartilages.
3 Extend this incision over the vault of the nostril down to the front of the septum.
4 Through this incision separate the skin on the top of the nose from the underlying septum.
5 Incise the mucosa along the roof of each nostril and divide the upper lateral cartilages from the septum.
6 Reduce the upper lateral cartilages as necessary.
7 Reduce the septal hump with a knife.
8 Remove the hump of the nasal bones with an osteotome and hammer.
9 Make a small incision in each pyriform fossa.
10 Insert a periosteal elevator through this incision on the lateral margin of the nose and elevate the periosteum from the lateral margin of each nasal bone.
11 Insert a nasal saw along each incision in turn and cut halfway through the nasal bone.
12 Insert an osteotome along each incision in turn and complete the nasal osteotomy.
13 Manipulate the nasal bones into the new position.
14 Rasp the nasal septum as necessary.
15 Through the intercartilaginous incision, evert the alar cartilages and reduce as necessary.
16 Expose the anterior margin of the nasal septum and adjust as necessary.
17 Suture the nasal mucosa with 3/0 absorbable thread.
18 Pack each nostril with paraffin gauze.
19 Dress with tape and a nasal splint.
20 Remove the nasal packs at 24 hours.
21 Remove the splint at 10 days.

BLEPHAROPLASTY

Appraise

1 This operation is carried out to reduce the skin and fat tissue in the upper and lower eyelids (Greek: *blepharon*=eyelid).
2 Identify before operation the site and volume of the underlying pads of fat.

Action

1 Under local or general anaesthesia, mark the excision margins of the skin of the upper eyelid as a crescent with an accessory tail laterally.
2 Mark the excision margin on the lower eyelid with a minimal reduction in height.
3 Infiltrate with local anaesthetic, if indicated.
4 Excise the skin from the upper eyelid and excise the underlying fat pads from beneath the orbicularis muscle if any are present. Achieve haemostasis and suture with subcuticular 5/0 polypropylene.
5 Raise the lower eyelid skin and, with a skin hook, pull the skin upwards and laterally.
6 Excise a triangle of skin at the lateral margin and a minimal amount of skin along the eyelid margin.
7 Reflect the skin flap and excise the fat pads from beneath the orbicularis muscle.
8 Suture the skin with 6/0 nylon.
9 Remove the sutures at 3–4 days.

CORRECTION OF PROMINENT EARS

Appraise

1 This operation is carried out to reduce the prominence of the ears, which may be due to a deep concha but is more commonly due to an absence of the anti-helical fold.
2 The principle of the operation is to remould the shape of the cartilage.
3 Operations that depend on skin and cartilage excision are unsatisfactory.
4 Defer surgery in children until the age of 6 years, as the cartilage is thin and children do not normally appreciate or suffer from any psychological problem before this age.

Action

1 Use general or local anaesthesia.
2 Infiltrate the pinna with local anaesthesia.
3 Mark the site of the proposed antihelical rim and tattoo the underlying cartilage by passing a needle covered with ink through the full thickness of the pinna at several points along this line.
4 Excise a narrow vertical ellipse of skin from the posterior surface of the pinna.
5 Incise the cartilage posteriorly along the tattoo marks.

6 Dissect the cartilage away from the anterior skin of the pinna.

7 Score the anterior aspect of the cartilage with circumferential and radial incisions, to allow the cartilage to fold backwards.

8 When you have obtained adequate reduction, re-drape the skin over the cartilage and suture the skin wound with subcuticular polypropylene.

9 Repeat the process for the opposite ear to provide symmetry.

10 Dress both ears with proflavine wool to ensure apposition of skin to cartilage.

11 Cover both ears with cotton wool and a supportive bandage.

12 Remove the dressing at 10 days and remove the sutures.

13 Maintain a protective dressing over the ears at night for 4 weeks.

BREAST AUGMENTATION

Appraise

1 Breasts can be augmented in size by inserting prostheses in the submammary plane or in the subpectoral plane.

2 The most common complication is the development of a fibrous capsule around the prosthesis. When this contracts appreciably, the prosthesis feels hard and uncomfortable and the breast becomes distorted.

3 The size of prosthesis to be used is dependent on the size of the patient and the breast size. A history of previous surgery, previous pregnancy and lactation and weight changes all influence the choice of the size of prosthesis to be used.

Action

1 Incise the skin along the submammary fold.

2 Dissect a pocket in the submammary plane sufficient to accommodate the prosthesis.

3 Insert the prosthesis.

4 Close the wound in layers.

5 Keep the breasts well supported in the postoperative phase and for the subsequent 3 months.

6 If a capsular contracture develops, carry out a closed capsulotomy by compression of the capsule in the first instance.

7 If this fails, carry out an open capsulotomy.

BREAST REDUCTION

Appraise

1 Breast reduction is carried out most commonly for physical symptoms.

2 Large breasts may be of sufficient weight to affect the posture of the patient and to cause backache.

3 Pressure marks over the shoulders may be evident where the straps of the brassiere rest.

4 The aim of surgery is to produce an aesthetic breast shape with a viable, sensitive nipple and areola. Preserve the areola on a vascular pedicle.

5 Breast feeding may be possible after breast reduction but warn the patient not to expect this.

6 There are many operations designed to reduce the mass of the breasts. The inferior pedicle technique devised by Robbins is described below.

Action

1 Mark the breasts preoperatively with the patient sitting.

2 Choose a suitable site for the new position of the nipple near the midclavicular line.

3 Use a keyhole-type breast reduction pattern based on this site and mark the lateral and medial skin flaps (Fig. 39.36).

4 Mark the medial and lateral ends of the submammary crease and the submammary crease itself.

5 Peroperatively, make an intradermal incision through the skin along the patterns marked out preoperatively so that the skin marks are not lost.

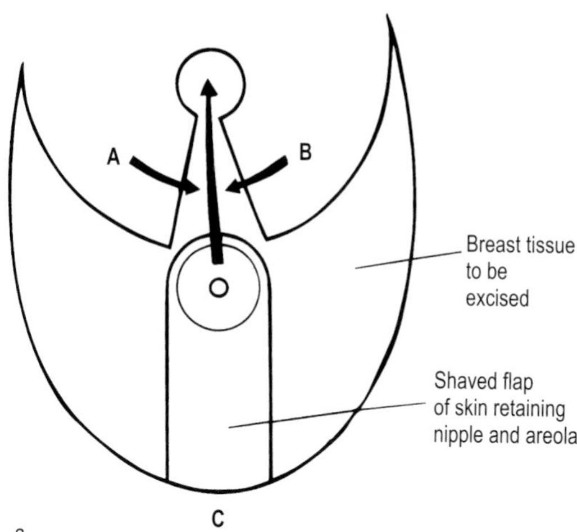

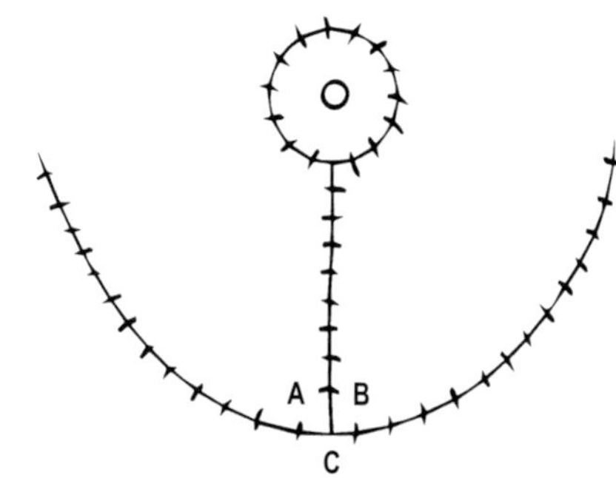

Fig. 39.36 Breast reduction—the inferior pedicle technique. The nipple and areola are preserved on a flap of skin in which the epidermis has been removed. This flap of skin helps to protect the underlying breast tissue which contains the vessels and nerves supplying the nipple. Breast tissue and overlying skin on either side and above this flap are excised (a). The nipple is transferred upwards and flaps A and B, after reflection outwards, are brought together in the midline below the nipple (b).

6 Shave off the epidermis from the skin between the normal areola and the inframammary fold, and from a rim of skin around the areola.

7 Excise the lateral and medial segments of skin between the lower margin of the skin flaps and the inframammary fold, together with the underlying breast tissue.

8 Excise breast tissue beneath the new site of the nipple and areola.

9 Dissect the inferior pedicle to its base.

10 Elevate the medial and lateral skin flaps with their underlying breast tissue.

11 Support the inferior pedicle by anchoring it to the pectoralis muscle superiorly.

12 Suture the nipple and areola into its new site.

13 Approximate the skin flaps in the midline below the new nipple site.

14 Insert a suction drain.

15 Close the wounds in layers, using subcuticular sutures to the skin.

16 Repeat the operation on the opposite side to provide symmetry.

17 Support the breast postoperatively with light dressings and remove the sutures at 3 weeks.

18 Keep the breasts well supported for 3 months postoperatively.

DERMAL MASTOPEXY

Appraise

1 The breasts of all women have a tendency to become ptotic with increasing age.

2 Ptosis tends to be greater when there has been considerable weight reduction or excessive involution following lactation. It is also marked when the breasts have not been supported with a brassiere over a long period.

3 Dermopexy or correction of the ptosis is appropriate when the nipple can be re-sited at a higher level and the skin envelope of the breast tissue can be reduced without any change in the volume of breast tissue.

Action

1 Mark the patient as for a breast reduction.

2 Carry out the stages as enumerated in a breast reduction, but do not excise breast tissue.

3 In advancing the inferior pedicle to its new site, incise breast tissue at the new site and undermine the skin edges around the new nipple site appropriately.

4 Manage the patient postoperatively as for a breast reduction.

ABDOMINAL REDUCTION

Appraise

1 An abdominal reduction or lipectomy is most appropriate when a patient has lax abdominal skin following multiple pregnancies or substantial weight loss.

2 It is not normally an operation to produce weight reduction.

Action

1 Mark out a symmetrical line traversing the lower abdomen. Start beneath the anterior superior iliac spine on one side and pass through the upper part of the site of the pubic hair to the other.

2 Incise along this mark and cut down to the fascia overlying the muscles.

3 Dissect upwards in this plane.

4 Incise the skin around the umbilicus and separate this from the skin flap.

5 Undermine the skin up to the costal margin on either side.

6 Stretch the skin downwards.

7 Excise the redundant skin and subcutaneous fat.

8 Identify the new site on the skin flap for the umbilicus and excise an oval piece of skin to accommodate it.

9 Break the operating table at the level of the pelvis to flex the hips.

10 Close the lower abdominal wound in layers and suture the umbilicus.

11 Insert a suction drain on each side.

12 Close the skin of the umbilical scar, if still present, in the vertical plane.

13 Postoperatively, keep the hips flexed to reduce tension on the lower abdominal wound for a few days.

14 Remove the sutures at 3 weeks.

LIPOSUCTION

Appraise

1 This technique of removing subcutaneous fat has a useful but limited place in aesthetic surgery.

2 It is occasionally used in refining a reconstructive procedure.

3 The technique is sometimes used alone but only a limited amount of fat can be removed without the need for excising further redundant skin.

4 The technique is often used as an adjunct to other surgery when skin is being removed, particularly in abdominoplasty and thigh and buttock reduction.

5 It can be used to remove lipomata from prominent sites on the trunk or limbs, avoiding an ugly scar and leaving a small discreet scar at some chosen distant inconspicuous site. In these circumstances excision is likely to be incomplete and the procedure may need repeating later for recurrence.

Action

1 Identify a suitable site for insertion of the liposuction cannula which is both discreet and within range of the area to be treated.

2 Make a small stab incision in the skin.

3 Through this insert the appropriate cannula and infiltrate the area with fluid made from adding 1 ml of 1/1000 adrenaline (epinephrine) and 20 ml of 0.25% bupivacaine to 500 ml of Hartmann's solution. Then wait at least 5 minutes.

4 Insert the chosen liposuction cannula and pass it into the deepest plane of subcutaneous fat.

5 Apply suction as the cannula is passed up and down the channel formed.

6 Repeat in multiple other deep subcutaneous channels.

7 Avoid passing the cannula superficially as this may cause pitting of the skin surface.

8 Suture the incision on removal of the cannula.

9 Apply a pressure garment immediately to the area treated and retain for 3 months.

LASER SURGERY

Lasers are being used to treat an increasing number of skin lesions. These fall into four principal groups.

- *Vascular lesions*. Many cutaneous vascular lesions can be eradicated without leaving any significant scarring. These include all types of telangiectasia, capillary haemangiomata, including port wine stains, pyogenic granulomata and other small vascular lesions. Many of the small lesions can be treated successfully with a single treatment with one of the pulsed dye lasers. While the larger lesions can be eradicated, treatment may leave a residual area of variable pigmentation.
- *Pigmented lesions*. Several lasers with short wavelengths, such as the Q-switched lasers, remove pigmented lesions limited to the epidermis and basal layer, such as lentigo simplex, solar lentigines and ephilides. They also remove pigment from the superficial dermis. Pigment in the deeper dermis requires a laser with a longer wavelength, but treatment of these lesions is less satisfactory and surgical excision may be the better option of treatment.
- *Tattoos*. Removal of professional as well as accidental tattoos with lasers is now much more effective than surgical excision because of the absence of scars. The Q-switched ruby, Nd-YAG and Alexandrite lasers are all effective in removing blue-black pigment, but complete excision can be difficult to achieve even with multiple treatments and pigmentation changes may occur.
- *Skin resurfacing*. The carbon dioxide laser in effect causes a predetermined superficial burn to the skin and has a similar effect to dermabrasion, which causes a physical burn, and a chemopeel, which causes a chemical burn. Treatment of wrinkles and irregular scarring of the skin surface with the carbon dioxide laser is more accurate and predictable than these treatments and is therefore replacing them. The occasional complication of a change in pigmentation remains unresolved.

ENDOSCOPIC PLASTIC SURGERY

Appraise

Endoscopic surgery was very limited until the development of fibreoptics and fibreoptic instruments. This allowed investigation and treatment of lesions of hollow viscera. By insufflation of air the peritoneal cavity becomes accessible to endoscopic surgery, and injection of saline into joints such as the knee has rendered these accessible to this type of surgery.

With refinements in the instrumentation it is now possible to explore soft tissues, allowing plastic surgeons to use the techniques that others have hitherto pioneered with the benefit of reducing the extent of scars on the skin surface. The latissimus dorsi muscle flap (see above) can now be raised and transposed into the breast area using only a small incision in the axilla and a periareolar incision. Nerve, vein or fascial grafts can be harvested. The carpal tunnel can be released and subcutaneous lesions can be removed. Tissue expanders and prostheses can be inserted. In the aesthetic field endoscopic brow lifts have replaced the conventional brow lift involving an extensive coronal scar and endoscopic surgery is used for some types of facelift.

PROSTHETIC IMPLANT MATERIALS

Appraise

1 All implants must be inserted under strict aseptic techniques.

2 Implants require good-quality soft tissue cover to prevent ulceration of the overlying skin.

3 If subsequently exposed, most implants will become infected and require removal. It may be possible to replace the implant when the infection has been eradicated.

4 All implants develop a surrounding fibrous capsule. This may be useful but is a disadvantage with a breast prosthesis as the fibrous capsule may contract and distort the prosthesis.

5 Several inert metals are used in reconstruction:
- Titanium plates are used in cranioplasty.
- Gold weights are inserted into the upper eyelid in facial palsy to improve function by assisting closure.
- Stainless steel, vitallium and tantalum are occasionally used.

6 Hard plastics used in reconstruction include: methyl methacrylate, used in cranioplasty; polyethylene, used as a mesh in abdominal wall repair; and polypropylene. Proplast, a combination of two polymers (polytetrafluoroethylene and pyrolytic graphite), is used to augment the cheek and the chin.

7 Silicone is a general term for a class of polymers with long chains of dimethylsiloxane units [$—CH_3—Si—O—CH_3$]. These are manufactured in many forms, including liquids, gels, resins, foams, sponges and rubbers.

8 Silicone implants are used in facial bone augmentation, small-joint replacement in the hand and as a stent to reconstruct tendon sheaths prior to tendon grafting.

9 Silicone implants are commonly used in breast augmentation or reconstruction. Some breast implants consist of a silicone gel contained within a silicone elastomer shell. Others are made using a cohesive gel that maintains their shape. A textured surface modifies the fibrous reaction of the body and capsule contracture is reduced. There is no scientific evidence to show that any silicone breast implant has a significant carcinogenic risk and although these implants may leak there is no evidence that the silicone that does leak causes any serious complication.

THE FUTURE

- When greater control of the immune response has been achieved, it will be possible to use many different parts of cadavers for reconstruction using microvascular surgery.
- Tissue culture is in an embryonic phase of development and has great potential in reconstruction. Cultured keratinocytes have been grafted on to open wounds.
- In utero surgery has been carried out and may have a role in treating congenital deformities.
- Better understanding and control of wound healing will improve the quality of plastic surgery and will help all branches of surgery.

FURTHER READING

Aston SJ, Beasley RW, Thorne CHM 1997 Grabb and Smith's plastic surgery, 5th edn. Lippincott-Raven, Philadelphia
A concise guide to clinical practice in plastic surgery in one volume. It is packed with information.

McCarthy JG 1990 Plastic surgery. Saunders, Philadelphia
Whilst this, in its eight volumes, remains the commonly accepted authoritative reference book in plastic surgery, it now requires updating.

McGregor AD, McGregor IA 2000 Fundamental techniques of plastic surgery and their surgical applications, 10th edn. Churchill Livingstone, Edinburgh
An excellent manual of basic techniques in plastic surgery, ideal for young trainees in the specialty and general surgeons.

Richards AM 2002 Key notes on plastic surgery. Blackwell, Oxford

Settle JAD 1996 Principles and practice of burns management. Churchill Livingstone, Edinburgh
A comprehensive guide to the management of patients with burns, indicating many of the difficulties and controversies in treating these cases.

Strauch B, Vasconez LO, Hall-Findlay EJ 1998 Grabb's encyclopaedia of flaps, 2nd edn. Lippincott-Raven, Philadelphia
Published in three large volumes, this is a comprehensive guide to flaps, with over 500 chapters each describing one or more flaps in detail.

40

Paediatric surgery

L. Spitz, I.D. Sugarman

CONTENTS

GENERAL CONSIDERATIONS IN NEONATAL SURGERY

INTRODUCTION

To obtain optimal results, neonatal surgery is best practised by fully trained paediatric surgeons working in large specialist centres. The concentration of clinical material in such centres offers experience in the management of a wide variety of congenital abnormalities and facilitates the organization of training and research programmes. Support is provided from experts in nursing, anaesthesia, radiology, pathology and paediatric medicine, all essential for a satisfactory outcome.

The neonatal period used to be defined as the first 28 days of extrauterine life, but this definition is obsolete now that babies are surviving birth at gestational ages as low as 22 weeks. Babies with a gestational age of less than 24 weeks or a birthweight of less than 750 g have a very high mortality rate, and survivors of very premature birth have an increased risk of multiple sensory and neurodevelopmental handicaps. Some of the survivors require surgery within the first 28 days of life whilst they still have very immature homeostatic mechanisms. Infants less than 44 weeks beyond conception (the current definition of the neonatal period) have a marked tendency to apnoea, especially during the first 24 hours of postoperative recovery. Day-case surgery in such infants is contraindicated.

The notion that the neonate is merely a scaled-down version of the adult is obsolete. The neonate differs widely from the adult in both structure and function. Full adaptation to independent life takes several weeks and during this time any severe stress may cause the ductus arteriosus to re-open and the circulation to regress to a 'persistent fetal circulation', resulting in shunting of deoxygenated blood into the systemic circulation. The resulting hypoxia may be difficult to correct. The neonatal circulation is unstable and any noxious stimulus may result in renal or intestinal ischaemia or intracranial haemorrhage. The ratio of surface area to weight in the neonate is twice that of the adult and this exposes the infant to genuine risks of dehydration from excessive insensible fluid loss accompanied by hypothermia, the latter enhanced by radiated losses, especially from the head. The neonatal kidney is immature and can only function within a limited homeostatic range. The diuretic response is weak and circulatory overload can easily occur following excessive intravenous fluid administration, which may also cause re-opening of the ductus arteriosus resulting in hypoxia and severe heart failure. Liver functions, particularly detoxifying enzyme systems, are restricted and hyperbilirubinaemia easily develops. Low immunoglobulin levels and reduced leucocyte activity result in poor resistance to infection, bacteraemia rapidly progressing to meningitis. Infection compounds any cardiac, renal or hepatic failure. Progressive multi-organ failure rapidly develops, the correction of which is difficult. Although techniques of assisted respiration have improved dramatically in recent years, haemodialysis and cardiac support still present difficulties.

RECOGNITION OF A CONGENITAL ANOMALY

External abnormalities are easily recognized at birth and do not merit further discussion, but there are a number of clinical features indicative of concealed anomalies that require further amplification.

- *Bilious vomiting.* Green bile in the vomitus indicates mechanical intestinal obstruction unless an alternative cause can be found (such as septicaemia).
- Respiratory distress merits an X-ray of the chest to exclude pneumothorax, diaphragmatic hernia, lobar emphysema or oesophageal atresia.
- Failure to pass meconium within 24 hours of birth in a full-term healthy infant suggests the possibility of Hirschsprung's disease.
- Failure to pass urine within 24 hours of birth may be due either to inadequate hydration or to urinary obstruction, such as posterior urethral valves.
- A lateral abdominal mass in a neonate is most likely to be a benign renal anomaly such as hydronephrosis or multicystic kidney, whilst a mass in the hypogastrium should suggest hydrocolpos in a girl or an enlarged bladder due to urethral valves in a boy. Tumours are uncommon at this age.

- The passage of blood in the stools may be caused by necrotizing enterocolitis or a strangulating type of intestinal obstruction, such as midgut volvulus.
- Congenital anomalies are frequently multiple. The pattern of associated anomalies is fairly constant, such as renal anomalies in association with anorectal malformations, congenital cardiac anomalies with exomphalos and duodenal atresia, and vertebral, anorectal, cardiac, tracheo-oesophageal fistula with oesophageal atresia, renal and limb anomalies (VACTERL association).

PRENATAL DIAGNOSIS

1 Advances in obstetrics, particularly in the widespread availability of ultrasound examination of the fetus, now detect a variety of abnormality before the baby is born.

2 Large structural abnormalities are most easily detected by ultrasound examination, so the conditions most commonly diagnosed include hydrocephalus, spina bifida, sacrococcygeal teratoma, exomphalos, gastroschisis, diaphragmatic hernia, duodenal atresia, severe congenital heart disease, urinary tract obstruction and ascites. Smaller abnormalities are now being picked up with more frequency (e.g. duplication or ovarian cysts).

3 Prenatal diagnosis facilitates planned obstetric management, including termination of the pregnancy, operative intervention on the fetus, or planned timing and method of delivery of the infant.

4 A combination of changes in natural incidence, termination of affected pregnancies and vitamin supplements (such as folic acid) for prospective mothers before conception have led to a dramatic decrease in the incidence of neonates with spina bifida.

5 Many urinary tract lesions, especially unilateral hydronephrosis, are diagnosed before birth and this has led to significant changes in the practice of paediatric urology, most patients now presenting during early infancy, before the onset of symptoms.

6 Prenatal diagnosis offers the opportunity for planning the management of the pregnancy and the timing and place of delivery as follows:
   - Detection of lethal abnormality (e.g. anencephaly, bilateral renal agenesis, severe chromosomal defect) would indicate termination of the pregnancy.
   - Detection of an abnormality that can be successfully treated after delivery. In these cases it is best to allow the pregnancy to continue to full-term and to treat the abnormality after birth.
   - Detection of an abnormality which may cause obstructive labour or may be damaged during delivery (e.g. sacrococcygeal teratoma, large exomphalos, cervical cystic hygroma)—recommend an elective caesarean section.
   - Detection of an abnormality in which progressive deterioration of function is likely to occur with ongoing pregnancy (e.g. gastroschisis)—consider early delivery.
   - At present in-utero correction of abnormalities is still experimental and its practice should be restricted to a limited number of research institutions.

NEONATAL TRANSPORT

1 Newborn infants can be transported safely over long distances provided adequate precautions are taken to maintain body temperature and the accompanying attendants are fully experienced and adequately equipped to deal with any cardiorespiratory emergency.

2 When resuscitation is required for shock, hypothermia, respiratory insufficiency, or disturbances of fluid, electrolyte or acid–base homeostasis, commence treatment at the base hospital. Delay transfer until the infant's condition has stabilized.

3 When surgery is urgently required, as for gastroschisis, intestinal volvulus, gastrointestinal perforation or profuse haemorrhage, continue resuscitation during transfer.

4 For the safe transfer of a surgical neonate ensure that:
   - The transport incubator is equipped with facilities for monitoring heart rate, body temperature and inspired oxygen concentration and has an in-built mechanical ventilator.
   - Cardiorespiratory resuscitation equipment, including paediatric laryngoscopes, endotracheal tubes, suction apparatus and chest drainage tubes plus a variety of inotropic and respiratory stimulant drugs are available.
   - Pass a nasogastric tube and leave it on free drainage. Have it regularly aspirated to keep the stomach empty to avoid the pulmonary complications of inhaled vomitus.
   - Send 10 ml of maternal blood to reduce the amount required from the infant for compatibility studies. All surgical neonates require blood to be available for transfusion at operation. The blood volume of a neonate is about 8% of body weight, and losses greater than 10 % need to be replaced, so that a 3000-g infant has a blood volume of 240 ml and losses above 24 ml require replacement with blood.
   - Send a valid consent form for operation.
   - Send copies of all records regarding the pregnancy, delivery and perinatal period, including biochemical results and X-rays.

Special precautions

- *Oesophageal atresia.* Keep the blind upper pouch empty to prevent aspiration of saliva. Apply continuous or frequent intermittent suction to an indwelling tube, preferably the double-lumen Replogle tube, size 10F. Place the infant in either the prone or lateral position to discourage gastric reflux.
- *Diaphragmatic hernia.* The majority of infants presenting after 24 hours of life can be managed in an oxygen-enriched environment. If the infant fails to respond, and for all those presenting with acute respiratory distress within 6 hours of birth, endotracheal intubation and mechanical ventilation are mandatory. Do not attempt ventilation with a face mask as this forces air into the intestines, further compromising respiration. Always pass a large *patent* nasogastric tube. Leave it draining freely to limit the amount of gas passing beyond the stomach. If there is any sudden deterioration during resuscitation or transfer, suspect the development of a tension pneumothorax. Immediately insert a hypodermic needle into the pleural space through the

second intercostal space anteriorly, on one or both sides, and aspirate the free air.

- *Exomphalos and gastroschisis.* The immediate problem is the loss of large quantities of fluid through the exposed intestine or thin covering membrane. Restrict these losses by wrapping the intestine or exomphalos sac in plastic film. Avoid using saline-soaked swabs because the water rapidly evaporates, causing severe hypothermia and circulatory collapse.

INTRAVENOUS FLUIDS

1 Use peripherally sited cannulas whenever possible. It may be tempting to use the umbilical vein but complications such as necrotizing enterocolitis and portal vein thrombosis limit its use except in an emergency.

2 Basic fluids for intravenous infusion should be 10% dextrose in 0.18% saline for neonates and 4% dextrose in 0.18% saline for infants and children.

3 Replace abnormal losses, as from nasogastric aspirate and enteric fistula, with 0.9% (normal) saline, adding 20 mmol potassium chloride per litre.

4 Calculate the daily requirements for intravenous fluid according to Table 40.1.

Postoperative fluid requirements

Neonates:

- First 48 hours after operation: one-half of maintenance requirements.
- Third and fourth days after operation: two-thirds of maintenance requirements.
- Fifth and subsequent days: full-volume maintenance requirements.

Infants and children:

- First 24 hours after operation: one-half of maintenance requirements.
- Second and third days after operation: two-thirds of maintenance requirements.
- Fourth and subsequent days: full-volume maintenance requirements.

Table 40.1 Daily intravenous fluid requirement

	Weight	Daily requirement
Neonates	Up to 1500 g	180 ml/kg
	1500–2500 g	150 ml/kg
	Over 2500 g	120 ml/kg
Infants and children	Up to 10 kg	100 ml/kg
	10–20 kg	1000 ml + 50 ml/kg for each kg above 10 kg
	Over 20 kg	1500 ml + 25 ml/kg for each kg above 20 kg

Examples:
An 8.0-kg infant requires 8.0 × 100 = 800 ml/day.
A 14.0-kg child requires 1000 ml plus 4 × 50 ml = 1200 ml/day.
A 25.0-kg child requires 1500 ml plus 5 × 25 ml = 1625 ml/day.

LAPAROSCOPY IN INFANTS AND CHILDREN

With instruments of suitable use in infants (including neonates) and children being widely available, many procedures—intra-abdominal (fundoplication, cholecystectomy, splenectomy, resection of Meckel's diverticulum and duplication cysts, pyloromyotomy, pull-through procedures, rectobladder fistula division in high anorectal malformations) and intrathoracic (lung cysts, bronchogenic cysts, mediastinal masses)—are being performed using minimally invasive surgery.

LAPAROTOMY IN INFANTS AND CHILDREN

Preoperative preparation

1 Cross-match 1 unit of fresh packed cells.

2 Administer vitamin K, phytomenadione 1 mg intramuscularly, if this was omitted in the immediate postnatal period.

3 Check the blood glucose using Dextrostix. Correct hypoglycaemia by giving 50% glucose intravenously.

4 Correct any fluid and acid–base imbalance (most acid–base imbalances will self-correct with adequate resuscitation).

5 In all emergencies, keep the stomach empty through a large (8FG) nasogastric tube.

6 Ensure good intravenous access through a cannula conveniently sited for the anaesthetist.

7 Use ECG, pulse, blood pressure and oxygen saturation monitors. Monitors for measuring partial pressures of oxygen and carbon dioxide in inspired and expired gases are also available.

8 For very sick infants, continuously record blood pressure through a transduced intra-arterial cannula that also facilitates intermittent blood gas analysis and assessments of serum electrolyte and haemoglobin concentrations.

9 Use a central venous cannula when blood loss is expected to be massive or when peripheral venous access is limited, but measurements of central venous pressure are of limited value in this age group.

10 Keep the infant normothermic. Radiant heat losses, especially from the head, must be limited by wrapping the head and limbs in aluminium foil and losses from convection must be limited by restricting the movement of personnel in the theatre and by swaddling the patient in warm gamgee. A thermostatically controlled warm air blanket should be placed below the patient. The ambient temperature of the theatre should be kept at 26°C with doors closed to prevent draughts.

THE ABDOMINAL OPERATION

KEY POINTS Incision

- Because of the relatively wide, truncated abdomen, greater access is afforded by transverse incisions than longitudinal incisions.
- A recommended 'general purpose' incision is a transverse, muscle-cutting, supra-umbilical incision extending across right and left rectus abdominus muscles.

Access

1 Place the prepared infant supine on the operating table.

2 Make a long, transverse skin incision, 1–2 cm above the umbilicus, with the scalpel.

3 Divide the subcutaneous fat and fascia with cutting diathermy to limit blood loss.

4 Similarly, divide the anterior sheath of left and right rectus abdominus muscles and then divide the muscle bellies.

5 Coagulate the superior epigastric vessels on the deeper surface of each rectus abdominus muscle.

6 Divide the posterior sheath and fascia down to the peritoneum.

7 Open the peritoneum on either side of the midline.

8 Identify, clamp and divide the relatively large umbilical vein. Ligate both ends of the vein with 0000 polyglycolic acid suture.

9 After assessment, the incision may be readily extended, using cutting diathermy, into the oblique muscles of the abdominal wall at either, or both, ends of the incision.

Closure

1 It is unnecessary to close the peritoneum separately.

2 Close the muscles and fascia en masse with either continuous or interrupted sutures of 000 or 0000 polyglactin, polyglycolic acid or polydioxanone.

3 Close the skin with a continuous subcuticular suture of 00000 polyglycolic acid, polydioxanone or polyglactin.

4 When wound infection is expected, omit the subcuticular suture and close with adhesive tapes, such as Steri-Strips.

5 Do not use tension sutures or through-and-through skin sutures because the cosmetic results are unacceptable.

ABDOMINAL WALL DEFECTS

Appraise

1 When present at birth, these are associated with longstanding evisceration of the abdominal contents into a hernial sac, thin external membrane, or the thoracic cavity. As a result, the abdominal cavity is relatively small, and repair of the defect causes:

- A rise in intra-abdominal pressure.
- Poor circulation in the lower parts of the body, kidneys and intestines resulting in oliguria, metabolic acidosis and intestinal ischaemia.

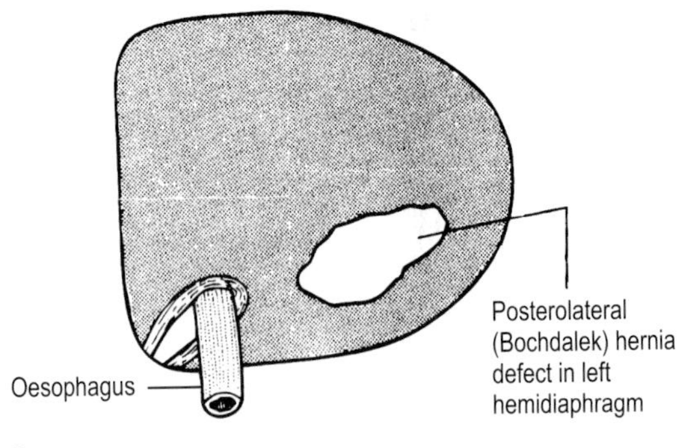

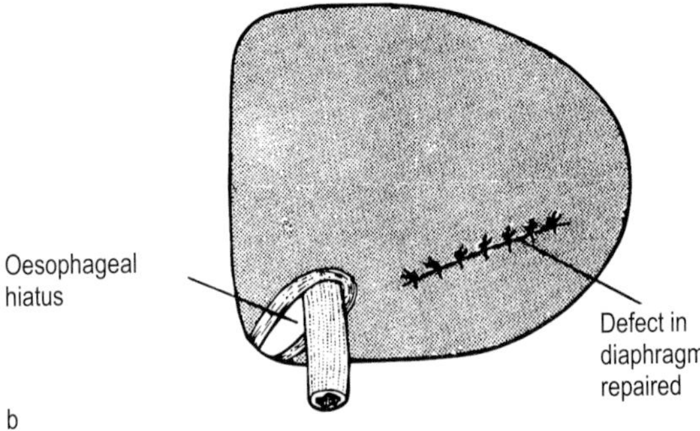

Fig. 40.1 Congenital diaphragmatic hernia before (a) and after (b) repair.

- Splinting of the diaphragm, causing respiratory acidosis and hypoxia.
- Hypoxia and pulmonary vasoconstriction, causing reopening of the ductus arteriosus and reversion to 'persistent fetal circulation' with increased shunting of deoxygenated blood into the systemic circulation, compounding the metabolic acidosis and hypoxia.

2 This vicious cycle of deterioration must be prevented by assisted endotracheal ventilation with high concentrations of oxygen, judicious use of plasma expanders, pulmonary vasodilator and inotropic drugs, and the careful timing of operative intervention.

CONGENITAL DIAPHRAGMATIC HERNIA (Fig. 40.1)

Appraise

1 The infant has respiratory distress with tachypnoea more than 60/minute, tachycardia more than 160/minute and cyanosis.

2 The infant is limp and using the accessory muscles of respiration in unsuccessful efforts to breathe.

3 A chest radiograph reveals intestinal gas shadows in the involved hemithorax with displacement of the mediastinal structures to the contralateral side.

Action

1 Pass an endotracheal tube and use positive-pressure mechanical ventilation.

2 Do not ventilate the infant with a face-mask as this will blow air down the oesophagus and into the intestine, resulting in rapid deterioration.

3 Pass a large (8FG) nasogastric tube to keep the stomach empty and to limit the amount of air passing into the intestine.

4 Ventilatory pressures should not exceed 12 cmH_2O to avoid alveolar rupture and pneumothorax. Treat tension pneumothorax by inserting a chest drain attached to an underwater seal.

5 Insert an intravenous cannula for expansion of circulating volume.

6 Insert an arterial cannula for estimations of blood gases.

KEY POINTS Resuscitation

- Once resuscitation is under way, arrange urgent rapid transfer to a regional surgical unit.
- Resuscitation must be undertaken rapidly and effectively, but operative intervention should not be performed until cardiorespiratory stability has been achieved.
- Respiratory support has developed significantly and now includes oscillatory ventilation, permissive hypercapnia, nitric oxide and liquid ventilation.
- The timing of operation is best assessed by an experienced regional team.

Principles

1 Laparotomy is performed using the 'general purpose' incision but confining it to the side of the hernial defect.

2 Withdraw the intestines, stomach and finally the spleen from the chest.

3 Identify the diaphragmatic defect and excise the sac if present.

4 If small, the diaphragmatic defect is primarily repaired with non-absorbable sutures.

5 If the defect is large that the diaphragm hardly exists, the defect must be repaired using a prosthetic patch of polypropylene or woven polyester (Dacron) and sutured with non-absorbable sutures to the chest wall.

6 Close the abdomen.

Aftercare

1 Postoperative assisted ventilation is mandatory.

2 Nurses experienced in neonatal intensive care are essential.

Prognosis

1 Infants developing symptoms after the age of 6 hours should all survive.

2 The survival rate for infants developing symptoms at birth is about 50%.

3 Infants presenting between the first and sixth hours of life have a survival rate of about 80%.

4 Death occurs almost entirely from pulmonary hypoplasia and hypertension.

5 A small number of infants with adequate lung size but refractory pulmonary hypertension may be saved by extracorporeal membrane oxygenation (ECMO).

EXOMPHALOS AND GASTROSCHISIS

Appraise

1 Exomphalos is herniation of abdominal viscera into the persistent fetal umbilical hernia. The viscera are covered by a thin transparent membrane consisting of an outer layer of amniotic membrane lined by peritoneum, with Wharton's jelly between the two.

2 Gastroschisis is evisceration of the intestine through a slit-like defect in the anterior abdominal wall immediately to the right of an apparently normal umbilical cord. The intestine rapidly becomes oedematous and exudes a proteinaceous fluid that cocoons and mats together the intestinal loops.

3 Exomphalos is often associated with other major abnormalities such as serious cardiac and renal defects. Lethal chromosomal abnormalities such as Patau and Edward's syndrome are not uncommon.

4 Gastroschisis is not associated with extra-abdominal anomalies but atresias may occur in the eviscerated intestine.

Transfer

KEY POINTS Abdominal wall closure?

- Neonates with gastroschisis and ruptured exomphalos have a better prognosis if the abdominal wall can be closed, or placed into a silo, within a few hours of birth.
- This implies either in-utero transfer or urgent transfer to the regional unit.

1 Before transfer, wrap the herniated bowel with Clingfilm to limit fluid losses and protect the intestine.

2 Insert an intravenous cannula and give the infant 20 ml/kg of plasma during the journey.

3 Pass a nasogastric tube and transfer as in neonatal transport, but with the baby on its side to prevent kinking of the blood supply to the bowel during transfer.

Principles

Exomphalos minor

1 If very minor (herniation into the umbilical cord), reduce the intestine into the abdominal cavity and ligate the base of the cord with a thick ligature, thereby avoiding operation.

2 If operative repair is necessary, close the defect with a purse-string suture of 000 or 0000 polyglycolic acid or polyglactin 910.

3 Radiological contrast studies of the upper gastrointestinal tract before the surgery as 30% of infants with intestinal malrotation will need a laparotomy and Ladd's procedure (see below).

Unruptured exomphalos major

1 Non-operative treatment is by applying an antiseptic such as povidone iodine or silver sulfadiazine (Flamazine) three times a day to the sac. Antiseptics are absorbed through the

membrane, so do not apply the toxic mercurochrome. Monitor thyroid function tests after prolonged application of povidone–iodine. After several weeks, the eschar separates leaving an epithelialized defect that grows at a slower rate than the rest of the infant. A large ventral hernia may result and this should be repaired during the second year of life.

2 Application of a Prolene mesh silo to cover the unruptured exomphalos, with gradual reduction of the contents over the subsequent days or weeks. The Prolene mesh is sutured to the abdominal muscles at the edges of the defect. When full reduction has been achieved the Prolene mesh is removed and the defect closed.

Ruptured exomphalos major

1 Primary repair is frequently impossible.

2 The most practical means of dealing with this difficult problem is to use prosthetic material, lyophilized dura mater or grafts of amniotic membrane to create coverings for the bowel to prevent peritonitis.

3 Once an artificial umbilical hernia has been created the management is similar to that of unruptured exomphalos.

Gastroschisis

1 During the first few hours after birth, primary repair can be performed in the majority. Return the eviscerated organs to the peritoneal cavity and close the defect in the abdominal wall longitudinally with 000 or 0000 polyglycolic acid or polydioxanone. An attempt should be made to recreate the umbilicus in the repair. Postoperative mechanical ventilation and parenteral nutrition are invariably required. Delayed repair of associated intestinal atresias may be necessary.

2 For those patients born with very matted bowel, or in whom this has been allowed to develop during the first few hours of extrauterine life, primary repair may not be possible without unacceptable deterioration in the circulatory and respiratory systems. Treatment consists of covering the eviscerated bowel with an artificial silo of flexible silicone rubber (there is one that is pre-made—Medicina Silo). The advantage is that a smaller defect is created with better cosmetic results. If this is not available, an artificial silo of flexible silicone rubber (Silastic), polytetrafluoroethylene (Teflon) or polypropylene mesh, as described by Schuster, is used. The patient is then treated as for unruptured exomphalos major. Some surgeons are now using the pre-made silo as their primary treatment, as it can be performed on the neonatal unit, thus removing the need for emergency surgery at a few hours of age.

Prognosis

1 In the absence of other serious anomalies, the prognosis for exomphalos minor is excellent.

2 The survival rate for gastroschisis is now over 90%. A small percentage of infants are born with loss of their herniated midgut ('closed gastroschisis') and these children have a much poorer outcome.

3 Because of operative difficulties and the presence of serious associated anomalies, the prognosis of exomphalos major is poorer.

INGUINAL HERNIA

Appraise

1 In the paediatric age range, inguinal hernia is generally due to failure of closure of the processus vaginalis. The hernia may be complete (to the scrotum) or incomplete (confined to the inguinal region). Operation is indicated in all cases.

2 Inguinal hernias become irreducible in up to 30% of infants, the peak incidence being between the ages of 6 and 12 weeks. Strangulation is rare in the neonatal period, but, when it does occur, there is appreciable postoperative morbidity and a high mortality rate.

3 If the hernia becomes irreducible, pressure upon the spermatic cord causes testicular ischaemia, and infarction may occur after as little as 4 hours. Up to 25% of neonates with an irreducible hernia develop severe testicular ischaemia.

4 Most 'irreducible' inguinal herniae can be reduced following sedation and 'taxis'—gentle to-and-fro pressure applied to the neck of the hernial sac at the level of the external inguinal ring. Following reduction, it is recommended that elective repair of the hernia is carried out about 48 hours later.

5 Premature babies are particularly prone to develop complications. Herniotomy should be carried out at a stage when the infant has gained sufficient weight to warrant discharge from hospital or as soon as complications occur. These small infants often have hydrocephalus following intraventricular haemorrhage and have bronchopulmonary dysplasia associated with the need for prolonged mechanical ventilation. The help of an experienced paediatric anaesthetist is invaluable and sometimes operation can be performed only by using spinal or epidural anaesthesia. These patients are prone to all of the complications associated with 'persistent fetal circulation', and postoperative deaths do occur, even with elective operation in a regional centre.

6 In infants under the age of 6 months, the tissues are thin and friable so operative difficulties are common. Treatment is best left to paediatric surgeons.

7 Before embarking upon operation for an inguinal hernia, ensure that the ipsilateral testis is in the scrotum, otherwise orchidopexy is indicated at the same time as herniotomy.

8 Performing an orchidopexy on an infant under the age of 6 months with an irreducible hernia is a particularly difficult operation that must not be attempted by a surgeon without special training unless there are exceptional circumstances.

9 Except in children with neuromuscular disorders, herniotomy rather than herniorrhaphy is the treatment of choice.

Herniotomy at the external ring

1 This was described by Mitchell Banks of Liverpool in 1882.

2 Make an incision, 2 cm long, in a skin crease over the external inguinal ring.

3 Dissect through the subcutaneous fat, Camper and Scarpa's fascia to reveal the spermatic cord as it passes from the external inguinal ring.

4 Split the external spermatic fascia and cremasteric fascia or muscle in the long axis of the cord.

4 Deliver the cord, surrounded by the internal spermatic fascia, from the wound.

5 Rotate the cord to bring its posterior surface into view.

6 Split the internal spermatic fascia longitudinally, allowing the vessels and vas to be separated from the sac.

7 Exert traction upon the sac, to withdraw as much of it as possible from within the inguinal canal, through the external inguinal ring.

8 Transfix and ligate the sac with a suture of either 0000 polyglycolic acid or polyglactin. Divide the neck of the sac distal to the suture.

9 Bring together the superficial fascia with one or two sutures of 0000 polyglycolic acid or polyglactin.

10 Close the skin with a subcuticular suture of polyglycolic acid or polyglactin. Alternatively, apply skin-closure tapes. Non-absorbable sutures or skin clips are not necessary and their removal causes unnecessary discomfort and anxiety.

? DIFFICULTY

1. Many surgeons in training find this a difficult operation. It is easy to lose the landmarks in the suprapubic fat pad of the young child.
2. It often appears that there are innumerable layers of fascia around the cord and in the confusion the sac may be missed altogether.
3. Having become 'lost' it is easy to find oneself dissecting the femoral canal or causing damage to the femoral vein.
4. It is possible to miss the spermatic cord altogether, dissect through the conjoined tendon and excise the lateral corner of the bladder, mistaking it for the peritoneal sac.
5. During the operation, the testis may emerge out of the scrotum and into the wound. It may be difficult to get the testis back into the scrotum in the correct layer. In these circumstances, convert the operation into an orchidopexy and secure the testis into a dartos pouch in the scrotum. Otherwise, the testis may be gradually expelled from the scrotum and become adherent to the scar tissue of the superficial inguinal pouch, necessitating a subsequent orchidopexy.
6. The concept of this operation depends on the belief that, in the infant, the external ring is placed almost immediately anterior to the deep ring, the inguinal canal being very short. Whilst this may be the case in absolute terms, the inguinal canal is relatively long in the infant and it is almost impossible to ligate the neck 'flush' at the deep ring when pulling the sac medially to the external ring. Hence, there is a small but definite recurrence rate from this operation, even in the most experienced hands. For these reasons, herniotomy is best performed through the inguinal canal, according to the method described first by Turner of Guy's Hospital in 1912 and subsequently by Potts in 1948.

Herniotomy through the inguinal canal

1 Make an incision 2 cm long in a skin crease midway between the deep ring and pubic tubercle.

2 Divide the subcutaneous fat and Camper's fascia using scissors.

3 Incise Scarpa's superficial fascia with scissors, and retract it.

4 Clear a small patch of external oblique aponeurosis over an area of 2 cm^2, at least 1 cm above the inguinal ligament.

5 Incise the external oblique aponeurosis with scissors or a scalpel and retract the edges. Do not open the external inguinal ring.

6 Dissect into the inguinal canal, keeping close to the posterior surface of the external oblique aponeurosis.

7 Soon the ilio-inguinal nerve will come into view, and this provides a useful landmark.

8 Using a mosquito artery forceps, split the fibres of the cremaster muscle overlying the spermatic cord just inferior to the ilio-inguinal nerve.

9 Gently grasp the internal spermatic fascia with a mosquito forceps and use this to deliver the spermatic cord from its bed whilst pushing away the adherent fibres of the cremaster muscle with a delicate non-toothed dissecting forceps.

10 Pass the index finger of the non-dominant hand behind the cord and use it and the thumb to rotate the cord so that its posterior aspect comes into view.

11 Using a non-toothed dissecting forceps, split the internal spermatic fascia overlying the vas and vessels in a longitudinal direction.

12 Gently sweep the vas and vessels away from the sac. Do not hold the vas or vessels with the forceps because a crush injury may occur.

13 Place an artery forceps across the sac, and divide the sac distal to the forceps. Allow the distal part of the sac to fall back into the wound.

14 Dissect the vas and vessels from the proximal part of the sac, until the inferior epigastric vessels are seen.

15 Rotate the artery forceps to twist the neck of the sac, so ensuring that there is no bowel or omentum within it.

16 Ligate the sac flush with the deep ring using a 0000 polyglycolic acid suture, and then transfix the sac just distal to this tie. Ligation prior to transfixation and ligation prevents the needle from causing a split in the sac that may spread across the deep ring and on to the peritoneum of the anterior abdominal wall, and prevents the escape of intestines or omentum at a difficult site to repair.

17 Allow the vas and vessels to drop back into the inguinal canal.

18 Close the inguinal canal with two or three sutures.

19 Approximate the Scarpa's fascia with one or two sutures.

20 Close the skin with a subcuticular stitch. If 0000 polyglycolic acid is used, the whole operation may be accomplished using but one suture. Alternatively, close the skin with adhesive skin tapes.

21 Gently pull the testis to the bottom of the scrotum to ensure that it does not become caught in the superficial inguinal pouch, necessitating an orchidopexy.

? DIFFICULTY

1. Do not panic: think rationally.
2. The ilio-inguinal nerve is a good landmark.
3. If lost, keep close to the deep surface of the external oblique, and track down to the inguinal ligament; the cord lies between the ligament and the ilio-inguinal nerve.
4. Remember that the inguinal canal has definite boundaries and the cord must lie between the external ring, which is palpable, and the deep ring that is delineated medially by the inferior epigastric vessels, which should be visible.
5. If still in doubt, check that you are in the inguinal canal, and check that the incision is placed between the landmarks of the deep and superficial inguinal rings.
6. As a last resort, extend the incision, identify the external inguinal ring and proceed from there, possibly by incising the ring and laying open the anterior inguinal wall.

Aftercare

1 Except in infants less than 44 weeks post-gestational age, the procedure is carried out on a day-case basis and there are no special postoperative precautions.

2 A slight fever on the first postoperative night is a normal response to surgery.

ORCHIDOPEXY

Appraise

1 Incidence of an undescended testis is approximately 3% at birth, falling to 1% at 1 year of age.

2 If either bilateral or unilateral associated with a hypospadias, perform chromosomes to rule out intersex.

3 If a testis is impalpable, laparoscopy is the investigation of choice to assess the presence or absence of the testis, and its site.

4 If there are bilateral impalpable testes that are confirmed at laparoscopy to be intra-abdominal, bring one testis down at a time. This can either be by a Fowler–Stephen's procedure (ligating the testicular vessels and relying on the spermatic fascia for vascularity of the testis) or microvascular transfer.

5 In the 'ascending testis', a testis that was normally sited in the scrotum 'ascends' with age. The incidence of this is unknown, but the condition is probably more common than suspected.

6 The operation for the undescended testis should be performed between the ages of 1 and 2 years.

Action for the palpable undescended testis

1 Make an incision 3–4 cm long in a skin crease midway between the deep ring and public tubercle.

2 Divide the subcutaneous fat and Camper's fascia using scissors.

3 Incise Scarpa's superficial fascia with scissors, and retract it.

4 Clear a small patch of external oblique aponeurosis over an area of 2 cm^2, at least 1 cm above the inguinal ligament.

5 Incise the external oblique aponeurosis with scissors or a scalpel. Extend the incision to open the external ring.

6 Ascertain the position of the testis. From the testis passing distally into the scrotum is the gubernaculum. Define this and divide it to allow free retraction of the testis.

7 On retracting the testis, gently grasp the internal spermatic fascia with a mosquito forceps and use this to deliver the spermatic cord from its bed whilst pushing away the adherent fibres of the cremaster muscle with a delicate non-toothed dissecting forceps.

8 Using a non-toothed dissecting forceps, split the internal spermatic fascia overlying the vas and vessels in a longitudinal direction.

9 Gently sweep the vas and vessels away from the sac. This is often more difficult than in a herniotomy as the sac invaginates itself around the vas and vessels.

10 Place an artery forceps across the sac, and divide the sac distal to the forceps. Allow the distal part of the sac to fall back into the wound.

11 Dissect the vas and vessels from the proximal part of the sac, until the inferior epigastric vessels are seen.

12 Rotate the artery forceps to twist the neck of the sac, so ensuring that there is no bowel or omentum within it.

13 Ligate the sac flush with the deep ring using a 0000 polyglycolic acid suture, and then transfix the sac just distal to this tie.

14 Assess the length of vas and vessels obtained in relation to placing the testis in the scrotum. Extraperitoneal dissection through the internal ring and division of flimsy adhesions to the testicular vessels is often necessary to achieve additional length of the vessels.

15 Once adequate length is achieved, make a 1-cm transverse incision, between the upper two-thirds and lower third of the scrotum. Using sharp dissection, develop the plane between dartos and skin. Once this pouch is large enough, push the mosquito through the dartos and up into the inguinal incision.

16 Grasp the testis in the mosquito and deliver it and its attachments into the dartos pouch. Make sure the vessels have not rotated during this move.

17 Close the scrotal skin with buried 00000 absorbable sutures, taking a pass through the testis with at least one suture.

18 Close the inguinal canal with two or three sutures.

19 Approximate the Scarpa's fascia.

20 Close the skin with a subcuticular stitch.

? DIFFICULTY

1. Freeing the vas and vessels from a very thin sac can be difficult. The sac may be opened and freed off the vas and vessels from inside, held with multiple mosquitoes until full control of the sac is achieved.
2. If inadequate length of vas and vessels is achieved, try dividing the lateral fibres (of Dennis Browne, 1892–1967, surgeon to Great Ormond Street Hospital for Sick Children), which may be tethering the vas, or gently sweep the peritoneum off the vas and vessels deep to the internal ring, or pass the vas, vessels and testis under the inferior epigastric vessels.

Aftercare

1 In a young child the procedure can be performed as a day case. With older children postoperative vomiting is not uncommon and may require an overnight stay.

2 Follow-up should be long enough to confirm the survival of the testis following the procedure.

OESOPHAGEAL ATRESIA

KEY POINTS Refer to specialist?

- Surgery for the repair of oesophageal atresia is seldom an emergency so there is adequate time for referral to a specialist centre.
- In the absence of other severe congenital anomalies (especially cardiac malformations) nearly all infants weighing over 1500 g survive.

APPRAISE (Fig. 40.2)

1 Establish the diagnosis with a plain X-ray to reveal arrest of a radio-opaque nasogastric tube in the upper oesophagus. Include the abdomen on the radiograph. Air in the stomach indicates a distal tracheo-oesophageal fistula, for which primary repair is usually possible.

2 Absence of an abdominal gas shadow usually indicates isolated oesophageal atresia in which the distance between the proximal and distal segments is too long to permit primary oesophageal anastomosis, so a feeding gastrostomy and an end cervical oesophagostomy may be required.

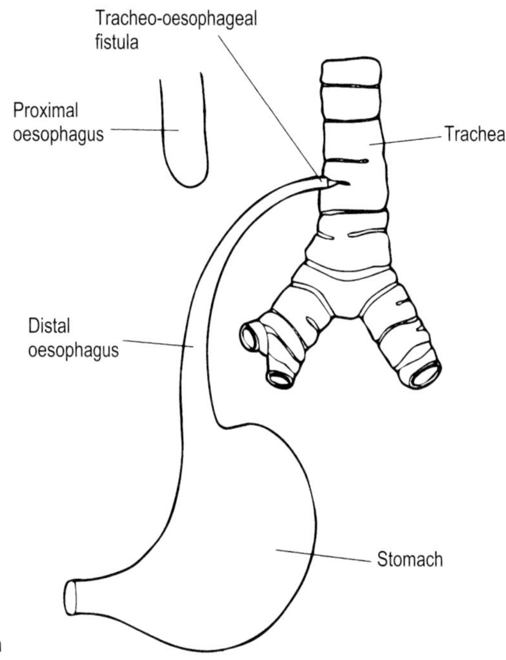

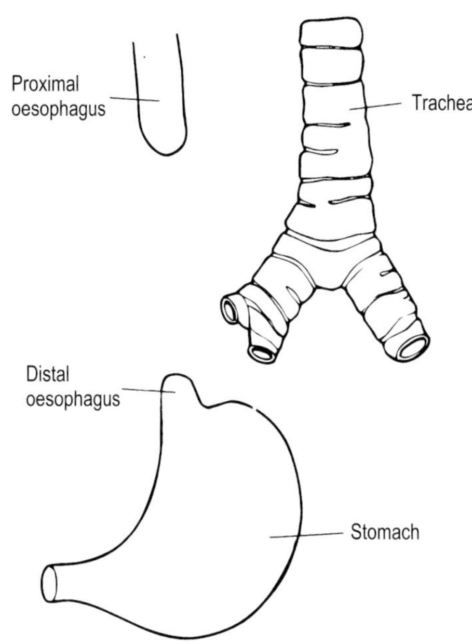

Fig. 40.2 The two main varieties of oesophageal atresia: (a) the most frequent (90%) condition with distal tracheo-oesophageal fistula; (b) the infrequent (5%) state of isolated oesophageal atresia.

GASTROSTOMY

STAMM GASTROSTOMY (Fig. 40.3)

Access

1 Make a transverse incision 3–4 cm long in the left hypochondrium, midway between the umbilicus and the costal margin.

2 Incise the subcutaneous tissues, muscles and peritoneum along the length of the incision using cutting diathermy.

Action

1 Identify the stomach and choose the site for the gastrostomy—on the anterior surface of the body of the stomach 0.5–1.0 cm away from the greater curvature.

2 Insert two purse-string sutures around the proposed site of the gastrostomy using an atraumatic 0000 polyglycolic acid suture. Avoid the gastroepiploic vessels.

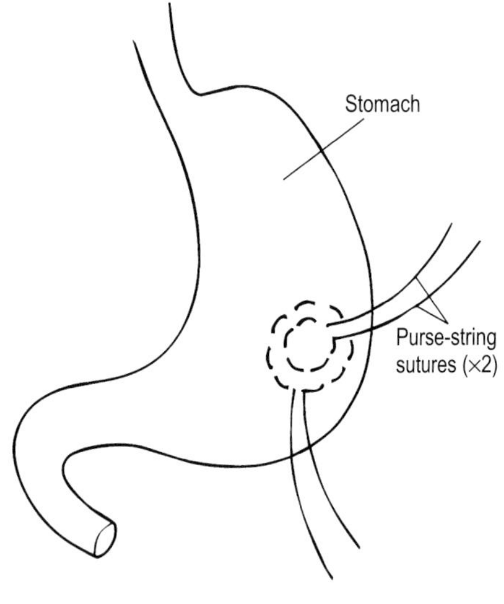

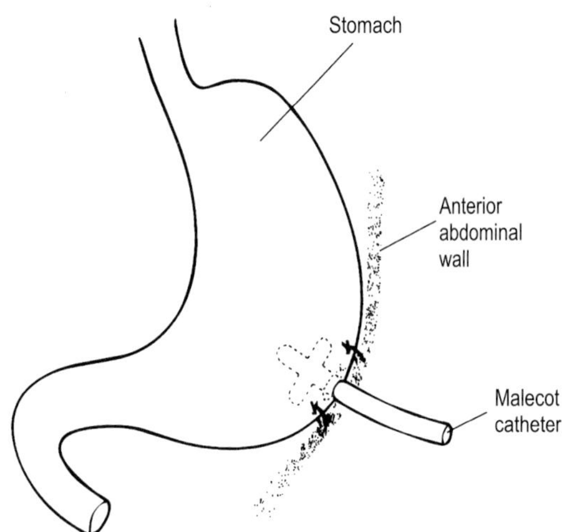

Fig. 40.3 The recommended technique of performing a Stamm gastrostomy.

3 Make a small incision in the stomach in the centre of the two purse-string sutures with a pointed scalpel blade and insert a no. 10–12 Malecot catheter into the stomach.

4 Tie first the inner and then the outer purse-string suture.

5 Bring the Malecot catheter out through a separate stab incision in the left upper quadrant.

6 Anchor the anterior wall of the stomach to the abdominal wall at the site of exit of the tube with three or four absorbable sutures. This will prevent retraction of the stomach from the abdominal wall and peritonitis from leakage of gastric content.

Closure

1 Close the wound en masse with 0000 polyglycolic acid suture. Suture the skin with an absorbable subcuticular suture.

2 Firmly anchor the tube to the skin of the abdomen with one or two silk sutures.

PERCUTANEOUS ENDOSCOPIC GASTROSTOMY

1 Percutaneous endoscopic gastrostomy (PEG) has become the preferred method of gastrostomy insertion as it avoids an 'open' procedure. This cannot be used in a child with an unrepaired oesophageal atresia.

2 The indications are mainly for long-term nutrition in the handicapped child or hyperalimentation in children with either cystic fibrosis or chronic renal failure.

Action: the 'pull' technique

1 Use general anaesthetic with the child supine.

2 An endoscope is passed into the stomach and directed anteriorly such that the light from the scope can be seen on the anterior abdominal wall.

3 The assistant pushes on the anterior abdominal wall at the site of illumination to confirm the position of the stomach underneath the light.

4 A small stab incision is made and then a needle with trocar is pushed firmly into the stomach.

5 The needle is removed and a guide-wire is passed into the stomach through the trocar. The guide-wire is grasped by endoscopic forceps and pulled up through the mouth.

6 The guide-wire is tied to the PEG tube which is then pulled back into the stomach and through the anterior abdominal wall incision.

7 The endoscope is re-passed into the stomach to check the position of the flange of the tube within the stomach.

8 The tube is then secured onto the anterior abdominal wall.

? DIFFICULTY

1. In a very obese child or a child with multiple scars it may be difficult to see the light of the endoscope on the anterior abdominal wall. Make sure you can see the assistant pressing on the stomach wall before they attempt to pass the needle.
2. If the stomach is overinflated it is possible to rotate the stomach and pass the needle through the transverse colon.
3. If you push the needle with trocar too gently it is possible to create a submucosal channel without actually breaching the stomach mucosa.

Aftercare

1 The tube can be used 6 hours after insertion.

2 The tube can remain in situ for up to 2 years, but needs to be changed under a general anaesthetic. It can be changed for a gastrostomy button. These do not require a general anaesthetic to change, but need to be changed every 3–6 months.

REPAIR OF OESOPHAGEAL ATRESIA

Only the principal steps are outlined. Repair requires special training and facilities.

Access

1 The incision is a right posterolateral thoracotomy.

2 Gain access via the third or fourth intercostal space.

3 Follow a retropleural approach to the mediastinum. This has distinct advantages over the transpleural approach in controlling an oesophageal leak.

4 Ligate and divide the azygos vein which crosses the oesophagus

Action

1 Identify the vagus nerve that courses on the surface of the distal oesophagus.

2 Trace the distal oesophagus to its proximal connection with the trachea.

3 Divide the oesophagus at this site and suture the defect in the trachea with interrupted 00000 or 000000 polypropylene, polyglactin 910 or polydioxanone sutures.

4 Identify the blind-ending upper oesophagus by asking the anaesthetist to apply pressure on the oro- or naso-oesophageal catheter.

5 Excise the tip of the blind-ending upper oesophagus.

6 Construct an anastomosis between the proximal and distal oesophagus using a single layer of interrupted 00000 or 000000 polyglactin, polypropylene or polydioxanone sutures. It is vital that each suture of the oesophageal wall includes the submucosa and mucosa (otherwise an anastomotic stricture will result), which tend to retract away from the cut ends.

Closure

Close the thoracotomy wound in layers with 00 pericostal and 000 tissue sutures of polyglycolic acid or polyglactin 910.

PYLORIC STENOSIS

Appraise

1 This occurs predominantly in male infants (male-to-female ratio=4:1) around the second to fourth week of life.

2 The cardinal features are projectile non-bilious vomiting, failure to thrive and constipation.

3 The diagnosis is established by palpating the pyloric 'tumour' in the right hypochondrium.

4 Confirmation by ultrasound examination is performed when doubt about the diagnosis remains after examination.

Prepare

1 Measure serum urea, electrolytes and acid–base status.

2 Correct hypochloraemia and hypokalaemia with intravenous infusion of half-normal saline adding potassium (10–15 mmol KCl per 500 ml of 0.45% saline).

3 It is unnecessary to correct the alkalosis, which resolves spontaneously with the saline infusion. Surgery should not be performed until the serum bicarbonate is 26 mmol/litre or less.

4 Prohibit all milk feeds and leave a nasogastric tube on free drainage, replacing losses millilitre for millilitre with normal saline and potassium (10 mmol KCl per 500 ml of 0.9% saline).

5 Check that serum potassium levels are above 3.5 mmol/litre before arranging operation.

> **KEY POINTS Resuscitate**
>
> - The operation for pyloric stenosis is NEVER an emergency.
> - Delay it for 24–48 hours until you have corrected dehydration and electrolyte disturbances.

Anaesthesia

Although local anaesthesia has been used for pyloromyotomy with great success in the past, general endotracheal anaesthesia by an experienced paediatric anaesthetist is superior.

Access

1 The infant lies supine on the operating table protected from cold.

2 There are two possible incisions:
- *Either* a transverse incision, 3–4 cm long, in the right hypochondrium midway between the costal margin and the palpable inferior margin of the liver; the medial end of the incision ends 1–2 cm from the midline.
- *Or* a supra-umbilical incision of adequate length to allow delivery of the 'tumour'.

3 Having incised the skin with the scalpel, divide the subcutaneous tissue and muscles using cutting diathermy to limit blood loss.

4 Open the peritoneum.

5 Retract the inferior margin of the liver superiorly by means of a broad malleable retractor protected by a moist gauze swab. Not required with a supra-umbilical incision.

6 Identify the greater curvature of the stomach directly or after applying gentle traction on the transverse mesocolon.

7 Do not attempt to withdraw the pyloric tumour by applying direct traction on the mass; this results in serosal tears and haemorrhage.

8 Deliver the greater curvature of the body of the stomach into the wound.

9 Apply gentle traction on the greater curvature until the firm, white, glistening pyloric tumour is brought into view. Ease it out of the peritoneal cavity and into the wound.

10 Identify the pyloric vein of Mayo. This marks the distal end of the pyloric canal.

Action (Fig. 40.4)

1 Make an incision 1–2 mm deep with a scalpel on the anterior surface of the pyloric tumour in the relatively avascular

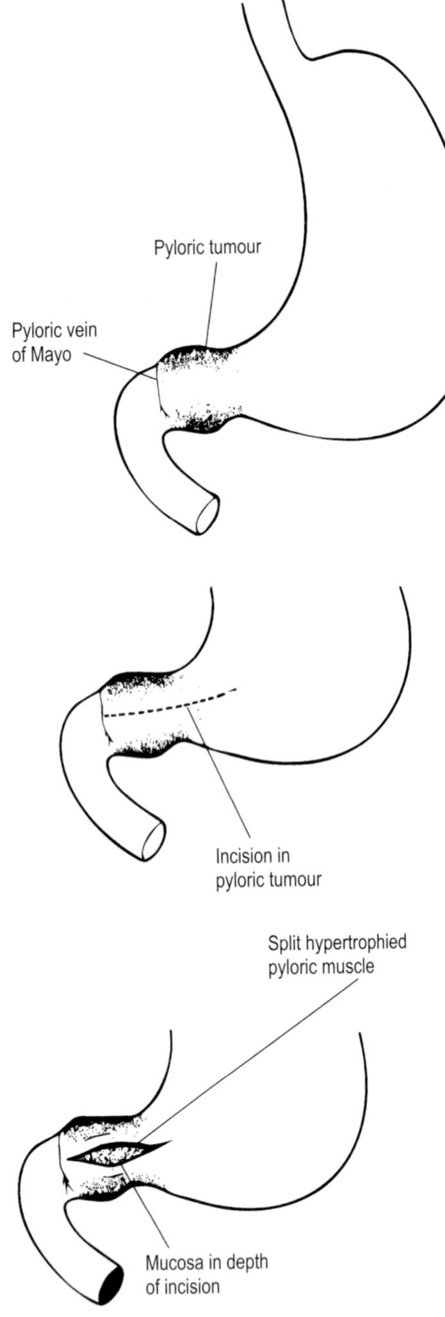

Fig. 40.4 Ramstedt's pyloromyotomy.

plane midway between the superior and inferior borders. Extend the incision from the pyloric vein of Mayo, through the pyloric canal and onto the hypertrophied body of the stomach.

2 Using firm but gentle pressure on the incised pylorus with a MacDonald dissector, the blunt handle of a scalpel or a blunt artery forceps, split the hypertrophied muscle down to the submucosa.

3 Split the pyloric mass from end to end using a pyloric spreader (Denis Browne) or blunt artery forceps. Ensure that all the fibres of the pyloric tumour are split.

4 Bubbles of air or bile at the duodenal end of the incision signify a perforation of the mucosa, most common in the duodenal fornix.

5 Close a perforation with a few interrupted 00000 absorbable sutures and cover with omentum.

6 Haemorrhage from the incised pylorus is mainly due to venous congestion. Bleeding usually ceases once the pylorus is returned to the abdominal cavity. If bleeding persists, use diathermy coagulation.

Closure

1 Close the wound en masse using interrupted 0000 polyglycolic acid sutures.

2 Approximate the skin with a continuous subcuticular 00000 absorbable suture.

Note: The operation can be performed laparoscopically with equally good results.

Aftercare

1 Many surgeons commence feeds within 4–6 hours of operation. There is evidence that gastric peristalsis is ineffective at this stage and vomiting is common.

2 Continue intravenous fluids for 12–24 hours.

3 Starting with 15–20 ml of milk, re-introduce feeds cautiously 12 hours after operation. Gradually increase the volume until normal milk feeds are being offered at 24–48 hours.

4 The infant should be ready for discharge from hospital on the second or third postoperative day.

5 If a perforation of the mucosa occurred, withhold feeds for 24 hours while continuing nasogastric decompression and intravenous fluids.

INTESTINAL OBSTRUCTIONS

The infant with intestinal obstruction is best managed in a specialist centre for paediatric surgery, not just for the operative treatment but especially for the postoperative care which often entails prolonged parenteral nutrition, particularly when massive resection results in 'short-bowel syndrome'.

Appraise

1 The main causes of intestinal obstruction are:

- Intraluminal causes—meconium ileus.
- Intramural causes—atresias, stenoses, necrotizing enterocolitis and Hirschsprung's disease.
- Extramural causes—malrotation with or without volvulus, duplication cysts, peritoneal bands, adhesions from necrotizing enterocolitis and tumours.
- Functional causes—ileus secondary to septicaemia, urinary infection, hypoglycaemia, hypocalcaemia, endocrine disorders, and prematurity.

2 Transfer as in neonatal transport, ensuring effective nasogastric decompression.

3 Neonates with intestinal obstruction can be safely transported over long distances (transcontinentally and intercontinentally) but local circumstances may dictate that operation has to be performed by a general surgeon. The principles of the operative procedure are described below.

Prepare

1 As for any neonatal operative procedure with special emphasis on adequate resuscitation and rehydration.

2 Use a broad-spectrum antibiotic (e.g. benzylpenicillin plus metronidazole plus amikacin or gentamicin).

Anaesthesia

1 General endotracheal anaesthesia is used.

2 The infant is in the supine position.

Access

The best exposure is the 'general purpose' incision for neonatal laparotomy.

Action

This depends upon the findings.

Meconium ileus

1 Identify the site of obstruction at the transition between dilated proximal and collapsed distal intestine. The terminal ileum and colon contain pellets of inspissated, tenacious mucus.

2 There may be associated small-bowel atresia or intestinal malrotation, or the condition may be complicated by perforation of the obstructed intestine.

3 Perform an enterotomy at the site of obstruction.

4 Endeavour to disimpact the distal intestine by irrigating with warm saline, Gastrografin or Tween 80. The latter two substances are strongly hygroscopic and must be used with considerable caution to avoid dehydration and shock. If lavage succeeds, the enterotomy may be closed.

5 If lavage fails, the Bishop–Koop chimney anastomosis is constructed by many paediatric surgeons, but the simplest and safest treatment is to perform a standard double-barrelled Mikulicz ileostomy.

6 The diagnosis of mucoviscidosis is established on preoperative immunoreactive trypsin levels, gene probes or sweat tests. Analysis of the sweat at the age of 4–6 weeks reveals sodium levels in excess of 60 mmol/litre. Since mucoviscidosis is a recessively inherited condition, the implications for the family are considerable.

Intestinal atresia

1 Identify the site of obstruction. There is an abrupt transition between dilated proximal intestine and the narrow, collapsed, 'un-used' distal bowel.

2 The bowel ends may be adjacent to one another, connected by a fibrous strand, or completely separate.

3 Resect the atretic segment with 1–2 cm distally, the proximal extent of the resection being dependent on the site of the atresia. In high jejunal atresia, resection cannot be carried out proximal to the duodenojejunal flexure. In mid-small-bowel atresia, resection can be performed into proximal intestine of fairly normal calibre. Avoid extensive resections if possible.

4 Test that the distal bowel is patent by injecting saline through a catheter introduced into the lumen.

5 Anastomose the ends using a single layer of interrupted 00000 or 000000 extramucosal sutures of polyglactin 910, polydioxanone or polypropylene. Perform an end-to-end or end-to-back anastomosis and avoid side-to-side anastomosis.

? DIFFICULTY

1. Grossly dilated proximal intestine may have to be 'tapered' in order to achieve an end-to-end anastomosis.
2. 'Tapering' is performed by excising an antemesenteric wedge of proximal bowel.

Hirschsprung' s disease

1 The diagnosis should have been confirmed prior to laparotomy by suction rectal biopsy.

2 Frozen-section histopathology should be available to identify the transition between proximal ganglionic and distal aganglionic colon.

3 Identify the transition between dilated and collapsed colon.

4 Perform a loop colostomy in the proximally dilated colon as described in the section on anorectal malformations.

5 Excise a narrow ellipse of full-thickness intestine at the site of the colostomy for identification of ganglion cells on paraffin sections.

6 The definitive treatment of Hirschsprung's disease is highly specialized and should only be performed by experienced paediatric surgeons with the assistance of expert histopathologists.

Note: The incidence of laparotomy for Hirschsprung's disease is falling as the majority of infants can be managed initially with rectal wash-out to decompress the obstructed colon, with the intention of performing a one-stage pull-through procedure in the first few months of life. The risk of Hirschsprung's enterocolitis is ever present and requires intensive resuscitation and frequent decompressing saline wash-outs. If this is unsuccessful, laparotomy and stoma formation is indicated.

Duplication cysts

1 These cysts are situated on the mesenteric border of the intestine and cause obstruction by stretching and compressing the lumen of the adherent normal bowel.

2 Identify the duplication cyst.

3 Resect the cyst en bloc with the adjacent intestine.

4 Perform an end-to-end anastomosis in one layer with interrupted 00000 or 000000 sutures of polypropylene, polydioxanone or polyglactin 910, using an extramucosal technique.

MALROTATION WITH OR WITHOUT MIDGUT VOLVULUS

Development

The midgut develops within the physiological umbilical hernia in early intrauterine life. Between the tenth and twelfth weeks of development, the midgut loop returns to the peritoneal cavity, rotating in an orderly manner beginning with the jejunum and ending with the ileocaecal region. The duodenum rotates into its C-loop and the ileocaecal loop undergoes counter-clockwise rotation of 270°, resulting in fixation of the proximal duodenum and ascending colon in the right retroperitoneum and the duodenojejunal flexure on the left. As a result, the root of the mesentery of the small intestine is obliquely attached across the posterior abdominal wall over a relatively long distance.

Malrotation results when this process of rotation and fixation is incomplete and has two effects:

- Formation of abnormal bands that cross, and may compress, the second part of the duodenum.
- A narrow base to the midgut that is prone to volvulus. Volvulus may occur at any age but it is particularly likely to occur during the first month of life.

Appraise

1. Consider the diagnosis of malrotation in any infant manifesting bilious vomiting, especially when this is intermittent, suggesting 'twisting' and 'untwisting' of the bowel.
2. Plain abdominal radiographs reveal a dilated stomach and duodenum with the rest of the abdomen relatively 'gasless' when volvulus has occurred.
3. Confirmation of the diagnosis can be made by means of upper gastrointestinal contrast radiography.
4. Treatment is urgent when volvulus has occurred, producing shock and gastrointestinal haemorrhage. The blood supply to the entire midgut may be obstructed and delay in treatment serves only to increase the amount and extent of intestinal necrosis. Nevertheless a short (1–2 hours) intensive period of active resuscitation to correct fluid and electrolyte loss and acid–base imbalance is worthwhile.

Prepare

1. Correct dehydration with intravenous plasma (20 ml/kg) as rapidly as possible.
2. Administer broad-spectrum antibiotics.
3. Effect urgent transfer to a specialized paediatric surgical unit, ensuring that full resuscitative measures continue en route.
4. Where specialized facilities are unavailable, operation will have to be performed locally.

Anaesthesia

Use general endotracheal anaesthesia with the infant in the supine position.

Access

Open the abdomen using the 'general purpose' incision.

Assess

1. Inspect the bowel for obvious areas of gangrene. These should be handled very gently as the intestinal wall is extremely friable and prone to perforation.
2. Assess the direction of rotation and untwist the volvulus. A counter-clockwise manoeuvre will release the volvulus.
3. Whilst awaiting return of circulation to compromised bowel, inspect the root of the mesentery for evidence of malrotation.
4. In a typical case, the root of the mesentery between the duodenojejunal flexure and the ileocaecal junction is very narrow and fibrotic. The caecum lies below the liver and may even be attached to the gallbladder by peritoneal bands.

Action

1. Ladd's procedure is recommended.
2. Divide the avascular peritoneal bands between the caecum and liver.
3. Once all the bands are divided, the caecum may be placed in the left upper quadrant of the abdomen.
4. See that the duodenojejunal flexure is to the right of the midline. Adhesions anchoring the duodenojejunal flexure may have to be divided.
5. Mobilize the duodenum by Kocher's manoeuvre and divide all peritoneal folds so that all kinks in the duodenum are straightened.
6. Incise what is now the anterior layer of peritoneum at the root of the mesentery and divide all fibrous bands so that the caecum may be moved as far to the left as possible, away from the duodenojejunal flexure, broadening the base of the mesentery.
7. Inspect the duodenum carefully, searching for areas of duodenal stenosis. This is uncommon except in patients presenting in early infancy. Correct duodenal stenosis by performing a duodenoduodenostomy. Do not incise the annular pancreas, as this increases the morbidity and mortality rates and does not relieve duodenal obstruction.
8. Return attention to the small bowel. Measure the length of the ischaemic bowel and assess the blood supply.
9. Resect all truly gangrenous areas unless this would leave the child with less than 30 cm of small bowel. Consider whether it would be better to perform a primary anastomosis or to bring out both ends as temporary stomata. If the ends of resected intestine are viable it is preferable to perform a primary anastomosis. Alternatively, in advanced countries, elect to perform enterotomies and maintain the child by parenteral nutrition until the general condition is improved. In this way it may be possible to preserve more intestine than would be possible with a primary anastomosis.
10. When most of the intestine is ischaemic, return it to the abdomen, having untwisted the volvulus and divided constricting bands and adhesions. Close the abdomen en masse. Continue intensive medical treatment, and re-explore after 24 hours.

At the 'second-look' laparotomy in young infants, one is often surprised at how the blood supply has improved. At the second operation, resect all bowel that is obviously gangrenous, but retain all bowel of doubtful viability. Bring the two ends out as temporary stomata. An anastomosis in compromised bowel is not advised as it is prone to disruption.

11 If all the bowel is viable, consider performing an appendicectomy, because the appendix would otherwise lie below the left costal margin and could cause diagnostic confusion at a later date. Appendicectomy is best performed by the inversion method so as not to spill intestinal bacteria in an otherwise 'clean' operation.

Closure

1 Close the abdomen en masse.

2 Suture the skin with subcuticular interrupted sutures.

Aftercare

1 Postoperative mechanical ventilation may be necessary in the infant with massive intestinal necrosis.

2 In such cases, close monitoring of arterial pressure and oxygenation is essential. Maintain the circulating volume by infusing plasma or fresh whole blood as required. Peripheral vasodilator drugs may be necessary. Administer diuretics to maintain an adequate urinary output (minimum of 1–2 ml/kg/hour).

3 In uncomplicated malrotation with or without volvulus, ileus commonly occurs for up to 2 weeks and parenteral nutrition is often necessary.

4 After massive intestinal resections, prolonged parenteral nutrition will be required. Oral nutrition is re-introduced with considerable caution as there is frequently intolerance to lactose, lipids and proteins.

NECROTIZING ENTEROCOLITIS

Appraise

KEY POINT Emergency

- Necrotizing enterocolitis is now the most common abdominal emergency in the neonatal intensive care unit.

1 The condition presents with bilious vomiting, rectal bleeding and radiological pneumatosis intestinalis caused by transmural inflammation of the intestine and is of unknown aetiology. It may affect any part of the gastrointestinal tract from stomach to rectum, most commonly the terminal ileum and splenic flexure.

2 The condition mainly affects premature babies in special care units and may occur in small epidemics.

3 Presentation may occur in the early acute phase with severe constitutional upset or in the recovery phase with intestinal obstruction caused by intestinal stricture or adhesion formation.

4 Management in the acute phase is non-operative. Discontinue enteral feeding. Maintain circulating volume and correct electrolyte imbalance with electrolyte solutions and colloids. Correct haemolytic anaemia with fresh blood. Give intravenous broad-spectrum antibiotics. Mechanical ventilation and inotropic support are often required.

5 Indications for operation include:
- Deterioration despite a short period of intensive medical treatment.
- Impending intestinal gangrene indicated by an erythematous abdominal wall, a loop of dilated intestine that remains static on X-rays for more than 24 hours, and a palpably tender loop of distended intestine.
- Inability to exclude a diagnosis of midgut volvulus.
- Free intestinal perforation indicated by a pneumoperitoneum.
- Inability to ventilate the infant because of gross abdominal distension.

6 During the subacute phase, indications for operation include:
- A localized perforation producing an abscess.
- Intestinal obstruction secondary to adhesion formation.
- Intestinal obstruction secondary to a stricture, usually in the left colon or terminal ileum.

Action

1 Intensive medical treatment is of paramount importance.

2 Operation is indicated only for specific surgical complications of condition.

Access

The 'general purpose' incision.

Assess

1 Pus should be aspirated and sent for bacteriological examination.

2 Gangrenous intestine should be resected.

3 Localized perforation in well-perfused bowel should be oversewn.

4 Extensive areas of perforation in ischaemic bowel should be resected.

5 If the resected ends have a good blood supply a primary anastomosis may be performed but otherwise the two ends should be exteriorized.

6 In very sick premature infants it may not be possible to do more than a proximal defunctioning enterostomy.

Prognosis

1 Overall, 80% of infants undergoing operation will survive.

2 About 20% of survivors will have 'short-bowel syndrome'.

3 15–20% of survivors will have permanent neurological disability.

4 Infants with severe systemic upset and poor peripheral circulation accompanied by pH below 7.2 will do badly, especially in the presence of thrombocytopenia and haemolytic anaemia with disseminated intravascular coagulation.

INTUSSUSCEPTION

Appraise

1 Between the ages of 6 months and 2 years, most intussusceptions are 'idiopathic', possibly caused by viral infections. The vast majority originate in the ileocaecal region. The condition is less common after the age of 2 years and rare in the neonatal period.

2 In the 'idiopathic age group', and in the absence of radiological evidence of intestinal obstruction or perforation, initial treatment is attempted using either pneumostatic or hydrostatic reduction, the latter by means of a barium enema. If this is unsuccessful, operation is required.

3 Outside the usual age range there is more likely to be a leading point such as a Meckel's diverticulum, polyp, duplication cyst or tumour causing the intussusception, and operation should be advised at an early stage.

4 The sick infant should be resuscitated and then transferred to a specialized unit, resuscitation continuing during the journey. These infants often deteriorate rapidly after operation and may not survive unless there are adequate facilities for intensive care.

5 If the infant is in good condition and local facilities are of high standard, prepare for operation.

Prepare

1 Set up a well-placed, adequately running, intravenous infusion.

2 Most infants will have reduced intravascular volume and will need preoperative rehydration. Many will require replacement of 10% or more of blood volume with plasma, plasma expanders or whole blood.

3 Once anaesthetized, the peripheral vascular resistance falls and the child may deteriorate suddenly.

4 Administer preoperative antibiotics.

5 Pass a large nasogastric tube.

Access

1 An expert may be able to reduce an intussusception through a short Lanz incision, as for appendicectomy.

2 In the absence of such skills, it is wise to use the 'general purpose' supra-umbilical transverse incision.

Assess

1 There should be an obvious sausage-shaped mass, usually in the midline, but possibly along the course of the left colon.

2 The anatomy of the right colon will be distorted, being drawn towards the transverse colon.

3 The appendix may not be visible.

Action

1 Withdraw the colon distal to the mass and gently attempt to push out the intussusceptum by squeezing the intussuscipiens in an antiperistaltic direction towards the caecum.

KEY POINT Gentleness

- Never try to pull out the intussusceptum by traction upon it, for if the bowel is ischaemic it will perforate or tear away in your hand.

2 Patience and gentleness will succeed in the majority of cases.

3 Reduction becomes increasingly difficult as it proceeds towards the starting point (apex), the last few centimetres being the most difficult. Proceed very slowly if the serosa of the intussuscipiens begins to split.

4 Continue assessment during reduction. If the reduced intussusceptum is obviously gangrenous or perforates, abandon the reduction and proceed to a limited right hemicolectomy.

5 If the reduction is successful, examine the distal ileum to ensure there is no ileo-ileal element to the intussusception. The antimesenteric border of the ileum 5–10 cm from the ileocaecal valve is the usual starting point of the intussusception and it is to be expected that there will be a thickened patch in the bowel wall 2–3 cm long at that site. This is not an indication for intestinal resection. This patch of oedematous bowel is an enlarged Peyer's patch and is not to be confused with a polyp or tumour.

6 If the bowel is viable, some surgeons perform an appendicectomy (especially if the Lanz incision is used), by either the inversion or the routine method. If there is doubt about the viability of the caecum, leave the appendix in situ and cover the intestine with hot packs for 5–10 minutes. If there is still doubt, it is probably safe to return the intestine to the abdominal cavity and suture the wound. The intestine has remarkable powers of healing in this age group.

7 If the bowel is non-viable, resect the affected areas. A standard right hemicolectomy is rarely necessary. Excise only the gangrenous areas and perform an end-to-end ileocolic anastomosis, using a one-layer anastomosis with sutures of polypropylene, polyglactin 910 or polydioxanone.

8 Check for a Meckel's diverticulum. If present, excise it and re-establish intestinal continuity with a one-layer anastomosis.

9 Ensure that there is no polyp, duplication cyst or tumour acting as a 'lead-point'.

Closure

As for neonatal laparotomy.

Aftercare

1 Observe closely for hypovolaemic or bacteraemic shock, following gangrenous intussusceptions.

2 Hyperpyrexia is not uncommon in the first 24–48 hours. Measures to reduce body temperature may be required.

ANORECTAL ANOMALIES

Appraise

1 It is essential to differentiate the high (supralevator) anomaly from the low (translevator) lesion. The high lesion requires

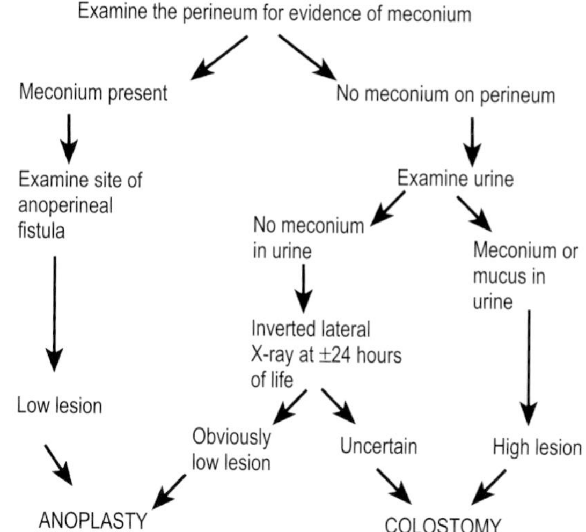

Fig. 40.5 Differentiation of low and high lesions in boys.

a preliminary colostomy whereas the low lesion can be managed successfully by anoplasty. A primary anorectoplasty in the neonatal period is performed by some surgeons for high anorectal anomalies.

2 In case of uncertainty perform a colostomy. Do not explore the perineum in search of the rectum as this may result in permanent incontinence.

3 In boys, plan treatment according to Figure 40.5.

4 In girls, determine the number of orifices present on the perineum: if three orifices are present, it is a low lesion requiring an anoplasty; if there are two orifices, or only one from which meconium is being passed, there is a high lesion, so perform a colostomy.

ANOPLASTY

Action (Fig. 40.6)

1 Make an inverted 'V' in the skin, the apex being centred on the pinhole opening on the perineum where meconium is visible.

2 Undermine the skin by sharp dissection.

3 Insert stay sutures and incise the rectal mucosa vertically for 1–2 cm.

4 Suture the skin flap into the rectal incision using 0000 sutures of polyglycolic acid.

5 The success of the operation depends upon the construction of a relatively large anus that may need to be dilated daily for 2 months. Failure to carry out regular dilatation results in anal stenosis and acquired megacolon which is extremely refractory to treatment.

COLOSTOMY

The technique to be described is based on the original description of a skin-bridge colostomy as recommended by Nixon. This avoids

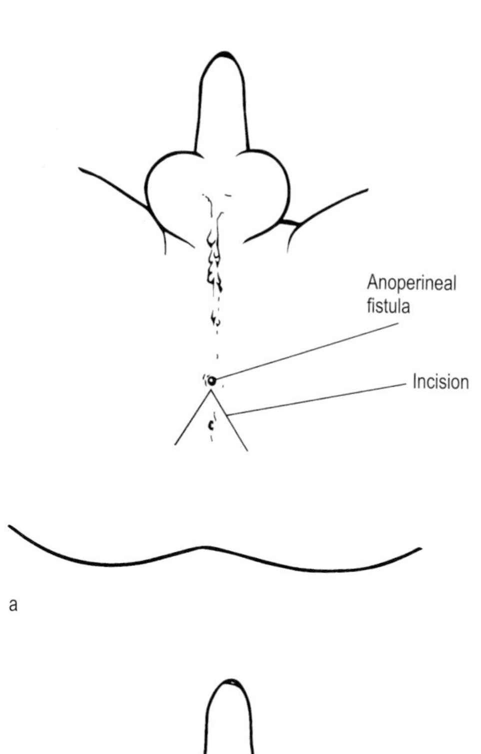

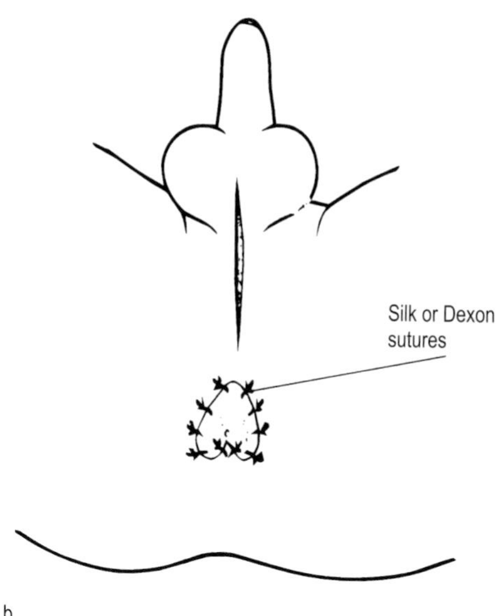

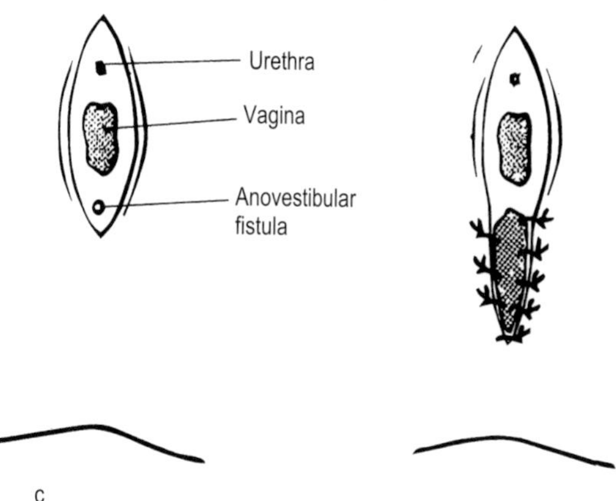

Fig. 40.6 Anoplasty procedures: male (a,b) and female (c) infants.

the use of a rod to prevent retraction of the intestine into the peritoneal cavity.

Action (Fig. 40.7)

1 Make a V-shaped incision, either in the left iliac fossa for a sigmoid colostomy, or in the right hypochondrium for a transverse colostomy. The latter colostomy has the advantage of leaving sufficient distal colon for secondary surgery to be performed without disturbing the colostomy.

2 Carry the V incision through skin and subcutaneous tissue.

3 Raise the flap of the V, exposing the underlying muscle.

4 Excise two shallow ellipses of skin and subcutaneous tissue immediately adjacent to the V flap to avoid compression of the colon immediately proximal and distal to the stoma.

5 Incise the muscle transversely, perpendicular to the V incision, using cutting diathermy.

6 Open the peritoneum in the same direction as the muscle incision.

7 Locate the part of the intestine that will form the colostomy. Remember that the sigmoid loop may be greatly dilated and may appear in the right upper quadrant where it is easily confused with the transverse colon. The lack of an omental attachment serves to differentiate it from the transverse colon.

8 Ensure that the bowel is not twisted as it is drawn to the surface. Twisting may produce intestinal obstruction.

9 Make a small opening in the colonic mesentery.

10 Pass the apex of the V skin flap through the mesenteric defect and suture it to its original position with two or three loosely tied 0000 polydioxanone sutures.

11 Suture the peritoneum or muscular fascia to the colonic serosa with a few interrupted 0000 polyglycolic acid sutures. This prevents herniation of small intestine alongside the colostomy.

12 Incise the colon longitudinally with cutting diathermy.

13 Suture the full thickness of the opened colon to the surrounding skin with interrupted 0000 polyglycolic acid sutures.

Aftercare

1 The infant should be referred to a specialized paediatric surgical unit for investigation to determine the precise anatomy of the anorectal malformation and to exclude additional congenital anomalies, particularly of the urogenital system.

2 The definitive pull-through procedure requires experience and skill if there is to be any chance of the child developing an acceptable degree of faecal continence.

MYELOMENINGOCELE

Appraise

1 Because of the naturally declining incidence and increased availability of termination of pregnancy, this has become an uncommon condition in Britain during the last 5 years, but remains common in other parts of Western Europe.

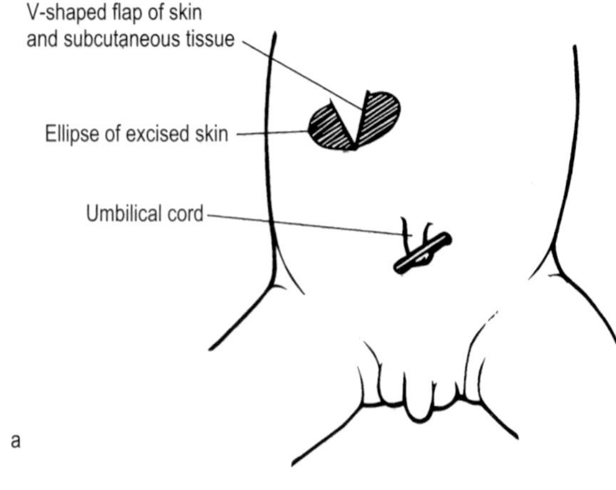

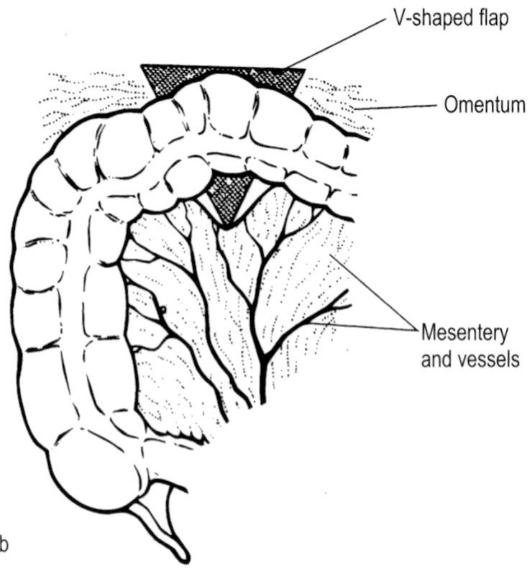

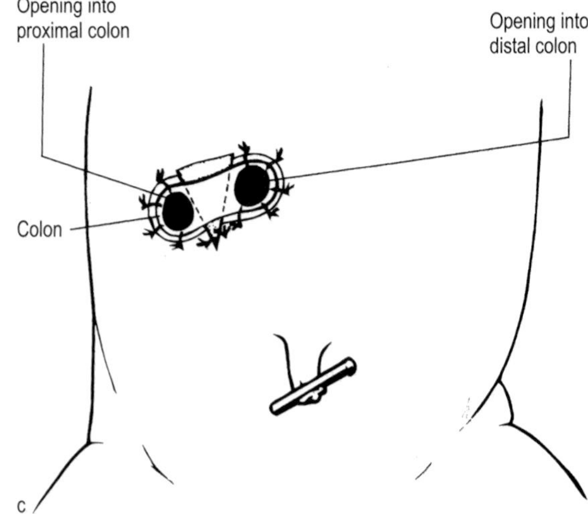

Fig. 40.7 Transverse loop skin-bridge colostomy.

KEY POINT Know your limitations

- There has never been a role for the occasional operator in the management of this condition and not all regional paediatric units have special facilities for these patients. In many centres this surgery is now performed by paediatric neurosurgeons.

2 All affected neonates should be referred to one of the dwindling number of specialized units for assessment and treatment. In these units there are paediatric surgeons experienced in urology, neurosurgery and orthopaedics, as well as nurses, physiotherapists, anaesthetists and radiologists with special skills.

3 The initial neonatal operation has little influence on the long-term prognosis, which depends upon the site and size of the myelomeningocele. The operation on the back simply rids the infant of the myelomeningocele, so facilitating nursing. It ensures more rapid healing of the lesion than would occur naturally. Whether or not the infant survives depends more on whether or not the associated hydrocephalus is treated.

4 Relative indications for operation are a small defect that is easily closed, absence of neurological deficit, or a robust infant with some neurological deficit. The parents may demand surgery despite knowing that the infant will have moderately severe handicaps.

5 Relative contraindications for operation are a large high lesion that will be difficult to repair, an infant in poor general condition, or the presence of other severe congenital anomalies. Operation is unlikely to be of benefit for a neonate in an underdeveloped country with inadequate facilities for treating hydrocephalus, urinary tract complications, or complex orthopaedic abnormalities.

6 An extensive neurological deficit, severe kyphoscoliosis, and gross hydrocephalus militate against aggressive treatment.

Action

1 Puncture the membrane between the neural plaque and the skin, allowing some of the cerebrospinal fluid to drain.

2 Using a scalpel, make an incision round the circumference of the neural plaque at its junction with the membrane, ensuring that there is no damage to the underlying nerve roots.

3 Having freed the neural plaque, excise the whole of the membrane back to healthy skin.

4 Make an incision round the outer limits of the dural layer of fascia, starting on either side and taking particular care in the midline both superiorly and inferiorly to avoid damage to the underlying spinal cord.

5 Close the dural layer with a continuous suture of 00000 polyglycolic acid or polydioxanone.

6 If the defect is relatively small, make an incision in the thoracolumbar fascia, on either side, at the medial borders of the bifid spinal processes. Elevate the muscles by blunt dissection and suture the fascia together in the midline using 00 polyglycolic acid. If the lesion is very wide it is wiser to omit this step.

7 Having brought the musculofascial layers together in the midline it is usually possible to do likewise with the skin edges. There is often a distinct fibrous ring round the edges of the defect and this can be sutured with a continuous stitch of 000 polyglycolic acid, so taking tension off the skin edges. Suture the skin with interrupted sutures of 00000 nylon or polypropylene. It should be seldom necessary to perform relaxing incisions in the flanks to achieve apposition of the skin over the defect.

Aftercare

1 Nurse the infant in the prone position until the wound has healed. Leave the skin sutures in situ for 10–14 days.

2 Measure the head circumference regularly to anticipate the early onset of hydrocephalus.

3 Fully investigate the urinary tract.

4 Long-term problems include urinary incontinence and/or renal damage, orthopaedic problems, complications of hydrocephalus and its treatment, psychosexual and education difficulties.

FURTHER READING

1. Spitz L, Coran AG (eds) 1995 Operative surgery: paediatric surgery, 5th edn. Chapman & Hall, London
2. Puri P (ed.) 2003 Newborn surgery, 2nd edn. Arnold, London
3. Beasley JW, Hutson JM, Myers NA (eds) 1993 Paediatric diagnoses. Chapman & Hall, London
4. Ashcraft KW, Holcolm GW III, Murphy JP (eds) 2005 Paediatric surgery, 4th edn. Elsevier Saunders, Philadelphia
5. Rowe MI, O'Neill JA, Fonkalsrud EW et al (eds) 1995 Essentials of pediatric surgery. Mosby Year Book, St Louis

41

Neurosurgery

R.S. Maurice-Williams

CONTENTS

GENERAL PRINCIPLES

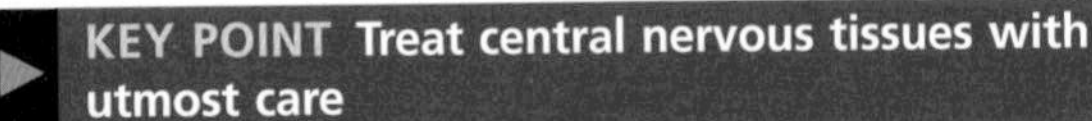

KEY POINT Treat central nervous tissues with utmost care

- Before operating on the brain or spinal cord, remember that central nervous tissue is easily damaged and, once damaged, cannot regenerate.

Although patients may make remarkable recoveries from injuries to the central nervous system, these recoveries are mediated by the compensatory action of intact neural tissue, rather than by local repair of the damaged areas.

These characteristics make neurosurgery different in several important respects from general surgery. You must not inflict any unnecessary damage on nervous tissue, so carry out every stage of the operation with meticulous care. You cannot afford any complications, even in the simplest neurosurgical procedure; a wound haemorrhage or infection may have appalling consequences. Achieve complete haemostasis. Packs cannot be used, drains can be inserted only for brief periods and to superficial tissue layers.

If possible, avoid neurosurgical operations. In most Western countries, telephoned expert neurosurgical advice can be obtained within minutes. Very few neurosurgical emergencies deteriorate while they are being transferred to a neurosurgical centre. Rapidly developing arterial extradural haemorrhage, however, is one emergency that will not travel and needs to be dealt with urgently. If you work in isolation however, you may need to carry out a wider range of neurosurgical operations.

Appraise

1 If the situation clearly demands neurosurgery on the spot, discuss the situation on the telephone with the neurosurgeon at the nearest available centre beforehand. You will avoid making elementary mistakes and have established a contact for further advice if necessary.

2 Do not rush. Carefully assess the clinical situation and decide what you hope to achieve by an emergency operation. Are further investigations or information required before you start operating? Is there any reasonable prospect of the operation benefiting the patient? Inappropriate over-treatment may result in an outcome for which no-one will thank you, particularly in the case of trauma to the brain. If the patient has clearly received a very severe primary brain injury from which a useful recovery is unlikely, there is no point in performing multiple exploratory burr holes. Patients with very severe head injuries commonly have extradural and subdural haematomas which are incidental to the main injury to the brain. The removal of an intracranial haematoma in such a patient may result in the survival of a hopelessly disabled person.

Prepare

1 Have adequate quantities of blood cross-matched; in inexperienced hands, intracranial operations are often accompanied by substantial blood loss and the patient may already have lost blood, either from scalp lacerations or injuries elsewhere.

2 Prefer general anaesthesia if possible. If you use local anaesthesia, a deeply unconscious patient may suddenly become restless and uncontrollable when intracranial tension is lowered by releasing a haematoma.

3 Ask the anaesthetist to have the patient paralysed and ventilated to lower the intracranial pressure, and be prepared to lower the blood pressure if necessary to control bleeding. However, systolic blood pressure should not fall below 70–80 mmHg or there is a risk of ischaemic cerebral damage, since control of the cerebral circulation is defective in the injured brain.

4 When the patient is prepared for anaesthesia, administer intravenous 250 ml of 20% mannitol for a teenager or an adult, or 100 ml for a child aged 3–10 years, given over 5–10 minutes. If it has crystallized out of solution, first warm the bottle to dissolve it. Mannitol lowers intracranial pressure for up to 3–4 hours, causing a brisk diuresis, so insert a urinary catheter. Intravenous mannitol is invaluable for 'buying time' if rising intracranial pressure causes rapid deterioration on the way to the theatre. If you have decided to operate, do

not be tempted to delay if the mannitol has produced a dramatic improvement of conscious level; when the effects wear off, the rebound rise in intracranial tension may cause sudden deterioration.

5 Position the patient supine with the head supported on a horseshoe-shaped ring for operation above the tentorium; turn the head from side to side to give access to either side. Rotation can be increased by placing a sandbag under the appropriate shoulder.

6 Reduce cerebral venous pressure to minimize cerebral swelling by tilting the patient feet-down by 20° but not more or there is a risk of producing air embolism if a major venous sinus is inadvertently opened. Do not twist the head sufficiently to cause compression of the neck veins or cerebral congestion is increased.

7 For access to the posterior fossa, position the patient prone, face lying in the head ring. Fully flex the neck to open up the atlanto-occipital angle, thus giving enough room to work in the posterior fossa. Ensure the eyes are well padded and not compressed by the head ring. Insert foam rubber padding between the ring and face and forehead to prevent disfiguring areas of pressure oedema and necrosis.

8 Shave the whole head; unexpected negative findings are common, demanding further exploratory burr holes elsewhere. Clip the hair then closely shave it, using a sharp blade in a holder of the type used for skin incision. Clean the whole scalp with an appropriate antiseptic solution such as Hibitane in spirit. Clear any debris from the scalp surface is cleared away. Cover the eyes with tulle gras, sealed with waterproof adhesive tape. Plug the ears with cotton wool to exclude antiseptic solution from damaging the drum.

9 Mark out intended incisions with a light scratch on the scalp, and then infiltrate the scalp beneath them with adrenaline (epinephrine) 1:200 000 in physiological saline. This reduces blood loss from the richly vascular scalp. Infiltrate the injection up the skull vault into the loose areolar tissue between the galea and the pericranium. If excessive force is required, then the needle tip is outside the galea; re-locate it.

10 Clean the head once more with antiseptic, dry it, towel up around the intended incision, securing the drapes to the scalp with towel clips. Place skin clips just above the eyebrows with their handles bridging the eyes to rest on the prominences of the cheeks, thus further shielding the eyes from inadvertent pressure.

Access to the brain

1 Burr holes can be carried out rapidly if preoperative computed tomography (CT) is not available, to establish whether there is any haematoma on the brain surface in that part of the head or whether the brain is under tension.

KEY POINTS Limitations of burr holes

- A burr hole exposes only a tiny part of the surface of the intracranial contents; nearby or deep pathology may not be detectable
- Burr holes seldom provide sufficient access for definitive treatment of important lesions.

2 Because of the limitations of burr holes, always place scalp incisions and burr holes so that they can be converted into an osteoplastic flap or craniectomy, to allow improved access. Apart from the use of multiple exploratory burr holes after a head injury, a single burr hole may be used to biopsy a cerebral tumour, drain a cerebral abscess or tap the lateral ventricles in acute hydrocephalus.

3 *Craniotomy*. An osteoplastic flap is turned and is replaced at the end of the operation (see p. 644). A craniotomy is the best way of exposing a wide area of the intracranial contents above the tentorium.

4 *Craniectomy*. A burr hole is extended by removing bone around it, leaving a defect which remains at the end of the operation. Avoid a craniectomy on the skull vault above the tentorium as the bone defect will require a plastic repair later. There are two situations where a craniectomy can be fashioned without the need for later surgery. A craniectomy is the usual mode of exposing the posterior fossa contents. The bone defect is covered over by the thick suboccipital muscles. The outer wall of the middle fossa may be removed by a 'subtemporal craniectomy', to provide access to an arterial extradural haematoma or a swollen temporal lobe. At the end of the operation the defect is concealed by suturing the temporalis muscle over it.

MULTIPLE EXPLORATORY BURR HOLES

Appraise

1 Multiple burr holes may be required after a head injury, when a deteriorating level of consciousness and/or the appearance of focal neurological signs leads you to suspect an expanding intracranial haematoma and a diagnostic CT scan is not available.

2 Even if the type and site of the haematoma seem certain, always mark out for multiple burr holes on each side of the head (Fig. 41.1). If a haematoma is present, it will not necessarily be on the side of the fracture or dilated pupil or contralateral to a hemiparesis. Furthermore, there may be bilateral haematomas.

Access (Fig. 41.2)

1 Mark with an indelible pencil the midline of the skull vault from the nasion (the median point of the frontonasal suture) to the external occipital protuberance.

2 Mark out three burr holes on each side.
- *Frontal*. Incise the scalp anteroposteriorly within the hairline and in line with the pupils when the eyes face forwards. Centre the skin incision 3.5 cm lateral to the midline and 10–11 cm back from the nasion.
- *Parietal*. Incise the scalp anteroposteriorly, over the parietal eminences, centred 6 cm lateral from a midline point, which lies 20–21 cm back from the nasion.
- *Temporal*. Gives access to the region of the squamous temporal bone where an arterial extradural haemorrhage often originates. Incise vertically to end just above the upper edge of the zygoma, 2.5 cm anterior to the external auditory meatus.

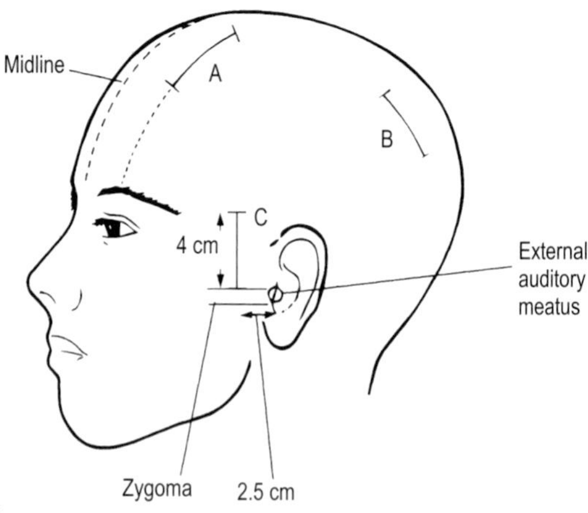

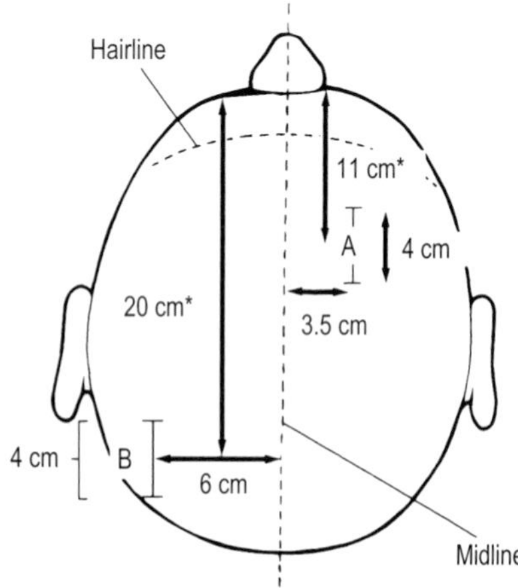

Fig. 41.1 Surface markings for exploratory burr holes: A, frontal; B, parietal; C, temporal.

> **KEY POINT Caution**
>
> - Avoid facial nerve branches.

3 If you prolong the incision further forwards or run it below the zygoma, you endanger branches of the facial nerve supplying orbicularis oculi. Incise down to bone through the scalp for 3–4 cm for each burr hole, then scrape the scalp away from the bone with a periosteal elevator. Separate the scalp edges widely with a self-retaining retractor to expose the bone surface. In the temporal region make the incision longer, as it needs to pass through the temporalis muscle to reach the bone.

4 Have the head held firmly while drilling and use the widest available diameter set of matching sized perforator and burr. A burr that is smaller than the perforator may break through into the intracranial contents.

5 First drill with the perforator in the Hudson brace (the perforator is the drill piece with the flat blade). Drill at 90° to the skull vault, cautiously but firmly, until you feel the tip of the perforator begin to wobble slightly. When this happens the tip of the perforator will have penetrated just inside the inner table, exposing a small patch of dura, perhaps covered with a thin flake of bone. Remove the perforator and check that this is so.

> **KEY POINTS Fracture line nearby?**
>
> - Drill cautiously.
> - The skull vault may suddenly give way, allowing the drill to penetrate deeply into the brain.

6 When you have confirmed that the perforator has penetrated the inner table, drill next using either the rose-shaped or conical burr until you feel the sensation that the burr is being gripped by the bone edge. Remove the burr and a wide area of dura should be exposed, slightly narrower in diameter than the outer part of the burr hole.

7 Clear bone dust from the incision. Arrest bleeding from the diploe by firmly applying bone wax. Surface dural bleeding may be stopped using diathermy coagulation but do not use a strong current or this will cut the dura, causing more bleeding.

Assess

1 An extradural haematoma is apparent immediately inside the bone when the burr hole is fashioned. A thin, 1–2-mm film of extradural clot is of no clinical significance.

2 An appreciable extradural haemorrhage is at least 1 cm deep and extrudes from the burr hole under pressure. The burr hole may allow the head of pressure from a tense extradural haemorrhage to reduce and thus 'buy time', but to evacuate it adequately and secure the source of bleeding, you need to convert the burr hole to a craniectomy if the extradural haemorrhage is in the middle fossa, or to a craniotomy if the extradural haematoma is situated elsewhere beneath the vault (see below).

> **? DIFFICULTY**
>
> - If there is no appreciable extradural haematoma, you must open the dura.

3 The dura is bulging and probably bluish in colour from a subdural haematoma. If it is slack following the removal of an extradural haematoma do not open it but if it remains tense, open it since there must be a co-existing subdural haematoma.

4 To open the dura, lift the central exposed disc of dura with a sharp hook and incise it with a sharp pointed blade. Now insert a dural guide between the dura and the brain surface and cut down on it to open the dura back to the bone in a cruciate fashion. Coagulate the tips of the four small dural flaps with diathermy, so they are well burned back to the bone surface.

5 If you find subdural blood, your action depends upon its consistency and how long it has been present. An acute subdural haematoma from a torn artery in a cortical laceration only shortly before may still be fluid; it may be possible to remove it through multiple burr holes alone. If the haematoma is partly or wholly clotted or bleeds briskly when you disturb the clot, convert the burr holes into a craniotomy so you can thoroughly clear the haematoma and secure the bleeding point. If you find a subacute subdural haematoma present for several days, most probably originating from a torn cortical bridging vein, it will be at least partly clotted, requiring

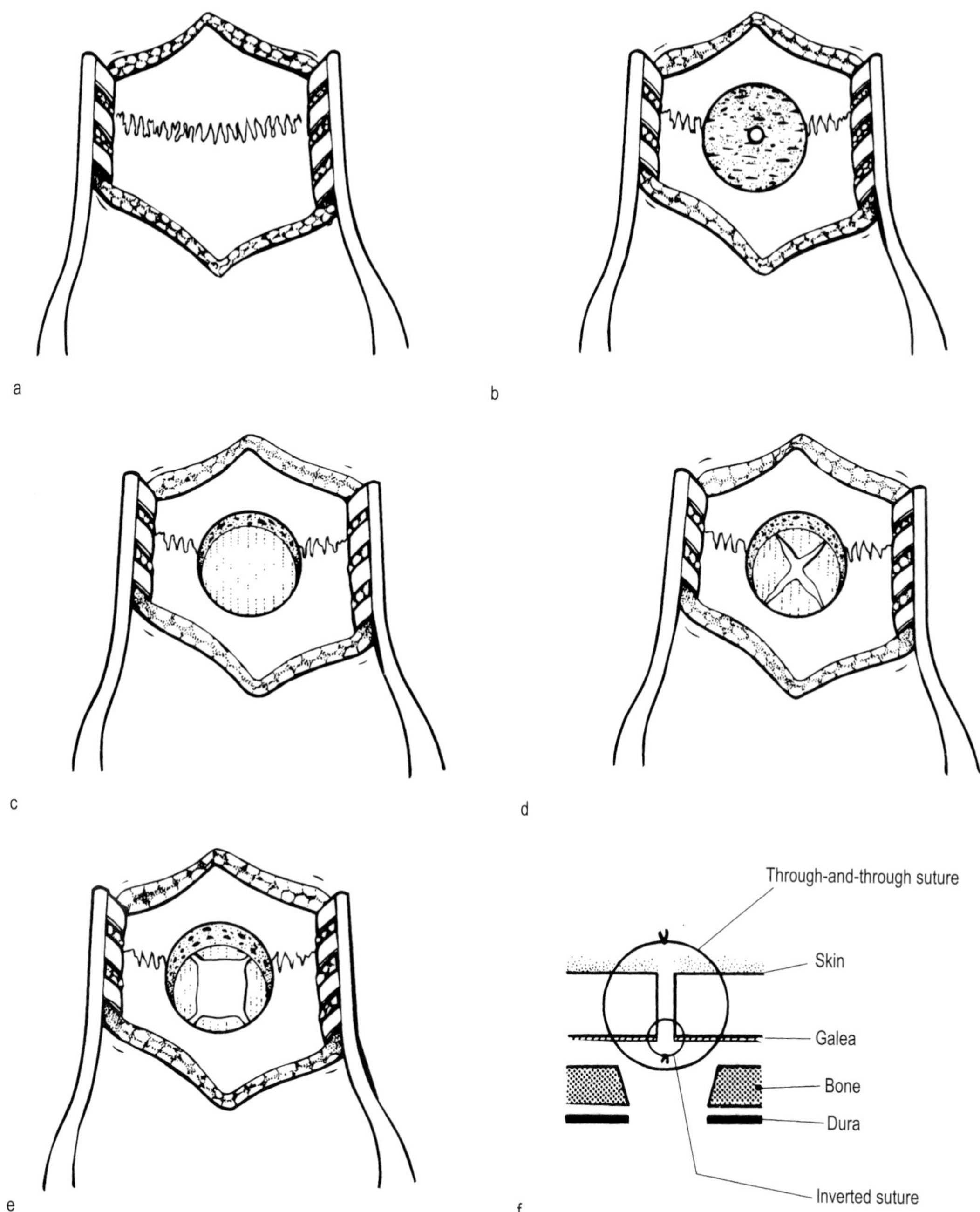

Fig. 41.2 Stages of making a burr hole: (a) scalp cut down to bone; (b) after use of perforator to expose a small area of dura; (c) after use of conical burr to expose dura more widely; (d) dura opened in cruciate fashion; (e) dura burnt back with the diathermy; (f) closure of the scalp.

conversion to a flap for thorough removal. A chronic watery subdural collection can usually be removed through burr holes alone.

Action

1 If burr holes alone appear adequate for evacuating a subdural haematoma, use a combination of suction and irrigation. Raised intracranial pressure usually forces out any fluid blood. Wash out any residual small clots from the subdural space with a firm jet of normal saline at or just below body temperature. Direct the saline through each burr hole in turn, thus achieving a fairly thorough wash-out of the subdural space. Do not suck on the brain directly. Keep the sucker tip just on the bone edge. To suck within the burr hole, first interpose a small square of lintine (a lintine patty) held in the tips of a pair of forceps, between the sucker tip and the brain surface. Ensure that the subdural space is in communication between the burr holes on each side. If the

burr holes communicate, saline squirted into one escapes through the others.

> **KEY POINTS Persistent subdural space**
>
> - After evacuating subdural haematoma the brain usually expands, largely obliterating the subdural space.
> - In a chronic watery subdural collection, expansion may not occur. The brain surface may remain well below the inside of the dura; left alone, the space may fill up again with fluid and the symptoms may recur.

2 To obliterate a persisting subdural space, try tipping the patient's head down on the operating table. If this does not work, insert a lumbar puncture needle into the lumbar sac and slowly inject normal saline at body temperature until the brain has re-expanded almost to the dura. Carry out this procedure only under direct vision, before you close the wounds. Usually 60–120 ml of saline are needed to re-inflate the brain.

3 If brisk bleeding continues from inside the dura after you have removed a subdural haematoma, convert the multiple burr holes into a craniotomy to reveal the bleeding point.

4 If multiple burr holes have revealed no surface haematoma and the brain surface is not tense, it is most unlikely that there is any intracranial pathology requiring surgical treatment, so close the wounds. If the brain surface is tense and bulging out through the burr holes then clearly there is some mass effect within the brain. Following trauma this is probably caused by diffuse or focal cerebral oedema, or a haematoma within the brain. There is no way in which you can differentiate between these possibilities without special investigation such as CT scan or cerebral angiography, available only in specialist centres. Therefore transfer the patient, if this can be done, and the patient's clinical condition justifies it.

Closure

1 Before closing ensure you have achieved perfect haemostasis. Arrest oozing from the brain surface with a patch of Surgicel laid inside the dura and pressed onto the brain surface with a wet piece of lintine. Stop bleeding from the dura with low-power diathermy current. Stop bleeding from the scalp vessels with through-and-through skin stitches.

2 Do not insert any drains.

3 Close the scalp in two layers of interrupted 3/0 silk sutures. Hold the wound edges together with galeal sutures, 1 cm apart, inverted so that the knots face inwards. Cut the loose ends very short so that they cannot work their way out through the skin. Insert skin sutures 1.0–1.5 cm apart, passed through all the layers of the scalp and tied fairly tightly to arrest bleeding from the scalp layers. Remove these sutures on the fifth postoperative day. Do not insert small sutures closer together than 1 cm or you may produce necrosis of the wound edges.

BURR HOLE FOR VENTRICULAR DRAINAGE

Appraise

This procedure is indicated for acute hydrocephalus.

Access

Make a burr hole in the right frontal region as described above.

Action

1 Open the dura. In acute hydrocephalus, the brain bulges out under tension.

2 Find a small area of cortical surface that is free of vessels and diathermize its surface for 2–3 mm.

3 Make a small cut in the coagulated cortex.

4 Run a brain cannula into the brain, holding it gently between thumb and index finger. Aim the needle slightly medially towards an imaginary line joining the external auditory meati.

5 At a depth of 4–5 cm inside the brain you will feel a slight 'give' as the needle enters the ventricle. Remove the stylette to check that the needle is within the ventricle; cerebrospinal fluid (CSF) should squirt out under pressure. Advance the cannula for another 1 cm into the ventricle and then remove it from the brain.

6 Insert a fine soft rubber catheter, maximum diameter 3 mm, along the needle track, introducing its tip for 2–3 cm into the ventricle. Check that CSF still flows out and then spigot the end of the catheter.

Closure

1 Close the wound around the catheter, while your assistant holds it firmly to prevent it retracting out of the ventricle. Alternatively, bring out the catheter through a stab incision separate from the main wound.

2 Suture the catheter to the wound so that it cannot pull out. Remove the spigot to make sure that CSF still flows from the catheter.

BURR HOLE FOR TAPPING CEREBRAL ABSCESS

Appraise

The diagnosis is supported by symptoms of raised intracranial pressure developing in a patient with neglected otitis media or frontal sinusitis.

Access

1 Make a burr hole according to the clinical situation, either through a vertical incision in the temporal region just above the top of the pinna in line with the external auditory meatus or through a horizontal incision in the forehead just above the line of the affected frontal sinus.

2 Frontal sinuses vary considerably in size and configuration, so have a preoperative anteroposterior skull X-ray available so you can place your burr hole avoiding entering the sinus.

Action

1 Diathermize the tense brain surface, avoiding any vessels, and incise the coagulated cortex.

2 Hold the widest available brain cannula between thumb and index finger and gently run it towards the expected position of the abscess. This is either just behind the frontal sinus or just above the tegmen tympani.

3 The wall of the abscess is rubbery offers a definite resistance to the cannula tip. Push the cannula through into the centre of the abscess.

4 Remove the stylette and gently suck out the pus, using moderate suction until no pus comes out freely. Inject 5 ml of normal saline containing dissolved 200 000 units of penicillin and 50 mg of streptomycin, into the empty cavity. Also inject 1 ml of sterile barium sulphate to outline the cavity.

Closure

Withdraw the cannula and close the scalp in two layers of interrupted silk as already described, without drainage.

SUBTEMPORAL CRANIECTOMY FOR EXTRADURAL HAEMATOMA

Indications

If an exploratory temporal burr hole reveals an appreciable extradural clot, you will need to extend the burr hole into a craniectomy to remove it.

Access (Fig. 41.3)

1 Extend the vertical temporal burr hole skin incision upwards to a total length of 8–9 cm, curving gently backwards above the tip of the pinna.

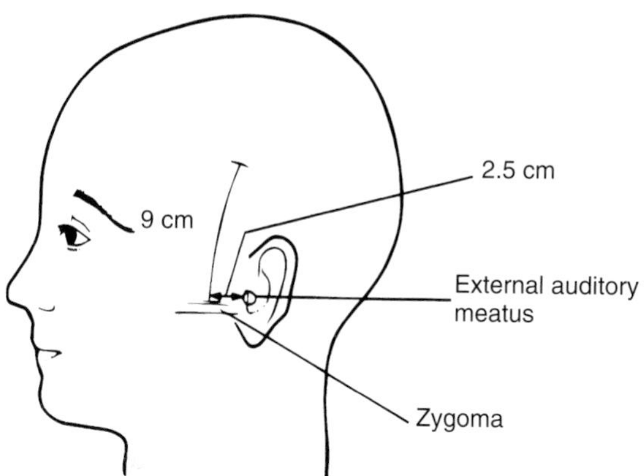

Fig. 41.3 Incision for extradural haematoma.

2 Hold the skin edges apart with two self-retaining retractors. Use diathermy coagulation to seal cut branches of the superficial temporal artery.

3 Incise the temporalis muscle to the bone in the line of the skin incision, using cutting diathermy. Scrape the muscle from the bone and re-insert the self-retaining retractors in the muscle incision to expose a wide area of the squamous temporal bone.

4 Nibble away the bone around the burr hole to produce a circular or oval bone defect 4–5 cm across. This usually involves removing the fracture line, which has crossed the path of the middle meningeal artery.

Action

1 Remove the extradural clot with the sucker, breaking it up by irrigation it with normal saline at body temperature.

2 Now the bleeding middle meningeal artery can generally be seen on the surface of the dura. Sometimes arterial bleeding has already been stopped by the pressure of the clot and arterial spasm. Stop bleeding from the meningeal vessels or the dura with diathermy coagulation but do not use too strong a current or it will cut through the vessel and produce more bleeding.

3 If you cannot stop the bleeding with coagulation, under-run the responsible dural vessel with a silk suture. If the bleeding arises from the artery where it enters the skull through the foramen spinosum, the matchstick tip of popular legend is of little use. Arrest the bleeding effectively by coagulating within the foramen, if necessary reinforced by a plug of bone wax firmly pushed into the foramen.

4 If the dura is tense and blue after removing the extra-dural haematoma, there may be an associated subdural haematoma. Lift the dura with toothed forceps and incise it to exclude subdural clot. If the dura is not tense or discolored, there is no need to open it. Stop residual oozing from the surface of the dura by covering the area with a sheet of cellulose mesh (Surgicel), leaving it in situ. Prevent further bleeding into the extradural space opened up by the haematoma, by suturing the dura to the temporalis muscle around the edge of the bone defect with interrupted 3/0 silk sutures at 2-cm intervals.

Closure

1 If the dura has been opened, close it with interrupted 3/0 silk sutures. It does not matter if the dural edges have retracted following diathermy coagulation, preventing a tight dural closure; merely cover the dural defect with Surgicel.

2 Approximate the separated fibres of the temporalis muscle with interrupted 3/0 silk sutures.

3 Close the scalp in two layers as described in the section on burr holes.

4 If haemostasis has been difficult and the dura was not opened, you may drain the extradural space for 24 hours using gentle suction through a drain tube brought out through a separate stab incision.

CRANIOTOMY

Appraise

1 This approach gives wide access to the intracranial contents above the tentorium.

2 Most traumatic intracranial haematomas require a craniotomy to remove them effectively.

Access (Figs 41.4, 41.5)

1 Mark out the scalp flap, in the shape of an inverted 'U'. Ensure that the base of the flap is the widest and nearest the base of the skull, since the scalp blood vessels come from below, and that the length of the flap does not exceed its width.

KEY POINT Caution

- Beware the frontal sinus and intracranial venous sinuses.

2 Place the flap so that the lines of the bone flap do not enter the frontal sinus or overlie the great sinuses—the superior sagittal and transverse sinuses. To avoid encroaching on the draining

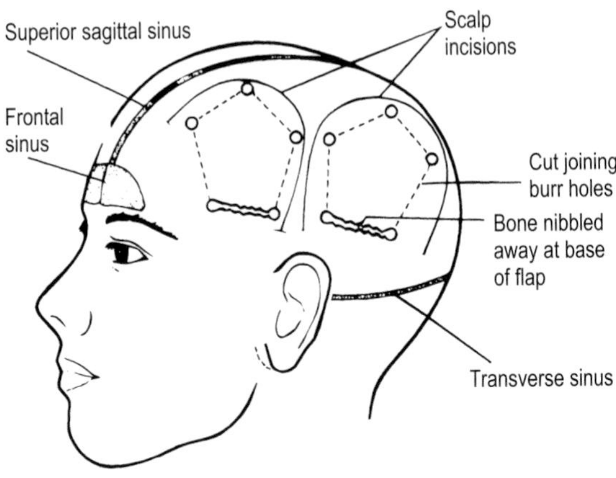

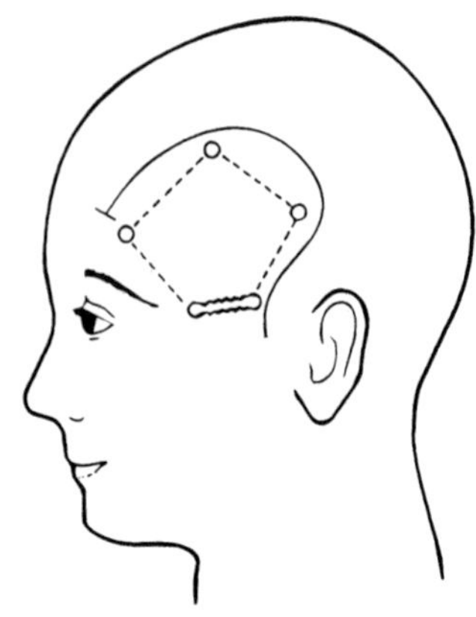

Fig. 41.4 Incisions for craniotomy: (a) frontal and parietal osteoplastic flaps; (b) flap to expose temporal lobe.

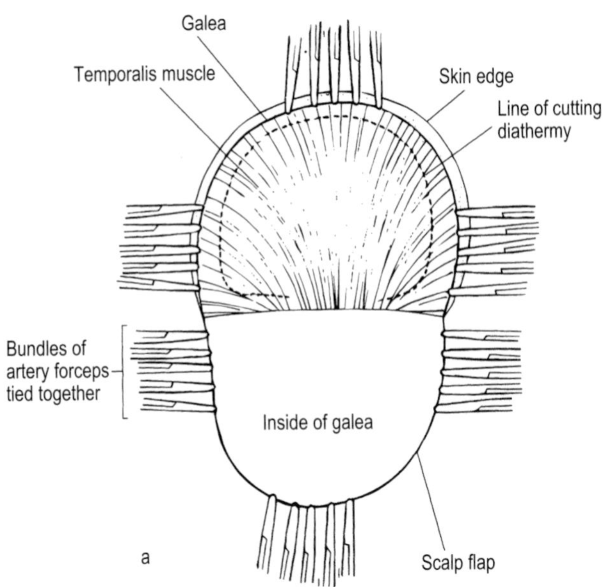

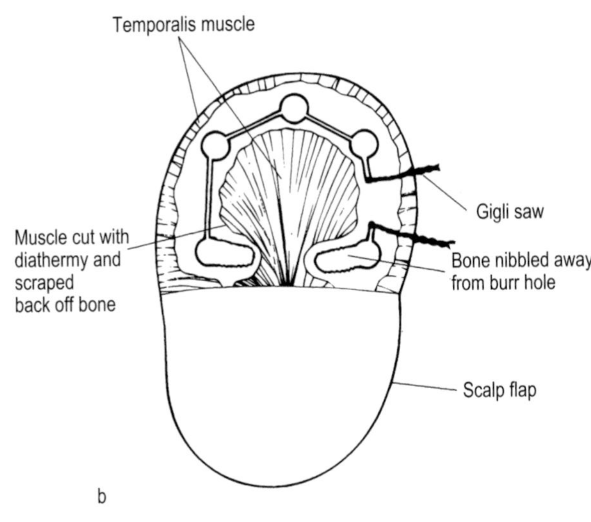

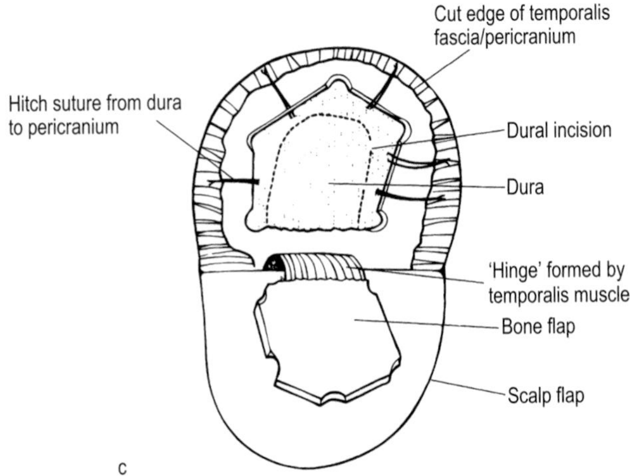

Fig. 41.5 Stages of osteoplastic flap: (a) scalp reflected-artery forceps on galea; (b) burr holes made and joined up by Gigli saw—basal burr holes connected by craniectomy; (c) bone flap reflected to expose dura.

veins and venous lakes which project from the sides of the superior sagittal sinus, mark out the scalp incision so that it does not come closer than 3 cm to the midline.

3 Incise each of the three sides of the scalp flap in turn, almost to the bone, while your assistant firmly compresses the scalp on each side with the fingertips to minimize bleeding.

4 As you cut, grasp the galea on each side at 2-cm intervals with the tips of artery forceps, securing any obvious bleeding points as you do so. The galea is a well-defined layer which you should have no difficulty in finding.

5 On each limb of the scalp flap, on either side of the incision, unite the handles of the artery forceps with rubber bands, allowing each bundle to fall back, everting the galeal edges and reducing bleeding.

6 Reflect the scalp flap by opening up, using sharp dissection, the plane of loose areolar tissue lying between the galea superficially and the contiguous pericranium and temporalis fascia deeply. Reflect the scalp flap, placing a rolled-up swab behind it, so that the bundles of attached artery forceps can turn back the edges of the galea. Secure the bundles of artery forceps to the surrounding drapes with towel clips.

7 Now fashion an osteoplastic (bone) flap, hinged on the temporalis muscle. Using cutting diathermy, cut to the bone a horseshoe-shaped flap of the conjoined pericranium and temporalis muscle, keeping intact a band of temporalis muscle 3–5 cm wide to form the hinge.

8 Scrape the pericranium and muscle back widely to expose the bone surface.

9 Drill the burr holes that are to be linked up to form the bone flap. Four or five holes will be needed, spaced according to the size of the defined flap with about 6–7 cm between the holes. Place the two burr holes that will be linked to form the base of the flap somewhat closer together, say 5 cm apart.

10 Carefully separate the dura from the bone between the burr holes by running an Adson's periosteal elevator against the inside of the bone surface from one hole to the next. If you are rough you may lacerate the dura.

11 Saw the bone between the burr holes using a Gigli saw. Run the blade of the saw between the burr holes on its special protective guide while keeping the blade fairly taut, to prevent it projecting sideways from the guide and tearing the dura. Make the cut so the bone flap is bevelled with the outer table extending outwards; this allows that the bone flap will slot into place at the end of the operation. Do not cut the bone between the two burr holes at the base of the flap with the Gigli saw, but nibble it away with bone cutters to complete the flap.

12 Hinge the bone flap backwards on the stalk of temporalis muscle to expose the dura. Suture the dura to the pericranium round the edges of the bone defect with interrupted 3/0 silk sutures at 3-cm intervals, to prevent bleeding into the extradural space around the flap.

13 Coagulate any large vessels on the dural surface.

14 Open the dura as a flap with its base towards the base of the skull.

15 Incise the dura after lifting it with a sharp hook or toothed forceps. Make a small cut in the raised area, so entering the subarachnoid space without damaging the cortex. Gently lift the dura, cutting it with fine scissors in sections. Before cutting each section, gently push a piece of wet lintine between the dura and the brain surface to separate them. When incising the dura near the great venous sinuses or at the frontal or temporal poles, make sure that you do not cut through a bridging vein.

16 Stop bleeding from vessels on the brain surface using diathermy coagulation or metal clips. Place patches of cellulose mesh (Surgicel) or fine muslin to stop oozing from areas of haemorrhagic contusion. Press them into place under patches of wet lintine. They may be left in place when the lintine is taken off.

Closure

KEY POINT Stop all bleeding

- Do not close any layer until you have achieved perfect haemostasis.

1 Close the dura with interrupted 3/0 silk sutures. Cover areas where the dural edges will not come together with Surgicel.

2 Replace the bone flap, holding it in place with interrupted 3/0 silk sutures to the pericranium/temporalis muscle layer.

3 Close the scalp in two layers.

4 If you have achieved good dural closure but still have troublesome bleeding below the scalp flap, drain the subgaleal space with a low-tension suction drain brought out through a separate stab wound and removed after 24 hours.

SCALP LACERATIONS

Appraise

1 An unsutured small scalp laceration can bleed profusely, so arrest bleeding from the scalp as soon as is practicable after injury, using a temporary single layer of through-and-through sutures.

2 If the patient has been struck on the head with a heavy object, X-ray the skull to ensure that the laceration does not cover a depressed skull fracture.

Action

1 Shave adequately and closely round the laceration before exploring it.

2 The scalp is vascular, heals well and seldom gets infected, so do not excise the contused edges of the laceration too enthusiastically and produce a scalp defect or require to appose the edges with tension.

3 If the galea has been breached, always close the scalp laceration in two layers, one for the galea and a second through-and-through skin layer, as previously described.

4 If possible, transfer a patient with severe scalp loss to a special unit where plastic and neurosurgical facilities are available.

DEPRESSED SKULL FRACTURE

Appraise

1 The purpose of elevating a depressed skull fracture is to reduce the risk of infection, so elevate only compound depressed skull fractures.

2 Leave alone depressed fractures with intact overlying scalp. Occasionally, the dislocation of the skull contour may be so great that elevation is required for cosmetic reasons, but these more severe injuries are invariably compound, so that the customary indication for operation is also present.

Access

1 Excise the overlying scalp laceration if it is badly contused. Extend the incision to give access to the whole depressed area. Scrape the scalp off the underlying bone and hold the incision wide open with self-retaining retractors.

2 Clear the pericranium away with a periosteal elevator to reveal the whole depressed area.

3 The inner table will have been driven in over a much wider area than the visible area of depressed outer table. Make a single burr hole just outside the edge of the visibly depressed region in order to expose dura not involved in the depression.

Action

1 Insert a periosteal elevator into the burr hole, slide it gently between the bone and the dura and ease out the depressed fragments so that the dura beneath them is fully exposed. Remove dirt, debris and any small flakes of bone from the wound and send them for bacteriological culture.

2 If the dura is intact, do not open it. If it is lacerated, carefully extend the laceration to inspect the brain beneath. If the brain surface is torn, probe gently in the tear for any in-driven debris and bone and remove them.

3 Remove pulped and clearly necrotic brain tissue by a combination of gentle suction and irrigation with normal saline at body temperature.

4 Coagulate bleeding points in the brain with low-intensity diathermy coagulation, and diffuse oozing by applying patches of Surgicel compressed into place beneath lintine strips.

5 If the depressed bone fragments have been driven through the dura, their removal may tear large cerebral vessels as the fragments are extracted. A large cerebral vessel, not visible on the brain surface, may be picked up and held in the tip of a fine sucker under fairly strong suction while it is coagulated with diathermy or occluded with a metal clip.

KEY POINTS Beware venous sinuses

- Be very cautious about elevating a depressed fracture overlying the superior sagittal or lateral sinus.
- If the dura over the sinus is torn there will be torrential bleeding as you remove the bone.

6 If a sinus is torn, do not try to close it with sutures. Reduce the pressure in the sinus by tilting the patient feet-down, then cover the sinus with several layers of Surgicel and hold them firmly in place under lintine strips for 5–10 minutes. When you release the pressure and remove the lintine, the bleeding does not recur. Do not now disturb the Surgicel.

? DIFFICULTY

If the bleeding is absolutely uncontrollable, you may suture a small piece of gauze in place beneath the scalp, which is closed over it, as a temporary measure to reduce bleeding while you arrange transfer of the patient to a special centre.

Closure

1 Before closing, irrigate the whole wound with hydrogen peroxide solution and 20 ml of normal saline containing 20 000 units of penicillin and 50 mg of streptomycin.

2 Close the dura with interrupted 3/0 silk sutures. Cover any gaps in the dura with two layers of Surgicel.

3 Unless the wound has been neglected and is obviously infected, replace the removed bone fragments on the dura to fill in the skull defect. Scrub them thoroughly in aqueous Savlon before replacing them.

4 Close the scalp in two layers without drainage.

MISSILE WOUNDS OF THE BRAIN

Appraise

1 The energy carried by the missile is related to the square of its speed. If the energy is transmitted to the object it strikes, even a small high-velocity missile may release an enormous quantity of energy as it passes through the body. This causes tissue destruction extending far outside its track. The small size of an entry hole may conceal massive disruption of the intracranial structures.

2 Decide whether active treatment is likely to lead to a worthwhile outcome. Through-and-through missile wounds of the brain are almost always fatal. The prognosis is very poor if the patient has been deeply unconscious with fixed dilated pupils from the time of the injury or has persistent hypotension which cannot be explained by blood loss, because these features suggest damage to the central structures of the brain.

3 Do not operate until the patient has been resuscitated and has a stable condition. Early bleeding into the intracranial contents is not a common complication of missile wounds of the brain, and a delay of 3–4 hours allows replacement of any blood loss, assessment of the extent of neurological damage, together with an interim assessment and treatment of other injuries.

4 As soon as the neurological assessment has been carried out, anaesthetize, intubate and hyperventilate the patient to reduce any cerebral oedema.

Prepare

1 Before performing an operation obtain good-quality skull X-rays to show the position of fragments of missile, bone and debris.

2 Cross-match adequate quantities of blood as the blood loss during surgery may be considerable.

3 Start a parenteral broad-spectrum antibiotic at high dosage, together with anticonvulsant medication.

Access

1 The underlying principle of treatment is to minimize the risks of infection and of cerebral swelling by removing all in-driven debris and all devitalized brain tissue. Primary debridement must be adequate.

2 Do not try to operate through an approach which limits access. Turn a generous scalp flap that encompasses the entry wound well inside its boundaries. This allows exposure of any damaged tissue and provides a scalp flap that can be turned at a later date for cranioplasty.

3 Turn a separate periosteal/temporalis muscle flap, based downwards like the scalp flap. Clear this flap away from the skull vault to expose the entry hole and the surrounding intact bone.

4 Drill a burr hole 3 cm from the edge of the entry hole in the bone to expose undamaged dura. From the burr hole nibble away damaged bone so as to produce a craniectomy extending 3–4 cm in each direction outwards from the entry point. This large craniectomy should provide adequate access to damaged tissue.

Action

1 Open the dura widely. Excise damaged dura. Pick out in-driven bone and debris. With the aid of saline irrigation and gentle suction, clear debris, bone fragments and pieces of missile from along the track. Clear surrounding pulped brain. Coagulate bleeding vessels. Leave very deeply in-driven missile fragments if they cannot be removed readily.

2 Irrigate the debrided track with hydrogen peroxide solution, 20 000 units of penicillin and 50 mg of streptomycin, dissolved in physiological saline.

3 Control cerebral swelling by hyperventilation and intravenous mannitol.

Closure

1 Close the dura with interrupted 3/0 silk sutures, replacing deficient dura with a patch of fascia lata sutured in place.

2 Excise any contaminated wound edges from the scalp and pericranial tissue.

3 Close the scalp wound edges and the scalp flap in two layers of 3/0 silk sutures.

Postoperative

1 Control cerebral swelling by continuing intubation, sedation and hyperventilation for at least 48 hours. This regime obscures the signs of postoperative intracranial bleeding, but oedema is the greater risk.

2 Continue giving a broad-spectrum antibiotic for at least 7 days.

3 Continue anticonvulsant medication: for an adult, phenytoin 150 mg twice daily or phenobarbital 45 mg twice daily.

REPAIR OF DEFECTS IN THE SKULL VAULT

1 Bone defects in the skull vault left by trauma or previous operation only require later repair if they are disfiguring or are so large as to leave the intracranial contents unprotected. To minimize the risk of infection, defer the repair for at least 6 months.

2 The defect is exposed by a scalp flap placed so that its edges are well clear of the defect. The defect may be covered by a premoulded titanium or tantalum plate, or by titanium strips. Holes in the metal permit it to be sutured to the surrounding pericranium. Alternatively, after the scalp flap has been reflected, a methyl methacrylate plate may be moulded to fit the defect and held in place by thick braided silk sutures. The sutures are passed through drill holes in the plate and the surrounding bone, after the bone edge round the defect has been cleared of tissue.

AFTERCARE FOLLOWING INTRACRANIAL SURGERY

1 Do not give opiate analgesics. Besides depressing the conscious level and thus interfering with postoperative assessment of the patient, they may also depress respiration and cause intracranial pressure to rise by retention of carbon dioxide. Cranial wounds are not very painful, and codeine phosphate in a dose for adults of 30–60 mg intramuscularly every 4 hours provides adequate analgesia.

2 The consequences of infection of an intracranial wound are so serious that broad-spectrum antibiotic therapy is a wise precaution. Start the antibiotic parenterally at the time of operation and continue it for 5 days postoperatively.

3 If there has been any injury to the cerebral cortex, give prophylactic anticonvulsants. Start the anticonvulsant by intravenous injection during the operation. Continue it postoperatively for 3 months and then discontinue it if the patient has been free of seizures. Suitable regimes are: for adults, phenytoin 150 mg b.d.; for teenagers, phenytoin 100 mg b.d.; and for children aged 3–10, phenytoin 50 mg b.d.

4 Sometimes status epilepticus follows intracranial surgery. The safest and most effective way to stop it is with intramuscular paraldehyde, 10 ml for a teenager or adult, 5 ml for a child aged 3–10 years. Intravenous diazepam is both ineffective and dangerous, for it may seriously depress respiration and cause rising intracranial pressure.

5 The most common complication of an intracranial operation is cerebral compression from bleeding or oedema at the operation site. The symptoms of this occurrence are three-fold. First, there is a steady deterioration of the conscious level. Second, there is the appearance and progression of a focal neurological deficit

appropriate to the site of compression. Thus compression of the left temporal lobe will give rise to dysphasia and a weakness of the right arm. Compression of the ipsilateral third nerve may give rise to a fixed dilated pupil on the side of the compression. Lastly, there will be a rise in blood pressure and a fall in the pulse rate. By the time these last features appear, cerebral compression will have reached an advanced stage.

To detect cerebral compression close observation should be kept on the patient in the early postoperative period. The following observations should be recorded by the nurse in attendance: conscious level (the most important parameter, which should be described in detail), the degree and extent of limb movements, the size, symmetry and reactions of the pupils, and the pulse and blood pressure. These observations should be performed every half-hour for the first 12 hours after operation and then, if the patient's condition is quite stable, they may be decreased to once-hourly for the next 12 hours. If there is anything to suggest cerebral compression, the patient must be taken back to theatre and the wound re-explored without delay.

6 Other complications such as wound infection or thromboembolism are rare after neurosurgical operations. In general, if a patient survives the first 24 hours after operation, his subsequent course is likely to be trouble-free.

7 Mobilize the patient from bed as soon as possible. This will generally be on the first postoperative day. Mobilization will lessen any postoperative periorbital or facial swelling.

8 Since intracranial operations do not give rise to ileus, free oral or nasogastric feeding can be started within 24 hours. The intravenous drip can be taken down as soon as it is certain that no intravenous agents such as blood or mannitol will be required.

9 If the scalp has been closed in two layers, the skin sutures can be removed at 5 days from supratentorial incisions and at 7 days in the case of posterior fossa incisions.

FURTHER READING

Collins REC, Cashin PA 1999 General surgeons and the management of head injuries. Annals of the Royal College of Surgeons of England 81:151–153

Connolly ES, McKhann GM, Huang J et al 2002 Fundamentals of operative techniques in neurosurgery. Thieme, New York

Greenberg MS 2001 Handbook of neurosurgery, 5th edn. Thieme, New York

Jennett WB, Lindsay KW 1994 An introduction to neurosurgery, 5th edn. Butterworth-Heinemann, London

This is a good basic guide to neurosurgery, suitable for the medical neurologist, general surgeon, or for the house officer on a neurosurgical unit.

42

Upper urinary tract

C.G. Fowler, I. Junaid

CONTENTS

INTRODUCTION

1 Urology has developed as a separate discipline in part due the sophistication of endoscopic procedures which demand specialist skills. In the UK, general surgeons no longer perform occasional urological procedures and urologists do not undertake general surgical emergencies. Major open operations for urological cancer, stone disease and reconstruction are increasingly performed by specialists.

2 In an emergency, or in the absence of specialist colleagues, you may, as a general surgeon, need to operate to save life or correct severe morbidity. Moreover, routine inguinoscrotal and genital procedures such as circumcision, hydrocele repair, orchidopexy and excision of epididymal cysts are performed by both urologists and general surgeons.

3 You should be capable of treating acute retention, impacted ureteric stone, torsion of the testes, priapism, urinary tract trauma and urinary extravasation in the absence of a specialist colleague. You may need to deal urgently, effectively and as simply as possible with ruptured urethra, with or without pelvic fracture, pending expert urological advice.

4 Be aware of the potential benefits of specialist procedures.

ACUTE PYONEPHROSIS (OBSTRUCTED INFECTED KIDNEY)

Appraise

1 An acutely ill patient is liable to die from septicaemia and its consequences. Underlying obstruction may be due to a stone, a congenital hold-up at the pelviureteric junction or, much less commonly, tumour within or outside the urinary tract. Diabetics and immunologically compromised patients are particularly at risk. Confirm the diagnosis with plain abdominal X-ray and ultrasound examination. Plain X-ray may show air in the collecting system. The urine contains organisms that can also be cultured from the blood.

2 Ultrasound-guided percutaneous nephrostomy is usually the best way to drain an obstructed infected kidney.

3 Aspiration of the tube helps to establish that it is in the correct position and also provides a specimen of pus for culture.

4 Initially, the rate of drainage may be disappointing. Output from the nephrostomy often increases as renal function recovers.

5 Open operation is indicated only if you are sufficiently expert, and it is impossible to introduce a satisfactory percutaneous drain or if the pus in the kidney is too thick to be aspirated through the small-calibre tube used for percutaneous nephrostomy. This is not a simple procedure, so do not undertake it lightly.

6 If you undertake open operation when the cause of obstruction is a calculus in the ureter or renal pelvis, remove it.

OPEN NEPHROSTOMY FOR ACUTELY OBSTRUCTED KIDNEY

Prepare

1 Promptly rehydrate the patient, and intravenously administer a broad-spectrum antibiotic. If necessary, manage a severely ill patient in an intensive care unit for monitoring, and respiratory and circulatory support.

2 Mark the side to be operated upon.

3 Position the patient yourself in a lateral position with the side to be operated on uppermost, before scrubbing up.

4 Have the break in the table under the 12th rib to open the flank fully. Flex the uppermost hip and knee and place a pillow between the legs. Maintain the position using a back support behind the thorax and fix the arm to an armrest with a wide adhesive bandage.

5 Check that the lowermost arm is not compressed by the patient's body.

Access

Make an incision below the 12th rib of sufficient length to expose the convex border of the kidney. Perirenal tissues appear oedematous and the kidney is swollen.

KEY POINTS Handle gently

- Tissues are friable and bleed easily on dissection.
- Take extra care to handle the tissues gently.

Action

1 Occasionally, the pus-filled calyces 'point' on the surface of the kidney like ripe abscesses. Make an incision through the parenchyma at this point, so releasing a satisfying gush of pus.

2 More commonly, the calyces are impalpable because the overlying renal tissue is stiff and oedematous. Try using a large-bore needle on a syringe to locate the pus-filled collecting system. This can be surprisingly difficult. If you find pus, incising into the calyx can be surprisingly difficult even when you follow the needle track.

3 A more certain method is to enter the collecting system through the renal pelvis. Follow the capsule over the convex posterior border of the kidney, keeping towards the lower pole. Find the renal sinus and gently clear away the fat by blunt dissection to reveal the posterior surface of the renal pelvis. It is not necessary to mobilize the kidney fully.

4 Make a small transverse pyelotomy (Greek: *pyelos*=trough, pelvis+*tome*=a cutting).

5 Introduce a malleable silver probe with an eyehole at the end, through the pyelotomy and manoeuvre it to puncture the cortex from within a lower pole calyx.

6 Tie the tip of a size 18F tube drain or a Foley catheter to the probe with a suture and pull it back into the renal pelvis (Fig. 42.1). Use a Willschner nephrostomy tube with a built-in malleable stylet if it is available.[1]

7 Close the pyelotomy using 3/0 or 4/0 absorbable sutures. Tie these sutures gently and with tension just enough to approximate the edges, as there is risk of these sutures cutting through. Anchor the catheter to the capsule using absorbable sutures.

KEY POINTS Anatomy

- Take care to puncture the renal parenchyma near the convex border of the kidney and not on the anterior or posterior surface.
- This minimizes the risk of injury to large intrarenal vessels.

8 Bring out the nephrostomy tube through the abdominal wall with as straight a course as possible, to facilitate changing the tube if necessary.

Aftercare

1 Perform gentle saline wash-outs if the percutaneous nephrostomy does not drain adequately, or insert a larger calibre tube after dilating the track.

2 If side-holes of the nephrostomy tube slip outside the parenchyma, urinary extravasation occurs. Re-adjust it under radiographic control.

3 A nephrostomy can be left in place for weeks or months, but it has a tendency to fall out, however carefully it is anchored.

4 As soon as possible, refer the patient to a urologist for definitive management.

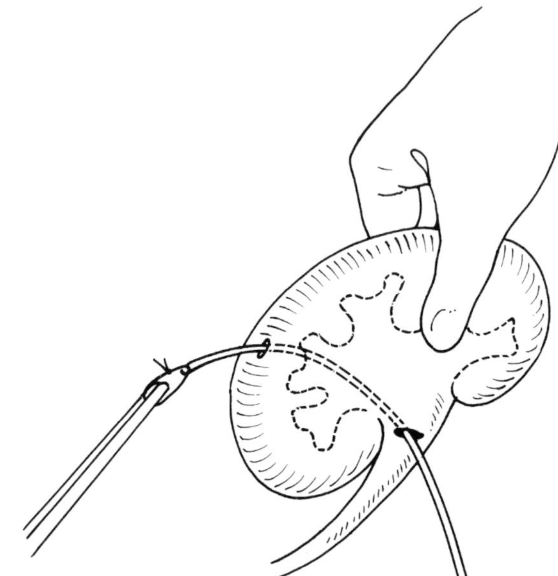

Fig. 42.1 Technique of open nephrostomy tube insertion.

REFERENCE

1. Noble M 1989 Miscellaneous renal operations. In: Novick AC, Streem SB, Pontes JE (eds) Stewart's operative urology, 2nd edn. Williams & Wilkins, Baltimore, pp 240–249

OBSTRUCTED KIDNEY CAUSED BY AN IMPACTED STONE

Appraise

1 Obstruction of a kidney for a few days does not usually cause serious harm. However, if there is infection or if there is no function in the contralateral kidney, there is an urgent need to drain the kidney.

KEY POINT Danger of septicaemia

- An obstructed infected kidney is a potent cause of septicaemia and represents a urological emergency.

2 The obstruction may be due to an impacted stone at the pelviureteric junction or in the lower ureter.

3 The diagnosis is usually made with a plain abdominal X-ray and ultrasound scan or an intravenous urogram. A patient with solitary obstructed kidney or with bilateral renal obstruction rapidly develops renal failure and uraemia.

4 An acutely obstructed kidney is best relieved using a percutaneous nephrostomy. If you do not have an expert radiologist available, perform an open nephrostomy.

5 For bilateral upper tract obstruction, urgently insert bilateral nephrostomy tubes to retrieve the patient from renal failure. If the patient is seriously ill with associated Gram-negative septicaemia, urgently transfer the patient to an intensive care unit or renal unit to save life.

6 Drain a solitary obstructed kidney as soon as possible before permanent renal damage develops.

7 Unilateral obstruction lasting for over 6 hours leads to gradual decrease in renal blood flow and after 24 hours it is reduced to 55%. Following relief of 7 days of unilateral ureteric obstruction, full recovery of renal function occurs within 2 weeks. However, obstruction of 14 days' duration results in a permanent decline in renal function to 70% of control levels. An obstructed kidney is at risk of infection and pyonephrosis (Greek: *pyon*=pus+*nephron*=kidney+*-osis*=production).

8 The current management of upper urinary tract stones is by extracorporeal shock-wave lithotripsy (ESWL), percutaneous nephrolithotomy (PCNL) with or without ESWL, and laser fragmentation of ureteric stones. These treatments are so successful that when they are available open procedures are rarely required.

9 Consider performing open ureterolithotomy to remove an impacted stone from the lower half of the ureter if urological help is not available. Operations for impacted calculi in the upper ureter, at the pelviureteric junction and very low at the vesicoureteric junction are potentially more difficult and the best course is probably to insert a percutaneous nephrostomy pending referral to a urologist.

URETEROLITHOTOMY FOR A LOWER URETERIC CALCULUS

Action

1 Select the appropriate incision for the location of the stone as shown on the X-ray. Make an oblique muscle-splitting or muscle cutting incision on the lateral side of the anterior abdominal wall down to peritoneum. You can extend the incision upwards or downwards if necessary (Fig. 42.2).

2 Sweep the peritoneum medially to expose the retroperitoneal structures. Identify the ureter and impacted stone within it. This can be surprisingly difficult, so take your time. It may help to first identify the gonadal vein in the vicinity. When dissecting the ureter, remember that it crosses over the common iliac vessels at the pelvic brim, so dissect carefully here. Try not to dislodge the stone while palpating it—it is easily done. When you find the calculus, place a wetted nylon tape around the ureter proximal to the stone to prevent it from slipping upwards towards the kidney. Even though it rarely escapes distally towards the bladder, be ready to place a second tape below the stone. Try not to strip the ureter of its adventitia and blood vessels.

3 Make a vertical incision in the ureter directly over the stone (Fig. 42.3), a few millimetres longer than the calculus and ease out the stone using a Watson–Cheyne dissector.

KEY POINTS Precaution

- There may be a second unsuspected stone.
- To guard against this, pass an 8F infant-feeding tube distally into the bladder and proximally to the renal pelvis to exclude any remaining obstruction.

4 Close the ureterotomy by loosely approximating the adventitia with a few interrupted, absorbable sutures. Leave a soft tube drain in the vicinity.

? DIFFICULTY

1. If the ureter is difficult to find, remember that it crosses the bifurcation of the common iliac artery, so search for it lower down.
2. The ureter may be adherent to the peritoneum so look for it under the retractor used to draw the peritoneum medially.

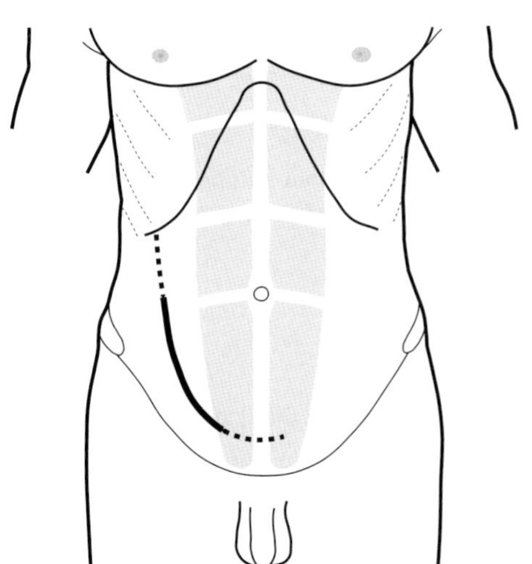

Fig. 42.2 Incision for lower ureteric calculus.

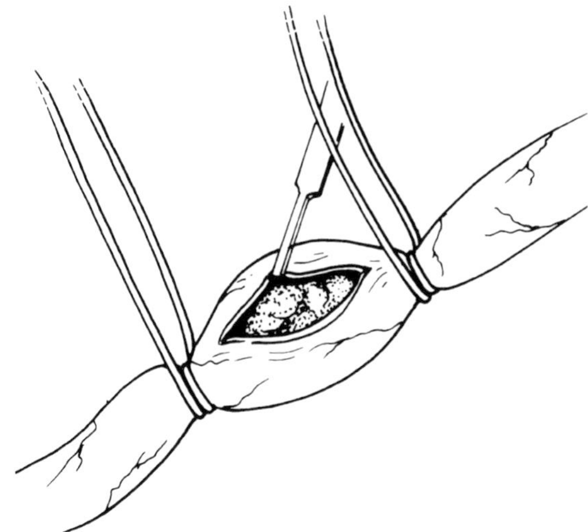

Fig. 42.3 Easing out the calculus from the ureter using a Watson–Cheyne dissector.

RUPTURE OF THE KIDNEY

Appraise

1 Renal trauma is associated with blunt or penetrating injuries. The majority of injuries result from blunt trauma resulting from falls, road traffic accidents and sports injuries. Penetrating injuries are associated with gunshot and stab wounds. These injuries are often multiple, with associated trauma to bowel, pancreas and spleen.

2 Resuscitate the patient and thoroughly assess the damage.

3 A history of trauma associated with haematuria is an indication for spiral computed tomography (spiral CT). If that is not available, order intravenous urography (IVU), combined with angiography if you suspect involvement of the renal pedicle. If the IVU is normal, then observe the patient with care. Most blunt injuries can be managed conservatively but penetrating injuries demand exploration.

4 If there is parenchymal disruption associated with extravasation of contrast from the collecting system, conservative management is still possible but be ready to operate quickly if the patient's condition deteriorates. Poor visualization, even on CT scan, suggests injury to the renal pedicle. If the patient is stable, perform angiography. Perform urgent surgical exploration if the patient is haemodynamically unstable.

KEY POINTS Surgical exploration

- If the patient has not had a preoperative IVU and you discover renal trauma at exploration, perform IVU on the operating table to determine the status of the uninvolved kidney.
- If you suspect associated bowel and pancreatic injury, perform a laparotomy through a midline incision. If the kidney is irretrievably damaged, remove it after ligating the renal artery and vein.
- Explore and complete the bowel, pancreatic, splenic and other intra-abdominal surgery (see Ch. 4) before opening the retroperitoneal space, provided there is no major bleeding.
- If you have excluded any other abdominal visceral injury preoperatively, you may explore the kidney through a loin incision. However, a transperitoneal approach through a midline incision gives excellent access to the renal pedicle and the great vessels in the abdomen.

Access

1 Place the patient in the supine position

2 Employ a midline transabdominal incision, which provides access to abdominal organs and kidneys.

3 Perform abdominal exploration and palpate the retroperitoneal structures. If you encounter a large pulsatile expanding haematoma, gain control of the renal pedicle before opening the perirenal fascia of Gerota. Eviscerate the small intestine and incise the peritoneum over the aorta, exposing the vena cava and aorta. Identify the renal artery(ies) and vein(s). Place vessel loops around the vessels of the injured kidney to gain control.

? DIFFICULTY

1. Bleeding can be terrifying. Do not blindly clamp vessels. You may cause collateral damage that is difficult to repair. Instead, insert a pack and apply direct pressure for 10 minutes or more before taking another look at the vessels.
2. When the anatomy is distorted and obscured by haematoma, you might commit the disastrous mistake of ligating the vessels of the undamaged, contralateral kidney in error. Take care!

4 When you have the bleeding under control, open the fascia of Gerota (Dumitru, 1867–1939, Professor of Surgery in Bucharest) and expose the kidney. If you have the necessary skill, and the parenchymal damage is not great, repair the kidney. Close the defects in the collecting system with continuous sutures of 4/0 Monocril or any other available absorbable suture. Carefully excise devitalized tissue, preserving as much capsule as possible. Fill large defects in the parenchyma with gelatin foam (Gelfoam or Surgicel) and place simple interrupted sutures through the capsule, parenchyma and Gelfoam with 3/0 Monocril or other absorbable suture. The renal parenchyma and capsule are both very fragile, so place sutures with a very light touch to avoid them cutting out. Insert shallow figure-of-eight sutures to transected vessels.

KEY POINT Drain?

- If the collecting system is injured, always leave a drain in the perinephric space.

5 Try to preserve the kidney if at all possible, but if it is badly traumatized perform nephrectomy.

6 If the contralateral kidney has been confirmed as intact, perform a nephrectomy rather than exposing the patient to unnecessary risk by attempting a difficult repair.

NEPHRECTOMY FOR TRAUMA

Assess

1 If it is not possible to repair and preserve the kidney, especially in an unstable patient, proceed to nephrectomy.

Action

1 Patient is already lying supine, with a midline abdominal incision.

2 Mobilize the bowel and peritoneum off the aorta and vena cava.

3 Place vessel loops around the renal artery(ies) and renal vein(s).

4 Double ligate the artery(ies) and the vein(s) with 2/0 Vicryl suture in continuity and then divide the vessels. If the right renal vein is very short, perform suture ligation using 2/0 Vicryl on a round-body needle for extra safety.

5 Carefully ligate and divide any adrenal vein and artery(ies) arising from the main renal vessels.

6 In the case of the left kidney, also ligate and divide gonadal vein draining into the renal vein.

KEY POINTS Anatomical variations

- A lumbar vein frequently drains into the left renal vein on the posterior aspect. Carefully ligate and divide it.
- Remember that accessory arteries are present in about 25% of people and that there are frequent variation of venous anatomy.

7 The fascia of Gerota has already been dissected off the kidney for exploration and assessment of renal injury. Complete any required remaining dissection to free the kidney from the surrounding tissues.

8 Remove the kidney by dividing the ureter between clamps. Ligate the distal ureteric stump with 2/0 Vicryl suture.

9 After removing the kidney, carefully check the haemostasis, particularly of the hilar vessels and the adrenal area. Control any bleeding by suture ligation.

10 Place a 20F Silastic tube drain with its tip in the most dependent point of the cavity.

11 Close the abdominal wound in a single layer using 1/0 looped monofilament PDS or nylon.

REPAIR OF A DAMAGED URETER

Assess

If you operate in the vicinity of the ureter, always check for damage. If you recognize inadvertent surgical ureteric injury at the operation, repair it immediately.

Action

1 Mobilize both ends of the divided ureter to make sure that they are accessible for anastomosis.

2 Place a double pigtail stent with one end in the renal pelvis and the other in the urinary bladder. If you do not have available a double pigtail stent, splint the anastomosis with a small-calibre (6F or 8F) paediatric feeding tube.

3 Open out the ends like a broad, flat-bladed spatula (Greek: *spathe*=broad blade) and hold the ends between stay sutures (Fig. 42.4). Anastomose them using fine interrupted sutures of 4/0 or 5/0 Monocril or any other available absorbable suture.

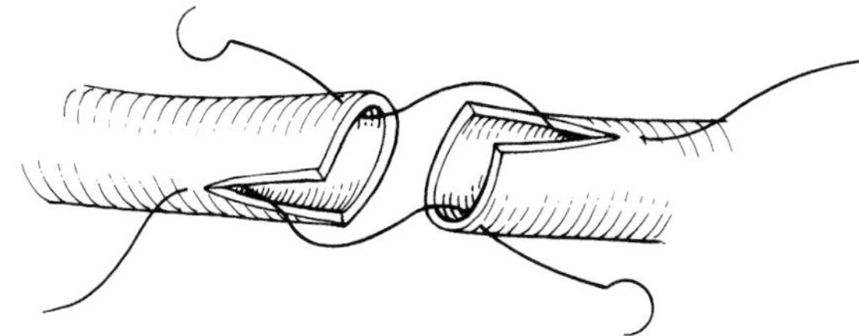

Fig. 42.4 Spatulated uretero-ureterostomy.

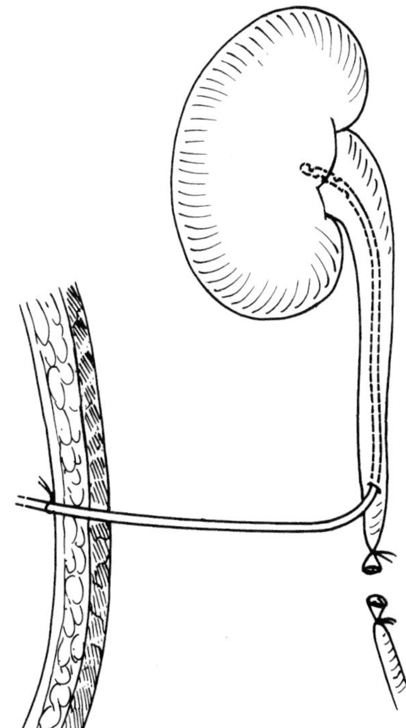

Fig. 42.5 Intubated ureterostomy.

? DIFFICULTY

1. If you cannot repair the ureter, and if the patient's prognosis is poor, perform nephrectomy, provided that the contralateral kidney is normal. It is sometimes safer in such patients to sacrifice the kidney than to be committed to multiple repair operations. It is a better option than tying off the proximal ureter and leaving the obstructed kidney in situ, although this is permissible in an emergency.
2. If the patient's prognosis is good, pass a simple tube through the proximal ureter into the renal pelvis, bringing it out through the skin (Fig. 42.5). Ligate the distal end with a marker suture for identification. When the patient has recovered, arrange a referral to a specialist centre for reconstruction.

4 Leave a size 18F tube drain in the vicinity of the ureteric anastomosis.

5 Remove the stent or tube splint after about 10 days.

DRAINAGE OF A PERINEPHRIC ABSCESS

Appraise

KEY POINTS Have you identified the cause?

- Is the patient diabetic? Immunocompromised? Debilitated?
- Is the patient suffering from renal cortical abscess or pyonephrosis?

1 The safest procedure is preliminary drainage followed by nephrectomy.

2 Percutaneous drainage by a trained interventional radiologist is the best option. If this is not available then undertake open drainage.

Action

1 Position the patient as for nephrectomy

2 Make a small incision below the 12th rib or where the abscess is pointing on the surface.

3 Deepen the incision to the perinephric space. Pus usually starts to pour out as you reach the space.

4 Sweep your forefinger around in the perinephric space to break down all the septa.

5 Leave a wide-bore soft plastic tube drain in the cavity and secure it to the skin.

6 Close the wound lightly with interrupted monofilament nylon sutures.

FURTHER READING

Camunez F, Echenagusia A, Prieto ML et al 1989 Percutaneous nephrostomy in pyonephrosis. Urologic Radiology 11:77

Corriere JN, Sandler CM 1982 The diagnosis and immediate therapy of acute renal and perirenal infections. Urologic Clinics of North America 9:219

Fernandez JA, Miles BJ, Buck AS et al 1985 Renal carbuncle: comparison between surgical open drainage and closed percutaneous drainage. Urology 25:142

Ghali AM, El-Malik EM, Ibrahim AI et al 1999 Ureteric injuries: diagnosis, management, and outcome. Journal of Trauma 46:150–158

Krane RJ, Siroky MB, Fitzpatrick JM (eds) 2000 Operative urology: surgical skills. Churchill Livingstone, London

Santucci RA, Wessells H, Bartsch G et al 2004 Evaluation and management of renal injuries: consensus statement of the Renal Trauma Subcommittee. BJU International. 93:937–954

43

Lower urinary tract

C.G. Fowler, I. Junaid

CONTENTS

URETHRAL DILATATION

Appraise

1 You may encounter an unforeseen urethral stricture when attempting urethral catheterization either to relieve acute urinary retention or as a prelude to major pelvic surgery.

2 Internal visual urethrotomy with the Sachse urethrotome is the urologist's preferred treatment for a newly diagnosed stricture but it requires specialist endoscopic skills. Urethral dilatation may be a satisfactory alternative especially for the relatively common short strictures just behind the urethral meatus or in the bulbar urethra. If the stricture is more extensive or complicated, however, or if you are insufficiently skilled, 'blind' dilatation can create false passages and periurethral fibrosis so severe that it will blight the patient's life for years.

KEY POINT Know your limitations

- When in doubt about your ability to dilate a stricture, abandon urethral instrumentation and insert a suprapubic catheter to drain the bladder.

Prepare

1 Whether you use local or general anaesthesia depends entirely on the situation. It is difficult to anaesthetize the terminal urethra effectively with local applications and studies have indicated that lidocaine gel 1–2% must be left in place for more than 10 minutes to numb the posterior urethra effectively.

2 The distance that an instrument or catheter will pass down the urethra gives an indication of the site of the stricture within the urethra. Urethroscopy gives information about the general state of the urethra but does not show the length or complexity of the stricture. An ascending urethrogram characterizes the stricture but is rarely available at the time the stricture is discovered.

3 *Instruments*. The most commonly used dilators are bullet-tipped curved metal rods, or 'sounds' described by the St Thomas' Hospital London surgeon Henry Clutton (1850–1909). Plastic or gum-elastic bougies (French: Bougie in Algeria, where candles are made; originally bougies were made from waxed linen) are flexible rods that are sometimes equipped with a screw-fitting at the distal tip to allow them to be attached to a pliable rod of small diameter called a 'filiform'. Dilators come in graduated sizes, usually described in 'French' (F) gauge which is the circumference of the widest part of the dilator in millimetres.

Action

1 Lay the patient supine with hips slightly abducted.

2 Clean and drape the penis.

3 For topical anaesthesia empty a tube containing 15–20 ml of 2% lidocaine gel into the urethra. Be gentle: it stings. Massage the gel back into the posterior urethra by stroking firmly backwards from the glans along the anterior surface of the penis before applying a penile clamp. Cover with a sterile drape and leave for at least 10 minutes.

4 While firmly elevating the penis with your left hand, insert the dilator into the urethra so that the concavity of its curve faces the patient's head.

KEY POINTS Avoid damage

- A small-gauge dilator has a sharp-pointed tip with which it is easy to make a false passage.
- Choose a medium-sized metal dilator.

5 Advance the dilator until you encounter the stricture. Now, with gentle manipulation, still holding the penis stretched with the left hand, try to feel your way through the stricture. Always make sure that the curve of the instrument follows the anatomical course of the urethra.

6 If you cannot pass the stricture, use a next smaller sized dilator with great care and be ready to abandon the attempt. For posterior strictures, as you pass the dilator through the bulbar urethra and into the membranous urethra, depress the handle of the dilator down between the patient's legs. It then easily slips into the bladder. You can confirm this by rotating the 'sound' very gently.

? DIFFICULTY

1. If you use force, you will almost certainly make a false passage.
2. If you encounter difficulty, stop. It is probably better to insert a suprapubic catheter that will drain the bladder until specialist help is available.
3. Avoid overdilatation. A 24–28F dilator is quite big enough.
4. For anterior urethral strictures, use shorter, straight 'female' dilators or the plastic bougies without filiforms.

Impassable stricture

1 If it is impossible to pass the metal dilators and for some reason suprapubic bladder drainage is not possible, try inserting a set of filiforms and followers.

2 The filiforms are so thin and flexible that it is difficult to cause serious damage to the urethra with them.

▶ KEY POINT Inserting a filiform

- Before you insert a filiform, make a shallow S-shaped bend or 'dog-leg' about 2 cm from the distal tip. This moves the tip off-centre so that you can control its position within the urethral lumen by rotating the shaft.

3 If you have a cystourethroscope, insert the filiform alongside the sheath of the instrument and guide the tip through the stricture under vision. If not, you may be fortunate enough to negotiate the filiform through the stricture by gentle probing.

4 The 'faggot' (French: *fagot*=bundle of sticks) method looks easy in textbooks but is difficult in practice. Hold the penis taut as before, and gently insert a number of filiforms into the urethra to the level of the stricture. Eventually, you hope that one will find its way through the tight stricture and you will feel it slide through into the bladder. You can then remove the others.

5 Once a filiform is in place, bougies of increasing size can be attached to it using a screw fitting. The filiform is soft and pliable enough to curl up within the bladder. As the bougie is advanced, its tip follows the filiform through the stricture.

6 If all these manoeuvres fail and the patient is in acute retention, perform some form of suprapubic drainage.

Aftercare

1 It is customary to leave a small urethral catheter in place for 48 hours after dilating a difficult stricture.

2 Administer an appropriate antibiotic if the urine is infected.

3 If the patient spikes a high temperature, either following the dilatation or when he next passes urine, then immediately start treatment as for Gram-negative bacteraemia.

SUPRAPUBIC CYSTOTOMY DRAINAGE

Appraise

1 A suprapubic tube can be used to drain the bladder if it is impossible or inappropriate to pass a urethral catheter.

2 A suprapubic cystostomy is often a routine alternative to urethral catheterization but is particularly indicated when the urethral route is closed by trauma causing urethral disruption, or stricture. Use local anaesthesia unless the patient is already under general anaesthetic or deeply unconscious.

▶ KEY POINTS Full bladder needed

- A 'stab' suprapubic cystostomy can be performed safely only if the bladder is full.
- If it is not palpable, order an ultrasound scan to check that the bladder contains urine.
- If the bladder is empty, wait until it fills.

Action

1 Prepare and drape the patient, who lies supine. Select a point 2–3 cm above the pubic symphysis. Infiltrate local anaesthetic through the skin, subcutaneous tissues and linea alba. There is a 'give' as the needle enters the bladder and clean urine can be drawn back into the syringe. This indicates the depth and direction of your suprapubic access to the bladder.

2 A variety of disposable suprapubic catheters come packaged with instructions for use. Some are threaded over a sharp obturator rather like a knitting needle. Advance the assembly of needle and catheter carefully until you feel a 'give' that indicates that the tip is in the lumen of the bladder. Confirm this by noting when urine flows back between the catheter and its introducer. Now advance the tube into the bladder before removing the needle.

Another type has a disposable plastic trocar and sheath which is used to establish a track into the bladder through which a catheter can be passed. With the patient lying flat, aim downwards and slightly caudally.

▶ KEY POINTS Careful control

- Be wary of the sudden loss of resistance that indicates that the end of the introducer is in the bladder.
- If you use too much force, you risk impaling the posterior wall of the bladder and may even penetrate the rectum!

3 When you reach the bladder, take care to thread a sufficient length of catheter into the bladder so that it stays in when the bladder collapses.

4 Secure the catheter. Many are equipped with a balloon or a preformed 'pigtail' end that curls up in the bladder. Even so, it is reassuring to know that the catheter is attached firmly to the skin with a suture.

5 With a very scarred suprapubic area, particularly when the bladder is not palpable, it may be preferable to formally expose the bladder and sew in the suprapubic catheter.

- Make a 3–4-cm transverse or vertical incision 3 cm above the symphysis pubis. Expose the anterior rectus sheath and incise the linea alba in the midline. Hold the rectus muscles apart with retractors and use your index finger to develop the space between the posterior surface of the pubic bone and the anterior bladder wall.
- Pick up the bladder with two tissue forceps. If there is retropubic scarring it may be difficult to identify the bladder. However, it is safe to continue in a downward and backward direction provided the bladder is distended. Confirm that you have correctly identified the bladder by withdrawing urine from it with a syringe and needle.
- Divide the bladder wall between the forceps and enter the bladder. Pass in a selected catheter such as a large Foley, and inflate the balloon. Close the bladder wall around the catheter with one or two all-coats 3/0 Monocril or any other absorbable suture.
- Appose the rectus muscles with absorbable sutures. It is permissible to bring the catheter out of the skin incision.
- Fix the catheter to the skin with a suture. Determine to have this suture taken out after 6–7 days.

CYSTOSCOPY

Appraise

1 There are really very few indications for you, as a general surgeon, to cystoscope a patient.

2 However, you may be forced to pass an instrument, usually a rigid one, in order to relieve clot retention. Therefore understand the technique of passing a rigid cystoscope. It is very similar to that of passing a metal urethral dilator.

Action

1 Place the patient in the lithotomy position.

2 Use general anaesthesia when possible.

3 Clean and appropriately drape the patient.

4 Check the cystoscope for lighting and irrigation.

5 Insert the cystoscope under direct vision, using a 0° or 30° rod-lens telescope, with the irrigation running. The whole of the urethra can be visualized as you insert the instrument and so you are less likely to cause damage. There is no justification for passing the cystoscope blindly. This is particularly important immediately following prostatectomy, when 'blind' passage of the cystoscope can be extremely difficult and its tip may well undermine the trigone.

6 If it is necessary to pass a large 27F resectoscope sheath in order to clear the clot, try to use a visual obturator so that you can insert it under vision. If this is not available and you have to insert the sheath 'blind', obtain a preliminary view of the urethral anatomy with the cystoscope to help you know where you are going.

PROSTATECTOMY

Appraise

1 Most prostatectomies are performed by transurethral resection. If you practise in isolation, you may need to perform a retropubic prostatectomy, usually for men in acute urinary retention.

2 Operative treatment is infrequently withheld in patients with acute retention resulting from prostatic hypertrophy. The alternative of a permanent indwelling catheter may be acceptable in some patients with dementia and those with severe Parkinson's disease, since they are at high risk of postoperative incontinence.

3 Operation is also required for patients with chronic retention and overflow, or chronic retention with back pressure on their upper urinary tracts. If renal impairment is significant, first pass a urethral catheter. The massive diuresis that sometimes occurs when the urinary system is decompressed can then be treated by appropriate fluid replacement before operation. Bleeding from the wall of the decompressed bladder can be alarming but usually settles spontaneously.

4 Consider symptomatic patients for operation according to their degree of disability. Beware of patients with urgency, frequency and urge-incontinence; such men often have primary bladder instability and are often not improved by operation. Ideally, such patients are assessed with urodynamic studies. In practice, however, neither surgery for symptomatic patients who are not in urinary retention, nor urodynamic studies are likely to be available in countries where open prostatic surgery is routinely performed by general surgeons.

5 Preliminary assessment of the upper urinary tract with intravenous urography is unrewarding in patients presenting in retention. Ultrasound examination demonstrates any dilatation of the upper tracts. Urine and blood analyses, uroflow studies and measurement of the volume of urine remaining in the bladder are components of the routine urological assessment of bladder outflow obstruction.

6 When in doubt about the advisability of surgery, it is almost always better not to operate. Such patients can be managed quite effectively by medical treatment using an α-adrenergic-receptor antagonist and/or 5α-reductase inhibitor drugs.

7 Trained urologists select transurethral resection (TUR) almost exclusively, reserving open procedures either for large glands weighing more than 100 g or when there are concomitant conditions that require treatment, such as a large hard stone. Some urologists perform a TUR even when the gland is large, preferring to perform an incomplete resection that relieves bladder obstruction rather than resort to open operation.

8 As a general surgeon, choose an open approach to the prostate via the retropubic or transvesical route, unless you are specifically trained in transurethral surgery. Occasional performance of TUR is hazardous and its complications may prove fatal.

9 Do not approach clinically malignant prostates through the open route. Unless you have resection experience, refer them to a specialist unit.

10 Very small prostates, often amounting only to a tight unrelaxing bladder neck, are far better approached transurethrally, so whenever possible refer them to a specialist centre.

KEY POINTS Caution

- Know your own limitations
- In case of doubt, refer patients to a specialist centre rather than to attempt potentially hazardous surgery.

RETROPUBIC PROSTATECTOMY

Prepare

1 Perform a preliminary cystourethroscopy to establish that the gland is suitable for enucleation and that there is no urethral or bladder pathology.

2 Position yourself on the left side of the patient; clean the lower abdomen, genitalia and upper thighs. Apply drapes so that you have access to the genitalia.

3 Place the patient in the Trendelenburg position.

Access

1 Make a Pfannenstiel incision, slightly convex downwards, 7–9 cm long, so that its lowest part crosses the upper margin of the symphysis pubis.

2 Expose the rectus sheath.

3 Excise the rectus sheath over each rectus muscle from one lateral margin to the other, so exposing each muscle belly.

4 Use curved dissecting scissors to enlarge each end of this incision laterally to include the external oblique aponeurosis.

5 Grasp the midline of the upper and lower borders of the rectus sheath with long artery forceps, and with finger dissection free the rectus sheath from both muscles. Use scissors for the linea alba; carry this downwards to the symphysis and upwards for about 6 cm, exposing the rectus muscles (Fig. 43.1).

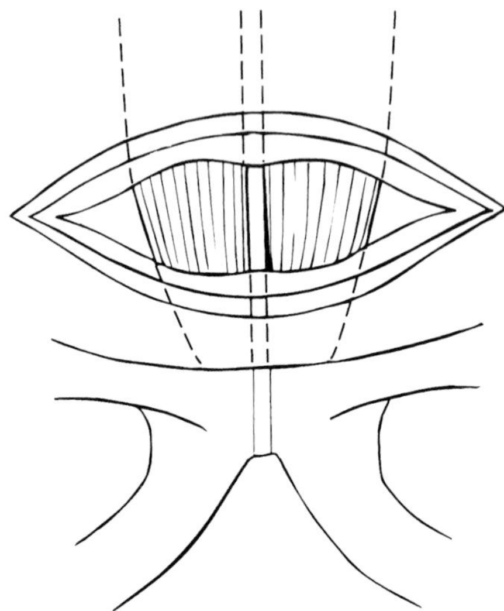

Fig. 43.1 Exposure of rectus muscles.

6 Gently dissect with scissors between the rectus muscles, developing the longitudinal gap between them.

7 Hook two index fingers into the space so formed and retract the two rectus muscles apart. This exposes the bladder with its overlying fat and areolar tissue.

8 Once the rectus muscles have been parted, sweep your right index finger beneath the symphysis and so clean the retropubic space. Position a long-bladed Millin self-retaining retractor that depresses the bladder while holding the wound open.

Action

1 With diathermy forceps, coagulate all the veins coursing across the prostatic capsule. After this, clean the capsule of fatty tissue.

2 Define the anterior capsule stretched over the prostate and in particular its upper border.

3 Have your assistant depress the lower part of the bladder downwards and backwards with a sponge in a sponge-holder, thus throwing into relief the upper border of the prostate gland (Fig. 43.2a).

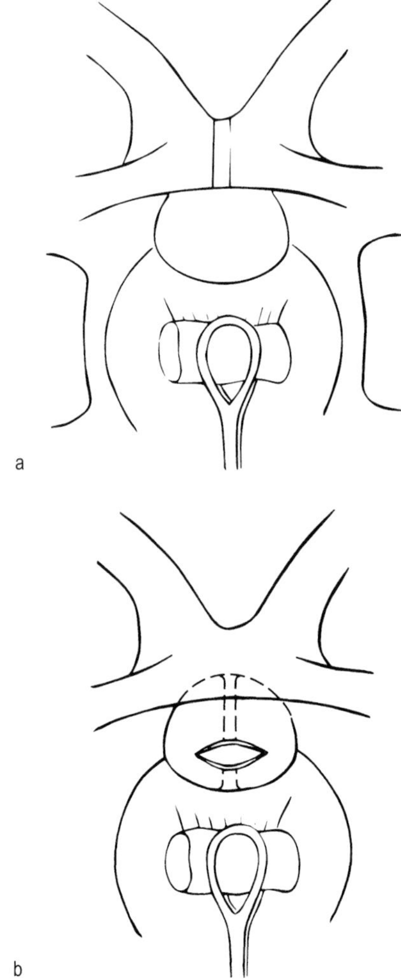

Fig. 43.2 (a) Exposure of prostatic capsule. (b) Incision into prostatic capsule.

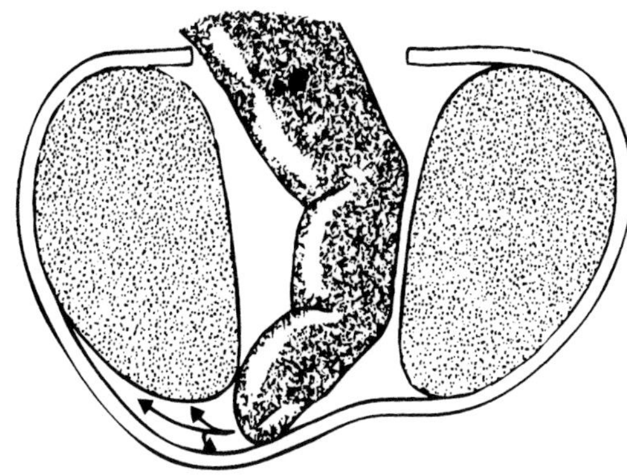

Fig. 43.3 Enucleation of prostatic 'adenomas'.

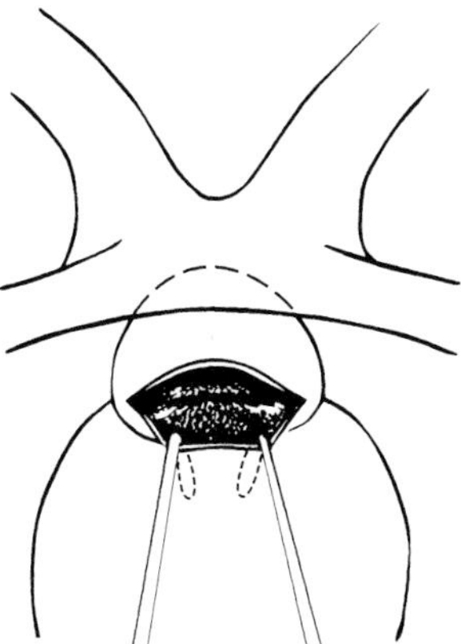

Fig. 43.4 Bladder neck retractor in position.

4 Make a 2-cm transverse incision through the capsule of the prostate just below the upper border, with a cutting diathermy point (Fig. 43.2b). The capsule may be up to 0.5 cm thick, and there are vessels within it that need to be coagulated. The two lobes of the prostate bulge into view.

5 Insert long dissecting scissors between the two lobes into the prostatic urethra and open them longitudinally. Remove the retractor and other instruments.

6 Insert your right index finger into the prostatic urethra. You feel it gripped between the two lobes. Now push your finger downwards until it reaches the back of the prostatic urethra and then curl it laterally towards yourself. You will be able to break into a plane between the urethra and the left lobe of the 'adenomatous' gland. Extend this plane to the apex of the prostate and backwards to the bladder neck (Fig. 43.3).

7 Next, come back to the apex (distal end) of the prostate. With your index finger under the lobe and your thumb on the outside of the capsule, you can nip through the apex and so free it. Now carry your index finger round the front and lateral border, so freeing the lobe completely except for that part attached to the bladder neck.

8 Repeat the process on the opposite lobe. It is often convenient to start mobilizing this lobe using your left index finger and complete it with your right one.

9 Dislocate the two lobes out of the capsule and nip them off at the bladder neck, using thumb and forefinger as pincers.

? DIFFICULTY

If there is a very large middle lobe, it is often easier to cut this off at the bladder neck, again with a diathermy cutter. This leaves the bladder neck behind, which can then be excised under direct vision. Sometimes, with a very large trilobed gland, the neck becomes insignificant.

10 Insert a bladder neck spreader into the bladder. The Badenoch spreader is one of the most satisfactory available. Get an assistant to hold it in position (Fig. 43.4). This throws into relief the bladder neck, and middle lobe if present, both of which must be totally excised. It is often useful to pack a swab into the prostatic cavity to prevent the field from being obscured by blood, and likewise into the bladder to stop the bladder urothelium folding upwards (Fig. 43.5). The bladder neck can now be grasped with long-toothed forceps and excised with a diathermy point. Do not be tempted to excise just a small 'V'.

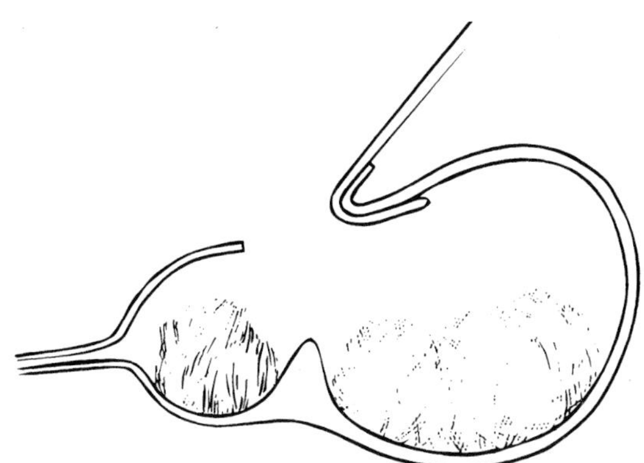

Fig. 43.5 Swabs in prostatic cavity and bladder, exposing the bladder neck to be excised.

11 Arrest all bleeding points with diathermy.

12 Insert a wide-bore (24F) three-way irrigating catheter, preferably one in which the walls do not easily collapse.

13 Close the prostatic capsule using a continuous suture of 2/0 Monocril or any other absorbable suture available. It is better to start the sutures from both ends of the incision in the prostatic capsule using two different lengths of the suture and meet in the middle tying the two together. Make sure both lateral angles are firmly secured. Use either a boomerang needle or a fish hook needle.

14 Wash out the bladder to ensure your suture line is watertight.

Closure

1 Close the recti, rectus sheath and skin as before but in this case always use a drain down to the retropubic space, either a Redivac or wide-bore perforated tube attached to a drainage bag.

2 Finally wash the bladder out, ascertaining that the irrigation fluid (normal saline) is running freely. Attach the catheter to a suitable Uribag.

Postoperative

What catheter, and whether to irrigate?

1 Your aim is to prevent blood loss and clot retention, which may be troublesome following open prostatectomy. A fast irrigation system with a three-way catheter is often required. Suprapubic irrigation is needed to cope with the expected bleeding following a transvesical procedure.

2 The advent of good, irrigating, non-collapsing catheters has diminished the problems of bleeding and clot retention.

3 If you decided to irrigate, start it as soon as the capsule is closed and continue it at a high rate until the effluent is just pink, then slow it down. This is better than waiting until troublesome bleeding ensues. It is much easier to prevent clot forming in the bladder than it is to deal with it.

4 Clot in the bladder and prostatic cavity prevents proper drainage and leads to increasing problems until the patient's bladder is thoroughly washed out. This may mean returning the patient to the operating theatre and thoroughly washing out the bladder under a general anaesthetic.

5 Maintain the irrigation until you are sure that active bleeding has stopped.

6 Remove the suprapubic catheter when fear of bleeding and clot retention has passed.

7 Following open prostatectomy, leave the urethral catheter for 10 days.

KEY POINTS Monitor the temperature

- Bacteraemia following open prostatectomy may lead to life-threatening septicaemia.
- Carefully monitor the temperature chart.

MANAGEMENT OF SUPERFICIAL URINARY EXTRAVASATION

Appraise

1 Superficial urinary extravasation may follow injury during urethral dilatation or develop behind an anterior urethral stricture.

2 Superficial extravasation of urine is relatively uncommon but extremely dangerous, producing extensive necrosis of subcutaneous tissues and eventually of the skin. Colles fascia, the lower and posterior extension of Scarpa's deep abdominal wall fascia into the perineum, which attaches to the ischiopubic rami and posterior edge of the perineal membrane, and the attachment of Scarpa's fascia to the fascia lata just below the inguinal ligament in the thighs, limit migration of fluid posteriorly and into the thighs. Urine therefore fills the subcutaneous tissue of the scrotum and the penile shaft and ascends up the anterior abdominal wall. The clinical context and the distribution of swelling distinguish it from the far more common dependent perineal oedema that is sometimes seen in cardiac failure.

3 If the urine is not already infected, the necrotic tissues will certainly become so.

Action

1 Divert the urinary stream by draining the bladder by the suprapubic route as described above.

2 Make as many incisions as are necessary in the perineum, scrotum, penile shaft and anterior abdominal wall to let out the infected urine and necrotic tissue. Never be afraid to open up the spaces widely.

3 Use a specific antibiotic if the microorganism is known, otherwise administer a broad-spectrum one.

KEY POINTS Fournier's gangrene

- Watch for the spreading, fulminating streptococcal gangrene described by Jean Fournier (1832–1914) the Parisian Professor of Dermatology.
- If present, you must radically excise all necrotic tissue and start an intensive course of antibiotic therapy in order to save the patient's life.
- Even in expert hands, the outlook is very poor.

Postoperative

Deal with the stricture when all inflammation and swelling has settled.

EMERGENCY TREATMENT OF RUPTURED URETHRA

Appraise

1 Such injuries are often seen in victims of multiple trauma. There are essentially two varieties:
- *Direct perineal injury.* This damages the bulbous or penile urethra. The injury may be partial or complete.
- *Associated with pelvic ring fracture.* This is either a partial or complete tear of the posterior urethra associated with fracture of the pelvic ring; a distracting force pulls the prostatic urethra away from the membranous urethra.

2 The first imperative is to save life; dealing with the urethral injury is subordinate to coping with other more immediately threatening conditions. The extent of the urethral injury can often be deduced from the pattern of bony injury to the pelvis. Wide distraction of the anterior part of the pelvic ring is very often associated with complete urethral disruption. If circumstances allow, gently perform an ascending urethrogram, using an aqueous contrast solution, to give useful information about the state of the urethra. If the contrast medium enters the bladder, then rupture is either insignificant or incomplete, and in this instance institute simple suprapubic drainage if the patient is unable to void.

RUPTURED BULBOUS URETHRA

Appraise

1 With 'falling astride' injuries, the patient's general condition is usually good and the ends of the damaged urethra are close

together. Seek the help of a specialist if at all possible. Intervention is necessary only if the patient cannot pass urine.

2 Very gentle attempts to pass a small-calibre urethral catheter risks converting a partial into a complete rupture. It is probably safer to avoid instrumentation of the urethra unless you have extensive experience and this is unlikely, since such injuries are relatively uncommon.

KEY POINT Know your limitations

- Under no circumstances operate on ruptured urethra if a urologist is available.

3 In case of need, insert a suprapubic tube into the bladder and refer the patient to a specialist.

RUPTURE OF THE POSTERIOR URETHRA

Appraise

1 Injuries to the urethra that result from pelvic trauma require expert attention if the patient is to avoid lifelong disability.

2 If the patient cannot pass urine following lower abdominal or pelvic trauma, the differential diagnosis lies between bladder rupture and posterior urethral injury. Urethral injury is more likely if there is significant bony deformity of the pelvis.

3 Stabilize the urinary tract condition by inserting a suprapubic catheter while life-threatening injuries receive attention.

4 The operative management of posterior urethral rupture is often complex so seek details in a urological text.

TRAUMATIC RUPTURE OF THE BLADDER

Appraise

1 Extraperitoneal rupture can follow blunt trauma to the lower abdomen when the bladder is full. It is easily diagnosed by a cystogram, using aqueous contrast medium, which also indicates the existence of associated urethral injury.

2 Extraperitoneal bladder rupture can be treated conservatively by inserting a urethral catheter, giving broad-spectrum antibiotics and monitoring the patient.

3 Operative repair of the bladder is indicated if there is a failure to drain urine through the catheter, increasing lower abdominal distension or evidence of intraperitoneal rupture.

4 Rupture of the bladder into the peritoneal cavity is an unusual injury in isolation, though it may occur as a complication of transurethral surgery to a bladder lesion. If it results from external trauma, there are commonly associated injuries that need attention.

Action

1 Expose the bladder intra- and extraperitoneally. This enables you to perform an exploratory laparotomy at the same time.

2 Clean the peritoneal cavity using saline lavage.

3 Open the bladder anteriorly to detect other bladder injuries that may have escaped notice.

4 Close the bladder incision and injuries in two layers using an absorbable suture. Drain the bladder urethrally if there is no urethral injury, and suprapubically if there is any doubt.

DRAINAGE OF PERIURETHRAL ABSCESS

Appraise

1 This usually results from a urethral stricture. It may be necessary, before draining the abscess, to establish adequate urinary drainage with a suprapubic catheter.

2 It is hazardous to use force to dilate the stricture under these conditions.

Action

1 Make an incision over the most prominent part of the abscess and lay it completely open.

2 Break down any loculi and pack the cavity with a Eusol or similar dressing.

3 Once healing is proceeding well, it is safe to pass a dilator and establish urethral drainage if necessary.

4 When healing is complete, perform a urethrogram to establish the extent of the stricture; use this information to decide on future management.

FURTHER READING

Blandy J 1986 Cystoscopy. In: Blandy J Operative urology, 2nd edn. Blackwell Scientific, Oxford, pp 6–9

Blandy J 1986 Dilatation of a stricture. In: Blandy J Operative urology, 2nd edn. Blackwell Scientific, Oxford, pp 216–219

Blandy J 1986 Suprapubic cystostomy. In Blandy J Operative urology, 2nd edn. Blackwell Scientific, Oxford, pp 117–120

Blandy J, Fowler C 1996 Bladder: trauma. In: Blandy J, Fowler C Urology, 2nd edn. Blackwell Scientific, Oxford, pp 265–271

Blandy J, Fowler C 1996 Urethra and penis: trauma. In: Blandy J, Fowler C Urology, 2nd edn. Blackwell Scientific, Oxford, pp 460–471

Chapple C, Barbagli G, Jordan G et al 2004 Consensus statement on urethral trauma [review]. BJU International 93:1195–2002

Millin R 1945 Retropubic prostatectomy: new extravesical technique. Report on 20 cases. Lancet ii:693

Nesbit RM 1943 Transurethral prostatectomy. Charles C Thomas, Springfield

Renvall S, Nurmi M, Aho A 1989 Rupture of the urinary bladder: a potentially serious condition. Scandinavian Journal of Urology and Nephrology 23:185

Webster GD, Mathes GL, Selli C 1983 Prostatomembranous urethral injuries: a review of literature and a rational approach to their management. Journal of Urology 130:898

44

Male genitalia

C.G. Fowler, I. Junaid

CONTENTS

CIRCUMCISION

Appraise

1 Circumcision is most commonly performed for cultural reasons. The strictly medical indications are few and include phimosis (Greek: =muzzling), paraphimosis, recurrent balanoposthitis (Greek: *balanos*=acorn, glans+*posthe*=prepuce+ -*itis*=inflammation) and carcinoma of the penis.

2 Phimosis may be:

- Infantile, which must be distinguished from the entirely normal failure of the foreskin to retract in early life because of physiological adhesions between the prepuce and glans penis.
- Seen in later life, almost invariably due to balanitis xerotica obliterans.

3 In some cultures, where circumcision has developed into a religious rite, carcinoma of the penis and balanitis are virtually non-existent. However, with good education and hygiene, the medical need for wholesale circumcision, with its inevitable morbidity and mortality, however small these may be, is questionable.

4 It is unethical to expose infants to unnecessary risk. There may be future medicolegal hazards to performing ritual surgery on infants unable to give consent. You must, however, make up your own mind when confronted with a request for infant circumcision.

Prepare

1 Circumcision in infants is traditionally performed without anaesthesia but the justification for this must be open to question.

2 The patient can be prepared with a penile ring block using a mixture of lidocaine and bupivacaine; adjust the local anaesthetic dose to the patient's body weight, and do not use adrenaline (epinephrine).

3 Alternatively, perform circumcision under general or spinal anaesthesia.

Action

1 Grasp the tip of the dorsal surface of the foreskin in the midline with a small artery forceps and gently pull it downwards until it is held on the stretch.

2 If phimosis is particularly severe, use a second pair of artery forceps as a dilator to enlarge the opening.

3 Using a silver probe in the infant, or artery forceps in the adult, gently free the foreskin from the glans so that it can be completely retracted, leaving no adhesions or inspissated smegma (Greek: =soap), behind. Wash it with non-spiritous solution.

4 Gently pull the foreskin down over the glans and apply two straight artery forceps side by side in the midline on the dorsal surface of the foreskin. Divide it between these two (Fig. 44.1a).

5 Continue the incision in the same direction with straight scissors about 3–6 mm short of the corona (Fig. 44.1b).

6 From the apex of this incision, cut laterally until the incision reaches the lateral border of the glans (Fig. 44.1c).

7 Now carry the incision towards the frenulum (Latin: *frenum*= bridle), making sure that both surfaces of the foreskin are cut together. This ensures that the undersurface of the glans is not denuded of skin (Fig. 44.1d).

Alternative method

1 A more elegant alternative method is particularly useful for adults.

2 Grasp the tip of the foreskin between two haemostats and gently stretch it over the glans.

3 Make a circumferential incision in the penile skin at the level of the corona using a blade, taking care not to sever the veins that lie just below the skin. Divide the veins between haemostats and ligate them.

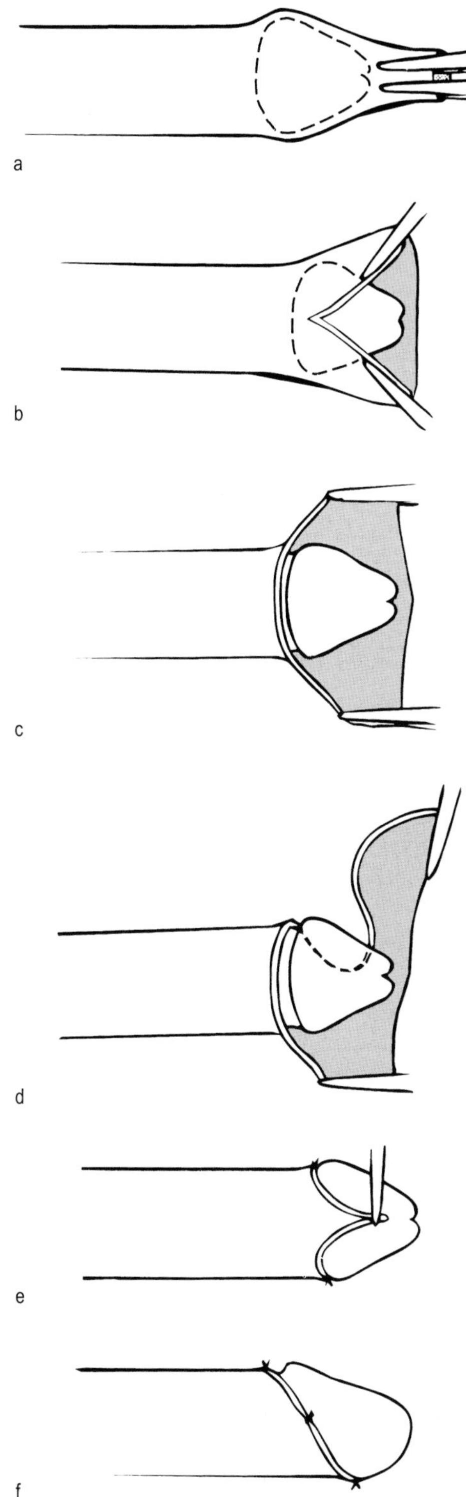

Fig. 44.1 Circumcision.

4 Make an incision through the dorsum of the foreskin to expose the glans penis followed by a second circumferential incision in the skin of the inside surface of the prepuce about the 0.5 cm from the corona. Free the foreskin by cutting the connective tissue that remains, until it is attached only by the frenulum.

5 Place a small artery forceps across the frenulum, so catching the inverted-V extension of skin and frenulum together, and excise the foreskin (Fig. 44.1e).

6 Transfix the frenulum and apex of the shaft skin with a fine synthetic absorbable stitch and tie it firmly, releasing the artery forceps. Leave one end of the suture long to act as a stay suture.

7 Search for, pick up and ligate with fine synthetic absorbable thread, all the bleeding vessels. There is usually an artery on each side of the shaft of the penis that tends to retract.

8 Bring the two layers of the foreskin together with absorbable sutures. Leave a long end to the suture placed at the dorsal position so it can also act as a stay stitch. Appose by gentle traction on the two stay sutures, the cut edges of the fore-skin, ready for suturing. Avoid using too many sutures (Fig. 44.1f).

? DIFFICULTY

1. Do not pull downwards too forcefully on the foreskin once the initial two artery forceps have been applied, or you will remove too much skin.
2. Never use monopolar diathermy for circumcision in a young boy. If the penis is small, the high density of diathermy current at its base can lead to coagulation of the blood supply and necrosis of the penis. Bipolar diathermy is safer.
3. An adherent foreskin may be very difficult to separate from the glans. It may even require sharp dissection, particularly with longstanding phimosis in adults following repeated infections, or in balanitis xerotica obliterans.
4. Always make sure all bleeding is stopped. Infants cannot tolerate blood loss.

Aftercare

1 Dressings usually fall off and are unnecessary. A loose dressing is all that is needed.

2 In particular, avoid sewing dressings in place. Baby boys have been known to lose the glans penis through ischaemia caused by tight dressings or by constricting threads from a dressing.

3 Permit gentle bathing from the second postoperative day.

4 Warn the patient, or parents, that it will take several weeks for the penis to heal and achieve the final cosmetic result.

PARAPHIMOSIS

Appraise

1 In paraphimosis (Greek: *para*=beyond; beyond the glans), the retracted foreskin causes a constriction that interferes with venous and lymphatic return from the glans penis. The resulting oedema makes it even more difficult to reduce the paraphimosis.

2 It is often possible to reduce it by gentle but prolonged squeezing of the swollen glans penis and manipulation of the foreskin.

3 If this fails, operate.

Prepare

It is usual to use general anaesthesia but the penile ring block described above works well.

Action

1 Hold the penis on the fingers of one hand, placing the thumb uppermost on the glans.

2 Depress the glans downwards to expose the constricting band. In longstanding paraphimosis the resulting oedema makes it exceedingly difficult to identify this ring clearly.

3 Transect the ring longitudinally with a small knife. This incision should be of sufficient length and depth to release the constriction and so enable the paraphimosis to be reduced.

4 Leave the incision wide open, covered with loose dressings.

5 Proceed to formal circumcision when all inflammation and oedema has settled.

MEATOTOMY

Appraise

1 The indications for this operation are meatal (Latin: *meare*=to go) stenosis or insufficient meatal size to allow free passage of endoscopic instruments.

2 In a urological department, the Otis urethrotome is the standard instrument for meatotomy. Make the incision dorsally, having introduced the urethrotome into the distal urethra, and open it to a 20–30F gauge. This dorsal incision heals perfectly and leaves no resulting stenosis.

3 Meatoplasty, using a skin flap to widen the urethra, corrects the misdirected stream or spraying that often complicates a standard meatotomy.

4 The operation most commonly performed in general departments is the standard meatotomy. If there is resultant spraying refer the patient to a specialist unit for meatoplasty.

Action

1 Gently dilate the meatus until one blade of a straight artery forceps can be introduced into the orifice.

2 Direct the forceps just to one side of the midline and introduce one blade until its tip lies in the fossa navicularis. Firmly clamp the forceps and leave it for 5 minutes (Fig. 44.2).

3 Remove the forceps and divide the crushed area with straight scissors. If there is any bleeding, use a fine absorbable suture to under-run the bleeding point.

4 Instruct the patient how to keep the cut edges apart. He should do this each time he passes urine and when he has a bath, until the wound is well healed. A small spigot may be inserted to act as a meatal dilator during healing.

Checklist

1 Have you opened far enough back into the urethra to reach normal tissue?

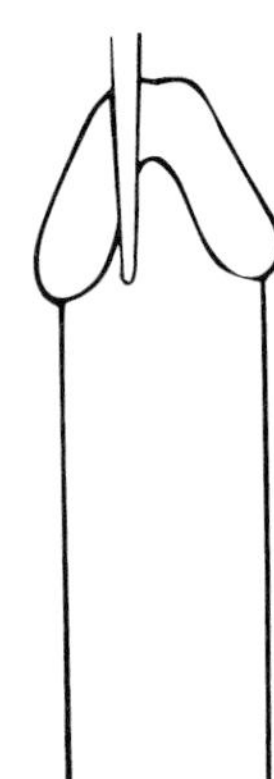

Fig. 44.2 Meatotomy.

2 Failure to keep the incision wide open until it has healed results in re-stenosis.

3 Loss of directional effect of the meatus may occur, with resultant spraying of the stream.

ADULT HYDROCELE

EXCISION OF HYDROCELE

This procedure is suitable for very large or thick-walled hydroceles.

Action

1 Grasp the scrotum firmly with one hand and stretch the skin over the hydrocele.

2 Choose an appropriate area between the vessels, which usually run transversely, to make a transverse skin incision. Carry the incision through all layers of the scrotum. Make the incision long enough so you can deliver the entire scrotal contents. The scrotal skin stretches easily, so this incision need not be of great length. Secure all bleeding points.

3 Using dissecting scissors, clean all the coverings off the hydrocele sac until its outer surface come into view.

4 Incise the sac and allow the fluid to escape. Continue the incision until you can deliver the testicle.

5 Excise the sac only, keeping close to the testicle.

6 Run a fine continuous haemostatic Monocryl or any other absorbable suture along the cut edge of the sac.

7 Secure all small bleeding points with fine absorbable sutures.

8 Return the testicle to the scrotum.

9 Grasp the dartos (Greek: =skinned or flayed) muscle at each end of the incision with tissue forceps. Elevate them to bring the muscle into view.

10 Approximate the dartos muscle with a continuous absorbable suture. This gathers the muscle together and with it the skin, obviating the need for skin sutures.

11 Apply a firm Litesome or similar scrotal support, or use a 10-cm crepe bandage to wind around the scrotum to minimize any subsequent swelling.

12 If the sac is adherent, requiring scissors dissection to free it from the scrotum, there may be some oozing. Do not hesitate to insert a drain.

13 An alternative technique is the operation described by Mathieu Jaboulay (1860–1913) of Lyon. Instead of running a haemostatic suture along the cut edge of the sac, suture the edges together behind the epididymis.

LORD'S PROCEDURE

Appraise

The procedure described by the contemporary Wycombe surgeon, Peter Lord, is particularly valuable when the sac is relatively thin-walled. It has the advantage of requiring only a small incision in the scrotal skin and in the hydrocele sac itself, minimizing bleeding.

Action

1 Incise the scrotum down to and including the hydrocele sac, securing all bleeding points in the incision.

2 Widen the incision only until it is big enough to deliver the testis.

3 Deliver the testis, everting the hydrocele sac behind it.

4 Using interrupted sutures, pick up the edge of the sac and gather up the sac wall with a series of bites according to the sac size, finally taking a bite of the tunica.

5 When all these sutures are in place, tie them, so bunching up and obliterating the hydrocele around the testis (Fig. 44.3).

6 Finally close the scrotal incision as described previously, with absorbable sutures.

7 Apply a scrotal support.

INFANTILE HYDROCELE

These hydroceles are hernias and should be treated as such. Do not attempt to excise the sac (see Ch. 40).

TORSION OF THE TESTICLE

Appraise

KEY POINTS Diagnosis

- A swollen painful testis in a boy is a torsion until proved otherwise.
- Never delay operation: every minute counts. Never be tempted to leave the good side for another time; the child may leave the district and never return to hospital.

Prepare

1 Carefully counsel the boy and his parents. Seek consent for exploration, orchidectomy if the testis is necrotic and fixation of the contralateral side.

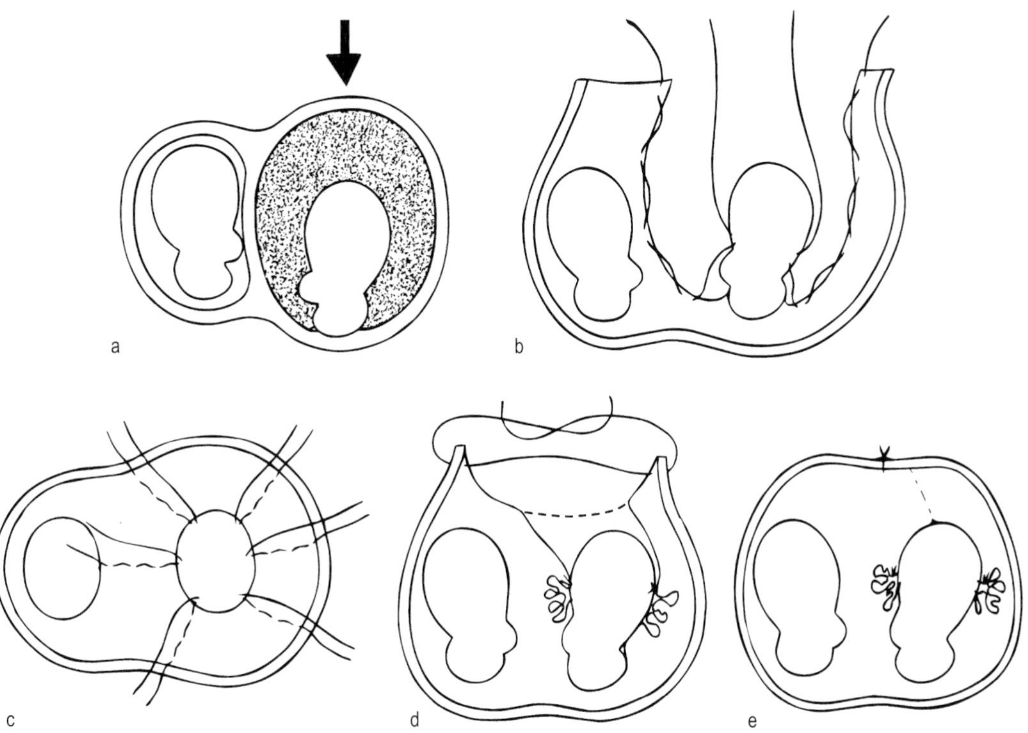

Fig. 44.3 Lord's hydrocele operation.

2 Counselling includes the information that the insertion of a testicular prosthesis can be considered in the future if the testis has to be removed.

Action

1 Incise the scrotum transversely as described for hydrocele operations. Continue the incision in depth until you can deliver the testicle and cord.

2 Untwist the torsion and wrap the testicle in a warm pack.

3 While you are waiting to see if the torted (Latin: *torquere*=to twist) testis recovers, make a similar incision in the other side of the scrotum and deliver the non-twisted testicle, noting any abnormal anatomy that may be present.

4 With a fine nylon stitch, take a firm bite of the tunica of the testicle and anchor it to the side-wall of the scrotum. It is advisable to place three sutures for fixation taking care to avoid the vas, the epididymus and the blood supply to testis.

5 Close the scrotal incision on the non-twisted side.

6 Remove the pack from the untwisted testicle and examine it carefully for viability. If it is obviously dead and remains black, remove it. Place a strong artery forceps across the cord and then remove the testicle and tie the cord with strong absorbable suture.

7 If the untwisted testis appears potentially viable, return it to the scrotum, fixing it with fine nylon sutures as described for the other side.

ORCHIDECTOMY

SIMPLE ORCHIDECTOMY

Appraise

The indications for simple orchidectomy are:

- Severe or recurrent attacks of acute epididymitis.
- Chronic epididymitis, including tuberculous epididymitis.
- Severe testicular trauma when the testis is not salvageable.
- Testicular infarction from a neglected torsion.
- In the management of advanced cancer of the prostate.

Prepare

Remember to discuss the possibility of inserting a testicular prosthesis.

Action

1 If the condition is inflammatory and involves the skin, then make the incision in the scrotum so as to excise the overlying attached infected skin. The incision therefore varies in shape and size according to the condition.

2 Leave the involved skin attached to the underlying structures. Enter the scrotal sac away from the inflamed area.

3 Deliver the testicle with the overlying attached area of skin. Do not hesitate to remove all the involved surrounding skin. The scrotal skin has amazing powers of regeneration.

4 Apply gentle traction to the testicle and clean the cord structures to free 4–6 cm of cord.

5 Cross-clamp the cord at this level with two strong artery forceps, dividing it between them. Do not pull on the testicle or the divided upper end may retract from view.

6 Tie the clamped upper end with strong absorbable suture, but do not release the forceps before applying a second tie. If the cord is very thick, tease it into two structures and cross-clamp each, to avoid creating a bulky tie.

7 Use finger dissection and traction on the lower divided cord to remove the testicle.

8 Leave the scrotal wound unsutured to drain freely if there is infection. Otherwise insert a few interrupted absorbable sutures to approximate the skin edges.

9 Apply loose dressings only.

TESTICULAR TRAUMA

Appraise

1 Given the exposed position of the scrotum, this is mercifully uncommon and is largely confined to sporting injuries and assaults.

2 The immediate pain may be excruciating, but in the excitement of a rugby match may be passed off as trivial and indeed may not manifest itself until some hours later.

KEY POINTS Misdiagnosis?

- Late discovery may lead to the diagnosis of testicular torsion.
- Since exploration is mandatory in both circumstances this error is of no consequence.

3 It is important to explore the scrotum when it is obvious that there is increasing size and pain. Otherwise simple support, rest and analgesics suffice. In the former circumstance there is a danger of increasing haemorrhage within the tunica vaginalis compressing and destroying the testicle; also, the pain of a disrupted testis can be so severe that exploration is necessary.

Action

1 If the testis is completely disrupted, perform simple orchidectomy.

2 However, the testis can often be salvaged by simply evacuating the haematoma and loosely tacking the split and torn tunica albuginea together. Allow plenty of space for the blood to escape. Be willing to insert a small drain.

3 Administer prophylactic antibiotics.

EXCISION OF EPIDIDYMAL CYSTS

1 Excise epididymal (Greek: *epi*=upon+*didymos*=twin; upon the testes) cysts only when they become uncomfortably large.

2 Removal of epididymal cysts is relatively contraindicated in young or unmarried males, as it may render that side sterile.

3 The condition is multiple, so warn patients that recurrent cysts are likely.

Action

1 Incise the scrotum as described for excision of a hydrocele sac.

2 Deliver the testicle along with its appendages, including the cysts. Remember that cysts are often multiple and commonly occur in the upper pole of the epididymis.

3 Combine blunt and scissors dissection. Hold the testicle with one hand, or have an assistant hold it, while you clean off all the adventitial tissue surrounding the cyst.

4 With scissors, completely excise the cyst or else marsupialize it by cutting off the whole protruding surface.

5 If there are very many cysts, excise that part of the epididymis bearing them. Oversew the raw area left following this, using fine absorbable sutures.

6 Return the testicle to the scrotum and continue as described for hydroceles.

EXCISION OF VARICOCELE

Appraise

1 Varicoceles, dilated veins of the spermatic cord, are common, particularly on the left side. Most of them do not require treatment.

2 When you discover a varicocele, as a precaution order an ultrasound scan of the kidneys to exclude the presence of a mass interfering with venous drainage from the affected side.

3 The evidence that varicoceles cause subfertility is questionable.

4 Testicular pain is common and the coincidence of a varicocele does not mean that it is the cause of the pain. Varicoceles can cause a dragging scrotal discomfort but many men have continuing scrotal pain despite curative varicocele surgery.

5 The testicular venous plexus rapidly regenerates and all types of treatment for varicocele have a high failure rate.

Action

1 Make an incision in the inguinal region as for a hernia.

2 Expose the external oblique aponeurosis and open it in the line of its fibres into the external ring.

3 Free the cord from the canal and deliver the testicle out of the scrotum.

4 Dissect out, tie off with fine absorbable thread, and remove all the enlarged and tortuous veins that make up the pampiniform (Latin: *pampinus*=tendril; resembling a tendril) plexus. Do this over the whole length of the cord. Do not be afraid to remove all the enlarged veins; leaving but a few prejudices the result.

5 Make sure that all bleeding points are secure, then return the testicle to the scrotum.

6 Close the external oblique aponeurosis with continuous 1 synthetic absorbable thread and close the skin.

7 Fit a Litesome or similar scrotal support.

8 In some specialist centres, high ligation has been superseded by laparoscopic ligation or percutaneous embolization. This is not, however, widely practised and the method described above gives reasonable results in general use.

VASECTOMY FOR STERILIZATION

Appraise

This operation results in more irritating, usually trivial, postoperative complaints leading to litigation in the courts, than any other urological procedure.

Prepare

1 Fully explain to the patient and his partner exactly what is entailed.

2 Warn that, if a local anaesthetic is unsatisfactory, the procedure must be abandoned and will be performed under a general anaesthetic at a later date.

3 Warn that any operation on the scrotum is liable to cause pain, swelling and infection. Very exceptionally this may be so severe as to necessitate re-exploration.

4 Warn that pain may continue well after the operation, because a small amount of sperm may leak, setting up an area of irritation in the scrotum, producing painful lumps. Exceptionally, these may need to be excised.

5 Sterilization is not immediate. The store of sperm must first be exhausted, which usually takes 2–3 months. To be certain, perform a seminal count at 3 months and 4 months; only when two consecutive completely negative counts are obtained a month apart is it safe to pronounce the patient sterile. If the counts are equivocal, be prepared to re-explore the procedure.

6 Warn that re-canalization can rarely occur, in between 1 and 2 per 1000 vasectomies. It can occur years later and is not the result of surgical error or omission. If the partner shows signs of pregnancy, she should seek appropriate advice. Early re-canalization can be deduced from the equivocal postoperative sperm counts.

KEY POINT Consent form

- Make sure the detailed consent form covers all these points, that it is understood and signed.

Action

1 Grasp the upper part of the scrotum between the first two fingers and the thumb so as to be able to roll the scrotal skin between them.

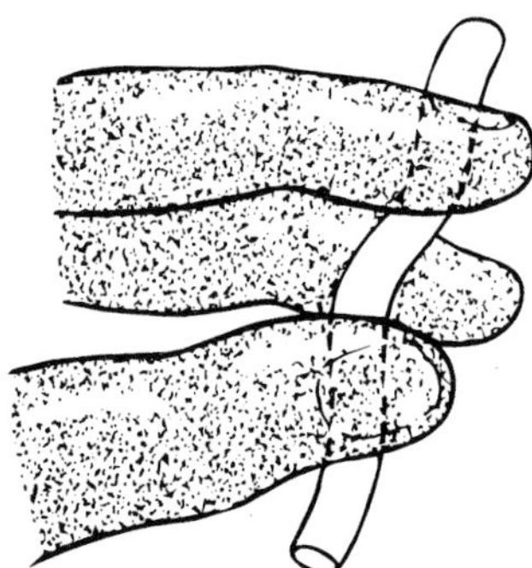

Fig. 44.4 Vasectomy: identifying the vas.

2 Identify the hard round structure of the vas and roll it away from the other structures of the cord (Fig. 44.4).

3 Grip the vas between the middle finger, which invaginates the scrotum, and the thumb on the outside. Move the index finger nearer to the thumb. Now spread the index finger and thumb apart, so holding the vas firmly across the invaginating middle finger. This presents the vas in relief.

4 Make a 1-cm cut into the scrotal skin in the direction of the vas and extending down to it, cutting through the covering adventitia.

5 Still firmly holding the vas, grasp it with tissue holding forceps such as Alliss or, even better, with ring forceps especially designed to encircle the vas. It helps to make a longitudinal cut through the immediate coverings of the vas to reveal its glistening white muscular coat, before enclosing it with the forceps.

6 Release the finger and thumb. The vas now protrudes from the incision, held by the forceps.

7 Force an artery forceps under the vas to separate a length of it from its coverings and to be doubly sure that it cannot escape back into the scrotum.

8 Apply artery forceps about 3 cm apart on the vas and excise the segment between them. Tie each end with no. 2 Vicryl suture, burying the lower end deep in the scrotum. Incorporate the tied upper end into the subcutaneous tissues when closing each wound. This separates the two ends as widely as possible.

9 Repeat the procedure on the other side.

10 Preserve the excised segments for histological confirmation.

? DIFFICULTY

1. Do not attempt this operation under local anaesthesia unless the patient, and the scrotum, are relaxed.
2. If you use local anaesthesia, ensure that both the skin and the tissues immediately around the vas are infiltrated and that you have allowed sufficient time for the local anaesthetic to take effect.
3. If you lose the vas in the scrotum, try again. Never be tempted to grope blindly for structures in the scrotum.
4. If the operation is difficult, do not be content with simple division. Stop and try again on another occasion, after explaining the reason to the patient.

ORCHIDOPEXY

Appraise

1 In adults, the testis is often atrophied, so consider whether orchidectomy is a better choice.

2 The testis is often palpable in the inguinal canal or neck of the scrotum. In case of doubt, confirm its presence by ultrasound or CT (computed tomography) scanning.

3 Maldescent of the testis (Greek: =orchis) should be detected soon after birth but sometimes presents in childhood or later in life.

KEY POINTS Expertise

- Paediatric surgery should be performed by experts.
- The management of testes high in the inguinal canal or above should be in the hands of a specialist.

4 Simple orchidopexy is within the scope of a general surgeon.

Action

1 Make a small inguinal incision centred over the external ring. In young and fat boys, Scarpa's fascia may be thick and can be mistaken for the external oblique aponeurosis.

2 Expose the external oblique over its medial third. In cases of ectopic testes, where the testis lies outside the external oblique, take care not to damage either the testicle or cord while exposing the external oblique.

3 If the testis lies in the superficial inguinal pouch, free it and the cord until the latter can be traced backwards into the external ring.

4 The testis and cord should now be lying free, but there is insufficient cord length to bring the testicle down into the scrotum. Open the external oblique in the line of its fibres into the external ring.

5 Free the cord from within the canal right up to the internal ring. This adds more length.

6 Gently insert your little finger under the cord and in through the internal ring, sweeping it gently from side to side. This frees the cord, vas and vessels from any posterior adhesions, again adding length.

7 Look for an indirect hernial sac lying in front of the cord. If so, grasp it and gently pull it laterally.

8 Hold the testis with one hand and apply gentle traction to the cord so that it is held taut. With fine non-toothed forceps, gently separate the vas and vascular pedicle from the adventitial bands that extend laterally to the hernial sac or retroperitoneum. Take care not to damage either the vas or vessels. This frees the maximum length of available cord.

9 Insert your forefinger into the scrotum, so widening the neck into it. This provides easy access to bring down the testis. Hold the scrotum stretched over the forefinger and make a small, 1-cm long, transverse cut in the scrotal skin over its most dependent part (Fig. 44.5).

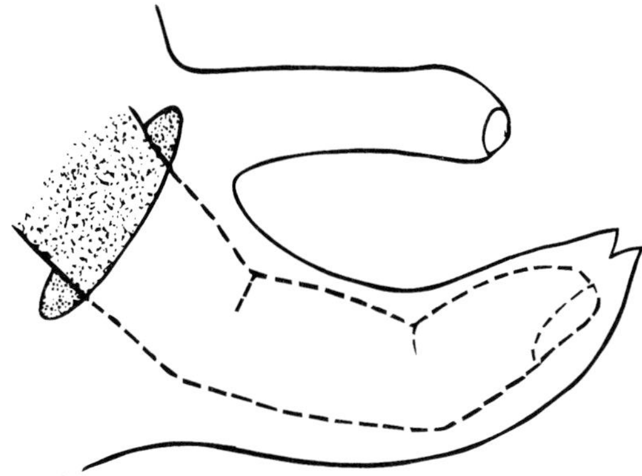

Fig. 44.5 Orchidopexy: skin incision for dartos pouch.

10 Incise the skin only, leaving the dartos muscle intact. Now, with fine curved dissecting scissors, create a subcutaneous pouch between skin and dartos muscle for a distance of about 1 cm all round the incision.

11 Thrust a fine artery forceps through the exposed dartos, out through the groin incision, and grasp the remains of the gubernaculum (Fig. 44.6).

12 Bring the testicle down through the scrotum and tease it out through the small hole in the dartos made by the forceps. Make sure the cord structures are not twisted. Place the testicle in the subcutaneous pouch and close the skin of the scrotum with fine synthetic absorbable thread (Fig. 44.7).

13 Using this technique of anchoring the testicle avoids any tension on the cord, which might endanger the vascular supply to the testicle.

14 Close the inguinal incision.

? DIFFICULTY 44.3

1. For undescended testis, which may lie within the canal or just within the internal ring, use exactly the same technique. However, for these the cord length is often shorter, so take great care to obtain as much length as possible without either damaging the vessels or applying traction.
2. When there is not enough cord to bring the testicle into the scrotum, leave it as low as you can and try again when the child is older.
3. If the testicle is of very small size, with little cord length, and the contralateral one is normal, then remove it.
4. If you cannot find the testicle and cord structures at all, then close the wound and refer the case to a specialist.
5. If the condition is bilateral, explore both sides at the same operation. It is unkind to submit the child to two procedures.

KEY POINT Preserve spermatogenesis

- Always bring the testes down before the age of 2 years. After this time spermatogenesis decreases.

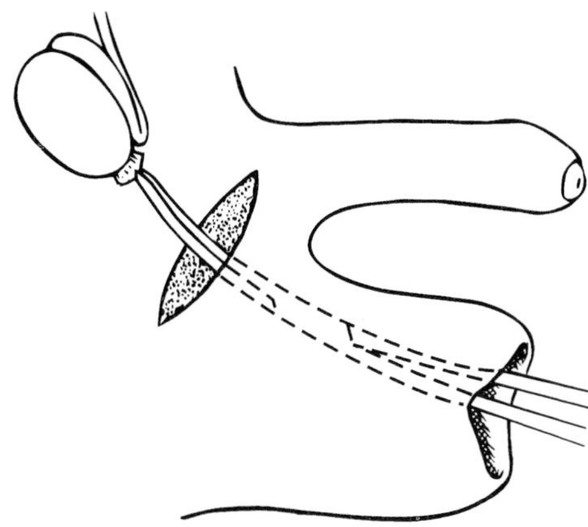

Fig. 44.6 Orchidopexy: manipulating testis into dartos pouch.

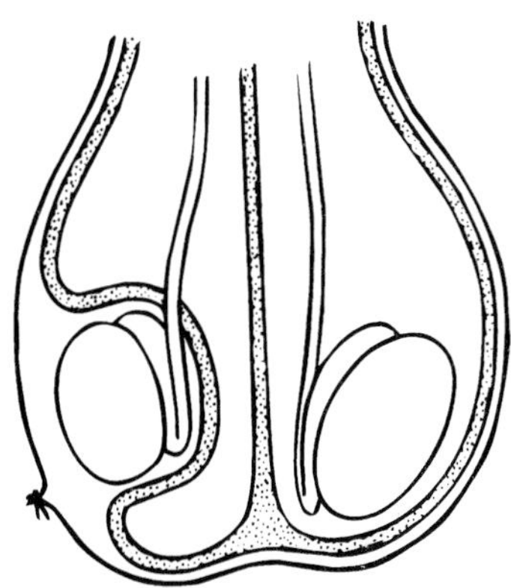

Fig. 44.7 Orchidopexy: testis in dartos pouch.

PRIAPISM

Appraise

1 Whatever the cause, commence treatment as soon as possible.

2 If there is delay, the resulting sludging of the blood in the corpora and eventual fibrosis lead to impotence. Even with early treatment, impotence is common.

3 Carry out the simplest procedure to obtain detumescence and then refer the patient to a specialist centre.

Irrigation

1 Pass a catheter as these patients have difficulty in voiding.

2 Either under local anaesthesia such as spinal or epidural, or preferably general anaesthesia, insert a wide-bore aspiration needle into the distal end of one corpus cavernosum and another into the proximal end of the opposite one.

3 Irrigate with 100–200 ml of physiological saline or heparin saline into the proximal needle.

4 After a while the fluid emerging from the opposite needle is reasonably clear. Each injection of fluid causes a considerable hardening of the priapism.

5 Massage the corpora to facilitate escape of the fluid, making them flaccid. If necessary insert four needles into the corpora.

6 For persistent priapism make up a solution of phenylephrine in normal saline (1 ml containing 10 mg, diluting it to 100 ml with normal saline). Inject 3–5 ml into the corpora, repeated at 10-minute intervals until the erection subsides. Monitor pulse and blood pressure.

7 Apply a firm bandage and return the patient to the ward.

8 It may be necessary to repeat this process three or four times over the ensuring 48 hours before the corpora remain flaccid.

FURTHER READING

Blandy J 1986 Radical cure of hydrocoele. In: Blandy J Operative urology, 2nd edn. Blackwell Scientific, Oxford, pp 246–247

Blandy J, Fowler C 1996 Circumcision. In: Blandy J, Fowler C Urology, 2nd edn. Blackwell Scientific, Oxford, pp 445–447

Blandy J, Fowler C 1996 Orchidopexy. In: Blandy J, Fowler C Urology, 2nd edn. Blackwell Scientific, Oxford, pp 553–556

Blandy J, Fowler C 1996 Torsion of the testis. In: Blandy J, Fowler C Urology, 2nd edn. Blackwell Scientific, Oxford, pp 569–571

Dittrich A, Albrecht K, Bar-Moshe O et al 1991 Treatment of pharmacological priapism with phenylephrine. Journal of Urology 146:323

Nilsson S, Edvinsson A, Nilsson B 1979 Improved fertility after varicocele correction: fact or fiction? Fertility and Sterility 51:591

Rickwood AMK 1999 Medical indications for circumcision. British Journal of Urology International 83 (Suppl 1):45–51

Tulloch WS 1955 Varicocoele in subfertility: results of treatment. British Medical Journal 2:356

45

Gynaecological surgery

M.E. Setchell

CONTENTS

GENERAL CONSIDERATIONS

Introduction

1 General surgeons may be called upon to perform gynaecological or even obstetric operations in certain circumstances. There may be an unexpected finding at an emergency operation, or there may be an incidental gynaecological lesion, or in an emergency there may be no gynaecologist available. Try, therefore, to become familiar with the gynaecological pathology that you are likely to encounter and learn how to deal with it. But remember that most elective gynaecological operations are of a specialized nature and should not be tried on an occasional basis.

2 When operating on women in the reproductive phase of life, be particularly careful and gentle in handling the pelvic organs. Careless surgery in the female pelvis will result in pelvic adhesions, which may drastically disturb a woman's fertility and affect the rest of her life and happiness.

3 Gynaecologists use the Pfannenstiel incision for many operations, but in emergencies dealt with by the general surgeon a midline or paramedian incision will often have been chosen because of the uncertain nature of the diagnosis.

4 Gynaecologists have used the laparoscope as a diagnostic tool in acute pelvic pain for many years, as do general surgeons. Both surgeons and gynaecologists now use the laparoscope and sophisticated minimally invasive instruments for a growing range of operative procedures.

5 The usefulness of ultrasound as a diagnostic aid in gynaecological conditions is now well established, and in many cases exploratory laparotomy and laparoscopy may be avoided.

Preoperative care

KEY POINTS Special considerations in gynaecology

- Nowhere is informed consent more important than in gynaecological surgery. Give a full explanation of the probable operative procedure and its consequences, particularly if future fertility is likely to be affected. If the woman wishes, keep the partner informed as well.
- Keep shaving of pubic and vulval hair to a minimum; it is particularly uncomfortable when it is re-growing.
- Patients should stop taking the oral contraceptive pill 6 weeks before elective major gynaecological surgery. Menstruation is not a contraindication to gynaecological surgery, nor indeed to thorough examination.
- Remember that pregnancy predisposes to thromboembolism, and use prophylactic heparin readily.

Prepare

1 *Positioning of patient.* Vaginal operations are carried out in the lithotomy position. Laparoscopy is best carried out with the patient in Lloyd-Davies stirrups, with steep head-down tilt. Abdominal operations are carried out with the patient supine and 5–10° of head-down tilt.

2 *Catheterization.* Empty the bladder by catheterization before all abdominal procedures, laparoscopy included. Separate the labia and swab the urethral meatus with antiseptic solution. Without allowing the labia to close again, pass a silver or plastic catheter well into the bladder. Now let the labia approximate and press firmly and continuously suprapubically. When the urine flow ceases, gradually withdraw the catheter, taking care not to allow air to be sucked into the bladder.

MINOR GYNAECOLOGICAL OPERATIONS

DILATATION AND CURETTAGE

Appraise

You may need to perform a diagnostic dilatation and curettage (D&C) on a patient with heavy or prolonged vaginal bleeding, or a therapeutic dilatation and curettage for bleeding associated with retained products of conception.

Prepare

1 Any woman in the reproductive age group (13–50 years) who has heavy bleeding could have an incomplete or missed abortion; order a preoperative β-hCG (beta-subunit of human chorionic gonadotrophin) pregnancy test on blood or urine and a transvaginal ultrasound scan of the uterus before she is taken to theatre. Also order a full blood count and group, and 'save serum'. Blood transfusion is rarely necessary.

2 Gynaecologists usually perform a hysteroscopy prior to a diagnostic D&C, but you are unlikely to gain sufficient experience to make this useful. If the D&C is for a miscarriage of greater than 10 weeks' gestation, ask the anaesthetist to give 5–10 units of synthetic oxytocin (Syntocinon) intravenously immediately before commencing the operation.

Access

1 Perform a bimanual examination to determine the size and axis of the uterus and to detect any adnexal swellings.

2 Insert a Sim's or Auvard's speculum into the vagina and grasp the cervix with two Volsellum (Latin: *vulsus*=to pluck) forceps.

Action

1 Gently pass a uterine sound to determine the length and direction of the uterus, but omit this step if you think there has been a recent pregnancy. The soft pregnant uterus is easily perforated by a sound.

2 Dilate the cervix progressively, increasing by 1 mm at a time, by passing metal dilators devised by Alfred Hegar (1830–1914, Professor of Gynaecology in Freiburg). You may need to press to pass through the internal cervical os, but then be careful to reduce the pressure as soon as you overcome the resistance. If it is difficult, go back to the previous dilator. An 8-mm-diameter dilator is adequate for a diagnostic D&C, 10 mm for a therapeutic one.

3 Pass a pair of polyp forceps, open them, twist through 90°, close them and withdraw any tissue present. Repeat two or three times in different planes or more frequently if there are retained products of conception.

4 Pass a curette, small and sharp in a non-pregnant woman, large and blunt in a patient who has been pregnant, until you reach the fundus of the uterus. With firm pressure on the uterine wall, withdraw the curette and collect the specimen on a swab. Repeat the manoeuvre, going round the whole surface of the uterine cavity. In a pregnant patient, make sure that the cavity is completely empty. Send the curettings for histology.

KEY POINTS Caution

- If you are unsure whether the uterus is anteverted or retroverted, pass the sound with great care.
- If you think you have perforated the uterus, as a rule perform laparoscopy to see whether any other structure has been damaged.
- If the uterus is bleeding, you can usually control it with diathermy in the non-pregnant uterus, but if the uterus was pregnant you usually need to perform a laparotomy to suture it.

Postoperative

1 In the absence of infection or bleeding, discharge the patient the same day.

2 If there is evidence of infection such as offensive tissue, pyrexia or raised white blood cell count, treat it with broad-spectrum antibiotics and keep the patient in hospital.

3 If there is endometrial hyperplasia or carcinoma, refer the patient as soon as possible to a gynaecologist.

BARTHOLIN'S CYST OR ABSCESS

Appraise

1 An abscess of the glands described in 1677 by the Copenhagen Professor Caspar Bartholin (1655–1738), is an acutely painful condition so deal with it as an emergency.

2 A cyst may be dealt with electively.

3 The operation of marsupialization (Greek: *marsyp(p)ion*=a pouch) is the procedure of choice since recurrence is very likely following simple incision and drainage.

Action

1 Make a vertical incision 1 cm long just inside the hymenal ring.

2 Remove a semicircle of skin and cyst wall from each side of the incision. Take a microbiological swab from the discharging pus.

3 Insert half a dozen or so fine synthetic absorbable sutures circumferentially to bring the cyst wall and skin into apposition, so leaving a wide ostium to the gland. Leave a gauze ribbon drain in the cavity for 1–2 days.

Postoperative

1 Discharge the patient home the same day, and encourage her to bath or shower regularly.

2 Administer antibiotics such as amoxicillin for 5 days, or doxycycline for 10 days if *Chlamydia* culture is positive.

3 Arrange for contacts to be traced if gonorrhoea or *Chlamydia* is confirmed.

LAPAROSCOPY

Appraise

1 This is a very useful and important diagnostic procedure in the diagnosis of pelvic pain, both acute and chronic. It is particularly valuable in cases of suspected ectopic pregnancy.

2 You may find diagnostic laparoscopy useful in many situations, including the acute abdomen, the diagnosis of ascites, for direct liver biopsy and for peritoneal biopsy.

3 Perform laparoscopy only if you are trained in the technique (see Ch. 5). It is contraindicated in the presence of generalized peritonitis, intestinal obstruction or ileus. Be particularly cautious when you suspect extensive adhesions. Pre-existing severe cardiovascular and respiratory disease may also be contraindications.

4 Do not attempt operative laparoscopy unless suitable equipment is available such as diathermy, laser and laparoscopic instruments, and you are appropriately trained.

Prepare

When you intend to perform laparoscopy for acute pelvic pain, first order a full blood count, β-hCG pregnancy test and preoperative transvaginal ultrasound scan.

Access

1 Place the patient in the semilithotomy position, with the legs in Lloyd-Davies stirrups.

2 Empty the bladder and perform a bimanual examination. Apply Volsellum forceps and a Spackman cannula to the cervix.

3 Make an incision in or just below the umbilicus; for a 5-mm diagnostic laparoscope a 5-mm incision is sufficient, but if operative laparoscopy is a possibility prefer a 10-mm laparoscope and incision.

? DIFFICULTY

If there are extensive lower abdominal scars from previous surgery, it may be safer to insert the Veress needle and trocar in the left upper abdomen just below the ribs in the midclavicular line (Palmer's point).

Action

1 Introduce the Veress needle almost vertically through the umbilical skin incision. As soon as the tip is through the abdominal wall, alter the direction towards the pelvis, and check that the needle point is free and mobile.

2 Aspirate the needle with a syringe to check that neither a blood vessel nor a viscus has been entered. Then attach a syringe with 10 ml of physiological saline and remove the plunger to check that the saline passes into the peritoneal cavity under the force of negative pressure alone.

3 Connect the needle to the carbon dioxide insufflator and introduce the gas initially at a flow rate of no more than 1 litre/minute. Provided the pressure remains below 25 mmHg, increase the gas flow to 3 litres/minute until approximately 3 litres have been instilled.

4 Remove the Veress needle and pass the large trocar and cannula into the peritoneal cavity, using the same direction as used for the Veress needle. It is helpful to hold up the abdominal wall between fingers and thumb to provide counter-pressure.

5 Remove the trocar and insert the telescope through the cannula; attach the fibrelight cable and, whenever possible, the video camera.

6 The uterus can be moved by an assistant grasping the Spackman cannula to facilitate visualization of all parts of the pelvis. Insert a second trocar suprapubically or laterally in order to pass a probe to assist in demonstrating pelvic anatomy clearly.

7 After thorough inspection of the pelvic organs, rotate the telescope in its cannula to inspect the upper abdomen and peritoneum. Remove any necessary biopsies with biopsy forceps, using diathermy coagulation to obtain haemostasis.

8 When the procedure is completed, let out as much of the carbon dioxide as possible, remove the trocar and insert one skin suture in each incision.

? DIFFICULTY

1. If the Veress needle has been misplaced, the pressure recorder shows a rise in pressure above 25 mmHg.
2. Remove and re-insert it, if necessary suprapubically, in order to obtain a satisfactory pneumoperitoneum.

Checklist

1 Ensure that both tubes, including the distal ends, and ovaries have been visualized, the pouch of Douglas, and anterior and posterior surfaces of the uterus.

2 If you detect no disease, look at the appendix, caecum and upper abdomen.

3 Make a decision as to whether operative laparoscopy, laparotomy or no further surgical procedure is necessary.

OVARIAN OPERATIONS

Appraise

1 You may be required to deal with an ovarian cyst that has caused acute abdominal pain because of rupture, torsion or haemorrhage. A preoperative ultrasound scan may have suggested the diagnosis; a transvaginal ultrasound gives better images than abdominal, and colour Doppler scan is useful to demonstrate the presence of neovascularization, which may be indicative of malignancy.

2 On other occasions you may discover a cyst when carrying out a laparoscopy or laparotomy for acute pain, or for another indication.

KEY POINTS Decision-making

- Perform a bimanual examination under anaesthetic if you suspect an ovarian cyst clinically or on ultrasound.
- If a diagnostic laparoscopy has revealed an ovarian cyst, consider removing it laparoscopically, but it is wise to call in a gynaecologist to help in the assessment.

Prepare

KEY POINT Importance of informed consent

- In no other gynaecological operation is fully informed consent more important, particularly when one or both ovaries may need to be removed once the abdomen is open and the clinical findings apparent.

Order preoperative full blood count and take blood for tumour markers such as CA125 and carcinoembryonic antigen (CEA), even if results may be available only postoperatively.

Access

1 Unless you have had considerable gynaecological experience, you need to remove most ovarian tumours by laparotomy.

2 Use a transverse suprapubic incision only if preoperative ultrasound or laparoscopy have provided strong evidence that the tumour is benign. In all other cases, employ a vertical incision.

Assess

1 It is of great importance for you to recognize the features of tumours that are likely to be benign and of those which signal malignancy. In a woman of reproductive age it is better to err on the side of conservatism, even if a further laparotomy will be required, rather than risk sacrificing healthy ovaries. In general, a smooth surface and the absence of ascites, peritoneal, omental or nodular metastases are features of benign tumours; bilaterality is no guide to the likelihood of malignancy.

2 You must distinguish a mature graafian follicle or a corpus luteum cyst from a neoplastic cyst. A luteal cyst may develop in early pregnancy; unnecessary removal can result in abortion.

3 Do not remove any ovarian cyst under 5 cm in diameter without good evidence either that it is neoplastic or that it has undergone haemorrhage or rupture, giving rise to acute abdominal pain.

4 Ovarian cystectomy is the preferred treatment for benign ovarian cysts. Carry out salpingo-oophorectomy:
- If there is evidence of malignancy.
- If the cyst has undergone torsion and is gangrenous.
- If the tumour is very large and little normal ovarian tissue can be conserved.

5 If you suspect malignancy, explore the whole abdomen, including the diaphragmatic surface of the liver and the undersurface of the diaphragm. Palpate the para-aortic nodes and biopsy them if they are enlarged. Send ascitic fluid or peritoneal washings for cytology. Further treatment depends upon accurate staging. If there are no metastases and the contralateral ovary is grossly normal, split it open and send a slice for histology or frozen section if it is available, before closing the ovary with fine absorbable synthetic or fine non-absorbable sutures.

6 If the ovarian tumour is obviously malignant, remove the uterus, both ovaries and tubes (see Hysterectomy, below), the omentum and as much metastatic tumour bulk as possible. The only exception to such radical surgery is in a young woman with disease confined to one ovary and no sign of abdominal metastases.

Action

Ovarian cystectomy

1 Separate the tumour from adhesions and draw it out of the wound.

2 Surround the operation site with large gauze packs, and have a sucker ready in case the cyst is accidentally ruptured.

3 Make an incision in the ovarian cortex around the base of the tumour (Fig. 45.1a).

4 Find the plane of cleavage and shell out the tumour, using scissors and gauze swab dissection (Fig. 45.1b). If the cyst ruptures, ensure that you remove all the cyst lining.

5 Repair the residual ovarian tissue, using 2/0 absorbable synthetic sutures or fine monofilament nylon; good haemostasis is important to prevent future adhesion formation.

Salpingo-oophorectomy

1 If you decide to remove the whole ovary, place one clamp across the ovarian pedicle (infundibulopelvic fold) and a second across the ovarian ligament and fallopian tube, adjacent to the uterus. Resect the ovary together with the tube and broad ligament between the clamps.

2 Doubly ligate each pedicle with 0 polyglactin 910. Use a transfixion suture or gently release and re-apply the clamp while tying the ligature. At the end of the operation check the pedicles before closing the abdomen.

Checklist

1 If you inadvertently rupture an ovarian cyst, thoroughly wash out the fluid from the peritoneum. Dermoid cyst fluid and endometrioma 'chocolate fluid' is highly irritant, and leakage of malignant cyst fluid may result in peritoneal metastases.

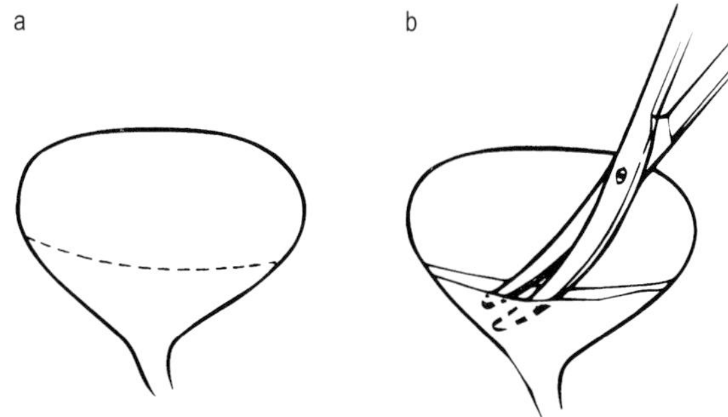

Fig. 45.1 Ovarian cystectomy: (a) circumcision; (b) separation of cyst from ovary.

2 If the ovarian cyst(s) look like endometriomas, remember to look for other signs of pelvic endometriosis, particularly on the uterosacral ligaments and peritoneum of the pouch of Douglas, and document their presence.

3 If the cyst has malignant features, carefully record the presence of any metastases.

Closure

1 Suture the peritoneum with 2/0 polyglactin 910 or similar material.

2 Close the rectus sheath with the same material for a transverse incision but use nylon to close a vertical incision.

3 Close the skin with sutures or clips.

Postoperative

1 If both ovaries have been removed, consider starting the patient on hormone replacement therapy (oestrogen±progesterone).

? DIFFICULTY

1. If you come across a malignant ovarian tumour that is fixed in the pelvis, perhaps with matted adherent omental metastases, it is better to remove a small biopsy and carefully record the site and size of the metastases and close up, rather than perform a very inadequate debulking operation. If at all possible, refer the patient to a gynaecological oncology team for full radiological investigation in order for decisions to be made regarding preoperative chemotherapy.
2. It is rarely necessary to remove an ovarian cyst laparoscopically in an emergency. A cyst that is less than 5 cm, has a smooth and regular surface and has not undergone torsion or rupture is best left alone. If it is larger than 5 cm and has undergone torsion or rupture, deal with it by laparotomy but, if it does not appear to be undergoing any acute process, refer the patient to a gynaecologist at a later date unless you have experience in differentiating different types of cyst.

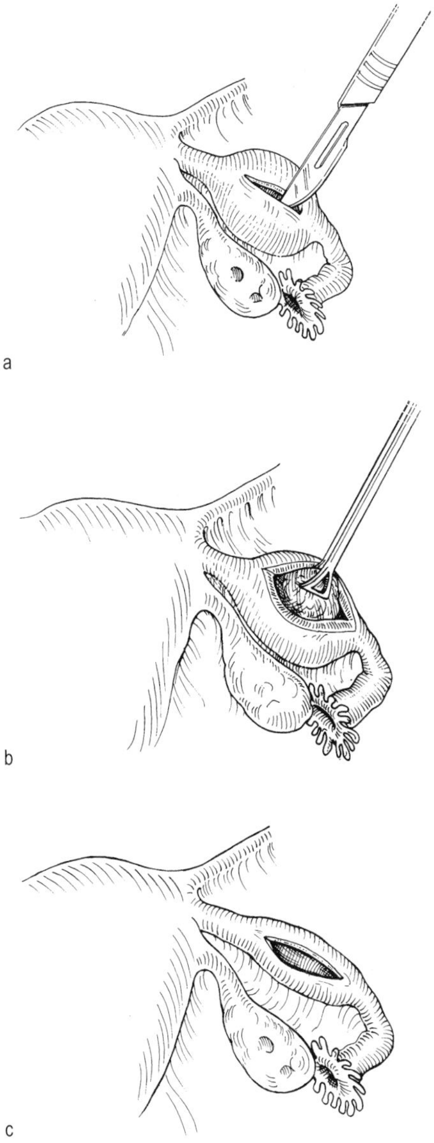

a

b

c

Fig. 45.2 Conservative management of an ectopic pregnancy; a similar technique applies to both a laparoscopic and an open approach: (a) incision over antimesenteric border of tube with needle diathermy; (b) removal of the trophoblast tissue with grasping forceps and suction/irrigation cannula; (c) salpingotomy left to heal without suturing after ensuring haemostasis.

SURGERY OF ECTOPIC PREGNANCY

Appraise

1 A classic ruptured ectopic pregnancy is easily diagnosed by the findings of severe abdominal pain, guarding and rebound, and hypovolaemic shock. A tubal abortion or slowly leaking ectopic pregnancy is less easy to diagnose, and ultrasound scanning, using a transvaginal probe, together with a rapid β-hCG assay, often helps to make the diagnosis.

2 Laparoscopy is not often required to confirm the diagnosis of ruptured ectopic pregnancy but is always required in the less acute forms of tubal abortion or slow leakage. In non-ruptured cases, laparoscopic salpingotomy and aspiration of the pregnancy may be the treatment of choice if future pregnancy is desired (Fig. 45.2). Very early ectopic pregnancies may be managed medically, with a single dose of methotrexate.

3 Once the diagnosis of ruptured ectopic has been made, take the patient to the operating theatre as soon as possible. Do not wait for blood to be cross-matched or hope that the patient's condition will improve. She will improve only when the fallopian tube is clamped.

Prepare

1 Order a full blood count, group and save serum if not cross-matching, and secure intravenous access as soon as you suspect ectopic pregnancy.

2 If the patient is shocked, take her to the operating theatre for immediate laparotomy. In less acute forms arrange for laparoscopy with a view to conservative laparoscopic surgery.

LAPAROSCOPIC SALPINGOTOMY OR SALPINGECTOMY

Access

1 Use a 10-mm laparoscope if available as this gives better visualization in the presence of a haemoperitoneum.

2 Ensure that a suction/irrigation device is available if you contemplate laparoscopic surgery.

3 Have monopolar electrodiathermy equipment available for incising the tube and if possible use bipolar diathermy for obtaining haemostasis.

4 Having introduced the laparoscope, insert a lateral port so that a probe or forceps can be used to demonstrate and manipulate the fallopian tube.

5 If there is copious blood in the peritoneal cavity, aspirate it using the suction/irrigation apparatus to improve the view of the tube.

Appraise

1 Make a careful inspection of the uterus and of both tubes and ovaries, in order to decide the most appropriate operation.

2 Decide whether to proceed to laparotomy or complete the operation laparoscopically. Laparotomy is appropriate if there is major bleeding preventing good visualization, the patient is shocked or you are not experienced in laparoscopic surgery.

3 The second decision is whether to perform a salpingotomy, conserving the tube, or salpingectomy. Salpingectomy is generally the preferred option, especially if:
- The contralateral tube is normal.
- The tube is badly damaged by the tubal rupture.
- The bleeding is substantial.
- The patient does not wish for future pregnancies.

Action, if laparoscopic removal of the ectopic pregnancy appears feasible

1 Insert a second lateral port in the other iliac fossa.

2 Grasp the affected tube as close as possible to the tubal swelling with grasping forceps near the uterine end.

3 Apply bipolar diathermy to the mesosalpinx, and coagulate the tissue with its blood vessels. Divide the mesosalpinx with laparoscopic scissors.

4 Alternatively the tube may be removed by using an Endoloop ligature to occlude the vessels, and then remove the tube with scissors.

5 Remove the fallopian tube through the 10-mm port, using a bag if necessary.

6 Irrigate and aspirate the peritoneal cavity to remove as much blood, clot and trophoblast as possible.

7 If you decide that salpingotomy and conservation of the tube is more appropriate make a 10-mm linear incision over the site of the tubal swelling, using diathermy needle, scissors or hook.

8 Use the suction/irrigation cannula to separate the trophoblast tissue from the tube and then remove the tissue with grasping forceps. If the ectopic pregnancy is close to the fimbrial end of the tube, it may be possible to aspirate and remove it through the fimbrial ostium, which is likely to be dilated.

9 Extract the tissue from the abdomen through a 10-mm port, unless it is very small, using an extraction bag if necessary.

10 It is not necessary to close the salpingotomy incision but, if there is any residual bleeding after applying pressure, use the diathermy forceps to complete haemostasis.

KEY POINTS Decisions

- It is usually better to perform a salpingectomy rather than a salpingotomy unless the contralateral tube is also damaged by chronic pelvic inflammatory disease or the ectopic pregnancy is very early and can be aspirated.
- If it is difficult to gain access to the tube because of adhesions, or copious blood, proceed to laparotomy.
- Inspect the contralateral tube and record its condition.

Closure

Close the laparoscopic incisions, using a deep suture if 10- or 12-mm operating ports have been used.

Postoperative

If salpingotomy and trophoblast aspiration have been carried out, perform follow-up serum β-hCG levels twice weekly until it is certain that levels are declining, because of the small risk of persistence of the trophoblast.

SALPINGECTOMY OR SALPINGOTOMY BY LAPAROTOMY

Appraise

1 This is the standard treatment for a ruptured ectopic pregnancy and is the method of choice unless you are skilled in laparoscopic surgery.

2 If the patient has appreciable signs of surgical shock, proceed to laparotomy forthwith.

Access

Make a generous incision, either midline or Pfannenstiel, provided you are used to this incision.

Action

1 As soon as the peritoneal cavity is open, aspirate blood with the sucker.

2 Pass a hand into the pelvis and bring the uterus with its appendages up into the wound. Identify the ruptured tube.

Place one or more clamps across the mesosalpinx and another clamp across the cornual end of the tube, then excise the damaged tube. In most cases it is neither necessary nor desirable to remove the ovary. Doubly ligate the pedicles beneath the clamps, using polyglactin 910.

3 You can decide to conserve the tube if the other tube is also damaged or has previously been removed, and the tubal pregnancy is small. The pregnancy can be removed by aspiration or salpingotomy.

4 If the ectopic pregnancy is small and distal you may aspirate it through the fimbrial end.

5 If not, create a salpingotomy with a 1-cm linear incision using a scalpel or needle diathermy over the swollen portion of the tube (see Fig. 45.2) and remove the pregnancy with a combination of forceps traction and hydrodissection. You do not need to close the tube but ensure that haemostasis is complete using diathermy coagulation.

6 Inspect the contralateral tube and ovary. The other tube may have a hydrosalpinx or haematosalpinx but do not be tempted to tamper with it. Bilateral tubal pregnancy is excessively rare. Carefully record the state of the pelvis.

7 Before closing the abdomen, aspirate and swab out as much blood as possible, and estimate the volume of blood loss. Washing the peritoneal cavity with Hartmann's solution may help to reduce adhesion formation.

KEY POINTS Inspect and react to findings

- If the tubal pregnancy is greater than 4 cm in diameter, elect to perform a salpingectomy rather than a salpingotomy.
- If the accessibility of the tube is difficult because of adhesions or copious blood, proceed to laparotomy.
- Inspect the contralateral tube and record its condition.

Postoperative

1 Obtain as accurate an estimate as possible of the amount of blood aspirated from the peritoneal cavity, and replace it with blood transfusion if the loss exceeds 1 litre.

2 Use central venous pressure monitoring to gauge blood and fluid replacement if there has been severe shock.

3 Administer prophylactic antibiotics such as cefradine and metronidazole or co-amoxiclav for three doses if tubal rupture and substantial haemoperitoneum have occurred.

TUBAL LIGATION

Appraise

1 You may be asked to carry out a sterilization procedure, either in the course of a caesarean section operation (see below) or as an additional procedure during the course of an abdominal operation. Obtain prior consent from the patient. Avoid sterilizing a woman under the age of 30 years unless there is a good medical reason to perform it.

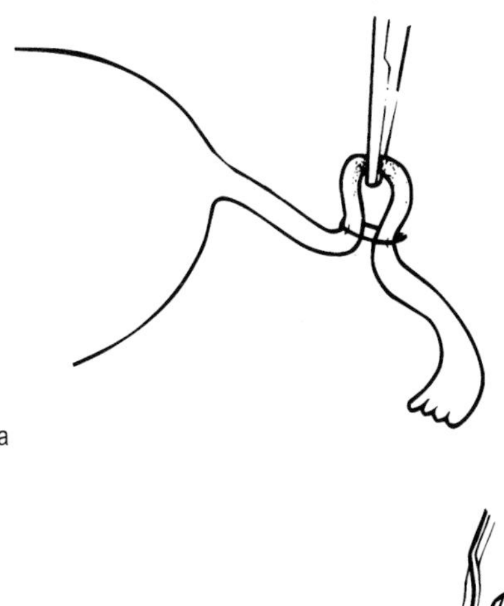

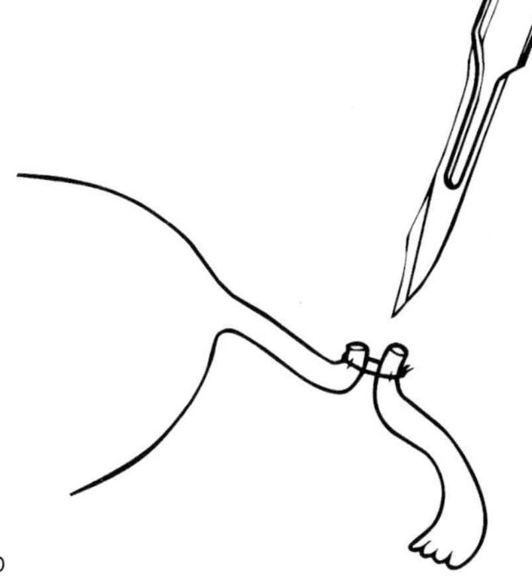

Fig. 45.3 Pomeroy sterilization: (a) ligature round loop of tube; (b) excision of loop of tube.

2 Sterilization may be carried out by one of the modifications of Pomeroy's method as described below, or by the application of Hulka or Filshie clips.

Action

1 Pick up a loop of fallopian tube with a Spencer Wells forceps 2–3 cm from the uterus (Fig. 45.3a).

2 Tie an absorbable synthetic ligature tightly around the base of the loop and excise the end of the loop. You may seal each end of the tube with the diathermy needle as an additional precaution (Fig. 45.3b).

HYSTERECTOMY

Appraise

1 You may need to perform a hysterectomy—for example, as part of a larger surgical procedure such as the removal of a rectal cancer, because of fibromyomata or other benign uterine disease causing severe menorrhagia, or for ovarian carcinoma that had not been diagnosed preoperatively. Do not be tempted to carry out a hysterectomy during the course of another operation because of the incidental finding of large uterine fibroids, unless you have discussed the possibility with the patient preoperatively.

2 Unless there is gynaecological malignancy, conserve at least one ovary whenever possible in premenopausal women.

3 Vaginal hysterectomy and radical hysterectomy, described in 1900 by the Viennese gynaecologist Ernst Wertheim (1864–1920), are not likely to fall within your competence.

Access

1 Empty the bladder by catheterization and cleanse the vagina with an antiseptic. Bonney's blue or methylthioninium chloride (methylene blue) dye has the advantage of staining the vaginal skin, making it more easily recognized at operation.

2 A Pfannenstiel incision is suitable for many hysterectomies, but avoid it if you suspect malignancy, if the uterus is larger than the size of a 16-week pregnancy or if the diagnosis is in doubt. In these cases use a vertical incision.

3 Carefully pack off the intestines, both large and small, to render the operation easier and safer. It is well worth spending a few minutes displacing all the intestines from the pelvis and packing them above the pelvic brim.

4 Insert a self-retaining retractor of the Gosset type, preferably one with a third blade.

Action

1 Place a strong straight clamp such as Kocher's or Rogers type as close to the uterus as possible across the fallopian tube, round ligament, ovarian ligament and upper part of the broad ligament. If these structures are held on the stretch, an avascular window is visible at a depth of about 3 cm into the broad ligament. Aim to put the tip of the clamp into this avascular window.

2 Place a second straight clamp just lateral to the first clamp, again with the tip in the avascular window.

3 Divide the tissue between the clamps down to their tips, and ligate the lateral pedicle with 1 absorbable synthetic suture material, doubly tied (Fig. 45.4).

4 Repeat this procedure on the opposite side.

5 Open the layers of the broad ligament below the sutured pedicle by inserting closed scissors and gently opening them. Incise the anterior leaf of the broad ligament and gradually continue opening the broad ligament, until you reach the loose fold of uterovesical peritoneum.

6 Now pass the closed scissors in a medial direction, open them and cut the loose uterovesical peritoneum. Carry out the same manoeuvre on the other side until the bladder peritoneum is completely incised in front of the cervix.

7 Pick up the bladder flap with dissecting forceps and apply tension. This manoeuvre displays the loose connective tissue between bladder and cervix, which can be carefully cut with scissors while keeping their points angled towards the cervix.

8 Now push the bladder off the cervix, either with a swab on a sponge-holder or with the swab wrapped around your thumb. Apply pressure on to the cervix rather than the bladder. Once

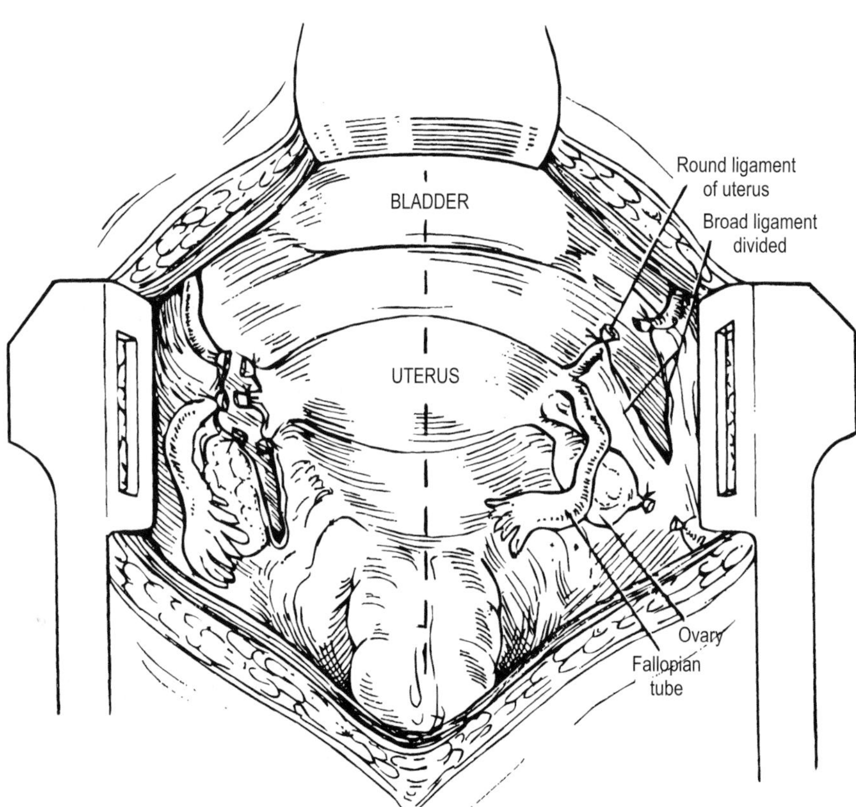

Fig. 45.4 Hysterectomy: incision of broad ligament, with conservation of adnexa (left), with adnexa removed (right).

the longitudinal fibres of the vagina are visible, no further displacement of the bladder is necessary. Adequate displacement of the bladder may also be checked by gripping the cervix between thumb and forefinger until you can feel that you are below the level of the cervix.

9 Using the two clamps that are still applied to the uterine cornu, pull the uterus up with as much tension as possible, so accentuating the fold of the uterosacral ligaments. Divide these with a scalpel and the uterus can now be lifted even higher out of the pelvis. If the uterosacral ligaments look thick and vascular, apply a Spencer Wells forceps to them before cutting them.

10 Now clamp the uterine vessels. Apply a strong straight or curved clamp at right-angles to the uterus just above the level at which the uterosacral ligaments have been divided. Make sure that the tips of the clamp are as close as possible to the uterus. Divide the uterine vessels by cutting with a knife close to the clamp, and continue cutting until you are just into the uterine wall.

11 Next, clamp the paracervical tissue by applying another straight clamp at right-angles to the uterine vessel clamp. The depth to which this clamp is applied depends upon the length of the cervix, but it is rarely necessary to apply it to a depth of greater than 1 cm. With the scalpel, cut the pedicle, keeping the direction of incision somewhat medial and towards the cervix.

12 Now open the vagina by inserting a scalpel in the midline through the vaginal fascia and then into the vagina itself. Pick up the anterior vaginal edge with Littlewood's forceps, and extend the vaginal incision circumferentially. Pick up each vaginal angle with another Littlewood's forceps, and place a fourth one posteriorly in the midline.

Closure

1 The most important sutures are at the vaginal angle. Place an interrupted suture just below the tip of the paracervical clamp so as to include the vaginal angle. Having tied the suture, apply a Spencer Wells forceps to the end of the suture to act as a holder (Fig. 45.5).

2 Close the vaginal vault with a series of interrupted absorbable sutures. Alternatively, leave it open and arrest oozing by inserting a running suture around the vault (Fig. 45.6).

3 Doubly ligate the uterine vessels with 1 synthetic absorbable thread.

4 Check that there is no bleeding from the vaginal vault or uterine vessels. Many surgeons now do not close the pelvic peritoneum provided haemostasis is good. If there is oozing it is worth tacking it across with continuous 0 synthetic absorbable stitch, starting at one ovarian pedicle and concluding at the other.

5 The parietal peritoneum need not be closed, but carefully close the rectus sheath with 0 or 2/0 polyglactin 910, before closing the skin with clips or sutures.

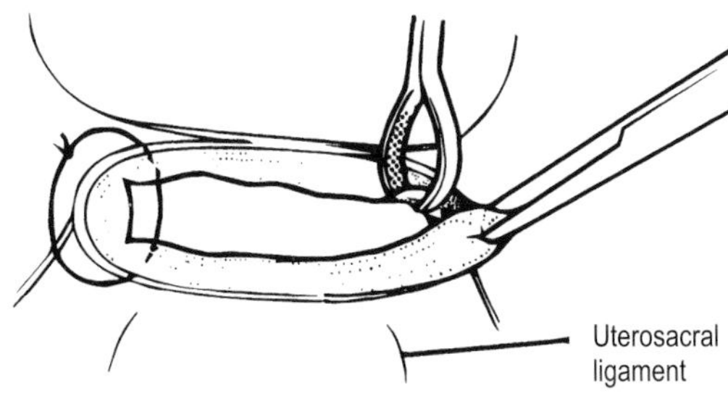

Fig. 45.5 Closure of vault: tying of vaginal angle.

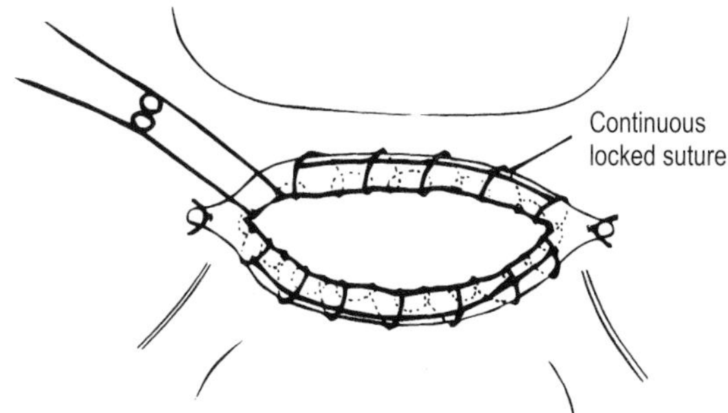

Fig. 45.6 Vaginal vault circumsuture, leaving vagina open for drainage.

Postoperative

1 Give a single dose of peroperative antibiotics and continue this if there were any signs of pelvic sepsis.

2 If both ovaries have been removed, discuss the use of hormone replacement therapy with the patient.

Complications

1 Reactionary or secondary haemorrhage from the vaginal angle may occur, and presents as profuse vaginal bleeding. It can be dealt with through the vagina, applying a figure-of-eight suture to the bleeding points.

2 Ureteric or bladder injury are unwelcome complications, which will present either as urinary leakage and fistula formation, or loin pain if the ureter is completely tied off. Get expert urological assistance if there is any suggestion of such complications.

? DIFFICULTY

1. Occasionally, if there are very dense pelvic adhesions and the uterus remains fixed in a deep pelvis, or if there is an extensive ovarian malignancy, it may be difficult to remove the cervix. It may then be safer to perform subtotal hysterectomy.
2. Proceed exactly as described, but there is no need to apply a clamp to the paracervical tissue (step 2). At this stage, cut across the stump to close the cervical canal. Cover the stump with the pelvic peritoneum.

MYOMECTOMY

Assess

1 As a general surgeon you are unlikely to be called upon to carry out this procedure. In a young patient with fibromyomata it may be preferable to remove the myomata, conserving the uterus. If

the fibroids are multiple, the operation can be more time-consuming and hazardous than hysterectomy. A solitary pedunculated subserous fibroid, which may have undergone torsion, is easily removed.

2 Remove as many fibroids as possible through one uterine incision. Try to avoid incisions in the posterior wall of the uterus, since these often give rise to small intestinal adhesions. You can often remove a posterior fibroid through an anterior incision and crossing the uterine cavity.

3 If you have to remove multiple fibroids, it is worth applying a Bonney's myomectomy clamp or tying a rubber sling around the cervix to reduce haemorrhage.

Action

1 Make an incision in the uterus, usually over the largest fibroid.

2 Grasp the fibroid with tissue-holding forceps. It is easy to identify a plane of cleavage and shell out the tumour, either with a finger or by opening and closing a pair of curved scissors.

3 Trim off any excess uterine muscle and insert deep synthetic absorbable sutures to obliterate the cavity left after removal of the fibroid. Several layers of sutures may be needed to achieve haemostasis.

4 Close the serous surface of the uterus with 0 or 00 polyglactin 910 or polypropylene sutures.

5 If the uterus falls back into retroversion, plicate the round ligaments with non-absorbable suture in order to antevert the uterus. This manoeuvre prevents adhesion formation.

INCIDENTAL GYNAECOLOGICAL CONDITIONS

PELVIC INFLAMMATORY DISEASE

1 Not uncommonly, a patient explored for suspected appendicitis is found to have acute salpingitis. The condition is almost always bilateral, although one tube may be more affected than the other. The tubes are oedematous and reddened, and pus is often seen dripping from the fimbrial end. Take a swab for bacteriological culture and close the abdomen. Start antibiotics at once, according to local antibiotic guidelines. This usually includes a cephalosporin and tetracycline to cover *Chlamydia trachomatis*, which is now the most common pathogen.

2 Sometimes, tubal infection may have progressed to the development of a tubo-ovarian abscess or a pyosalpinx. Alternatively, a pelvic abscess may have developed. Adhere to the usual surgical principle of draining pus, preferably inserting a drain through a separate abdominal incision. Send swabs for culture, and give appropriate antibiotics.

FIMBRIAL CYST AND PAROVARIAN CYST

1 Small cysts may be seen in relation to the distal end of the fallopian tube or broad ligament. They arise in remnants of the mesonephric (wolffian) duct and occasionally undergo torsion to produce acute abdominal pain.

2 Remove them only if they have undergone torsion. Tie the pedicle before excision.

ENDOMETRIOSIS

1 This condition may involve the ovaries forming chocolate cysts, or the pelvic peritoneum when it appears as small purple or dark-brown nodules. Rupture of a chocolate cyst produces acute abdominal pain. Occasionally it involves the intestine, when the appearance may mimic a carcinoma. In the large intestine it may produce subacute obstruction and can be extremely difficult to differentiate from carcinoma.

KEY POINTS Endometriosis or carcinoma?

- Make sure you differentiate them. Excision of an endometrioma can be more limited than for a carcinoma.
- Rarely, endometriomas may be seen in an abdominal scar.

2 Many patients with endometriosis are now treated medically with hormones or by laparoscopic diathermy or laser, so do not try to be radical if you unexpectedly find pelvic endometriosis.

? DIFFICULTY

Endometriosis results in dense adhesions, often distorting anatomy, particularly of the ureter, so take particular care to identify the course of the ureter during pelvic dissection for endometriosis.

CAESAREAN SECTION

Appraise

1 You may be asked to perform a caesarean section (said to have been the method of delivery of Julius Caesar) if you work in a hospital where there is no specialist obstetrician. It is likely that the patient has been in labour for some hours, although occasionally it is necessary to perform the operation on a patient who is bleeding heavily from a placenta praevia.

2 The lower segment operation is almost universally employed nowadays, being associated with less bleeding and fewer postoperative complications than 'classical' section.

Prepare

1 Cross-match at least 2 units of blood preoperatively.

2 Perform the operation under general or epidural anaesthesia; the latter carries a lower mortality in most circumstances.

3 Apply about 15° of lateral tilt to the operating table, to avoid compression of the inferior vena cava during the operation. Either tilt the operating table or place a wedge under the patient's buttocks.

4 Empty the bladder by catheterization and leave the catheter in place during the operation.

5 Give a single dose broad-spectrum antibiotic, such as co-amoxiclav or cefradine.

6 Give prophylactic subcutaneous heparin if there are any other risk factors such as obesity, age more than 35 years, antenatal bed rest, or smoking.

Access

1 A Pfannenstiel incision is suitable, but if you are inexperienced you may find a vertical subumbilical midline incision easier.

2 After opening the peritoneal cavity, place a large Doyen retractor into the lower edge of the wound.

Action

1 Identify the loose fold of uterovesical peritoneum. Pick it up with dissecting forceps and incise it with scissors in the midline. Extend the incision laterally almost to the broad ligament on each side.

2 Push the bladder downwards with a swab and replace the Doyen retractor over the bladder to retract it well away from the lower uterine segment.

3 Incise the lower segment transversely, beginning in the midline. The lower segment may be very thin, especially if the patient has been in labour for a long time, so take care not to cut too deeply. Once the incision is large enough to admit two fingers, insert the index finger of each hand and extend the incision laterally by stretching until the incision is approximately 11 cm in length (Fig. 45.7).

4 Rupture the exposed membranes with scissors while your assistant aspirates liquor and blood with a sucker.

5 Insert your right hand into the uterus below the presenting part, easing it out of the pelvis.

6 Deliver the fetal head into the wound. Once the face is exposed, aspirate the infant's nose and throat. Now ask your assistant to apply fundal pressure while you gently withdraw the baby from the uterus. Once the head is delivered, have the anaesthetist give an intravenous injection of synthetic oxytocin (Syntocinon) 10 units.

7 Lay the baby on the mother's thighs and apply two clamps to the umbilical cord. Divide the cord and hand the baby to the midwife.

8 Grasp the lateral ends of the uterine incision with Green–Armytage forceps and also place two of these forceps on the upper and lower flaps of the uterine incision. This controls most of the bleeding from the uterus.

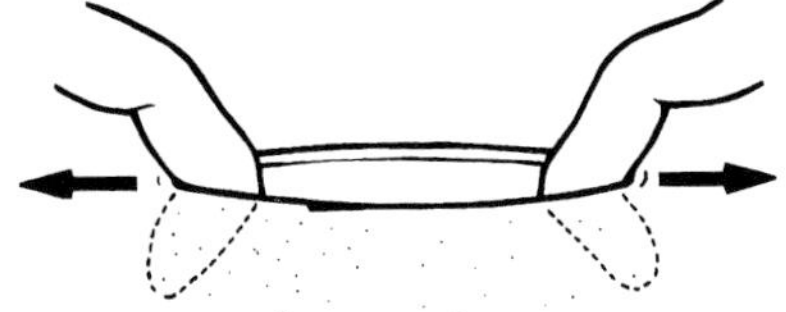

Fig. 45.7 Caesarean section: digital enlargement of incision.

9 Deliver the placenta by applying gentle cord traction and light fundal compression.

? DIFFICULTY

1. If the fetal head is deeply wedged in the pelvis, ask to have the table tilted head-down.
2. If this still does not facilitate delivery of the head, have the head pushed up vaginally by an assistant.

Closure

1 Replace the Doyen's retractor.

2 Using an atraumatic 0 or 1 synthetic absorbable suture, insert a stitch in one angle of the uterine incision and close the incision with a continuous running suture. If there is sufficient thickness of uterine muscle, do not include the full thickness in this first layer of sutures. Insert a second continuous running suture to invaginate the first, so closing the uterus in two layers.

3 Apply a swab firmly over the uterine incision for 2 minutes. When it is removed there may be one or two small bleeding vessels, which need to be dealt with by individual stitches.

4 Closure of the uterovesical peritoneum with absorbable synthetic sutures is optional.

5 Swab out any blood or liquor from the paracolic gutters on each side.

6 Close the abdominal incision.

? DIFFICULTY

1. In exceptional circumstances it may be necessary to carry out a 'classical' upper segment caesarean section. This may be necessary if there is an anterior placenta praevia (Latin: *previus* = leading the way), or a fibroid over the lower segment, or if the operation is being performed at an early stage of pregnancy. In this case use a vertical skin incision and make a large midline incision in the upper segment of the uterus. The uterine wall is much thicker in the upper segment and three layers of sutures are needed to close it.
2. Sometimes the uterine incision may extend, either laterally to involve the uterine vessels or downwards, where the ureter or bladder may be jeopardized if sutures are inserted hastily to try and secure haemostasis. It is often helpful to deliver the uterus through the incision to obtain better access to insert additional sutures.

Postoperative

1 Maintain intravenous fluids for 12 hours, but start oral fluids as soon as the patient ceases to feel nauseated.

2 Leave a Foley catheter in place for 12–24 hours.

3 Encourage breastfeeding as soon as possible after delivery.

4 The patient should be ready for discharge 3–6 days postoperatively.

Complications

1 Pyrexia may be due to urinary infection, breast engorgement or infection, wound infection or endometriosis. Take appropriate microbiological samples before starting antibiotics.

2 Broad ligament haematoma is a rare but important problem. Suspect it if there is excessive pain, fall in haemoglobin and pyrexia, possibly with a mass in the iliac fossa.

PREGNANCY AND EMERGENCY SURGERY

The presence of a pregnancy may cause considerable confusion in the diagnosis of an acute abdomen and may make access more difficult at laparotomy. It should not, however, deter you from performing emergency abdominal operations when necessary.

APPENDICITIS

The appendix is pushed upwards and outwards during pregnancy, so that the physical signs of appendicitis may be considerably altered. Because the large pregnant uterus may prevent the normal walling-off of acute appendicitis, generalized peritonitis occurs more readily. Make a gridiron incision above and lateral to the normal site, or consider a right paramedian incision if there is doubt about diagnosis.

CHOLECYSTITIS

Acute cholecystitis and biliary colic are not uncommon in pregnancy, but the symptoms may be atypical, simulating hyperemesis or indigestion of pregnancy. If you make the diagnosis of gallbladder disease in pregnancy, prefer to wait until after delivery before carrying out cholecystectomy. If you need to perform the operation during pregnancy, prefer to do so in the middle trimester.

RED DEGENERATION OF A FIBROID

Pregnancy and fibroids often co-exist, and a fibroid growing rapidly during pregnancy may undergo red degeneration. This is an extremely painful condition; sometimes the pain is so severe that exploratory laparotomy is carried out.

KEY POINTS Danger of myomectomy in pregnancy

- Once you diagnose fibroids do not attempt to remove them.
- Myomectomy in pregnancy risks catastrophic haemorrhage and loss of the fetus.
- The only exception to this rule is if a pedunculated fibroid has undergone torsion and is gangrenous.

PLACENTAL ABRUPTION

1 The condition of abruptio placentae—premature detachment of the placenta—results in severe abdominal pain and uterine tenderness, which may or may not be accompanied by vaginal bleeding.

2 A major degree of abruption causes profound shock and usually results in fetal death. Lesser degrees may cause diagnostic difficulty.

3 Tenderness is localized over the uterus, and in the severe form the uterus acquires a characteristic woody/hard feel to it.

4 Unless labour occurs spontaneously, induce it with prostaglandins and amniotomy—puncture of the fetal membranes.

RENAL AND URETERIC CALCULI

Urinary tract calculi may occur during pregnancy. Manage them as in a non-pregnant patient, with analgesics and a high fluid intake, resorting to surgical management if this fails.

PYELONEPHRITIS AND URINARY TRACT INFECTION

These are particularly common in pregnancy because of stasis produced by uterine pressure on the bladder, and progesterone-induced ureteric dilatation. The symptoms may not be typical, so include an MSU (midstream urine) specimen whenever you investigate an obscure abdominal pain in pregnancy. Avoid antibiotics that are known to have an adverse effect on the fetus.

RECTUS SHEATH HAEMATOMA

Occasionally, a spontaneous haematoma occurs in the rectus sheath as a result of spontaneous haemorrhage from the inferior epigastric vessels in pregnancy. A tender mass appears in the abdominal wall. Treat the condition conservatively.

FURTHER READING

Berek JS, Hacker NF 2000 Practical gynecologic oncology, 3rd edn. Lippincott, Williams and Wilkins, Philadelphia
Burghardt E, Monaghan JM 1989 Operative treatment of ovarian cancer. Best Practice & Research Clinical Obstetrics and Gynecology 3:1–215
Hudson CN, Setchell ME 2004 Shaw's textbook of operative gynaecology, 6th edn. Elsevier, New Delhi
Setchell ME, Cass PL 1990 In: Williamson RCN, Cooper JM (eds) Emergency abdominal surgery. Churchill Livingstone, Edinburgh
Shaw RW, Soutter WP, Stanton SL 1997 Gynaecology, 2nd edn. Churchill Livingstone, Edinburgh
Sutton CJ, Diamond MP 1998 Endoscopic surgery for gynaecologists. Saunders, Philadelphia

46

Ear, nose and throat

M.P. Stearns

CONTENTS

INTRODUCTION

Otolaryngological emergencies need to be managed on occasion by generalists. You may need to decide if that treatment can await later specialist care (e.g. a foreign body in the ear canal), or may even be unnecessary. Avoid acting inexpertly in such circumstances. Remember the maxim *'Primum non nocere'* (Latin: =First do no harm).

If a patient presents a challenge outside your personal experience but the operative techniques are familiar to you, then you may feel equipped to proceed if qualified aid is unavailable. If these conditions are not met, it may be wiser to accept the role of general practitioner and temporize. If you are a generally trained surgeon, lacking ENT training and with no ENT colleague at hand, you may find some of the procedures described are within your competence, such as incision of retropharyngeal abscess, removal of foreign bodies from the throat and relief of upper airway obstruction.

As a junior doctor faced with an ear, nose or throat condition in the Accident and Emergency Department, you may be able to remove a foreign body from the nose or ear and control nasal bleeding, and initial management of a fractured nose.

FOREIGN BODY IN THE EAR

Appraise

1 The patient, usually a child, may complain of pain in the ear if the foreign object is irritating or has caused infection in the external ear canal.

2 A live insect may cause noise in the ear.

3 Most foreign bodies in the external auditory canal are found by chance.

Action

1 Remove insects to relieve pain. Fill the ear with olive oil to asphyxiate it, or kill it with alcohol. Gently remove it by syringing the ear with water at body temperature.

2 Inanimate foreign bodies may yield to gentle syringing, but those that occlude, or nearly occlude, the meatus cannot be removed by syringing so they need to be extracted with an instrument. Commonly inserted small pieces of sponge rubber can be removed using crocodile forceps if they lie close to the external auditory meatus. Unless you are expert, do not attempt to remove solid foreign bodies, since you risk damaging the middle ear, including the ossicular chain. A general anaesthetic may be required.

3 If the child is co-operative, examine the ear in a good light, initially without, then with, an auroscope. When the child is relaxed and quiet, touch the foreign body with a fine probe to confirm its shape and texture. You may not need to insert an aural speculum to do this. Look for a graspable edge; if you can seize it with very fine Hartmann's crocodile forceps you may be able to remove it.

? DIFFICULTY

1. If the object is smooth and rounded, such as a bead, do not apply forceps; they cannot grasp the object, and risk pushing it deeper into the meatus, through the drum, ossicular chain, facial nerve and labyrinth.
2. The safest way to remove an occluding foreign body is under general anaesthesia, using an operating microscope. If this is not available, use illuminating loupes and the largest aural speculum the meatus will accept. Insinuate a stapedectomy hook beyond the object unless there is an obvious space above it, turn the hook to engage it, and ease it out by rolling or sliding. Alternatively, try the effect of using a small sucker.
3. *Golden rules*:
   - Do nothing that could push the foreign body further into the ear canal.
   - Pass hooks or probes anteroinferiorly, where the obliquity of the tympanic membrane allows you to insert the instrument more deeply without risk of injury.

REMOVAL OF NASAL FOREIGN BODY

Appraise

1 Suspect a self-inserted foreign body in any young child with unilateral nasal discharge, which is usually foul smelling, obstruction or bleeding.

2 The foreign body is commonly a screwed-up fragment of paper, vegetable matter, a plastic or metal bead, or plastic sponge.

Prepare

1 As with aural foreign bodies, first gain the child's co-operation. You may succeed if the foreign body is graspable and if you have appropriate instruments, clear visibility, a headlight, and are skilful in using a nasal speculum. If any of these are lacking, it needs to be removed under general anaesthesia by a specialist with oral, not nasal, intubation.

2 Ask the anaesthetist to avoid inflating the lungs with a face-mask, since this could force a nasal foreign body backwards.

3 Alternative positions:

- Place the patient in the tonsillectomy position which is supine with the neck extended. Use a Boyle–Davis gag to prevent the foreign body slipping backwards into the nasopharynx, where it will stay because this is the most dependent part.
- Alternatively, insert a firm oropharyngeal pack around the tube to entrap the foreign body if it slips backwards. Have the head of the table raised so that you can look along the floor of the nose.

4 If the object is graspable use fine forceps, otherwise use a small hook that can be passed above the foreign body, easing it downwards and forwards for delivery.

KEY POINT Do not operate 'blind'

- Retain full visibility throughout.

MANIPULATION OF FRACTURED NOSE

Appraise

1 Realignment of displaced nasal bones is not only a cosmetic operation. Nasal fractures are frequently associated with nasal obstruction and many nasal fractures have an associated fracture of the nasal septum.

2 Nasal fractures may be associated with other facial injuries such as a fractured maxilla or 'blow-out' fracture of the orbit. Do not fail to examine the patient for other facial injuries.

3 Try to manipulate nasal fractures within 2 weeks of the injury. The most suitable times to do so are either very early, before there has been much nasal swelling, or after about 5–10 days to allow much of the swelling around the fracture site to subside. If you try to manipulate the nasal bones while there is much swelling, it is difficult to see whether or not the nose is straight.

Action

1 It may be possible to straighten the nose by digital pressure, easing the nasal skeleton back into the midline. You can often manipulate it without anaesthesia within the first hour or two after injury. Alternatively re-align the nasal bones under local anaesthesia. You may feel a click as the fragments move into place.

2 If you cannot reduce the fracture in these ways you need the aid of general anaesthesia.

KEY POINTS General anaesthetic precautions

- You must either have the patient intubated or have the facility of using a laryngeal mask.
- Without these precautions sudden heavy bleeding into the airway puts the patient at great risk.

3 First, attempt manual reduction, pressing with your thumbs against the more prominent of the nasal bones. If this succeeds, over-reduce the fracture, and then mould the mobilized fragments into the desired symmetry.

4 If this fails, insert one blade of a Walsham's forceps into the nostril and grasp one nasal bone. The rubber cuff on the other blade of Walsham's forceps should lie on the skin, protecting it from damage by the forceps. Rotate and displace the nasal bone laterally to disimpact the fractured nasal bone. Then grasp the other nasal bone with the other Walsham's forceps and rotate it laterally also. The nasal fragments are now mobile and can be centralized with digital moulding. Take great care to protect the skin from injury during manipulation with these instruments.

5 If the septum is displaced, or the bridge-line is depressed, pass the blades of Asche's forceps into the nostrils, grasp the septum, and bring it into the midline, while lifting up the dorsum.

KEY POINT Gentleness

- Use only minimal force or the nasal mucosa will be torn, causing bleeding which may even requiring nasal packing.

Postoperative

1 If the reduced fracture is stable do not cover it with a splint.

2 Grossly comminuted, unstable fractures require a plaster-of-Paris splint secured with adhesive strapping. Mould the splint and the underlying nose beneath, while the plaster sets. Leave the splint in place for 7 days.

FOREIGN BODIES IN THE THROAT

Appraise

1 Fish bones lodge at any level, often in the tonsil or vallecula (diminutive of Latin: *vallis*=valley). More substantial bones (e.g. from chicken, rabbit or chops) usually stick in the postcricoid region or upper oesophagus.

2 Rarely, occluding foreign bodies such as sweets or a meat bolus can cause airway obstruction, leading to sudden death.

3 Dentures, which are often broken, impact in the mid-oesophagus.

4 A benign or malignant stricture may become occluded by a small bolus, such as a pea or piece of potato.

Action

1 Inspect the throat carefully, using a headlight and tongue depressor. Look for the tip of a buried fish bone in the tonsil or base of tongue. Remove it with a fine pair of angled forceps, if necessary anaesthetizing the throat with a lidocaine topical spray.

2 If you cannot see the foreign body directly, use a laryngeal mirror, in the same manner as in indirect laryngoscopy, to examine the back of tongue and laryngopharynx. You can often retrieve a bone in these sites under indirect vision, using angled forceps. Have the patient grasp his own tongue with a gauze swab and draw it forward as far as possible. Hold the mirror in your non-dominant hand and the forceps in your dominant hand.

KEY POINT Do not operate 'blind'

- You must grasp the foreign body in the forceps under vision or you risk causing serious damage.

3 If on examination with a mirror you see the foreign body deep in the pyriform fossa or postcricoid space, or if a radiograph demonstrates that it is in the hypopharynx or upper oesophagus, then you need to remove it by direct endoscopy under general anaesthesia. Use a laryngoscope or short oesophagoscope and suitable forceps to bring the foreign body into the lumen of the endoscope. Take care not to push a sharp object through the visceral wall. Try to rotate it so that its most traumatic aspect is disimpacted and either trails harmlessly or can be drawn within the endoscope as it is withdrawn.

? DIFFICULTY

1. Do not attempt to remove a denture bearing exposed sharp hooks from the oesophagus. Safe removal may be facilitated by passing a cutting forceps through the endoscope and cutting the denture into pieces.
2. In some cases the foreign body can be removed safely only by thoracotomy and oesophagotomy (see Ch. 33).

INCISION OF QUINSY (PERITONSILLAR ABSCESS)

Appraise

1 Suspect the diagnosis of quinsy (Greek: *kynos*=dog+*anchien*= to throttle) or peritonsillar abscess from a history of an extremely sore throat in a toxic patient. The patient has trismus (Greek: *trizein*=to grate, gnash) and dysphagia for solids and liquids, often with drooling because swallowing saliva is too painful.

2 Although inspection may be difficult because of the trismus, a swelling of the soft palate may be seen in association with a contralateral tonsillitis.

3 Although incision of peritonsillar abscess is frequently described in textbooks, it is rarely performed because it usually responds to versatile systemic antibiotics. Treat early disease with high dosage given intravenously, and reviewed after 24–36 hours. Incise it only if the swelling is not subsiding or if there is a fluctuant peritonsillar abscess.

Action

1 Inject local anaesthetic into the palatal mucosa at the intersection of a horizontal line through the base of the uvula with a vertical line along the anterior pillar of the fauces. Preferably use a dental syringe and needle with 2% lidocaine and 1:80 000 adrenaline. Allow at least 5 minutes for it to take effect.

2 Use a Bard–Parker handle with a no. 15 blade which can be wrapped in adhesive tape with the last 1 cm only exposed, preventing too deep penetration of the pharynx. Insert the knife blade backwards through the mucosa to a depth of 1 cm (Fig. 46.1). When pus gushes out, widen the track with sinus forceps.

3 Take a swab for culture. Quite often, however, no pus is obtained, because the quinsy is not sufficiently mature.

KEY POINT Caution

- Do not insert the blade more deeply than 1 cm, or you risk damaging the internal carotid artery.

4 As an alternative to incising the abscess use a large-bore hypodermic needle. You can dispense with local anaesthesia.

INCISION OF RETROPHARYNGEAL ABSCESS

Appraise

1 As a cause of acute illness with respiratory obstruction in infants and toddlers, this abscess tends to be to one side of the midline.

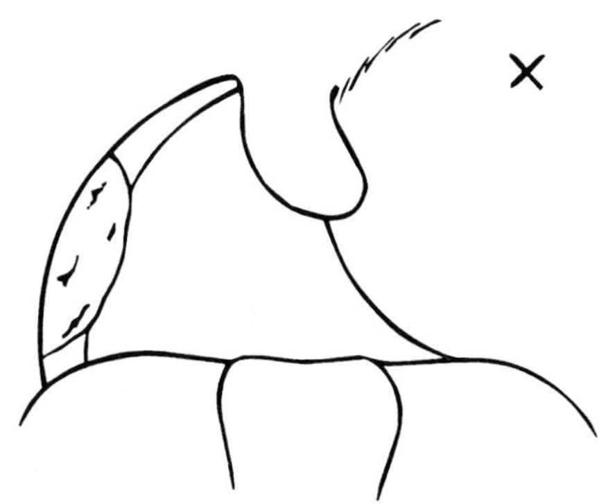

Fig. 46.1 Quinsy. 'X' shows the point of incision.

2 In older patients the abscess may be truly prevertebral, strictly midline and, usually, tuberculous in nature, secondary to tuberculous osteomyelitis of a cervical vertebra, in which case treatment is not primarily surgical.

3 If significant respiratory obstruction develops in spite of intravenous versatile antibiotic treatment in a young child or infant, you should incise a pyogenic abscess.

4 Lateral retropharyngeal abscesses in particular are often associated with a foreign body. Consequently carry out a careful search for one when incising the abscess.

Action

Lateralized pyogenic abscess

1 Have the child anaesthetized by an experienced anaesthetist because, if the abscess is ruptured during intubation, the patient may inhale the pus. Have the patient held in a head-down position when being intubated and until the airway is protected by a cuffed endotracheal tube.

2 When the tube is in place the abscess contents can be aspirated with a per-oral needle. Alternatively, it can be incised through a pharyngoscope or using a Boyle–David gag.

3 Having incised the abscess send specimens of the abscess wall for histology and culture.

RELIEF OF UPPER AIRWAY OBSTRUCTION

Appraise

1 Immediately relieve respiratory obstruction from major facial or laryngeal trauma, laryngopharyngeal tumours and impacted foreign bodies.

2 Ensure that there is a clear airway of the patient is comatose. If necessary assist respiration with mouth-to-mouth breathing, Ambi bag, a laryngeal mask or endotracheal intubation. If necessary, ventilate the patient.

3 An obstructed airway can frequently be expanded using positive pressure by mouth-to-mouth respiration or through a face-mask or oral tube, thus providing an adequate passage for air or oxygen.

KEY POINTS Managing airway obstruction

- Identify the cause of obstruction.
- Eliminate the cause if possible.
- Or pass an endotracheal tube through or past it.
- Or perform laryngotomy or tracheotomy to get below the obstruction.
- A totally obstructed patient can be partially relieved by inserting one or more large-bore hypodermic needles through the cricothyroid membrane.

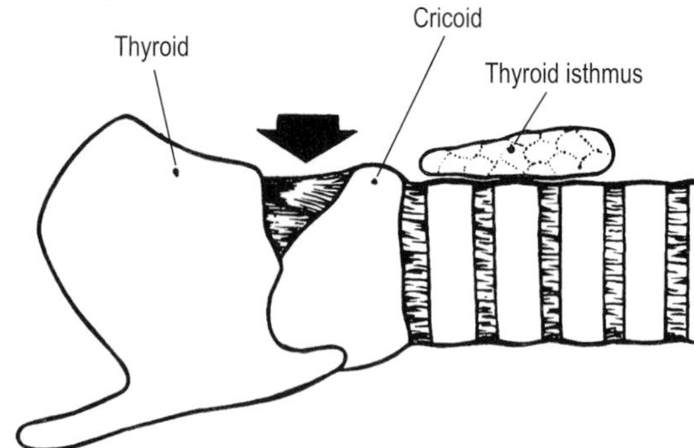

Fig. 46.2 Emergency laryngotomy: incision through cricothyroid membrane.

LARYNGOTOMY

1 Lie the patient supine with extended neck.

2 Make a horizontal stab incision between the cricoid and thyroid cartilages. Press the blade backwards until you feel the point enter the airway and air begins to hiss in and out through the wound with respiration (Fig. 46.2).

3 With no loss of time, remove the knife and insert a small tube, curved downwards, inside the tracheal lumen. A correctly designed laryngotomy tube is flattened somewhat, so as to lie neatly between the cartilages, but if none is available use any type of tube—metal, rubber or plastic—even unsterile, if it maintains the airway.

4 An improvised tube is difficult to keep in a correct position so control it manually until you can establish a stable airway.

5 Unless the cause of acute asphyxia is quickly curable by removing an impacted foreign body or reducing angioneurotic oedema, perform an elective tracheostomy within 48 hours and close the laryngotomy incision.

EMERGENCY TRACHEOSTOMY

Appraise

1 Always prefer laryngotomy to tracheotomy because can be performed more quickly, with less haemorrhage.

2 Rarely, if, for example, a subglottic lesion makes it impossible to perform laryngotomy and defies attempted incubation even through a rigid bronchoscope, you must perform emergency tracheostomy.

Prepare

1 Lie the patient supine with extended neck by placing a sand bag or a 1-litre bag of fluid for intravenous infusion beneath the shoulders. Ensure the head is in a central position.

2 Deliver oxygen by face-mask to give a few more minutes of operating time.

3 If there is time, inject local anaesthetic such as 1% lidocaine with 1:100 000 adrenaline (epinephrine).

Action

1 Cut vertically from the lower border of the thyroid cartilage in the midline, to the suprasternal notch. Deepen the incision and extend it between the strap muscles. Feel the first tracheal ring with the left index finger.

2 Then divide the thyroid isthmus to expose the anterior tracheal wall. Control bleeding, which can be profuse, by pressure from an assistant. Decide quickly whether there is time to clamp major bleeding points before incising the trachea vertically through the second, third and fourth rings.

3 Insert a tracheal dilator to secure an airway. Introduce a tracheostomy tube. A cuffed tube prevents further aspiration of blood and allows ventilation, but is slightly more difficult to insert.

4 Now control the worst of the bleeding. Use a tracheal suction catheter through the tube to clear blood that has already been aspirated into the trachea.

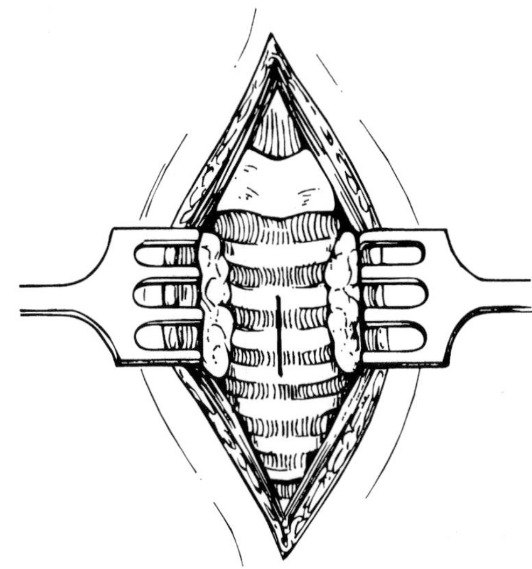

Fig. 46.3 Elective tracheostomy.

Postoperative

1 Subsequent decisions and procedures depend upon the cause of the obstruction and the patient's general condition.

2 Monitor respiration and pulse during, and for several hours after, such a crisis.

3 Institute assisted ventilation and/or cardiac resuscitation immediately postoperatively if necessary.

ELECTIVE TRACHEOSTOMY

1 This procedure is considerably easier to perform, in controlled conditions on an appropriately prepared and anaesthetized patient. Use either local or general anaesthesia.

2 Ensure that you have available a correct-sized tracheostomy tube. If it has a cuff, test it for leaks. If you intend to ventilate the patient, use a plastic cuffed tube, not a metal one. Check the patency and security of connections from tube to anaesthetic equipment.

Action

1 Inject the surgical area with a solution of 1:200 000 adrenaline (epinephrine) to help achieve haemostasis. Make a horizontal skin crease incision halfway between the cricoid cartilage and the suprasternal notch.

2 Separate the pretracheal muscles vertically and divide the thyroid isthmus between artery clips. Seal with diathermy the pretracheal vessels just below the cricoid. Ligate the inferior thyroid veins, since diathermy is unreliable. Ligate or oversew the edges of the thyroid isthmus and expose the anterior tracheal wall.

3 Having established haemostasis, make a 1–2-cm vertical incision, centred on the third or fourth tracheal ring (Fig. 46.3). Do not excise segments or cut flaps because there is a risk of subsequent stenosis. In addition, a tracheal flap may obstruct the passage of a tube.

KEY POINTS Avoid extubation

- If a patient is accidentally extubated and the tube cannot be rapidly replaced, fatal respiratory obstruction can occur.
- Insert a strong stitch through the cut tracheal edge on each side and leave the ends long, protruding through the skin wound. These can be used to draw the trachea forwards and open the incision in it, to facilitate the re-introduction of a tube. This is particularly useful in paediatric tracheostomies.

4 Hold the tracheal incision open with a tracheal dilator. Ask the anaesthetist to remove the endotracheal tube to the subglottic level. Now insert, for example, a cuffed plastic tracheostomy tube. Inflate the cuff just sufficiently to prevent leakage around it when the anaesthetist inflates the patient's lungs. Overinflation of the cuff can lead to subsequent tracheal stenosis. The anaesthetist can now connect the tubing to the tracheostomy tube and withdraw the endotracheal tube. Have the endotracheal tube left until now, so that if there is any difficulty in inserting the tracheostomy tube, or, if the cuff bursts, the anaesthetist can continue to ventilate the patient through the endotracheal tube.

5 Close the skin loosely around the tube. Loose suturing allows drainage of any blood and also helps prevent air emphysema around the incision.

Complications

1 Haemorrhage can occur from the thyroid isthmus and the inferior thyroid veins. Ensure that the surgical field is dry before closing up.

2 In young infants the brachiocephalic vein may rise above the suprasternal notch, so take care to avoid injuring it.

47

Oral and maxillofacial surgery

I.M. Laws

CONTENTS

GENERAL PRINCIPLES OF ORAL SURGERY

This chapter is limited to oral surgical procedures that you may need to perform when an appropriately trained colleague is not available. Whenever possible obtain the advice of a maxillofacial surgeon.

KEY POINTS Can you see and manoeuvre within the mouth?

- The oral cavity is small, dark, sensitive and has a slippery surface.
- Patients may be nervous. They may tend to move their tongue or close their mouth at an inopportune moment.
- Anxious patient? Consider giving intravenous sedation in adults.

Preparation

1 Ensure you have good illumination.

2 Arrange for adequate suction apparatus.

3 Make sure your assistant is efficient and can anticipate possible difficulties.

Anaesthesia

KEY POINTS Anaesthesia

- For general anaesthesia, an endotracheal tube and a throat pack are required to prevent inhalation of blood and debris.
- Remember to remove the pack at the end of the operation.

1 Most minor procedures such as tooth extraction, biopsy, removal of salivary calculi and suturing of lacerations can be carried out using local analgesia. Local anaesthetics are available in 2-ml glass cartridges, the most common of which contain 2% lidocaine with adrenaline. Use 3% prilocaine with felypressin for patients sensitive to adrenaline. These cartridges fit into a syringe with a disposable needle.

2 In the upper jaw, deposit 1.5 ml of solution over the apex or apices of the offending tooth on the buccal side and about 0.5 ml on the palatal side. In the lower jaw, a similar technique may suffice for the anterior teeth. For the posterior teeth, an inferior alveolar and lingual nerve block is required at the lingula of the mandible, along with a long buccal nerve block at the anterior edge of the ramus of the mandible. Regional nerve block can also be used in the maxilla but, before attempting this, refer to appropriate literature.

KEY POINTS Failure of local anaesthesia?

- Test the tissues at the operation site and ask the patient if the area feels numb.
- Adequate analgesia may not be achieved in the presence of inflammation.
- If so, try depositing a few drops of anaesthetic solution into the periodontal membrane of the tooth.

3 General anaesthesia is often preferable in the treatment of children, patients who have fluctuant abscesses and if there is a history of allergy to local anaesthetic.

4 Hold the jaws apart with a prop or gag and stabilize the head in a rubber ring or horseshoe. Do not dislocate the jaw or scuff the lips, which tend to be dry following preoperative anticholinergic drugs.

5 Lightly coat the lips with petroleum jelly or keep them moist.

Haemostasis

1 Remove excess clot. Suture tightly across the socket and repair any lacerations. Apply pressure with a gauze pad for 10 minutes, timed by the clock.

2 If bleeding continues, lightly press a resorbable haemostatic material, such as oxidized cellulose, into the socket.

3 Sit the patient up at least 45° and if necessary give a sedative.

4 Control secondary haemorrhage with pressure, treat infection with systemic and/or local antibiotics and prescribe 6% hydrogen peroxide mouthwashes.

5 Treat medical causes for prolonged bleeding appropriately, such as haemophilia, thrombocytopenia or hepatic cirrhosis. Give haemophiliacs and patients taking warfarin 5% tranexamic acid as a mouthwash. Flush the socket with the liquid then insert

some oxidized cellulose and suture the socket. Prescribe the mouthwash four times a day for 5 days.

6 If the prothrombin time is within the normal therapeutic range, you need not stop the warfarin in order to remove only a few teeth.

KEY POINTS Post-extraction haemorrhage?

- Post-extraction bleeding is often due to torn mucosa or unsupported mucosa.
- Did you identify and correct pre-existing medical causes of bleeding?

Suturing

1 Use a half-circle 22–24-mm needle with a reverse cutting edge.

2 Use 000 sutures. Silk is easy to use but must be removed. Nylon is uncomfortable and also needs to be removed. Polyglactin 910 remains intact in the mouth for 3–4 weeks and produces minimal reaction but the knots and ends are irritating.

3 Use a needle-holder with a ratchet to avoid dropping the needle into the pharynx.

4 Insert the needle into the mucosa 3–5 mm from the edge, taking greater care on the more friable lingual edge.

5 The mucosal edges can rarely be approximated over a socket without excessive removal of bone. If you wish to apply even tension, insert mattress sutures.

6 Tie knots with the needle-holder rather than fingers. This is easier if you keep the end of the suture material short.

7 Remove non-resorbable sutures after 5–7 days.

Aftercare

1 Warn the patient that, until healing is complete, there may be constant discomfort because of the need to eat, swallow and speak.

2 If necessary prescribe moderate analgesics. Aspirin mixture, used as a gargle, relieves a sore throat caused by an endotracheal tube and packing and ensures more comfortable swallowing. Ice packs applied to the skin for the first 4–6 hours reduce the swelling and subsequent discomfort.

3 Advise the patient that there may be difficulty in opening the mouth wide, chewing may be painful so that a soft diet may be beneficial.

4 Patients who have had their fractured jaws fixed together require special care in the early postoperative hours to avoid inhaling vomit. Swallowed blood may cause vomiting. To avoid this ensure that the stomach is empty preoperatively and administer an anti-emetic. Keep a suction machine and wire-cutters by the bedside and show the nurses which wires to cut in an emergency.

5 When carrying out an operation on bone, many surgeons prescribe prophylactic antibiotics.

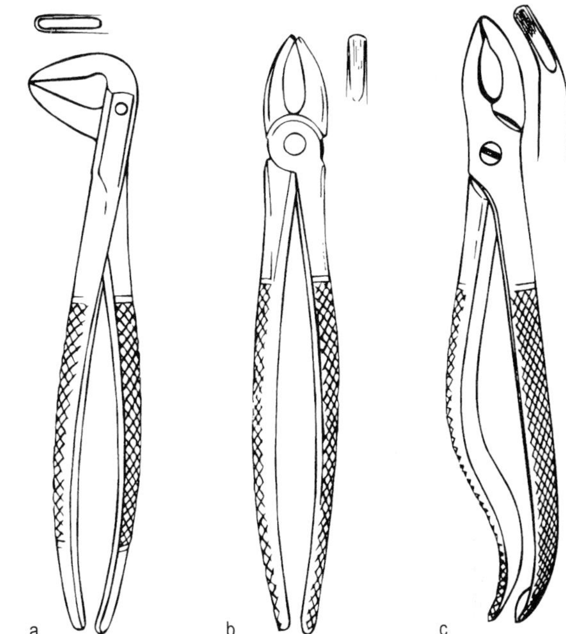

Fig. 47.1 Extraction forceps: (a) for mandibular teeth; (b) for maxillary anterior teeth; (c) for maxillary posterior teeth.

TOOTH EXTRACTION

Appraise

1 Is the extraction urgent or will antibiotics give relief until a specialist is available?

2 Tooth removal is indicated when there is a large cavity in a painful tooth, a painful loose tooth resulting from periodontal infection, an alveolar abscess or a loose tooth following trauma that could be inhaled.

Prepare

1 Extraction forceps: there are three basic pairs (Fig. 47.1), although many more specialized forceps are available.

2 Elevators (levers) enable you to remove broken roots or to loosen teeth before using forceps.

3 Prepare yourself by obtaining a radiograph before removing them to display unfavourable root patterns such as buried roots, impacted teeth and latent pathology.

4 As a rule have the patient seated, although the supine position is sometimes appropriate. Use local or general anaesthesia.

Action

1 Stand in front of the patient for most extractions. If you are right-handed, it is most convenient to stand behind the patient's right shoulder to remove lower right teeth.

2 Position the forceps blades on the buccal and lingual aspects of the tooth and push them under the gum as far as they will go along the root.

3 Grip the tooth and move it to expand the socket.

4 Deliver the tooth in the direction of the weakest wall—generally the buccal.

> **KEY POINTS Gently as possible**
>
> - Avoid excessive force or you will fracture the jaw.
> - Tooth extraction varies enormously in difficulty and root removal can be unexpectedly complicated.

5 Squeeze the socket with your fingers to reduce the dead space and position a gauze pad for the patient to bite on until the clot has formed.

6 Instruct the patient to avoid touching the clot for 24 hours, then bathe the wound frequently with warm saline until it heals.

7 Leave small broken roots but attempt to remove large superficial roots using fine forceps or elevators.

8 If possible, refer patients with unerupted or impacted teeth to a specialist. Extraction may necessitate removing sufficient bone to allow elevation of the tooth. Use a chisel or drill to remove the bone.

Aftercare

1 Inspect the socket if infection and pain develop a few days following extraction.

2 If the blood clot has disappeared, the empty socket fills with debris and pus.

3 Syringe out the socket and insert an antiseptic which usually cures the osteitis. Although the socket closes slowly, a protective epithelial layer soon covers it.

JAW INFECTIONS

DENTAL ABSCESS

1 Once pus has escaped from bone, its direction of spread is influenced by gravity and muscle attachments.

2 Antibiotics given before there is significant fluctuation may suppress it.

3 Order radiographs.

Action

1 If there is no swelling, remove the tooth. Antibiotics are rarely required.

2 Treat a non-fluctuant swelling with antibiotics. The bacteria may be anaerobic.

3 Remove the source of infection if you can provide adequate anaesthesia.

4 When the tooth is partly erupted, clean the underside of the gum flap with an antiseptic solution or 6% hydrogen peroxide.

5 A sharp upper wisdom tooth may traumatize the cheek or the gum over a lower tooth. Removal of the upper is usually simple and gives relief of pain until the more complex lower can be extracted.

6 When fluctuation is present in the mouth, remove an accessible tooth and incise the swelling in the buccal sulcus or palate to release pus that has not emptied into the socket.

7 Pus around the muscles of mastication produces trismus and prevents easy access to posterior teeth. This usually presents as a submandibular abscess. Under endotracheal anaesthesia, incise the skin of the neck at the most dependent point of the swelling and parallel to the lower border of the mandible. Extend the wound by blunt dissection then open up the loculi. Pass a pair of sinus forceps to the full depth of the cavity. Open the jaws of the forceps and remove them to enlarge the opening. Repeat this manoeuvre in a plane at right-angles to the original. In large cavities, the septae can be broken down with a finger.

8 Insert a drain for 24–48 hours. If the abscess is extensive, pass the drain from the skin through the abscess cavity and lingual mucosa into the mouth lateral to the submandibular duct. Draw it out of the mouth and fix it to the other end of the drain.

9 Remove the diseased tooth when the acute phase is over.

CELLULITIS

1 Cellulitis involving the sublingual and submandibular spaces and the cervical fascial plane is named Ludwig's angina after the German surgeon who described it. It is usually caused by streptococcal infection, making breathing and swallowing difficult.

2 Inspect an X-ray of the neck and mediastinum looking for gas bubbles.

Action

1 Administer parenteral penicillin which will produce rapid improvement in early cases.

2 If the infection is established, you may need to make multiple superficial incisions of the skin of the neck to relieve pressure on the glottis.

3 Perform tracheostomy if dyspnoea threatens. If the source of infection is accessible, remove it. If gas is present in the tissues, administer metronidazole.

OSTEOMYELITIS OF THE JAW

1 This rarely occurs in well-nourished populations.

2 The maxilla is not usually involved after infancy except in the immunocompromised.

3 Most patients respond to long-term treatment with antibiotic therapy, but if the infection persists operation may be required.

Action

1 In the acute phase, expose the lateral cortex of the mandible through a submandibular incision. Remove the cortex with a dental drill. If a large drill is not available, make multiple perforations and prise off segments with a chisel. Remove loose sequestra. Insert drains and close the wound.

2 In the chronic stage, expose the outer cortex of the mandible and dissect out the inferior alveolar neurovascular bundle. Remove the area of involved bone in a block and plan to graft

the defect at a later date. Gentamicin beads or foam may be helpful.

FACIAL SINUS

1 A sinus on the face, such as the chin, cheek or nasolabial fold, may be caused by a low-grade dental infection. Multiple or recurring sinuses suggest the possibility of actinomycosis.

2 Clinical and radiographic examination usually shows a tooth is involved.

Action

1 If the sinus is recent, remove the tooth.

2 Excise the sinus with an ellipse of skin if it is retracted. Encourage a small sinus to heal by cauterizing the track with a crystal of silver nitrate.

3 If you suspect actinomyces infection, give an antibiotic such as penicillin for 6 weeks.

FACIAL FRACTURES

Appraise

1 Facial injuries involve the nose, maxilla, zygoma and mandible. Fractures of the nose are dealt with in Chapter 46.

2 *Respiration*. Posterior and inferior displacement of the maxilla and blockage of the nose with blood clot causes respiratory distress. Bilateral fractures of the body of the mandible may result in lack of support for the tongue, which then falls back against the pharynx if the patient lies on his back.

3 Bleeding from facial injuries may appear copious but is rarely life-threatening. If there are signs of shock, check other injured sites such as ruptured internal organs and fractured limbs. Fixation of fractures reduces haemorrhage.

KEY POINTS Exclude other injuries

- Fractures of the skull and other bones are often associated with facial injuries.
- Cervical fractures are also often present.

Emergency action

1 Respiratory obstruction from displacement of the maxilla will be relieved by pulling the maxilla forwards with a finger hooked around the back of the palate.

2 Relieve obstruction following bilateral mandibular fractures by placing the patient in the recovery position. This allows the tongue to fall forward under gravity and prevents blood and debris from being inhaled. If necessary, insert a tongue stitch to pull the bulk of the tongue forwards.

3 Remove foreign bodies, such as broken teeth or dentures, from the mouth and pharynx. Plastic dentures are radiolucent and may not be apparent on a chest X-ray.

4 Unconscious patients with severe facial injuries generally require an elective tracheostomy.

5 Control persistent bleeding from the nose with posterior nasal packs.

Assess

1 Mandibular fractures are often bilateral. Unilateral condyle neck fractures may not require treatment if the occlusion can be maintained. Bilateral condyle neck fractures combined with a fractured maxilla may require complex treatment.

2 Most fractures through the tooth-bearing areas are compound.

3 Carefully look for deformity or loss of facial symmetry.

4 Assess the number and position of teeth, and note any wear facets, in order to determine if the relationships have been altered.

5 Note the proximity of a fracture line to apex of tooth as a devitalized tooth may become infected and delay healing.

6 Identify and record the presence and site of skin lacerations.

7 Test for sensory loss to assess the possibility of nerve damage, including loss of smell, indicating possible olfactory nerve damage.

8 Look for possible complications of fractures, such as diplopia and trismus.

9 Carefully check for cerebrospinal fluid leakage from the nose or ear.

Appraise

1 If the teeth meet correctly, the mandibular fractures are probably reduced.

2 Maxillary fractures need to be splinted to the skull or zygomatic arches if they are intact.

3 Intermaxillary fixation of maxillary fractures needs to maintained for 3 weeks and 4–6 weeks for the mandible.

4 Remove teeth if they are in the line of the fracture.

5 Give appropriate antibiotics.

6 Treat the patient under general anaesthesia unless the displacement is minimal.

7 If a general anaesthetic is administered remember to remove the throat pack before finally tightening the intermaxillary fixation.

8 Consider the need for anti-emetics and nasogastric tube gastric aspiration.

MANDIBLE

Appraise

Plating is rigid and reduces the need for intermaxillary fixation and time off work. The technique is not difficult but intraoral access can make it complex. The plates are placed across the fracture line and where possible along the known stress lines in the jaw. Titanium is more malleable than steel but is less rigid. Neither needs to be removed unless it becomes infected or exposed. The plate, drill, screws and screwdriver must be made of the same metal to avoid electrolytic action.

> **KEY POINTS Plating fractured facial bones**
>
> - Plating is the method of choice, but you should not attempt it unless you are properly trained in the various techniques and a specialist is not available.
> - The anatomy of the area may be distorted by haematoma and the displacement of bone fragments. Identify the large neck blood vessels which may have been displaced.
> - The inferior alveolar neurovascular bundle is easily damaged when manipulating the jaw or when drilling into the bone.
> - Avoid the roots of teeth and main nerves. Drilling or inserting a screw into a tooth root risks loss of vitality, loss of the tooth and infection in the fracture line.

Action

1 *Plating*:
- If appropriate, expose the fracture through the mouth or a skin laceration.
- Remove an unerupted posterior tooth if it is in the fracture line.
- Reduce the fracture.
- Apply temporary intermaxillary fixation to hold fragments accurately.
- Mould the plate to lie flush against the bone, with at least two holes on each fragment. In atrophic mandibles apply the plate external to the periosteum to minimize damage to an already compromised blood supply.
- Drill holes, starting with an end one.
- Insert screws (Fig. 47.2).
- Close the wound.
- Remove the intermaxillary fixation at the end of the operation for safety, replacing it for a few days when the patient is fully conscious.

2 *Eyelet wiring*. This may be possible when there are sufficient occluding teeth. Stretch soft, stainless steel wire of 0.5 mm diameter by 10%. Fold 15 cm of wire in half and bend round the shaft of a dental burr to form a loop in the middle. Pass the two ends between adjacent teeth so that the eyelet is on the buccal side. Separate the ends and pass them around each tooth. Thread one end through the eyelet and twist off with the other. The wire should be between the gum margin and the most bulbous part of the tooth (Fig. 47.3). When sufficient wires have been placed in both jaws and on all fragments, place the teeth in occlusion. Pass a tie wire through an eyelet in the lower jaw and one in the upper jaw and twist them together. Ensure the ends of the twisted wires are tucked between a pair of teeth to protect the lips and cheeks (Fig. 47.4). By convention all wires are twisted in a clockwise direction. Take care when using wires to avoid a needle-stick injury.

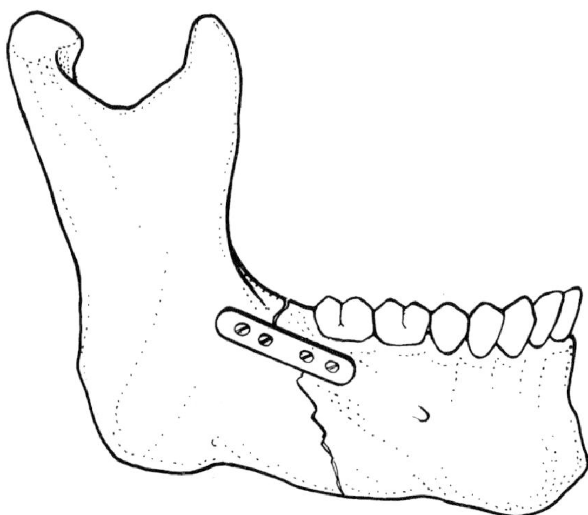

Fig. 47.2 Bone plate in position across mandibular fracture.

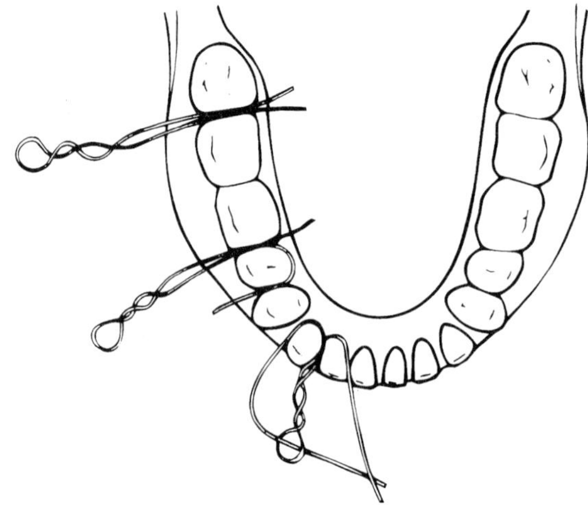

Fig. 47.3 Steps in the placement of eyelet wires.

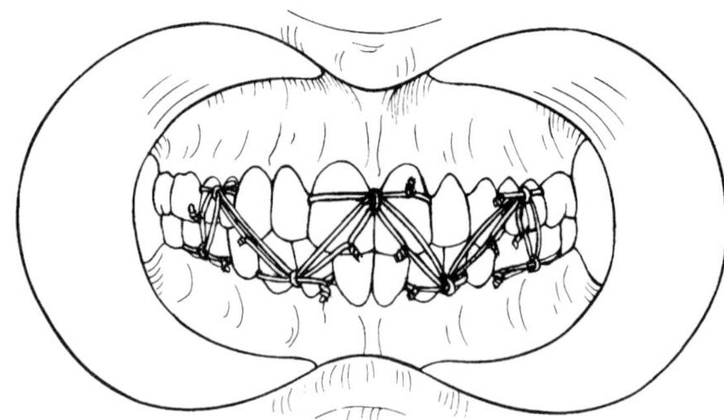

Fig. 47.4 Eyelet wires and intermaxillary wires in place.

3 *Arch bars*. These are an alternative to eyelets, especially when there are missing teeth. Commercially prepared bars are available with loops or cleats attached. Cut a sufficient length of bar and apply it to all the teeth in one jaw. The loops point towards the roots of the teeth. Fix the bar to the jaws with wire twisted round each tooth and the bar. Carry out a similar procedure in the other jaw. Place the teeth in occlusion and twist the wire around the opposing loops of the arch bars (Fig. 47.5).

4 *Gunning splints*. Use these for edentulous patients. Obtain the help of a maxillofacial technician. The splints are made from impressions of the patient's mouth or from dentures if available. The splints or dentures are wired to the jaws after reduc-

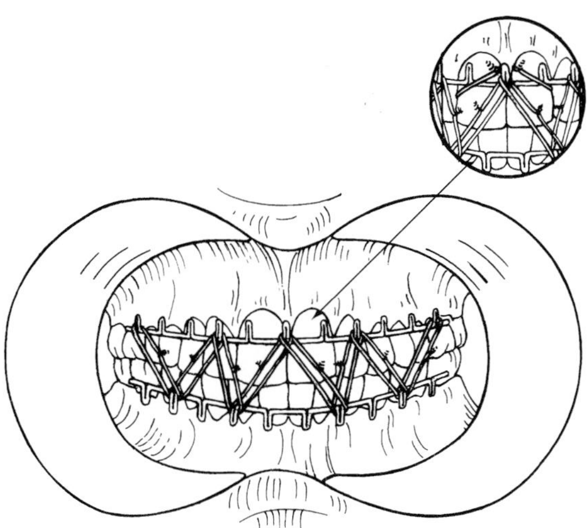

Fig. 47.5 Arch bars and intermaxillary fixation. The inset shows the intermaxillary wires and some of the wires fixing the arch bar to the teeth.

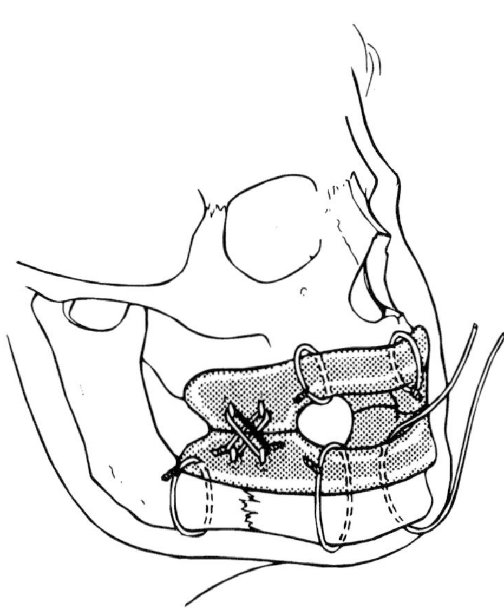

Fig. 47.6 Gunning splints fixed to jaws.

ing the fractures. The wires are passed round the splint and the mandible. In the upper jaw the wires are looped round the denture and through the alveolar ridge. A large hole in the palate of the splint makes this easier. The wires are placed using an awl with a hole near the trocar point in which the wire can be held (Fig. 47.6). Take care not to let the wire enter the fracture or damage the submandibular ducts.

5 *Barrel bandage*. This is normally used only as a temporary measure before the patient can receive the correct treatment. The bandage should be non-stretch material. Apply it to hold the lower jaw against the upper and not to pull the chin backwards (Fig. 47.7). Ensure there is adequate space for easy observation of the pupils and lips.

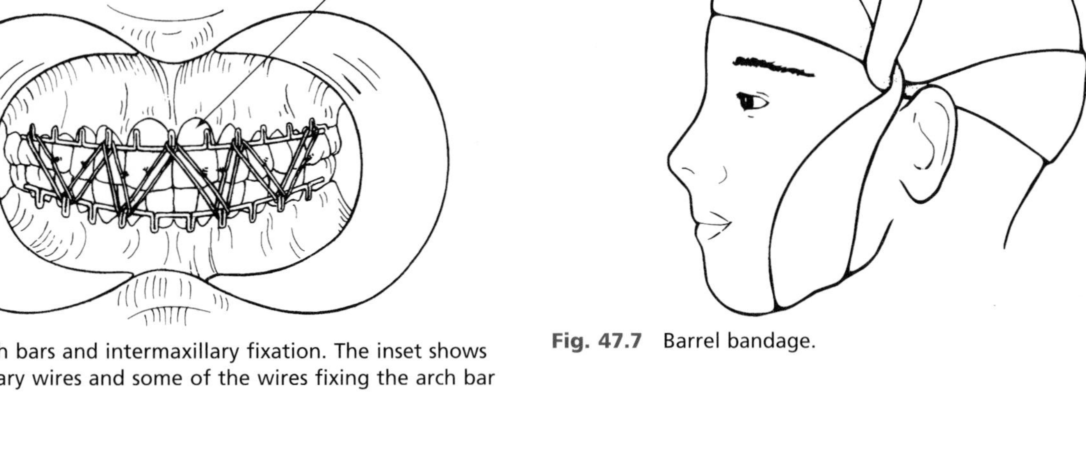

Fig. 47.7 Barrel bandage.

MAXILLA

1 A fractured maxilla is displaced posteriorly and inferiorly.

2 Disimpaction involves moving the maxilla in the opposite directions after freeing it with disimpaction forceps.

3 After disimpaction, fix the teeth in occlusion with a few wires round upper and lower teeth.

4 By applying pressure under the mandible, reduce the fracture between the maxilla and skull.

5 Cranial fixation is then normally applied.

? DIFFICULTY

1. Reduction of the fracture may be difficult because of impaction of the bones and oedema. Access is easier after 3–4 days when the oedema has subsided.
2. Inadequate reduction results in a concave profile that is difficult to correct.

Fixation

1 *Plating*. Do not embark on this unless you have had special training in the use of plates and are familiar with the anatomy of the maxilla and nose. Plates can be used to fix a fractured maxilla, reducing the need for intermaxillary fixation. They are placed across the fracture lines using a suitably shaped plate. The bone over the zygomatic buttress is thick and will hold a relatively long screw but the anterior wall of the maxilla is thin and the thread of the screw may strip the bone. Avoid placing a screw into the maxillary antrum or a tooth root. Metal plates can interfere with CT (computed tomography) scans. Titanium causes less interference and can be used round the orbit, on the frontal bone and nose.

2 *Halo frame*. This is easy to use, versatile and firm but you should not attempt to use it unless you have had special training. The same warnings apply to the use of pins and screws.

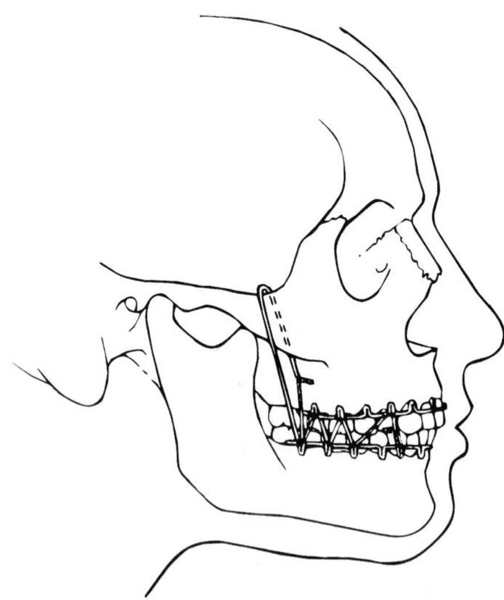

Fig. 47.8 Circumzygomatic wires fixed to arch bars on teeth.

3 *Internal fixation* may be within your capabilities. Using an awl or lumbar puncture needle, pass a loop of wire round the zygomatic arch and into the mouth in the molar region. Pass one end through an eyelet or round a cleat on splints or arch bar in the upper or lower jaws and twist it with the other end (Fig. 47.8).

Aftercare

1 Administer prophylactic antibiotics where there are compound fractures around the mouth. Consider giving a sulfonamide if you suspect cerebrospinal fluid leakage.

2 If you have used a general anaesthetic remove the anaesthetist's throat pack.

3 Patients with intermaxillary fixation need close supervision postoperatively in case they inhale vomit. Keep a suction machine and wire-cutters by the bedside and instruct the nurses how to use them.

4 Give anti-emetics at the end of the general anaesthetic.

5 Elastic bands are safer than wires for intermaxillary fixation but need replacement.

6 Give a fluid or semifluid diet. Six small meals are easier to take than three large ones.

7 Keep the mouth clean with mouthwashes in a syringe and a small toothbrush.

ZYGOMATIC COMPLEX (MALAR)

These are best treated within a week of injury, but allow excessive periorbital oedema to subside first.

Access

1 Use Gillies's temporal approach. Make a 2.5-cm incision in the hairline between the main branches of superficial temporal vessels. Cut nearly parallel to the zygomatic arch.

2 When you reach glistening temporalis fascia, incise it carefully to avoid damaging the temporalis muscle.

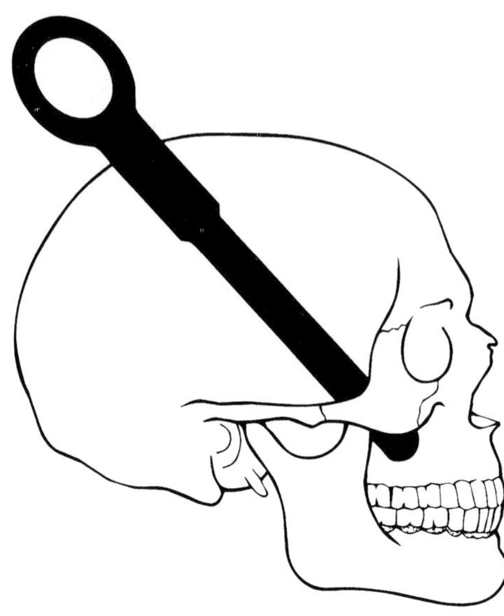

Fig. 47.9 Elevator under zygomatic arch.

3 Slide a Howarth's periosteal elevator or similar shaped instrument under the fascia until it is beneath the zygomatic arch. You should not feel any resistance until you reach the arch.

Action

1 Exchange the Howarth for a Bristow's elevator or one of the modifications (Rowe zygomatic elevator) and lift the displaced bone with an anterior and lateral motion. A slight lateral rotation may also help. Do not lever against the middle cranial fossa. The bone usually jams into place with a click (Fig. 47.9).

2 Suture the skin.

3 Mark the affected cheek and instruct nurses not to lay the patient on that side. Pressure on the bone at this stage may easily displace it.

? DIFFICULTY

1. The reduced fracture may be unstable. Do not attempt to insert plates or wires unless you are specially trained. If you attempt wiring, look for and protect the infraorbital nerve as it comes out of the foramen. The fracture often runs through it. Protect the eye when drilling the holes (Fig. 47.10).
2. Support can be provided by placing a pack into the antrum, but do not attempt to insert a pack into the antrum through a Caldwell–Luc approach unless you have had special training.
3. If there are trapped orbital contents and the patient displays marked diplopia with unequal pupil levels, you should make every effort to obtain specialist help and advice.

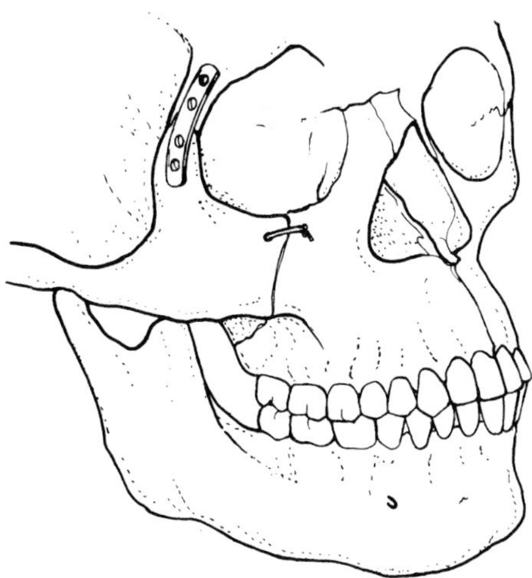

Fig. 47.10 Interosseous wires and bone plate in unstable zygomatic bone fractures.

FURTHER READING

Banks P, Brown A 2000 Fractures of the facial skeleton. Wright, Oxford

Burkitt HG, Quick CRG 2002 Essential surgery, 3rd edn. Churchill Livingstone, Edinburgh

Ferraro JW 1997 Fundamentals of maxillofacial surgery. Springer, New York

Hawkesford J, Banks JG 1994 Maxillofacial and dental emergencies. Oxford University Press, Oxford

Hutchison I, Lawlor M 1990 Major maxillofacial injuries. British Medical Journal 301:595-599

Kaban LB, Pogrel MA, Perrott DH 1996 Complications in oral and maxillofacial surgery. Saunders, Philadelphia

Langdon JD, Patel M 1998 Maxillofacial Surgery. Chapman & Hall Medical, London

McGowan DA 1999 An atlas of minor oral surgery: principles and practice. Martin Dunitz, London

Miloro M 2004 Peterson's principles of oral and maxillofacial surgery, 2nd edn. Marcel Decker

Moore UJ 2000 Principles of oral and maxillofacial surgery, 5th edn. Blackwell Science, Oxford

Moore JR, Gilbe GV 1991 Principles of oral surgery, 4th edn. Manchester University Press, Manchester

Pedlar J Frame JW 2001 Oral and maxillofacial surgery. Churchill Livingstone, Edinburgh

Robinson PD, Pitt Ford TR, McDonald F 2000 Local Anaesthesia in dentistry. Wright, Oxford

Ward-Booth P, Hausaman J, Schendel SA 1999 Maxillofacial surgery. Churchill Livingstone, Edinburgh

Wray D, Stenhouse D, Lee D et al 2003 Textbook of general and oral surgery. Churchill Livingstone, Edinburgh

48

Ophthalmology

J.D. Jagger, B. Mulholland

CONTENTS

INTRODUCTION

The procedures described here are semi-expert but do not require extraordinary technical skills. Appraisal of particular cases that might indicate the need for these procedures is likely to take place without the full examination facilities available to the ophthalmologist. On the other hand, they would be undertaken by the non-specialist only in emergency circumstances; these indications will perforce be obvious even on unsophisticated examination.

KEY POINT Anatomy

- Do not embark on ophthalmic procedures without first revising the anatomy.

Prepare

1 Many of the procedures described in this chapter can be carried out with small instruments available in a general surgical theatre.

2 Ideally, however, a selection of special instruments will render these eye operations easier to perform:

- *Lid specula*: right and left, guarded, to keep the eyelashes away.
- *Forceps*: plain (Moorfields); 1-in-2 (Lister's); 1-in-2 fine (Jayle's or St Martin's); 2-in-3 fixation forceps; iris forceps (Barraquer's).
- *Scissors*: straight iris scissors; blunt-nosed straight and curved or spring conjunctival scissors; corneal scissors; De Wecker's iris scissors.
- *Knives*: disposable knife for entry into the anterior chamber (Alcon or Becton Dickinson) or diamond knife if available; Bard Parker handles with no. 11 and 15 blades.
- *Needle-holder*: coarse (Castroviejo); fine (Barraquer's).
- *Sutures*: black silk 3/0, 4/0, 6/0; 4/0, 6/0; synthetic absorbable such as Vicryl 4/0, 6/0, 8/0; nylon 9/0, 10/0; all these are available on atraumatic needles.
- *Muscle hooks*.
- *Iris repositors*.
- *Eyedrops and ointments*: antibiotics are chloramphenicol 0.5% and ofloxacin drops 0.3%, and fusidic acid (Fucithalmic) ointment 1% in gel; local anaesthetic drops are tetracaine (amethocaine) 1% and cocaine 4%, or proxymetacaine 0.5% (does not sting).

REMOVING AN EYE

Appraise

1 The main indications for removal of an eye are irreparable injury with loss of sight, total or near total, severe pain in an already blind eye, or neoplasms such as a choroidal malignant melanoma that is too large for local irradiation.

2 There are two surgical approaches: enucleation and evisceration. In the former. the eyeball is removed from within Tenon's capsule—the sheet of connective tissue beneath the conjunctiva that covers both the eye and the insertion into it of the ocular muscles. In evisceration, the eyeball is not removed as a whole but the structural wall—the sclera—is left in situ, the contents being removed; access is obtained by removing the cornea.

3 Evisceration is often reserved for blind eyes with obvious gross intraocular infection but with no evidence of malignancy. Mobility of the prosthetic eye is better following evisceration than following enucleation.

ENUCLEATION

Prepare

1 Decide how sophisticated an operation you are going to do.

2 A general anaesthetic is usual but, in severely ill patients, local anaesthesia, including a retrobulbar injection (see Relief of pain), may be adequate.

Action

1 Sit at the head of the table and put in an eye speculum to separate the lids. Most specula are sprung. Keep the lids about 20 mm apart by tightening the screw.

2 Carry out a peritomy (incision of the conjunctiva around the rim of the cornea) by first opening the conjunctiva close to the

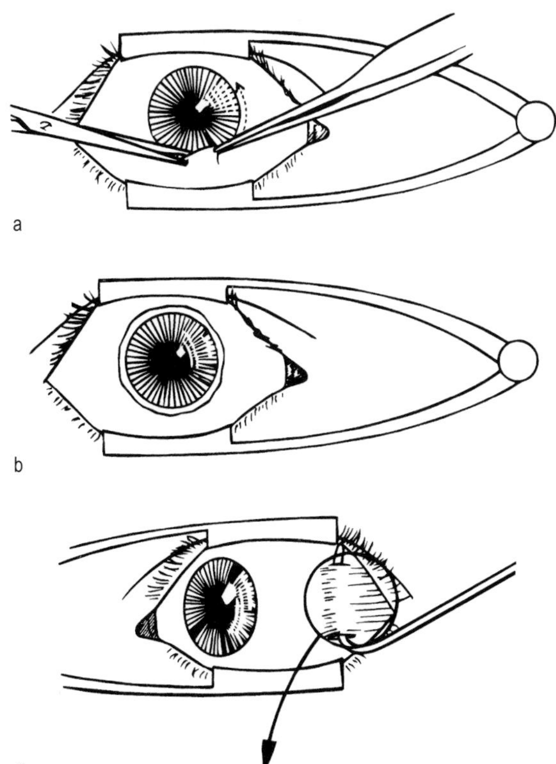

Fig. 48.1 Enucleation: (a) opening the conjunctiva; (b) conjunctiva freed; (c) tenting Tenon's capsule.

edge of the cornea. Pick up a fold at 6 o'clock on the corneal dial (Fig. 48.1a) with plain forceps (Moorfields) and cut it with sharp-pointed scissors.

3 Undermine both away from the cornea and towards the left (if you are right-handed), keeping close to the cornea. Cut the conjunctiva close to this edge, undermine some more and proceed snipping right round the cornea. The conjunctiva should now be free from the globe (Fig. 48.1b) and sufficiently undermined backwards for you to explore and open Tenon's capsule.

4 This is best done in the lower nasal quadrant, below the medial rectus muscle. If Tenon's capsule is thick you may not be able to see the muscles at all at this stage. If you have opened the correct part of Tenon's capsule you will expose the sclera. This is a lustrous grey-white colour, and you should satisfy yourself that you are really down to it by cutting away any other loose fascial planes (e.g. episcleral tissue) that can be picked up.

KEY POINT Bleeding?

- Achieve perfect haemostasis using bipolar diathermy forceps. Clear visualization is essential.

5 Next expose and cut off the extraocular muscles, starting with the medial rectus. Take a muscle hook and pass it upwards through the opening in Tenon's capsule, with its blunt point against the sclera deep to this muscle. Test that you have caught the muscle by pulling the hook anteriorly, when it will be stopped short at the insertion and will then move the whole eye. With the point above the level of the muscle, rotate the hook so as to tent Tenon's capsule (Fig. 48.1c).

6 Cut down on this and then brush back Tenon's fascia with a small swab so as to expose a length of the muscle tendon. Cut this off with blunt-nosed scissors, 3–5 mm behind the insertion, in order to leave a stump of muscle.

7 Through the gap in Tenon's capsule above the medial rectus, pass a hook laterally to engage the superior rectus and cut this off, using the same steps described for the medial rectus; then carry on round to the lateral and the inferior recti. Cut off the tendons of the superior, lateral and inferior recti flush with the globe instead of leaving a stump attached to the globe as was done with the medial rectus.

8 If you have any idea where the inferior and superior oblique muscles are, and they can be found, divide them. Usually, however, no formal search need be made for them as they can be dealt with as the globe is removed.

9 Once the rectus muscles have been dissected from the globe, test whether the globe rotates freely by grasping the stump of the medial rectus. If it does not do so, explore backwards beneath Tenon's fascia with blunt-nosed scissors and divide any structures that resist the rotation.

10 Next, dislocate the globe forwards. Loosen the screw on the eye speculum and, holding it so as to keep it about 25 mm apart, press it back towards the apex of the orbit (i.e. towards the floor). The eyeball should now come forwards with something of a jerk; its equator will be in front of the plane of the speculum. Now slightly close the speculum and tighten its screw so that the globe is kept in its forward dislocated position. This stretches its remaining attachments, making it easier to divide them.

11 Divide the optic nerve. There are special scissors for this, but any short, but tough, blunt-nosed scissors, preferably slightly curved, will do. First rotate the globe outwards by grasping the stump of the medial rectus with 2-in-3 fixation forceps. Probe the region of the optic nerve, which you cannot yet see, by passing the points of closed scissors from the nasal side to where it should be. Move the scissor tips up and down to feel the cord-like structure. Do this two or three times to make sure of its location. Now withdraw the scissors about 5 mm, open the blades widely enough to flank the nerve, then advance the blades to engage it, making sure you are far enough in to section the nerve with one cut.

KEY POINT Optic nerve section

- Avoid too flush a section of the nerve or, even worse, an amputation of the posterior pole of the eye.

12 While the scissors are in position embracing the nerve, dip them about 15° so that the tips of the blades go slightly deeper into the orbit. In this position close the blades, boldly cutting through the nerve.

13 The globe now comes forwards very easily. Trim away from it any remaining attachments such as the oblique muscles and posterior ciliary vessels, allowing you to remove it completely.

14 Bleeding is usually brisk at this stage so proceed immediately to pack the socket with gauze wrung out in hot saline. Keep two or three fingers' pressure on this for 1 minute. Inspect it then and reapply a fresh pack and pressure until bleeding stops. Direct haemostasis is virtually never needed. While applying pressure, inspect the enucleated eye for completeness of removal, especially in the region of the optic nerve. In the most unsophisticated enucleation, simply put on some antibiotic powder, line the conjunctival sac with tulle gras, cover the lids similarly and apply a pressure dressing—two eyepads and a crepe bandage. Fold the deeper pad double.

Suturing the conjunctiva and Tenon's fascia

Do this if it worries you not to do so. Always do it, however, if you implant anything in the orbit (see below). Use a continuous 8/0 synthetic absorbable suture, either in a continuous keyhole or over-and-over pattern; tie at each end.

Orbital implants

Modify your technique as follows.

1 Insert sutures into each of the rectus muscles before cutting them off the globe. If you intend to use an implant to which the muscles will actually be attached, use 6/0 synthetic absorbable sutures. If the implant is simply a ball (glass or plastic) then use 4/0 black silk.

2 The sutures should be 'whipped' or tied so as to give a better grip of the tendons (Fig. 48.2).

3 In all cases where an implant is to be used, dissect back under Tenon's capsule to make a definite layer that can be sutured over the front of the implant. The capsule, described by the Parisian surgeon in 1806, is the connective tissue sheath of the eyeball.

4 If a ball is to be used, after removing the eye and securing reasonable haemostasis, put the implant in and lift up the muscles by their silk sutures. Then sew a purse-string suture of 6/0 absorbable to close Tenon's capsule over the ball and include the muscle tendons in the purse-string. Remove the black silk sutures. Finally, close the conjunctiva as a separate layer with 6/0 or 8/0 synthetic absorbable suture.

5 If the muscles are to be attached to the implant, do this and then pull Tenon's capsule forwards to cover it. Dissect it well enough to avoid much tension. Sew up Tenon's capsule using a continuous 6/0 absorbable suture for both, starting with Tenon's right to left and then coming through to the conjunctiva proceeding left to right.

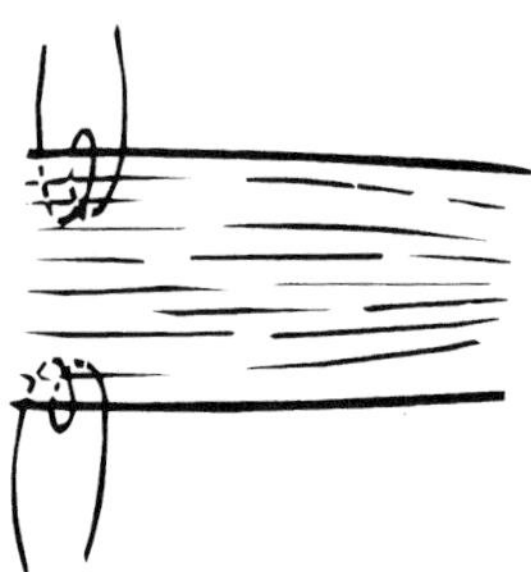

Fig. 48.2 Suturing the rectus muscles when using an implant.

> **KEY POINT Capsular closure**
>
> - Failure to close Tenon's capsule in a separate layer results in late extrusion and infection.

6 The best cosmesis is obtained by suturing the muscles to a hydoxyapatite orbital implant covered in polyglactin 910 mesh or a Vicryl ball implant covered in Mersilene mesh.

PROTECTING THE EYE: TARSORRHAPHY

Appraise

1 Stitching the lids together may be done either centrally, which of course obscures vision, or laterally, where the protection given is due to the shortening and consequent narrowing of the palpebral fissure.

2 Reserve central tarsorrhaphy for inability to close the lids (lagophthalmos) is a serious danger to the covering of the cornea, or when ulceration is actually present. This type of tarsorrhaphy is indicated also when severe or protracted ulceration occurs for other reasons, for example in a numb cornea.

3 In mild dysthyroid disease, and ectropion of the lower lid, in particular that occurring in facial palsy, a lateral tarsorrhaphy suffices.

Assess

1 First decide if a tarsorrhaphy proper is really necessary. Strapping the lids, or supergluing the lashes together, may well suffice if the protective covering is required for a short period only.

2 If strapping looks to be insufficient, a temporary tarsorrhaphy may be performed, sutures being inserted as detailed below but without denuding the surfaces of the lid margins.

3 If a bandage soft contact lens is available, try this, but copious lubricants and daily observation are required.

4 Temporary protection of the cornea can be achieved by inducing a ptosis. Inject 100 pg of botulinum A toxin into the levator palpebrae superioris through the upper lid, entering above the tarsal plate. Keep close to the orbital roof to avoid injecting the toxin into the superior rectus muscle, which would cause diplopia.

5 Superglue closure is dangerous to use except by experienced experts.

Action

1 In all cases, use local anaesthesia with tetracaine (amethocaine) 1% drops to the conjunctiva and 1% lidocaine with adrenaline (epinephrine) infiltration into the lid substance, both subcutaneously and subconjunctivally.

2 In tarsorrhaphy proper, raw surfaces of the lid margins are prepared. The easiest way to do this is simply to divide the lid into anterior and posterior layers through the 'grey line' (Fig. 48.3a). This is the midline of the edge of the lid between the roots of the eyelashes in front and the mouths of the meibomian glands

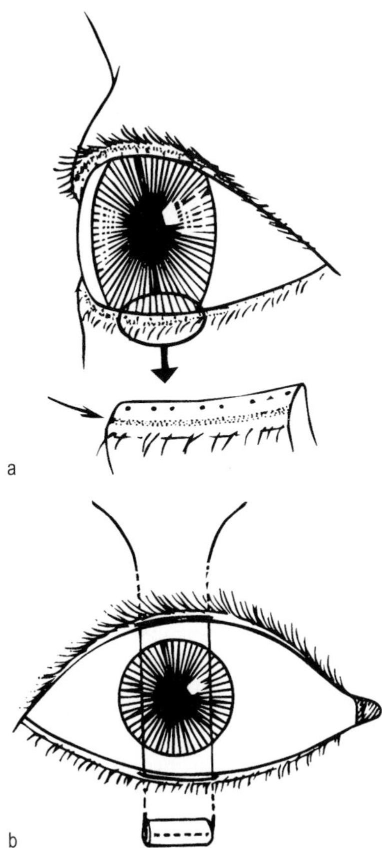

Fig. 48.3 (a) Tarsorrhaphy: (a) division through the 'grey line'; (b) inserting the sutures.

behind. The trouble is that in many patients it does not exist as a defined line, and when preparing the lid it is important to keep away from the roots of the lashes as this could distort them and lead to their growing inwards.

3 Start with the lower lid. Hold it up vertically with toothed forceps while an assistant holds it up with similar forceps some way along. Sink the blade (no. 15BP) of a scalpel in about 3–4 mm through the grey line in the plane of the lid, and take the cut the required length along the lid. If the initial stretch of lid grasped by yourself and your assistant is not long enough, both of you move along and continue the incision. Deal similarly with the upper lid opposite the raw area in the lower. In a lateral tarsorrhaphy make sure the two raw areas are continuous round the outer canthus.

4 Now insert the sutures (Fig. 48.3b). Use double-armed 4/0 black silk and pass the needle through the bore of a 3-mm length of rubber tube so as to prevent it cutting out. Grasp the edge of the lower lid with one blade of the toothed forceps in the raw area in the lid margin, the other in the substance of the lid 3–4 mm from the margin. Enter the needle through the skin 4 mm from the lid margin and come out in the raw area. Now grasp the upper lid similarly and pass this needle through the raw area and out on the skin 4 mm from the lid margin. Repeat this procedure with the other needle, entering the skin of the lower lid about 4 mm laterally or medially from the entry of the first.

5 Now pass one needle through a second similar piece of rubber tube and either tie it or, according to the length of lid closure required, put in as many more of these mattress sutures as are indicated.

6 Before tying, wipe away any clot from the raw edge of the lids. Do not buckle the lids when tying; moderately firm apposition is all that is needed as postoperative swelling will add further tension.

7 Put on antibiotic ointment and bandage the eye over paraffin gauze or non-adherent dressing and a pad only if bleeding has been excessive. Uncover the next day. Inspect again in a week and remove the sutures after 2 weeks.

EYELID INJURIES

1 Lacerations heal well, but there are important points to remember.

2 If the lid margin is involved, try to appose the edges as accurately as possible. Use 6/0 Vicryl for the skin but try to insert a suture of 6/0 silk through the lid margin itself. Enter the needle on one side through the grey line 2–3 mm from the cut edge, emerging in the latter a similar distance down the cut and then in reverse through the other edge. After tying the suture, leave the ends 3 cm long and strap them down, then check that they do not abrade the cornea. Use the skin sutures to tie over the long ends of the lid margin sutures to keep them out of the eye.

3 If the lids are widely split, suture the tarsal plate before tackling the skin. Do this with interrupted 6/0 absorbable stitches. Insert the sutures at 2-mm intervals, placing the knots anteriorly in the substance of the lid, not facing backwards where they will be uncomfortable and again may abrade the cornea.

4 In cases where the inner third of the lower lid is lacerated, or there is a deep horizontal cut of the upper lid, call in the experts immediately. Restoration of continuity of a possibly divided lower lacrimal canaliculus or levator repair is too specialized a procedure to be covered here.

5 Massive loss of the substance of the lids may give rise to an immediate problem of ocular (particularly corneal) protection. A protective contact lens may be indicated. Immediate plastic procedures may be advisable if possible, finishing with some form of tarsorrhaphy or even a purse-string conjunctival flap to protect the cornea. This creates a moist chamber. This entails making a circular incision around the ocular conjunctiva well away from the limbus, mobilizing the ocular conjunctiva off the sclera, then inserting a purse-string suture around the margin, drawing it together to form a closed chamber protecting the cornea.

INJURIES OF THE GLOBE

LACERATIONS

Appraise

1 *Conjunctiva*. Leave small cuts (less than 5 mm) alone. Suture larger ones under local anaesthesia with interrupted 8/0

synthetic absorbable at 4-mm intervals, removing any prolapsed Tenon's capsule if excessive, or burying it.

2 *Cornea and sclera*. Insert a speculum, and find and remove foreign bodies. Glass from windscreens is especially difficult. Put a drop of fluorescein in the eye; it may help to show small particles as well as corneal epithelial loss.

KEY POINT Foreign bodies

- For removal of metal foreign bodies, see page 701, but always X-ray a lacerated eyeball as a matter of routine.

3 If obvious foreign bodies are present in the anterior chamber only, attempt to remove them with the finest small-bladed forceps under high magnification after reforming the anterior chamber with Viscoelastic. Do this only during a procedure for a lacerated cornea. There is no substitute for Viscoelastic, so do not attempt to re-form the anterior chamber if none is available.

4 Cut off any prolapsed iris, ciliary body, lens remnants or vitreous. Pick them up with iris forceps and withdraw a little in an attempt to free them from an incarcerated position in the wound. Make a cut with De Wecker's scissors to remove the tissue, flush with the plane of the globe at the site of the penetration. Gently replace any intraocular tissue remaining in the wound, using an iris repositor. In an emergency, leave alone incarcerated material that is not prolapsed externally, particularly if the anterior chamber is not lost.

Closure

1 Wound closure varies in difficulty. Insert sutures into clean lacerations of less than 5 mm only if aqueous humour is leaking.

2 As a general surgeon you may not wish to undertake direct corneal or scleral suture. If you do undertake it, however, remember that, although the stitches should be almost full thickness, they must not penetrate into the eyeball (Fig. 48.4). Use magnification, if it is available, to ensure this.

KEY POINT Placing sutures

- You must place the stitches in, but not through, the tissue.

3 Enter and emerge about 1–1.5 mm from the wound edge. Grasp each edge lightly with the finest-toothed forceps you have, such as Jayle's, St Martin's, or finer. Use 9/0 or 10/0 nylon and keep the sutures in a line perpendicular to the wound. In suturing scleral wounds it may be necessary to dissect the conjunctiva back from the edge.

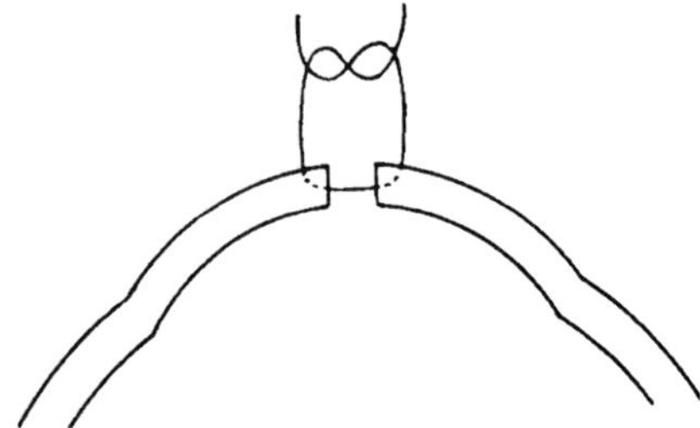

Fig. 48.4 Corneal and scleral sutures.

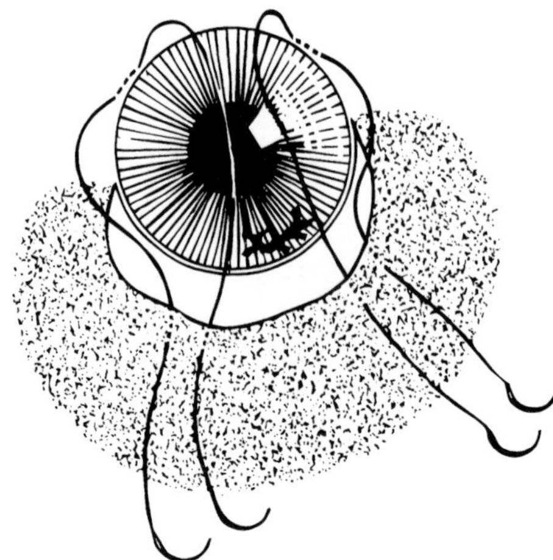

Fig. 48.5 Conjunctival flap.

4 It may, however, be unwise to attempt direct suture, either because you lack experience or because the wound is too irregular. In such cases, and particularly if the anterior chamber is shallow or absent, prefer to cover the wound with a conjunctival flap. In a corneal wound, for example, carry out a partial peritomy (see p. 697). Thus if, for example, the wound is in the 4 o'clock meridian, cut the conjunctiva at the limbus (Latin: =border; between the sclera and the cornea) from 1 o'clock to 7 o'clock in the lower left half of the globe (Fig. 48.5). If it is possible to choose the origin and direction of the flap, remember that the upper and temporal conjunctiva is the loosest and easiest to mobilize. Undermine the conjunctiva so freed back, for at least 15 mm. Insert one needle of a double-armed 8/0 absorbable suture in the paralimbal connective tissue at 8 o'clock and, using a second suture, do the same at 12 o'clock.

5 To insert these sutures, try to get a reasonable bite without going right through the sclera into the eye. Aim for a 2-mm track, parallel to and 1 mm from the limbus. To steady the eye use fine-toothed forceps such as Jayle's, to grasp the episcleral tissue close to the point of suture insertion.

6 Now put the two arms of one suture through the edge of the freed conjunctiva at an appropriate place and repeat this with the other suture. Figure 48.5 indicates suitable insertion points. Tie each suture while an assistant, using two pairs of plain forceps, draws the edge of the flap well over the site of the penetration. If the penetration is central, it should still be possible to cover it in this way.

7 Finally, give a subconjunctival injection of cefuroxime 125 mg in 1 ml of water. Supplement the injection with Mydricaine, if it is available, otherwise insert topical drops of atropine. Use a fine (25G) needle and give the injection by passing the needle tangentially through the conjunctiva in a horizontal direction 1 cm back from the limbus, into the quadrant opposite to that of the penetrating injury.

BLUNT INJURIES

EVACUATION OF HYPHAEMA

Appraise

1 Hyphaema (Greek: *hypo*=under+*haima*=blood; bleeding into the anterior chamber) is invariably treated conservatively initially, with bed rest and topical steroids to reduce the risk of further bleeding, such as dexamethasone (Maxidex) 0.1% four times a day. Cover the eye with a shield.

2 Paracentesis of the anterior chamber is therefore very rarely indicated. Undertake it only when:
- The anterior chamber is full of blood.
- There is a considerable rise in the intraocular pressure, which is unresponsive to acetazolamide (Diamox) and oral glycerol or mannitol infusions over a 3-day period.
- The patient is in severe pain.

Action

1 Anaesthetize the eye with topical 4% benoxinate, tetracaine (amethocaine) or cocaine drops given at 5-minute intervals. A general anaesthetic is unnecessary.

2 Insert an eye speculum. Have available a disposable or diamond knife, otherwise use a Bard Parker scalpel with a no. 11 blade.

3 Grasp the medial rectus muscle with a 2-in-3 forceps and gently lift the eye ceiling-wards, to fix its position. Hold the knife like a pencil and steady your hand by placing your fourth and fifth fingers on the patient's temple. Pass the tip of the blade through the cornea 2 mm inside the limbus (corneoscleral junction) with the plane parallel to the presumed plane of the iris, which you cannot see.

KEY POINTS Correct plane

- Keep in the plane of the limbal 'ring' (the corneoscleral junction; Fig. 48.6).
- Enter at 3 o'clock or 9 o'clock on the corneal dial.

4 You cannot see the tip of the knife once it is within the anterior chamber because it disappears in blood. Do not push on any further than 2 mm once this happens. Withdraw the knife gently but rapidly in its own plane. If you withdraw it correctly, nothing escapes from the anterior chamber even if the ocular tension is very high.

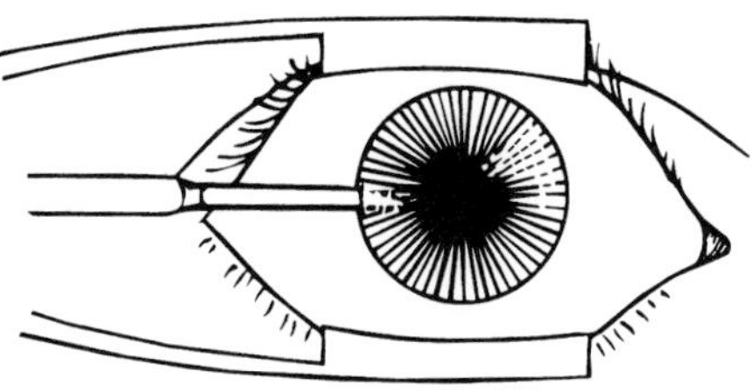

Fig. 48.6 Evacuation of hyphaema. Fixation of globe not shown.

5 Now press gently on the posterior (peripheral) lip of the incision and some bloodstained aqueous should escape. Do not press for longer than a second at a time initially, since a rapid drop in intraocular pressure may re-start the bleeding. Repeat intermittent pressure until you note some clearing of the anterior chamber. Do not persist until all blood has been evacuated.

6 Inject subconjunctival cefuroxime, remove the speculum and cover the eye with a plastic shield.

7 Very little blood may appear if the anterior chamber contains a solid clot. You may try the effect of urokinase irrigation but this is speculative.

8 Paracentesis is also a standard emergency procedure for arrest of the retinal circulation (central retinal artery occlusion). Carry it out within 2–3 hours of the onset. This condition justifies a much more rapid evacuation of the clear normal aqueous humour.

RUPTURED GLOBE

Appraise

1 A totally disrupted eyeball may require enucleation, either immediately or within a few days of the injury, and the same applies to badly lacerated and collapsed eyes.

2 Take the decision for enucleation, bearing in mind the possibility of the dreaded complication of sympathetic ophthalmia. Months, or even years later, the unaffected eye develops panuveitis with sight-threatening sequelae including glaucoma and cataract.

3 Smaller posterior ruptures with some preservation of function may be diagnosed by the finding of a deep anterior chamber and chemosis from loss of the vitreous humour. An ophthalmic surgeon might explore the eye. You should manage the rupture conservatively.

FOREIGN BODIES

Appraise

Intraocular foreign bodies

KEY POINTS Management

- These require specialist intervention if it is available.
- It is important that you recognize the possibility of the condition.

1 A foreign body is easily missed when the entry wound is small and the initial disturbance minimal.

2 If there is a history of something going into the eye, especially while hammering and chiselling, and you cannot detect a foreign body on superficial inspection, promptly order an X-ray of the orbit.

3 Most small intraocular foreign bodies are sterile. Be willing to wait if this allows more favourable conditions for treatment.

4 A large foreign body may cause a penetrating injury that requires to be dealt with in itself.

Subtarsal foreign bodies

1 Remove these by everting the upper eyelid after instilling proxymetacaine, tetracaine (amethocaine), oxybuprocaine or cocaine. Have a cotton-wool swab to hand before starting. Ask the patient to look down and keep doing so. Grasp the upper lid lashes with the thumb and forefinger of one hand and pull the lid down and forwards. With an orange stick, press the upper edge of the tarsal plate downwards (some 4 mm from the lid margin) and then lift the lashes so as to rotate the lid over the orange stick, which pushes the tarsal plate down and under the lid margin at the same time.

2 Once the eyelid is everted, keep hold of the lashes and press them against the eyebrow, instructing the patient meanwhile to keep looking down. Remove the orange stick and use your freed hand to remove the foreign body with the cotton-wool swab. Return the lid to its normal position by withdrawing both hands and asking the patient to look up.

Corneal foreign bodies

1 If you suspect the foreign body to be deep within the cornea, manipulation may push it into the anterior chamber. Unless you are expert, with available equipment, avoid tackling it.

2 Superficial corneal foreign bodies can be removed after anaesthetizing the eye. Make sure you have a good light focused on the cornea, and magnification.

3 Very superficial foreign bodies may be brushed off with a cotton-wool swab. Embedded foreign bodies require to be needled out. Insert a 19G disposable needle tangentially to the cornea to get behind the foreign body. Do not insert the needle directly at the foreign body but enter the cornea a little to the side. Lever the foreign body out. If any rust is left behind, attempt to pick it out, but do not persist too long. Rust that is slight and milk-chocolate in colour will disappear itself. Remove as much dark rust as can be delivered easily. You may be able to remove more after a few days of softening up, inserting chloramphenicol ointment, three times a day.

4 Pad the eye after putting in an antibiotic ointment. Put in a mydriatic drug (a pupil dilator) according to the degree of required manipulation. If it was easy, no mydriatic is required; if it was moderately easy, homatropine 2% drops suffices; if it was very difficult, insert atropine 1% drops. Monitor the patient daily until it has healed and no longer stains with fluorescein.

BURNS

1 *Chemical burns*. Immediately concentrate on removing any matter mechanically and, in particular, copiously irrigate the eye using any harmless fluid you have at hand. Do not hunt for specific antidotes. If the cornea is affected, apply antibiotic/steroid ointments such as Maxitrol, containing dexamethasone 0.1%, neomycin sulphate 0.35%, hypromellose 0.5%, polymyxin B sulphate 6000 IU drops, or Sofradex containing dexamethasone 0.05%, framycetin sulphate 0.5% and gramicidin 0.005% drops, and atropine. Keep the conjunctival fornices patent to prevent symblepharon (Greek: *syn*=together+*blepharon*=eyelid; adhesion of the eyelids to the eyeball), by twice-daily passing a glass rod between the lids and the eyeball after anaesthetizing the eyeball with oxybuprocaine 0.4% (Benoxinate) or tetracaine (amethocaine) hydrochloride 0.5% drops. Always admit patients with lime burns for observation as the effects may be delayed and you may need to institute half-hourly drops including vitamin C in high dosage. Also encourage the patient to eat citrus fruits, since vitamin C is an antioxidant and a cofactor in collagen synthesis.

2 *Thermal burns*. Treat those affecting the lids as skin burns elsewhere, but problems of ocular protection may arise. If there is loss of skin following a thermal burn, the ocular surface may also be severely damaged by the injury. If there is exposure of the cornea, apply lubricants such as hypromellose 1.0% and try to produce a moist chamber. In the longer term it will be necessary to reconstruct the lids using tissue from elsewhere, such as skin from behind the ear and hard palate grafts to recreate the tarsal plate.

INFECTIONS AROUND THE EYE

PYOGENIC INFECTIONS

Appraise

1 These usually arise in the lids. A stye is an infection of a sebaceous gland of the lid. Meibomian cysts, described by the German physician Heinrich Meibom in 1666, result from inflammation of glands on the under surface of the lids. Inflammation in the tear ducts—the lacrimal (Latin: *lacrima*=tear) apparatus—is termed acute dacryocystitis (Greek: *dacryon*= tear). Rarely, cellulitis within the orbit may point.

2 Avoid incision wherever possible but, in the presence of a tense abscess causing pain, release it.

3 A local anaesthetic may not be necessary for treating acute dacryocystitis if it is obviously pointing. Incise it from below the inner palpebral (Latin: =eyelid) ligament/medial central tendon, downwards and outwards for 15 mm, parallel to the orbital margin. You do not need to drain it.

4 Infections of the eyeball itself may be localized, as for example a pyogenic corneal ulcer, or widely disseminated, as when a metastatic infection lodges in the choroid, spreading thence to the vitreous and all parts of the eye.

5 A corneal ulcer may perforate and require a conjunctival flap to cover it and help it to heal. It may also be accompanied by pus in the anterior chamber (hypopyon); if this is unresponsive to intensive local and systemic chemotherapy, you may need to perform paracentesis to obtain a specimen for microscopy and culture. Application of superglue may provide emergency treatment of corneal perforation. Anaesthetize the eye first with amethocaine. Apply 2–3 drops of superglue to the perforation after drying the cornea with a sterile swab. Cover the eye with a bandage contact lens.

6 Treat severe destructive infection or endophthalmitis with local and systemic chemotherapy and steroids. Failure to control it may require removal of the eye.

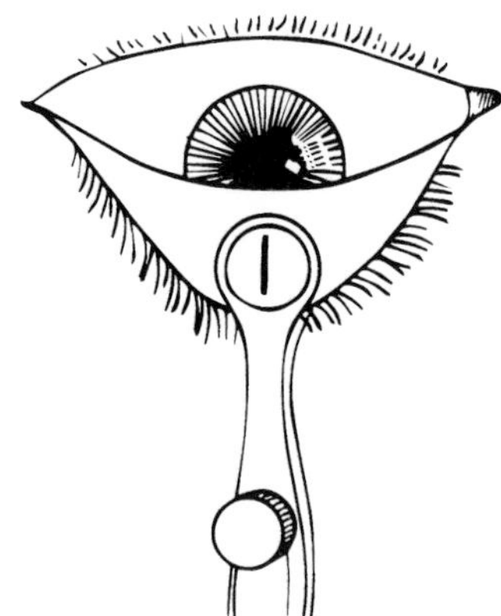

Fig. 48.7 Everting the lower lid, with a chalazion clamp.

Action

Whenever possible, incise lid abscesses from the inner aspect. Anaesthetize the lid (see Tarsorrhaphy, above). Evert the lid (Fig. 48.7) and incise it at right-angles to its margin, through the tarsal plate. Do not curette any meibomian granulations as you would do for a non-infected cyst.

EVISCERATION

Appraise

1 If the vital internal structures of the eye are destroyed by infection, with loss of vision, evisceration is indicated rather than enucleation, since mobility is better following evisceration.

2 If you have any suspicion of an intraocular tumour, however, choose enucleation.

Action

1 Insert a speculum to separate the eyelids.

2 Cut off the cornea. This may be difficult if the eye is very soft, following, for example, perforation of an infected corneal ulcer. Steady the eye by grasping the insertion of a rectus muscle with toothed forceps. Now cut through the periphery of the cornea circumferentially over a 5-mm length by progressively deepening a scalpel incision. Use the belly of a Bard Parker no. 15 blade or ophthalmic blade.

3 Once you have entered the anterior chamber, cut right round the edge of the cornea with corneal scissors, if they are available; alternatively, use any narrow-bladed, blunt-nosed scissors.

4 Having topped the eye, scoop out all its contents—lens, iris and retina as well as the humours. It is important to do this thoroughly. A special scoop is available, but a large and not-too-sharp curette is adequate. End by wrapping gauze round it to wipe away all the remnants of the uvea (Latin: *uva*=grape. Galen likened the choroid and iris as resembling a grape with the stalk torn out). Inspect the cavity to make sure that all that is left is sclera. Recent practice is to sever the optic nerve, split the posterior sclera and insert the implant behind the scleral remnant to reduce the risk of extrusion—a technique for the specialist.

5 Finally, pack the socket with paraffin gauze, apply a pad and bandage. Dress in 48 hours. No suture is required.

GLAUCOMA

Appraise

1 Chronic open-angle glaucoma is difficult for a non-specialist to recognize. Acute glaucoma produces sudden pain, loss of vision, headache, nausea and vomiting. It may be preceded by episodes of seeing haloes in the evenings. The eye appears red, with a swollen conjunctiva and the pupil may be mid-dilated and unresponsive to light. The corneal reflex is often cloudy or glassy in appearance.

2 Surgical intervention is infrequently necessarily indicated because of the availability of effective medications. Treat acute angle-closure glaucoma with miotics (Greek: *myein*=to blink, close; hence, causing pupillary closure), such as pilocarpine 4% 1 drop every hour, the beta-blocker timolol maleate 0.5% (Timoptol-LA) twice daily, dexamethasone 0.1% (Maxidex) four times a day. Oral acetazolamide (Diamox) 500 mg may be given orally twice daily; it may be administered intravenously if the patient has severe nausea and vomiting. When ophthalmological facilities are available, a YAG laser is used to produce a peripheral iridotomy. Since patients with chronic open-angle glaucoma are asymptomatic they may be managed with timolol maleate 5% or prostaglandin analogues such as latanoprost (Xalatan) 1 drop each day.

3 In primary acute closed-angle glaucoma the pressure can usually be lowered adequately, if temporarily, by acetazolamide (Diamox), 500 mg intravenously, miotic drops and osmotic agents. For this reason, classic iridectomy for glaucoma is hardly ever employed as an emergency procedure. In ophthalmic units laser iridectomy is performed several hours or days after the acute attack has been controlled and the eye is 'quiet', the pressure having been controlled with miotics such as pilocarpine 4%.

Relief of pain

1 Intractable glaucoma with severe pain is one example of the blind, painful eye, and for this sort of glaucoma some relief may be given by a retrobulbar alcohol injection if removal of the eye is impracticable.

Retrobulbar alcohol injection

1 Put 1.5 ml of 1% xylocaine with 1:200 000 adrenaline (epinephrine) in a 2-ml syringe and fit a retrobulbar needle or a 40-mm 23G or 25G needle.

2 Clean the skin of the lower lid after determining the site of entry of the needle, which should be the lower outer angle of the bony orbit.

3 With the patient lying down, ask him to keep his eyes open and to look straight ahead.

4 Insert the needle through the skin in the intended direction, which is backwards, and slightly medially and upwards (Fig. 48.8), towards the opposite superoparietal area. There is a

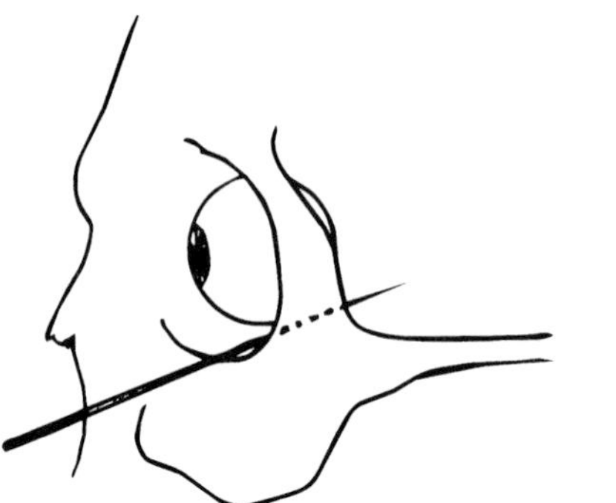

Fig. 48.8 Retrobulbar alcohol injection.

tendency to avoid getting too close to the globe for fear of penetrating it; but, if you keep too far away, you will miss the muscle cone, which you want to penetrate through Tenon's capsule between the lateral and inferior recti.

5 Inject very slightly as you go in. You will probably feel resistance when Tenon's is about to be penetrated and you may see the eye roll slightly down and out at this point. Be resolute and push on; the eye will resume its former position. Inject the bulk of the local anaesthetic. When it has had time to work there will be some relief of pain.

6 Now leave the needle in place and detach the syringe. Draw up 1 ml of 75% alcohol and after an interval of 1 minute inject this through the retrobulbar needle still in situ. Withdraw needle and syringe.

7 Warn the patient that relief may not be very long-lasting (it does, however, often last months), and also warn of the possibility of ptosis of the upper lid, which again may not be permanent.

NEOPLASMS

Appraise

The most common important ocular neoplasms affect the lids and the uveal tract.

Small benign lesions of the lid

These can be removed by cautery or a variety of methods of excision under local anaesthetic or even lidocaine 2.5%, prilocaine 2.5% (EMLA) cream.

Larger benign and malignant lesions of the lid

1 Carefully decide upon the surgical approach after noting the size of the lesion and its position in relation to the lid margins. You need to remove at least 3 mm beyond the visible margin of the lesion of a malignant lesion, to allow for possible microscopic extension.

2 For larger lesions away from the lid margin, you may excise the lesion and arrange a local skin flap. Alternatively, insert a free graft of skin from the contralateral upper lid. As you distend the skin with the preoperative anaesthetic injection of 2% lidocaine with added adrenaline (epinephrine) to reduce bleeding, you can ensure that the graft is of adequate size, and also that you can close the donor site.

3 For lesions of the lid margin, employ a pentagonal excision, provided that the gap can be simply closed by direct suture. If this will cause too much tension, facilitate closure by making an outer canthal incision, dividing the lateral canthal tendon mobilizing the lid and gaining horizontal laxity. This allows the lateral portion of the lid to be easily approximated. This is also helpful when shortening the lower lid for senile ectropion. Local anaesthesia is all that is required.

4 Make the excised pentagon at least 2 cm in height with the tarsal edges vertical, the apex being angled. Closure is effected in two layers as described in the section on lid injuries.

5 Major reconstructive surgery of the eyelids is beyond the scope of this section. Intraocular malignancies are again a matter for the specialist, but the general principle applies that, for lesions of any size (which to the non-specialist means any degree of obviousness), enucleation is indicated.

FURTHER READING

Collin JRO 1993 A manual of systematic eyelid surgery. Churchill Livingstone, Edinburgh
Leatherbarrow B 2002 Oculoplastic surgery. Martin Dunitz. London
Tyers AG, Collin JRO 1997 Colour atlas of ophthalmic plastic surgery. Butterworth-Heinemann, Oxford
Willshaw H 1993 Practical ophthalmic surgery. Churchill Livingstone, Edinburgh

INTERNET WEB SITE

www.eyetext.net

Index

A

B

C

D

E

F

G

H

I

J

K

L

O

P

Q

R

T

U

V

W

X

Z